Accessing the E-book edition

Using the VitalSource® ebook

Access to the VitalBook™ ebook accompanying this book is via VitalSource® Bookshelf – an ebook reader which allows you to make and share notes and highlights on your ebooks and search across all of the ebooks that you hold on your VitalSource Bookshelf. You can access the ebook online or offline on your smartphone, tablet or PC/Mac and your notes and highlights will automatically stay in sync no matter where you make them.

1. **Create a VitalSource Bookshelf account at** ***https://online.vitalsource.com/user/new*** or log into your existing account if you already have one.
2. **Redeem the code provided in the panel below to get online access to the ebook.** Log in to Bookshelf and select **Redeem** at the top right of the screen. Enter the redemption code shown on the scratch-off panel below in the **Redeem Code** pop-up and press **Redeem**. Once the code has been redeemed your ebook will download and appear in your library.

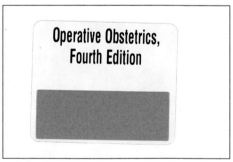

Operative Obstetrics,
Fourth Edition

No returns if this code has been revealed.

DOWNLOAD AND READ OFFLINE

To use your ebook offline, download BookShelf to your PC, Mac, iOS device, Android device or Kindle Fire, and log in to your Bookshelf account to access your ebook:

On your PC/Mac

Go to ***https://support.vitalsource.com/hc/en-us*** and follow the instructions to download the free **VitalSource Bookshelf** app to your PC or Mac and log into your Bookshelf account.

On your iPhone/iPod Touch/iPad

Download the free **VitalSource Bookshelf** App available via the iTunes App Store and log into your Bookshelf account. You can find more information at ***https://support.vitalsource.com/hc/en-us/categories/200134217-Bookshelf-for-iOS***

On your Android™ smartphone or tablet

Download the free **VitalSource Bookshelf** App available via Google Play and log into your Bookshelf account. You can find more information at ***https://support.vitalsource.com/hc/en-us/categories/200139976-Bookshelf-for-Android-and-Kindle-Fire***

On your Kindle Fire

Download the free **VitalSource Bookshelf** App available from Amazon and log into your Bookshelf account. You can find more information at ***https://support.vitalsource.com/hc/en-us/categories/200139976-Bookshelf-for-Android-and-Kindle-Fire***

N.B. The code in the scratch-off panel can only be used once. When you have created a Bookshelf account and redeemed the code you will be able to access the ebook online or offline on your smartphone, tablet or PC/Mac.

SUPPORT

If you have any questions about downloading Bookshelf, creating your account, or accessing and using your ebook edition, please visit ***http://support.vitalsource.com/***

OPERATIVE OBSTETRICS

SERIES IN MATERNAL-FETAL MEDICINE

Published in association with the

Journal of Maternal-Fetal & Neonatal Medicine

Edited by

Gian Carlo Di Renzo and Dev Maulik

Howard Carp, *Recurrent Pregnancy Loss*, ISBN 9780415421300

Vincenzo Berghella, *Obstetric Evidence Based Guidelines*, ISBN 9780415701884

Vincenzo Berghella, *Maternal-Fetal Evidence Based Guidelines*, ISBN 9780415432818

Moshe Hod, Lois Jovanovic, Gian Carlo Di Renzo, Alberto de Leiva, Oded Langer, *Textbook of Diabetes and Pregnancy, Second Edition*, ISBN 9780415426206

Simcha Yagel, Norman H. Silverman, Ulrich Gembruch, *Fetal Cardiology, Second Edition*, ISBN 9780415432658

Fabio Facchinetti, Gustaaf A. Dekker, Dante Baronciani, George Saade, Stillbirth: *Understanding and Management*, ISBN 9780415473903

Vincenzo Berghella, *Maternal–Fetal Evidence Based Guidelines, Second Edition*, ISBN 9781841848228

Vincenzo Berghella, *Obstetric Evidence Based Guidelines, Second Edition*, ISBN 9781841848242

Howard Carp, *Recurrent Pregnancy Loss: Causes, Controversies, and Treatment, Second Edition*, ISBN 9781482216141

Moshe Hod, Lois G. Jovanovic, Gian Carlo Di Renzo, Alberto De Leiva, Oded Langer, *Textbook of Diabetes and Pregnancy, Third Edition*, ISBN 9781482213607

Vincenzo Berghella, *Maternal–Fetal Evidence Based Guidelines, Third Edition*, ISBN 9781841848228

Vincenzo Berghella, *Obstetric Evidence Based Guidelines, Third Edition*, ISBN 9781841848242

Eyal Sheiner, *The Long-Term Impact of Medical Complications in Pregnancy: A Window into Maternal and Fetal Future Health*, ISBN 9781498764674

Joseph J. Apuzzio, Anthony M. Vintzileos, Vincenzo Berghella, Jesus R. Alvarez-Perez, *Operative Obstetrics, Fourth Edition,* ISBN 9781498720564

OPERATIVE OBSTETRICS

FOURTH EDITION

Joseph J. Apuzzio, M.D.
Professor, Department of Obstetrics, Gynecology and Women's Health
Director of Maternal Fetal Medicine
Professor of Radiology
Director of Maternal Fetal Medicine
Rutgers New Jersey Medical School
Newark, New Jersey

Anthony M. Vintzileos, M.D.
Chair, Department of Obstetrics & Gynecology
Winthrop University Hospital, Clinical Campus of
Stony Brook University School of Medicine, Mineola, New York
Professor of Obstetrics, Gynecology & Reproductive Medicine
Stony Brook University School of Medicine
Stony Brook, New York

Vincenzo Berghella, M.D.
Professor, Department of Obstetrics and Gynecology
Director, Division of Maternal–Fetal Medicine
Thomas Jefferson University
Philadelphia, Pennsylvania

Jesus R. Alvarez-Perez, M.D.
Director of Obstetrics and Perinatal Diagnostics for the Women's Hospital Services
Hackensack University Medical Center
Hackensack, New Jersey

Editor Emeritus: **Leslie Iffy, M.D.**
Professor, Obstetrics, Gynecology & Women's Health (retired)
Rutgers New Jersey Medical School
Newark, New Jersey

CRC Press
Taylor & Francis Group
Boca Raton London New York

CRC Press is an imprint of the
Taylor & Francis Group, an **informa** business

CRC Press
Taylor & Francis Group
6000 Broken Sound Parkway NW, Suite 300
Boca Raton, FL 33487-2742

Printed on acid-free paper
Version Date: 20161109

International Standard Book Number-13: 978-1-4987-2056-4 (Pack - Book and Ebook)

Visit the Taylor & Francis Web site at
http://www.taylorandfrancis.com

and the CRC Press Web site at
http://www.crcpress.com

This book is dedicated to my family—my parents, Ann and Ralph, who gave me the ideals that I have; my brothers, Lou and Ralph, who made my path in life enormously easier as I followed them; my wife, Marili, who is the most courageous person that I know; my daughter, Leila, who is always there for me, and my 21-year-old son, Kevin, who is my hero and a true American hero. Kevin was a Rutgers University student and EMT/volunteer fireman who gave his life while trying to save a woman from her burning home. My family has inspired me, and their love and support have carried me through life.

Joseph J. Apuzzio

To my sister, Elisavet; to my "brother" Spyros; and to my wife, Cathy, with all my love and gratitude.

Anthony M. Vintzileos

To my wife, Paola; my sons, Andrea and Pietro; my parents, Andrea and Tita; my sister, Anna, and my brother, Pietro, for all the love and support throughout my life. You all made it happen for me.

Vincenzo Berghella

I dedicate this book to my family, especially my wife, Robyn, and to my children, Susito, Christopher, and Grace—each one has been a God blessing in my life. With love—Daddy

Jesus Alvarez-Perez

Acknowledgments from the Editors

The editors wish to express their gratitude for the support and cooperation provided by Taylor & Francis Group and, in particular, by Mr. Robert Peden and the production staff of Taylor & Francis Group.

Contents

Contributors

Tracy Adams
Division of Maternal–Fetal Medicine
Department of Obstetrics and Gynecology
Winthrop University Hospital
Clinical Campus of Stony Brook University School of Medicine
Mineola, New York

Abdulla Al-Khan
Department of Obstetrics, Gynecology, and Women's Health
University of Medicine and Dentistry of New Jersey Newark,
New Jersey

Jesús R. Alvarez-Perez
Department of Obstetrics and Perinatal Diagnostics for the
Women's Hospital Services
Hackensack University Medical Center
Hackensack, New Jersey

Maria Andrikopoulou
Department of Obstetrics and Gynecology
Winthrop University Hospital
Clinical Campus of Stony Brook University School of Medicine
Mineola, New York

Stephanie Andriole
Comprehensive Genetics, Fetal Medicine Foundation
of America
Mt. Sinai School of Medicine
New York, New York

Joseph J. Apuzzio
Department of Obstetrics, Gynecology, and Women's Health
Rutgers New Jersey Medical School
Newark, New Jersey

Robert H. Ball
Obstetrix of the Mountain States
Salt Lake City, Utah

Nicholas Behrendt
Division of Maternal Fetal Medicine
Department of Obstetrics and Gynecology
Children's Hospital Colorado
Aurora, Colorado

Michael A. Belfort
Department of Obstetrics and Gynecology
Departments of Surgery and Anesthesiology
Baylor College of Medicine
and
Texas Children's Hospital
Texas Medical Center
Houston, Texas

Vincenzo Berghella
Department of Obstetrics and Gynecology
Division of Maternal–Fetal Medicine
Thomas Jefferson University
Philadelphia, Pennsylvania

Robyn T. Bilinski
Department of Obstetrics, Gynecology, and Women's Health
Rutgers New Jersey Medical School
Newark, New Jersey

Isaac Blickstein
Department of Obstetrics and Gynecology
Kaplan Medical Center
Rehovot, Israel

Rupsa Boelig
Department of Obstetrics and Gynecology
Division of Maternal Fetal Medicine Thomas Jefferson
University Hospital
Philadelphia, Pennsylvania

David W. Britt
Fetal Medicine Foundation of America
Mt. Sinai School of Medicine
New York, New York

Vance Broach
Memorial Sloan–Kettering Cancer Center
New York, New York

Haywood L. Brown
Maternal– Fetal Medicine
Duke University
Durham, North Carolina

Martin R. Chavez
Division of Maternal–Fetal Medicine
Department of Obstetrics and Gynecology
Winthrop University Hospital
Mineola, New York
and
Stony Brook University School of Medicine
Stony Brook, New York

Frank A. Chervenak
Department of Obstetrics and Gynecology New York
Presbyterian Hospital New York, New York

Ravi P. Chokshi
Department of Anesthesiology
University of Florida College of Medicine
Gainesville, Florida

Bernadette M. Cracchiolo
Department of Obstetrics and Gynecology
Division of Gynecologic Oncology
Rutgers New Jersey Medical School
Newark, New Jersey

Timothy M. Crombleholme
Division of Pediatric General, Thoracic, and Fetal Surgery
Children's Hospital Colorado
Aurora, Colorado

Elaine K. Diegmann
Nurse Midwifery Educational Program
University of Medicine and Dentistry of New Jersey
Newark, New Jersey

James Edwards
Duke University
Durham, North Carolina

Mark I. Evans
Comprehensive Genetics, Fetal Medicine Foundation of America
Mt. Sinai School of Medicine
New York, New York

Shara M. Evans
Comprehensive Genetics, Fetal Medicine Foundation of America
Mt. Sinai School of Medicine
New York, New York

Márta Gávai
Gynaecology and Obstetrics
North Denmark Regional Hospital
Thisted, Denmark

Shimon Ginath
Department of Obstetrics and Gynecology
Wolson Medical Center
Holon, Israel
and
Sackler Faculty of Medicine
Tel Aviv University
Tel Aviv, Israel

Lisa N. Gittens-Williams
Division of Maternal Fetal Medicine
Rutgers New Jersey Medical School
Newark, New Jersey

Abraham Golan
Department of Obstetrics and Gynecology
Sackler Faculty of Medicine
Tel Aviv University
Tel Aviv, Israel

Gregory Grimberg
Department of Surgery
Rutgers New Jersey Medical School
Newark, New Jersey

George F. Guirguis
Division of Maternal Fetal Medicine
Rutgers New Jersey Medical School
Newark, New Jersey
and
Hackensack University Medical Center
Division of Maternal Fetal Medicine and Surgery
Hackensack, New Jersey

Torre L. Halscott
Department of Anesthesiology and Critical Care Medicine
Division of Adult Critical Care Medicine
The Johns Hopkins University School of Medicine
Baltimore, Maryland

Christopher R. Harman
Department of Obstetrics, Gynecology and Reproductive Sciences
University of Maryland School of Medicine
Baltimore, Maryland

Karen Houck
Gynecologic Oncology Division
Temple University
Lewis Katz School of Medicine
Philadelphia, Pennsylvania

Rebecca Jackson
Department of Obstetrics and Gynecology
Thomas Jefferson University
Philadelphia, Pennsylvania

Soheila Jafari
Department of Anesthesiology
New York Methodist Hospital
Brooklyn, New York

Mark P. Johnson
The Center for Fetal Diagnosis and Therapy
Children's Hospital of Philadelphia
Philadelphia, Pennsylvania

John P. Keats
The David Geffen School of Medicine at UCLA
University of California, Los Angeles
Los Angeles, California

Sundeep G. Keswani
Texas Children's Fetal Center
Texas Children's Hospital
Houston, Texas

Wendy L. Kinzler
Department of Obstetrics and Gynecology
Winthrop University Hospital
Mineola, New York
and
Stony Brook University School of Medicine
New York City, New York

David Kulak
Obstetrics, Gynecology, and Women's Health
Rutgers New Jersey Medical School
Newark, New Jersey

Nadia B. Kunzier
Division of Maternal–Fetal Medicine
Department of Obstetrics and Gynecology
Winthrop University Hospital
Clinical Campus of Stony Brook University School of Medicine
Mineola, New York

Gene T. Lee
Department of Obstetrics and Gynecology
University of Kansas Medical Center
Kansas City, Missouri

Mario M. Leitao
Department of Gynecology Service
Memorial Sloan–Kettering Cancer Center
New York, New York

Pierre F. Lespinasse
Department of Obstetrics, Gynecology, and Women's Health
Rutgers New Jersey Medical School
Newark, New Jersey

Babak Litkouhi
Division of Gynecologic Oncology
Smilow Cancer Center
Yale School of Medicine
New Haven, Connecticut

Anna Locatelli
University of Milano Bicocca
and
Vittorio Emanuele III Hospital-Carate Brianza (MB)
Milan, Italy

Mark Martens
Department of Obstetrics and Gynecology
Jersey Shore University Medical Center
Neptune, New Jersey

George A. Mazpule
Department of Surgery
Division of Advanced Laparoscopic Surgery/Robotics/Bariatric Surgery
Hackensack University Medical Center
Hackensack, New Jersey

Donald A. McCain
Department of Surgical Oncology
Hackensack University Medical Center
and
Department of Gastrointestinal Oncology
John Theurer Cancer Center
Hackensack, New Jersey

Ana Monteagudo
Department of Obstetrics and Gynecology
NYU Langone Medical Center
New York University School of Medicine
New York, New York

Owen C. Montgomery
Department of Obstetrics and Gynecology
Drexel University College of Medicine
Philadelphia, Pennsylvania

Sara S. Morelli
Department of Obstetrics, Gynecology, and Women's Health
Rutgers New Jersey Medical School
Newark, New Jersey

Diana El-Neemany
Department of Obstetrics and Gynecology
Jersey Shore University Medical Center
Neptune, New Jersey

Rhonda Nichols
Department of Obstetrics and Gynecology
University of Medicine and Dentistry of New Jersey
Newark, New Jersey

Yinka Oyelese
Atlantic Maternal Fetal Medicine
Atlantic Health System
Morristown, New Jersey

Zoltán Papp
Maternity Department of Obstetrics and Gynecology
Semmelweis University
Budapest, Hungary

Sriram C. Perni
Department of Obstetrics and Gynecology
Mercy St. Vincent Medical Center
Mercy Health System
Toledo, Ohio

Armando Pintucci
Department of Obstetrics and Gynecology
University of Milano Bicocca
and
Department of Obstetrics and Gynecology
Vittorio Emanuele III Hospital-Carate Brianza (MB)
Milan, Italy

Lauren A. Plante
Departments of Obstetrics and Gynecology, Anesthesiology
Drexel University College of Medicine
Philadelphia, Pennsylvania

Maria Lyn Quintos-Alagheband
Pediatric Critical Care
Winthrop University Hospitals' Children's Medical Center
Mineola, New York
and
State University of New York
Stony Brook University Medical School
Stony Brook, New York

Johanna Quist-Nelson
Department of Obstetrics and Gynecology
Thomas Jefferson University
Philadelphia, Pennsylvania

Joanne Ramos
Department of Obstetrics and Gynecology
New York University School of Medicine
New York, New York

E. Albert Reece
Department of Obstetrics, Gynecology, and Reproductive Sciences
School of Medicine
University of Maryland
College Park, Maryland

John R. Roost
Department of Obstetrics and Gynecology
Mercy St. Vincent Medical Center
Mercy Health System
Toledo, Ohio

Charbel Salamon
Division of Urogynecology and Pelvic Reconstructive Surgery
Fellowship in Female Pelvic Medicine and Reconstructive Surgery
Atlantic Health System
Morristown, New Jersey

Alireza A. Shamshirsaz
Department of Obstetrics and Gynecology
Baylor College of Medicine
Houston, Texas

Genevieve B. Sicuranza
Department of Obstetrics and Gynecology
Winthrop University Hospital
Mineola, New York
and
State University of New York
Stony Brook University Medical School
Stony Brook, New York

Neil S. Silverman
Department of Medicine
University of Massachusetts Medical School
Worcester, Massachusetts

Maria Small
Department of Obstetrics and Gynecology
Duke University
Durham, North Carolina

Toghrul Talishinskiy
Department of Surgery
Division of Advanced Laparoscopic Surgery/Bariatric Surgery
Hackensack University Medical Center
Hackensack, New Jersey

Patrice M.L. Trauffer
Capital Health Regional Medical Center
Trenton, New Jersey

Ilan E. Timor-Tritsch
Department of Obstetrics and Gynecology
New York University School of Medicine
New York, New York

Sevan A. Vahanian
Department of Obstetrics and Gynecology
Stony Brook University Medical Center
Stony Brook, New York
and
Department of Obstetrics and Gynecology
Winthrop University Hospital
Mineola, New York

Arthur Jason Vaught
Department of Obstetrics and Gynecology
Division of Maternal–Fetal Medicine
Department of Surgery
Division of Surgical Critical Care
The Johns Hopkins University School of Medicine
Baltimore, Maryland

Anthony M. Vintzileos
Department of Obstetrics and Gynecology
Winthrop University Hospital
Clinical Campus for Stony Brook University School of Medicine
Stony Brook, New York

Ronald J. Wapner
Department of Obstetrics and Gynecology
Columbia University Medical Center
New York, New York

Jonathan David Weinberg
Department of Anesthesiology
New York Methodist Hospital
Brooklyn, New York

Carl P. Weiner
Department of Obstetrics, Gynecology, and Reproductive Sciences
Department of Physiology
University of Maryland School of Medicine
Baltimore, Maryland

Gerson Weiss
Department of Obstetrics, Gynecology, and Women's Health
Rutgers New Jersey Medical School
Newark, New Jersey

Shauna F. Williams
Department of Obstetrics, Gynecology, and Women's Health
Rutgers New Jersey Medical School
Newark, New Jersey

R. Douglas Wilson
Department of Obstetrics and Gynecology
University of Calgary
Calgary, California

Ruofan Yao
Department of Maternal–Fetal Medicine
University of Maryland
Baltimore, Maryland

Joel Mann Yarmush
Department of Anesthesiology
New York Methodist Hospital
Brooklyn, New York

Anatomy of the anterior abdominal wall, uterus, and pelvic organs

1

BERNADETTE M. CRACCHIOLO and JOSEPH J. APUZZIO

CONTENTS

A complete and thorough knowledge of female abdominal and pelvic anatomy is important for specialists in obstetrics and gynecology since patient safety in the operating room during surgery is critically dependent on this knowledge along with the appropriate functioning of the operating room team.[1] Therefore, this chapter reviews anatomy of the female pelvis with emphasis on avoiding anatomic complications of laparotomy and/or laparoscopic and robotic pelvic surgery[2] and on structures important in pelvic organ support and urinary continence.[3,4]

ANTERIOR ABDOMINAL WALL

Boundaries and surface landmarks

The anterior abdominal wall is bound above by the xiphisternal junction in the midline and the arching margin of the lower costal cartilages (costal margin) laterally. Below, it is bound by the symphysis pubis in the midline and laterally by the pubic crest, inguinal (Poupart's) ligament, and iliac crest (Figure 1.1). There are no bony structures laterally, the wall being limited by a vertical line from the middle of the axillary depression (midaxillary line) that crosses the 10th rib to the iliac crest. Additional

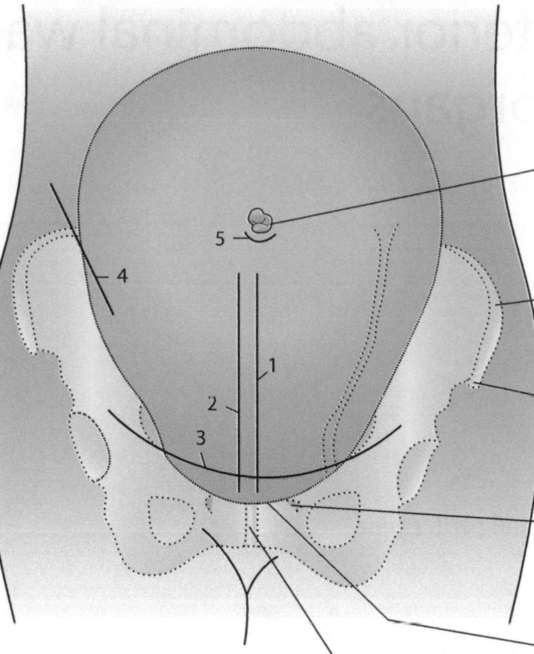

Figure 1.1 Surface landmarks and the sites of popular incisions for obstetric surgery: (1) vertical median incision, (2) vertical paramedian incision, (3) transverse incision, (4) oblique incision, and (5) umbilical incision.

bony landmarks are the xiphoid process in the midline above, the pubic tubercle located below at the lateral end of the pubic crest, and the anterior superior iliac spine at the anterior end of the iliac crest. The inguinal ligament courses from the pubic tubercle to the anterior superior iliac spine, separating the abdominal wall from the thigh. The pubic bone and symphysis pubis separate the wall from the genitalia.

In addition to the above bony landmarks, several soft tissue landmarks are apparent, their degree of visibility largely dependent upon the amount of fat in the subcutaneous tissue. Most obvious is the umbilicus, which lies in the midline about two-thirds of the distance between the suprasternal (jugular) notch and the symphysis pubis[5] at approximately the level of the lumbar (L3–4) intervertebral disk. The aponeuroses of the lateral abdominal muscles unite in the midline with their equivalent on the other side, forming the linea alba, which runs from the xiphoid process to the symphysis pubis. The linea alba is usually the strongest point in the aponeurotic part of the wall. In lean, muscular subjects, it is represented on the surface as a vertical midline depression. On each side the lateral margin of the rectus muscle is evident in similar subjects, appearing as a slightly curved, vertical depression called the linea semilunaris.

The surface markings and contour of the anterior abdominal wall vary considerably with age, body mass index (BMI), muscular status, parity, and period of gestation. The normal landmarks mentioned above usually are present during pregnancy, and, in some instances, the umbilicus and linea alba may be more intensified because of the distention of the wall by the expanding uterus. Abdominal contents sometimes protrude through a weak umbilicus, resulting in an umbilical hernia. The distention during pregnancy also may widen the linea alba, thereby separating the rectus muscles and creating diastasis recti of varying degrees. In severe cases, the uterus is covered only by skin, a thin layer of fascia, and peritoneum. A brown-black pigment frequently is deposited in the midline skin, forming the linea nigra.

Skin and subcutaneous tissue

Usually the skin of the abdomen is smooth, very elastic, and firmly attached to the deeper tissue in the midline. The cleavage lines of the skin (Langer's lines) mainly run transversely.[6] Transverse incisions through the skin course mainly parallel to the lines of tension, whereas vertical incisions cut perpendicular to them. The cutaneous lips of vertical incisions, therefore, tend to retract. In the latter months of pregnancy about one-half of all pregnant women develop reddish, slightly depressed streaks (striae gravidarum) in the abdominal skin. In addition to reddish striae, the abdominal skin of multiparous women frequently exhibits glistening, silvery, vertical lines that represent cicatrices of previous striae.

The subcutaneous tissue (superficial fascia) of the anterior abdominal wall, like other areas of the body, is composed mainly of fat and connective tissue and contains cutaneous blood vessels, lymphatics, and nerves (Figure 1.2). The quantity of fat in this region varies remarkably from one individual to another. In fatty subjects, the outer portion of the superficial fascia in the lower abdominal wall appears more fatty in texture than the deeper portions, where sheets (lamellae) of

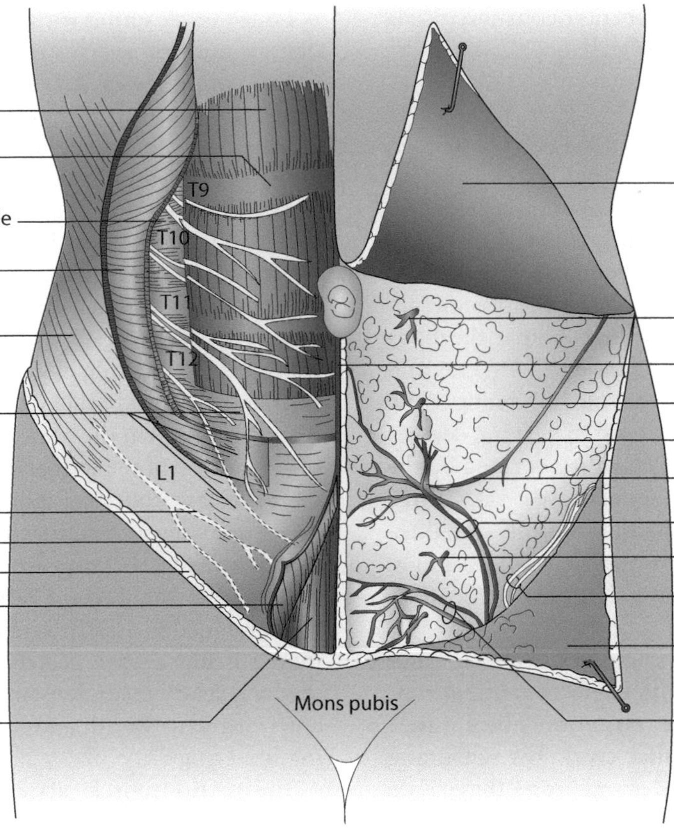

Figure 1.2 Front view of the layers and components of the infraumbilical part of the anterior abdominal wall. The more superficial subcutaneous layer is exposed on the left side of the body; the deeper muscular layer and the anterior rectus sheath are shown on the right side.

overlapping fibrous connective tissue tend to concentrate.[7] The fibrous sheets do not always form on the deep surface of the fat. Often they are enclosed in fat themselves and, on occasion, may comprise more than one layer.[8,9] In thin individuals, it may be impossible to demonstrate distinct fatty and fibrous portions. The subcutaneous tissue is continuous inferiorly into the labia majora and perineum. Often a vertical, thickened, fibrous band is present in the midline in the lower abdominal wall which is adherent to the linea alba. It represents the fundiform ligament, which usually is described only in the male. On each side of the midline the subcutaneous layer is loosely separated from the deep fascia over the lower part of the external abdominal aponeurosis. This fascial cleft is quite definite and is continuous below with a similar cleft in the perineum.

The superficial (subcutaneous) arteries arise from various sources and freely anastomose with each other in the subcutaneous layer. Most of the skin below the umbilicus is supplied by three small branches that ascend from the femoral artery passing superficial to the inguinal ligament: the superficial epigastric courses obliquely toward the umbilicus and then rises upwards approximately 4 cm lateral to the midline, the superficial circumflex iliac passes laterally just above the iliac crest, and the superficial external pudendal runs medially, superficial to the round ligament of the uterus to the perineum and lower-most part of the wall (Figure 1.2). The superficial (subcutaneous) veins accompany the arteries but are more numerous and form extensive anastomoses. Below the umbilicus they course mainly downward, also crossing superficial to the inguinal ligament to empty into the great saphenous vein in the upper thigh. The subcutaneous veins in the lower abdominal wall anastomose with those draining the upper wall. When the deeper, main venous drainage of the lower limb is obstructed, these anastomoses enlarge, forming a large venous channel, the thoracoepigastric vein that connects the great saphenous vein with the axillary vein. The superficial (subcutaneous) lymph vessels generally follow the course of the veins. Below the umbilicus they course downward to the superficial inguinal nodes located just below the inguinal ligament. The cutaneous nerves arise from the lower six thoracic nerves and the first lumbar nerve (T7–12 and L1). The seventh thoracic nerve supplies the skin over the xiphoid process, the tenth thoracic nerve courses to the umbilicus, and the eleventh and twelfth thoracic nerves and the iliohypogastric nerve (L1) innervate the skin of the infraumbilical portion of the wall. The nerves to the skin on each side of the midline are arranged in two vertical rows, a small, anterior, cutaneous series that pierce the anterior rectus sheath a short distance from the midline, and a larger, lateral, cutaneous series that enter the subcutaneous layer near the midaxillary line.

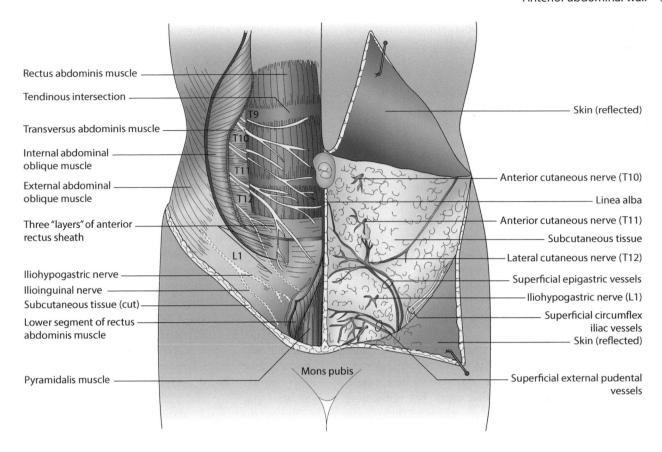

The anterior branches of the lateral cutaneous series supply a large segment of the anterior wall.

Muscles and rectus sheath

The anterior abdominal wall contains five pairs of muscles that support and protect the abdominal viscera in front and laterally (Figure 1.2). The muscles are mainly attached above and laterally to the sternum and lower ribs, and below to the pelvic bone. Three of the muscles are located laterally and superimpose as sheets one on the other. From superficial to deep, they are the external oblique, the internal oblique, and the transversus muscles. The rectus and pyramidalis muscles make up the medial group lying adjacent to the linea alba and enclosed in varying degrees by the rectus sheath. The rectus sheath is formed by the fusion of the sheet-like tendons (aponeuroses) of the three lateral muscles as they course to the midline. The linea alba might be considered the common area of decussation of the aponeuroses of the three lateral muscles rather than their insertion.[10]

The external oblique muscle originates from the outer surface of the lower eight ribs, its fibers coursing downward and forward. The more posterior fibers insert directly on the outer lip of the iliac crest. The remaining muscle fibers give rise to a broad aponeurosis that passes in front of the rectus muscle to attach to the linea alba. Above, the aponeurosis attaches to the sternum; below, it attaches to the anterior superior iliac spine, pubic tubercle, and symphysis pubis. The lower border of the aponeurosis is thickened and folded back on itself to form the inguinal (Poupart's) ligament between the anterior superior iliac spine and the pubic tubercle. The inguinal ligament is bound down to the deep fascia of the thigh (fascia lata). A small oval opening in the external oblique aponeurosis, the superficial inguinal ring, is located about 2.5 cm above and lateral to the pubic tubercle. Its inferior margin lies close to the inguinal ligament. The round ligament of the uterus passes through the ring into the labium majus, where it attaches to the subcutaneous tissue.

Immediately deep to the external oblique is the internal oblique muscle. Its fibers arise from the lateral half of the inguinal ligament, iliac crest, and lumbodorsal fascia. The posterior fibers run upward and forward to insert into the lower ribs and their cartilages. The anterior fibers course medially and give rise to an aponeurosis. Most of the fibers of the external and internal oblique muscles run at right angles to each other, an arrangement that contributes strength to the wall. The internal oblique aponeurosis divides at the lateral border of the rectus into anterior and posterior lamellae. The anterior lamella joins the aponeurosis of the external oblique to form the anterior rectus sheath in front of the rectus and pyramidalis muscles. In the upper three-fourths of the wall, the posterior lamella joins the aponeurosis of the transversus muscle to form the posterior rectus sheath, passing deep to the rectus muscle to attach in the midline to the linea alba (Figure 1.3). Approximately midway between the umbilicus and the symphysis pubis, the entire aponeurosis of the internal oblique muscle unites with the aponeurosis of the external oblique and transversus muscles, and together they pass in front of the lowest part of the rectus muscle in the anterior rectus sheath. The posterior rectus sheath, therefore, is lacking below this point, its lower border referred to as the arcuate line (semilunar line of Douglas).

The deepest of the lateral muscles is the transversus muscle. Like the internal oblique, its fibers originate from the inguinal ligament, iliac crest, and lumbodorsal fascia, but it has an additional origin from the inner aspect of the lower six costal cartilages. Its fibers are directed mainly transversely, coursing medially to give rise to an aponeurosis at the lateral border of the rectus muscle. Its aponeurosis helps to form the posterior rectus sheath in the upper three-fourths of the wall and the anterior rectus sheath in the lower one-fourth. The lowermost fibers of the transversus muscles join similar fibers of the internal oblique muscle and together they arch inferiorly and medially over the inguinal canal as the falx inguinalis. More medially, the combined fibers give rise to the conjoined tendon that inserts below on the pecten of the pubis. The conjoined tendon blends medially with the lowermost part of the anterior rectus sheath and lies just deep to the superficial inguinal ring.

The rectus muscle arises from the xiphoid process and the anterior surface of the fifth, sixth, and seventh costal cartilages. Passing inferiorly as a thick, flat, strap-like muscle, it inserts on the front of the pubic bone and symphysis pubis. It is broad and thin above, narrow and thick below. The rectus muscle is enclosed by the rectus sheath except posteriorly in its lower one-fourth. Above the umbilicus, the muscle is attached to the anterior rectus sheath at approximately three levels by transverse bands called tendinous intersections or inscriptions (Figure 1.2).

The pyramidalis muscle lies deep in the lowest part of the anterior rectus sheath in front of the rectus muscle (Figure 1.2). It arises from the pubic crest and courses superiorly and medially to insert into the lower part of the linea alba. This muscle is absent approximately 10%–20% of the time; it is more frequently missing in whites than African-Americans and is usually missing bilaterally.[11,12]

The muscles of the anterior wall are innervated mainly by the lower six thoracic nerves (T6–12) (Figure 1.2). The iliohypogastric and ilioinguinal branches of the first lumbar nerve (L1) are primarily cutaneous nerves. The lower five intercostal nerves and the subcostal nerve enter the anterior wall after giving off lateral cutaneous branches. They spiral forward and inferiorly between the internal oblique and transversus muscles, sending motor branches to them and the external oblique muscle. The nerves then enter the lateral aspect of the rectus sheath, innervate the rectus muscle, and terminate by piercing the anterior rectus sheath as anterior cutaneous nerves. The lateral border of the rectus muscle, therefore, cannot be easily freed and retracted medially without injuring its nerve supply. It can be retracted safely laterally, however. The infraumbilical portion of the rectus muscle usually is innervated by the 10th, 11th, and 12th thoracic nerves. The pyramidalis

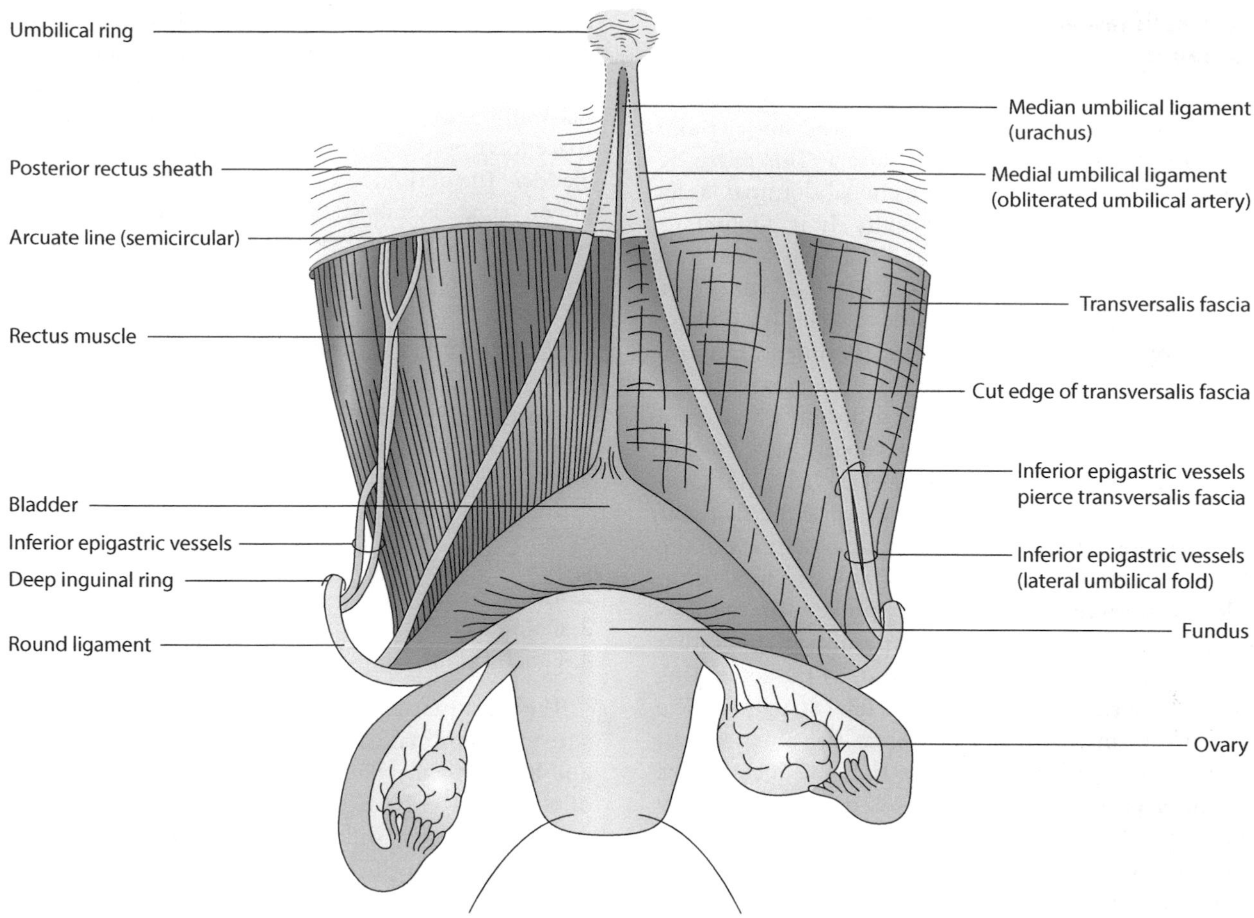

Figure 1.3 Posterior view of the infraumbilical part of the anterior abdominal wall. The parietal peritoneum and extraperitoneal (preperitoneal) tissue are removed from the right side, exposing the layer of transversalis fascia. On the left side, the transversalis fascia is removed, revealing the deep surface of the rectus muscle, below the arcuate line, and the posterior rectus sheath, above the arcuate line.

muscle receives its motor innervation from the subcostal nerve (T12). The iliohypogastric and ilioinguinal nerves often arise in common with the first lumbar nerve and enter the anterior wall in series with the lower thoracic nerves. They divide close to the iliac crest but do not enter the rectus sheath. The ilioinguinal nerve may send a branch to the lower part of the internal oblique muscle and then passes through the inguinal canal to emerge through the superficial ring to supply cutaneous branches to the labium majus. Injuries can occur with extended transverse or laparoscopic incisions and can present with neuropathic pain which is usually burning or sharp in quality and is sometimes associated with neurothesias.

The deep arteries to the anterior wall include branches of the lower five intercostal arteries and the subcostal artery that accompany their respective nerves. They sometimes enter the rectus sheath, where they anastomose with the superior and inferior (deep) epigastric arteries. The smaller superior epigastric artery is the inferior continuation of the internal thoracic (mammary) artery. It passes downward behind the seventh costal cartilage, enters the rectus sheath, and becomes buried in the deep portion of the rectus muscle. The larger inferior epigastric artery arises from the external iliac artery behind the middle of the inguinal ligament. It courses medial to the deep inguinal ring and then runs diagonally upward and medially between the transversalis fascia and peritoneum (Figure 1.3). Close to the lateral border of the rectus muscle, the inferior epigastric artery pierces the transversalis fascia and enters the rectus sheath by passing in front of the arcuate line. It ascends on the deep surface of the rectus muscle, gradually becoming buried in it. In only about one-half the cases studied did the superior and inferior epigastric arteries anastomose to form a vertically coursing channel within the rectus sheath.[13] The course of the inferior epigastric vessels can be more difficult to identify in overweight patients at laparoscopy.[14] The lower lateral part of the anterior wall is supplied by branches of the deep circumflex iliac artery. This vessel also arises from the external iliac artery and ascends between the internal oblique and transversus muscles.

The veins draining the deeper portions of the anterior wall correspond to the arteries. Below the umbilicus they course downward to the external iliac vein, but above this level they pass upward to the internal thoracic vein and laterally to the intercostal veins.

Transversalis fascia, extraperitoneal tissue, and peritoneum

The fascia deep to the transversus muscle is better developed than it is between the abdominal wall muscles and it is referred to as the transversalis fascia. This relatively strong fascial layer is a part of the endoabdominal fascia that lines the entire abdominal cavity. It is continuous with that of the other side in the midline deep to the linea alba and lies adjacent to the deep surface of the rectus muscle in the lower one-fourth of the anterior wall, where the posterior rectus sheath is absent (Figure 1.3). Above the arcuate line, it lies adjacent to the deep surface of the posterior rectus sheath. Superiorly, it becomes the fascia on the underside of the diaphragm. Inferiorly, it attaches to the pubis, but more laterally in the pelvis it helps form the femoral sheath and is continuous with the iliopsoas fascia. Posteriorly, the transversalis fascia blends with the fascia on the anterior surface of the quadratus lumborum muscle. The transversalis fascia is separated from the peritoneum by loose extraperitoneal (preperitoneal) tissue that contains a variable quantity of fat and, in the lower portion of the anterior wall, remnants of fetal structures. The peritoneum forms the deepest layer of the anterior wall and is the serous membrane lining the peritoneal cavity. In the lower part of the anterior wall, it extends laterally on the deep side of the inguinal canal and reflects superiorly to line part of the iliac fossa on each side. Inferiorly, the parietal layer of peritoneum becomes visceral by continuing onto the superior surface of the bladder into the vesicouterine pouch to the anterior aspect of the uterus. In the infraumbilical part of the anterior wall, there may be little or no fat in the extraperitoneal layer or there may be a considerable quantity. The ligamentous remnants of fetal structures course superiorly within this layer to the deep side of the umbilicus (Figure 1.3). In or near the midline is the single median (middle) umbilical ligament that represents the remains of a tubular structure called the urachus. The urachus connected the fetal bladder to the body wall at the umbilicus. The proximal part of the ligament retains its tubular structure and attaches to the apex of the bladder. Its distal segment is a fibrous cord that usually divides into three strands as it approaches the umbilicus.[15] This ligament is often hypertrophied during pregnancy and is sectioned during mobilization of the bladder. Located farther laterally on either side is the medial (formerly called lateral) umbilical ligament, a remnant of the distal part of the umbilical artery. It sometimes is referred to as the obliterated umbilical or hypogastric artery. During fetal life the umbilical artery arose as a large, rounded trunk from the uppermost part of the internal iliac artery. It actually represented the main stem of the parent artery that continued along the lateral pelvic wall, up the deep side of the anterior abdominal wall to the umbilicus, and then through the umbilical cord to the placenta. The definitive branches of the internal iliac artery during fetal life were relatively small. Thin sheets of connective tissue that stretch between the medial umbilical ligaments have been observed in the extraperitoneal tissue but are of little clinical importance. Of more importance is the fact that the extraperitoneal tissue in the lower anterior abdominal wall continues below to the prevesical or retropubic space (cave of Retzius), allowing for easy separation of the bladder. The peritoneum in the lower anterior wall in the gravid female is mobilized in an extraperitoneal cesarean section by the development of this space from the suprapubic approach (Figure 1.4).

Abdominal surgical incisions

The main abdominal incisions used in obstetric surgery are in the infraumbilical portion of the abdominal wall and are as follows (Figure 1.1):

1. Vertical
   a. Median (1)
   b. Paramedian (2)
2. Transverse (3)
3. Oblique (4)
4. Umbilical (5)

The ideal incision is one that affords maximum exposure with minimal damage to the tissue, especially nerves and blood vessels. Sites that predispose to the formation of postoperative hernias should be avoided whenever possible. Many factors influence the surgeon's choice.

Perhaps the most commonly used is the median vertical incision. It has the advantage of a good exposure and comparative avascularity, cuts through no muscle fibers or nerves, and can be repaired to produce a strong abdominal wall. The linea alba is incised, using the pyramidalis muscles as a guide to the midline (Figure 1.2). The medial margins of the rectus muscles are exposed and retracted laterally. The rectus muscles lie in close proximity, unless diastasis has occurred. The deeper median umbilical ligament usually is pushed to one side (Figure 1.3).

The paramedian vertical incision is made through similar layers as in the median incision, except that the anterior rectus sheath is cut rather than the linea alba. The rectus muscle may be retracted medially or laterally; medial retractions tend to jeopardize its nerve supply. In muscle-splitting incisions, the rectus muscle is dissected vertically along the length of the wound. When the posterior rectus sheath is divided, the inferior epigastric vessels are retracted laterally (Figure 1.3). Since the posterior rectus sheath is absent, the transversalis fascia is encountered immediately below the arcuate line (semicircular line of Douglas).

The transverse incision is made in a curved manner two finger breadths above the symphysis pubis just below the hairline to avoid bladder entry.[16] The anterior rectus sheath is cut transversely on both sides. The median sagittal septum (linea alba) that separates the rectus muscles is freed above and below the cut. The rectus muscles are retracted laterally, and the peritoneal cavity is entered by a vertical incision through the transversalis fascia, extraperitoneal tissue, and peritoneum. When additional exposure is

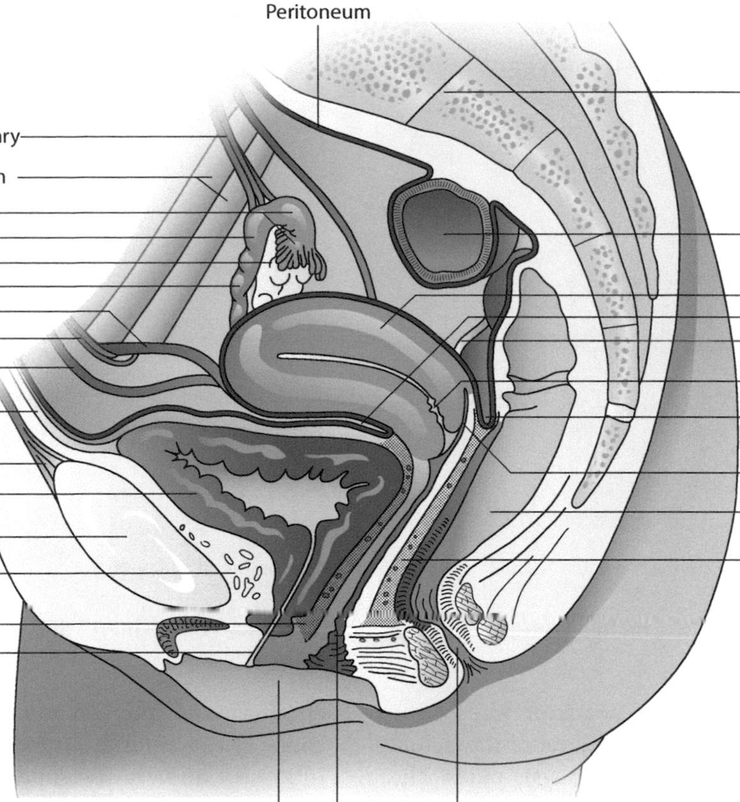

Figure 1.4 Midsagittal view of the female pelvis, showing the relations of the viscera to each other and the peritoneal cavity.

required, the rectus muscles are cut transversely (Maylard or Mackenrodt technique) or their insertion on the symphysis pubis is detached.[17] When the need for even greater exposure is anticipated, the skin incisions may extend from one anterosuperior iliac spine to the other (Mackenrodt's approach). As the rectus muscles are cut transversely in this approach, the inferior epigastric vessels are ligated and cut. The transversalis fascia, extraperitoneal tissue, and peritoneum also are cut transversely.

The oblique incision (McArthur or McBurney incision) is a muscle-splitting incision in the lower lateral part of the anterior wall, providing good postoperative support because of the grid type of closure. The three flat abdominal muscles (external oblique, internal oblique, and transversus) are divided in the direction of their fleshy and tendinous fibers. The aponeurosis of the external oblique muscle is encountered first and is separated inferiorly and medially in the direction of its fibers. The internal oblique and transversus muscles are then encountered and separated in the direction of their fibers. Last, the incision is made through the underlying transversalis fascia, extraperitoneal tissue, and peritoneum. In the pregnant patient, consideration must be given to the possible upward and lateral displacement of the underlying viscera by the gravid uterus. The more advanced the pregnancy, the higher must be the incision in the abdominal wall for exposure of the appendix and uterine adnexa.

The umbilical incision is a short semilunar incision made at the lower edge of the umbilicus. The incision is made through stretched skin and the underlying subcutaneous layer. Transversely cutting the underlying transversalis fascia and peritoneum is now preferred to the initial vertical incision.

UTERUS

Parts and relations of the nongravid uterus

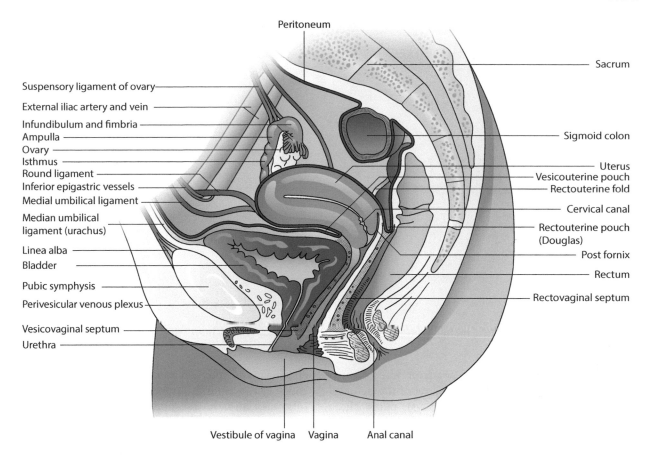

The nongravid uterus is a hollow, flat, pear-shaped, muscular organ located in or near the midline of the pelvis between the bladder and small intestine, in front, and the rectum and sigmoid colon, behind (Figure 1.4). It is best divided into three major parts: an upper triangular portion, the body; a lower, tubular portion, the cervix; and an intervening, short, constricted segment, the isthmus (Figure 1.5). The dome-shaped portion of the body, above the entrance of the uterine tubes, is the fundus. The cervix is continuous inferiorly with the vagina, the wall of which attaches to the cervix along an oblique line dividing it into supravaginal and vaginal segments. The nongravid uterus usually has an anteverted and anteflexed position with the convex fundus directed anteriorly. The anterior surface of the body is flat and rests on the superior surface of the bladder. Its posterior surface is convex and lies close to the rectum and sigmoid colon. The cervix is directed downward

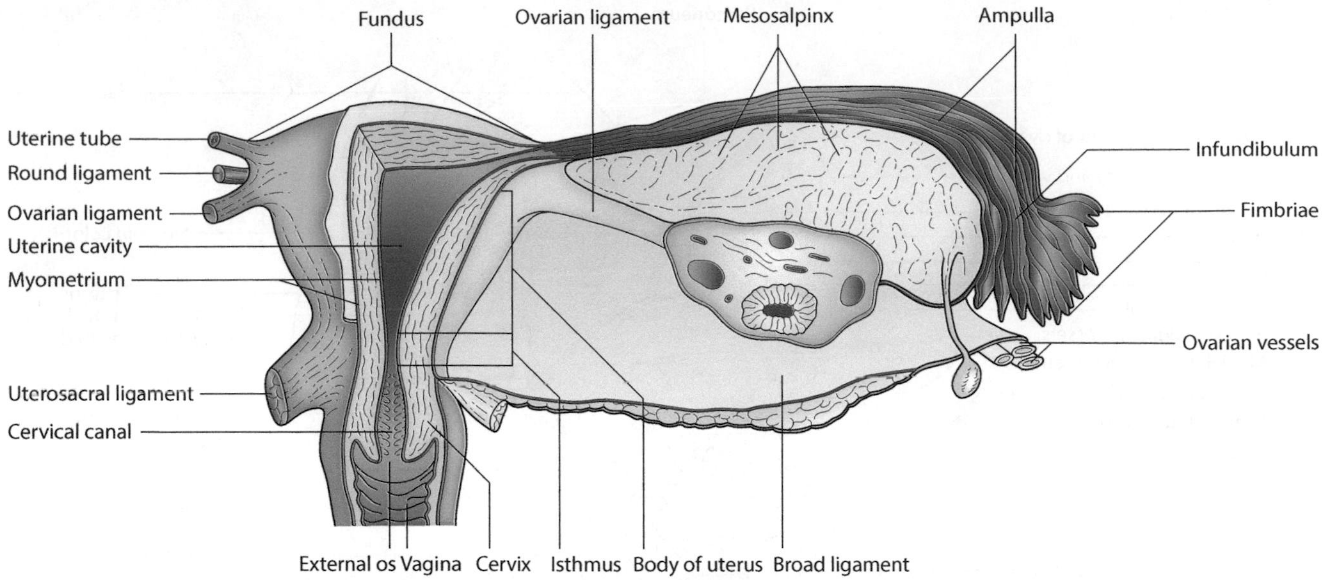

Figure 1.5 Posterior view of the mature, nongravid uterus and adnexa. Part of the uterus and the right uterine tube and ovary are frontally sectioned.

and backward, resting against the posterior wall of the vagina. Its external os lies at about the level of the ischial spine and the upper border of the symphysis pubis. The ureter lies immediately lateral to the cervix, making it very susceptible to injury at this level (Figures 1.6 through 1.8). The fundus and body are covered by peritoneum that is reflected anteriorly at the level of the isthmus to the upper surface of the bladder, forming the vesicouterine pouch (Figure 1.4). Posteriorly, the peritoneum extends farther inferiorly, covering the isthmus, supravaginal cervix, and posterior fornix of the vagina before reflecting to the rectum to form the rectouterine pouch of Douglas.

Size and positional changes of the gravid uterus

First trimester

The dimensions of the nongravid uterus vary considerably. The body averages approximately 5 cm in length, 5 cm at its widest part, and 3–4 cm in thickness (anteroposteriorly). The isthmus and cervix together measure about 2.5 cm in length and 3 cm in diameter. The uterus that has accommodated a previous pregnancy is usually slightly larger than the one that has not. For the first few weeks of pregnancy, the original pear shape is maintained. By the end of the second month of gestation, the uterus triples in size and changes from the typical flat pear shape to a rounded form, a shape it retains throughout the second trimester. Because of the rapid increase in size and weight during the second month, the uterus may assume exaggerated positions of anteflexion, retrocession, and retroversion. By the end of the first trimester, the fundus usually can be palpated above the symphysis (Figure 1.9).

Second and third trimesters

During the second trimester, the uterus expands superiorly out of the pelvic cavity, through the superior pelvic aperture, and into the abdominal cavity (Figure 1.9). It contacts the anterior abdominal wall and displaces the intestines laterally and superiorly. Midway through pregnancy (20 weeks gestation), the fundus is at the level of the umbilicus. By 8½ months, the fundus reaches the level of the xiphoid process, but during the last month it recedes slightly when the presenting part of the fetus descends into the pelvis (lightening). At the beginning of the third trimester, the uterus assumes an ovoid shape, the vertical axis increasing more rapidly than either the transverse or anteroposterior axis.[18] The pregnant uterus is quite mobile and tends to rotate to the right with the left side moving anteriorly toward the midline. Rotation to the right is considered to result from the pressure of the sigmoid colon in the left side of the pelvic cavity. Occasionally, rotation of the uterus to the left occurs when there is a pelvic or lower abdominal mass on the right side. In the erect standing position, the abdominal wall supports the uterus. In the supine position, the uterus lies backward, resting upon the aorta and inferior vena cava.

The myometrium during pregnancy

The wall of the uterus is composed of a thin outer covering of peritoneum (serosa), a thick, intermediate layer of variable proportions of muscle and connective tissue (myometrium), and an inner mucosal layer (endometrium). The body of the uterus contains the most muscle, with the content of muscle fibers diminishing below as the cervix is approached. The cervix is composed mainly of connective tissue and only about 10% muscle fiber.[19] The arrangement of the muscular fibers within the myometrium of the body is complex as a result of its development from the fused portion of the paramesonephric (Müllerian) ducts (Figure 1.10), but generally they can be divided into three layers. The external longitudinal layer

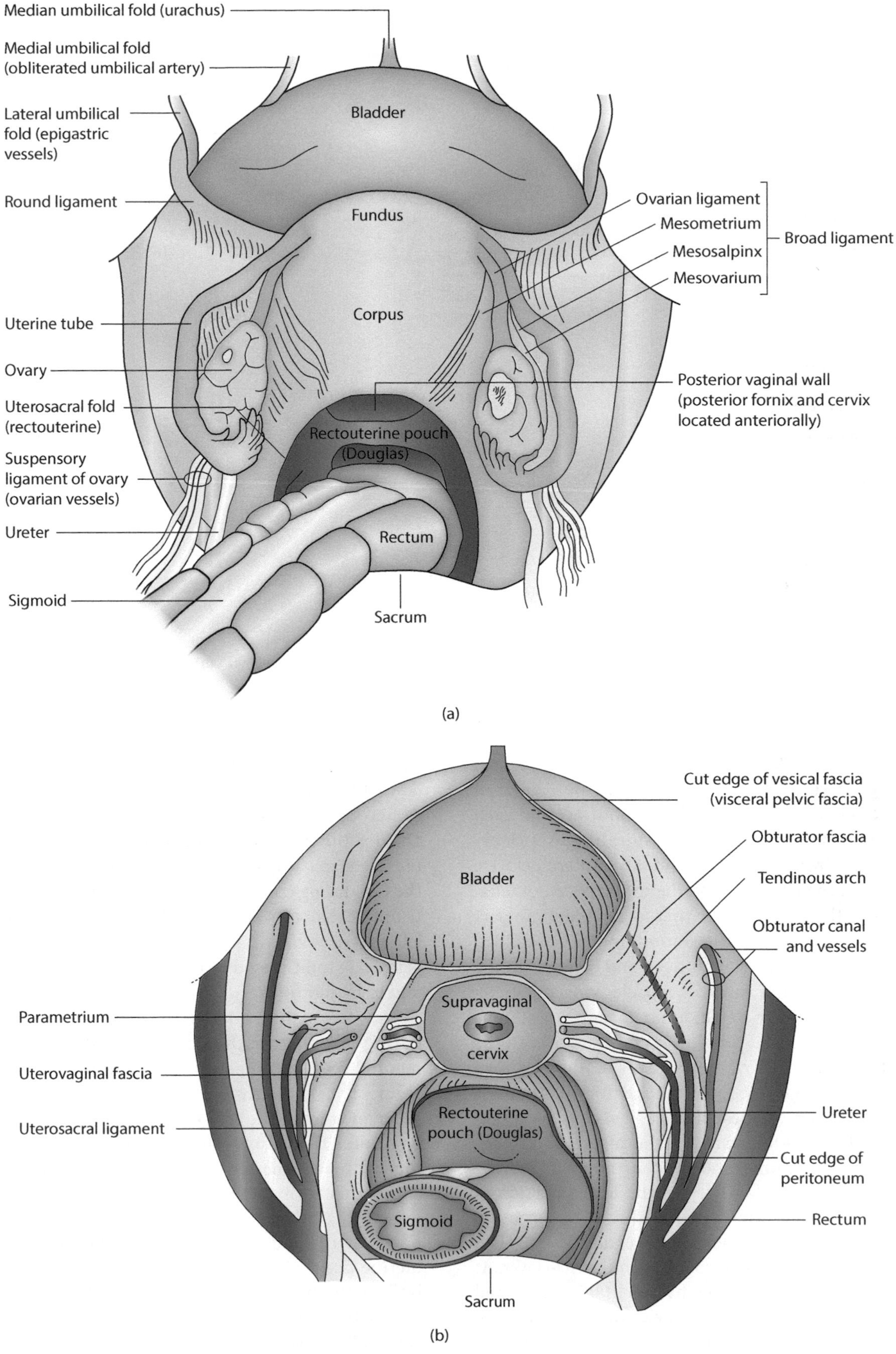

Figure 1.6 Female pelvis viewed from above at three different levels. (a) Highest level showing the relations of the nongravid uterus, adnexa, bladder, and rectum to the peritoneal cavity. (b) Middle level showing the course of the ureters and their relations to the supravaginal part of the cervix and uterine vessels. *(Continued)*

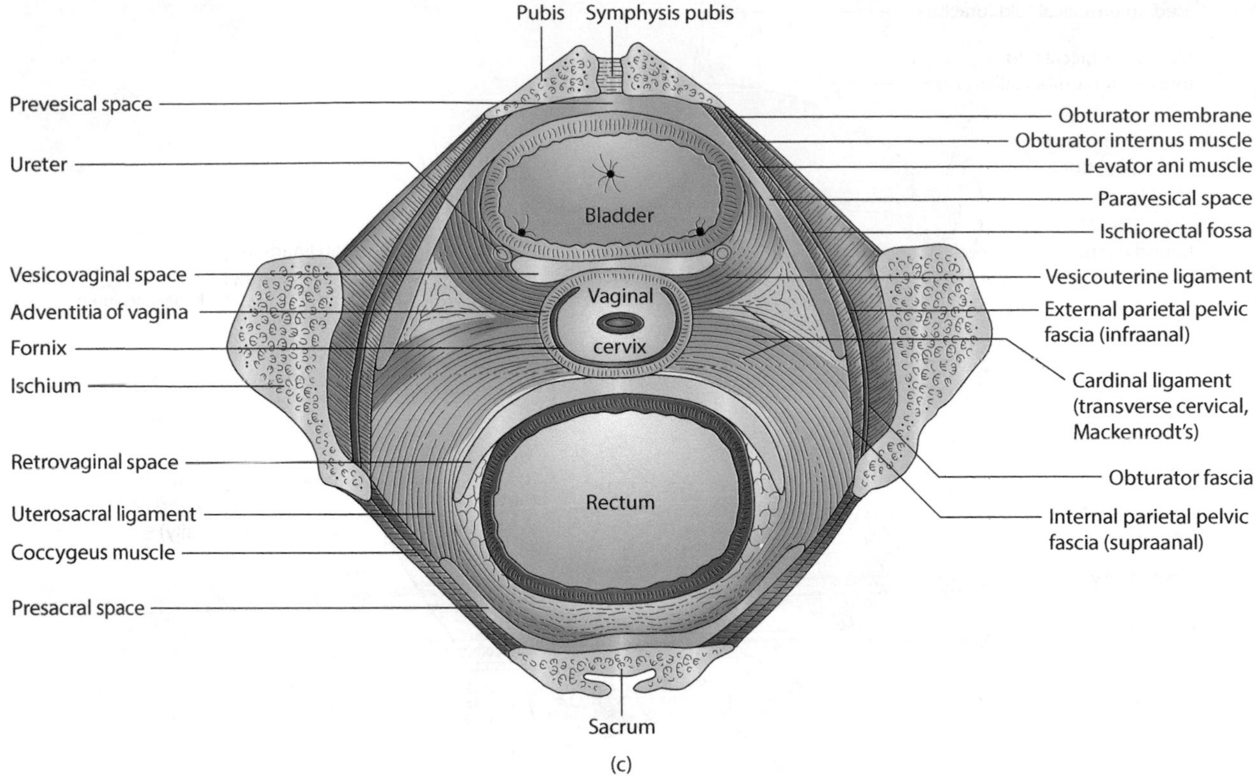

Figure 1.6 (*Continued*) Female pelvis viewed from above at three different levels. (c) Lowest level showing the relations of the fascial ligaments and spaces to the cervix and upper vaginal wall.

of the uterine tube blends with the outer layer of vertical fibers of the uterus.[20] Muscle fibers in the outer part of the inner circular layer of the tube spiral around each tube and continue into the uterus, spiraling in a clockwise direction from the right and a counterclockwise direction from the left. This interlacing network of muscle fibers is in the middle layer that forms the main part of the uterine wall. Bundles of smooth muscle contained in the supportive ligaments interlace and blend with the middle layer. The inner layer of muscle consists of circularly arranged, sphincter-like fibers at the isthmus and, at the orifices of the tubes, it is continuous with the inner portion of the inner circular layer of the tube. Two muscle bundles, the fasciculi cervicoangulares, are present at the lateral aspect of the uterus, bridging the cervix and fundus. The bundles may serve as a system for conduction or coordination of muscle contraction.[21] During pregnancy, the muscle fascicles in the lower portion of the uterus overlap one another like shingles on a roof.

Uterine enlargement during pregnancy involves stretching and marked hypertrophy of the muscle layer. At term the body of the uterus weighs over 1000 g compared to approximately 70 g in the nongravid state. Since mitotic activity is rarely observed in the myometrium, the smooth muscle cells are considered to undergo hypertrophy rather than hyperplasia. The new muscle cells which do form likely originate from growth of the media of the myometrial arteries and veins.[22] Hypertrophy of the myometrium begins during the first few weeks and overall increases 5- to 10-fold, mainly during the third month. Increases in fibrous and elastic tissue accompany the hypertrophy. During the second and third trimesters, the increased uterine size is caused mainly by the pressure exerted by the expanding conceptus. In early pregnancy the myometrium of the body is 2–3 cm thick but thins to 1–2 cm in late pregnancy. Thinning of the uterine wall may be exaggerated in multigravid women, during multiple pregnancy and in hydramnios.

The musculature in the wall of the isthmus must dilate during labor rather than contract and, after the second month, makes up the major portion of the lower uterine segment. It is poorly defined during the early weeks of pregnancy when the area feels softer than either the body or cervix. The isthmus hypertrophies like the body during the first trimester, and its canal triples in length to approximately 3 cm (Figure 1.11). During the second trimester, the isthmus becomes incorporated into the body of the uterus and the isthmic canal becomes part of the uterine cavity.[23–25] Since the wall of the isthmus and the wall of the body are approximately the same thickness during this time, their junction region no longer is visible externally. This condition persists until the middle of the last trimester, when a transverse linear depression appears in the junction region. The musculature above the depression is thicker than that below. The transverse depression forms just below the vesicouterine pouch and is thought

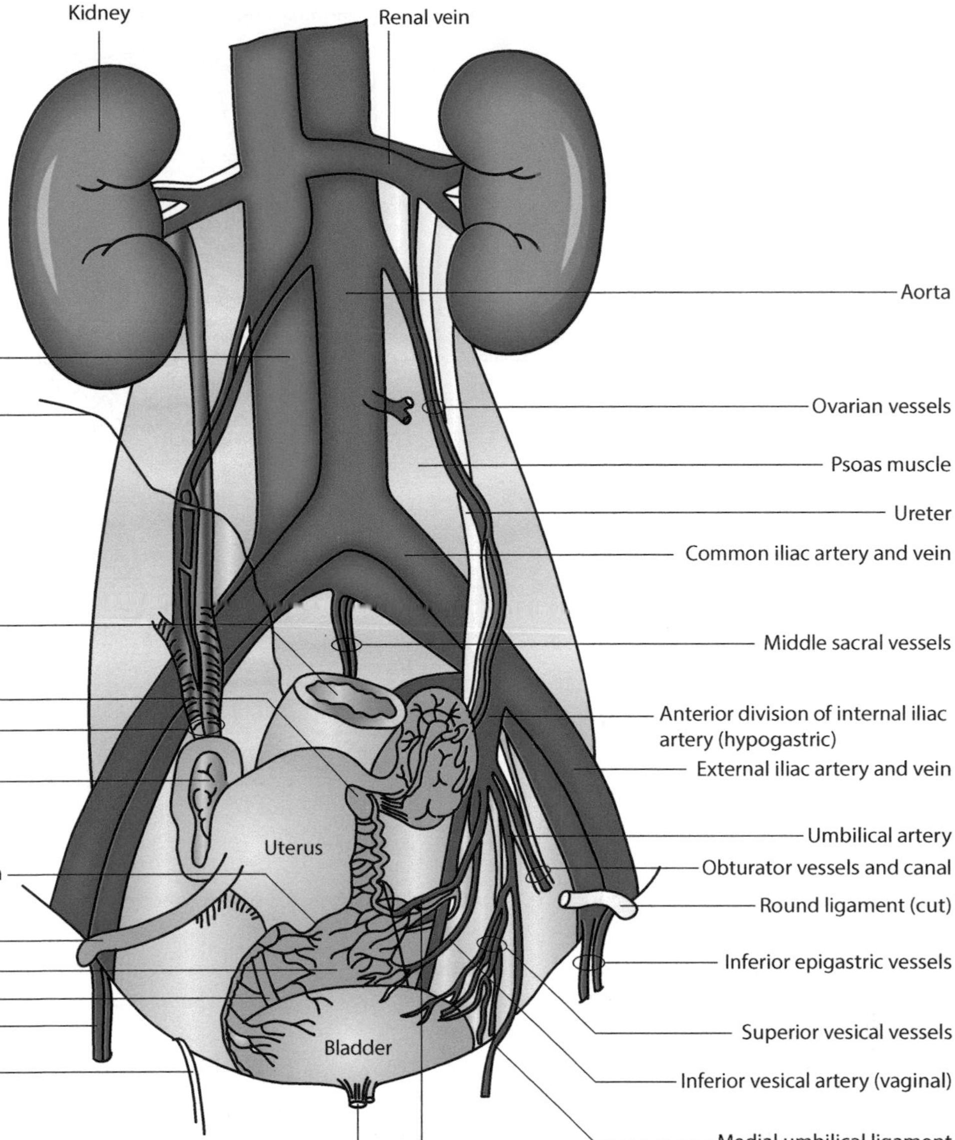

Figure 1.7 Anterior view of the origin, course, and relations of the ureter and the ovarian and uterine vessels on the left side.

to correspond to the level of the anatomic internal os. It is sometimes referred to as the physiologic contraction ring, which rises to a higher level during labor. After delivery the ring appears as a marked constriction between the body and the cervix.

The cervix of the gravid uterus

The size of the cervix in relation to the body of the uterus varies with age and parity. The cervix is twice the size of the body in a young child, about equal in nulliparous women, and about one-third the size of the body in a multiparous woman. It then regresses to its prepubertal state in menopause. It is composed mainly of collagen-rich connective tissue and only approximately 10% is muscle.

The cervix undergoes profound changes during pregnancy and labor. Two of the earliest signs of pregnancy are cervical softening and cyanosis caused by increased vascularity and edema. Soon after conception, the cervical glands secrete a very thick mucus into the cervical canal, forming a plug that closes off the canal during the gestation period. In the nonpregnant state, the glands usually comprise only a small fraction of the cervical mass. They undergo such remarkable proliferation during pregnancy that by term they make up approximately one-half its mass. There is no appreciable change in the muscle content of the cervix during pregnancy. The cervix dilates during labor as a result of collagen dissociation. The incompetent cervix dilates painlessly during the second or early third trimester, resulting in rupture of the membranes, followed by the delivery, usually, of a previable fetus. Previous cervical trauma from such procedures as dilation, curettage, and cauterization appears to be a major causative factor. The ratio of muscle to collagen has been reported to change, resulting in more abundant muscle fibers. Cervical

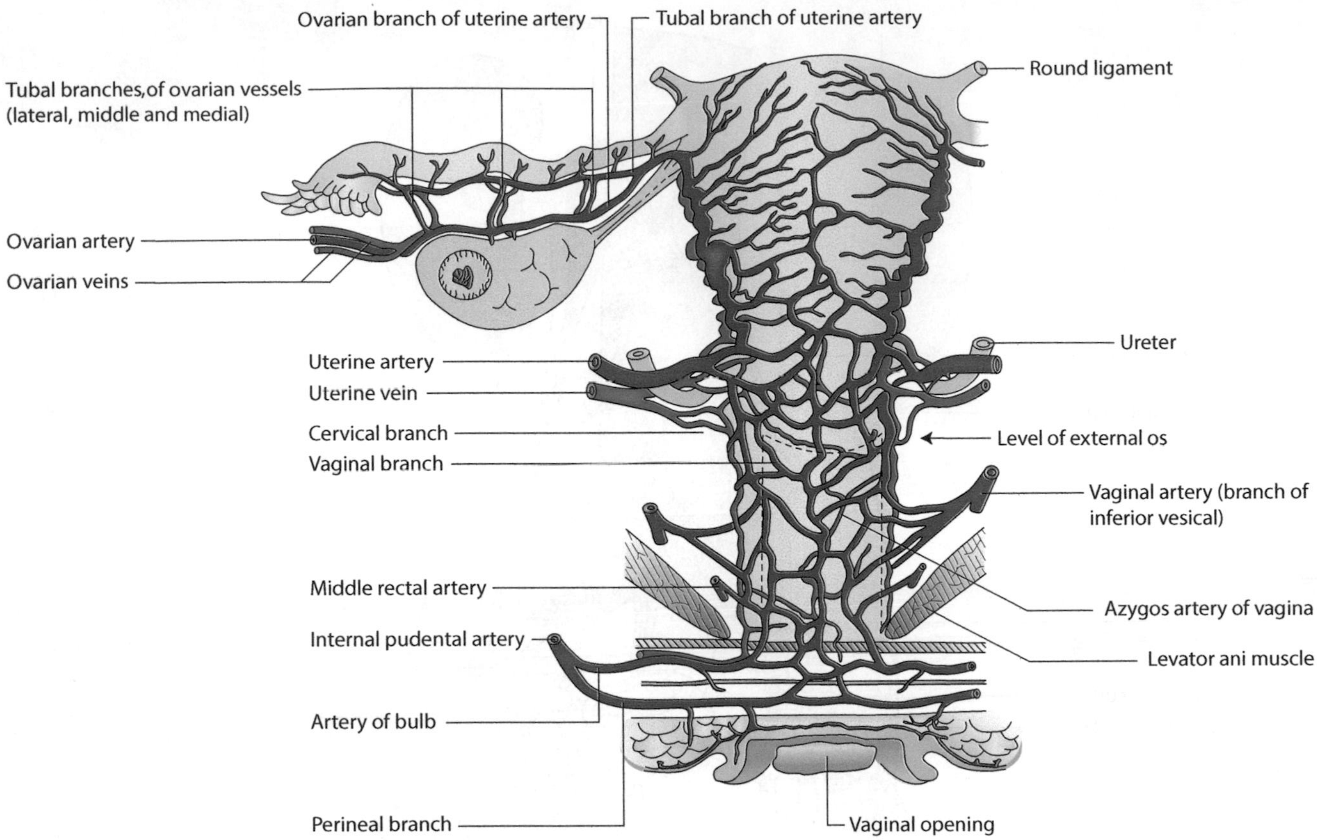

Figure 1.8 Posterior view of the course, relations, and anastomoses of the ovarian and uterine vessels.

weakness is reinforced surgically by the placement of a purse-string suture around the vaginal cervix after the first trimester but before significant dilation occurs.

Changes in the uterine cavity during pregnancy

The uterine cavity in the nongravid state is little more than a slit, when viewed laterally, with close anterior and posterior walls (Figure 1.4). From the front, the cavity has the shape of an inverted triangle with a base superiorly, where it is continuous on each side with the lumen of the uterine tube, and an apex inferiorly, where it is continuous with the canal through the isthmus and cervix (Figure 1.5). The cervical canal is slightly expanded in its middle and opens into the vagina through the external os. It is continuous superiorly with the constricted canal of the isthmus, which may be 6–10 mm long (Figure 1.11). The point where the lower end of the isthmic canal widens into the cervical canal is known as the histologic internal os, as it is the point where an abrupt microscopic change occurs in the mucosa. Its upper end widens into the uterine cavity at the anatomic internal os. The uterine cavity in the gravid condition enlarges as the myometrium hypertrophies. Initially, its rate of enlargement is greater than the growth rate of the conceptus. Later, during the early part of the second trimester, the uterine cavity becomes completely filled by the rapidly expanding conceptus. Uterine enlargement is not symmetric but is sometimes most marked in the fundus and other times in the body below the tubes. This probably is influenced greatly by the location of the implantation site.

FALLOPIAN TUBE

A long, narrow, trumpet-shaped uterine (fallopian) tube extends laterally from each side of the uterine body, arching over the upper pole of the ovary and then downward on the posterior part of its medial surface (Figures 1.4 through 1.6). Its canal runs from the superior angle of the uterine cavity to the ovary and gradually increases in diameter as it courses laterally. When straightened, the tube in the nongravid state measures approximately 10 cm long. It can be divided into four parts. The intramural portion passes through the uterine wall and has the smallest lumen diameter (1 mm or less). The portion that extends laterally from the uterus is the narrow isthmus. It continues laterally into a broad, sometimes tortuous, portion called the ampulla. The ampulla terminates near the ovary as the funnel-shaped infundibulum. Finger-like fimbriae extend from the periphery of the infundibulum surrounding the abdominal ostium. One or more fimbriae are in contact with the ovary (ovarian fimbria). The wall of the uterine tube is made up of three layers: an outer serosa, an intermediate smooth muscle layer (myosalpinx), and an inner mucosal lining (endosalpinx). The endosalpinx is arranged into longitudinal folds that become highly branched in the ampullary segment. The uterine tube occupies the upper border of the broad ligament and stretches with it as tension is exerted on

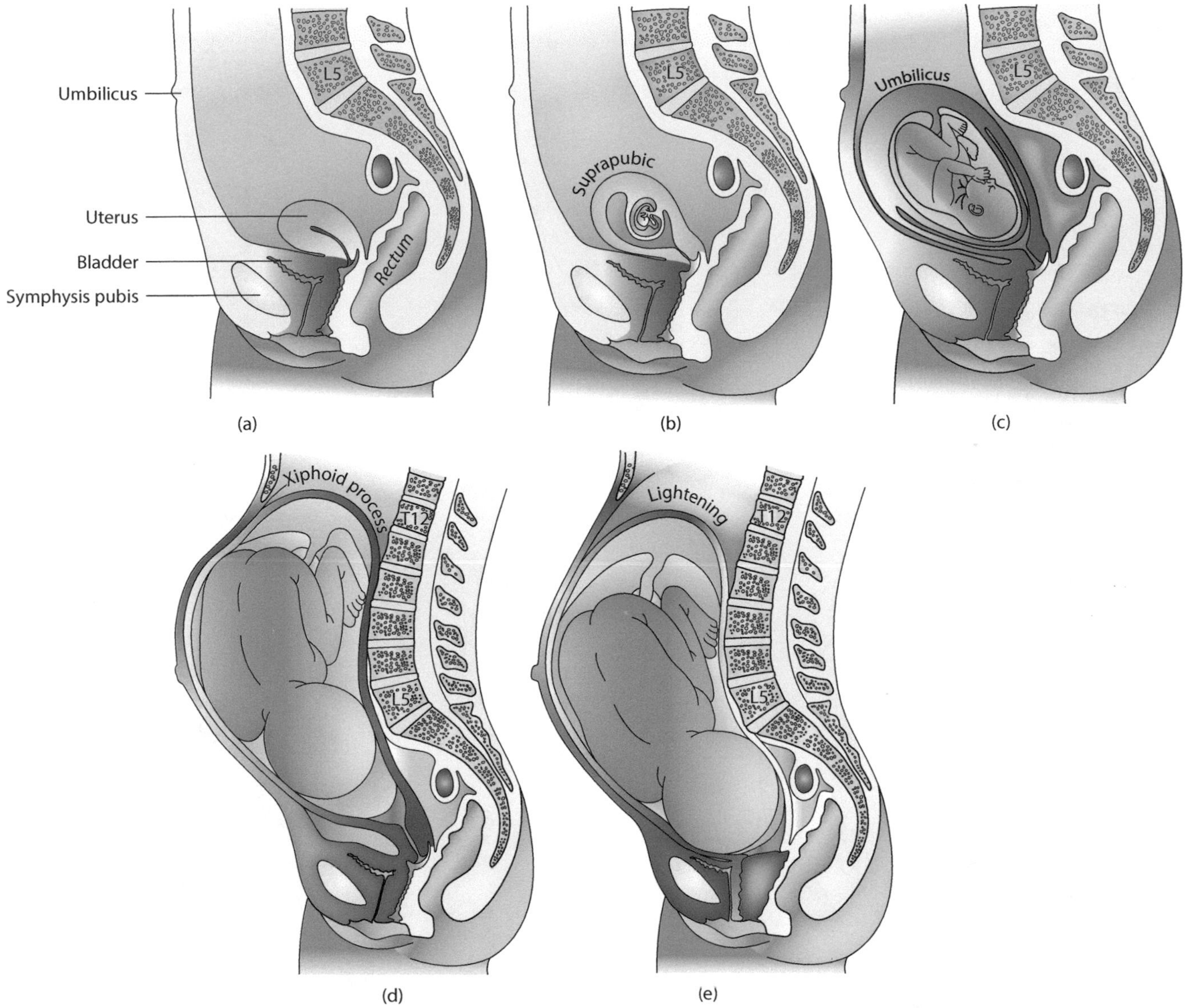

Figure 1.9 Relations of the body of the uterus and superior extent of the fundus at different periods of gestation: (a) nonpregnant, (b) first trimester, (c) second trimester, (d) third trimester, and (e) term.

them by the rising, gravid uterus. It becomes hyperemic but undergoes little hypertrophy during pregnancy.

OVARY

Medial to the curved segment of the uterine tube on each side lies the solid, almond-shaped ovary (Figures 1.4 through 1.6). Each ovary measures approximately 4 cm long, 2 cm wide, and 1 cm thick and usually has a grayish-pink color and a puckered, uneven surface. Its long axis is nearly vertical, with the upper pole located close to the uterine tube and the lower pole nearer the uterus. One surface faces medially, and the other laterally. Its posterior border is free, but its anterior border is attached to the broad ligament by a short, two-layered fold of peritoneum, the mesovarium, through which vessels and nerves pass to the hilum of the ovary. The ovary in the nulliparous woman usually lies in the upper part of the pelvic cavity in a slight depression on the lateral pelvic wall between

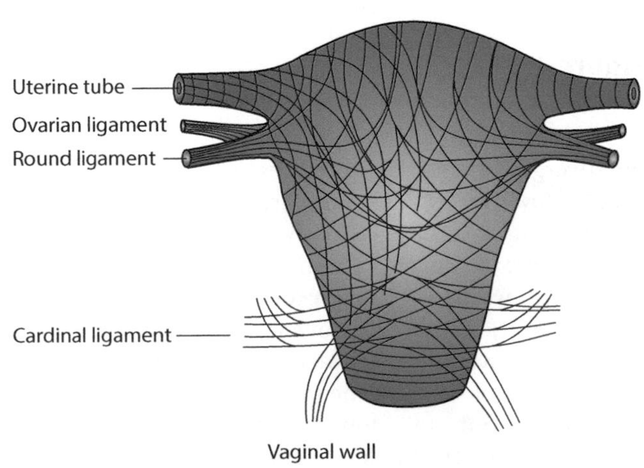

Figure 1.10 Course and arrangement of smooth muscle fibers in the myometrium and their continuities with those in the uterine tube, vaginal wall, and lateral ligaments.

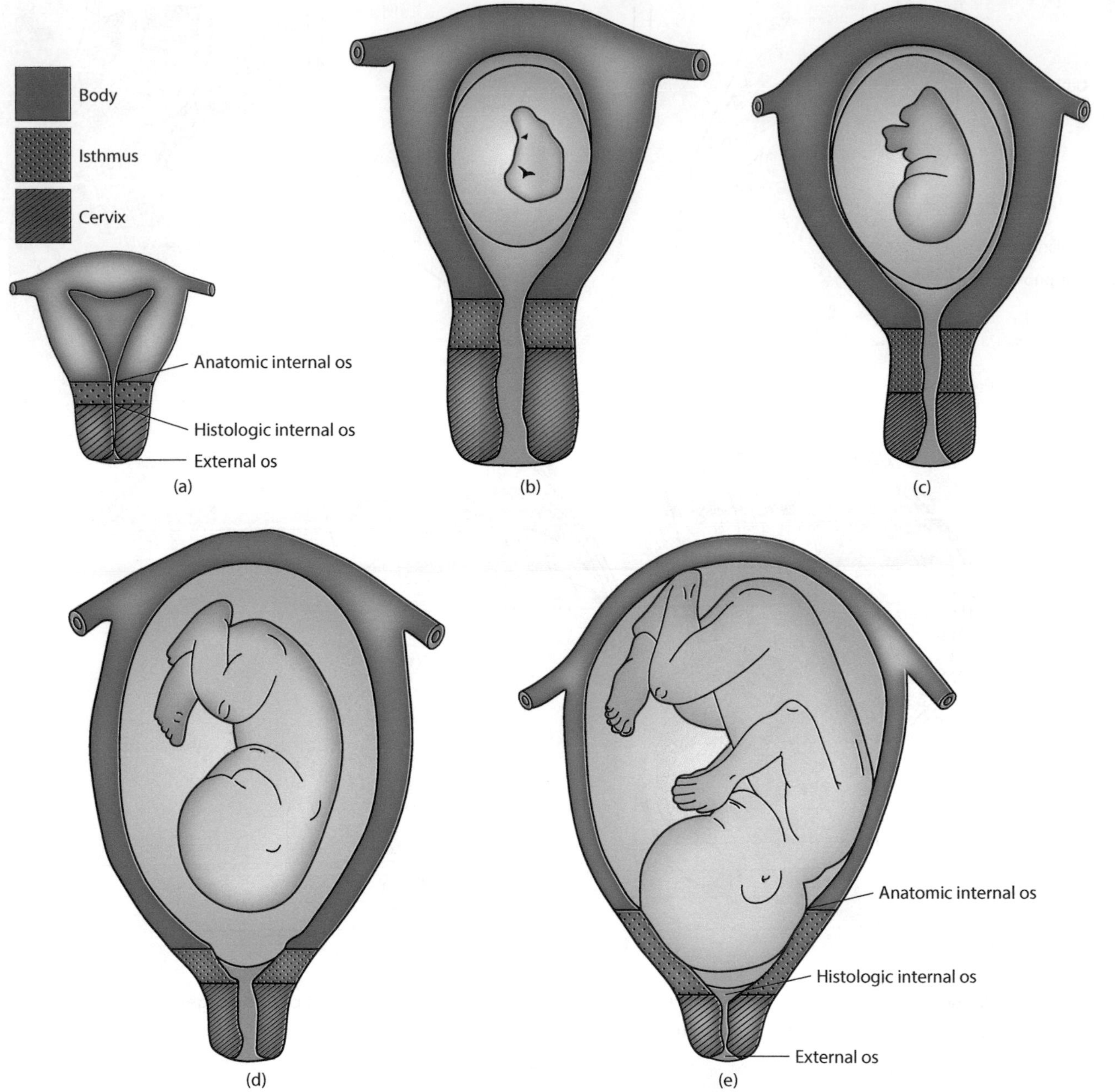

Figure 1.11 Location and extent of the three parts of the uterine wall at different periods of gestation: (a) nonpregnant, (b) first trimester, (c) first trimester (late), (d) second trimester, and (e) third trimester.

the diverging external and internal iliac vessels (ovarian fossa). However, in the multiparous woman, it may lie anywhere against the lateral pelvic wall and sometimes in the rectouterine pouch.[26] During the first pregnancy, the ovary becomes displaced and probably never returns to its original position. In nulliparous women, the upper pole of the ovary lies near the external iliac vein, and attached to it is a vascular fold of peritoneum, the suspensory ligament of the ovary (infundibulopelvic), containing the ovarian vessels and nerves. The lower pole is attached to the lateral angle of the uterus behind the uterine tube by a round cord, the ligament of the ovary that is made up mainly of fibrous tissue but also contains some smooth muscle fibers.

During the first month of pregnancy, the ovary enlarges, and the corpus luteum reaches its maximal size of 2–2.5 cm in diameter. After the second month, the ovary becomes smaller and its surface often is covered by patches of the reddish-appearing decidual reactions in the underlying stroma. Regressive changes appear in the corpus luteum within 2–3 weeks after implantation. Parts of the corpus luteum persist until the middle of pregnancy, but eventually it involutes and becomes the corpus albicans.

As pregnancy progresses, the adnexal structures move superiorly. An adnexal mass may present in the upper abdominal quadrant during the last trimester.

LIGAMENTS OF THE UTERUS

The broad ligament is the mesentery of the uterus, uterine tube, and ovary. It is formed by extensions laterally of the peritoneum on the anterior and posterior surfaces of the uterus to the lateral pelvic wall (Figures 1.5 and 1.6a). Enclosed between the two peritoneal layers are important structures related to the uterus, tubes, and ovaries. A reflection from the posterior surface of the broad ligament forms the mesovarium portion. That part above the mesovarium containing the tube in its free border is the mesosalpinx, while the part below this level is the mesometrium. The suspensory ligament of the ovary and its contained vessels and nerves continue into the lateral aspect of the broad ligament. The ligament of the ovary lies within the broad ligament as it courses to the lateral border of the uterus. The base of the broad ligament encloses the uterine vessels and nerves and part of the uterus (Figure 1.6b). As the gravid uterus enlarges and rises, it exerts tension on the broad ligament and the structures within it.

The connective tissue and smooth muscle within the broad ligament are referred to as the parametrium. The parametrium is scant medially near the uterus and superiorly near the tube where the two layers of the ligament are close. Laterally and inferiorly, the ligament thickens, and the parametrial tissue is more abundant. The connective tissue in the base of the ligament is continuous with the connective tissue of the pelvic floor. Its densest portion is referred to as the cardinal ligament (transverse cervical or Mackenrodt's) that blends medially with the supravaginal portion of the cervix and upper vaginal wall and laterally with the fascia on the lateral pelvic wall (Figure 1.6c). The cardinal ligament is the main supportive structure of uterus and divides the paravesicular space from the pararectal space. Continuous with the posterior aspects of the cardinal ligament is another fascial condensation known as the uterosacral ligament. It extends posterolaterally from the supravaginal portion of the cervix, encircles the rectum, and becomes continuous with the fascia over the second and third sacral vertebrae. It is covered by peritoneum forming the uterosacral fold, which is the lateral boundary of the rectouterine pouch (Figure 1.6). While the cardinal and uterosacral ligaments have long been regarded as important supports of the uterus, they are considered primarily perivascular sheaths or simple condensations of intrapelvic fibrous tissue rather than distinct anatomic ligaments.[27] The uterosacral fold does not contain thick fibrous tissue. In nulliparous women, pregnancy is associated with increased pelvic organ prolapse.[28,29]

The round ligament of the uterus is attached to the lateral uterine border in front of the attachment of the ovarian ligament. It passes laterally through the broad ligament to reach the pelvic wall. There it ascends over the external iliac vessels, enters the deep inguinal ring, and passes through the inguinal canal to anchor in the tissue of the labium majus. The round ligament of the uterus is composed of smooth muscle fibers and connective tissue, and it has a diameter of 3–5 mm. As the gravid uterus rises, the round ligament of the uterus increases substantially in both length and diameter (Figures 1.3, 1.4, and 1.6a).

UTERINE BLOOD VESSELS, LYMPHATICS, AND NERVES

Arteries

Knowledge of the origin, course, and branching pattern of the vessels that supply the uterus is important in controlling bleeding during surgery. The uterine artery is the main blood supply to the uterus, although the ovarian artery assists through its large anastomoses with the uterine artery (Figures 1.7 and 1.8). The uterine artery arises in a variable manner from the anterior division of the internal iliac (hypogastric) artery.[30] Nearly half of the time, it arises independently from the internal iliac artery, but very often it may originate from the umbilical artery.[30] Origins from the internal pudendal, inferior vesical, vaginal, and a stem in common with two other anterior division vessels have been observed, as well as doubling of the artery. From its origin, the uterine artery courses along the lateral pelvic wall downward, forward, and medially, passing in front of and above the ureter, to which it may send a branch. It turns sharply medially in the base of the broad ligament running toward the cervix. The surrounding connective tissue binds it to the accompanying veins, the ureter, and the cardinal ligament (Figures 1.6b and c). As the uterine artery approaches the cervix, it supplies the cervix with several tortuous, penetrating branches that allow for rapid cervical expansion. It then divides into a large, very tortuous ascending branch and one or more smaller descending branches to the upper vaginal wall and adjacent portions of the bladder (Figure 1.8). The ascending or main branch courses superiorly along the side of the uterus supplying arcuate branches to the body of the uterus. The arcuate arteries circle the uterus just beneath the serosa and, at intervals, give off radial branches that penetrate directly inward, passing between interlacing muscle fibers of the myometrium. When the muscle fibers contract after delivery, their interlacing arrangement constricts the radial branches, thus acting as ligatures. The arcuate arteries rapidly diminish in size as they pass toward the midline. This arrangement explains why midline sections of the uterus bleed relatively less than lateral ones.

As the ascending branch of the uterine artery approaches the uterine tube, it turns laterally in the upper part of the broad ligament, where it divides into tubal and ovarian branches (Figure 1.8). The tubal branch courses laterally in the mesosalpinx close to the uterine tube, which it supplies through a series of branches. The ovarian branch passes into the mesovarium, where it forms a broad anastomosis with the ovarian artery proper from the abdominal aorta. The anastomotic channel supplies the ovary and gives a series of tubal branches through the mesosalpinx that anastomose with the tubal branch of the uterine artery.

Both the uterine and ovarian arteries undergo marked enlargement during pregnancy, the latter vessel bringing blood to the uterus through its broad anastomosis with the ovarian branch of the uterine artery. The tortuous arrangement of the ascending branch of the uterine artery allows the vessel to elongate and accommodate to the growth of the uterus during pregnancy. The unspiraled descending branches are felt easily along the lateral side of the cervix at vaginal examination as a result of their increased size during pregnancy. A vast ipsilateral and contralateral arterial anastomotic network forms throughout the uterus.[31] There is an increase in the size and degree of arborizations of the arcuate arteries in and around the implantation site.

Veins

The uterine venous plexus drains inferiorly and the vaginal venous plexus drains superiorly into a plexiform arrangement of uterine veins that surround the uterine artery lateral to the cervix (Figures 1.7 and 1.8). Near the lateral pelvic wall, the uterine veins unite to form usually two trunks that drain into the internal iliac vein. The major portion of venous blood from the uterus is drained by way of the uterine veins. The remainder drains through the ovarian or pampiniform plexus. On the right, the ovarian plexus drains superiorly through the suspensory ligament of the ovary, crosses the right ureter obliquely, and then empties into the inferior vena cava. On the left, the ovarian plexus drains into the left renal vein and usually does not cross the ureter on that side. The ovarian veins on both sides dilate to enormous size during pregnancy and are possible routes for thrombus formation. They can be injured by external trauma and occasionally rupture spontaneously. The diameter of the ovarian vascular pedicle nearly triples during pregnancy.[32,33] The veins surrounding the uterus (plexus of Santorini), including those beneath the bladder, within the broad ligament, and around the cervix and upper vagina, become greatly enlarged during pregnancy.

Dissection during cesarean section must remain near the midline to avoid excessive bleeding from these dilated venous plexuses. Those veins in the broad ligament appear medusa-like and may be 1 cm or more in diameter. The ovarian and uterine veins are devoid of valves, so that constant venous pressure within the uterus is probably maintained by their expansion and contraction. Hypervascularity of the uterine wall during pregnancy may occur 20% of the time, probably representing dilation of myometrial veins.[34,35] Hypervascularity of the anterior uterine wall may cause excessive bleeding during invasive procedures. Collateral circulation is extensive and can occur through the internal iliacs, lumbar, sacral, hemorrhoidal, and systemic branches.

Lymphatics

Lymph channels are especially numerous in the walls of the female genital tract.[35] Intramural plexuses drain both the endometrium and myometrium into a subserous plexus from which efferent vessels arise. Studies on the rhesus monkey show the intramural plexuses much enlarged during pregnancy.[36] Efferent vessels from the lower uterus empty mainly into sacral nodes and nodes along the external, internal, and common iliac vessels. Some empty into lower lumbar nodes around the aorta, and a few empty into superficial inguinal nodes. Most of the lymphatics from the upper uterus pass laterally in the broad ligament, where they join those from the uterine tube and ovary. Together, they leave the pelvis by coursing superiorly through the suspensory ligament of the ovary, accompanying the ovarian vessels on the posterior body wall to empty into nodes along the lower part of the abdominal aorta.

Nerves

Nerves to the uterus and vagina are derived from the pelvic plexus (Frankenhauser's ganglion) and consist of afferent and sympathetic fibers but few, if any, parasympathetic fibers. The uterovaginal portion of the plexus passes medially toward the cervix around the uterine vessels in the upper part of the cardinal ligament. Most of the nerves accompany the branches of the uterine artery, with the cervix supposedly receiving more fibers than the body of the uterus. During pregnancy, the nerve supply to the uterus hypertrophies and is accompanied by an increase in size of the pelvic plexus. The function of the motor supply to the uterus is not well understood and is not essential to normal activity at parturition. Catecholamines exert a greater inhibiting effect on the pregnant than the nonpregnant uterus,[37] and norepinephrine can both excite and inhibit the musculature of both the uterus and uterine tube.[38]

Preganglionic sympathetic fibers to the uterus course from the aortic plexus through the hypogastric plexus just below the sacral promontory to the pelvic plexus, where they synapse in ganglia contained within the plexus. Afferent pain fibers from the body apparently travel also through the hypogastric plexus and lumbar sympathetic trunk to enter the spinal cord through the T11 and T12 nerves. Pain in cancer of the uterus has been relieved by blocks of the first three lumbar sympathetic ganglia,[38] and hypogastric resection makes biopsy of the fundus painless.[39] Sensory pain fibers from the cervix and upper vagina pass through the pelvic nerves to enter the spinal cord through the sacral (S2, S3, and S4) nerves.

PELVIC PORTION OF URETER

The course and relations of the pelvic ureter can be clearly demonstrated by endovaginal magnetic resonance imaging. Both ureters can usually be identified with laparoscopy even in overweight patients.[14] As the ureter enters the pelvis, it crosses the common or external iliac artery, coursing medial to the ovarian vessels (Figure 1.7). The base of the pelvic mesocolon lies between the left ureter and the midline. In the pelvis the ureter on both sides passes medial to the internal iliac artery, its branches, and the obturator nerve (Figures 1.6b and 1.7). It courses in a curved manner just posterior to the ovary on the upper part of the pelvic wall where it lies just beneath the peritoneum (Figure 1.6a). If the uterus is elevated anteriorly by traction, the course of the ureter frequently can be seen clearly through the transparent peritoneum and posterior leaf of the broad ligament to below the cervical level without involving dissection.[40] Or found by entering the retroperitoneal space by dividing the round ligament and opening the posterior leaf of the broad ligament lateral to the suspensory ligament. Its course can then be traced on the medial side of the posterior leaf of the broad ligament. The ureter is in close proximity to the suspensory ligament of the ovary through which the ovarian vessels course (Figures 1.5 and 1.6). It adheres to the undersurface of the peritoneum and may be accidentally drawn into the jaws of artery forceps if traction is placed on the peritoneum when the suspensory ligament is clamped. Dissection of the bladder off the anterior surface of the supravaginal cervix displaces the ureter downward and laterally. As the uterosacral fold is approached, the ureter loses its peritoneal relation by passing deeply lateral to the connective tissue of the uterosacral and cardinal ligaments at the base of the broad ligaments of the uterus. Here it passes obliquely medially, behind and beneath the uterine artery (Figures 1.7 and 1.8). The ureter and uterine artery are closely related for 1–2.5 cm of their length[41] and are enclosed in a common connective tissue sheath. At this point the ureter lies approximately 1.5–2 cm lateral to the cervix, varying 1–4 cm.[42] This segment of the ureter is most susceptible to injury during surgery, its ligation common accident, but ligation of the uterine vessels also may produce injury.[42] Identification of the cord-like medial umbilical ligament (obliterated hypogastric or umbilical artery) and following it to its lateral origin help locate the distal ureter.[43,44]

After the ureter leaves the base of the broad ligament, it inclines medially and downward in front of the upper vaginal wall through the ureteric tunnel. It then runs through the inferior portion of vesicouterine ligament. This segment is eminently palpable. At the posterior wall of the bladder, the ureters are approximately 5 cm apart. Their slit-like openings inside the bladder are only 2.5 cm apart approximately because of their very oblique downward and medial course through the thick wall of the empty bladder. The oblique course of the ureter through the bladder wall is important in preventing reflux. It is unclear whether or not reflux, which may occur with chronic bladder distention, causes the hydroureter that often accompanies pregnancy. The connective tissue sheath that encloses the lower one-third of the ureter and uterine vessels hypertrophies during pregnancy. This, together with the accompanying massive enlargement of the uterine vessels, would favor urinary stasis and dilation of the upper portion of the ureter. After the pregnant uterus rises completely out of the pelvis (fourth month), it may compress the ureter at the pelvic brim, also producing hydroureter. Ureteral dilation above the pelvic brim is usually more marked on the right side.[45,46] The right ovarian vein, which becomes greatly dilated during pregnancy, obliquely crosses the right ureter, possibly contributing to dilation on the right side.[47] The pressure of the enlarged uterus frequently causes lateral displacement and elongation of both the abdominal and pelvic portions of the ureter.

The chief arterial supply to the pelvic portion of the ureter arises close to the pelvic brim from the common, external, or internal iliac arteries rather than descending with it from higher levels.[47–49] Since this branch reaches it from the lateral side, the pelvic ureter should be exposed from its medial side. The lower end of the ureter close to the bladder regularly receives a branch from the uterine and inferior vesical arteries. As many as 10–15% of ureters may have inadequate anastomoses in their pelvic portions.[50,51] Interruption of one of the supplying vessels in such cases may damage the ureter.

Nerves to the pelvic portion of the ureter are limited to a few branches from the hypogastric nerve and the pelvic plexus. Although ureteric peristalsis is not dependent upon a nerve supply, the lower part of the ureter receives both sympathetic and sacral, parasympathetic fibers.

BLADDER AND URETHRA

Bladder

The bladder is a hollow, muscular organ lined with a mucous membrane and covered superiorly with peritoneum (Figures 1.4 and 1.6). The shape and relations of the bladder vary, depending upon its state of distention. The place when empty, the bladder has a pyramidal shape with an apex directed forward and slightly upward, a base (fundus) directed backward and slightly downward, and a superior and two lateral surfaces. The place where the two lateral surfaces meet the base is the neck, which lies on the superior layer of the urogenital diaphragm and is continuous with the urethra. The apex is continued superiorly as the median umbilical ligament, which runs to the umbilicus in the extraperitoneal tissue between the peritoneum and transversalis fascia. Below the vesicouterine pouch, the base of the bladder is related to the cervix and the anterior vaginal wall, from which it is separated by a concentration of connective tissue called the vesicovaginal septum. This region contains a large venous plexus (vesical, pudendal, or Santorini's) that drains the posterior surface of the bladder, the cervix, and upper vagina. An awareness of these veins is important during low cervical cesarean section and total hysterectomy. Toward the end of pregnancy, the base of the bladder is moved superiorly out of the pelvis by the enlarging uterus to a position in the lower abdomen. The pressure of the presenting part may impair the drainage of blood and lymph from the base of the bladder, causing the area to swell and become traumatized. During parturition, the anterior vaginal wall is enlarged and is the site of possible vesicovaginal fistulas.

The superior surface of the bladder is covered by peritoneum and, when empty, is flat or concave and in contact with the body of the nongravid uterus which lies directly upon it (Figure 1.4). When the bladder fills, the superior surface becomes convex and comes into close relation with coils of small intestine. As the pregnant uterus expands, it compresses the superior surface from above. The lateral surfaces are separated from the symphysis pubis and pubic bones by a loose connective tissue space called the prevesical or retropubic space (of Retzius) that allows for easy separation of the bladder from the pubis. The space may contain a large amount of fat and extend around the sides of the bladder, upward through extraperitoneal tissue to the umbilicus. An extraperitoneal cesarean section is performed through the upper part of this space with mobilization of the peritoneum over the bladder.[52] More laterally, the lateral surface of the bladder lies close to the levator ani and obturator internus muscle (Figure 1.6c); between these muscles and the bladder passes the obliterated umbilical artery that courses forward and upward on the anterior abdominal wall as the medial umbilical ligament.

Adjacent to the bladder wall and surrounding it is a loose layer of visceral pelvic fascia allowing for great distention. Between the bladder and the cervix, there are sometimes thickened bands of parietal pelvic fascia (called the vesicouterine or pubocervical ligament) that course obliquely anteriorly to the symphysis pubis as the pubovesical ligament. The bladder is supported by this fascia and the underlying pelvic floor.

The mucous membrane lining the interior of the bladder is loosely attached to the muscular coat and appears folded when the bladder is empty. Only in a smooth triangular area at the base of the bladder (called the trigone) is the lining smooth. Here the mucous and muscular layers are bound firmly. The lateral angles of the trigone are formed by the orifices of the ureters. Underlying muscle fibers between the ureteral orifices raise the mucosa into an interureteric ridge. After the fourth month of pregnancy, the bladder becomes hyperemic, the trigone elevates, and the interureteric ridge thickens. The trigone region progressively deepens and widens until the end of pregnancy.

Urethra

The female urethra is a short tube approximately 3–4 cm long that extends from the bladder neck to the external urethral orifice (meatus) in the vestibule of the vagina (Figure 1.4). The upper end begins at the level of the middle of the symphysis pubis, where it is surrounded by dense fascia and the vesical plexus of veins. It extends downward and forward in a gentle curve to terminate posterior to the lower border of the symphysis pubis. Intact pubourethral ligamentous and muscular attachments aid in stabilizing the urethra to its normal anatomic position and help maintain continence.[53] Posteriorly, the urethra is applied closely to the anterior vaginal wall, from which its upper half is separated by dense connective tissue and blood vessels. Its lower half is actually embedded in the anterior wall of the vagina. While superiorly the bladder and vagina are separated from each other by a cleavage plane, called the vesicovaginal septum, this plane does not extend inferiorly to separate the urethra and vagina. The urethra pierces the urogenital diaphragm where it is surrounded by the sphincter urethrae muscle. Its mucosa is arranged into longitudinal folds that contribute to the ease with which the female urethra can be dilated.

The arteries to the bladder vary in origin, number, and branching pattern. One to four superior vesical arteries usually arise from the proximal, patent segment of the umbilical artery and supply the apex and superior and lateral surfaces of the bladder. In about 10% of the cases, a superior vesical artery arises from the uterine artery. Anastomoses occur with the inferior epigastric artery in the extraperitoneal tissue, but none were found in the bladder wall. The usually single inferior vesical artery has a variable origin directly or indirectly from the internal iliac artery to supply the base and neck of the bladder and the upper part of the urethra and vagina (Figure 1.8). The vesical plexus of veins around the neck of the bladder drains most of the bladder wall, receives the deep dorsal vein of the clitoris, and communicates with the vaginal plexus. It drains laterally by three channels into the internal iliac vein.[54,55] Lymphatics from the bladder drain laterally into the external and internal nodes.

The nerves to the bladder are derived from the superior hypogastric plexus, the sacral sympathetic trunk, and the pelvic splanchnic nerves, all of which join together in the pelvic plexus. The vesical plexus of nerves is an anteroinferior continuation of the pelvic plexus that turns medially toward the bladder. Numerous cholinergic (parasympathetic) nerves supply the bladder neck and the proximal urethra,[56] although there are few adrenergic (sympathetic) nerves in these areas except in the trigone area, where they are abundant.[57] The connective tissue lateral to the bladder containing the arteries, veins, and nerves to the bladder and the terminal part of the ureter is known as the lateral (true) ligament of the bladder. The connective tissue blends inferiorly and laterally with the fascia on the upper surface of the levator ani muscle. It sometimes thickens to form the vesicouterine ligament, which laterally binds the shallow vesicouterine pouch (Figure 1.6c). No muscular connections are found between the levator ani muscle and the pelvic organs.[57] A layer of fascia is always interspersed between them.

SIGMOID COLON, RECTUM, AND ANAL CANAL

Sigmoid colon

The sigmoid (pelvic) colon is the continuation of the descending colon, beginning in the left iliac fossa near the pelvic brim and ending in front of the third sacral vertebra by becoming the rectum. The course of the sigmoid colon is S-shaped, entering the true pelvis by passing over the medial border of the left psoas major muscle, crossing the midline in front of the sacrum, and then swinging back to the left and inferiorly to become the rectum in the posterior pelvic wall. The uterus, uterine tubes, and ovaries are anterior to this segment of the colon (Figure 1.4). Structures crossing the left pelvic brim are posterior to the sigmoid colon, including the left ovarian vessels, left ureter, and left common iliac vessels (Figure 1.7). In the midline the sacral promontory and first three sacral vertebrae are posterior. The sigmoid colon is covered completely with peritoneum and is suspended by the sigmoid mesocolon. After pelvic surgery, the sigmoid colon sometimes is used to cover the operative site and thereby prevent adhesions to the small intestine.

Rectum

At the level of the third sacral vertebra, the sigmoid colon loses its mesentery and becomes the rectum. The rectum is approximately 10 cm long and extends downward and forward in the back of the true pelvis, following the curve of the sacrum and coccyx (Figure 1.4). Below the coccyx, it turns sharply backward to become the anal canal. The highest one-third of the rectum is covered with peritoneum on its front and sides. Only the front of the middle one-third is covered with peritoneum where it is reflected upward in the floor of the rectouterine pouch onto the posterior fornix of the vagina and supravaginal cervix. The lowest one-third of the rectum has no peritoneal covering and is sometimes dilated, forming the ampulla. Posterior to the rectum are located the lower sacrum, coccyx, and anococcygeal raphe. Related laterally are, from above downward, the sigmoid colon in the pararectal fossa, the sacral plexus, and the piriformis, coccygeus, and levator ani muscles. Anteriorly, the upper part of the rectum usually is separated from the cervix and posterior fornix of the vagina by coils of intestine that fill the rectouterine pouch. The posterior vaginal wall is directly anterior to the lower part of the rectum, from which it is separated by a thin layer of fascia named the rectovaginal septum. Although its existence has been controversial, the rectovaginal septum can be separated from the rectum by a cleavage space but is associated more closely with the vaginal fascia.[58,59]

Anal canal

The anal canal is the terminal segment of the large intestine, beginning at the lower flexure of the rectum as the intestinal tract passes through the pelvic diaphragm between the pubococcygeus portions of the levator ani muscles (Figure 1.4). The canal is 3–4 cm long, extending downward and backward to end at the anus. It is separated from the ischiorectal fossa by the levator ani muscle and is surrounded by an upper, involuntary internal anal sphincter and a lower, voluntary external anal sphincter. Anorectal varicosities or hemorrhoids are very frequent during pregnancy and arise from the venous plexus just deep to the surface lining of the anal canal. The upper part of the plexus drains into the hepatic portal system by the superior rectal (hemorrhoidal) vein. There are no valves in this system of veins, and the plexus therefore is affected particularly by the pressure from the growing uterus.

Obesity in pregnancy

A special note must be made about obesity in pregnancy. Depending upon the body mass index of the patient, the site of surgical incisions into the abdomen should be carefully selected. For example, the umbilicus in a morbidly obese patient with a pendulous abdomen will often be just above the public symphysis. So if a transverse abdominal incision for a cesarean delivery is made using the umbilicus as a landmark, it will be too low to allow entry into the abdominal cavity. So great care must be taken with obese patients, since the usual anatomic landmarks may be distorted by adipose tissue. However, the optimal skin incision for cesarean delivery (vertical compared to transverse) in obese patients has not been determined.[60]

ACKNOWLEDGMENT

The authors acknowledge that this chapter contains material from the previous chapter authored by Raymond F. Gasser.

REFERENCES

1. American College of Obstetricians and Gynecologists. Patient Safety in the Surgical Environment. Committee Opinion No. 464. Reaffirmed 2014. *Obstet Gynecol* 2010; 116: 786–90.
2. Bedaiwy MA, Zhang A, Falcone H, Soto E. Surgical anatomy of supraumbilical port placement and implications for robotic and laparoscopic surgery. *Fertil Steril* 2015; 103: e33.
3. Kluteke CG, Siegel CL. Functional female pelvic anatomy. *Urol Clin North Am* 1995; 22: 487–98.
4. Strohbehn K. Normal pelvic floor anatomy. *Obstet Gynecol Clin North Am* 1998; 25: 683–705.
5. Johnson MM. A study in surface anatomy with special reference to the position of the umbilicus. *Anat Rec* 1911; 5: 461–71.
6. Cox HT. The cleavage lines of the skin. *Br J Surg* 1941; 29: 234–40.
7. Tobin CE, Benjamin JA. Anatomic and clinical re-evaluation of Camper's, Scarpa's and Colles' fascia. *Surg Gynecol Obstet* 1949; 88: 545–59.
8. Forster DS. A note on Scarpa's fascia. *J Anat* 1937; 72: 130–1.
9. Howell AB. Anatomy of the inguinal region. *Surgery* 1939; 6: 653–62.
10. Rizk NN. A new description of the anterior abdominal wall in man and mammals. *J Anat* 1980; 131: 373–85.
11. Chouke KS. The constitution of the sheath of the rectus abdominis muscle. *Anat Rec* 1935; 61: 341–9.
12. Beaton LE, Anson BJ. The pyramidalis muscle: Its occurrence and size in American whites and negroes. *Am J Phys Anthropol* 1939; 25: 261–9.
13. Milloy FJ, Anson BJ, McAfee DK. The rectus abdominis muscle and the epigastric arteries. *Surg Gynecol Obstet* 1960; 110: 293–302.
14. Nezhat CH, Nezhat F, Brill AI, Nezhat C. Normal variations of abdominal and pelvic anatomy evaluated at laparoscopy. *Obstet Gynecol* 1999; 94: 238–42.
15. Begg RC. The urachus: Its anatomy, histology and development. *J Anat* 1930; 64: 170–83.
16. Pfannenstiel J. Über die Vorteile des suprasymphysaren Fascien—Querschnitts für die gynakologischen

Koliotomien, zugleich ein Beitrag zu der Indikationsstellung der Operationswege. *Samml Klin Vortr (Neue Folge) Gynaekol* 1900; 97: 1735–56.
17. Cherney LS. A modified transverse incision for low abdominal operations. *Surg Gynecol Obstet* 1941; 72: 92–5.
18. Gillespie EC. Principles of uterine growth in pregnancy. *Am J Obstet Gynecol* 1950; 59: 949–59.
19. Schwalm H, Dubrauszky V. The structure of the musculature of the human uterus—Muscles and connected tissue. *Am J Obstet Gynecol* 1966; 94: 391–404.
20. Kipfer K. Das Muskelsystem des menschlichen Eileiters. *Schweiz Med Wochenschr* 1948; 78: 65–7.
21. Toth A. Studies on the muscular structure of the human uterus. *Obstet Gynecol* 1977; 49: 190–6.
22. Schwarz OH, Hawker WD. Hyperplasia and hypertrophy of the uterine vessels during various stages of pregnancy. *Am J Obstet Gynecol* 1950; 60: 967–76.
23. Danforth DN. The fibrous nature of the human cervix and its relation to the isthmic segment in gravid and nongravid uteri. *Am J Obstet Gynecol* 1947; 53: 541–60.
24. Danforth DN, Ivy AC. The lower uterine segment: Its derivation and physiologic behavior. *Am J Obstet Gynecol* 1949; 57: 831–41.
25. Danforth DN, Chapman JCF. The incorporation of the isthmus uteri. *Am J Obstet Gynecol* 1950; 59: 979–88.
26. Waldeyer W. Topographical sketch of the lateral wall of the pelvic cavity, with special reference to the ovarian groove. *J Anat Physiol* 1897; 32: 1–10.
27. Tamakawa M, Murakami G, Takashima K et al. Fascial structures and autonomic nerves in the female pelvis: A study using microscopic slices and their corresponding histology. *Anat Sci Int* 2003; 78: 228–42.
28. O'Boyle AL, Woodman PJ, O'Boyle JD et al. Pelvic organ support in nulliparous pregnant and nonpregnant women: A case control study. *Am J Obstet Gynecol* 2002; 187: 99–102.
29. Ramanah R, Berger MD, Parrotte DM, Delaney J. Anatomy and histology of apical support concerning the cardinal and uterosacral ligaments. *Int Urogynecol J* 2012; 23; 1482.
30. Moore KL, Dalley AF, Agur AM. *Clinically Oriented Anatomy* (7th edition), Philadelphia, PA: Lippincott, Williams and Wilkins, 2013.
31. Roberts WH, Krishingner GL. Comparative study of human internal iliac artery based on Adachi classification. *Anat Rec* 1967; 158: 191–6.
32. Itskovitz J, Lindenbaum ES, Brandes JM. Arterial anastomosis in the pregnant human uterus. *Obstet Gynecol* 1980; 55: 67–71.
33. Hodgkinson CP. Physiology of the ovarian veins during pregnancy. *Obstet Gynecol* 1953; 1: 26–37.
34. Hadlock FP, Deter RL, Carpenter R et al. Hypervascularity of the uterine wall during pregnancy: Incidence, sonographic appearance and obstetrical implications. *J Clin Ultrasound* 1980; 8: 399–403.
35. Baggish M. Introduction to pelvic anatomy In: Baggish MM, Karrman M (eds), *Atlas of Pelvic Anatomy and Gynecologic Surgery* (3rd edition). Philadelphia, PA: Elsevier Saunders, 2011.
36. Wislocki GB, Dempsey EW. Remarks on the lymphatics of the reproductive tract of the female rhesus monkey (*Macaca mulatta*). *Anat Rec* 1939; 75: 341–63.
37. Nakanishi H, McLean J, Wood C et al. The role of sympathetic nerves in control of the nonpregnant and pregnant human uterus. *J Reprod Med* 1969; 2: 20–33.
38. Nakanishi H, Wansbrough H, Wood C. Postganglionic sympathetic nerve innervating human fallopian tube. *Am J Physiol* 1967; 213: 613–19.
39. Pereira A de S. A basis for sympathectomy for cancer of the cervix uteri. *Arch Surg* 1946; 52: 260–85.
40. Meigs JV. Excision of the superior hypogastric plexus (presacral nerve) for primary dysmenorrhea. *Surg Gynecol Obstet* 1939; 68: 723–32.
41. Skinner D. The pelvic ureter. *J R Soc Med* 1978; 71: 541.
42. Brundenell M. The pelvic ureter. *J R Soc Med* 1977; 70: 188–90.
43. Hollinshead WH. *Anatomy for Surgeons. The Thorax, Abdomen, Pelvis* (3rd edition), Vol. 2. New York, NY: Harper Collins, 1982.
44. Burch JC, Lavely HT. Avoidance of ureteral injury by routine palpation during total hysterectomy. *Am J Surg* 1950; 79: 819.
45. Niceley EP. Injuries of the ureters following pelvic surgery. *J Urol* 1950; 64: 283–9.
46. Rubi RA, Sala NL. Ureteral function in pregnant women. III. Effect of different positions and of fetal delivery upon ureteral tonus. *Am J Obstet Gynecol* 1968; 101: 230–7.
47. Schulman A, Herlinger H. Urinary tract dilatation in pregnancy. *Br J Radiol* 1975; 48: 638–45.
48. Bellina JH, Dougherty CM, Mickal A. Pyeloureteral dilation and pregnancy. *Am J Obstet Gynecol* 1970; 108: 356–63.
49. Meigs N. The Wertheim operation for carcinoma of the cervix. *Am J Obstet Gynecol* 1945; 49: 542–53.
50. Michaels JP. Study of ureteral blood supply and its bearing on necrosis of the ureter following the Wertheim operation. *Surg Gynecol Obstet* 1948; 86: 36–44.
51. Daniel O, Shackman R. The blood supply of the human ureter in relation to ureterocolic anastomosis. *Br J Urol* 1952; 24: 334–43.
52. Ricci JV. Simplification of the Physick–Frank–Sellheim principle of extraperitoneal cesarean section. *Am J Surg* 1940; 47: 33–40.

53. Cruikshank SH, Kovac SR. The functional anatomy of the urethra: Role of the pubourethral ligaments. *Am J Obstet Gynecol* 1997; 176: 1200–3.
54. Shehata R. The arterial supply of the urinary bladder. *Acta Anat* 1976; 96: 128–34.
55. Shehata R. Venous drainage of the urinary bladder. *Acta Anat* 1979; 105: 61–4.
56. Gosling JA, Dixon JS, Lendon RG. The autonomic innervation of the human male and female bladder neck and proximal urethra. *J Urol* 1977; 118: 302–5.
57. Ek A, Alm P, Andersson KE, Persson CG. Adrenergic and cholinergic nerves of the human urethra and urinary bladder. A histochemical study. *Acta Physiol Scand* 1977; 99: 345–52.
58. Frohlich B, Hotzinger H, Fritsch H. Tomographical anatomy of the pelvis, pelvic floor, and related structures. *Clin Anat* 1997; 10: 223–30.
59. Milley PS, Nichols DH. A correlative investigation of the human rectovaginal septum. *Anat Rec* 1969; 163: 443–51.
60. American College of Obstetricians and Gynecologists. Obesity in pregnancy. Practice Bulletin 156. *Obstet Gynecol* 2015; 126: e112–26.

Topographic anatomy of the perineum, vulva, vagina, and surrounding structures

2

KAREN HOUCK

CONTENTS

VULVA

The region of the external genital organs, known as the vulva (or pudendum), lies in front of and below the pubis (Figure 2.1). It is the term applied to the mons pubis and labia majora, and the structures that lie between the labia (i.e., labia minora, vestibule of the vagina, clitoris, bulbs of the vestibule, and greater vestibular glands).

Mons pubis

The mons pubis is a rounded, median elevation lying anterior and inferior to the pubic bone. It consists mostly of a pad of fat. After puberty, the overlying skin is covered by coarse hair. The suspensory ligament of the vagina attaches to the subcutaneous tissue of the mons pubis.

Labia majora

The labia majora are two large folds of skin that run downward and backward from the mons pubis. These elongated folds enclose between them the median pudendal cleft and are largely filled with subcutaneous fat. After puberty, their outer aspects are overlaid by pigmented skin that contains sweat and sebaceous glands and are covered by coarse hair. Their interval aspects are hairless and smooth. Anteriorly, the labia majora meet in the midline at the anterior labial commissure. They are not united posteriorly, but the forward projection of the tendinous center of the perineum into the pudendal cleft gives the appearance of a posterior labial commissure. Each labium majus contains the termination of the round ligament of the uterus.

Clinical Correlate: Because the round ligament terminates in the labia majora, inguinal hernias can rarely present as labial masses. In pregnancy, varicosities of the round ligament can readily be mistaken for inguinal hernias. Color Doppler sonography can be useful in making the diagnosis.[1]

Labia minora

The labia minora are fleshy, smaller lips located between the labia majora at either side of the opening of the vagina. The two lips are without hairs and are in contact with each other. There is wide variation in size and shape of normal labia minora. Posteriorly, the labia minora may be united by a small fold of the skin called the frenulum of the labia.

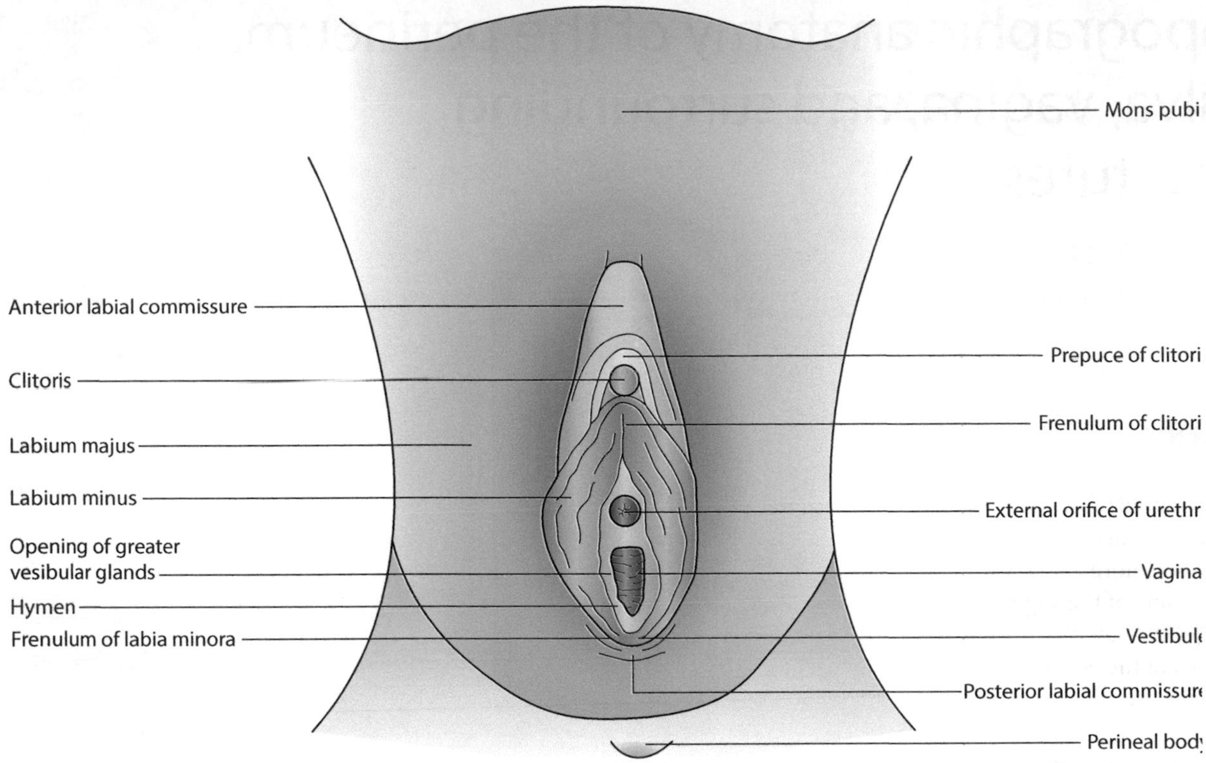

Figure 2.1 Vulva showing mons pubis, labia majora, labia minora, vestibule, glans clitoris, and the opening of the greater vestibular glands.

Anteriorly, each labium minus divides into a lateral and a medial part. The lateral part joins the corresponding one from the opposite side to form the prepuce of the clitoris. The medial parts unite below the clitoris to form the frenulum of the clitoris.

Clinical Correlate: Partial or complete removal of the labia minora and/or majora due to female genital mutilation is increasingly seen in the United States. Recent reports estimate that up to 507,000 females in the United States have undergone or are at risk for genital cutting.[2] Infibulation, or narrowing of the vaginal orifice by cutting and apposing the minor and or majora can increase the risk of obstructed labor, postpartum hemorrhage, and cesarean delivery. Antepartum defibulation may have a role in the care of these patients.[3]

Vestibule of the vagina

The vestibule of the vagina is the space between the labia minora. It contains the orifices of the urethra, vagina, and ducts of the greater vestibular glands. The external urethral orifice (meatus) is located about 2 cm or more behind the glans clitoris and immediately in front of the vaginal orifice. It is usually a median slit with slightly everted margins. The vaginal orifice is considerably larger than the urethral one and is also a median cleft. Its appearance and size depend upon the condition of the hymen, which is a thin fold of mucous membrane that partially or sometimes wholly occludes the vaginal orifice. It varies much in shape and extent.

Clitoris

The clitoris lies between the anterior ends of the labia minora. The parts of the labia minora lying anterior to the clitoris form the prepuce of the clitoris, whereas the parts lying posterior to it form the frenulum. The clitoris consists mainly of erectile tissue and is capable of enlargement like the penis as a result of engorgement with blood. It is composed of two corpora cavernosa which form the body of the clitoris, which is about 2.5 cm long. The corpora cavernosa are enclosed by a fibrous envelope and are separated from each other by an incomplete septum. The body of the clitoris separates posteriorly into two crura, each of which is attached to its respective ischiopubic ramus. The glans of the clitoris is the small elevation on the free end of the body. It also is composed of erectile tissue and, like the glans of the penis, is covered by sensitive epithelium. The suspensory ligament of the clitoris connects the organ to the front of the pubic symphysis.

Bulbs of the vestibule

The bulbs of the vestibule are two elongated masses of erectile tissue, one lying at each side of the vaginal opening under the bulbospongiosus muscle. They are narrow in front where they unite with each other to form a thin strand which is connected to the underside of the glans clitoris. Their posterior ends are broad and in contact with the greater vestibular glands.

Greater vestibular glands

The greater vestibular glands, commonly referred to as Bartholin glands, are small ovoid bodies, one located on each side of the vaginal vestibule posterolateral to the vaginal orifice at 4 and 8 o'clock. The duct of each gland opens into the groove between the labium minus and the attached margin of the hymen. During sexual intercourse, the greater vestibular glands are compressed and secrete mucus which lubricates the vagina. There are many smaller, lesser vestibular glands on each side of the vestibule which open between the urethral and vaginal orifices.

Clinical Correlate: Cysts and abscess of the gland are not uncommon. Cysts can be managed expectantly in women under 40 years old. Ascending infections have been described with bartholin abscess in pregnant women. The infections are typically polymicrobial with *Escherichia coli* being the most common isolate.[4] Because of its location in the vestibule, bartholins abscesses will often appear with vulvar masses. When incising a bartholin abscess, the incision should be made at, or proximal to, the hymen.

PERINEUM

The perineum is a diamond-shaped area which forms the most inferior part of the trunk (Figure 2.2). It extends from the symphysis pubis, anteriorly, to the sacrum and the tip of the coccyx, posteriorly, with an ischial tuberosity on each lateral side. Its superior limit is the pelvic diaphragm consisting of the levator ani and coccygeus muscles. It is restricted to the region immediately around and between the anal and vaginal orifices. The perineum is divided into two parts, the urogenital region and the anal region. The urogenital region is anterior to an imaginary horizontal line joining the midpoints of the two ischial tuberosities. The anal region is posterior to this line.

The *perineal body* or tendinous center of the perineum is a fibromuscular mass that is located in the median plane between the anal canal and the lower vagina. It contains smooth and skeletal muscle fibers bound with elastic and collagenous tissue. Attached to it are the superficial and deep transverse perineal, the bulbospongiosus, the levator ani, and the anal sphincter muscles. The anal sphincter muscles include an external sphincter, which is a thick ring of predominately striated muscle, and an internal anal sphincter. The internal sphincter is found deep to the external sphincter and extends approximately 1 cm superior to external sphincter, along the anal canal. The superficial and deep perineal fasciae and the superior and inferior fasciae of the urogenital diaphragm blend with it.

Clinical Correlate: Lacerations or episiotomies in the midline may involve the anal sphincter and the rectum. Command of the anatomy in this region is imperative to safely and successfully repair these defects. Particular attention should be placed to restoring the both the internal and external anal sphincters, if involved, as they perform roles in anal continence.

Urogenital region

The urogenital region contains the external genital organs and the associated muscles and glands. This region is divided into a superficial and a deep perineal compartment.

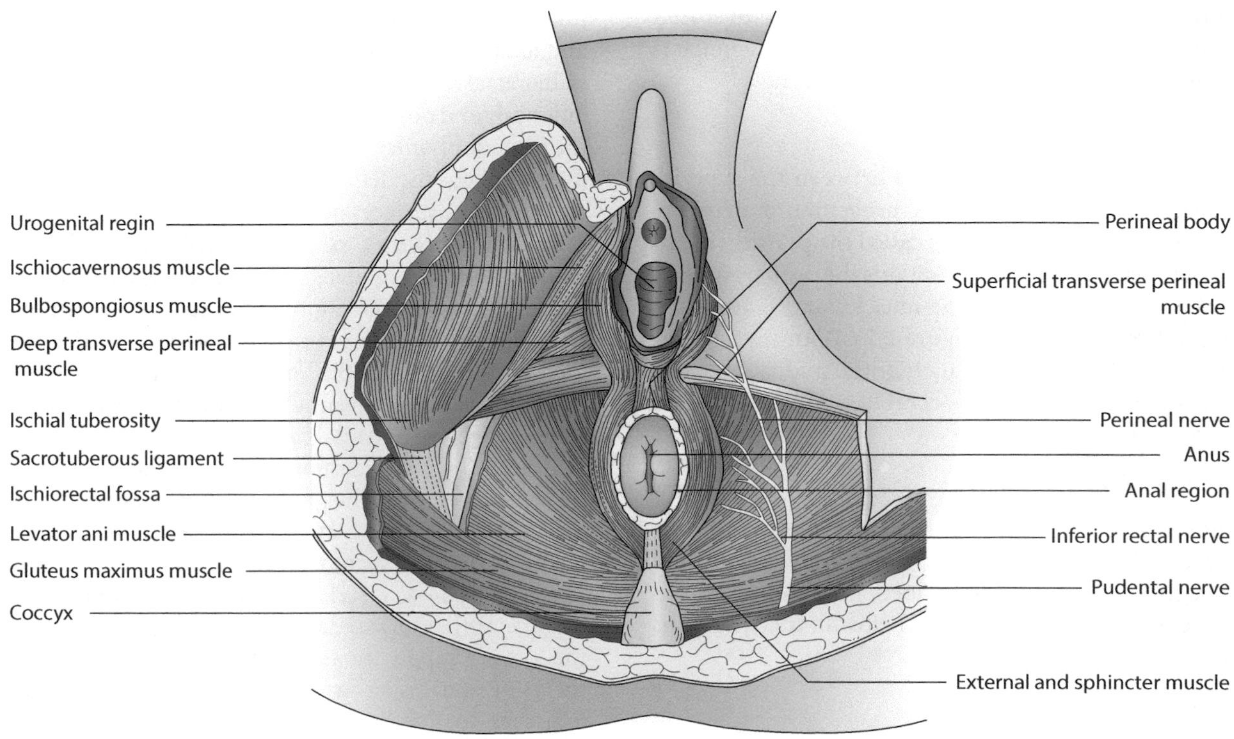

Figure 2.2 Female perineum showing urogenital and anal regions.

Superficial perineal compartment

The superficial compartment lies superficial to the inferior layer of fascia of the urogenital diaphragm and contains on each side the bulbospongiosus muscle with the underlying bulb of the vestibule, the ischiocavernosus muscle with the underlying crus of the clitoris, the superficial transverse perineal muscle, and the greater vestibular gland. All of the muscles in the superficial compartment are supplied by the perineal branch of the pudendal nerve.

Bulbospongiosus muscle

This muscle arises from the tendinous center of the perineum and passes forward around the lower part of the vagina covering the bulb of the vestibule. It is inserted partly into the side of the pubic arch and partly into the dorsum and body of the clitoris. The muscle with its counterpart on the other side constricts the vagina. This muscle is sometimes referred to as bulbocavernosus.

Clinical Correlate: This muscle is often disrupted in second degree vaginal lacerations and mediolateral episiotomies. Care should be taken to reapproximate it when repairing these defects.

Ischiocavernosus muscle

This muscle originates from the inner surface of the ramus of the ischium and inserts on the lower and medial aspects of the crus of the clitoris. It helps to maintain erection of the clitoris by compressing the crus and thus retarding the flow of blood from the clitoris.

Superficial transverse perineal muscle

This muscle arises from the lower part of the inner surface of the ramus of the ischium adjacent to the tuberosity and inserts into the tendinous center of the perineum. It is poorly developed, and its action is insignificant.

Deep perineal compartment

The deep compartment is enclosed between the superior and inferior layers of fascia of the urogenital diaphragm. The inferior layer of fascia also is called the perineal membrane. The deep compartment contains the deep transverse perineal and sphincter urethrae muscles and is traversed by the urethra and vagina (Figure 2.2). Both muscles are innervated by the perineal branch of the pudendal nerve. Their arrangement varies considerably, and often they are poorly developed.

Deep transverse perineal muscle

This muscle arises from the inner surface of the ramus of the ischium. Its anterior fibers insert into the lateral wall of the vagina, and its posterior fibers insert into the tendinous center of the perineum. It helps fix the tendinous center.

Sphincter urethrae muscle

This muscle arises from the inner surface of the inferior ramus of the pubis. Most of its fibers insert into the lateral wall of the vagina, but a few pass in front of the urethra and between the urethra and vagina. Since the urethra and vagina are fused inferiorly, the fibers of the sphincter urethrae muscle do not surround the urethra completely.

The superior fascia of the urogenital diaphragm is indistinct, but the inferior fascia is relatively dense and strong. The deep compartment contains the internal pudendal vessels, the dorsal nerve of the clitoris, and branches of the perineal nerve that supply the two muscles located there.

Anal region

The anal region contains the anus, the external anal sphincter muscle, and the ischiorectal fossa (Figure 2.1). The anal canal passes through the pelvic diaphragm and opens onto the surface of the perineum as the anus. The skin around the anus is pigmented and contains sweat and sebaceous glands.

The external anal sphincter muscle surrounds that part of the anal canal which is located in the anal triangle below the pelvic diaphragm. This muscle forms a broad band on each side of the anal canal and is divided into three parts: subcutaneous, superficial, and deep. The external anal sphincter muscle is under voluntary control and is supplied mainly by the inferior rectal nerve. The anterior portion of the muscle is innervated by the perineal division of the pudendal nerve. An additional innervation may be the perineal branch of the forth sacral nerve. The coccygeal nerve can be found near the posterior part of the external anal sphincter muscle close to where this muscle attaches to the coccyx. It is sensory to the skin over the coccyx.

The ischiorectal fossa is a wedge-shaped space located between the skin of the anal region below and the levator ani muscle above. It is filled with fat, which allows the rectum and anal canal to distend during the passage of feces. The ischiorectal fossa is not limited to the anal region but extends anteriorly and posteriorly. Anteriorly, when the fossa reaches the posterior border of the urogenital diaphragm, it extends forward above the diaphragm but below the levator ani muscle. When the surfaces of these two structures meet near the symphysis pubis, the fossa is obliterated. Posteriorly, the fossa extends above the gluteus maximus muscle to the sacrotuberous ligament. Laterally, it is limited by the ischium and the fascia covering the inferior part of the obturator internus muscle. The fossa extends medially into the levator ani and external anal sphincter muscles, which separate the fossa from the rectum and anal canal.

In addition to the ischiorectal pad of fat, the ischiorectal fossa contains branches of the internal pudendal vessels and pudendal nerve that run in its lateral wall in a channel through the obturator fascia called the pudendal canal. Posteriorly, these vessels and this nerve give off the inferior rectal (hemorrhoidal) vessels and nerve, which cross the fossa to supply the external anal sphincter muscle and the skin and fascia around the anus. Other cutaneous branches, such as the perforating branch of the second and third sacral nerves and the perineal branch of the fourth sacral nerve, also pass through the ischiorectal fossa.

Nerves and vessels of the perineum

The pudendal nerve is the principal nerve to the perineum and divides into three terminal branches. The nerve contains fibers from S2, S3, and S4 spinal cord segments and leaves the pelvis through the greater sciatic (ischiatic) foramen. It passes behind the spine of the ischium and enters the ischiorectal fossa through the lesser sciatic (ischiatic) foramen. The pudendal nerve divides near the ischial spine into three branches: (1) the inferior rectal nerve, which crosses the ischiorectal fossa and innervates the external anal sphincter muscle, the skin around the anus, and the lining of the anal canal below the pectinate line; (2) the perineal nerve, which enters the urogenital region and divides into superficial and deep branches (the superficial perineal branch gives posterior labial branches to the labia majora and lower vagina, whereas the deep perineal branch supplies the levator ani and external anal sphincter muscles, the muscles of the superficial and deep perineal compartments, and the bulb of the vestibule); and (3) the dorsal nerve of the clitoris, which runs forward in the urogenital diaphragm, and then passes through the inferior layer to the dorsum of the clitoris.

The internal pudendal artery is the principal artery to the perineum, where it gives off many branches. It arises from the internal iliac artery and leaves the pelvic cavity by passing out the greater sciatic foramen. It crosses behind the spine of the ischium and enters the pudendal canal in the lateral wall of the ischiorectal fossa through the lesser sciatic foramen. Its inferior rectal branch crosses the ischiorectal fossa to the muscles and skin around the anal canal. The perineal branch enters the superficial perineal compartment to supply the structures there and continues as posterior labial branches to the labium majus and minus. The internal pudendal artery enters the deep perineal compartment, where it gives branches to the bulb of the vestibule, urethra, and greater vestibular gland. It terminates near the pubic symphysis by dividing into the deep and dorsal arteries to the clitoris.

The veins primarily accompany the arteries and drain into the internal iliac vein. An exception is the deep dorsal vein of the clitoris, which passes entirely or mainly into the pelvis through a gap in the perineal membrane to the vesical venous plexus.

The lymph vessels from the perineum course mainly to the superficial inguinal lymph nodes, but some also pass to the deep inguinal nodes. A few lymph vessels from the clitoris follow the deep dorsal vein to join lymphatics from the upper part of the urethra and bladder to empty into the internal iliac nodes.

Clinical Correlate: Because the majority of the perineum and perineal body is served by the pudendal nerve, pudendal block at the level of the level of the ischeal spines can provide adequate anesthesia for repair of most obstetrical lacerations and episiotomies. With increasing availability of epidural anesthesia, use of the pudendal block has decreased, but it remains a valuable tool in certain settings.

VAGINA

The vagina is the female organ of copulation, extending from the uterus to the vestibule. Its walls are distensible and serve as the lower end of the birth canal. The upper part of the vagina is located in the pelvic cavity and the lower part lies in the perineum. The longitudinal axes of the vagina and uterus are almost at right angles. The vagina extends forward and downward in a plane parallel to that of the pelvic inlet. This plane is about 60° from the horizontal. The vagina forms an angle of about 90° with the uterus.

The anterior and posterior walls of the vagina are in contact with each other below the entrance of the cervix. The anterior wall is about 7 cm in length; the posterior wall is 2.5–3 cm longer. The lateral walls are attached above to the cardinal ligament and below this to the pelvic diaphragm. The vaginal lumen surrounding the cervix forms a recess called the fornix. Since more of the posterior part of the cervix enters the vagina than the anterior part, the posterior fornix is deeper than the anterior fornix. The vaginal recess lateral to the cervix is called the lateral fornix.

The opening of the vagina into the vestibule is partially covered by the hymen. After the hymen ruptures, small fragments remain attached to its margin called hymenal caruncles.

Relationship to surrounding structures

Anteriorly

The upper part of the vagina is related to the base of the urinary bladder, the terminal parts of the ureter, and the urethra, whose lower half is actually embedded in the vaginal wall. The vagina is connected to the pubis by the pubovesical ligament.

Posteriorly

The upper third of the vagina lies close to the rectouterine peritoneal pouch (pouch of Douglas); below this, it is adjacent to the ampulla of the rectum. The lower part is related to the tendinous center of the perineum, which separates it from the anal canal.

Laterally

The ureter and uterine vessels are closely related to this part of the vagina. More inferiorly, the pubococcygeal portion of the levator ani muscle, the greater vestibular gland, the bulb of the vestibule, and the bulbospongiosus muscle are near. The levator ani muscles together act as a sphincter of the vagina by decreasing the size of the lumen about 3 cm above the orifice.

The uppermost part of the vagina is supplied by a branch of the uterine artery. The lowermost part has a blood supply from the internal pudendal artery. The middle portion of the vagina may be supplied by vaginal branches from the internal iliac, inferior vesical, and middle rectal arteries. The vessels anastomose on and in the vaginal wall, forming a longitudinal channel anteriorly and posteriorly known as the azygos artery. All the arteries to the vagina directly or indirectly originate from the internal iliac artery.

The veins from the vagina drain into a vaginal venous plexus, then upward to the uterine plexus, and then to the internal iliac vein. The lymphatics from the upper part of the vagina accompany the uterine artery and drain to the external and internal iliac nodes. From the middle part, the lymph vessels accompany the vaginal artery and drain to the internal iliac nodes. Lymph from the lower part of the vagina adjacent to the hymen drains into the superficial inguinal nodes.

The nerves to the upper vagina are derived from the uterovaginal portion of the hypogastric plexus. Parasympathetic, sympathetic, and afferent fibers pass through this plexus to supply the cervix and superior part of the vagina. The lowermost part of the vagina receives its innervation from the pudendal nerve, which has its origin from the same sacral nerves (S2, S3, and S4) that supply the viscera in the pelvis.

For a more extensive review of the anatomic relationships of the female reproductive organs, see Clemente,[5] Hollinshead,[6] Leeson and Leeson,[7] Moore,[8] and Snell.[9]

ACKNOWLEDGMENT

The author acknowledges the author of the previous edition of this chapter, Shamshad H. Gilani.

REFERENCES

1. Lechner M, Fortelny R, Ofner D, Mayer F. Suspected inguinal hernias in pregnancy—Handle with care! *Hernia* 2014; 18(3): 375–9.
2. Mather M, Feldman-Jacobs C. Women and Girls at Risk of Female Genital Mutilation/Cutting in the United States. http://www.prb.org/Publications/Articles/2015/us-fgmc.aspx, 2016. Accessed September 19, 2016.
3. American College of Obstetrics and Gynecology. *Guidelines for Women's Health Care* (3rd edition), p. 243. Washington, DC: ACOG, 2007.
4. Kessous R, Archa-Tamir B, Sheizaf B et al. Clinical and microbiological characteristics of Bartholin gland absesses. *Obstet Gynecol* 2013; 122(4): 794–9.
5. Clemente CD. *Gray's Anatomy* (30th edition). Philadelphia, PA: Lea & Febiger, 1985.
6. Hollinshead WH. *Textbook of Anatomy* (5th edition). Baltimore, MD: Lippincott Williams & Wilkins, 1997.
7. Leeson CT, Leeson TS. *Human Structure* (2nd edition). New York, NY: Elsevier, 1989.
8. Moore KL. *Clinically Oriented Anatomy* (4th edition). Baltimore, MD: Lippincott Williams & Wilkins, 1999.
9. Snell RS. *Clinical Anatomy* (7th edition). Baltimore, MD: Lippincott Williams & Wilkins, 2003.

Clinical pelvimetry

3

ELAINE K. DIEGMANN and RHONDA NICHOLS

CONTENTS

Power, passenger, and passage; this is the triad that controls the birth process. Unaffected by the ebbs and tides of modern technology, the dimensions of the bony pelvis remain constant. Therefore, it is of utmost importance to understand the role of the pelvis and to commit to memory the types, the dimensions, and prognosis for birth of the basic pelvic types, since the practitioner will be making decisions regarding the route of birth that may have significant consequences for mother and infant. Therefore, this chapter will focus on the bony pelvic structures, the best predictors of birth outcomes. Knowledge of pelvic adequacy is an essential component in the decision to allow a trial of labor and plan for a vaginal birth.

PELVIC ANATOMY

The pelvis is composed of the two innominate bones (each of which is further divided into the ilium, the ischium, and the pubis): the sacrum and the coccyx (Figure 3.1).

Each innominate bone has several points of obstetric significance. The ilium contains the greater sacrosciatic notch between the inferior iliac spine and the ischial spine. The ischium contains the ischial spine, the landmark for the smallest pelvic diameter; the ischial tuberosity, located at the lowest border of the ischium; and the lesser sacrosciatic notch housed between them. The side walls of the ischium can be slightly convergent in the normal pelvis.

The pubis joins the two innominate bones anteriorly to form the symphysis pubis, the lower border of which serves as the apex of the pubic arch. The inferior pubic rami form the side walls of this significant anatomic structure, the angle of which is a predictor of successful vaginal birth.

The sacrum comprises the posterior pelvic boundary. It has five fused vertebrae, the angle and inclination of which predict the birth outcome. The sacral promontory is the anterior surface of the first sacral vertebra. It is a significant obstetric landmark of the pelvis.

The coccyx, composed of four vestigial vertebrae, forming the "tail bone," articulates with the sacrum.

Four joints articulate with the pelvic bones. Laterally, the sacroiliac joints join the sacrum to the two innominate bones at the iliac portions. Anteriorly, the symphysis connects the pubic portions of the innominate bones. Posteriorly, the sacrococcygeal joint joins the sacrum and the coccyx.

The sacrospinous ligament spans the greater sacrosciatic notch from the junction of the fifth sacral and first coccygeal vertebrae to the ischial spine. The sacrosciatic notch is a landmark in determining the posterior capacity of the pelvis. The sacrotuberous ligament is attached to the level of the third, fourth, and fifth sacral vertebrae posteriorly and to the ischial tuberosities anteriorly. The two ligaments form the side walls of Alcock's canal, through which the pudendal nerve passes.

THE OBSTETRIC PELVIS

The pelvis is divided into the false and the true pelvis. The linea terminalis, also known as the iliopectinal line, is the structural boundary which separates the two. The false pelvis provides support for the abdominal and pelvic organs and has no obstetric significance. The true pelvis is located beneath the false pelvis and is of paramount importance to the birth process. As the fetus enters the pelvis, the pelvic axis curves gradually downward and backward. Once the fetus traverses the midpelvis, the axis is gradually directed downward and forward.

There are four planes of the pelvis through which the passenger (fetus) must pass: the pelvic inlet, the plane of greatest pelvic dimensions, the plane of least pelvic dimensions, and the pelvic outlet.

The pelvic inlet is shaped like a rounded heart. Its boundaries are the sacral promontory, the iliopectinal line, and the upper aspect of the symphysis pubis. The anteroposterior diameter, known as the anatomic (true) conjugate, extends from the top of the symphysis to the sacral promontory and measures 11.5 cm. It has no obstetric relevance, since it is not the smallest diameter of the inlet. The anteroposterior diameter, known as the obstetric conjugate, is the shortest distance between the sacral promontory and the posterosuperior surface of the symphysis pubis. It should measure at least 10 cm and is the shortest anteroposterior diameter of the pelvis through which the presenting part must pass. Since this distance cannot be measured clinically, the diagonal conjugate is

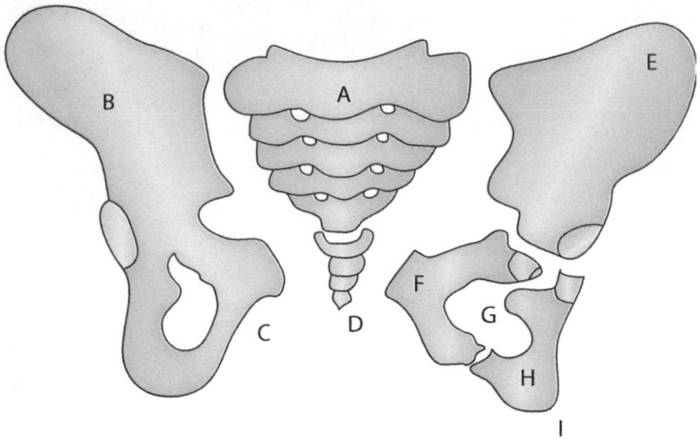

Figure 3.1 Pelvic bones: (A) sacrum, (B) innominate bone, (C) inferior rami, (D) coccyx, (E) ilium, (F) pubis, (G) ischial spine, (H) ischium, and (I) ischial tuberosity.

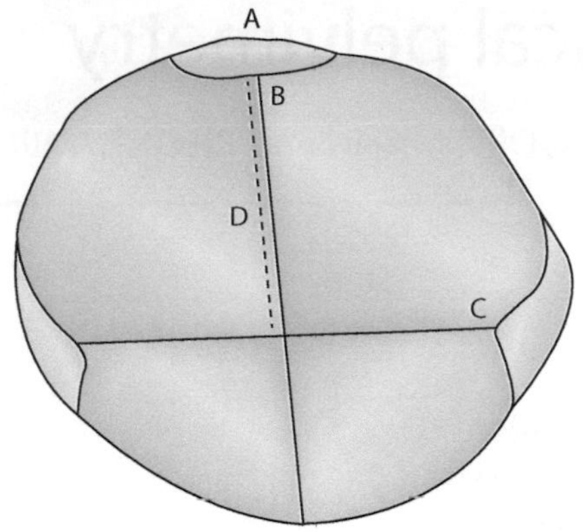

Figure 3.2 Pelvic midplane: (A) sacrum, (B) anteroposterior diameter, (C) bispinous diameter, and (D) posterosagittal diameter.

used to estimate it. The diagonal conjugate, which can be determined by bimanual examination, is measured from the lower margin of the symphysis to the sacral promontory. It usually measures 12.5 cm or more. By subtracting 1–1.5 cm (depending on the inclination of the symphysis), the obstetric conjugate can be estimated. The normal transverse diameter is 13 cm or more at the inlet. The average oblique diameter is 12.5 cm. Right/left designation of the oblique diameters is determined by the sacral crest.

The midpelvis has two planes. The plane of greatest dimensions runs from the middle of the symphysis through the second and third sacral vertebrae. It is the roomiest plane and, therefore, does not have obstetric significance. On the other hand, the plane of least dimensions is very important obstetrically, since it is the smallest plane of the pelvis, accounting for most cases of arrest of labor. This plane circles at the level of the ischial spines, the apex of the pubic arch, and the fourth and fifth sacral vertebrae (Figure 3.2).

The anteroposterior diameter of the midpelvis extends from the fourth and fifth sacral vertebrae to the lower margin of the symphysis. It usually measures 11.5 cm. The transverse diameter, also known as the bispinous diameter, is the smallest midplane measurement through which the fetus must travel. A less than 10.5 cm measurement of this diameter may have adverse effects on the birth progress. The posterior segment of the midpelvis is predictive of the birth outcome. This diameter extends from the midpoint between the ischial spines to the junction of the fourth and fifth sacral vertebrae. It should measure 4.5 cm or more.

The pelvic outlet is diamond shaped. It has been described as two triangles with the bituberous diameter as the common base.

Anteriorly, the landmarks are the lower margin of the symphysis pubis, the pubic rami, and the tuberosities. Posteriorly, the landmarks are the sacrotuberous ligaments and the sacrococcygeal joint. Again, there are two anteroposterior diameters which must be addressed. The anatomic anteroposterior diameter is measured from the apex of the pubic arch to the tip of the coccyx. This diameter measures only about 9.5 cm but is not considered in the determination of pelvic capacity, since the coccyx is mobile and is pushed backward at the time of birth. Of clinical significance is the obstetric anteroposterior diameter. It extends from the lower border of the symphysis to the sacrococcygeal joint and measures 11.5 cm. The transverse (or bituberous) diameter is the distance between the ischial tuberosities. It measures an average of 11 cm. In the pelvic outlet, both the anterior and posterior sagittal diameters are important. The posterior sagittal diameter extends from the midpoint between the ischial tuberosities to the sacrococcygeal joint and measures 9 cm. The anterior sagittal diameter extends from the same point to the apex of the pubic arch and measures 6 cm.

PELVIC SHAPES

There are four basic pelvic shapes classified by Caldwell and Moloy,[1] who are recognized authorities on pelvic architecture.[2] The four types are gynecoid, android, anthropoid, and platypelloid.[3]

The gynecoid pelvis is the typical female type configuration. Its inlet is rounded in shape. The measurements of this pelvic type reflect the optimum dimensions of the pelvic planes. The average inlet measurements include the obstetric conjugate (11 cm), the diagonal conjugate (12.5 cm), and the transverse diameter (13 cm). The midplane measurements include the anteroposterior diameter (12 cm), the transverse diameter (bispinous) (10.5 cm), and the posterosagittal diameter (4.5 cm). The greater sacrosciatic notch is wide and short, the ischial spines are blunt and not encroaching, and the sacrum is concave and inclined backward. The side walls of the pelvis are straight. The posterosagittal diameter is spacious, encouraging the passage of the fetus through the midpelvis without obstruction. The measurements of the outlet include the anteroposterior diameter (11.5 cm) and the transverse diameter (bituberous) (11 cm). The pubic arch is wide: about 90° at its apex. The inferior rami are short and gently splay outward. The fetal head typically enters this pelvic type in the transverse diameter. Labor usually progresses without complications and culminates in spontaneous vaginal birth (Figure 3.3).

The android pelvis is the male-type configuration. Its inlet is wedge shaped, with the sacral promontory deeply encroaching on the anteroposterior diameter of this plane, reducing the posterosagittal diameter as well. The transverse diameter is usually adequate, but the anterior pelvis is sharply angulated. In the midpelvis the anteroposterior and the transverse diameters are reduced. The spines are usually prominent and encroaching. This further reduces the already small midpelvic diameter. The side walls are convergent. This reduces the capacity of the midplane as well as that of the outlet. The sacrum is flat, narrow, thick, and inclined forward. The greater sacrosciatic notch is narrow and high. This combination reduces the capacity of the posterior midpelvis and diminishes the posterosagittal diameter. Coupled with the angulation of the anterior pelvis, the dimensions of the midpelvis are so reduced that the fetal head may not be able to engage. The measurements of the outlet may also be reduced. The anteroposterior diameter is short, due to the flatness of the sacral curve. The transverse or bituberous diameter is decreased. The pubic arch is narrow, and the inferior rami are long and straight. The angle of the arch is less than 90°. Occipitoposterior and transverse rotations of the vertex are common with this pelvic type. In occipitoposterior positions, especially because the head is often not well flexed until it hits the pelvic floor, engagement is difficult. Thus, the progression of labor may be delayed. If the head negotiates the inlet in the transverse position, deep transverse arrest in the midplane is common. The android pelvis frequently is the source of labor dystocia, requiring operative delivery (Figure 3.4).

The anthropoid pelvis is commonly known as the apelike pelvis. Its inlet is a long oval. All the planes of this pelvis are adequate. The anteroposterior diameter of the inlet usually is long. The transverse diameter tends to be the least adequate. The sagittal diameters are deep. In the midplane, again, the anteroposterior diameter generally is long and the transverse diameter adequate. The posterosagittal measurement is deep. The greater sacrosciatic notch is wide and long, and the sacrum is narrow, long, and inclined backward. The spines are variable, and the side walls usually are straight. The measurements of the outlet are also adequate. The anteroposterior measurement is the longest. The pubic arch may be somewhat narrow, depending upon the length and angulation of the inferior rami. The fetal head often engages in the oblique diameter. Occipitoposterior rotation of the vertex is common. Face presentation is prevalent in this pelvic type. The progress of labor is usually normal, and the prognosis for vaginal birth is good (Figure 3.5).

The platypelloid pelvis is commonly known as the flat pelvis. Its inlet is a horizontal oval. The anteroposterior diameter is short, and the antero- and posterosagittal diameters are shallow. The transverse diameter is wide. The midplane has the same characteristics: a short anteroposterior diameter, a long transverse diameter, and reduced antero- and posterosagittal diameters. The greater sacrosciatic notch is wide and shallow. The sacrum is wide and deeply curved, with sharp angulation. The sacral vertebrae tend to be thick. The side walls are straight or divergent.

The outlet measurements mirror the other planes, the anteroposterior diameter being short, and the pubic arch wide. The inferior pubic rami are also wide, with decreased angulation. The fetal head engages in transverse rotation, but, due to the reduced anteroposterior dimensions, cannot rotate to complete the mechanisms of labor. Thus, deep transverse arrest often occurs. The prognosis for vaginal birth is unfavorable, and cesarean section is a frequent mode of delivery (Figure 3.6). The above-quoted

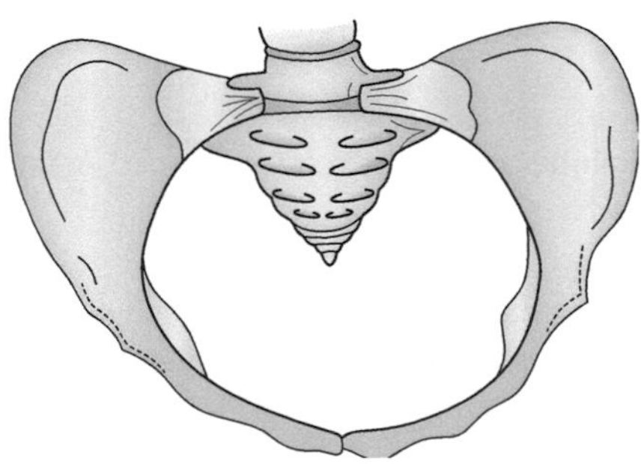

Figure 3.3 Gynecoid pelvis.

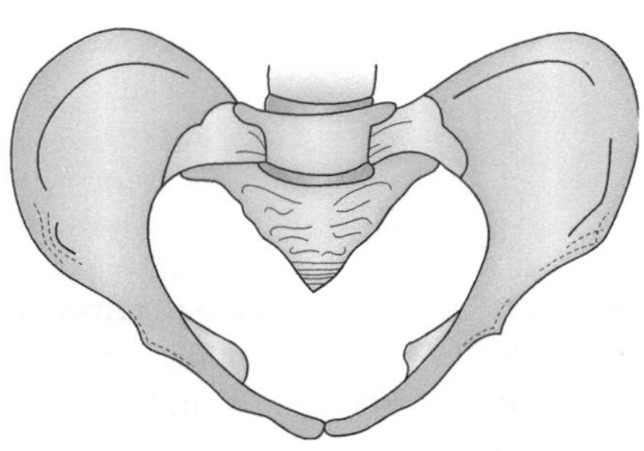

Figure 3.4 Android pelvis.

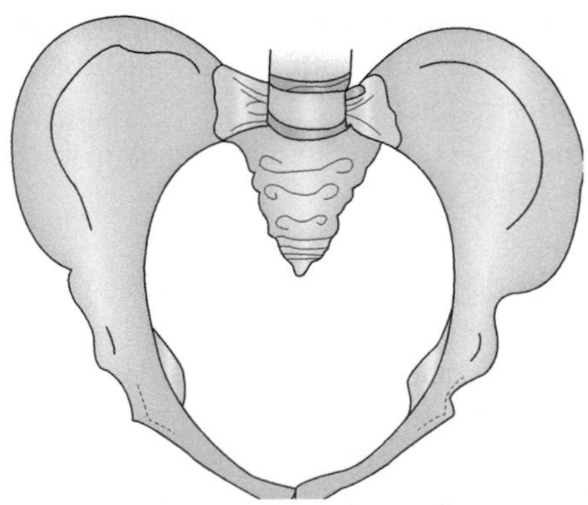

Figure 3.5 Anthropoid pelvis.

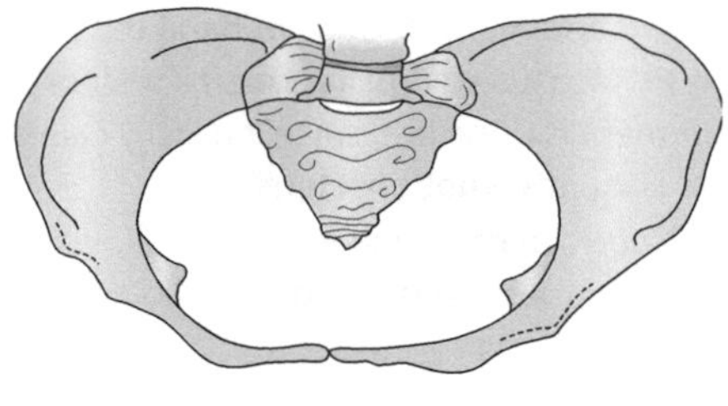

Figure 3.6 Platypelloid pelvis.

pelvic configurations represent the pure prototypes. In any individual gravida, these types may be mixed to various extents.

CLINICAL PELVIMETRY

Due to the potential hazards associated with x-rays, radiologic examinations have little place in obstetric practice today. Computed tomography (CT) scanners can be utilized to calculate pelvic measurements, with negligible amounts of radiation to mother and fetus, but at great expense.[4] However, the obstetrician and the nurse midwife have at their fingertips an effective and readily available tool with few working parts to break down: clinical pelvimetry.[5–7] All the clinician needs is a pair of gloves and awareness of a few measurements.

It is important to measure from the angle of the thumb to the third finger for the determination of the diagonal conjugate. The measurement should be made in centimeters. The width of the fist of the examining hand should also be measured in centimeters. This measurement will assist in determining the bituberous diameter.

There are several sequences for doing a clinical pelvimetry. One's preference is the main prerequisite for choosing a particular sequence. As with all procedures, the clinician should choose one and refine his or her skills. An explanation to the patient both before and during the examination is of paramount importance. The patient should empty her bladder prior to the examination and be instructed not to hold her breath or lift her head during the procedure in order to avoid tension of the vaginal muscles. Table 3.1 illustrates one effective technique. Documentation for clinical pelvimetry should be succinct as follows:

- Pubic arch
- Angle of symphysis
- Notch
- Spines

Table 3.1 Sequence for performing clinical pelvimetry.

Technique	Findings
1. Slide the index and middle fingers into the vagina and evaluate the width of the subpubic arch in FB. Then slide fingers up along the *symphysis* to determine the angle of the pubic bones (separate fingers slightly to "splint" urethra, thereby eliminating discomfort).	Slide arch: average about two FB. Angle of the symphysis: about 90°.
2. Next outline the sacrosciatic notch. Feel the *sacrospinous ligament* by placing the gloved fingers between the ischial spine and the lateral edge of the sacrum.	Sacrosciatic notch: note depth; it gives clue to pelvic type. Sacrospinous ligament: short, average, or long.
3. Continue down to the back until reaching the *ischial spine*. Determine its prominence.	Ischial spines: blunt, defined, palpable, prominent, sharp, encroaching.
4. Proceed either to left or right and palpate the side walls to determine their splay. The splay is determined by following a line from the point of origin of the widest transverse diameter of the inlet downward to the inner aspect of the tuberosity. (Placing the thumb or the examining hand on the patient's buttocks over the tuberosity may increase spatial conceptualization.)	Side wall slope: convergent, straight, divergent.
5. Sweep the fingers down the sacrum, noting its curvature. Note angle and mobility of coccyx.	Straight, concave or convex, forward, or backward inclination. Coccyx mobile or rigid.
6. Measure the diagonal conjugate. Keep vaginal hand relaxed by placing your corresponding foot on a stool and rest your arm against your thigh or hip if comfortable. Exert downward pressure on the perineum and keep away from the symphysis to prevent undue discomfort to the patient. With the examining fingers directed upward at an acute angle toward the upper sacrum and with the longest finger touching the sacral vertebrae, walk up the sacrum until the promontory is reached or fingers lose contact with the sacrum. Raise fingers to the symphysis. Drop elbow and mark off on your hand the point that touches the symphysis. Measure this distance on a ruler or centimeter scale. This measurement is done last, since it usually causes discomfort and may increase patient's emotional tension.	Exact measurement in centimeter if reached. Greater than your measurement limit if not reached.
7. The *ischial tuberosities* are measured by following the descending rami down to the tuberosities and placing your fist between them.	Average, 10 cm. Note exact measurement in centimeter if your fist fits snugly between the tuberosities. Chart greater-than-fist measurement if there is room between your fist and the bones.

Abbreviation: FB, finger breadth.

- Side walls
- Sacrum
- Coccyx
- Diagonal conjugate measured by the examining finger
- Obstetric conjugate (calculated)
- Bituberous diameter measured by the fist

Knowledge of pelvic measurements and a sequential technique for clinical pelvimetry should facilitate the assessment of pelvic capacity and the formulation of a prognosis for vaginal birth. The size of the examiner's hand and the length of the fingers probably have little effect on the accuracy of clinical pelvimetry. If they do, one's reach can be extended by the placement of a thimble on the middle finger under the glove. Knowledge of pelvic architecture and expertise in recognizing the pelvic landmarks are important. The practitioner who has small hands must be more inventive in hand placement and must learn to position patients to the best advantage. One should remember that, when positioning the hand to begin the examination, the middle and index fingers should be straight, with the thumb extended at greater than 90°. The ring finger and the pinky should be flexed across the palm, with the first and second joints extended. This position decreases the angulation of the hand between the extended middle finger and the flexed first and second fingers, allowing partial admission of these two fingers posteriorly into the vagina to increase the reach of the examining fingers. When positioning the patient, ask her to place her fists under her buttocks. This will decrease the angle between the pelvis and the examining table and thus increase the efficiency of the small examining hand.

Until the 1950s, assessment of the gravida's pelvic capacity by external measurements was a routine procedure. It was discarded almost overnight when an anonymous "expert" declared that "the size of the dining room cannot be determined by measuring the outside walls of the house." Members of the profession overlooked that, whereas a house may contain as many as 20 chambers, the various pelvic bones surround only one. Thus, in keeping with the experience of early twentieth-century obstetricians, external pelvic measurements may provide useful information about a woman's pelvic dimensions. When the technique was discarded, x-ray pelvimetry was a routine procedure and accurate enough to make external pelvimetry unnecessary. Today, since x-ray pelvimetry is not considered appropriate in current practice, only practitioners who have mastered the technique of clinical pelvimetry can perform accurate pelvic assessments. Therefore, the obstetric calipers may deserve to be reintroduced into clinical practice as a practical method for assessing a woman's pelvis with acceptable accuracy (Figure 3.7).

The external pelvic diameters to be measured are indicated in Table 3.2. The tips of the arms of the instrument are to be placed onto the quoted anatomic points. Representing the best palpable pelvic prominence (anterosuperior spines) and the most distant points of the pelvic side walls (iliac crests), the critical anatomic landmarks are easily identifiable. The same is true for the

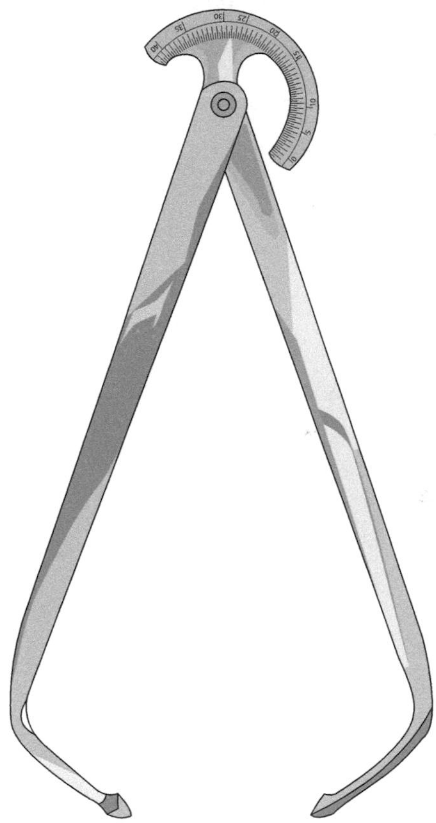

Figure 3.7 Obstetric calipers.

Table 3.2 External pelvic diameters.

Measurable pelvic diameter	Normal pelvis	Borderline pelvis	Contracted pelvis
Distance between the anterosuperior iliac spines	26 cm or more	23–25 cm	Less than 23 cm
Distance between the iliac crests	29 cm or more	26–28 cm	Less than 26 cm
Distance between the middle of the symphysis and the deepest point of Michaelis's rhomboid	20 cm or more	18–19 cm	Less than 18 cm

Note: With considerable approximation, these pelvic measurements permit the identification of various pelvic types as well as pelvic adequacy or inadequacy for an average size fetus.

anteroposterior diameter. The predictive value of "normal," "borderline," and "contracted" pelvic measurements approaches that obtainable by internal manual pelvimetry performed by an experienced examiner. This alternative method can be helpful for those accoucheurs who are not comfortable with their manual skills in clinical pelvimetry as well as for those who may utilize it to check their accuracy. It can be invaluable in a clinical situation when a previously unregistered gravida is hospitalized after premature rupture of the membranes, prior to the onset of labor, a situation which renders manual pelvimetry contraindicated.

REFERENCES

1. Caldwell WE, Moloy HC. Anatomical variations in the female pelvis and their effect on labor with a suggested classification. *Am J Obstet Gynecol* 1933; 26: 479–505.
2. Cunningham GF, Leveno K, Bloom S, et al. *Williams Obstetrics* (24th edition), pp. 51–60. New York, NY: McGraw Hill, 2014.
3. King T, Brucker M, Kriebs J, Fahey J, Gegor C, Varney H. *Varney's Midwifery* (5th edition), pp. 711–14. Burlingon, MA: Jones & Bartlett Learning, 2015.
4. Kordi M, Alijahan R. The diagnostic accuracy of external pelvimetry to predict dystocia in nulliparous women. *Zahedan J Res Med Sci* 2012: 36–38.
5. Korhonen U, Taupole P, Heinonen S. Assessment of the bony pelvis and vaginally assisted deliveries. *ISRN Obstet Gynecol* 2013: 5. Article ID 763782.
6. Posner G, Jessica D, Amanda B, Griffith J. *Oxorn-Foote Human Labor & Birth* (6th edition), pp. 38–52. New York, NY: McGraw Hill, 2013.
7. Steer C, Moloy HC. *Moloy's Evaluation of the Pelvis in Obstetrics*, pp. 793–833. New York, NY: Plenum Medical Books, 1975.

First-trimester embryofetoscopy

4

E. ALBERT REECE and ANTHONY M. VINTZILEOS

CONTENTS

INTRODUCTION

First-trimester embryofetoscopy is a technique that allows visualization and access to the developing embryo/fetus and its environment. The procedure can be performed by the introduction of an endoscope into the extracelomic space transcervically or transabdominally. The procedure uses a high-resolution fiber-optic equipment attached to a camera for direct visualization of the embryo/fetus. The need for first-trimester embryofetoscopy has been created by the recent technological advances of ultrasound for first-trimester prenatal diagnosis. Improved high-resolution of transvaginal ultrasound has made possible the morphologic evaluation of a developing embryo/fetus. Certain fetal anomalies cannot be diagnosed with certainty by using ultrasound alone. Therefore, the direct visualization of the fetus may be necessary to confirm some ultrasonically diagnosed fetal anomalies in the first trimester of pregnancy, and also to help in the management in selected families affected by recurrent genetic syndromes with recognizable external fetal abnormalities. An additional reason for introducing first-trimester embryofetoscopy is its potential for early in utero therapy, opening the way for a new era of early pregnancy intervention.

HISTORY

Transcervical fetal visualization in three early pregnancies was first reported by Westin in 1954 using the McCarthy panendoscope.[1] The gestational ages were not stated by the author, and measurements of fetal length suggested that these pregnancies were in the second trimester. It is unclear, however, whether fetal size had been overestimated by the varying magnification factor of the fiber-optic scope. Westin described the exploration of "the space between the uterine wall and the membranes up to the site of the placenta," a description which is suggestive of the unobliterated extracelomic cavity of the first trimester. In the 1960s, several groups of investigators performed transcervical chorion villus biopsy under endoscopic guidance; however, fetal anatomy and development were not a main focus. In 1974, MacKenzie described his experience with transcervical fetoscopy between 8 and 20 weeks gestation in 28 patients; he used a 5-mm, flexible-tip bronchofiberscope, which was introduced through an undilated cervix and without anesthesia or sedation.[2] Gallinat et al. reported in 1979 on transcervical embryoscopy using a hysteroscope and CO_2 inflation of the uterus; pregnancies that were intended to be terminated at 12 weeks gestation were followed weekly from 5 weeks gestation and gross fetal anatomy was described.[3] Roume et al.[4] and Dumez[5] from the Port Royal Maternity Hospital in Paris incorporated embryoscopy into their prenatal diagnosis program in 1979 and reported on the utility of this tool in the diagnosis of limb abnormalities. The largest study in noncontinuing pregnancies was reported in 1990 by Cullen et al.[6] They confirmed the utility of embryoscopy in the detection of fetal anomalies other than limb abnormalities. In

1990, Reece et al. demonstrated the accessibility of the embryonic blood circulation.[7]

Because the number of cases warranting fetal surgery remain low, specialized instruments for visualization of the embryo were not developed in earnest until the mid- to late 1990s.[8] Today's embryofetoscopes are designed to have the smallest diameter possible while still allowing sufficient image quality, available in lengths of 20–30 cm and diameters of 1.0–3.8 mm.[9]

TECHNIQUE

The technique of first-trimester embryofetoscopy consists of fiber-optic endoscopy, and it can be performed as early as 5 weeks menstrual age transcervically or transabdominally.[6] The first attempts of early embryofetoscopy were performed transcervically with rigid fiber-optic endoscopes 30 cm in length, with diameters 2–3.5 mm and angle lengths of 0° or 30°.[6] Under continuous sonographic guidance, the endoscope is passed through the cervix into the extracelomic cavity with extreme care, so that the amnion is not ruptured. The chorion is identified by its opaque character, and it is bluntly penetrated by the tip of the endoscope. The site of penetration is very carefully chosen to avoid the placenta and also areas where the chorion and amnion are juxtaposed (Figure 4.1).

Another technique of first-trimester embryofetoscopy uses the transabdominal approach. This approach was developed in recent years, and it is also performed under continuous sonographic guidance.[7] Instrumentation consists of a 0.8-mm fiber-optic endoscope and a 27-gauge needle, which are accommodated by a specially designed 16-gauge, double-barrel instrument sheath. Under the sonographic guidance, the endoscope and needle are passed transabdominally into the extracelomic or amniotic cavity. The morphology of the fetus, as well as any blood-sampling procedures, is viewed through a video camera and recorded. Only limited movement of the endoscope tip can be used to prevent intra-amniotic bleeding, which can occur in 10%–15% of pregnancies.[9] The procedure is very similar to performing an amniocentesis, and it avoids the potential risk of fetal trauma and introduction of infection that are associated with the transcervical route.

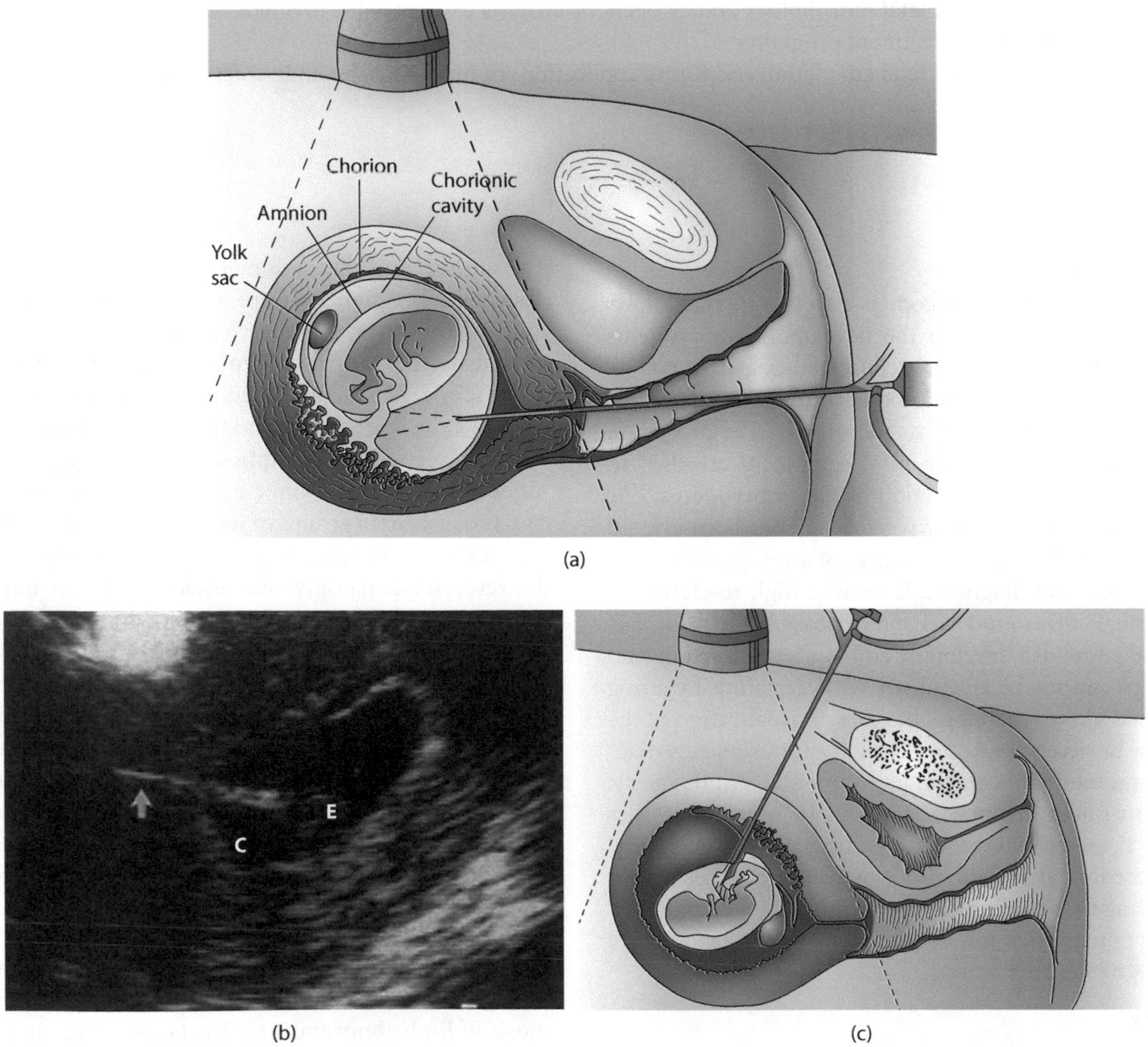

Figure 4.1 (a) Schematic representation of transcervical embryofetoscopy, (b) ultrasound image of transcervical embryofetoscopy, and (c) access to the umbilical cord via transabdominal embryofetoscopy.

APPLICATION

First-trimester embryofetoscopy has several current applications: (a) documentation of normal early human development; (b) confirmation or exclusion of first-trimester ultrasound findings; (c) evaluation of embryonic morphology and cytogenetic analysis in early failed pregnancies, recurrent miscarriages, and fertility treatment programs. Future applications may involve access to the fetal circulation for early fetal therapy.

Documentation of normal early human development

Embryoscopy can be a valuable tool for the primary diagnosis of congenital anomalies in the first trimester and for the confirmation of ultrasonographically suspected anomalies. Because this technique can be used as early as five menstrual weeks and allows for direct visualization of normal and abnormal development, it is of significant importance to our understanding of human embryology. Much of our knowledge of early human development has been based on the investigation of human abortuses or animal research, which only provides close approximations to normal human fetal growth. Embryoscopy visualizes the human embryo in vivo unaffected by any pathology of the uterine environment. The embryonic period, during which all major external and internal structures develop, extends from conception to 8 weeks (or 10 menstrual weeks). This is the period of greatest susceptibility to the effects of teratogens. At the end of this early development, the fetus has all external features of the human species.

The head and neck

The endoscopic view of the fetal face at 6 conceptual weeks reveals a prominent forehead, widely spaced eyes, and confluent oral and nasal cavities. At 8 conceptual weeks and beyond, greater facial detail is seen. Some congenital malformations of the head and neck can be visualized in early pregnancy. These include anencephaly, acrania, hydrocephaly, microcephaly, and macrocephaly. However, the most likely diagnosable malformations include anencephaly and acrania. Potentially diagnosable anomalies of the face include micrognathia and cleft lip.

The trunk

Development of the gut occurs at a time when the abdominal cavity is still small; hence, herniation occurs in the body stalk at about 5 weeks gestation. The gut remains extruded until about 10 weeks gestation, when reinsertion occurs, followed by complete closure of the ventral wall. These normal developmental events can be documented by embryoscopy. The ventral hernia is seen as early as 4 conceptual weeks, and by 8 conceptual weeks the hernia is almost completely resolved. It is likely, therefore, that dorsal and ventral wall defects are diagnosable by embryoscopy.

The neural tube

The neural tube is seen with the cephalic end open at about 5 conceptual weeks. By about 7 conceptual weeks, the complete closure of the neural tube is visible (Figures 4.2 and 4.3), unless malformations have occurred.

The limbs

The normal development of the limb buds is manifested first as lateral swellings or paddle-shaped structures in the late fourth week after conception (Figure 4.4). At 7 weeks gestation, a fully developed hand is seen (Figures 4.5 and 4.6). Foot paddles and well-developed feet are usually visible 2 weeks later than the equivalent in the upper extremities (Figure 4.7). Because the limbs can be clearly visualized by embryoscopy, this technique is likely to diagnose limb anomalies such as hemimelia, phocomelia, sirenomelia, missing digits, lobster claw, polydactyly (Figure 4.8), syndactyly, brachydactyly, clubhand, and clubfoot.

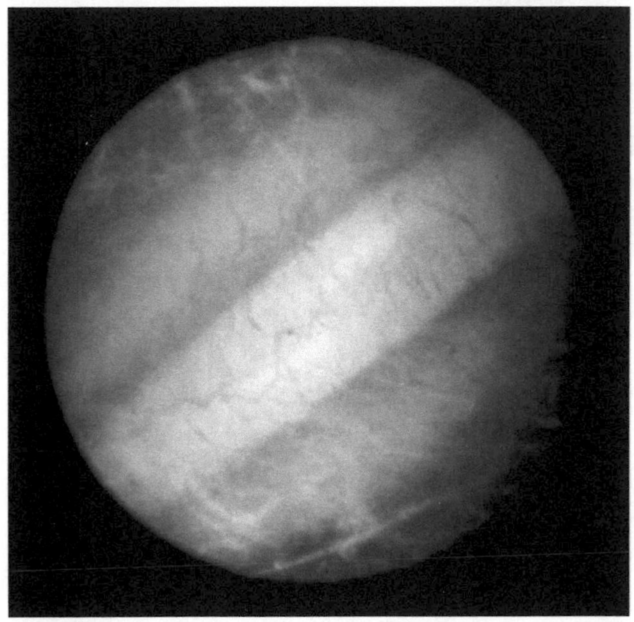

Figure 4.2 Completely closed neural tube is seen at 7 conceptual weeks.

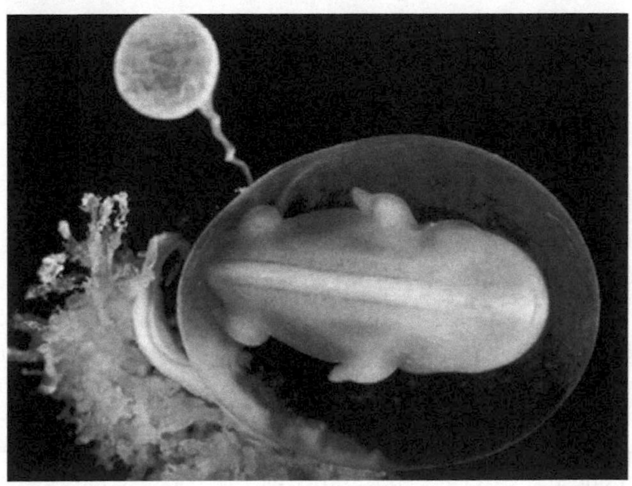

Figure 4.3 Posterior view of neural tube at 7 conceptual weeks.

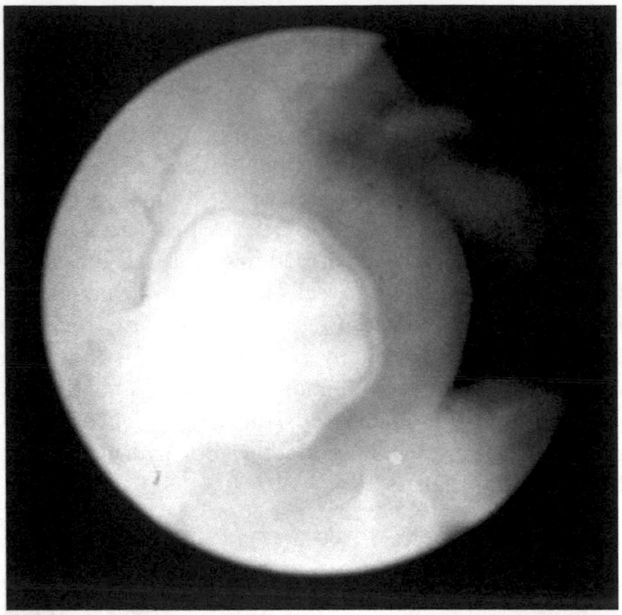

Figure 4.4 Hand paddle at 4 conceptual weeks with subtle demarcations of finger rays.

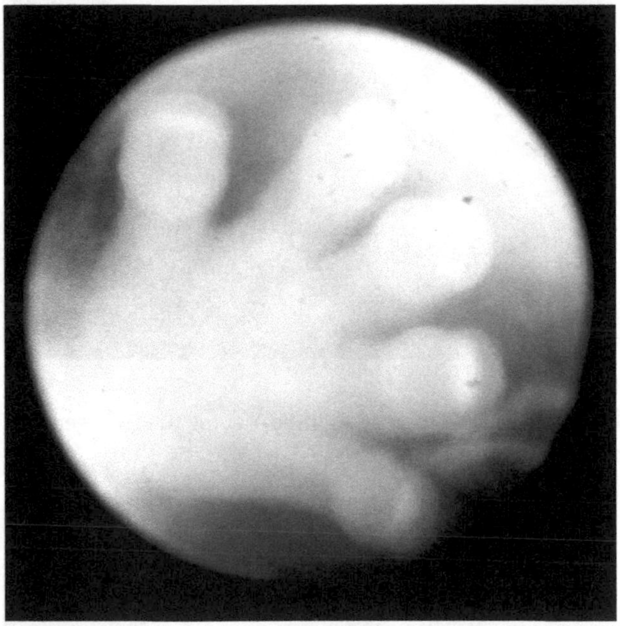

Figure 4.5 Hand at 7 conceptual weeks.

Other structures

The yolk sac can be visualized as early as 5 weeks gestation. Embryoscopically, the early yolk sac has a confluent and prominent vasculature in contrast to the yolk sac at 10 conceptual weeks, which contains smaller, more numerous, but less prominent vessels. The anomalous development and external appearance of the yolk sac have been described under experimental conditions and have been associated with embryonic malformations. It is likely that similar changes of yolk sac morphology will be detected

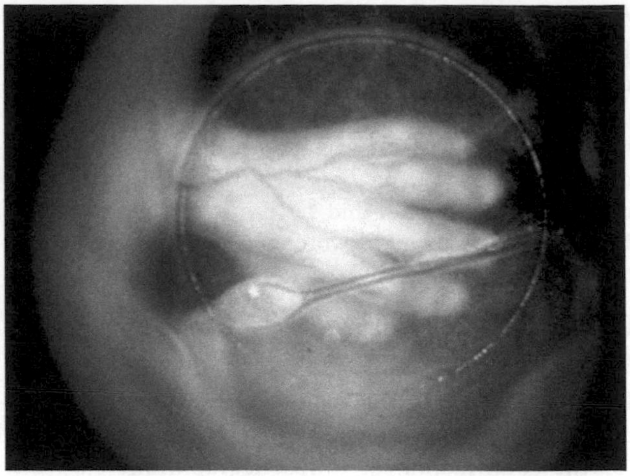

Figure 4.6 At 9 conceptual weeks, a fully developed hand is observed without webbing.

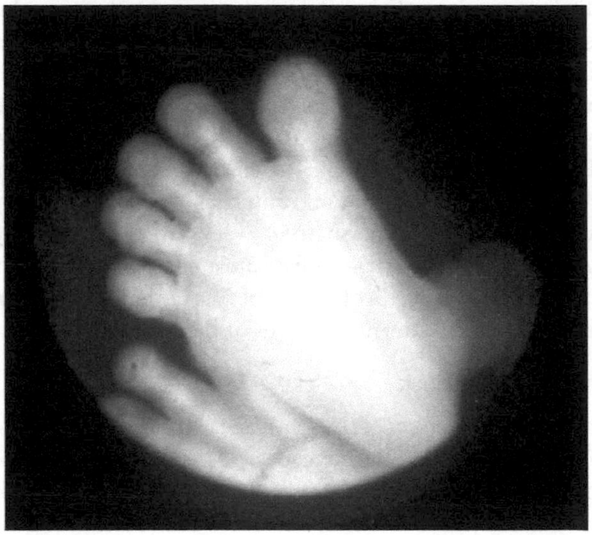

Figure 4.7 Well-developed fetal foot at 9 conceptual weeks with well-developed toes without webbing.

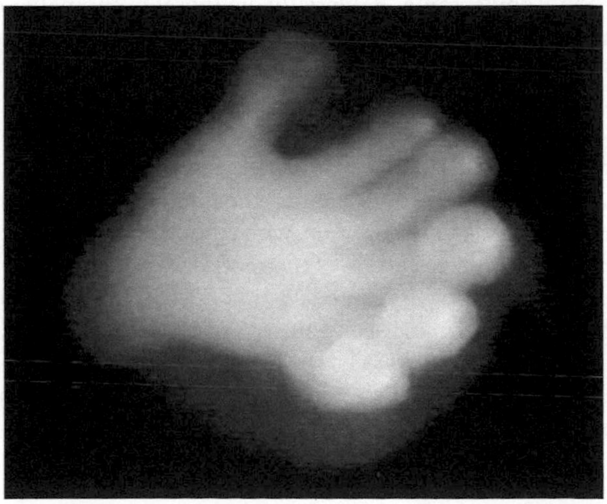

Figure 4.8 Hand at 7 conceptual weeks shows polydactyly.

by embryoscopy and correlated with pathologic states. The genitalia can also be seen to develop from a "nonspecific" genital ridge to typical male genitalia.

Utility and safety

According to Reece et al., first-trimester embryofetoscopy takes approximately 5 minutes, and fetal visualization is achieved in approximately 90% of the cases.[7,10] The risk of infection, uterine perforation, or any other maternal morbidity related to the procedure is very small. The possibility of trauma to the amnion is the least between 7½ and 11 menstrual weeks gestation and increases with gestational age. Other investigators have reported similar success rates of visualization.

Dumez reported using transcervical embryofetoscopy in over 60 continuing pregnancies.[5] Although he observed six pregnancy losses as a result of using transcervical embryofetoscopy, after introducing the transabdominal approach in 20 cases, there were no additional adverse outcomes. Quintero et al. reported their experience with transabdominal embryofetoscopy using an 18- or 19-gauge, thin-wall needle and a 0.7-mm endoscope in 18 patients undergoing first-trimester or early second-trimester pregnancy termination.[11] They obtained a thorough visualization of fetal anatomy from 7 to 13 weeks in 85% of cases. Ville et al. reported that the procedure-related risk of transabdominal, first-trimester embryofetoscopy is approximately 12%.[12] Yin et al. reported on 12 pregnant women scheduled for the legal termination of pregnancy at 6–12 weeks gestation.[13] A flexible fiber-optic endoscope was used transcervically under ultrasound guidance. Complete visualization of the embryo/fetus was accomplished in 50% of the cases. There were no procedure-related complications. Greco et al. reported on their experience with nine cases at 10–14 weeks gestation, using transabdominal embryofetoscopy.[14] They reported complete visualization of the embryo/fetus in all cases, and they concluded that fetal examination was easier at 10–12 weeks of gestation than at 13–14 weeks. Surbek et al. performed transabdominal embryofetoscopy in 14 patients scheduled for termination of pregnancy, using a 1-mm, semirigid, fiber-optic telescope with an 18-gauge examination sheath and a single-chip digital camera.[15] A 25-gauge needle was inserted through a 21-gauge side port to access the fetal circulation. The fetal head, face, abdomen, and complete upper and lower limbs were visualized in over 80% of the cases. However, the fetal back and external genitalia were visualized in only 35.7% and 64.3% of the cases, respectively. Injection of 10–20 mL of saline improved the visibility in 43% of the cases. The investigators attempted successful funipuncture in two of three attempts. Zwinger and Krofta attempted transabdominal embryofetoscopy at 7–8 postconceptional weeks and were successful in all seven cases.[16] Miliou-Paouleskou et al. attempted transabdominal embryofetoscopy during the first 12 weeks of pregnancy in 20 women prior to pregnancy termination.[17] A complete methodological survey of the embryo/fetus was possible in all cases. Access to embryonic circulation was attempted, and a small quantity of blood was obtained in 71.4% of the cases. The average length of the procedure was approximately 15 minutes. There were no maternal complications.

As an invasive procedure, embryofetoscopy carries the risk for preterm premature rupture of membranes (PPROM). In two recent reviews, Beck et al. examined the rates of PPROM following fetoscopy as reported in the literature, and found a trend in rupture rates and the diameter of the endoscope.[9,18]

Confirmation or exclusion of first-trimester ultrasound findings

The introduction of high-resolution vaginal sonography has tremendously improved our ability to diagnose fetal anomalies in the first trimester of pregnancy. However, when congenital anomalies are diagnosed at such an early stage of pregnancy and patients choose to terminate the pregnancy, pathologic confirmation, and anatomic studies are not possible due to the destructive nature of first-trimester induced abortions. First-trimester embryofetoscopy prior to pregnancy termination can be used to confirm prenatally diagnosed anomalies and ensure accurate patient counseling for subsequent pregnancies. In addition, embryofetoscopy can be used in cases where the ultrasound diagnosis is not certain or an ultrasound diagnosis may not be possible, depending upon the type and nature of the genetic disorder. In several cases, embryofetoscopy was used for early pregnancy prenatal diagnosis. In 1993, Quintero et al. diagnosed a case of Meckel–Gruber syndrome at 11 weeks menstrual age by visualizing postaxial polydactyly and occipital encephalocele.[11] Dommergues et al. used embryofetoscopy to diagnose a case of van der Woude's syndrome at 11 weeks menstrual age, allowing for early pregnancy termination.[19] Also, Rankine et al. were able to confirm the diagnosis of acrania at 12 weeks gestation by using transcervical endoscopy; in addition, they were able to demonstrate other abnormalities, including a small omphalocele, hexadactylism on both sides, and bilateral clubfoot.[20] More recently, Di Spiezio Sardo et al. reported on the embryofetoscopic diagnosis of Pentalogy of Cantrell by visualizing an omphalocele with ectopia cordis.[21]

Embryofetoscopy has also been used not only to confirm suspicious ultrasound findings but also to exclude congenital anomalies in continuing pregnancies. Reece et al. used transabdominal embryofetoscopy to rule out a suspected neural tube defect based on suspicious ultrasound findings.[22] In addition, Robert's syndrome was ruled out in a mother who had previously given birth to an affected infant; complete visualization of the embryo was achieved in this case, and no limb or facial abnormalities were seen.[23] Similarly, Hobbins et al. ruled out Smith–Lemli–Opitz type 2 syndrome in a patient at risk by using transabdominal embryofetoscopy after transvaginal ultrasound had suggested polydactyly; embryofetoscopy revealed a normal fetal hand and the patient chose to continue with the pregnancy, resulting in a healthy, normal baby at birth.[24]

Lee et al. ruled out short rib-polydactyly syndrome, type II (Majewski), at 13 weeks gestation by demonstrating the absence of limb and facial abnormalities by embryofetoscopy.[25] The same investigator reported on six patients who had embryofetoscopy performed between 12 + 6 and 14 + 6 weeks of gestation to rule out recurrent major and minor (cleft lip/palate) genetic abnormalities.[26] Satisfactory visualization was achieved in five of the six cases (83%) and the procedures lasted between 15 and 40 minutes. One pregnancy was terminated because the diagnosis of Meckel–Gruber was made, two pregnancies were terminated because of amniotic fluid leakage after the procedure, and the remaining three pregnancies resulting in full-term infants with no abnormalities.[26] The authors stressed the need to establish efficacy and safety of embryofetoscopy by large multicenter studies.

In summary, first-trimester embryofetoscopy has been used by various clinicians and investigators in patients who have already decided for a pregnancy termination if fetal anomalies are found and also in patients who wish to continue their pregnancies if fetal anomalies are excluded.

Evaluation of embryonic fetal morphology and cytogenetic analysis in early failed pregnancies in recurrent miscarriage or fertility treatment programs

One of the applications of embryofetoscopy is to evaluate the morphology of the embryo/fetus in early failed pregnancies. In such cases, the embryofetoscopy is performed transcervically to assess fetal morphology and obtain material directly from fetal tissues, so that successful fetal cytogenetic analysis is possible. Guida et al. used embryofetoscopy to make the diagnosis of spinal dysraphism in an early missed abortion in the first trimester of pregnancy; a dorsal cystic lesion was visualized, which was biopsied and proved to be meningeal tissue.[27] Yin et al. reported on transcervical embryoscopic diagnosis of conjoined twins in a 10-week missed abortion.[28]

Philipp and Kalousek reported on the use of transcervical embryofetoscopy in diagnosing localized and systemic defects in the embryonic morphogenesis of missed abortions in a population of 24 women.[29] They used the rigid hysteroscope, which was passed transcervically into the amniotic cavity. An embryo was visualized in 80% of the cases, and half of the embryos showed multiple developmental defects. Philipp et al. also reported on the use of transcervical embryofetoscopy in the evaluation of structural defects in four first-trimester, monochorionic twin, intrauterine deaths.[30] One case was diagnosed with trisomy 21, a second with thoracophagus twins, and a third with acardiac twins, while a fourth case was remarkable because of the concordance of limb reduction defects.

Philipp et al. subsequently reported on 272 patients with missed abortion in whom transcervical embryofetoscopy was used prior to dilation and curettage to study the morphology of the embryo/fetus and also to perform cytogenetic analysis of chorionic villi by either standard, G-banding cytogenetic techniques or comparative genomic hybridization in combination with flow-cytometry analysis.[31] Visualization of the embryo or early fetus was successful in 86% of the cases, and a successful karyotype was obtained in 81% of the cases. Approximately 75% of the cases had an abnormal karyotype, 18% had a morphologic defect with a normal karyotype, and no embryonic or chromosomal abnormality could be found in 7% of the cases. The authors concluded that transcervical embryofetoscopy for the evaluation of missed abortions provides valuable information for genetic counseling in planning for future pregnancies.

Ferro et al. used embryofetoscopy prior to curettage in 68 women with missed abortions between 4 and 19 weeks gestation to obtain direct embryo and chorion biopsies for chromosomal analysis; biopsies suitable for chromosomal analysis were obtained in 97% of the cases and all "46,XX misdiagnoses" of the conventional curettage karyotype due to maternal contamination (22%) were identified.[32] Paschopoulos and colleagues performed 42 embryofetoscopies in missed-abortion pregnancies, using the transcervical approach and leaving the amnion intact during visualization.[33]

It appears that the use of transcervical embryofetoscopy in accurate evaluation of embryonic morphology and cytogenetic analysis can be a helpful tool for understanding the reasons for early pregnancy failure; most importantly, it may provide extremely useful information for genetic counseling and planning for future pregnancies.

Access to the embryonal/fetal circulation and future applications of first-trimester embryofetoscopy

Cannulation of the vitelline and umbilical blood vessels under direct embryofetoscopic guidance is feasible. Reece et al. were the first to attempt fetal blood sampling by using first-trimester, transabdominal needle embryofetoscopy.[7,10] These investigators were able to infuse indigo carmine dye into the circulation of three patients at 8–12 weeks gestation prior to pregnancy termination. Surbek et al. reported on the use of transabdominal, first-trimester embryofetoscopy as a potential approach to early in utero stem-cell transplantation and gene therapy, since they succeeded in funipuncture in two of three attempts in patients prior to pregnancy termination.[15]

The best results in achieving access to the embryonal/fetal circulation during the first trimester of pregnancy were reported by Miliou-Paouleskou et al., who attempted first-trimester, transabdominal embryofetoscopy in 20 women.[17] Access to the embryonic circulation was attempted in 14 cases and was performed successfully in 10 (success rate 71.4%). There is no question that such high success rates, if confirmed by other investigators, would provide the vehicle for early intravascular stem-cell transplantation.

The prospects of human gene and cell therapy have become excellent in recent years. First-trimester embryofetoscopy allows accessibility to the circulation of the developing embryo/fetus at a time when it is immunologically naive, and, therefore, more receptive to grafts. The early in utero application of this technology may be advantageous in genetic diseases that produce irreversible damage by the time of birth. At present, the only technique that can be used effectively for gene transfer is bone marrow. In the near future, however, more should be learned about how to package DNA and make it tissue specific. If so, the use of embryofetoscopy for intravenous injection of genetic material will hold great promise. Although fetal gene therapy is still experimental, the availability of first-trimester embryofetoscopy brings fetal gene therapy within our reach, and this therapy may be proven in the future to be critical in preventing irreversible perinatal disease manifestations in many inherited conditions. However, it is prudent to investigate this approach extensively, first in animal models in order to improve the technological aspects of the procedure and assess the efficacy of gene expression, as well as possible side effects, before application in humans is considered.

Chan et al. have used embryofetoscopy to obtain fetal blood between 7 + 2 and 13 + 4 weeks gestation for ex vivo viral transduction of cultured human fetal mesenchymal stem cells, thus leading to possible ex vivo fetal gene therapy.[34] The same group of investigators showed that intrauterine transplantation of first-trimester fetal human mesenchymal stem cells repaired bone and reduced fractures by two-thirds in osteogenesis imperfect mice, thus putting forward the scientific basis for similar treatment of affected human fetuses.[35]

Another future application of first-trimester embryofetoscopy is research on the role of the human yolk sac. A major question awaiting elucidation is the role of the yolk sac in early human development. The yolk sac provides blood cell precursors, gonadocytes, and epithelia of the digestive and respiratory tracts and has been demonstrated to be structurally altered when exposed to high glucose concentrations in embryo culture experiments.[36] Therefore, the yolk sac may play an essential role in the pathogenesis of congenital anomalies in the fetuses of diabetic mothers. Direct observation of the yolk sac by embryoscopy, as well as aspiration of its contents for laboratory analysis, could enhance our understanding of human malformations considerably.

ETHICAL CONSIDERATIONS

Patients undergoing embryofetoscopy for either fetal diagnosis or therapy should be selected very carefully. The risks versus benefits should be carefully weighed in each individual case. The ability to treat terminal or debilitating congenital disorders before birth will lead to complex ethical questions with respect to the rights of the mother and fetus. The hospital ethics committee and other noninvolved physicians should be consulted in difficult or controversial cases.

CONCLUSION

In recent years, prenatal diagnosis has focused on the first trimester of pregnancy due to the improved resolution of transvaginal ultrasound and other first-trimester screening techniques such as nuchal translucency evaluation. We now have the ability to diagnose many fetal anomalies in the first trimester of pregnancy, and the opportunity may be given for early intervention in terms of termination of pregnancy or fetal therapy, depending upon the particulars of each situation and the parents' wishes. Soon the availability of first-trimester embryofetoscopy may routinely allow access to the embryo/fetus for early diagnosis and be coupled with potential therapeutic interventions. At the present time, however, early embryofetoscopy is typically considered in patients with early failed pregnancies for the evaluation of embryonic morphology and for fetal tissue retrieval for cytogenetic analysis.

REFERENCES

1. Westin B. Hysteroscopy in early pregnancy. *Lancet* 1954; 2: 872–5.
2. MacKenzie IZ. Transcervical fetoscopy. *Lancet* 1974; 2: 346–7.
3. Gallinat A, Lueken RP, Lindemann HJ. A preliminary report about transcervical embryoscopy. *Endoscopy* 1978; 10: 47–50.
4. Roume J, Aubry MC, Labbe F et al. Diagnostic prénatal des anomalies des membres et des extrémités. *J Genet Hum* 1985; 33: 457–61.
5. Dumez Y. Embryofetoscopy and congenital malformations. In: *Proceedings of International Conference on Chorionic Villus Sampling and Early Prenatal Diagnosis*, 28–29 May 1990. Athens, Greece.
6. Cullen MT, Reece EA, Whetham J et al. Embryofetoscopy: Description and utility of a new technique. *Am J Obstet Gynecol* 1990; 162: 82–6.
7. Reece EA, Goldstein I, Chatwani et al. Transabdominal needle embryofetoscopy: A new technique paving the way for early fetal therapy. *Obstet Gynecol* 1994; 84: 634–6.
8. Deprest J, Jani J, Lewi L et al. Fetoscopic surgery: Encouraged by clinical experience and boosted by instrument innovation. *Semin Fetal Neonatal Med* 2006 Dec; 11(6): 398–412.
9. Beck V, Pexsters A, Gucciardo L et al. The use of endoscopy in fetal medicine. *Gynecol Surg* 2010; 7(2): 113–25.
10. Reece EA. First trimester prenatal diagnosis: Embryoscopy and fetoscopy. *Semin Perinatol* 1999; 23: 424–33.
11. Quintero RA, Abuhamad A, Hobbins JC et al. Transabdominal thin-gauge embryofetoscopy: A technique for early prenatal diagnosis and its use in the diagnosis of a case of Meckel–Gruber syndrome. *Am J Obstet Gynecol* 1993; 168: 1552–7.
12. Ville Y, Khalil A, Homphray T et al. Diagnostic embryofetoscopy and fetoscopy in the first trimester of pregnancy. *Prenat Diagn* 1997; 17: 1237–46.
13. Yin CS, Liu JY, Yu MH. Transcervical flexible endoscopy for first trimester embryonic/fetal evaluation. *Int J Gynaecol Obstet* 1996; 54: 149–53.

14. Greco P, Vimercati A, Bettocchi S et al. Endoscopic examination of the fetus in early pregnancy. *J Perinat Med* 2000; 28: 34–8.
15. Surbek DV, Tercanli S, Holzgreve W. Transabdominal first trimester embryofetoscopy as a potential approach to early in utero stem cell transplantation and gene therapy. *Ultrasound Obstet Gynecol* 2000; 15: 302–7.
16. Zwinger A, Krofta L. Embryofetoscopy—Present possibilities of endoscopy in obstetrics. *Ceska Gynekol* 2000; 65: 3–6.
17. Miliou-Paouleskou D, Antsaklis A, Papantoniou N et al. First trimester transabdominal embryo fetoscopy. *Early Pregnancy* 2001; 5: 36–7.
18. Beck V, Lewi P, Gucciardo L, Devlieger R. Preterm prelabor rupture of membranes and fetal survival after minimally invasive fetal surgery: A systematic review of the literature. *Fetal Diagn Ther* 2012; 31(1): 1–9.
19. Dommergues M, Lemerrer M, Couly G et al. Prenatal diagnosis of cleft lip at 11 menstrual weeks using embryoscopy in the van der Woude syndrome. *Prenat Diag* 1995; 15: 378–81.
20. Rankine M, Hafner E, Schuchter K et al. Ultrasound and endoscopic image of exencephaly (acrania) in the 12th week of pregnancy. *Z Geburtshilfe Neonatol* 2000; 204: 236–8.
21. Di Spiezio Sardo A, Paladini D, Zizolfi B et al. Pentalogy of Cantrell: Embryofetoscopic diagnosis. *J Minim Invasive Gynecol* 2013; 20: 248–51.
22. Reece EA, Homko CJ, Wiznitzer A et al. Needle embryofetoscopy and early prenatal diagnosis. *Fetal Diagn Ther* 1995; 10: 81–2.
23. Reece EA, Homko CJ, Koch S et al. First-trimester needle embryofetoscopy and prenatal diagnosis. *Fetal Diagn Ther* 1997; 12: 136–9.
24. Hobbins JC, Jones OW, Gottesfeld S et al. Transvaginal ultrasonography and transabdominal embryofetoscopy in the first-trimester diagnosis of Smith–Lemli–Optiz syndrome, type II. *Am J Obstet Gynecol* 1994; 171: 546–9.
25. Lee K, Lee JW, Chay DB et al. transabdominal embryofetoscopy for the detection of short rib-polydactyly syndrome, type II (Majewski), in the first trimester. *J Korean Med Sci* 2006; 21:165–8.
26. Lee K, Kim CM, Seo SK et al. Transabdominal embryofetoscopy: 6 cases of first trimester prenatal diagnosis for congenital anomalies. *Ultrasound Obstet Gynecol* 2005; 26: 429–30.
27. Guida M, Di Spiezo Sardo A, Carbone MM et al. Spinal dysraphism in an early missed abortion: Embryofetoscopic diagnosis. *J Minim Invasive Gynecol* 2009; 16: 768–71.
28. Yin CS, Chen WH, Wei RY et al. Transcervical embryoscopic diagnosis of conjoined twins in a ten-week missed abortion. *Prenatal Diagn* 1998; 18: 626–8.
29. Philipp T, Kalousek DK. Transcervical embryoscopy in missed abortion. *J Assist Reprod Genet* 2001; 18: 285–90.
30. Philipp T, Separovic ER, Philipp K et al. Transcervical fetoscopic diagnosis of structural defects in four first-trimester monochorionic twin intrauterine deaths. *Prenat Diagn* 2003; 23: 964–9.
31. Philipp T, Philipp K, Reiner A et al. Embryoscopic and cytogenetic analysis of 233 missed abortion factors involved in the pathogenesis of developmental defects of early failed pregnancies. *Human Reprod* 2003; 18: 1724–32.
32. Ferro J, Martinez MC, Lara C, Pellicer A, Remohi J, Serra V. Improved accuracy of hysteroembryoscopic biopsies for karyotyping early missed abortions. *Fertil Steril* 2003; 80: 1260–4.
33. Paschopoulos M, Meridis EN, Tanos V et al. Embryofetoscopy: A new "old" tool. *Gynecol Surg* 2006; 3(2): 79–83.
34. Chan J, Kumar S, Fisk NM. First trimester embryofetoscopic and ultrasound-guided fetal blood sampling for ex vivo viral transduction of cultured human fetal mesenchymal stem cells. *Hum Reprod* 2008; 23: 2427–37.
35. Guillot PV, Abass O, Bassett JHD et al. Intrauterine transplantation of human fetal mesenchymal stem cells from first-trimester blood repairs bone and reduces fractures in osteogenesis imperfect mice. *Blood* 2008; 111: 1717–25.
36. Reece EA, Pinter E, Leranth C et al. Yolk sac failure in embryopathy due to hyperglycemia: Horseradish peroxidase uptake in the assessment of yolk sac function. *Obstet Gynecol* 1989; 74:755.

Chorionic villus sampling

5

PATRICE M.L. TRAUFFER, NEIL S. SILVERMAN, and RONALD J. WAPNER

CONTENTS

INTRODUCTION

The diagnosis of fetal cytogenetic abnormalities in the first trimester of pregnancy by chorionic villus sampling (CVS) has been a routine part of obstetrical care for over three decades. In the last 20 years, based on its proven safety and ability to provide a diagnosis earlier in pregnancy than amniocentesis, CVS has become the primary prenatal diagnostic approach in many centers. However, due to the continued improvement in noninvasive aneuploidy screening the use of all diagnostic procedures, including CVS, has decreased by over 33% to more and 50% in the last 5 years.[1,2] Despite this decrease in routine use, the procedure remains a valuable technique for the diagnostic evaluation of screen positive patients, for diagnosing disorders not amenable to noninvasive screening, and for providing an option for couples who desire to maximize the available cytogenetic information about the pregnancy.

CVS entails aspiration of a sample of placental villi represented by microscopic, finger-like projections emanating from the chorion frondosum. The procedure is most often performed between 9 and 12 weeks from the last menstrual period: a time when the developing gestational sac has not yet filled the entire uterine cavity offering an ideal opportunity for the passage of a sampling instrument transcervically into the developing placenta. The chorion layer has begun its differentiation into the chorion frondosum, which will become the placental site, and the smooth chorion laeve, from which the villi have already begun to degenerate (Figure 5.1).

The chorion frondosum contains the mitotically active villi cells and is, therefore, the area to be biopsied. At this early gestational age, the villi float relatively freely in the intervillous space and are anchored loosely to the underlying decidua, making aspiration minimally traumatic. The individual villi have a distinctive branched appearance with an outer single-cell layer, the syncytiotrophoblast, bordering on the proliferative cytotrophoblast. The mesenchymal core of the villi contains macrophages (Hofbauer cells) and fibroblasts. Fetal capillaries are present within the mesenchymal core of the villus (Figure 5.2). The mitotically active cytotrophoblast buds provide tissue for a rapid direct karyotype preparation. Tissue culture techniques analyze mesenchymal core cells and this is the approach most commonly used for clinical testing.

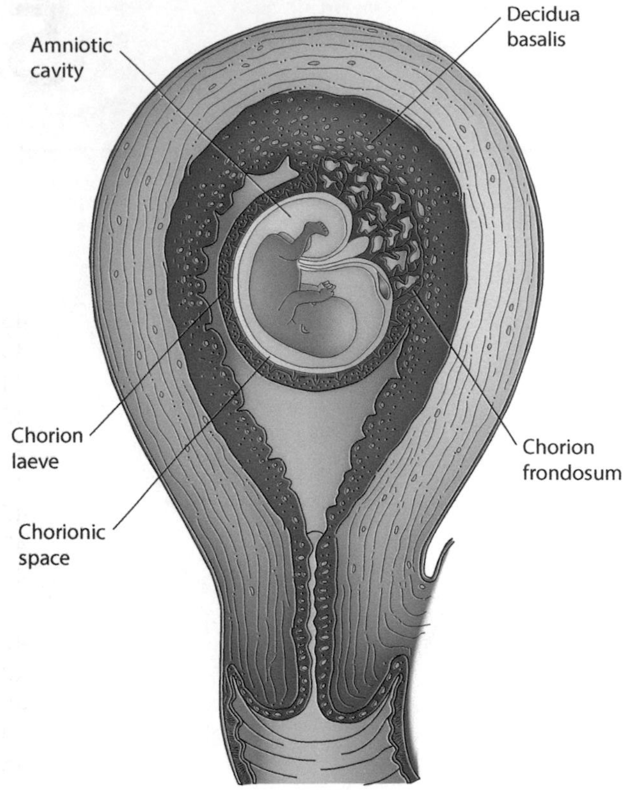

Figure 5.1 Chorionic villus sampling (CVS) is performed at 9–11 weeks' gestation. At this stage of gestation, the chorion has already differentiated into the frondosum, in which the villi are present, and the chorion laeve, in which the chorionic villi have degenerated. The chorionic space remains since the amnion and the chorion have not yet fused.

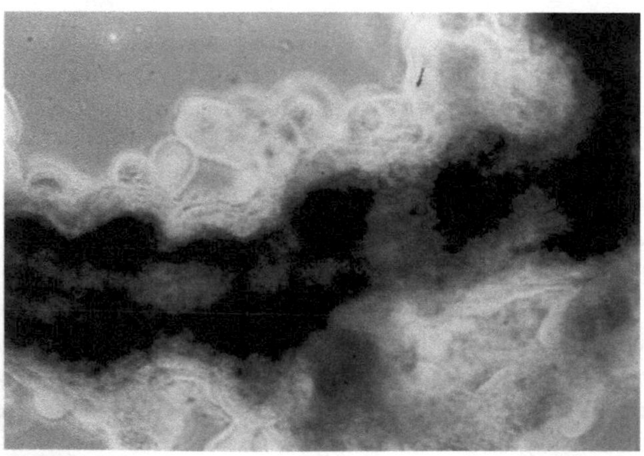

Figure 5.2 A high-power view of the chorionic villus. Cytotrophoblast buds are seen emanating from the villus core. Within the mesenchymal core of the villus, fetal blood vessels are easily identified.

THE SAMPLING PROCEDURE

Transcervical sampling

Before sampling, real-time abdominal or vaginal ultrasound is used to evaluate the pregnancy.[3] Fetal cardiac activity is documented. Measurements of the fetal crown–rump length (CRL) and gestational sac size are taken and compared with expected values for the gestational age by menstrual dates. Over 10% of our patients have had blighted ova diagnosed on this initial scan. Scheduling the procedure after 10 weeks' gestation appears to eliminate much of the potential early pregnancy loss and prevent sampling of karyotypically abnormal embryos destined to perish spontaneously.[4] Most importantly, sampling after 70 days from the last menstrual period eliminates the risk of fetal limb defects seen with earlier sampling (see Safety of CVS, below).

Ultrasound is used to map out the chorion frondosum, which is recognizable as a homogeneous, hyperechoic area. Visualization of the cord insertion can be used as confirmation of the correct location. The relative relationship of the uterus and cervix to the proposed sampling path should be noted and may be altered, to assist sampling, by distention or emptying of the maternal bladder, though overfilling, in an attempt to modify uterine anteversion. This can prevent uterine mobility, which is a requisite for safe sampling. Uterine contractions are frequently encountered and on occasion can interfere with the passage of the catheter (Figure 5.3). Waiting 10–20 minutes for dissipation or relocation of the contraction will make the procedure easier and therefore safer.

Once the conditions for sampling are satisfactory, the patient is placed in the lithotomy position; a speculum is inserted; the vulva, vagina, and cervix are aseptically prepared with a povidone-iodine (Betadine) solution.

The distal 3–5 cm of the 1.5-mm diameter sampling catheter is bent into a slight curve (Figure 5.4) and passed through the cervix under ultrasound visualization until loss of resistance is detected at the internal orifice of the cervix uteri (internal os). At this point, the operator waits until the tip of the catheter is clearly seen on ultrasound, then directs the catheter, under continuous ultrasound guidance, to the sampling site well in the substance of the chorion frondosum. A combination of up and down movement of the speculum to change the angle of approach, rotation of the catheter, and, if required, manipulation of the cervix with the tenaculum is used to guide the catheter into place. The catheter must be inserted slowly, without excessive force, along the unresisting tissue plane provided by the freely floating villi. Excessive force against resistance may cause the disruption of the underlying vessels or injury to the chorionic membrane. The catheter is inserted parallel to the axis of the chorion frondosum and passed almost to its distal end (Figure 5.5). The flexible obturator is then removed, the outer plastic catheter is held in place, and a 20-mL syringe containing 5 mL of nutrient medium with added heparin is attached to the catheter. Approximately 15–20 mL of negative pressure is applied through the syringe as the catheter and attached syringe are withdrawn slowly. Once the catheter is removed, the aspiration fluid is visually examined to confirm the retrieval of adequate villi, which are seen within the syringe as white, branched structures. If inadequate material is obtained on the first pass, up to three passes, each with a fresh catheter may be attempted. Although the risk of adverse outcome appears

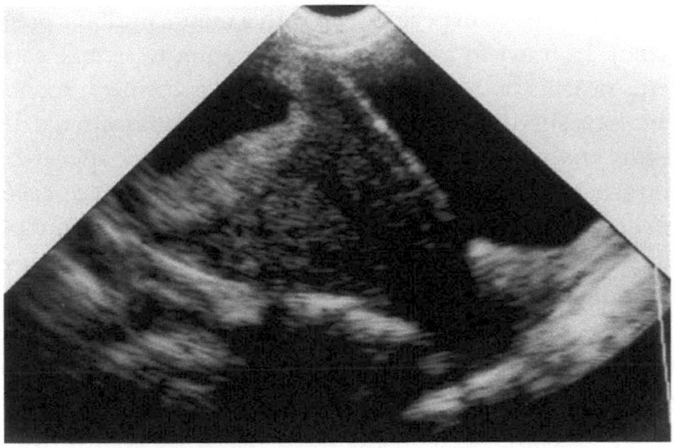

Figure 5.3 A uterine contraction is seen in the lower uterine segment displacing the sac upward. Waiting 15–20 minutes will frequently allow the contraction to dissipate and make sampling easier.

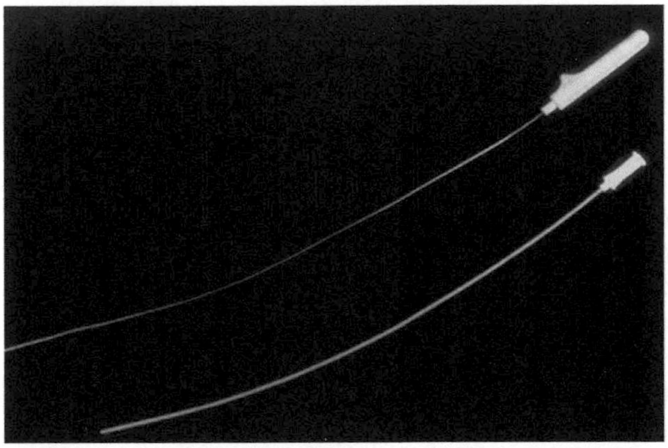

Figure 5.4 The catheter used for transcervical sampling includes a stainless steel inner stylet, which is easily malleable. The polyethylene outer sheath is also seen.

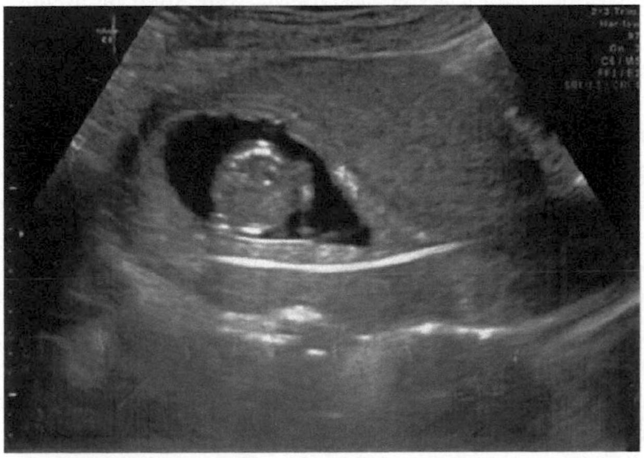

Figure 5.5 The CVS catheter is seen well within the chorion frondosum. The catheter is inserted into the distal end of the frondosum in order to maximize sample size.

to be proportional to the number of passes required, two or occasionally three appear to be safe and are sometimes needed to obtain a diagnosis.[5]

Once the technique is mastered, one can achieve sufficient tissue retrieval with one or two insertions in about 97% of the cases. After an adequate sample is obtained, the patient is discharged home with no required recovery period, except for mild reduction of activity for the first 24 hours. She is instructed to contact the sampling center if heavy bleeding or fever develops, though mild to moderate spotting or cramping is not uncommon up to 1 week after the procedure.

Transabdominal sampling

Though accumulated data suggest the safety and reliability of transcervical CVS for the first-trimester prenatal diagnosis, the technique has two major imitations. First, not all patients are appropriate candidates for a transcervical procedure. For example, that approach would be difficult or relatively contraindicated in women with active genital herpes, large cervical polyps, or a severely retroverted uterus. Second, many practitioners, because of experience gained by performing amniocenteses, are more comfortable with a transabdominal than with a transcervical approach. Two techniques for transabdominal CVS have been described. In one, a two-needle technique, using a larger outer needle as a trocar, through which a thinner sampling needle is inserted to obtain a suction biopsy is used.[6] Alternatively, a single-needle, "free-hand" method, using a 20-gauge spinal needle, under direct ultrasound guidance can be used.[7] Although the two-needle technique has the advantage of allowing reinsertion of the sampling needle without requiring a second skin puncture if sufficient tissue is not initially aspirated, the single-needle procedure is quicker, less uncomfortable, and able to retrieve adequate tissue with minimal number of insertions. In our center the single-needle approach for transabdominal sampling is used exclusively.

As with the transcervical technique, a careful ultrasound evaluation is performed before the procedure. The biopsy path is selected by ultrasound so that the needle will be inserted parallel to the chorionic plate while taking care to avoid accidental passage through the bowel. In most cases, a relatively empty bladder is preferred so that the uterus is closer to the abdominal wall, minimizing the possibility of an inadvertent visceral injury. Povidone-iodine preparation of the skin of the abdominal wall is performed, as in amniocentesis. We do not employ local anesthesia as a rule, though some centers do. At our center, an ultrasound biopsy guide is used to direct insertion of the needle tip into the myometrium just above the chorionic sampling site. Other centers prefer not to use a biopsy guide. Either approach appears to be equally successful, depending upon the operator's preference.[8] Once the needle is in place the needle is removed from the guide, the stylet is withdrawn, a syringe is placed into the needle's luer lock, and, while applying continuous negative pressure from the syringe, the biopsy needle is moved up and down three or four times through the entire length of the chorion before removal. If the sample is inadequate, a new needle is reinserted and the procedure is repeated. As with the transcervical technique, no recovery period is required. Patients experience little, if any, bleeding after transabdominal CVS but significantly more transient cramping than with the transcervical approach.

Because of the success with transabdominal CVS for diagnosis in the first trimester, investigators have suggested extending its use to rapid karyotyping in the second and third trimesters as well. Pijpers et al.[9] reported successful chromosomal analysis beyond 13 weeks' gestation. This confirmed the work by others[10,11] who advocated second-trimester transabdominal CVS for the rapid chromosomal evaluation of at-risk fetuses. A recent study demonstrated the efficacy of the procedure performed in the second and third trimesters and showed its special value in oligohydramnios, where amniocentesis was technically unfeasible.[12] Exact determination of the pregnancy loss rates associated with these placental biopsies is difficult, since many procedures are performed for abnormal pregnancies. Documented losses occurred in less than 1% of the reported cases within 2 weeks of the procedures.

Choosing the transcervical or transabdominal CVS approach

The transabdominal and transcervical approaches to villus sampling are equally safe when performed by individuals equally skilled in both.[13,14] In most cases, either approach can be used. But in about 3%–5% of cases, one approach is clearly more appropriate. For example, a posterior placenta will be more easily approached by the transcervical route, whereas a fundal or anterior placenta may be better sampled transabdominally. For this reason, operators should be capable of performing a CVS by both approaches, leaving them the option of sampling each patient by the most appropriate and hence safest procedure.[15]

Twin gestations

It has been demonstrated that CVS can be performed successfully and safely in twin gestations.[16–18] However, occasional studies have suggested a slight increase in pregnancy loss. There are a number of potential pitfalls that are not present when a singleton is sampled. Whereas dye can be injected into the amniotic sac of one twin to allow confirmation that each fetus has been sampled at the time of amniocentesis, no such marker is available for CVS. Therefore, the operator must be certain that each placental site is separately identified by ultrasound and individually sampled. It is recommended that once the sampling instrument is in place the operator pauses to allow the sonographer to confirm accurate catheter/needle placement. A combination of both sagittal and transverse scanning will maximize the accuracy.

Ultrasound is important in determining whether monochorionic or dichorionic placentation is present. The presence of the "twin peak" sign along with a thick well-defined membrane separating the two fetuses is a reliable indicator in the first trimester of a dichorionic pregnancy.[19] The absence of a membrane or a thin, wispy membrane without an identifiable twin peak is seen with a monochorionic pregnancy. In order to avoid errors, we attempt to sample each fetus near its placental cord insertion site whether a monochorionic or dichorionic placentation is demonstrated by ultrasound. Sampling both fetuses even if they appear by ultrasound to be monochorionic is important since cases of dizygotic monochorionic pregnancies with discordant karyotypes have been reported, especially following assisted reproductive technology.[20] Postzygotic nondisjunction can also occur leading to discordant monochorionic twins. Both of these occurrences are exceedingly rare so that monochorionic cases in which sampling both twins appears inordinately difficult may undergo one pass. In cases in which a membrane is not demonstrated, only one sample is retrieved. In our experience of hundreds of chorionic villus samplings in multiple gestations, utilization of this sampling technique has consistently led to correct information.

Cases in which the operator is not convinced that both fetuses within a dichorionic pregnancy have been independently sampled should have zygosity testing performed to confirm appropriate independent samples. Although monozygotic dichorionic twins cannot be differentiated from sampling one twin twice, it is advisable to offer amniocentesis in these cases. With experience, this should occur in less than 1% of cases.

Contamination of one tissue sample with villi from the other fetus is not uncommon and can lead to misinformation when the laboratory is not aware of this possibility. Clinically, this is usually not a problem when karyotype alone is to be analyzed, since the presence of an abnormal cell line in one fetus will be identified even if some of these villi are contaminating the other sample. However, this can lead to a completely inaccurate result when biochemical enzyme analysis is performed. Contamination is best avoided by choosing sampling routes that do not pass through both frondosums. Combinations of both abdominal and cervical sampling make this possible. For biochemical testing, analysis of individual villi rather than combining all villi in one sample will also diminish the possibility of an error. Most molecular analysis includes testing for maternal cell contamination, which will identify tissue from the coexisting twin.

The need for selective termination will occur when multiple gestations are tested. In our experience, 1%–2% of pregnancies in advanced maternal age patients will have at least one fetus with a karyotype abnormality. Fortunately, reduction or selective termination can be performed safely in early gestation.[21] However, the need to occasionally perform this procedure mandates that an accurate and detailed graph of fetal position be drawn at the time of sampling so that the aneuploid fetus can be identified 1–2 weeks later. In cases in which uterine rotation makes identification of the affected fetus inconclusive, a repeat CVS with a 1- to 3-hour direct preparation to confirm the karyotype is suggested.

Since twins present unique difficulties, it is suggested that only experienced operators sample these gestations. Multiple gestations of higher order such as triplets and quadruplets have also been successfully sampled, but in these cases the patient must be informed of the potential additive risks of the procedure.

Neural tube screening after CVS

Patients with either singleton or twin gestations who have first-trimester CVS should receive neural tube screening by either ultrasound examination or maternal serum alpha-fetoprotein (AFP) at 15–18 weeks' gestation. If the maternal serum AFP is elevated, the CVS need not be regarded as the cause of this elevation, these patients should have the appropriate workup to explain the high maternal serum AFP. Patients who have undergone selective termination are not candidates for maternal serum AFP screening because the residual fetal tissue will elevate the AFP; they should receive targeted ultrasound for malformation screening.

LABORATORY ASPECTS OF CVS

Tissue preparation

The average sample from a transcervical CVS contains 15–30 mg wet weight of villus material for analysis. Transabdominal samples are slightly smaller, on average, but are adequate for routine procedures.[22] The sample, once in the processing laboratory, is aseptically transferred to a Petri dish and inspected under an inverted microscope, where contaminating maternal tissue adherent to the villi is teased away with a fine forceps and discarded. Free-floating decidual tissue may also be present and likewise should be discarded. In contrast to the villi which have a frond-like branching appearance, decidua is amorphous. To avoid erroneously analyzing maternal tissue, atypical appearing villi should be discarded and only those with a classical appearance saved. Cleaned villi are then transferred to a balanced salt solution, gently washed with a swirling motion, and transferred again to smaller dishes for tissue culture, incubation, or further preparation and analysis for biochemical or DNA diagnoses.

Cytogenetic analysis

Processing of the villi for cytogenetic analysis may be performed by two distinct methods. The "direct" method described by Simoni et al.[23] makes use of the actively mitotic cytotrophoblast cells in the buds of the villi and may give a result in as little as 2 hours. In clinical practice, most laboratories use an overnight incubation and report results 3–4 days after the procedure. The second approach is to culture the cells of the villous mesenchymal core in standard monolayer cultures for about 5–8 days. Though the direct method is rapid and rarely plagued with decidual contamination, tissue culture is superior in identifying and evaluating discrepancies between the cytotrophoblast and the actual fetal state, which is more closely represented by the cells of the mesenchymal core.

SAFETY OF CVS

Evaluation of the risks of CVS has focused on the issues of fetal loss, particularly in regard to spontaneous abortion (Table 5.1). Procedure-related spontaneous abortion has generally been defined as spontaneous fetal loss or diagnosed intrauterine fetal death prior to 28 completed weeks of gestation. However, calculating procedure-induced losses is complicated by the background pregnancy loss rate. Investigators have demonstrated that 2%–5% of pregnancies shown by ultrasound to be viable at 7–12 weeks' gestation were either nonviable when rescanned at 18–20 weeks prior to amniocentesis[30–33] or were lost spontaneously prior to 28 weeks' gestation. The rate of spontaneous loss increases with maternal age and is highest in women whose age places them at particular risk of chromosomal abnormalities and thus in need of prenatal diagnosis.[31,33,34] Overall, these spontaneous losses appear to occur predominantly in early pregnancy, with losses after 16 weeks occurring uncommonly.[35] The largest compilations of data regarding the risks of CVS have come from two collaborative reports. In early 1989, the Canadian Collaborative CVS-Amniocentesis Clinical Trial Group performed a prospective randomized comparison of CVS and second-trimester amniocentesis and demonstrated no significant difference in the risk of pregnancy loss (relative risk [RR] 1.10; 95% confidence interval [CI] 0.92, 1.30).[24] Maternal complications were infrequent in each group.

Table 5.1 CVS and pregnancy loss.

Reference	Total procedures (technique used)	Induced abortions (%)	Spontaneous abortions (%) (losses upto 28 weeks/ continuing pregnancies	Procedural success (%)
Rhoads et al.[5]	2248 (TC)	45 (2.0)	77 (3.5)	97.8
Brambati et al.[16]	1159 (TA)	71 (6.1)	25/716 (3.5)[a]	99.7
Canadian Group[24]	1191 (TC)	26 (2.2)	57 (4.9)	98.5
Ward et al.[25]	163 (TC)	43 (26.3)	13 (10.8)	96.8
Green et al.[26]	940 (TC)	27 (2.9)	23 (2.5)	99.4
Wade and Young[27]	714 (TC)	29 (4.1)	31 (4.5)	N/A
Jahoda et al.[28]	1550 (TC)	101 (6.5)	73 (5.0)	97.8
Clark et al.[29]	211 (TC)	8 (3.8)	6 (2.9)	N/A
	8029	350/8176 = (4.3%)	305/7454 = 4.1%	

Abbreviations: CVS, chorionic villus sampling; N/A, not applicable; TA, transabdominal CVS; TC, transcervical CVS.

[a] Includes only completed pregnancies.

An American collaborative report described a prospective but nonrandomized trial of over 2200 women who had chosen either transcervical CVS or second-trimester amniocentesis for prenatal diagnosis.[5] As in the Canadian study, advanced maternal age was the primary indication for the procedures. When the losses were adjusted for group differences in gestational age and maternal age, an excess pregnancy loss of 0.8% referable to CVS, over amniocentesis, was calculated, which again was not significant.

Multiple single-center reports have confirmed the results of these collaborative trials regarding the safety and accuracy of transcervical CVS.[25–29,36] After adjustments for background loss, no significant increases in pregnancy losses were related to CVS, though a procedural "learning curve" was observed. The latter must be taken into account with any new technical development. Data from all studies show that loss rates increase with the number of insertions required to obtain an adequate sample and that the number of insertions is inversely proportional to the expertise of the operator.

Transabdominal CVS is equally safe with comparative trials demonstrating no significant difference in loss rates between the two approaches.[13,22] In the United States with over 1000 patients in each arm of the study, procedural success (over 99%) and total pregnancy loss rates were equivalent for both groups.[22] In addition, for a comparable numbers of patients only one attempt was required to retrieve the tissue (87%), some had unsuccessful procedures (less than 1%). These results were confirmed by others who also suggested that because of preexisting operator experience with transabdominal invasive procedures that approach might be the method of first choice for most CVS.[37]

Contemporary studies continue to confirm the safety of CVS. A recent meta-analysis and systematic review evaluated relevant citations reporting procedure-related complications of CVS.[38] Only studies reporting data on more than 1000 procedures were included to minimize the effect of bias from smaller studies. This analysis included 207 losses in 8899 women who underwent CVS. The risk of miscarriage prior to 24 weeks in women who underwent CVS was 2.18% (95% CI, 1.61%–2.82%). The background rate of miscarriage in women from the control group that did not undergo any procedures was 1.79% (95% CI, 0.61%–3.58%). The weighted pooled procedure-related risk of miscarriage was 0.22% (95% CI, -0.71% to 1.16%).

In conclusion, in experienced centers, CVS is safe with a procedure-related loss rate of approximately 1 in 500, a risk similar to that of second-trimester amniocentesis. However, the impact of operator experience cannot be underestimated. CVS, particularly the transcervical approach, has a relatively prolonged learning curve. Saura et al.[39] suggested that over 400 cases may be required before safety is maximized. The role of experience is further demonstrated by three sequential National Institute of Child Health and Human Development (NICHD) sponsored trials in which the majority of operators remained relatively constant. The postprocedure loss rate following CVS fell from 3.2% in the initial trial performed from 1985 to 1987,[5] to 2.4% for the trial performed from 1987 to 1989,[14] and to only 1.3% in their most recent experience from 1997 to 2001.[40] Most recently, Caughey et al.[41] confirmed the continuing improvement seen with experience. When outcomes from their center were analyzed in 5-year time intervals the overall postprocedure loss rate decreased from 4.4% in the interval 1983–1987 to 1.9% in the interval 1998–2003.

Complications of CVS

The incidence of post-CVS chorioamnionitis is low. One study found an incidence of 0.3% prior to 20 weeks' gestation,[42] while another reported only two clinically detected infections in 1000 procedures.[43] These results were confirmed by the large CVS collaborative series.[5,24] In our own series of over 8000 patients, we have observed no case of chorioamnionitis requiring uterine evacuation. We do not prescribe prophylactic antibiotics periprocedurally. Among our pregnancy losses, the suspected incidence of periabortion chorioamnionitis was 0.08%, about the same as seen in a series of spontaneous abortions that had not been previously sampled.[31,33]

Risk of fetal abnormalities after CVS

An association between exposure of a pregnancy to CVS sampling and fetal limb reduction defects (LRD) initially led to a significant concern about the safety of the procedure. In a series of 539 CVS-exposed pregnancies, Firth et al.[44] identified five infants with severe limb abnormalities, all of which came from a cohort of 289 pregnancies sampled at 66 days' gestation or less. Four of these infants had oromandibular-limb hypogenesis syndrome and the fifth had a terminal transverse LRD. Oromandibular-limb hypogenesis syndrome occurs with a birth prevalence of 1 per 175,000 live births[45] and LRD occur in 1 per 1,690 births.[46] In this initial report, all of the limb abnormalities followed transabdominal sampling performed at 55–66 days' gestation. Subsequent to this initial report, others added supporting cases,[47] while other case-control studies did not find an association.[4]

More contemporary studies have demonstrated that the risk of LRD from CVS exposure is limited to procedures performed in very early gestation. Most notably, Brambati et al.,[48] an extremely experienced group that found no increased risk of limb defects in patients sampled after 9 weeks, observed that patients sampled at 6 and 7 weeks had a 1.6% incidence of severe defects. This rate decreased to 0.1% for sampling at 8–9 weeks.

A review of almost 140,000 CVS procedures reported to a World Health Organization (WHO) registry has demonstrated no increase in the overall incidence of LRD after CVS performed beyond 63 days' gestation or in any specific type or pattern of defects.[47] Table 5.2 summarizes the studies evaluating the association between CVS and fetal limb defects for procedures performed after 63 days of gestation and confirms the findings of the registry.

In conclusion, present data demonstrate that performing CVS in the standard gestational window of 10–13

Table 5.2 Studies evaluating the association of CVS and LRDs: procedures performed after 63 days of gestation.

No association			Association		
Author	**No. of post-CVS live births**	**No. of LRD**	**Author**	**No. of CVS**	**No. of LRD**
Jahoda et al.[49]	3,973	3	Burton et al.[50]	394	4
Halliday et al.[51]	2,071	3 U	Mastroiacovo et al.[52]	2,759	3
Canadian Group[24]	905	0	Bissonnette (A)[53]	507	5
Schloo et al.[54]	3,120	2			
Monni et al.[55]	2,752	2			
Blakemore et al.[56]	3,709	3			
Silver et al.[57]	1,048	1 U			
Mahoney–U.S. NICHD[58]	4,588	8			
Jackson et al.[59]	12,863	5			
Smidt-Jensen et al.[60]	2,624	0			
Bissonnette (B)[53]	269	0			
Case–control studies	**OR**	**CI**		**OR**	**CI**
Eurocat[4]	1.8	0.7–5	Italian multicenter <76 days[61]	19	9–37
U.S. Multistate[62]			U.S. Multistate[62]		
Overall LRD	1.7	0.4–6	Terminal digital LRD	6.4	1.1–38
Transverse LRD	4.7	0.8–28			

Abbreviations: CI, confidence interval; LRD, limb reduction defects; OR, odds ratio; U, uncertain association.

weeks does not increase the risk of LRD. Sampling before 10 weeks is not recommended, except in very unusual circumstances, such as when a patient's religious beliefs may preclude a pregnancy termination beyond a specific gestational age.[63] These patients, however, must be informed that the incidence of severe LRD could be as high as 1%–2%.

Bleeding

Vaginal bleeding or spotting is relatively uncommon after transabdominal CVS procedures but not unusual after transcervical CVS. Most centers report this occurrence in 15%–20% of transcervically sampled patients, though heavy bleeding occurs in only a small percentage. Subchorionic hematoma formation immediately after sampling was seen in 4% of sampled pregnancies and was associated with up to 7 days of vaginal bleeding.[43] The hematoma usually disappeared before week 16 of pregnancy and was rarely associated with an adverse outcome. The heavy bleeding and resulting hematoma formation result from accidental placement of the transcervical catheter into the vascular decidua basalis underlying the chorion frondosum. In many of these cases, a distinct "pop" is felt prior to the bleeding and a gritty feeling indicates penetration into the decidual layer. In extreme cases, the development of a hematoma can be seen on ultrasound and its expansion charted (Figure 5.6). Careful attention to the feel of the catheter, which is gained with experience, can prevent many of these hemorrhagic episodes.

Rh sensitization

An acute and consistent rise in maternal serum AFP levels after CVS has been reported, implying a detectable degree of fetal maternal bleeding.[64–66] In Rh-negative women, this fact is critical, since Rh-positive cells in volumes as low as 0.1 mL can cause Rh sensitization.[67] The risk of fetal–maternal bleeding has been shown to be independent of CVS method (transcervical or transabdominal), and dependent on the amount of tissue aspirated, though all women with even a single pass by either method had detectable rises in AFP.[66] For these reasons, all Rh-negative nonsensitized women undergoing CVS, receive Rho (D) immunoglobulin subsequent to the procedure. The risk of worsening the already existing Rh immunization in previously sensitized women has been described and presents a relative contraindication to CVS in this population.[68]

Rupture of the membranes

Acute rupture of the membranes, documented either by obvious gross fluid leakage or by a decrease in amniotic fluid volume on ultrasound, is a very rare complication of CVS. In a collaborative review of over 6000 procedures from three centers, acute membrane rupture was not observed. In fact, attempts intentionally to rupture membranes with a transcervical catheter in pregnancies scheduled for termination have confirmed that the chorion can withstand significant pressure without rupturing.

Rupture of the membranes days or weeks after the procedure may occur, however, either from injury to the chorion allowing exposure and damage of the amnion or as a result of low-grade chorioamnionitis. Various groups have reported a 0.3% incidence of delayed rupture of the membranes after CVS.[42,43] A significant finding confirmed by our own experience is the presence of oligohydramnios in the second trimester in 6 of 1000 sampled patients, in the absence of clinical evidence of fluid leakage.[42] In one of our cases, blue dye injected transabdominally into the

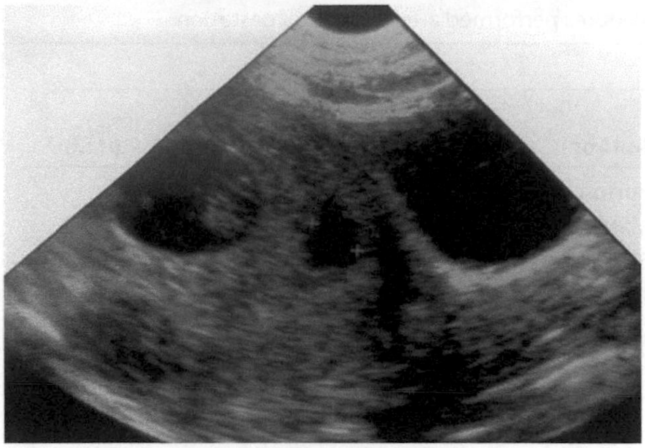

(a)

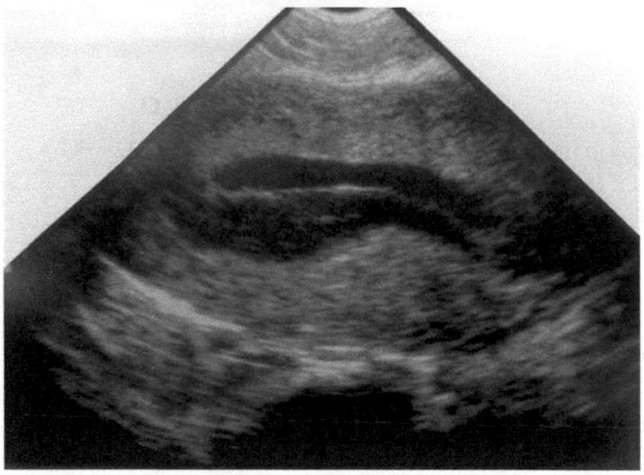

(b)

Figure 5.6 (a) Demonstrates a small subchorionic hematoma seen shortly after transcervical chorionic villus sampling. (b) Demonstrates a much larger hematoma found at the 16-week follow-up scan. Both of these hematomas resolved spontaneously and were not visible at follow-up scanning at 20 weeks.

amniotic sac was subsequently detected transvaginally, confirming the leak.

Perinatal complications

Absence of an increase in the rate of congenital abnormalities after CVS was noted in the large collaborative series and in our own experience of over 6000 deliveries. Prolonged follow-up of 53 children born after placental biopsy found all of them in good health, with normal development and school performance.[69] No series to date has demonstrated late perinatal complications. There has been no reported increase in preterm labor, premature rupture of the membranes, and small-for-date infants.[70] There have been reports of an increased risk of preeclampsia following CVS, which theoretically may occur because of an increased exposure of the mother to fetal tissue.[71,72] Other studies have not observed this increase.[73]

ACCURACY OF CVS

CVS is a highly reliable method of prenatal diagnosis with a 99.7% rate of successful cytogenetic diagnosis.[74] However, errors most often from maternal cell contamination or misinterpretation of mosaicism confined to the placenta can occur.

Maternal cell contamination

Chorionic villus samples frequently contain both villi and decidua. Even when specimens are inspected under a dissecting microscope, some maternal cells may remain and grow in the culture.

Contamination of samples with significant amounts of maternal decidua is rare but almost always due to the retrieval of a limited number of villi, making selection of appropriate tissue difficult. In experienced centers in which adequate quantities of villi are available, this problem is minimal.[75] Therefore, if the initial aspiration is small, a second pass should be performed rather than risk inaccurate results.

Confined placental mosaicism

Although the fetus and placenta have a common ancestry, the karyotype from chorionic villus tissue may not always reflect that of the fetus.[74,76–78] This usually is associated with confined placental mosaicism in which the CVS will demonstrate both a euploid and an aneuploid cell line with the abnormal cell line not being confirmed in the fetus. On rare occasions, the villi will have only aneuploid cells. 0.6%–1.3% of CVS samples will be mosaic, with approximately three-quarters being isolated to the placenta.[5,24,79]

Mosaicism can occur through two possible mechanisms.[80] In one, a meiotic error initially leads to a trisomic conceptus. On subsequent mitotic divisions, some of the cells loose one of the trisomic chromosomes resulting in a disomic cell line within the morula. Cells in the morula will then segregate to either the inner cell mass becoming the embryo or proceed to the trophoblast cell lineage. Because only a small proportion of cells are incorporated into the inner cell mass, involvement of the fetus will depend on the random distribution of the aneuploid progenitor cells. If only euploid cells comprise the fetal cell lineage "confined placental mosaicism" occurs in which the trophoblast will have aneuploid cells and the fetus will be euploid.

Mitotic postzygotic errors can also result in confined placental mosaicism with the distribution and percent of aneuploid cells depending on the timing and location of nondisjunction. If mitotic errors occur early in development, affected cells may segregate to the inner cell mass resulting in true fetal mosaicism or alternatively only to the trophoblast. Mitotic errors occurring after primary cell differentiation and compartmentalization will lead to cytogenetic abnormalities in only one lineage.

In most cases, if the mosaic results are confined to the placenta, fetal development will be normal, but if the mosaic cell line involves the fetus, significant phenotypic consequences are possible. When placental mosaicism is discovered, amniocentesis should be performed to elucidate the extent of fetal involvement. Under no circumstances should a decision to terminate a pregnancy be based entirely on a CVS mosaic result. Alternatively, no guarantees should be made if the amniocentesis is normal since a low-grade fetal mosaic result can be missed. Management of confined placental mosaicism is complex and patient counseling will vary depending on the chromosome involved and the percentage of abnormal cells present. Further testing such as ultrasound, fetal blood sampling, or even fetal skin biopsy is occasionally required to evaluate the risk of an abnormal fetal phenotype. Collaborative management with an experienced genetic specialist is recommended.

Depending on the chromosome involved, confined placental mosaicism may be a marker for fetal uniparental disomy (UPD) and inheritance of a pair of chromosomes from a single parent. In these cases delineation of the parental origin of the remaining disomic chromosomes may be necessary. UPD may have clinical consequences if the chromosomes involved carry imprinted genes in which expression is based on the parent of origin. For example, Prader–Willi syndrome may result from uniparental maternal disomy for chromosome 15. Therefore, a CVS diagnosis of confined placental mosaicism for trisomy 15 may be the initial clue that UPD could be present and lead to an affected child.[81,82] In addition to chromosome 15, chromosomes 7, 11, 14, and 22 are believed to be imprinted and require similar follow-up.[83] Overall, women with confined placental mosaicism can be generally reassured regarding the course of pregnancy and infant health and development.[84]

Confined placental mosaicism (unassociated with UPD) can alter placental function and lead to fetal growth failure or perinatal death.[80,85–90] The exact mechanism by which abnormal cells within the placenta alter function is unknown, but the effect is limited to specific chromosomes. For example, confined placental mosaicism for chromosome 16 leads to severe intrauterine growth restriction, prematurity, or perinatal death, with less than 30% of pregnancies resulting in normal, appropriate-for-gestational-age, full-term infants.[91–95]

ESTABLISHING A CVS PROGRAM

Although CVS has been demonstrated to be safe and efficacious in the hands of experienced operators, gaining this experience has proven difficult for a number of centers. Since transabdominal sampling utilizes skills that many operators already have, studies have demonstrated that trainees gain experience under the guidance of experienced operators so that they can use their skills safely and effectively.[96]

Ultrasound-guided transcervical sampling requires the learning of a new approach. However, the availability of both techniques dramatically improves the ability to retrieve tissue safely and easily. Transcervical sampling is best learned on pretermination patients. In general, 25–50 such procedures should be performed prior to beginning sampling on continuing pregnancies. It is suggested that the operator continue to practice sampling until he or she is able to retrieve sufficient villi from over 95% of patients. If pretermination procedures are unavailable, sampling in patients with blighted ova is useful and has the added advantage of offering the patients karyotype information on the abnormal pregnancy. At the present time, CVS sampling should be performed in centers in which samplers and cytogeneticists are in close proximity to each other, working as a single system. This allows the tissue to be reviewed prior to the discharge of the patient and permits a comprehensive and complete service for the patient.

ACCEPTANCE OF CVS

Initial experiences reporting on the technical feasibility of first-trimester sampling of the placenta for the purposes of prenatal diagnosis were followed by large-scale series that confirmed the safety of the procedure.[5,24,97] Still to follow were reports on the acceptability of the method by patients presenting for genetic diagnosis. Once the feasibility and acceptance of first-trimester diagnosis was established, aneuploid screening quickly moved from the second to the first trimester. Prenatal diagnosis in the first trimester has now found almost universal approval.

The major advantage of CVS is the privacy inherent in an earlier procedure. Psychologic studies on populations of women undergoing prenatal diagnosis demonstrate that first-trimester procedures lower maternal anxiety levels earlier and more consistently than traditional midtrimester amniocentesis. Measurable and significant decreases in anxiety scores are seen after normal results are available. CVS results, logically, produce lower scores earlier than did amniocentesis.

Women undergoing CVS report greater attachment to the pregnancy during the second trimester than women undergoing amniocentesis, assessed in terms of both attachment between mother and fetus and self-comparison to attachment perceived by other pregnant women.[98] The increased acceptance of prenatal diagnosis earlier in pregnancy has made researchers realize that, as earlier procedures become available, they quickly become the preferred choice making CVS the standard against which the safety and accuracy of even newer technologies have to be measured.

REFERENCES

1. Williams J, 3rd, Rad S, Beauchamp S et al. Utilization of noninvasive prenatal testing: Impact on referrals for diagnostic testing. *Am J Obstet Gynecol* 2015; 213: 102.e1–6.
2. Wax JR, Cartin A, Chard R et al. Noninvasive prenatal testing: Impact on genetic counseling, invasive prenatal diagnosis, and trisomy 21 detection. *J Clin Ultrasound* 2015; 43: 1–6.
3. Popp LW, Ghirardini G. The role of transvaginal sonography in chorionic villi sampling. *J Clin Ultrasound* 1990; 18: 315–22.
4. Dolk H, Bertrand F, Lechat MF. Chorionic villus sampling and limb abnormalities. The EUROCAT Working Group. *Lancet* 1992; 339: 876–7.
5. Rhoads GG, Jackson LG, Schlesselman SE et al. The safety and efficacy of chorionic villus sampling for

early prenatal diagnosis of cytogenetic abnormalities. *N Engl J Med* 1989; 320: 609–17.
6. Smidt-Jensen S, Hahnemann N, Jensen PKA, Therkelsen AJ. Experience with transabdominal fine needle biopsy from chorionic villi in the first trimester: An alternative to amniocentesis. *Clin Genet* 1984; 26: 272–4.
7. Brambati B, Oldrini A, Lanzani A. Transabdominal chorionic villus sampling: A freehand ultrasound-guided technique. *Am J Obstet Gynecol* 1987; 157: 134–7.
8. Nicolaides KH, Soothill PW, Rodeck CH et al. Why confine chorionic villus (placental) biopsy to the first trimester? *Lancet* 1986; 1: 543–4.
9. Pijpers L, Jahoda MG, Reuss A et al. Transabdominal chorionic villus biopsy in second and third trimesters of pregnancy to determine fetal karyotype. *BMJ* 1988; 297: 822–3.
10. Hogdall CK, Doran TA, Shime J et al. Transabdominal chorionic villus sampling in the second trimester. *Am J Obstet Gynecol* 1988; 158: 345–9.
11. Holzgreve W, Miny P, Basaran S et al. Safety of placental biopsy in the second and third trimesters. *N Engl J Med* 1987; 317: 1159.
12. Holzgreve W, Miny P, Gerlach B et al. Benefits of placental biopsies for rapid karyotyping in the second and third trimesters (late chorionic villus sampling) in high-risk pregnancies. *Am J Obstet Gynecol* 1990; 162: 1188–92.
13. Brambati B, Terzian E, Tognoni G. Randomized clinical trial of transabdominal versus transcervical chorionic villus sampling methods. *Prenat Diagn* 1991; 11: 285–93.
14. Jackson LG, Zachary JM, Fowler SE et al. A randomized comparison of transcervical and transabdominal chorionic-villus sampling. The U.S. National Institute of Child Health and Human Development Chorionic-Villus Sampling and Amniocentesis Study Group. *N Engl J Med* 1992; 327: 594–8.
15. Copeland KL, Carpenter RJ, Jr., Fenolio KR, Ledbetter DH. Integration of the transabdominal technique into an ongoing chorionic villus sampling program. *Am J Obstet Gynecol* 1989; 161: 1289–94.
16. Brambati B, Lanzani A, Oldrini A. Transabdominal chorionic villus sampling. Clinical experience of 1159 cases. *Prenat Diagn* 1988; 8: 609–17.
17. Wapner RJ, Johnson A, Davis G et al. Prenatal diagnosis in twin gestations: A comparison between second-trimester amniocentesis and first-trimester chorionic villus sampling. *Obstet Gynecol* 1993; 82: 49–56.
18. Agarwal K, Alfirevic Z. Pregnancy loss after chorionic villus sampling and genetic amniocentesis in twin pregnancies: A systematic review. *Ultrasound Obstet Gynecol* 2012; 40: 128–34.
19. Sepulveda W, Sebire NJ, Hughes K et al. Evolution of the lambda or twin-chorionic peak sign in dichorionic twin pregnancies. *Obstet Gynecol* 1997; 89: 439–41.
20. Miura K, Niikawa N. Do monochorionic dizygotic twins increase after pregnancy by assisted reproductive technology? *J Hum Genet* 2005; 50: 1–6.
21. Wapner RJ, Davis GH, Johnson A et al. Selective reduction of multifetal pregnancies. *Lancet* 1990; 335: 90–3.
22. Wapner RJ, Davis GH, Johnson A. A prospective comparison between transcervical and transabdominal chorionic villus sampling, Abstract No. Society of Perinatal Obstetricians Meeting. Houston, TX, 1990.
23. Simoni G, Terzoli G, Rossella F. Direct chromosome preparation and culture using chorionic villi: An evaluation of the two techniques. *Am J Med Genet* 1990; 35: 181–3.
24. Canadian Collaborative CVS-Amniocentesis Clinical Trial Group. Multicentre randomised clinical trial of chorion villus sampling and amniocentesis. First report. *Lancet* 1989; 1: 1–6.
25. Ward RH, Petrou M, ModellBM et al. Chorionic villus sampling in a high-risk population—4 years' experience. *Br J Obstet Gynaecol* 1988; 95: 1030–5.
26. Green JE, Dorfmann A, Jones SL et al. Chorionic villus sampling: Experience with an initial 940 cases. *Obstet Gynecol* 1988; 71: 208–12.
27. Wade RV, Young SR. Analysis of fetal loss after transcervical chorionic villus sampling—A review of 719 patients. *Am J Obstet Gynecol* 1989; 161: 513–8; discussion 8–9.
28. Jahoda MG, Pijpers L, Reuss A et al. Evaluation of transcervical chorionic villus sampling with a completed follow-up of 1550 consecutive pregnancies. *Prenat Diagn* 1989; 9: 621–8.
29. Clark BA, Bissonnette JM, Olson SB, Magenis RE. Pregnancy loss in a small chorionic villus sampling series. *Am J Obstet Gynecol* 1989; 161: 301–2.
30. Cashner KA, Christopher CR, Dysert GA. Spontaneous fetal loss after demonstration of a live fetus in the first trimester. *Obstet Gynecol* 1987; 70: 827–30.
31. Gilmore DH, McNay MB. Spontaneous fetal loss rate in early pregnancy. *Lancet* 1985; 1: 107.
32. Simpson J, Bombard A. Chromosomal abnormalities in spontaneous abortion, frequency, pathology, and geneticcounseling. In: Edmonds K, Bennett M (eds). *Spontaneous and Recurrent Abortion*, p. 51. London: Blackwell, 1987.
33. Wilson RD, Kendrick V, Wittmann BK, McGillivray BC. Risk of spontaneous abortion in ultrasonically normal pregnancies. *Lancet* 1984; 2: 920–1.
34. Warburton D, Stein Z, Kline J. Chromosome abnormalities in spontaneous abortion: Data from the New York City study. In: Porter I, Hook E (eds). *Human Embryonic and Fetal Death*, p. 261. New York, NY: Academic Press, 1980.
35. Simpson JL. Incidence and timing of pregnancy losses: Relevance to evaluating safety of early prenatal diagnosis. *Am J Med Genet* 1990; 35: 165–73.

36. Gustavii B, Claesson U, Kristoffersson U et al. [Risk of miscarriage after chorionic biopsy is probably not higher than after amniocentesis]. *Lakartidningen* 1989; 86: 4221–2.
37. Brambati B, Lanzani A, Tului L. Transabdominal and transcervical chorionic villus sampling: Efficiency and risk evaluation of 2,411 cases. *Am J Med Genet* 1990; 35: 160–4.
38. Akolekar R, Beta J, Picciarelli G et al. Procedure-related risk of miscarriage following amniocentesis and chorionic villus sampling: A systematic review and meta-analysis. *Ultrasound Obstet Gynecol* 2015; 45: 16–26.
39. Saura R, Gauthier B, Taine L et al. Operator experience and fetal loss rate in transabdominal CVS. *Prenat Diagn* 1994; 14: 70–1.
40. Philip J, Silver RK, Wilson RD et al. Late first-trimester invasive prenatal diagnosis: Results of an international randomized trial. *Obstet Gynecol* 2004; 103: 1164–73.
41. Caughey AB, Hopkins LM, Norton ME. Chorionic villus sampling compared with amniocentesis and the difference in the rate of pregnancy loss. *Obstet Gynecol* 2006; 108: 612–6.
42. Hogge WA, Schonberg SA, Golbus MS. Chorionic villus sampling: Experience of the first 1000 cases. *Am J Obstet Gynecol* 1986; 154: 1249–52.
43. Brambati B, Oldrini A, Ferrazzi E, Lanzani A. Chorionic villus sampling: An analysis of the obstetric experience of 1,000 cases. *Prenat Diagn* 1987; 7: 157–69.
44. Firth HV, Boyd PA, Chamberlain P, et al. Severe limb abnormalities after chorion villus sampling at 56–66 days' gestation. *Lancet* 1991; 337: 762–3.
45. Hoyme HE, Jones KL, Van Allen MI et al. Vascular pathogenesis of transverse limb reduction defects. *J Pediatr* 1982; 101: 839–43.
46. Froster-Iskenius UG, Baird PA. Limb reduction defects in over one million consecutive live births. *Teratology* 1989; 39: 127–35.
47. Froster UG, Jackson L. Limb defects and chorionic villus sampling: Results from an international registry, 1992. *Lancet* 1996; 347: 489–94.
48. Brambati B, Simoni G, Travi M et al. Genetic diagnosis by chorionic villus sampling before 8 gestational weeks: Efficiency, reliability, and risks on 317 completed pregnancies. *Prenat Diagn* 1992; 12: 789–99.
49. Jahoda MGJ, Brandenberg H, Cohen-Overbeek et al. Terminal transverse limb defecta and early chorionic villus sampling: Evaluation of 4,300 cases with completed follow-up. *Am J Med Genet* 1993; 46: 483.
50. Burton BK, Schulz CH, Burd LI. Limb anomalies associated with chorionic villus sampling. *Obstet Gynecol* 1992; 79: 726.
51. Halliday J, Lumley J, Sheffield LJ et al. Limb deficiencies, chorion villus sampling, and advanced maternal age. *Am J Med Genet* 1993; 47: 1096.
52. Mastroiacovo P, Tozzi AE, Agosti S et al. Transverse limb reduction defects after chorion villus sampling: A retrospective cohort study. *Prenat Diagn* 1993; 13: 1051.
53. Bissonnette JM, Busch WL, Buckmaster JG, et al. Factors associated with limb anomalies after chorionic villus sampling. *Prenat Diagn* 1993; 13(12): 1163–5.
54. Schloo R, Miney P, Holzgreve W et al. Distal limb deficiency following chorionic villus sampling? *Am J Med Genet* 1992; 42: 404.
55. Monni G, Ibba RM, Lai R et al. Limb-reduction defects and chorion villus sampling. *Lancet* 1991; 337: 1091.
56. Blakemore K, Filkins K, Luthy DA et al. Cook obstetrics and gynecology catheter multicenter chorionic villus sampling trial: Comparison of birth defects with expected rates. *Am J Obstet Gynecol* 1993; 169: 1022.
57. Silver RK, Macgregor SN, Muhlbach LH et al. Congenital malformations subsequent to chorionic villus sampling: Outcome analysis of 1048 consecutive procedures. *Prenat Diagn* 1994; 14: 421.
58. Mahoney MJ for the USNICHD Collaborative CVS StudyGroup.Limb abnormalities and chorionic villus sampling. *Lancet* 1991; 337: 1422.
59. Jackson LG, Wapner RJ, Brambati B. Limb abnormalities and chorionic villus sampling. *Lancet* 1991; 337: 1423.
60. Smidt-Jensen S, Permin M, Philip J et al. Randomized comparison of amniocentesis and transabdominal and transcervical chorionic villus sampling. *Lancet* 1992: 340: 1237.
61. Mastroiacovo P, Botto LD. Chorionic villus sampling and transverse limb deficiencies: Maternal age is not a confounder. *Am J Med Genet* 1994; 53: 182.
62. Olney RS, Khoury MJ, Alo CJ et al. Increased risk for transverse digital deficiency after chorionic villus sampling: Results of the United States Multistate Case–Control Study, 1988. *Teratology* 1995; 51: 20–9.
63. Wapner RJ, Lewis D. Genetics and metabolic causes of stillbirth. *Semin Perinatol* 2002; 26: 70–4.
64. Blakemore KJ, Baumgarten A, Schoenfeld-Dimaio M et al. Rise in maternal serum alpha-fetoprotein concentration after chorionic villus sampling and the possibility of isoimmunization. *Am J Obstet Gynecol* 1986; 155: 988–93.
65. Brambati B, Guercilena S, Bonacchi I et al. Feto-maternal transfusion after chorionic villus sampling: Clinical implications. *Hum Reprod* 1986; 1: 37–40.
66. Shulman LP, Meyers CM, Simpson JL et al. Fetomaternal transfusion depends on amount of chorionic villi aspirated but not on method of chorionic villus sampling. *Am J Obstet Gynecol* 1990; 162: 1185–8.
67. Zipursky A, Israels LG. The pathogenesis and prevention of Rh immunization. *Can Med Assoc J* 1967; 97: 1245–57.

68. Moise KJ, Jr., Carpenter RJ, Jr. Increased severity of fetal hemolytic disease with known rhesus alloimmunization after first-trimester transcervical chorionic villus biopsy. *Fetal Diagn Ther* 1990; 5: 76–8.
69. Angue H, Bingru Z, Hong W. Long-term follow-up results after aspiration of chorionic villi during early pregnancy. In: Fracaro M, Simoni G, Brambati B (eds). *First Trimester Fetal Diagnosis*, p. 1. New York, NY: Springer-Verlag, 1985.
70. Williams J, 3rd, Medearis AL, Bear MB, Kaback MM. Chorionic villus sampling is associated with normal fetal growth. *Am J Obstet Gynecol* 1987; 157: 708–12.
71. Daskalakis G, Papapanagiotou A, Antonakopoulos N et al. Invasive diagnostic procedures and risk of hypertensive disorders in pregnancy. *Int J Gynaecol Obstet* 2014; 125: 146–9.
72. Silver RK, Wilson RD, Philip J et al. Late first-trimester placental disruption and subsequent gestational hypertension/preeclampsia. *Obstet Gynecol* 2005; 105: 587–92.
73. Khalil A, Akolekar R, Pandya P et al. Chorionic villus sampling at 11 to 13 weeks of gestation and hypertensive disorders in pregnancy. *Obstet Gynecol* 2010; 116: 374–80.
74. Ledbetter DH, Martin AO, Verlinsky Y et al. Cytogenetic results of chorionic villus sampling: High success rate and diagnostic accuracy in the United States collaborative study. *Am J Obstet Gynecol* 1990; 162: 495–501.
75. Elles RG, Williamson R, Niazi M et al. Absence of maternal contamination of chorionic villi used for fetal-gene analysis. *N Engl J Med* 1983; 308: 1433–5.
76. Karkut I, Zakrzewski S, Sperling K. Mixed karyotypes obtained by chorionic villi analysis: Mosaicism and maternal contamination. In: Fraccaro M, Brambati B, Simoni G (eds). *First Trimester Fetal Diagnosis.* Heidelberg, Germany: Springer-Verlag, 1985.
77. Battaglia P, Baroncini A, Mattarozzi A et al. Cytogenetic follow-up of chromosomal mosaicism detected in first-trimester prenatal diagnosis. *Prenat Diagn* 2014; 34: 739–47.
78. Grati FR, Malvestiti F, Ferreira JC et al. Fetoplacental mosaicism: Potential implications for false-positive and false-negative noninvasive prenatal screening results. *Genet Med* 2014; 16: 620–4.
79. Vejerslev LO, Mikkelsen M. The European collaborative study on mosaicism in chorionic villus sampling: Data from 1986 to *Prenat Diagn* 1989; 9: 575–88.
80. Wolstenholme J. Confined placental mosaicism for trisomies 2, 3, 7, 8, 9, 16, and 22: Their incidence, likely origins, and mechanisms for cell lineage compartmentalization. *Prenat Diagn* 1996; 16: 511–24.
81. Cassidy SB, Lai LW, Erickson RP et al. Trisomy 15 with loss of the paternal 15 as a cause of Prader-Willi syndrome due to maternal disomy. *Am J Hum Genet* 1992; 51: 701–8.
82. Purvis-Smith SG, Saville T, Manass S et al. Uniparental disomy 15 resulting from "correction" of an initial trisomy *Am J Hum Genet* 1992; 50: 1348–50.
83. Ledbetter DH, Engel E. Uniparental disomy in humans: Development of an imprinting map and its implications for prenatal diagnosis. *Hum Mol Genet* 1995; 4 Spec No: 1757–64.
84. Baffero GM, Somigliana E, Crovetto F et al. Confined placental mosaicism at chorionic villous sampling: Risk factors and pregnancy outcome. *Prenat Diagn* 2012; 32: 1102–8.
85. Worton RG, Stern R. A Canadian collaborative study of mosaicism in amniotic fluid cell cultures. *Prenat Diagn* 1984; 4 Spec No: 131–44.
86. Kalousek DK, Dill FJ, Pantzar T et al. Confined chorionic mosaicism in prenatal diagnosis. *Hum Genet* 1987; 77: 163–7.
87. Kalousek DK, Howard-Peebles PN, Olson SB et al. Confirmation of CVS mosaicism in term placentae and high frequency of intrauterine growth retardation association with confined placental mosaicism. *Prenat Diagn* 1991; 11: 743–50.
88. Goldberg JD, Porter AE, Golbus MS. Current assessment of fetal losses as a direct consequence of chorionic villus sampling. *Am J Med Genet* 1990; 35: 174–7.
89. Johnson A, Wapner RJ, Davis GH, Jackson LG. Mosaicism in chorionic villus sampling: An association with poor perinatal outcome. *Obstet Gynecol* 1990; 75: 573–7.
90. Wapner RJ, Simpson JL, Golbus MS et al. Chorionic mosaicism: Association with fetal loss but not with adverse perinatal outcome. *Prenat Diagn* 1992; 12: 347–55.
91. Breed AS, Mantingh A, Vosters R et al. Follow-up and pregnancy outcome after a diagnosis of mosaicism in CVS. *Prenat Diagn* 1991; 11: 577–80.
92. Post JG, Nijhuis JG. Trisomy 16 confined to the placenta. *Prenat Diagn* 1992; 12: 1001–7.
93. Kalousek DK, Langlois S, Barrett I et al. Uniparental disomy for chromosome 16 in humans. *Am J Hum Genet* 1993; 52: 8–16.
94. Phillips OP, Tharapel AT, Lerner JL et al. Risk of fetal mosaicism when placental mosaicism is diagnosed by chorionic villus sampling. *Am J Obstet Gynecol* 1996; 174: 850–5.
95. Benn P. Trisomy 16 and trisomy 16 mosaicism: A review. *Am J Med Genet* 1998; 79: 121–33.
96. Monni G, Pagani G, Illescas T et al. Training for transabdominal villous sampling is feasible and safe. *Am J Obstet Gynecol* 2015; 213: 248–50.
97. Goldsmith MF. Trial appears to confirm safety of chorionic villus sampling procedure. *JAMA* 1988; 259: 3521–2.
98. Spencer JW, Cox DN. A comparison of chorionic villi sampling and amniocentesis: Acceptability of procedure and maternal attachment to pregnancy. *Obstet Gynecol* 1988; 72: 714–8.

Amniocentesis

6

SRIRAM C. PERNI, JOHN R. ROOST, and FRANK A. CHERVENAK

CONTENTS

HISTORICAL BACKGROUND

Amniocentesis is the most commonly performed invasive prenatal diagnostic test. Over a century ago, initial reports of extracting amniotic fluid from the gravid uterus appeared for the treatment of polyhydramnios.[1] Over the past few decades, indications for its use have significantly evolved. Amniocentesis was performed in the 1930s to identify the placental location and for the purpose of pregnancy termination by the instillations of dye and hypertonic saline, respectively.[2] Subsequently, in the 1950s, amniocentesis was utilized to monitor the progression of rhesus isoimmunization[3] and for fetal sex determination.[4] It was not until the 1960s that amniocentesis was used for the prenatal diagnosis of fetal abnormalities,[5] including the evaluation of metabolic derangements.[6] In the 1970s, amniocentesis was used to assess fetal lung maturity[7] and as an adjunct in the diagnosis of fetal neural tube defects with the amniotic fluid alpha-fetoprotein assay.[8] Currently, the diagnostic capabilities for invasive amniocentesis in the field of prenatal diagnosis are vast. However, the utility of this genetic test has evolved with the result of novel screening algorithms and with the advent of noninvasive screening technologies.[9]

GENETIC AMNIOCENTESIS

Trends

With the emergence of first-trimester risk assessment protocols, and the proven clinical utility of these algorithms in clinical practice, further options are available to expectant mothers outside of historic invasive genetic testing based on advanced maternal age alone.[10] Reduced utilization rates of invasive diagnostic testing have been observed recently, especially in women over the age of 35 years, secondary to the proven clinical value of first-trimester screening for aneuploidy risk assessment and also noninvasive screening technologies.[9,11] The first-trimester aneuploidy risk assessment was triggered by nuchal translucency screening which led to a reduction in the incidence of invasive diagnostic testing.[11] Prenatal screening using first- and second-trimester ultrasound and biochemical markers have been well established.[12,13] Studies have shown a consistent decline in the performance of genetic amniocentesis, as well as chorionic villus sampling, with the robust use of these screening algorithms.[14]

As noninvasive prenatal testing (NIPT) methodologies, using cell-free fetal DNA, have come to fruition there has been a further steady decline in the clinical application of these invasive prenatal diagnostic technologies.[9] A significant decrease in the usage of genetic amniocentesis (e.g., from 5.9% to 4.1% in patients with an increased risk for a fetal aneuploidy) was also validated in a study by Pettit et al.[15] Since 2011, NIPT has been corroborated to be a viable option for those women who are at increased risk of fetal aneuploidy, whose only previous option was invasive genetic testing.[16] Thus, NIPT, along with first-trimester risk assessment, significantly altered the clinical landscape for genetic amniocentesis.

Despite the capabilities of NIPT technology in women at an increased risk for fetal aneuploidy, genetic amniocentesis remains the gold standard for prenatal diagnosis.[15] NIPT should not replace invasive diagnostic testing, especially in the presence of ultrasound fetal anomalies, since it has significant limitations and shortcomings in identifying all fetal chromosome abnormalities.[17] NIPT may not capture the less common chromosomal abnormalities, which may otherwise be identified only with invasive genetic amniocentesis. Furthermore, although there has been a decline of genetic amniocentesis as a result of these noninvasive technologies, NIPT has not been validated to be a diagnostic test.[9]

Indications

Invasive prenatal diagnosis remains the reference standard for diagnosis in pregnancies at high risk of fetal aneuploidy, genetic disorders, and metabolic derangements. Amniocentesis is a safe and accurate procedure and can be selectively performed by the clinician to identify conditions after collecting amniocytes. Midtrimester amniocentesis continues to be the most common procedure performed in invasive prenatal diagnosis.[18,19] Patients at high risk for fetal aneuploidy, or those who have a finding of a fetal structural anomaly, are candidates for amniocentesis. If a structural fetal anomaly is identified on ultrasound evaluation, further invasive diagnostic testing and genetic counseling should be offered to the patient.[17]

Indications for genetic amniocentesis include advanced maternal age at the time of delivery, a pregnancy previously affected by aneuploidy, parental carriage of a balanced chromosomal translocation, a phenotypically normal mother with known sex chromosomal mosaicism, a female carrier of a sex-linked recessive condition, heterozygous parental carriers of a single-gene mutation disorder, evaluation of fetal neural tube defects in conjunction with maternal serum alpha-fetoprotein levels and fetal anatomic survey by ultrasonography, abnormal multiple serum marker biochemical screening, maternal request, and confirmation of the diagnosis of fetal aneuploidy suspected on NIPT, and remains the only consistent proven clinical way to diagnose fetal aneuploidy in multifetal gestation.[17,20] The most common of these indications for amniocentesis is a maternal age greater than or equal to 35 years of age at the time of delivery,[18] although the clinical use of an age cutoff has been questioned.[21]

Timing

Genetic amniocentesis is usually performed at 15–20 weeks of gestation.[19,20,22] At this gestational age, there should be a sufficient amount of amniotic fluid surrounding the fetus to allow for adequate collection. As fetal size and micturition steadily increase with advancing gestational age, approximately 100 cc of fluid is present at 14 weeks' gestation, and greater than 300 cc surrounds the fetus by 17 gestational weeks.[23] In addition, midtrimester results from the amniocentesis will be available to offer the patient the option of pregnancy termination. Fetal cells exfoliated from gastrointestinal and urogenital tracts, from the skin, and from the amnion are used for genetic analysis. Since these cells are not actively proliferating, they are cultured. Culture failure rates are low, owing to the fact that there are 1.2×10^4 cells/mL of amniotic fluid collected; however, culture failure is more likely if the fetus is abnormal.[24] Cell culture production for genetic analysis is undertaken by setting up multiple flask cultures or by allowing amniocytes to settle individually on a slide and form discrete colonies.[20] However, conclusive results may take weeks. Amniocentesis performed at this gestational age yields greater than 99% diagnostic accuracy.[25,26] The amniotic fluid collected can be used to test for fetal chromosomes, alpha-fetoprotein, and acetylcholinesterase levels, as well as fetal metabolic disorders when indicated.

Due to the significant recent advances in ultrasound visualization and laboratory techniques, efforts have been made to shift prenatal diagnosis into the first trimester of pregnancy to provide parents with an earlier diagnosis. The diagnostic options available in the first trimester for fetal karyotyping include chorionic villus sampling (CVS) and early amniocentesis (EA). A few studies have demonstrated the possibility of performing amniocentesis at 11–14 weeks of gestation,[27,28] the so-called EA. The primary concerns that the clinician faces when performing an EA are the reliability in obtaining a specimen and the potential for culture failure. A study evaluating EA in 600 patients demonstrated that a specimen could not be obtained in only 1.6% of patients.[29] Another study, however, demonstrated a higher culture failure rate with EA than in later gestational ages.[30] In our opinion, EA should not be performed. CVS is a safer alternative for earlier diagnosis.

Most new information on the safety and efficacy of EA comes from the Canadian Early and Midtrimester Amniocentesis Trial (CEMAT), a large, prospective, randomized clinical trial, of over 4000 pregnant women, with significant power to detect clinical outcome differences.[26,31,32] In this trial, EA was associated with a higher rate of total fetal loss, an increase in the incidence of talipes equinovarus, and a higher incidence of postprocedural amniotic fluid leakage compared with the midtrimester amniocentesis group. However, culture success (97.7%) and accuracy (99.8%) rates were high for the patients in the EA group; culture of EA fluid required one more day than the midtrimester amniocentesis group.

Studies have also evaluated and compared CVS with EA. These studies have also demonstrated a higher incidence of talipes equinovarus in the EA than in the CVS group.[33,34] In addition, higher rates of fetal loss after EA have also been demonstrated compared with CVS[33,35] and a higher rate of repeat testing was required in the EA group due to culture and sample failure.[35]

There are a few other technical considerations that make EA challenging to the clinician. Membrane tenting may be more likely to occur with EA due to the incomplete fusion of the amnion and chorion. With EA, the presence of physiologic gut herniation or bladder exstrophy between the abdominal wall and uterus makes the procedure difficult and potentially dangerous. We believe EA should not be performed in any situation.

FETAL LUNG MATURITY TESTING

Utilization of amniocentesis for determination of fetal lung maturity is usually performed in the mid-to-late third trimester of pregnancy. It usually is indicated at various late gestational ages depending on the maternal, fetal, and obstetric conditions that are involved. A variety of diagnostic laboratory tests are available to determine the relative concentrations of the surfactant-active phospholipids. Prior to 34 weeks' gestation, lecithin and sphingomyelin are present in similar concentrations in the amniotic fluid. However, after 34 weeks' gestation, the relative concentration of lecithin to sphingomyelin begins to increase. Some clinicians, in contrast, utilize the presence of phosphatidylglycerol in amniotic fluid as the definitive test to ensure fetal pulmonary maturity. A myriad of other tests, including the foam stability, lamellar body counting, surfactant-to-albumin ratio, and infrared spectroscopy tests, may also be performed by various reference laboratories on amniotic fluids obtained by amniocentesis.[22,36–38] This is an important procedure, especially in cases of poorly dated pregnancies; however, it should not be used to guide the timing of delivery in well-dated pregnancies.[39]

ISOIMMUNIZATION IN PREGNANCY

Hemolytic disease of the newborn resulting from rhesus alloimmunization was previously a major contributor to perinatal morbidity and mortality. Since the widespread availability of rhesus immunoglobulin (RhoGam), the prevalence of this condition has substantially decreased to one to six cases per 1000 live births.[40] Today, alloimmunization is more likely to result from the "atypical" antibodies (e.g., anti-Kell or non-D Rh antigens). Invasive diagnostic technologies, such as amniocentesis, have been regularly used historically in the management of pregnancies complicated by alloimmunization. However, with the advent of noninvasive ultrasound technology, an indirect methodology for evaluation for fetal well-being can be ascertained with evaluation of the fetal middle cerebral peak-systolic velocity Doppler waveforms.[41] Therefore, as a result, the utilization of amniocentesis for such pregnancies has substantially declined [41] and it is almost nonexistent in centers with the appropriate ultrasound expertise.

In situations where the appropriate ultrasound expertise for noninvasive evaluation for fetal anemia is available, amniocentesis with spectophotometric examination of the amniotic fluid can be used to assess for fetal anemia.[42] Amniotic fluid bilirubin, derived from fetal pulmonary and tracheal secretions, is quantified by spectrophotometrically measuring its absorbance at the 450-nm wavelength (change in optical density [ΔOD_{450}]). Care must be taken to shield the amniotic fluid specimen from light. Fetal status is estimated by plotting the results from the ΔOD_{450} measurement on the Liley curve and assessing which zone (i.e., zone I lowest, zone II middle, zone III uppermost) the measurement falls in. Amniocentesis is repeated as indicated, usually every 3–4 weeks if it is in zone I and every 1–4 weeks if it is in zone II.

TECHNIQUE OF AMNIOCENTESIS

Before amniocentesis is performed, the patient should be counseled. Since most amniocenteses are performed for genetic reasons today, such counseling is best done by a genetic counselor. A careful assessment of the patient's medical history and family pedigree analysis will provide useful information for both the patient and the obstetric caregivers. This time will also allow for a discussion regarding the risks and benefits involved in the amniocentesis procedure itself. At the initial encounter, the patient's laboratory tests (ABO blood type and indirect Coombs' tests status) should be verified to assess the need for RhoGAM after the amniocentesis. An ultrasound evaluation should also be performed prior to the procedure to document the viability, number, complete fetal anatomic survey, gestational age, and position of the fetus(es) and to identify the placental location. Only clinicians familiar with its indications and technique should perform amniocentesis.[43]

High rates of infection and failure to obtain amniotic fluid have been reported with amniocentesis performed transvaginally.[1] This technique also potentially causes greater patient discomfort and requires appropriate patient positioning. Thus, transabdominal amniocentesis is the approach of choice for this prenatal diagnostic technique.

Initially, transabdominal amniocentesis was performed without ultrasound guidance.[44] Later, static and real-time ultrasound was utilized during amniocentesis. The possibility of continuous ultrasound guidance during amniocentesis was first reported in the early 1980s.[45] Studies have demonstrated the superiority of continuous ultrasound visualization of the needle during amniocentesis to "blind" amniocentesis, in which ultrasound is performed prior to the procedure, with subsequent removal of the transducer and immediate sampling. Continuously monitored amniocentesis resulted in a lower number of dry and bloody taps of the first needle insertion, a decrease in the number of patients requiring multiple attempts, and a reduction in the number of spontaneous losses following the procedure.[46,47] Other studies have also corroborated the safety and efficacy of continuous visualization of the needle during amniocentesis.[48]

After the maternal abdomen is prepped in a sterile manner (e.g., Betadine), the transducer should be placed into a sterile plastic bag, sheath, or glove with gel. Sterile gel can then be applied to the abdomen for improved sonographic visualization of the intrauterine environment. Alternatively, the transducer can be held at a 90° angle outside the sterile field.

After the initial ultrasonic evaluation, the obstetrician locates an appropriate site for the needle insertion. An area that does not contain fetal parts (especially the head) or the umbilical cord, has an adequate volume of amniotic fluid, and avoids the lower uterine segment and placental tissue should be selected, if possible (see Figure 6.1).[19] Utilization of a local anesthetic agent (e.g., 1% lidocaine without epinephrine) prior to needle insertion is at the individual discretion of the physician and patient. Some would argue that this is an unnecessary step because the site of the initial needle insertion may change if the fetus moves; therefore, the anesthetic would have to be applied to another site. In addition, this may actually increase patient discomfort because an extra skin puncture would be required.

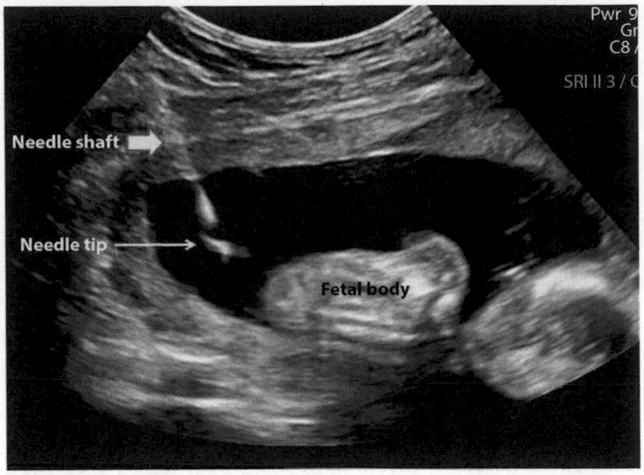

Figure 6.1 Ultrasound picture showing the appropriate placement of the needle (shaft and tip), away from the fetal body, during amniocentesis.

A variety of spinal needles can be utilized for amniocentesis. The procedure has been reported to use an 18-, 20-, or 22-gauge spinal needle.[1,19,20] The 18-gauge needle is used the least. We prefer to use a 22-gauge needle to minimize maternal discomfort and maintain uterine quiescence if possible. However, some clinicians prefer a 20-gauge spinal needle to the 22-gauge because of the decreased resistance to amniotic fluid flow, increased resistance to bending, and more echogenic visibility of the tip on real-time ultrasound. Needle guidance can adequately be performed with a linear or curvilinear transducer, and great care must be taken to ensure that the echogenic needle tip is always visualized by the clinician, and does not go outside the beam of the ultrasound. In addition, minimal pressure should be applied to the transducer so as not to distort the spatial relationship between the maternal abdomen and uterine cavity. Some obstetricians also prefer to use a needle guide during the procedure; however, there is a limited range of motion compared with the free-hand technique (Figure 6.1).

After meticulous asepsis of the maternal abdomen is completed and the puncture site has been selected after ultrasonic evaluation, the spinal needle is introduced into the maternal skin. After dermal and uterine penetration, the amniotic sac is perforated, with a characteristic "pop" or loss of resistance being perceived by the obstetrician. During this time, careful attention is paid to continuous visualization of the needle tip. Upon confirmation of appropriate entry into the amniotic cavity, the needle stylet should be removed. A 5-mL syringe can be attached and approximately 2–3 mL of amniotic fluid is aspirated and discarded to minimize the potential of maternal cell contamination of the specimen. Maternal cell contamination is much more pronounced in women with anterior placentas than in posterior placentation.[49] This most likely is the result of introduction of maternal cells from placental bleeding into the amniotic fluid cavity. Some investigators have evaluated different techniques of amniocentesis and their impact on maternal cell contamination; one study found no difference between amniocentesis technique and maternal cell contamination.[50] For the initial syringe application, a 5- or 10-mL syringe should be chosen for easier removal of amniotic fluid under less tension. If no fluid is aspirated, the needle should be slowly rotated. This "dry tap" is not uncommon in early gestation and may result from a tenting of the membranes. In the 1980s, two techniques were introduced to overcome tenting. The first technique involved withdrawing the needle tip back into the myometrium and reinserting it with a forceful thrust.[51] The second involved further needle penetration into the posterior myometrium under ultrasound guidance and then withdrawing the needle into the amniotic fluid pocket in an attempt to displace physically the obstructing membrane.[52] In 1996, a modified stylet technique was introduced to relieve membrane tenting.[53] In this technique, the membrane can be entered by using a stylet that is made longer than the inserted needle by advancing the stylet tip 10 mm beyond the needle tip.

After initial removal of the 2–3 mL of amniotic fluid to be discarded, a second syringe is attached. This is usually a 20- or 30-mL syringe. The amount of amniotic fluid to be aspirated depends on the indication for the procedure. A volume of 15–40 mL of amniotic fluid is usually required for chromosomal and alpha-fetoprotein analysis.[19,20] The amount of amniotic fluid to be removed depends on the gestational week in which the procedure is being preformed. In general, earlier in gestation, less fluid is removed. If large quantities of amniotic fluid are being removed in cases of polyhydramnios to alleviate maternal symptoms, a gravitational drainage system, multiple syringe aspirations, or a negative-pressure vacuum bottle aspiration system can be used safely to remove amniotic fluid at a rate of 89 mL/minute.[54] If amniotic fluid is required for assessment of fetal lung maturity, a smaller volume of amniotic fluid (10–15 mL) is sufficient.

After obtaining the appropriate volume of amniotic fluid, the stylet should be reinserted and the needle removed under continuous ultrasound visualization. If no fluid is obtained after more than two attempts, the patient should be offered the opportunity to repeat the procedure after 1 week. Fetal cardiac activity should be verified after the completion of the amniocentesis, whether successful or not. The patient can be discharged after the appropriate postprocedural counseling is completed and the results of the indirect Coombs test are confirmed.

AMNIOCENTESIS IN A MULTIFETAL GESTATION

Multifetal gestations have increased over the past decade owing to an increase in absolute number and proportion as a result of assisted reproductive technologies and women delaying childbirth.[55] The twin birth rate has increased 50% over the past two decades in the United States and risen 2% to 33.7 per 1000 in 2013.[56]

The first genetic amniocentesis in a multifetal gestation was performed in the 1970s.[57] Prenatal diagnosis of chromosomal abnormalities in multifetal gestation requires the sampling of two or more gestational sacs. Great care must be taken to ensure that all gestational sacs have been sampled. The clinician can instill 1 mL of a dilute indigo carmine dye solution (1 mL indigo carmine/9 mL normal saline) into the first gestational sac after amniotic fluid has been removed. In this manner, with sampling of the second sac, the amniotic fluid should be clear and colorless. If the fluid is not clear, this may indicate that the same sac was sampled twice. Methylene blue dye is contraindicated for this purpose because of the potential for fetal hemolysis. This technique usually requires two different skin puncture wounds under continuous ultrasound guidance.

Other techniques have been described for amniocentesis in a multifetal gestation. Two techniques were described in the early 1990s. In the first technique described, two separate needles are introduced sequentially into two different gestational sacs with visualization of the dividing membrane without altering the position of the transducer. This technique permits verification of the sampling of two different sacs without introduction of a foreign dye substance.[58] The second technique requires a single-needle insertion, does not require dye, and can potentially be performed quicker than the other techniques. In this technique, an amniotic fluid pocket is identified that contains the dividing membrane. Once fluid is aspirated from the first sac, the needle is guided to penetrate the dividing membrane, and fluid is removed from the second sac.[59] This technique cannot be encouraged at this point until larger studies evaluating the possibility of cross-contamination are adequately addressed. A recent study, however, utilizing quantitative fluorescent polymerase chain reaction assays of amniotic fluid samples obtained by the single-needle technique allowed detection of all aneuploid fetuses quickly and had great sensitivity in detecting small traces of contaminating cell lines.[60] In our opinion, amniocentesis in a multifetal gestation is best performed by the two separate skin punctures technique.

COMPLICATIONS OF AMNIOCENTESIS

As previously mentioned, amniocentesis is an invasive diagnostic procedure, which should be performed only after careful patient counseling for an appropriate indication. Due to the nature of the procedure, there are minimal risks, to both the mother and fetus, which the patient must understand. Amniocentesis is generally safe for both the mother and her fetus. Maternal risks, overall, are much less than fetal risks.

Although a major common concern for a patient undergoing amniocentesis is the risk of spontaneous abortion,[61] maternal factors also need to be addressed prior to performing amniocentesis. Maternal complications occur in approximately 1 in 1000 procedures.[62] The risk of developing chorioamnionitis after the procedure is 0%–1% and subclinical infection may complicate under 0.5% of pregnancies requiring repeated sampling.[19,62,63] Chorioamnionitis should be suspected if the patient presents with fever, with or without chills, and diffuse abdominal pain 24–72 hours after the procedure. If chorioamnionitis is diagnosed, expeditious delivery is advised with utilization of the appropriate broad-spectrum, intravenous, antibiotic regimen. Significant maternal sequelae can occur, including septic shock and death, if chorioamnionitis is not promptly handled. There are reports of maternal septicemia with *Escherichia coli* after midtrimester amniocentesis that resulted in septic shock, multiorgan failure, and ultimate demise.[62] The incidence of amniotic fluid leakage after amniocentesis has been reported to occur in 1%–2% of patients.[64] This usually does not represent frank rupture of the membranes, but rather a transient condition of extraovular leakage of fluid that should spontaneously resolve in 2–3 days. Other maternal complications, such as premature rupture of the membranes, preterm delivery, fetomaternal transfusion, and placental abruption, are rare. There has been a report that women undergoing amniocentesis more often had an operative vaginal delivery and opted for elective cesarean delivery.[61]

The most common and concerning fetal complication of amniocentesis is spontaneous loss. A spontaneous loss rate of 1.0% has been reported from randomized, controlled, prospective clinical trials.[65,66] However, lower loss rates have been reported.[62] Accepted reports of pregnancy loss associated with amniocentesis approach 1 in 300–500.[15] The fetal loss rate has been reported to be higher (2.7%) when amniocentesis is performed in a multifetal gestation.[67] Although it is impossible to predict which pregnancies will end in a fetal loss, certain variables have been identified that could increase the spontaneous loss rate, including older maternal age, uterine myoma, multifetal gestation, and earlier gestational age.[68] A review of 4600 amniocentesis procedures by one clinician over a 28-year period demonstrated that the indications for amniocentesis and the technique used have evolved over time; however, the procedure-related fetal loss rate did not improve significantly with increasing operator experience.[69] The reported loss rate in this study (0.95%) is consistent with loss rates described in other large series.

Before continuous ultrasound guidance was used for amniocentesis, fetal injuries, such as gangrene of the fetal limb and porencephalic cysts,[70,71] were reported to be due to direct needle trauma. Other reported neonatal morbidities with amniocentesis include potentially higher rates of pneumonia, respiratory distress syndrome, and ear infections.[1,68]

With the increase utilization of NIPT technologies, there has been concern with the practitioners ability to maintain their technical expertise in performing invasive tests.[9] This sentiment was corroborated, as there has been a decline in "hands-on" training for practitioners.[14]

CONCLUSION

Amniocentesis is the most common invasive procedure used in the field of prenatal diagnosis. It is a very accurate and safe technique that today is mostly used to diagnose many genetic and metabolic conditions. The procedure should be performed by experienced operators and only after careful patient counseling.

REFERENCES

1. Chervenak JL, Chervenak FA. Amniocentesis. In: Iffy L, Apuzzio JJ, Vintzileos AM (eds), *Operative Obstetrics* (2nd edition), pp. 64–9. New York, NY: McGraw-Hill, 1992.
2. Menees TO, Miller JD, Holly LE. Amniography: Preliminary report. *Am J Roentgenol Radiat Ther* 1930; 24: 363–6.
3. Liley AW. The technique and complications of amniocentesis. *Aust N Z J Med* 1960; 59: 581–6.
4. Fuchs F, Riis P. Antenatal sex determination. *Nature* 1956; 117: 330.
5. Jacobsen CB, Barter RH. Intrauterine diagnosis and management of genetic defects. *Am J Obstet Gynecol* 1967; 99: 796–807.
6. Nadler HL, Gerbie AB. Role of amniocentesis in the intrauterine detection of genetic disorders. *N Engl J Med* 1970; 282: 596–9.
7. Gluck L, Kulovich MV, Borer RC, Jr, Keidel WN. The interpretation and significance of the lecithin/sphingomyelin ratio in amniotic fluid. *Am J Obstet Gynecol* 1974; 120: 142–55.
8. Brock DJH, Sutcliffe RG. Alphafetoprotein in the antenatal diagnosis of anencephaly and spina bifida. *Lancet* 1972; 2: 197–9.
9. Williams J, III, Rad S, Beauchamp S et al. Utilization of noninvasive prenatal testing: Impact on referrals for diagnostic testing. *Am J Obstet Gynecol* 2015; 213: 102.el–6.
10. Perni SC, Predanic M, Kalish RB et al. Clinical use of first-trimester aneuploidy screening in a United States population can replicate data from clinical trials. *Am J Obstet Gynecol* 2006; 194: 127–30.
11. Chasen ST, McCullough LB, Chervenak FA. Is nuchal translucency screening associated with different rates of invasive testing in an older obstetric population? *Am J Obstet Gynecol* 2004; 190: 769–74.
12. Wapner R, Thom E, Simpson JL et al. First-trimester screening for trisomies 21 and 18. *N Engl J Med* 2003; 349: 1405–13.
13. Malone FD, Canick JA, Ball RH et al. First-trimester or second-trimester screening, or both, for Down's syndrome. *N Engl J Med* 2005; 353: 2001–11.
14. Robson SJ, Hui L. National decline in invasive prenatal diagnostic procedures in association with uptake of combined first trimester and cell-free DNA aneuploidy screening. *Aust N Z J Obstet Gynaecol* 2015; 55: 507–10.
15. Pettit KE, Hull AD, Korty L et al. The utilization of circulating cell-free DNA testing and decrease in invasive diagnostic procedures: An institutional experience. *J Perinatol* 2014; 34: 750–3.
16. Palomaki GE, Kloza EM, Lambert-Messerlian GM et al. DNA sequencing of maternal plasma to detect Down syndrome: An international clinical validation study. *Genet Med* 2011; 204(3): 205.el–11.
17. American College of Obstetricians and Gynecologists. Committee Opinion No. 640. Cell-free DNA screening for fetal aneuploidy. *Obstet Gynecol* 2015; 126:e31–7.
18. Wilson RD. Amniocentesis and chorionic villus sampling. *Curr Opin Obstet Gynecol* 2000; 12: 81–6.
19. D'Ercole C, Shojai R, Desbriere R et al. Prenatal screening: Invasive diagnostic approaches. *Childs Nerv Syst* 2003; 19: 444–7.
20. Robinson A, Henry GP. Prenatal diagnosis by amniocentesis. *Annu Rev Med* 1985; 36: 13–26.
21. Druzin ML, Chervenak F, McCullough LB et al. Should all pregnant patients be offered prenatal diagnosis regardless of age? *Obstet Gynecol* 1993; 81: 615–18.
22. Cunningham FG, Gant NF, Leveno KJ et al. *Williams' Obstetrics* (21st edition), pp. 989–92. New York, NY: McGraw-Hill, 2001.
23. Fuchs F. Volumes of amniotic fluid at various stages of pregnancy. *Clin Obstet Gynecol* 1966; 9: 449–60.
24. Persutte WH, Lenke RR. Failure of amniotic-fluid-cell growth: Is it related to fetal aneuploidy? *Lancet* 1995; 345: 96–7.
25. NICHD National Registry for Amniocentesis Study Group. Midtrimester amniocentesis for prenatal diagnosis. *JAMA* 1976; 236: 1471.
26. The Canadian Early and Mid-Trimester Amniocentesis Trial (CEMAT) Group. Randomized trial to assess safety and fetal out come of early and midtrimester amniocentesis. *Lancet* 1998; 351: 242–7.
27. Evans MI, Drugan A, Koppitch FC et al. Genetic diagnosis in the first trimester: The norm for the 1990s. *Am J Obstet Gynecol* 1989; 160: 1332.
28. Elejalde BR, de Elejalde MM. Early genetic amniocentesis, safety, complications, time to obtain results and contraindications. *Am J Hum Genet* 1988; 43: A232.
29. Godmillow L, Weiner S, Dunn LK. Early genetic amniocentesis: Experience with 600 consecutive procedures and comparison with chorionic villus sampling. *Am J Hum Genet* 1988; 43: A234.
30. Sundberg K, Jorgensen FS, Tabor A et al. Experience with early genetic amniocentesis. *J Perinat Med* 1995; 23: 149–58.
31. Winsor EJT, Tompkins DJ, Kalousek D et al. Cytogenetic aspects of the Canadian early and mid-trimester amniotic fluid trial (CEMAT). *Prenat Diagn* 1999; 19: 620–7.
32. Johnson JM, Wilson RD, Singer J et al. Technical factors in early amniocentesis predict adverse outcome. Results of the Canadian early (EA) vs mid-trimester amniocentesis (MA) trial (CEMAT). *Prenat Diagn* 1999; 19: 732–8.
33. Nicolaides KH, Brizot ML, Patel F et al. Comparison of chorion villus sampling and early amniocentesis for karyotyping in 1,492 singleton pregnancies. *Fetal Diagn Ther* 1996; 11: 9–15.

34. Sundberg K, Bang J, Smidt-Jensen S et al. Randomised study of risk of fetal loss related to early amniocentesis versus chorionic villus sampling. *Lancet* 1997; 350: 697–703.
35. Cederholm M, Axelsson O. A prospective comparative study on transabdominal chorionic villus sampling and amniocentesis performed at 10–13 weeks' gestation. *Prenat Diagn* 1997; 17: 311–17.
36. Anceschi MM, Piazze Garnica JJ, Unfer V et al. A comparison of the shake test, optical density, L/S ratio (planimetric and stechiometric) and PG for the assessment of fetal lung maturity. *J Perinat Med* 1996; 24: 355–62.
37. Carlan SJ, Gearity D, O'Brien WF. The effect of maternal blood contamination on the TDx-FLM II assay. *Am J Perinatol* 1997; 14: 491–4.
38. Liu K, Dembinski TC, Mantsch HH. Rapid determination of fetal lung maturity from infrared spectra of amniotic fluid. *Am J Obstet Gynecol* 1998; 178: 234–41.
39. American College of Obstetricians and Gynecologists. Committee Opinion No. 560. Medically indicated late-preterm and early-term deliveries. *Obstet Gynecol* 2013; 121: 908–10.
40. Moise KJ. Management of rhesus alloimmunization in pregnancy. *Obstet Gynecol* 2002; 100: 600–11.
41. Mari G. Noninvasive diagnosis by Doppler ultrasonography of fetal anemia due to maternal red-cell alloimmunization. *N Engl J Med* 2000; 342: 9–14.
42. American College of Obstetricians and Gynecologists. Management of isoimmunization in pregnancy. Washington, DC: ACOG, 1996; ACOG Technical Bulletin No. 227.
43. Verp MS, Gerbie AB. Amniocentesis for prenatal diagnosis. *Clin Obstet Gynecol* 1981; 24: 1007–21.
44. Crandon AJ, Peel KR. Amniocentesis with and without ultrasound guidance. *Br J Obstet Gynecol* 1979; 86: 1.
45. Jeanty P, Rodesch F, Romero R. How to improve your amniocentesis technique. *Am J Obstet Gynecol* 1983; 146: 593–6.
46. Romero R, Jeanty P, Reece EA et al. Sonographically monitored amniocentesis to decrease intraoperative complications. *Obstet Gynecol* 1985; 65: 426–30.
47. De Crespigny LC, Robinson HP. Amniocentesis: A comparison of 'monitored' versus 'blind' needle insertion technique. *Aust N Z J Obstet Gynecol* 1986; 26: 124–8.
48. Benacerraf BR, Frigoletto FD. Amniocentesis under continuous ultrasound guidance: A series of 232 cases. *Obstet Gynecol* 1983; 62: 760–3.
49. Nuss S, Brebaum D, Grond-Ginsbach C. Maternal cell contamination in amniotic fluid samples as a consequence of the sampling technique. *Hum Genet* 1994; 93: 121–4.
50. Steed HL, Tompkins DJ, Wilson DR. Maternal cell contamination of amniotic fluid samples obtained by open needle versus trocar technique of amniocentesis. *J Obstet Gynaecol Can* 2002; 24: 233–6.
51. Platt LD, DeVore GR, Gimovsky ML. Failed amniocentesis: The role of membrane tenting. *Am J Obstet Gynecol* 1982; 144: 479.
52. Bowerman RA, Barclay ML. A new technique to overcome failed second-trimester amniocentesis due to membrane tenting. *Obstet Gynecol* 1987; 70: 806–8.
53. Dombrowski MP, Isada NB, Johnson MP et al. Modified stylet technique for tenting of amniotic membranes. *Obstet Gynecol* 1996; 87: 455–6.
54. Dolinger MB, Donnenfeld AE. Therapeutic amniocentesis using a vacuum bottle aspiration system. *Obstet Gynecol* 1998; 91: 143–4.
55. Kalish RB, Vardhana S, Gupta M et al. Interleukin-4 and -10 gene polymorphisms and spontaneous preterm birth in multifetal gestations. *Am J Obstet Gynecol* 2004; 190: 702–6.
56. Martin JA, Hamilton BE, Osterman MJK et al. *Births: Final Data for 2013. National Vital Statistics Reports*, vol. 64, no. 1. Hyattsville, MD: National Center for Health Statistics, 2015.
57. Toth-Pal E, Papp C, Beke A et al. Genetic amniocentesis in multiple pregnancy. *Fetal Diagn Ther* 2004; 19: 138–44.
58. Bahado-Singh R, Schmitt R, Hobbins JC. New technique for genetic amniocentesis in twins. *Obstet Gynecol* 1992; 79: 304–7.
59. Jeanty P, Shah D, Roussis P. Single-needle insertion in twin amniocentesis. *J Ultrasound Med* 1990; 9: 511–17.
60. Cirigliano V, Canadas P, Plaja A. Rapid prenatal diagnosis of aneuploidies and zygosity in multiple pregnancies by amniocentesis with single insertion of the needle and quantitative fluorescent PCR. *Prenat Diagn* 2003; 23: 629–33.
61. Cederholm M, Haglund B, Axelsson O. Maternal complications following amniocentesis and chorionic villus sampling for prenatal karyotyping. *Br J Obstet Gynaecol* 2003; 110: 392–9.
62. Elchalal U, Shachar IB, Peleg D. Maternal mortality following diagnostic 2nd-trimester amniocentesis. *Fetal Diagn Ther* 2004; 19: 195–8.
63. Terzic MM, Plecas DV, Stimec BV et al. Risk estimation of intraamniotic infection development after serial amniocentesis. *Fetal Diagn Ther* 1994; 9: 35–7.
64. Crane JP, Rohland BM. Clinical significance of persistent amniotic fluid leakage after genetic amniocentesis. *Prenat Diagn* 1986; 6: 25.
65. Tabor A, Philip J, Madsen M et al. Randomised controlled trial of genetic amniocentesis in 4606 low-risk women. *Lancet* 1986; 1: 1287–93.

66. Bettelheim D, Kolinek B, Schaller A et al. Complication rates of invasive intrauterine procedures in a centre for prenatal diagnosis and therapy. *Ultraschall Med* 2002; 23: 199–22.
67. Yukobowich E, Anteby EY, Cohen SM et al. Risk of fetal loss in twin pregnancies undergoing second trimester amniocentesis. *Obstet Gynecol* 2001; 98: 231–4.
68. Papp C, Papp Z. Chorionic villus sampling and amniocentesis: What are the risks in current practice? *Curr Opin Obstet Gynecol* 2003; 15: 159–65.
69. Horger EO, Finch H, Vincent VA. A single physician's experience with four thousand six hundred genetic amniocenteses. *Am J Obstet Gynecol* 2001; 185: 279–88.
70. Lamb MP. Gangrene of a fetal limb due to amniocentesis. *Br J Obstet Gynaecol* 1975; 82: 829.
71. Youroukos S, Papadelis F, Matsaniotis N. Porencephalic cysts after amniocentesis. *Arch Dis Child* 1980; 55: 814.

Fetal transfusion

7

CHRISTOPHER R. HARMAN

CONTENTS

Treatment of fetal anemia may be the most complete example of the concept of fetal therapy that has been achieved so far. Detecting the fetus at risk, evaluating the extent of disease, and delivery of transfusion blood by ultrasound-guided intrauterine transfusion (IUT), all continue to improve. The combination of maternal testing, ultrasound parameters, refinement of the application of fetal blood sampling, and mechanisms for reducing disease severity have all impacted the roles of IUT, with increased application, better safety, and better, more detailed results.

Fetal transfusions were developed to address the staggering perinatal mortality of severe Rhesus (Rh) disease. Strict adherence to Rh prophylaxis produced a marked drop in the number of such cases, but IUT remains a critical resource for severe alloimmune anemia, as well as many other congenital and acquired causes. This chapter highlights the evolution of IUT, emphasizing fetal evaluation and transfusion techniques.

MECHANISMS OF FETAL ANEMIA

Alloimmunization

Maternal sensitization to foreign paternal–fetal red blood cell (RBC) antigens commonly follows transplacental hemorrhage (TPH). TPH occurs in many pregnancies, including over 50% at delivery and at least 15% antenatally.[1] Volumes are usually inconsequential, but Rh-negative "high responders" may immunize with as little as 0.01 mL of Rh-positive fetal blood.[2] Rh prophylaxis is indicated in routine pregnancies at 28 weeks and after delivery of an Rh-positive fetus, and in virtually all unusual pregnancies where TPH before 28 weeks is a concern.[3] Infrequently, TPH is so large that sensitization would not be prevented by standard treatment, and additional Rh immunoglobulin may be required.[4]

While universal prophylaxis has dramatically decreased the incidence of severe Rh disease, maternal D-alloimmunization remains a major cause of severe fetal anemia requiring IUT. Causes of serious anti-D alloimmunization include failure to provide prophylaxis for obstetric events, failure to administer the routine 28-week dose, inadequate Rh immunoglobulin for TPH, misidentification of Rh-negative women, absent prenatal care, and patient refusal.[5] Sources outside pregnancy are unusual, because RhD crossmatching for transfusion is routine. However, maternal intravenous drug abuse may produce extremely potent alloimmunization before any pregnancy.[6]

Non-D Rh disease is important, as transfusion blood is not typically matched for other Rh system components (CcEe). Anti-c disease is just as dangerous as classic Rh disease and is monitored and treated by similar protocols.[7,8] Anti-C disease is rarer, with less hydrops, but may require invasive testing and treatment in the third trimester.[9] Anti-E is more common, but milder still, while isolated anti-e virtually never causes fetal disease. Many other RBC antigens may induce maternal sensitization and (in subsequent pregnancies) fetal anemia due to transplacental immunoglobulin G (IgG)[10] (Figure 7.1).

IgG is the critical vector of fetal disease. It crosses the placenta by facilitated transport, reaches high concentration in the fetus, binds to paternal/fetal antigens, and induces fetal immune-mediated trapping of these antibody-labeled RBCs. Immune-based microphagocytosis and extravascular hemolysis rapidly eliminate labeled cells. Anemia and corresponding waste products result. Ultimately, severe Rh disease demands extreme erythropoietic effort, with release of many immature forms; hence, the term "erythroblastosis fetalis."

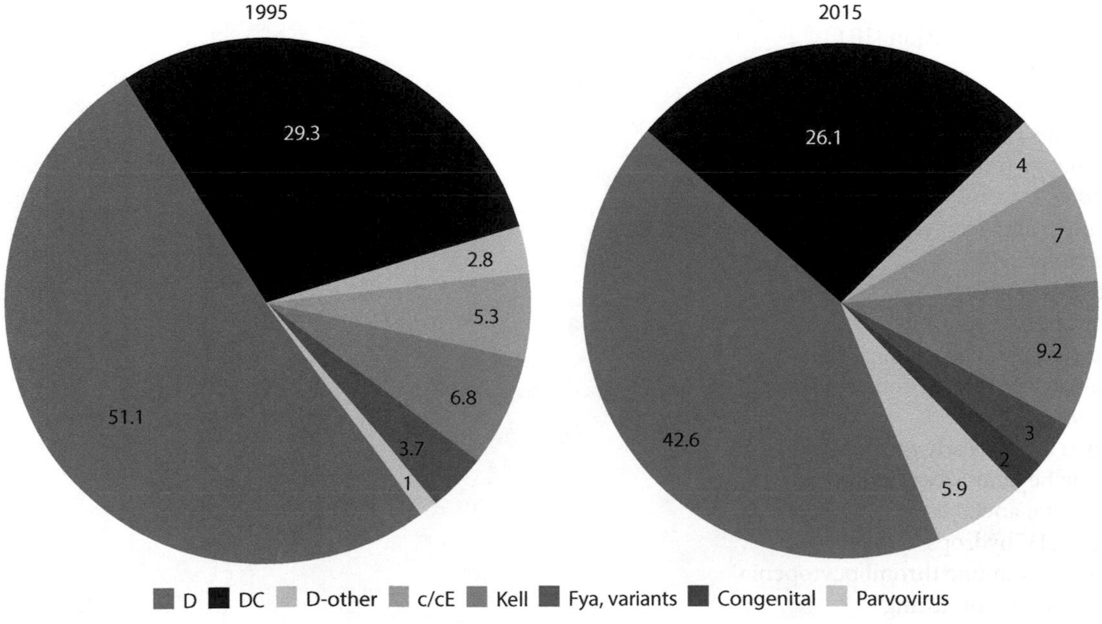

Figure 7.1 Distribution of sources of fetal anemia requiring intrauterine transfusion (IUT). Note the shift in the frequency of Kell alloimmunization and parvovirus, emergence of congenital category.

Kell alloimmunization has an additional complement-fixing mechanism, inducing hemolysis intravascularly and within fetal bone marrow.[11] The Kell antigen is an active RBC membrane component, and immunization may also inhibit cell division and erythropoietin response.[12] The result is more complete hemolysis, hemolysis of progenitor cells, and unexpectedly profound and sudden fetal anemia. For all alloimmune anemias, since the fetus simply produces more RBC with the same offending antigen, an accelerating process is inevitable.

Immune responsiveness is important. Up to 30% of Rh-negative women and 20%–30% of Kell-negative women immunized by mismatched blood transfusion will not produce antibody sufficient to cause fetal disease.[1]

Anemia due to fetal infection

Fetal infection may produce anemia in varying patterns: (1) hydrops with profound anemia, potentially remediable by serial IUT (e.g., parvovirus B19) and (2) hydrops with moderate anemia without improvement despite maintenance of normal hemoglobin levels by IUT (most other infections and even some parvovirus).

Parvovirus generates aplastic anemia by specific mechanism. The P antigen on RBC precursors facilitates integration of virus into the cellular genome, arresting cell division of colony-forming erythroid precursors (CFU-E) and more primitive burst-forming units (BFU-E).[13] Fetal RBC production is halted, almost absolutely.[14] There is no direct viral effect on circulating cells, although the RBC half-life may be shorted by associated hepatitis and myocarditis.[15] As erythropoiesis stops, natural attrition of 1%–2% per day results in progressive anemia. Immunity, acquired from the mother transplacentally, reverses this viral suppression. Reactivation of BFU-E and CFU-E takes some time, and recovery may be further complicated by liver failure with hypoproteinemia, and/or cardiac failure with nonanemic hydrops. In some fetuses, serious anemia lasts only a few days, and the disease is self-limited. In other fetuses, absent RBC production is so profound and sustained that recovery starting with release of very immature forms (another example of erythroblastosis) is too little, and hydropic stillbirth results. Lifesaving serial transfusions may be necessary in up to 50% of such fetuses.[16]

Other infections generate fetal anemia by chronic debilitation, induced hemolysis by hepatosplenomegaly, and sequestration in the enlarged placenta. In some cases of congenital syphilis, listeriosis, and coxsackie infection, fetal anemia may be severe enough to warrant transfusion, but, in general, anemia is a rather modest manifestation of hydrops, not a cause.

Congenital anemias

An increasing number of reports give information about successful management of various congenital causes of severe fetal anemia, including dyserythropoietic anemia of all types, previously lethal hemoglobinopathies such as α-thalassemia major, red cell membrane abnormalities, asplastic anemias such as Diamond–Blackfan, anemia syndromes such as Fanconi's anemia, and so on. In many cases, successful fetal treatment leads to stem cell or bone marrow transplant, so the result is true treatment.

Hydrops fetalis

As anemia worsens, physical manifestations become apparent, paralleling different patterns of response. In the fetus compensating, effectively for low-grade hemolysis with increased reticulocytosis and elevated production of bilirubin, yielding a very slow rate of anemia, physical changes may be limited to increased liver diameter (due to extramedullary erythropoiesis), modest cardiovascular changes (slight cardiac chamber dilation, increased peak systolic velocities in cerebral and systemic circulations, increased cardiac output, and increased heart rate—"hyperdynamic" fetal circulation) and increased amniotic fluid volume (increased cardiac output leads to increased fetal glomerular filtration rate).[17]

More severe anemia results in localized endovascular hypoxemia, with vasodilation in major vascular beds. RBC decline yields decreased blood viscosity, potentiating increased velocity, the basis for Doppler prediction of anemia. Fetal liver and, after 26–28 weeks, fetal kidney are potent sources of oxygen-dependent erythropoietin release. Erythropoietin acts not only on intramedullary BFU-E but also on dormant lines within liver, spleen, and other organs. Once erythropoietin rises, extramedullary RBC production displaces normal hepatic function. Hypersplenism, low production in bone marrow congested with hematopoiesis, and oxygen-sensitive shortened life span, may produce associated thrombocytopenia. Kell hemolysis leads to an almost-vacant marrow, so does not seem to be associated with thrombocytopenia.[18] Devotion of hepatic architecture to erythropoietic cells results in metabolic defects, including hypoproteinemia, disordered fixed acid buffering, and mechanical obstruction of venous cardiac return. Lymphatic blockade by the enlarged liver, decreased oncotic pressure due to hypoproteinemia, increased peritoneal vascular permeability from hypoxemia, and increased venous pressure all combine to produce ascites as hydrops begins. Worsening hypoproteinemia, venous congestion, and hypoxemic tissue fluid mishandling result in progressive anasarca, serous accumulations in pleural spaces and pericardium, and scalp and subcutaneous edema. The placenta also becomes increasingly edematous.[19] This full-blown picture is hydrops fetalis (Figure 7.2). Further decline features loss of heart rate variability and biophysical variables, as anemia becomes lethal. Once blamed for the onset of hydrops, fetal heart failure is now understood to be terminal, caused by hypoxemic myocardial malfunction. Classification of ultrasound hydropic manifestations (Table 7.1) serves as a system for description of fetal compromise.[20] There are direct hematologic correlates (Figure 7.3). Disease severity described by this classification also reflects prognosis.

These physical manifestations reflect pathophysiology, within limits. For instance, small pericardial effusions are

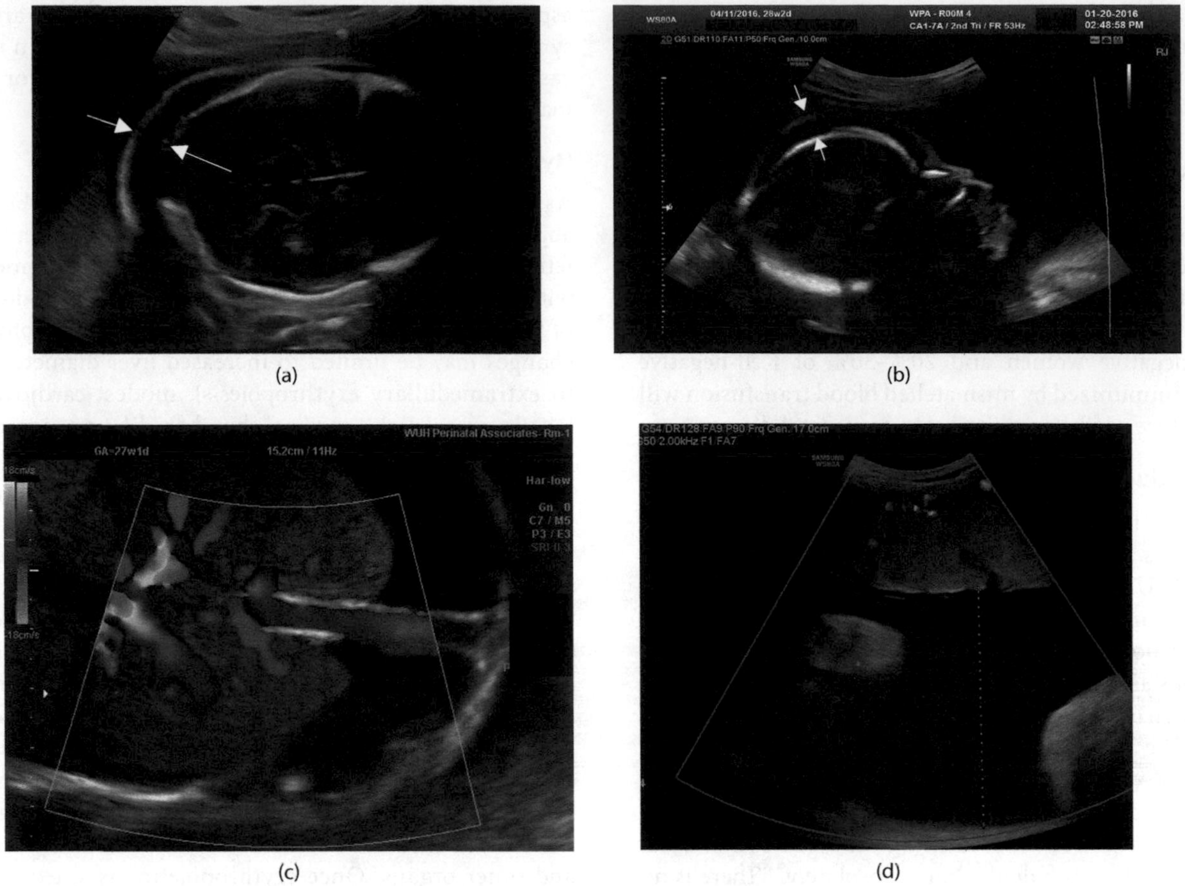

Figure 7.2 Ultrasound images of hydrops fetalis showing scalp edema (between arrows): (a) transverse view; (b) sagittal view; (c) massive ascites with umbilical cord stretched from the edematous abdominal wall to its insertion at the base of the fetal liver and (d) polyhydramnios (largest pocket between calipers=10 cm) and thick placenta at 30 weeks gestation.

Table 7.1 Ultrasound classification of fetal alloimmune disease.

Class	Elevated MCA Doppler	Placentomegaly	Ultrasound appearance ascites	Effusion	Anasarca	Abnormal BPS <4/10
0	–	–	–	–	–	–
I	+	+	–	–	–	–
II	+	+	+	–	–	–
III	+	+	+	+	+	–
IV	+	+	+	+	+	+

–, absent; +, present; BPS, biophysical profile score; MCA, middle cerebral artery.

common in mild to moderate anemia. Large pericardial effusions in end-stage hydrops are components of anasarca, not cardiac malfunction, while pericardial effusions seen with parvovirus may follow anemia and/or viral myocarditis. Often, onset of hypdrops is apparent only on serial observations by experienced operators in terminal fetal disease. Especially in midtrimester, ambient fetal P_{O2} is very high, so hydropic changes may be modest and, due to mechanical effects. The hypoxemic abnormalities readily inducible in third-trimester anemic fetuses do not usually occur prior to 22 weeks' gestation unless the fetus is preterminal. Thus, physical changes in anemic fetuses are important correlates of disease, but are too complex to use as sole determinants of therapy.

The present of fetal hydrops on ultrasound mandates immediate blood sampling. With known etiology (e.g., alloimmunization, parvovirus), starting transfusing before the opening hemoglobin value is known, may be appropriate. However, in many cases of nonimmune hydrops, comprehensive fetal testing is important before transfusion with adult donor cells permanently obscures diagnosis. High-level ultrasound examination and careful planning of sample requirements are imperative before the procedure is started.

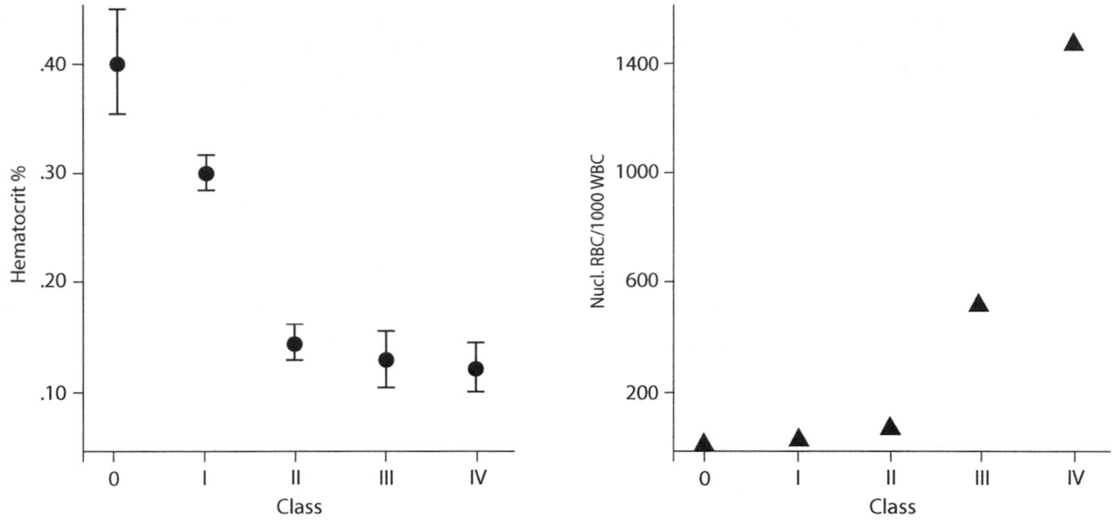

Figure 7.3 The relationship between disease severity by ultrasound classification (Table 7.1) and fetal hematologic parameters measured at the time of cordocentesis. There is a significant reflection of disease severity and prognosis.

Subjective "prehydropic" changes may have relevance to preprocedure monitoring in patients at very early gestational ages. For instance, abdominal circumference may accelerate before hydrops appears (Figure 7.4). Amniotic fluid volume and placental thickness, subjective appearance of fetal organs outlined by fluid, and minor reductions in fetal heart rate (FHR) variability determined by computerized interpretation are all features which may predict hydrops. Fetal middle cerebral artery (MCA) Doppler velocimetry predicts fetal anemia accurately enough to render these subjective elements less critical.

Noninvasive monitoring of fetal anemia

History

In alloimmune disease, the timing of invasive testing depends on the onset and severity of previous disease, as subsequent antigen-positive fetuses are often more severely affected. Recurrence is not invariable and not always as severe, so historical factors are always weighed against more relevant evidence from the index pregnancy.

Maternal antibody titers

The concept of "critical titer" is important. For each regional laboratory and for each antibody, there is a threshold concentration below which fetal disease is unlikely (Table 7.2).[21–23] Local standards may range from 1:16 to 1:128 depending on the test and control antigen-positive cells used. Typical titers at our institution (anti-D 1:16, anti-C 1:32, anti-K 1:4–8; direct antiglobulin test) may not apply to the reader's experience.[23,24] Serial titrations, done by the same laboratory using identical cell lines, performed monthly (sooner with important obstetric events) provide the most accurate assessment, but this remains controversial.[25] Reaching the critical tier, or a rise of two dilutions, mandates enhanced surveillance, but not invasive testing.

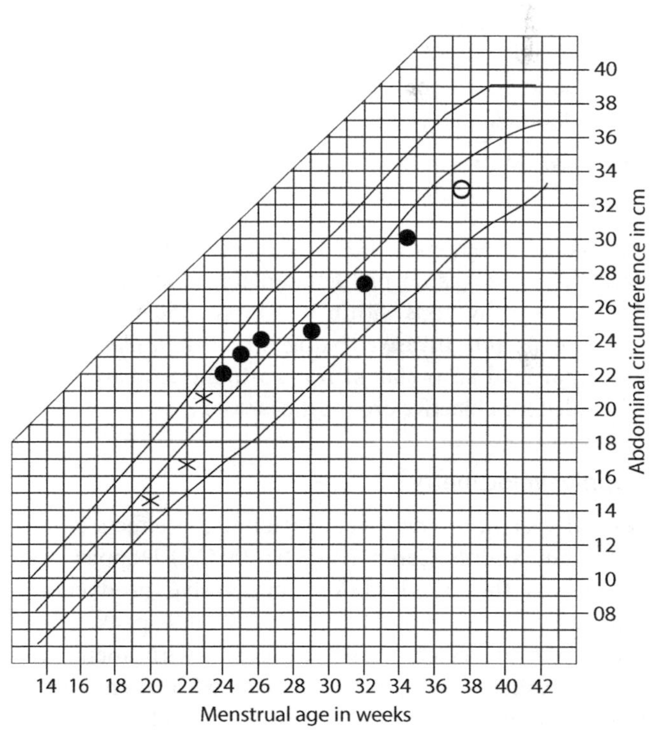

Figure 7.4 The relationship between abdominal circumference (AC) measured by ultrasound and disease progression. Asterisks show AC in a severely affected fetus without ascites, before treatment. Rapid increase in AC is a result of gross hepatosplenomegaly. With treatment by intravascular transfusion (IVT), liver size and, therefore AC, are reduced to previously established percentiles. Open circle represents AC at delivery.

Fetal anatomic survey

Ultrasound fetal anatomic survey provides interesting data on disease progression, but may incompletely reflect the onset of anemia. Many fetuses with hemoglobin under the 10th percentile have normal ultrasound. Among fetuses

Table 7.2 Assessment of alloimmunization.

Is the antibody dangerous?	
Antibody specificity	
Frequent	D, c, E C^{W}, K
Uncommon	C, e, Kp^{a}, Kp^{b}, Fy^{a}, Cellano, s, M, U
Antibody strength	
D	Titer 16
	Absolute level ≥6 IU/mL
Kell	Indirect Coombs titer ≥4
All others	Indirect Coombs titer ≥16
Recent two-dilution rise from any level	
Is this fetus at risk?: Determine fetal blood type	
Fetal DNA in maternal serum (D only—see text)	
Amniocentesis DNA (all Rhesus antigens, Kell)	
Fetal typing by cordocentesis	
Previous affected fetus, 2-dilution titer rise	
Is this fetus anemic?	
Serial middle cerebral artery Doppler looking for peak systolic velocity (PSV) >1.5 MOM	
Ultrasound examination abnormal	
Fetal blood sampling by cordocentesis	

Abbreviation: MOM, multiples of the median.

referred for emergency IUT, 15% had procedures deferred because "there was normal fetal anatomic survey," only to develop overt hydrops within 10–14 days.[5] Suspicious findings may prompt invasive testing *earlier* than planned, but a normal fetal scan should not postpone invasive testing scheduled for objective prognostic factors.[17]

Doppler velocimetry

Several vascular beds reflect regionalized effects of anemia,[17] but Middle Cerebral Artery (MCA) Doppler velocimetry is the standard for noninvasive production.[26] Mari et al.,[27] correlating anemia with MCA peak systolic velocity in untreated fetuses, in fetuses with anemia following transfusion,[28] and in fetuses with anemia other than alloimmune causes,[29] provide a solid experiential basis for application in prospective management of fetuses at risk (100% for detection of moderate to severe anemia, 95% confidence interval [CI] 86%–100%).[30] In fetuses with mild anemia, MCA Doppler velocimetry has a significant false-positive rate (up to 30% in unselected patients undergoing fetal blood sampling for nonanemic reasons) and a more concerning false-reassuring rate of about 5%—a rate which has declined, but persists, with substantial experience. In the latter case, normal MCA peak systolic velocity may delay invasive testing. When a significant rise finally occurred, fetal hemoglobin levels were below 5.0 g/dL.[31]

Some investigators have not duplicated Mari et al.'s high level of accuracy in predicting anemia. However, in all studies, the detection of fetal anemia improves as disease becomes more severe. Several factors may interact in this relationship. In mild anemia, blood viscosity may singly influence MCA changes (thinner blood is easier to push, volume cardiac output increases, and peak systolic velocity rises). With worsening anemia, additional mechanisms, including vasodilation due to endovascular hypoxemia, optimized ejection fraction due to mild cardiac dilation, increased sympathetic tone, and advancing gestational age, may interact, enhancing the accuracy of MCA peak systolic velocity.

The MCA is readily accessible, the Doppler angle is usually optimal, and adding color Doppler imaging helps in differentiating from other intracranial arterial waveforms. Gestational age variation appears predictable and thresholds for invasive testing seem applicable to all forms of fetal anemia. IUT produces Doppler changes concurrent with measured hematocrit (Figure 7.5). Incorporated in a routine of fetal physical and functional assessment, MCA Doppler velocimetry has become the standard in the noninvasive evaluation of fetal anemia.

Noninvasive fetal blood typing by cell-free DNA

In the past, calculations of likelihood, based on C/E antigen distribution, guided treatment with a heterozygous father. For D-alloimmunization such approximations are no longer necessary because fetal D-status is reliably obtained in >99.3% of patients by 12 weeks' gestation using cell-free fetal DNA from maternal serum.[32]

As noted earlier, many other antigens may be implicated in fetal hemolytic disease. Testing for C, c, E, and K antigen-determining fetal DNA has been established in some jurisdictions, but is currently under investigation before broad application in the United States.[33,34] D-typing is reliable by 10 weeks, essentially 100% by 12 weeks,[35] as are other Rhesus DNA types, while Kell is less reliable until 20 weeks.[34] There are limitations to this approach. (1) Not all antigens' DNA has been sequenced so that further research is needed to address less common sources of anemia. (2) There are many D-variants, some with D-expression at very low or even absent levels. (3) Maternal gene expression may be absent due to abnormal DNA regulation—her DNA may be normal D-positive DNA, but unexpressed due to promoter–region defect. This will result in a positive plasma DNA test in a serologically negative, alloimmunized mother, creating a paradoxical false positive.[36] (4) The method remains expensive, so it is not cost effective for D-determination in guiding postpartum prophylaxis versus routine cord blood typing.[37]

Despite these minor considerations, the accurate guidance of pregnancy management by knowing fetal blood type is a leap forward in fetal treatment. Currently for D, and soon for many others, fetal blood typing by using cell-free DNA should be a routine *maternal* blood test in all sensitized first-trimester pregnancies.

Invasive monitoring of fetal anemia

Invasive procedures require caution because of their potential aggravation of existing disease. Transplacental amniocentesis causing TPH may provoke maternal antibody production.[38] Cordocentesis for fetal blood typing with subcritical sensitization may convert a benign

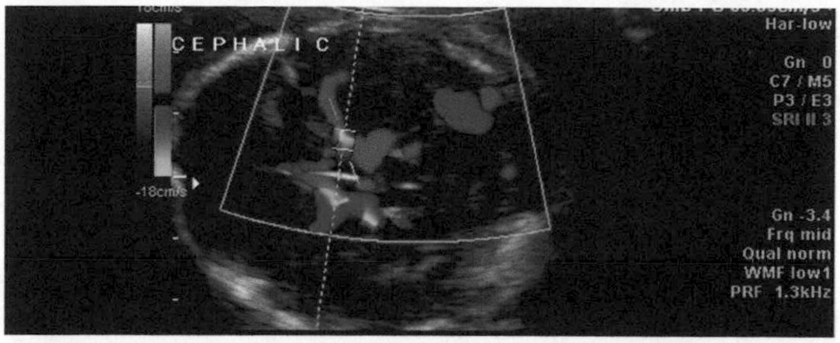

(a)

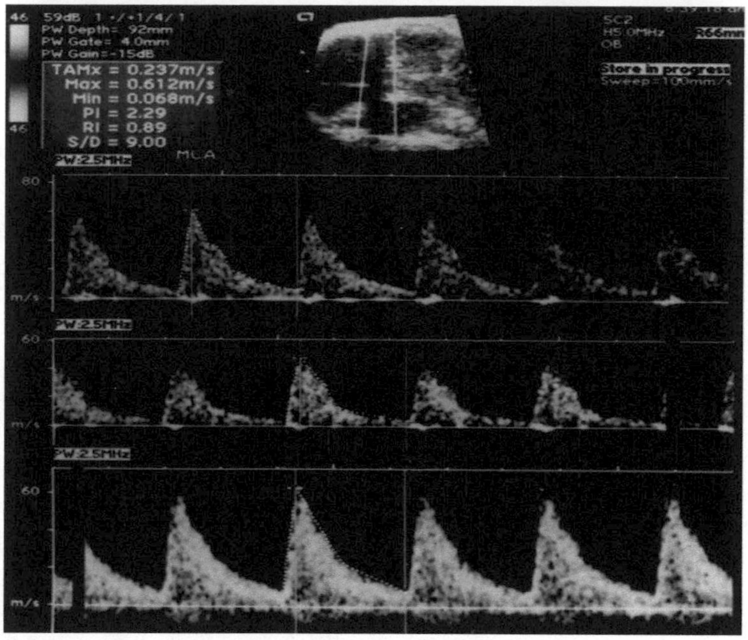

(b)

Figure 7.5 Serial Doppler waveforms from the middle cerebral artery (MCA) of a fetus severely affected by Rh disease. Top panel: MCA peak velocity is 61.2 cm/s, more than two standard deviations above the mean; fetal hemoglobin = 5.7 g/dL. Middle panel: post-IVT, MCA peak systolic velocity is 38.5 cm/s; fetal hemoglobin = 13.4. Bottom panel: 3 weeks later, pre-IVT MCA peak systolic velocity is 72.9 cm/s, as predicted by the post-IVT hemoglobin; the pretransfusion level is 6.0.

situation into one needing repetitive early IUT.[39] The goal of testing must be clear. If the father is a known homozygote, there is no reason to perform an invasive procedure for blood typing alone. In known alloimmunized pregnancies, when hydrops is present, cordocentesis for fetal blood sampling without transfusion is equally pointless.

Fetal blood typing

Knowing whether the fetus is at risk is extremely important in planning the treatment. In cases where cell-free fetal DNA testing is not applicable, direct determination may be indicated. If the father is heterozygous, 50% of the fetuses will be antigen negative, and completely unaffected. Fetal blood typing for Kell and non-D Rh system antigens requires simple amniocentesis only.[40,41] Standard DNA technology, as early as 14–16 weeks, can mandate ongoing surveillance (positive fetuses) or make it irrelevant (negative fetuses). The same methodology allows typing of fetal platelets for critical antigens in neonatal alloimmune thrombocytopenia (NAIT).[42] Currently, alloimmune disease from other sources requires fetal blood typing from RBCs obtained at cordocentesis. Again, rapid progress in noninvasive techniques likely will eliminate invasive blood typing in all but the most unusual situations.

Amniocentesis for ΔOD_{450}

The endpoint of hemolytic degradation is bilirubin. As hemolysis increases, much is transported across the placenta, fetal serum bilirubin levels are modestly elevated and amniotic fluid bilirubin also rises. Amniotic fluid bilirubin normally changes over gestation, requiring specific norms (Figure 7.6). Amniocentesis is generally easy to perform, it is within the technical range of most obstetricians, and it does not require specialized laboratory services. Amniocentesis done under continuous ultrasound guidance, through a placenta-free window, a sterile procedure, can provide safe reassurance in most cases. Limitations include contamination from blood and meconium, difficult interpretation before 22 weeks, a false alarm of about 10%, and a life-threatening false-reassuring rate of 3%–5%. The reliability of MCA

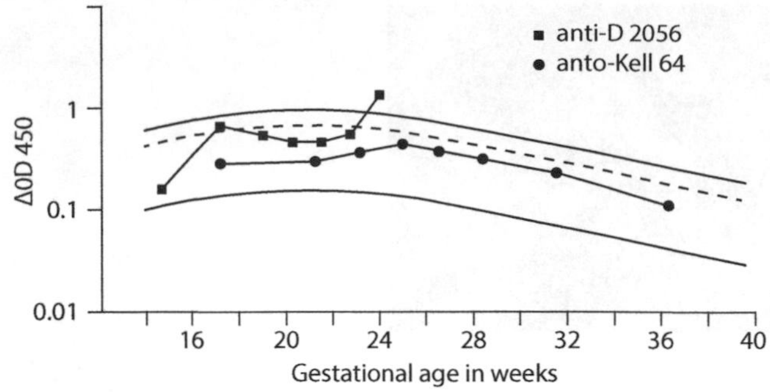

Figure 7.6 Gestational age application of ΔOD_{450} shows a curvilinear relationship. Depicted are two patients with significant alloimmunization. Upper profile in an Rh-alloimmunized woman shows a sudden rise in ΔOD_{450} at 24 weeks, associated with ultrasound evidence of accelerating hydrops (class II). This fetus survived intact with four IVT. ΔOD_{450} measurements in Kell disease may not accurately reflect disease severity; therefore, in this case (shown by circles), amniocenteses were performed frequently from 18 to 36 weeks. Serial results did not cross 80% zone II line, fetal blood sampling was not utilized, no IVT was done, and a healthy baby was delivered at 37 weeks, requiring only exchange transfusions for elevated bilirubin.

Doppler in predicting onset of severe fetal anemia has eliminated OD_{450} testing as a routine assessment tool.[43]

Fetal blood sampling

Cordocentesis for fetal blood typing alone has essentially no role. Sampling without intravascular transfusion (IVT) may be appropriate in several circumstances, and in others the need for transfusion is clear, so a separate cordocentesis procedure would not be indicated (Table 7.3).

Cordocentesis for fetal blood sampling without IVT is not considered for hydropic fetuses with known etiology. In nonhydrops, blood sampling is performed separately with IVT readily available. With suspicious history, ultrasound findings, rising antibody titers, or difficulty in obtaining rare donor blood types, a combined procedure (cordo-IVT) is prepared, but infusion of blood is withheld until the hemoglobin value is known at bedside. Here, the portable hemoglobin machine is invaluable, saving donor blood, but at the same time avoiding a repeat procedure, if transfusion is necessary.

Cordocentesis procedure

For simple cordocentesis, maternal sedation, prophylactic antibiotics, hospital admission, and antenatal steroids are not used. Meticulous identification of an umbilical vein target often takes as long as the procedure itself. The ideal image shown in Figure 7.7 is not always available. Alternative targets include umbilical vein within the fetal abdomen, free cord loop which can be pinned against adjacent uterine or placental surfaces, umbilical cord at its fetal abdominal skin incision, and fetal cardiac puncture, in the order of preference. Mother or fetus can be manipulated to improve target imaging. Only when a safe

Table 7.3 Cordocentesis for investigation of fetal anemia.

Cordocentesis alone
MCA PSV 1.5 MOM—2.0 MOM, known alloimmune
Late-gestation planning (>35 weeks)
Elevated MCA PSV with no known cause for anemia
Alloimmune IUGR fetus
Rare, hard to obtain donor blood
Ready to transfuse pending bedside Hb
Nonhydrops MCA PSV > 2.0 MOM, known alloimmune
Hydrops without known cause of anemia
Suspect accelerated hemolysis
Gestational age <24 weeks
Transfusion without waiting
Alloimmune or parvovirus hydrops
Subsequent IVT
Difficult access, maternal, fetal, vessel factors
Rare donor

Hb, hemoglobin; IVT, intravascular transfusion; IUGR, intrauterine growth restriction.

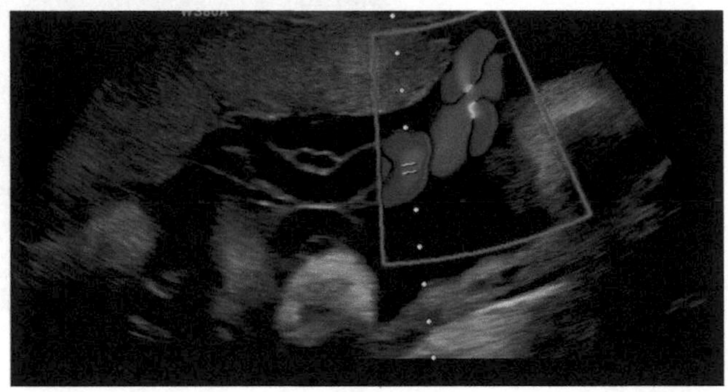

Figure 7.7 Sonogram of the insertion site of the umbilical cord on the surface of an anterior placenta. The umbilical vein, the prime target for IVT, is well visualized.

approach is identified, not traversing surface placental vessels or maternal vascular compartment, should cordocentesis proceed. Other prerequisites are shown in Table 7.4.

Cordocentesis is performed under continuous ultrasound visualization, with a 22-gauge spinal needle of appropriate length. Once the needle is positioned on the vessel, it is inserted with a vigorous "pop," and the tip should be readily seen within the lumen of the vessel (Figure 7.8). An initial sample is aspirated for immediate hemoglobin measurement, and further samples are slowly withdrawn while the reading is taken. Blood typing, direct Coombs test, hematologic values in duplicate, and biochemistry normally require 3.0 mL. Once samples are secured, a small "puff" of sterile saline identifies the vessel sampled, to validate results.

The following critical values may indicate proceeding directly to fetal transfusion:

1. *Hemoglobin concentration:* This rises throughout gestation; therefore, an age-correlated curve is used (Figure 7.9). Transfusing at the fifth percentile helps

Table 7.4 Prerequisites for performing invasive fetal testing/therapy.

Detailed indication
Informed consent
Experienced team
High-resolution ultrasound
Accessible target
Bedside testing
Detailed blood typing laboratory
Transfusion blood available
Fetal monitoring capability[a]
Emergency obstetric services[a]
Tertiary-level neonatal intensive care[a]
Maternal/family support systems

[a] Usually applicable only when gestation is >25–26 weeks.

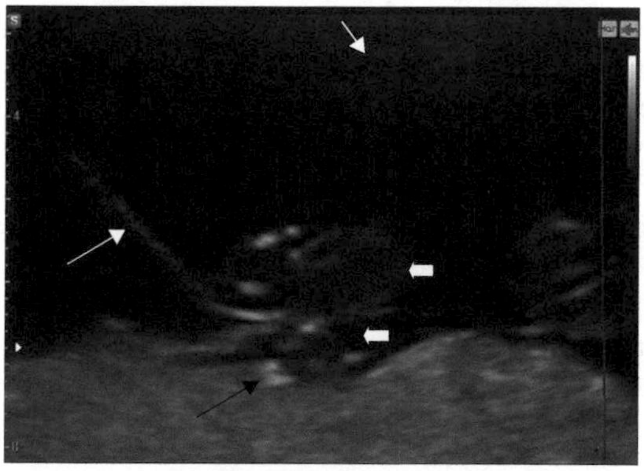

Figure 7.8 With a posterior placenta, the needle traverses the amniotic fluid, with the shaft indicated by the upper (white) arrow. The needle tip (lower black arrow) is within the umbilical vein (double arrow heads) during transfusion.

avoiding unnecessary transfusion of fetuses not requiring it (some have simplified this to a threshold of 9.0 g/dL for all gestations).

2. *Serum bilirubin*[44]: In hemolytic disease, clearance from the fetal compartment is rapid, but not complete. Total bilirubin over 80 mmol/L indicates potential hemolytic crisis and normal hemoglobin is interpreted cautiously—it may fall rapidly. Bilirubin 60–80 mmol/L indicates accelerated hemolysis. In this intermediate group, an elevated reticulocyte count may indicate adequate erythropoietic response.[45] For bilirubin under 40 mmol/L, hemolysis is most likely mild and timing of repeat cordocentesis is based on hemoglobin concentration and other clinical inputs.
3. *RBC precursors:* Some authors have evaluated nucleated red blood cell (NRBC) counts[46] (in our experience, NRBC vary with technical difficulties and may remain elevated for days following difficult cordocentesis), reticulocyte count[45] (in our experience, only levels under 2% predict anemia), and mean corpuscular volume (MCV), which rises as earlier/younger RBCs are elaborated. In the latter instance, microphagocytosis of older RBC produces smaller damaged forms, tending to lower MCV.[5]
4. *Blood gases/pH*: Most fetuses show minor changes in P_{O2} through mild to moderate anemia. Tissue hypoxemia responsible for local perfusion changes is not usually detectable in blood gas analysis.[47] Increased concentration of carboxyhemoglobin may indicate intravascular oxygen depletion, but is very difficult to measure clinically.

Preparing for IUT: amniocentesis versus cordocentesis

Some authors have suggested that geographic isolation, unavailable subspecialty resources, or inadequate ultrasound resources, may allow for amniocentesis as a means to assess alloimmunization until IVT is "necessary."[48] Our team agrees with the Society for Maternal-Fetal Medicine

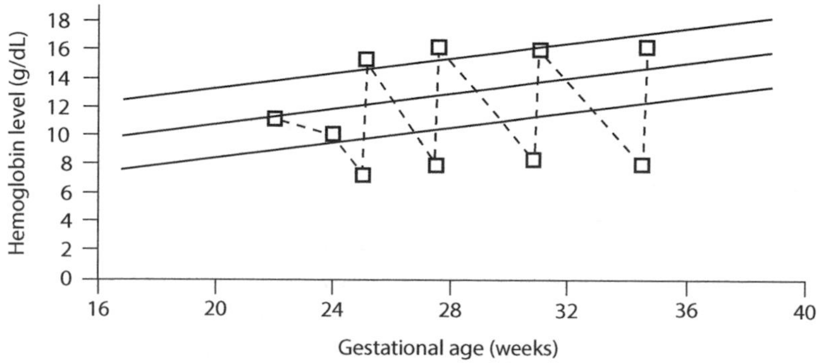

Figure 7.9 Normal hemoglobin concentration rises throughout gestation, depicted by lines indicating the 95th, 50th, and 5th percentiles. The case was that of a sensitized Rhesus (Rh)-negative woman in her third pregnancy, undergoing invasive testing, starting 3 weeks earlier than the severe anemia that had occurred in the second pregnancy. Serial cordocentesis, begun at 21.5 weeks, showed declining hemoglobin levels, reaching threshold for transfusion at 24+ weeks. Four transfusions, shown by rapid rise in hemoglobin concentration, allowed continuation of pregnancy until induction and vaginal delivery at 37+ weeks, with delayed cord clamping and newborn hemoglobin level of 11.8 g/dL.

(SMFM)[43] that amniocentesis ΔOD_{450} has no place in the monitoring of the antigen-positive fetus in a seriously alloimmunized pregnancy: referral to a center capable of accurate serial MCA monitoring and identification of resources for fetal blood sampling and IVT are in order.

Amniocentesis is easier than cordocentesis but provides relatively modest information of imperfect accuracy. Cordocentesis provides greatly superior data. Amniocentesis may be chosen primarily to avoid aggravation of mild to moderate maternal disease. As well as making existing conditions worse, cordocentesis may alloimmunize against other RBC antigens (e.g., Kell or Duffy in an Rh-negative woman), causing fetal disease, and at the least, complicating the crossmatching process. These considerations, in the context of noninvasive fetal blood typing, and reliable noninvasive determination of anemia mean that not only is amniocentesis eliminated but also cordocentesis alone is also much less frequent.

Invasive treatment of fetal anemia

Goals of transfusion

The goals of transfusion are as follows:

1. Restore hemoglobin concentration and, therefore, oxygen-carrying capability
2. Suppress production of (fetal) antigenic RBCs
3. Elevate hemoglobin concentration enough to allow significant interval between procedures, while minimizing the risk of high-volume infusion

Preoperative evaluation

Patients are counseled according to the likelihood of intact survival (Table 7.5). Maternal cooperation is critical; in selected patients, premedication with narcotic analgesic and mild sedation is used. However, much has become simplified in our experience with over 1000 IUTs. Nowadays, in the ultrasound era, maternal sedation, prophylactic antibiotics, and tocolytics are rarely used. Once viability is attained, mothers are NPO from midnight, and have an intravenous started. Prolonged hospital admission is rarely required.

Transfusion blood

Fresh RBC, group O, antigen negative, human immunodeficiency virus (HIV)-/hepatitis negative, buffy coat poor, and fully crossmatched with mother are irradiated immediately prior to the procedure. Centrifugation for approximately 10 minutes at 4000 revolutions per minute (rpm) achieves donor hematocrit 80%–85%. With class IV

Table 7.5 Likelihood of intact survival with fetal IVTs.

	Nonhydropic	Hydrops
First IVT		
<24 weeks	95%	70%
First IVT		
>24 weeks	99%	88%

hydrops (including parvovirus hydrops) platelet concentrate is also obtained for suspension of the packed RBCs. We usually order 30–40 mL more than the target volume to account for tubing, residue, and sampling losses.

Intravascular transfusion

The history of fetal transfusion includes hysterotomy and open cannulation of fetal vessels, repetitive transfusion via indwelling catheters, fetal exchange transfusions, IVT, and combined (intravascular and intraperitoneal) transfusions.[49,50] All had detailed justifications, and most had some success. It has become clear, however, that the shortest, simplest procedure, giving high-volume, highly concentrated RBCs in 20-mL aliquots, sampling halfway and at completion of the target volume, maximizes therapeutic effect and minimizes complications. Uterine tone and maternal complications, such as emesis, supine hypotension, and anxiety, are time dependent. Quickly reaching a high concentration of donor (adult) blood meets therapeutic targets. There appears no measurable advantage to giving extra blood intraperitoneally or fetal exchange transfusion because these do increase the time, technical difficulties, and complications.

Maternal operative preparation

Standard Betadine prep, maternal tilt, and 1% xylocaine infiltration directly above the targeted vessel are used. On the rarest occasion, for example, near term in a woman requiring difficult cesarean section (should urgent delivery be required), spinal epidural anesthesia may be initiated.

Needle insertion

A 22-gauge spinal needle is used, 20-gauge after 28 weeks. If needle removal is required, "a new needle is used" to preserve maximum sharpness. We do not use "echo tip" needles for this same reason. We have not found a rigid needle "guide" necessary for stability. The needle is directed under continuous ultrasound guidance to the umbilical vein, the picture format is zoomed, and gentle bouncing indents the vein wall. Vessel entry is characterized by a "pop." Just pressing forward does not enter the vessel cleanly; a 3-mm staccato advance achieves the necessary motion. Without follow-through, drag on the needle penetrating the vessel wall will usually stop it in the ideal position. The stylet is removed, and blood wells into the hub. Only light aspiration pressure is required—aspirating too hard may pull the vessel wall up against the needle. The vein is preferred—larger lumen, turbulence along the cord (vs. on the placental surface), no risk of vascular spasm—but we have performed over 50 full-volume intra-arterial IVT without complication. If blood return is not achieved, the stylet should not be reinserted above the target, as this may obscure the approach with air bubbles. After preliminary sampling, proper cannulation is confirmed by injecting 0.4–0.6 mL of sterile saline. This produces intravascular turbulence, confirming free placement (Figure 7.10). The first sample is used for bedside hemoglobin level. After correct vessel placement is

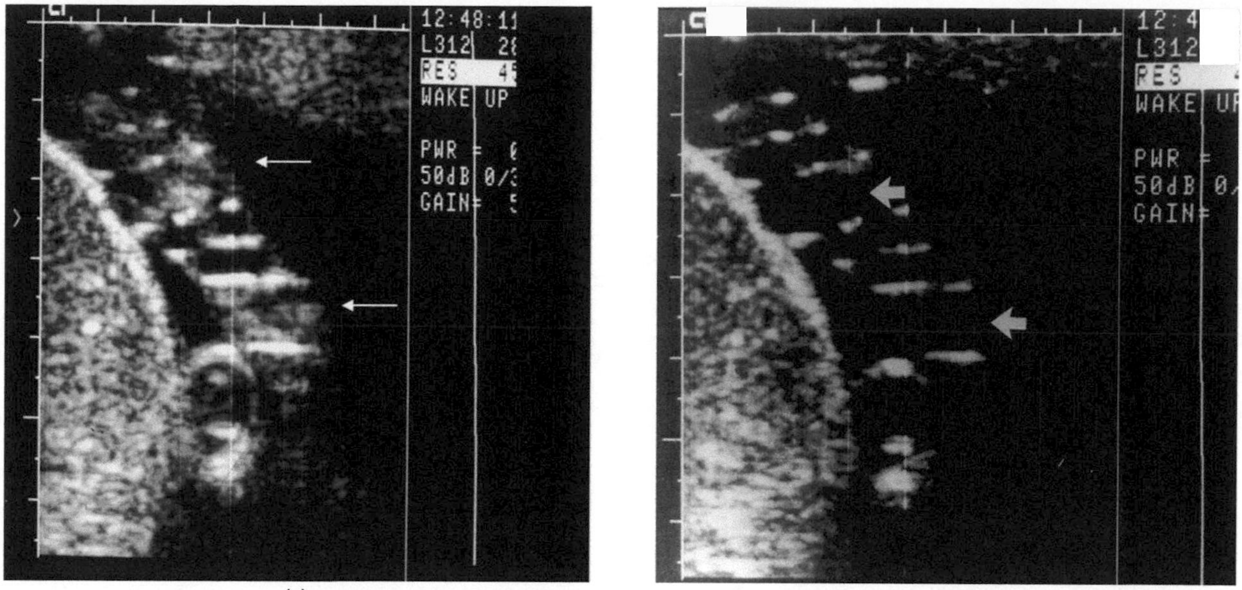

(a) (b)

Figure 7.10 The umbilical vein is infused with concentrated donor red blood cells (RBCs), producing turbulence during infusion (a), which stops immediately when the infusion stops (b) well shown by ultrasound.

ensured, it is common to inject 2–4 mg rocuronium for fetal paralysis. We use this approach in most transamniotic procedures and in about one-third of transplacental procedures in order to avoid needle displacement by fetal movement. In our region, availability of pancuronium is unreliable; vecuronium (causes frequent fetal arrhythmia) and atracurium (has shorter onset and duration) have not worked as well. Postprocedure monitoring is more complicated when the fetus is paralyzed, as an initial period of pseudosinusoidal heart rate follows paralysis and movement may not resume for up to 2 hours.

Transfusion volume

Pressuring the donor blood bag facilitates filling the 20-mL syringe connected via stopcock. The blood volume used aims to raise fetal hemoglobin concentration to approximately 16.0 g/dL.[5] However, for hydropic fetuses with pre-IVT hemoglobin under 4.0 g/L, or previously transfused fetuses with pre-IVT hemoglobin over 10.0 g/L, such blood volumes may not be tolerated. Sampling halfway verifies that the total volume will reach the desired target. If the needle is dislodged, it is reinserted, and target volume attained, unless one of the following occurs: there is a significant change in FHR (monitored by audible pulsed wave (PW) Doppler), there is severe maternal supine hypotension, over 75% target volume is reached, or visualization declines. Blood should never be injected if intravascular turbulence is absent.

Needle removal

When the total volume has been administered, the intravenous tubing is disconnected and the posttransfusion sample is obtained (Figure 7.11). This is not always simple. After large transfusions, dense blood coats the inner lumen and aspiration may be difficult; uterine tone may increase and preclude needle manipulation; visualization may decline; and all these may prevent post-IVT sampling. Calculation (versus measurement) of posttransfusion hemoglobin is approximate, but correlates with midpoint sampling and posttransfusion MCA Doppler.[51] We do not reinsert the needle just for a posttransfusion value. Back-bleeding after needle removal is common, but may be reduced if vessel penetration is via cord substance, and if the needle is removed very gradually. In severe hydrops, combination of elevated intravascular pressure and thrombocytopenia may result in excessive bleeding.[52] Arterial back-bleeding averages about 25% longer than venous.[53] In either case, it is watched until cessation. The threshold for cardiovascular collapse due to blood loss is 300 seconds (5 minutes) and this may indicate an immediate repeat procedure. Since tiny volumes of blood leaking from vessel punctures are detectable by ultrasound, it is common to overestimate blood loss. Blood loss during IVT in the intra-abdominal portion of the umbilical vein will ultimately be reabsorbed, so perhaps not truly "lost." Periodic checks of FHR, cardiac filling, cord artery, and MCA Doppler waveforms provide ample reassurance of circulating volume stability.

Complications

Most complications occur during the IVT (Table 7.6). Cord tamponade may be lethal, so IVT over 24 weeks is done on the delivery suite, with emergency cesarean section available. In 10 cases (1.1%), post-IVT monitoring was abnormal enough to prompt emergency cordocentesis, but the most common finding was normal post-IVT hemoglobin, and normal pH and blood gases. Since MCA PSV has been shown to return to more-normal levels very soon after transfusion, its role in immediate posttransfusion

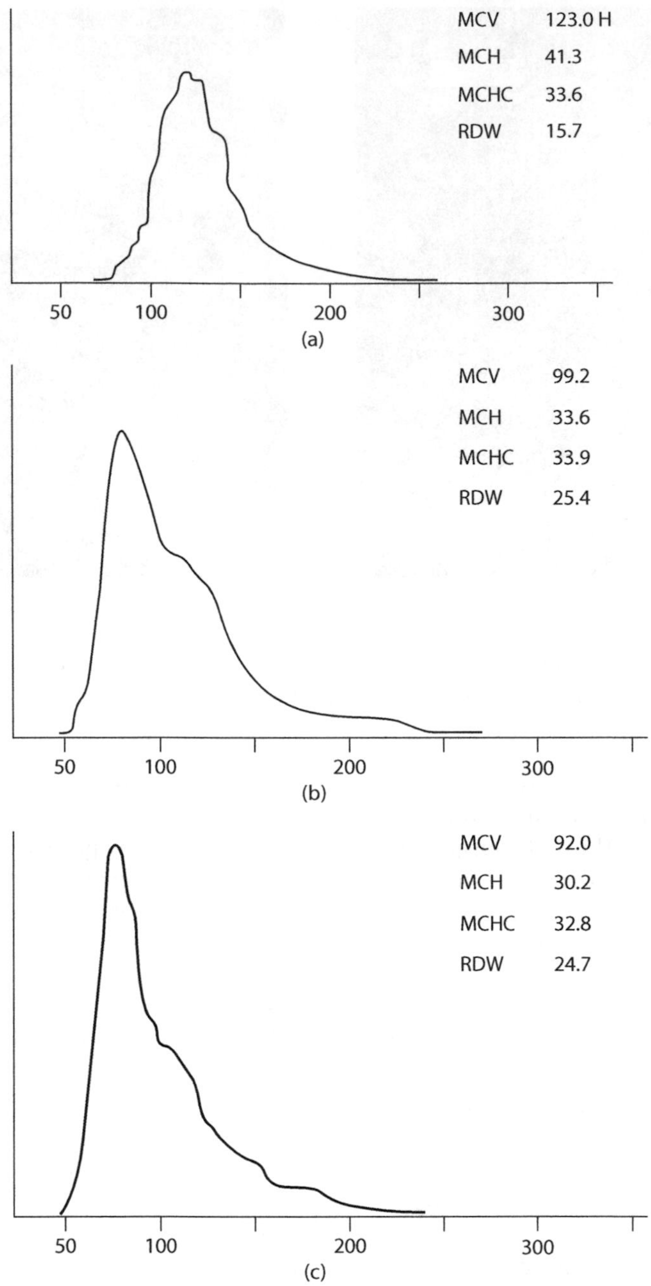

Figure 7.11 Serial RBC histograms taken during an IVT. Top panel: pretransfusion shows high mean corpuscular volume (MCV) (123.0) typical of an anemic fetus. Middle panel: bimodal curve demonstrates substantial addition of adult (donor) RBCs, lowering average MCV to 99.2. Lower panel: posttransfusion final MCV of 92 reflects the addition of donor hemoglobin, raising the initial pre-IVT hemoglobin value of 4.8 g/dL to a post-IVT value of 11.4 g/dL.

fetal assessment (e.g., slow recovery from paralysis, apparently excessive back-bleeding on needle removal) should be investigated.[54] Deaths of hydropic fetuses not improving with serial IVTs have occurred despite retransfusion within 12 hours of first IVT.

In general, the frequency and severity of procedural complications has declined, with better ultrasound, greater experience, centralization to fetal treatment centers, and earlier detection of severe fetal anemia with improved MCA Doppler surveillance. As discussed below, an emerging additional factor may be the use of IVIG to ameliorate disease, allowing transfusion at later (technically easier) gestational age. Complications are more common <24 weeks, with procedures in free cord loops (vs. either intra-abdominal or placental insertion, which do not differ), and are more often fatal in fetuses with hydropic disease.[55–57]

Intraperitoneal transfusion (IPT)

Transfusion blood is absorbed from the peritoneal cavity via subdiaphgragmatic and intrathoracic lymphatics. Absorption is directly related to volume, duration after transfusion, and presence of fetal diaphragmatic and

Table 7.6 Complications of 966 fetal IVTs.

Survivors Class I	141/144	98%
Survivors Class II–III	65/74	88%
Survivors Class IV	27/37	73%
Incomplete procedures[a]	44	4%
Compressive hematoma	10	1%
Bradycardia, unknown case	38	3.9%
Severe bradycardia	6	6.2%
Exsanguinating bleed	19	2%
Rupture of membranes	5	0.5%
Supine hypotension	32	3.3%

[a] 00%–49% of planned target transfusion volume given.

body movements.[58] Poor response of hydropic fetuses to IPT relates to dilution of transfused blood by ascites and, importantly, absence of fetal breathing movement accompanying low biophysical profile scores.[59] When fetal blood vessels are too small to cannulate, only under 17 weeks, IPT is used in hydrops. IPT (without fetal blood sampling) is less precise than IVT. Transplacental IPT is hazardous, featuring fetal mortality of up to 5% per procedure.[60]

Preparation

In addition to the prerequisites indicated for all transfusions, mandatory IPT criteria include:

1. Nonhydropic fetus
2. Ideal fetal position
3. Team experience in IPT
4. Posterior placenta

Further, IPT application is generally limited to times when fetal vascular access is not available, for example, very early in gestation when vessels are too small, or very late in gestation when fetal size, spine anterior, blocks vascular access.

Technique

Classical IPT uses a 16-gauge Tuohy needle with curved lumen, inserted into the peritoneal cavity, allowing threading of a no. 18 epidural catheter. Placement of the catheter free within the abdomen is confirmed by infusion of radiopaque dye (Figure 7.12).[61] A simpler procedure is to visualize by ultrasound the turbulence produced by pushing saline to prove free placement (Figure 7.13). However, many fetal complications may result from inadvertent injection of highly packed donor blood (prepared as for IVT) into a confined space. Considerable force is required to push this thick blood through the catheter in 10-mL aliquots. FHR is monitored throughout, showing characteristic tachycardia, probably indicating pain as the peritoneum distends. Bradycardia, failure of transfused blood to produce a fluid interface on ultrasound, and maternal complications are the most common reasons for terminating IPT before target volume.[62] Post-IPT monitoring is extended, as traumatic fetal bleeding may take time to produce detectable effects. Timing of repeat IPT is similar to IVT, averaging 3–4 weeks, but serial IPTs are seldom used.

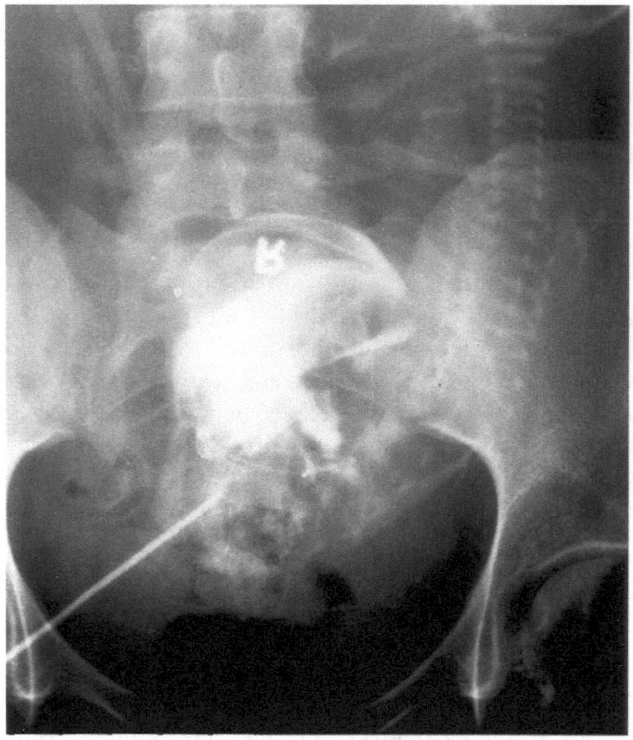

Figure 7.12 Radiograph of the fetal abdomen after injection of 3 mm of 76% Renografin via intraperitoneal catheter. The fetus, in a breech position, shows radiopaque dye along the dome of the diaphragm. Lower in the fetal abdomen, dye dispersed between loops of fetal bowel causes discrete scalloping confirming that the catheter tip is free within the peritoneal cavity.

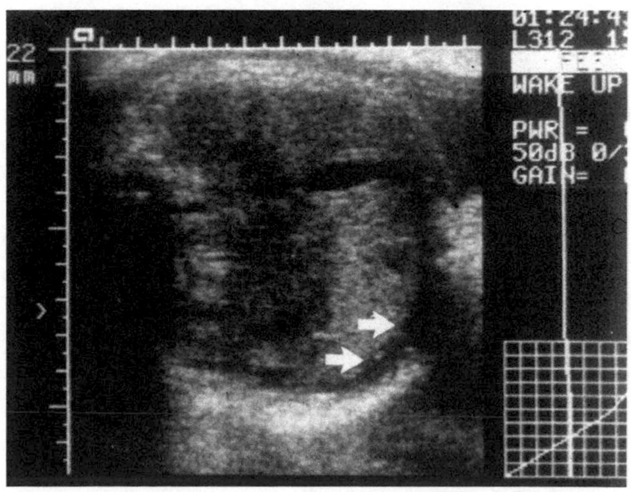

Figure 7.13 Intraperitoneal transfusion with ultrasound verification of proper placement. With ideal fetal position (spine at 11 o'clock position), a 20-gauge spinal needle was used to enter the peritoneal cavity, and placement free in the abdomen was confirmed with agitated saline. Arrows show intraperitoneal fluid rim forming (infused blood), at the 50-mL point in the transfusion.

IPT versus IVT

Theoretically, it might be easier to place a needle within the fetal peritoneal cavity than into a vessel. Also, more blood can be delivered intraperitoneally, according to the following formula.[62]

$$\text{IPT volume in milliliters} = (\text{weeks gestation} - 20) \times 10$$

The major drawback of IPT, in addition to limited ability to treat fetal hydrops, is fetal trauma. This is worse at premature gestation and with anterior placenta. Death from laceration of a major vessel, cardiac penetration, and neurologic injury have been reported. While these are decreased with continuous ultrasound guidance, data from a matched control trial display dramatic differences in safety and efficacy, all favoring IVT (Table 7.7).[63]

Fetal exchange transfusion

This topic includes modern revival of an original approach. Exchange transfusion takes much longer, involves many more dangerous excursions in fetal central perfusion, and has no apparent advantages.[64] Similarly, the combination of IVT and IPT to deliver a greater total volume of transfused RBC has no apparent advantage—except perhaps when intravascular access is tenuous, in order to complete an adequate volume. As a routine procedure, it does not prolong the interval until the next transfusion (all the transfused RBC will degrade on the same time-line) and adds the increased risks of IPT. In our view, the increased risks of IPT are far more significant than the occasional extra IVT that may be required because of less than full-volume IVT.

Intracardiac transfusion (ICT)

In severe early disease treated with IVT, fetal exsanguination occasionally occurs due to vessel trauma and/or thrombocytopenia. In such critical situations, the opportunity for resuscitation may pass in seconds. Vascular collapse makes repeating venous puncture impossible and fetal death is probable. ICT in such circumstances may be lifesaving. Even more rarely, ICT may be the only means of transfusing very early hydrops.[65]

Our experience includes 18 ICTs in 17 fetuses. Ten of these fetuses were exsanguinating. Twelve fetuses survived the acute event after successful intracardiac resuscitation (Figure 7.14). Intracardiac blood sampling and transfusion were semielective in two Rh-positive fetuses whose mothers had hydropic demise at 16 weeks in prior pregnancy.[5] Without life-threatening hypovolemia, ICT is relatively straightforward. The rigidity of a 20-gauge needle may allow improved maneuverability. While the right ventricle seems most appropriate, it is usually not easy to be that selective. IVT principles are utilized, with blood return and "puffs" of saline confirming placement and RBC infusion under continuous ultrasound visualization. Turbulence should be visible in umbilical arteries exiting the fetus. The initial response to severe hypovolemia is profound bradycardia. After the first few milliliters of intracardiac infusion. FHR rises to normal and then to tachycardia. Cold blood straight from the blood bank produces cardiac slowing and ventricular dysfunction. Therefore, one should warm several capped, 5-mL syringes of donor blood under running water. The catheter should not be removed from the needle hub for repeated sampling. We simply give 50% of anticipated IVT volume, sample once, and remove the needle. In fetuses recovering from this procedure, it is perhaps surprising that only one had a significant pericardial effusion. All class III or class IV hydropic fetuses have the potential for thrombocytopenia, vessel wall edema, and exsanguination at IVT. It is useful before starting IVT for such severe illness, to perform a complete anatomic survey of the fetal heart.[17] Cardiac puncture may be a routine way of obtaining early fetal blood samples, but has rarely been reported in nonemergent fetal treatment.[66]

Noninvasive management of fetal alloimmune disease

Especially prior to intravascular techniques, this consideration featured prominently in scholarly work about serious fetal anemia—the risks of IPT were so significant and

Table 7.7 Choice of management (IVT vs. IPT) (matched control trial—1990)

Factor	IPT	IVT	*p*
Number of procedures	2.4	3.9	.03
Attempts/transfusions	1.8	1.2	.02
Procedural complications	38%	10%	.004
Traumatic death	18%	3%	.001
Delivery (GA)	31	34	.011
Exchange transfusions	1.8	0.8	.007
ICN days	8.2	6.1	.044
Nonhydrops alive	83%	98%	NS
Hydrops alive	48%	86%	.01
Class IV alive	0/6	4/6	

Source: Harman CR et al., *Am J Obstet Gynecol*, 162, 1053–1059, 1990.

Abbreviations: GA, mean gestational age; ICN, intensive care nursery; IPT, intraperitoneal transfusion; NS, nonsignificant.

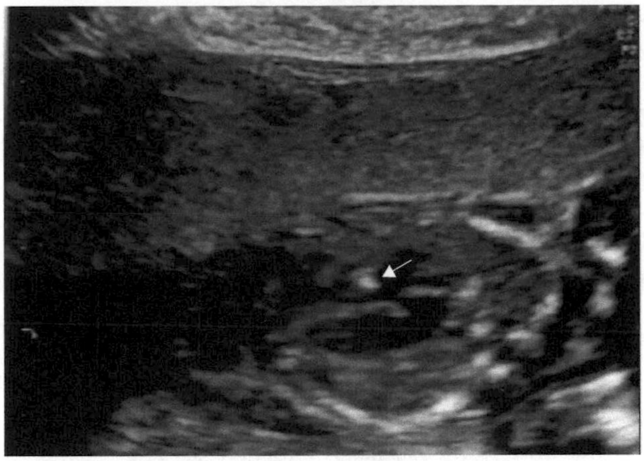

Figure 7.14 Intracardiac transfusion visualized by ultrasound. The needle enters the fetal chest, and the tip sits in the right ventricle (arrow) for intracardiac transfusion of an anemic hydropic fetus at 17 weeks gestation. The ICT was lifesaving. At last follow-up, this child was 2 years old, and developmentally normal.

benefits so delayed in gestation, that many maneuvers were considered, to delay or reduce the use of IPT. Now, the focus is on cases too early to manage safely with IVT (especially before 18–20 weeks), but emerging information suggests that these methods may not only delay the onset of intrauterine treatment, but obviate it altogether in some cases.

Plasmapheresis

In an infusion center, maternal whole blood is withdrawn, centrifuged to remove plasma, reconstituted, and transfused back to the mother. Typically, this is repeated to account for twice the maternal circulating blood volume (double volume plasma exchange). This lowers maternal IgG levels abruptly, with decreased anti-D titers of four dilutions, up to 15 IU/mL. The drop is transient, no longer than 5–7 days, and the process is arduous and expensive. Our team's experience is all pre-1985 (pre-IVT) and suggested that the onset of disease could be delayed, but never prevented.[62] Modern experience with plasmapheresis alone is confined to individual cases managed successfully until immunoglobulin-G infusion (IVIG), fetal transfusion, or both, were started. While the logic of reducing maternal antibody levels makes sense, the value of this demanding process has not been proven.[67,68]

High-dose IVIG

IVIG done weekly, with or without preceding plasmapheresis may be another story. Including several series and neonatal case–cohort evidence, IVIG may be associated with a significant delay (80%–90% delayed by at least 6 weeks compared with previous IVT treated pregnancies) or in some (up to 40% of women with critical titers and prior fetuses requiring IVT) avoiding IVT altogether.

Our experience includes 17 highly selected pregnancies in women with critical titers to D (16) or Kell (1), antigen-positive fetuses demonstrated before 16 weeks by cell-free DNA in maternal serum and poor history—hydrops <22 weeks, hydropic still birth, permanent perinatal injury. None required transfusion before 24 weeks, none were hydropic, and only 10 of 17 required any IVT. All were intact survivors, delivered at 36–39 weeks and had moderate neonatal disease (6/10 nontransfused) or minimal effects. Recognizing that these data are difficult to control (subsequent pregnancies are not always as severely affected), that the reliability of MCA Doppler surveillance generates fewer procedures than in prior practice, and that precise mechanism(s) have not been completely defined, the reader is justifiably skeptical.

IVIG is administered by protocol 1.0 Gm/Kg maternal weight intravenously, weekly, starting at 12–14 weeks' gestation. It is continued until fetal transfusions are required according to MCA PSV cutoff, or 36 weeks, whichever comes first. It is expensive, and thus reserved for fetuses proven antigen-positive and at high risk (regardless of maternal titer). Since Kell positivity is predicted less reliably <20 weeks, and the mechanism of Kell anemia is different from Rh antigens, recommendation of this technique is currently focused on anti-D disease.[69,70] The mechanisms of action are not proven, but placental Fc blockade appears most likely the most important. For this reason, we emphasize maintaining elevated maternal Ig levels by sticking to a weekly schedule.

There is no reliable evidence that direct fetal IVIG administration (without maternal therapy and/or IUT) can treat significant alloimmune disease.[71] On the other hand, neonatal therapy with IVIG appears quite effective in babies with untreated hemolysis.[72] This is in further support of the concept of placental blockade.

Disorder-specific issues

Transplacental hemorrhage

Chronic anemia due to blood loss may follow fetomaternal hemorrhage (FMH) which may occur either spontaneously or following trauma. IUT to replace blood loss has been successful in FMH, but chronic hemorrhage often continues. Because donor cells are adult, Kleihauer–Betke testing cannot assess post-IVT fetal bleeding. MCA Doppler and serial cordocenteses should be used in this situation.[73] In many cases, delivery is a better option once viability has been reached.

Twin-to-twin transfusion syndrome

In twin-to-twin transfusion syndrome (TTTS), IVT has been suggested for the donor twin after laser ablation of placental anatomoses when Twin Anemia Polycythemia Sequence (TAPS) is suspected.[74] This practice assumes that the TTTS donor is anemic due to fetofetal blood loss. However, donors have contracted intravascular volume that will eventually re-expand if placental function is adequate and, except in the minority, still have enough hemoglobin for oxygenation. IVT in TTTS is currently undergoing active research.

Parvovirus

Parvovirus hydrops with profound anemia is quite treatable with IVT. An average of 2.2 transfusions is enough to raise the hemoglobin and sustain it until fetal erythropoiesis resumes. Results will vary, as parvovirus may cause permanent deficits in cardiac function, hepatic function, cerebral function, and growth. Cautious counseling about the potential for permanent injury in other systems should accompany transfusion therapy in parvovirus.[75]

Anemia at very early gestational age

The majority of fetuses treated at this difficult stage have been managed successfully with the intravascular approach.[76,77] This probably is due to several factors—rarity of disease this severe, skill of the teams reporting this experience, and the time it takes (6–10 weeks following onset of high-capacity transplacental transport of maternal IgG at about 10 weeks gestation) for disease to outstrip fetal production. Early treatment by IPT is limited to 16 weeks and later as the fetal abdominal wall lacks the epithelialization to retain transfusion blood before this. It seems likely that a combination of maternal IVIG and delicate IVT will address these issues in the future.

Anemia beyond 32 weeks

In most centers, 32 weeks marks a watershed between mortality and morbidity of the neonate. Should one deliver the anemic fetus for transfusions in the neonatal intensive care unit (NICU) rather than "risking" IVT? For experienced teams, IVT up to 36 weeks has measurable advantages. The *neonate* challenged with rapid, high-volume transfusion may suffer cardiac failure and pulmonary edema. Due to the distensability of fetoplacental vasculature, the *fetus* simply makes volume corrections into the maternal space and amniotic cavity, tolerating large, rapid transfusion without compromise.[78] For the nonhydropic fetus, arrhythmia, NICU accidents, operator experience with exchange transfusion, and infectious issues may mean that a simple IUT is safer than multiple neonatal exchange transfusions.[5,58,79]

Lethal fetal anemias

Inherited hemoglobinopathies and RBC membrane disorders may cause severe fetal anemia and/or anemic hydrops. Serial fetal transfusions are timed similarly to those in Rh disease, suppressing production of abnormal RBCs, and allowing recovery from RBC breakdown products, while maintaining homeostasis. Hemosiderosis is a significant problem with potentially lethal complications in childhood. Advances in transfusion medicine, iron chelation, and bone marrow and liver transplantation in infancy have salvaged small numbers.[80,81] This demonstrates the potential for early and sustained fetal transfusion.[82,83]

Class III/IV hydrops

In such compromised fetuses, rapid transfusion to usual target volumes leads to cardiovascular collapse, due to the already high intravascular pressures, poor placental respiratory function caused by edema, and direct overload of the compromised cardiac function.[84] One gives 50%–60% target volume for gestational age, and 3–5 days later, the same volume is repeated. Response to the first two transfusions is a highly predictive of outcome (Figure 7.15). In Class IV disease, with abnormal biophysical profile, maternal oxygen is started preprocedure, and maintained until fetal heart rate and activity are normal. Rarely, thrombocytopenia is so severe that fetal platelet transfusion is required, Usually, a short,

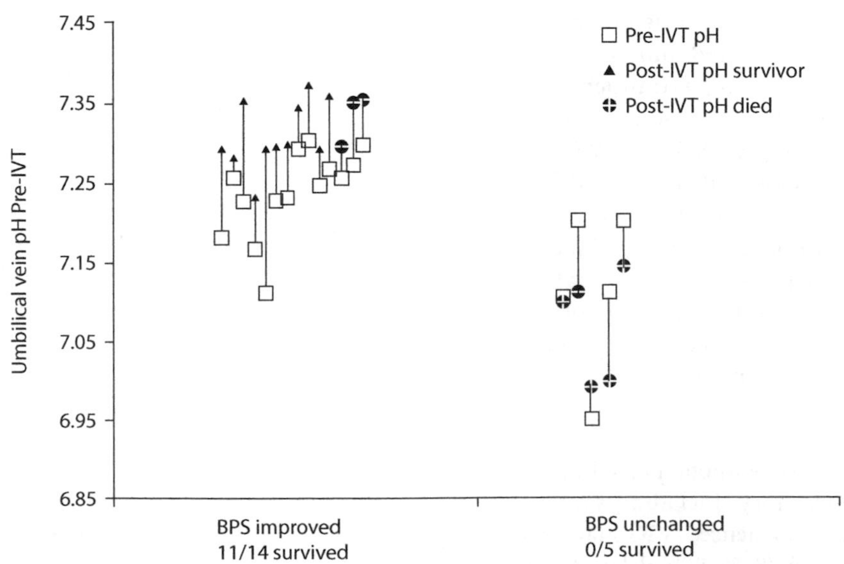

Figure 7.15 Initial response to fetal transfusion indicates prognosis in moribund class IV hydrops. On the left, 14 fetuses showed improvement in biophysical profile score (BPS) between first and second transfusions. Eleven of 14 survived. On the right, five fetuses, equally sick, showed no improvement in pH, and no return of fetal activity, and all died during or after the second transfusion. The return of normal behavior after the transfusion, even when the physical findings are severe, is reassuring.

single-puncture procedure restoring hemoglobin concentration to 6.0–8.0 g/dL produces a rapid return to normal neurologic function and normal vascular integrity (called "reanimation"), although physical changes of hydrops may take weeks to regress.

Neonatal alloimmune thrombocytopenia

This is a significant source of transfusion patients, meriting attention here. Maternal sensitization against platelet antigens (primarily PLA1 and Bak[a]) causes alloimmune destruction of fetal platelets via transplacental antiplatelet IgG. High-dose maternal IgG therapy may treat up to 70% of these fetuses at risk of intracranial hemorrhage antenatally. However, the problem with NAIT in its most severe form is that not all cases respond to IV IgG and the worst may have platelet counts so low that intracranial hemorrhage is probable.[85] Thus, after a significant course of therapy (starting at 14 weeks gestation, and extending for 6–8 weeks, until placental and fetal receptors are saturated with IgG), fetal blood sampling for platelet count may be appropriate to confirm therapeutic effect. However, there is controversy about this approach because bleeding after cordocentesis depends not only on thrombocytopenia but also on the fact that the offending antigen is present on fetal endothelial cells.[86] Both vascular integrity and platelet count and function are impaired, and both remain impaired in the 30% treatment failures. Exsanguination from uncomplicated cordocentesis in PLA1 disease caused our only fetal losses in hundreds of procedures. Because of this danger, every blood-sampling procedure for NAIT includes a fetal platelet transfusion. The platelets are fresh, moderately concentrated, at 10 mL/kg of anticipated fetal weight. The transfusion technique is similar, with a 25- or 22-gauge needle in the intrahepatic umbilical vein. If cord needling is utilized, it is in midcord where Wharton's jelly may assist in closing the puncture. Adjunctive, high-dose dexamethasone and early delivery further maximize therapeutic results. In our experience of 28 severely thrombocytopenic fetuses, of the 19 survivors, only 2 required serial fetal platelet transfusion.[87]

Posttransfusion monitoring

In class IV hydrops, FHR monitoring is continuous with maternal oxygenation until the biophysical profile score is normal. In less severe disease, oxygen is not used and the mother is discharged when FHR reactivity and fetal movement have returned and there are no uterine contractions. Weekly MCA Doppler and biophysical profile scoring are performed until the next transfusion. The next transfusion is intended to be when the pre-IVT donor hemoglobin has dropped to 80–90 g/dL. This is calculated by subtracting 0.3 g/dL per day from post-IVT donor level (e.g., if closing level is 16.6 g/dL, 10% residual fetal, repeat IVT in 20–24 days). This interval lengthens as gestational age advances and is modified by MCA results, noting that some authors have found this imprecise,[88] and others have had variable post-IVT response.[89] In our long-standing practice, calculation based on posttransfusion final sample, using 0.3 g/dL per day, is accurate within 1.0 g/dL >90% of the time.

Outcome studies

The results of our transfusion program are shown in Table 7.8.[5,17] We have seen substantial improvement in IVT technique and outcome statistics since its first inception, with renewed focus on preventing prematurity and related morbidity.

In our series, the factors most highly associated with perinatal mortality were Class IV hydrops (relative risk [RR] 4.53 CI 1.4–9.2) and first IVT <24 weeks (RR 1.8 CI 0.96–2.08, nonsignificant [NS]). Reports by many other centers are similar: survival rate >90%, normal long-term outcome in the majority (almost always in nonhydrops) and similar paucity of pretransfusion predictive factors.[90–92] The LOTUS study is the largest long-term follow-up study of children who were transfused as fetuses, identifying hydropic disease, early-onset disease (via increased procedural complications), and possibly parvovirus infection causing hydrops, as primary determinants of long-term developmental deficit.[93]

Long-term follow-up is key, whenever fetal therapy is considered. For many intrauterine interventions, infancy and childhood are marked with multiple complications and a very challenging course. However, in general, this is not the case for survivors of fetal transfusion, regardless of severity of disease. In class IV hydrops, with poor fetal behavior, outcomes include 10% incidence of cerebral palsy.[94] Other than this discrete group, long-term results are excellent, with very low incidence of permanent handicap.

In the short term of neonatal life, most babies who had serial IVT have delayed erythropoietic response.[95] In the transfused fetus, erythropoietin levels have been suppressed for weeks or months prior to delivery. Donor cells have a reduced half-life in the newborn. With this combination of delayed response and rapid attrition, it is very common for IVT survivors to have two or more neonatal "top-up" transfusions, typically at 6 and 10 weeks. In many cases, this is the only hematologic manifestation of disease. The fully transfused neonate has normal bilirubin, ample iron to make new RBC, and an excellent birth hemoglobin level if cord clamping is delayed, and often needs no transfusion during its short NICU stay. For many fetal transfusion teams, these neonatal benefits clearly justify the application of transfusion therapy until late in gestation.

Table 7.8 IVT (1986–2015).

	IVT	Fetuses	Survival
	966	255	91%
Class 1	508	144	98%
Class 2	121	35	88%[a]
Class 3	143	39	
Class 4	194	37	73%[a]

[a] There was no significant difference in survival between causes of hydropic hemolytic disease (anti-D, anti-Kell, parvovirus) when hydrops of comparable severity is compared.

SUMMARY

Access to the fetal circulation has made precise monitoring and pretransfusion evaluation routine. Cell-free fetal DNA in maternal serum has the potential to identify fetuses at risk, and to exclude antigen-negative fetuses from dangerous management, with accelerating precision. Data obtained by cordocentesis have validated noninvasive Doppler techniques using MCA Doppler velocimetry, reliably identifying fetuses at risk of anemia, while reliably excluding fetuses not yet anemic. Fetal IVT techniques have been simplified and now account for almost all IUT procedures. This has resulted in a high level of success, even in the presence of fetal hydrops. The success of these techniques has led to the application of IVT in many other areas with promising results. Against a background of continued vigilance to prevent alloimmunization by proper transfusion and prophylaxis techniques, IUT stands as a model of successful fetal therapy.

REFERENCES

1. Harman CR, Manning FA. Alloimmune disease. In: Pauerstein CJ (ed), *Clinical Obstetrics*, pp. 441–69. New York, NY: Wiley, 1987.
2. Bowman JM. Blood group immunization in obstetric practice. *Curr Probl Obstet Gynecol* 1983; 7: 1–61.
3. Bowman JM. The prevention of Rh immunization. *Transfusion Med Rev* 1988; 2: 129–50.
4. Bowman JM. Suppression of Rh isoimmunization. *Obstet Gynecol* 1978; 52: 385–93.
5. Harman CR. Invasive techniques in the management of alloimmune anemia. In: Harman, CR (ed), *Invasive Fetal Testing and Treatment*, pp. 107–91. Boston, MA: Blackwell Scientific, 1995.
6. Bowman JM, Harman CR, Manning FA et al. Intravenous drug abuse causes Rh immunization. *Vox Sang* 1991; 61: 96–8.
7. Bowell PJ, Brown SE, Dike AE et al. The significance of anti-c alloimmunization in pregnancy. *Br J Obstet Gynaecol* 1986; 93: 1044–8.
8. Hackney DN, Knudtson EJ, Rossi KQ et al. Management of pregnancies complicated by anti-c isoimmunization. *Obstet Gynecol* 2004; 103: 24–30.
9. Bowman JM, Pollock JM, Manning FA et al. Severe anti-C hemolytic disease of the newborn. *Am J Obstet Gynecol* 1992; 166: 1239–43.
10. Bowman JM. Maternal blood group immunization. In: Creasy RK, Resnick R (eds), *Maternal-Fetal Medicine: Principles and Practice* (2nd edition), pp. 613–49. Philadelphia, PA: Saunders, 1989.
11. Bowman JM, Pollock JM, Manning FA et al. Maternal Kell blood group alloimmunization. *Obstet Gynecol* 1992; 79: 239–44.
12. Vaughan JI, Manning M, Warwick RM et al. Inhibition of erythroid progenitor cells by anti-Kell antibodies in fetal alloimmune anemia. *N Engl J Med* 1998; 338: 798–803.
13. Norbeck O, Tolfvenstam T, Shields LE et al. *Parvovirus B19* capsid protein VP2 inhibits hematopoiesis in vitro and in vivo: Implications for therapeutic use. *Exp Hematol* 2004; 32: 1082–7.
14. Corcoran A, Doyle S. Advances in the biology, diagnosis and host-pathogen interactions of *Parvovirus B19*. *J Med Microbiol* 2004; 53(Pt 6): 459–75.
15. Vogel H, Kornman M, Ledet SC et al. Congenital *Parvovirus* infection. *Pediatr Pathol Lab Med* 1997; 17: 903–12.
16. Crane J. *Parvovirus B-19* infection in pregnancy. *J Obstet Gynaecol Can* 2002; 24: 727–43.
17. Harman CR. Ultrasound in the management of the alloimmunized pregnancy. In: Fleischer AC, Manning FA, Jeanty P, Romero R (eds), *Sonography in Obstetrics and Gynecology: Principles and Practice* (6th edition), pp. 683–709. New York, NY: McGraw-Hill, 2001.
18. van den Akker ES, Klumper FJ, Brand A et al. Kell alloimmunization in pregnancy: Associated with fetal thrombocytopenia? *Vox Sang* 2008; 95(1): 66–9.
19. Harman CR. Specialized applications of obstetric ultrasound: Management of the alloimmunized pregnancy. *Semin Perinat* 1985; 9: 184–97.
20. Harman CR. Fetal monitoring in the alloimmunized pregnancy. *Clin Perinatol* 1989; 16: 691–733.
21. Moise KJ Jr. Management of rhesus alloimmunization in pregnancy. *Obstet Gynecol* 2002; 100: 600–11.
22. Moise KJ Jr, Perkins JT, Sosler SD et al. The predictive value of maternal serum testing for detection of fetal anemia in red blood cell alloimmunization. *Am J Obstet Gynecol* 1995; 172: 1003–9.
23. Walsh CA, Doyle B, Quigley J et al. Reassessing critical maternal antibody threshold in RhD alloimmunization: A 16-year restrospective cohort study. *Ultrasound Obstet Gynecol* 2014; 44: 669–73.
24. Nicolaides KH, Rodeck CH. Maternal serum anti-D antibody concentration and assessment of rhesus isoimmunization. *BMJ* 1992; 304: 1155–6.
25. Clark DA. Red-cell antibodies in pregnancy: Evidence overturned. *Lancet* 1996; 347: 485–6.
26. Mari G, Detti L, Oz U et al. Accurate prediction of fetal hemoglobin by Doppler ultrasonography. *Obstet Gynecol* 2002; 99: 589–93.
27. Mari G, Adrignolo A, Abuhamad AZ et al. Diagnosis of fetal anemia with Doppler ultrasound in the pregnancy complicated by maternal blood group immunization. *Ultrasound Obstet Gynecol* 1995; 5: 400–5.
28. Mari G, Rahman F, Olofsson P et al. Increase of fetal hematocrit decreases the middle cerebral artery peak systolic velocity in pregnancies complicated by rhesus alloimmunization. *J Matern-Fetal Med* 1997; 6: 206–8.
29. Hernandez-Andrade E, Scheier M, Dezerega V et al. Fetal middle cerebral artery peak systolic velocity in the investigation of non-immune hydrops. *Ultrasound Obstet Gynecol* 2004; 23: 442–5.

30. Mari G, Deter RL, Carpenter RL et al. Noninvasive diagnosis by Doppler ultrasonography of fetal anemia due to maternal red-cell alloimmunization. *N Engl J Med* 2000; 342: 9–14.
31. Kush ML, Baschat AA, Weiner CP et al. When should you investigate elevated middle cerebral artery Doppler? *Am J Obstet Gynecol* 2004; 19: S149.
32. Clausen FB, Damkjaer MB, Dziegiel MH. Noninvasive fetal RhD genotyping. *Transfus Apher Sci* 2014; 50(2): 154–62.
33. Rieneck K, Bak M, Jonson L et al. Next-generation sequencing: Proof of concept for antenatal prediction of the fetal Kell blood group phenotype from cell-free fetal DNA in maternal plasma. *Transfusion* 2013; 53(11): 2892–8.
34. Finning K, Martin P, Summers J, Daniels G. Fetal genotyping for the K (Kell) and Rh C, c, and E blood groups on cell-free fetal DNA in maternal plasma. *Transfusion* 2007; 47(11): 2126–33.
35. Chitty LS, Finning K, Wade A et al. Diagnostic accuracy of routine antenatal determination of fetal RHD status across gestation: Population based cohort study. *BMJ* 2014; 349: g5243.
36. Wagner FF. RHD PCR of D-negative blood donors. *Transfus Med Hemother* 2013; 40: 172–81.
37. Hawk AF, Chang EY, Shields SM, Simpson KN. Costs and clinical outcomes of noninvasive fetal RhD typing for targeted prophylaxis. *Obstet Gynecol* 2013; 122(3): 579–85.
38. Bowman JM, Pollock JM. Transplacental fetal hemorrhage after amniocentesis. *Obstet Gynecol* 1985; 66: 749–54.
39. Bowman JM, Pollock JM, Peterson LE et al. Fetomaternal hemorrhage following funipuncture: Increase in severity of maternal red cell alloimmunization. *Obstet Gynecol* 1194; 84: 839–43.
40. Lee S, Bennett PR, Overton T et al. Prenatal diagnosis of Kell blood group genotypes: KEL1 and KEL2. *Am J Obstet Gynecol* 1996; 175: 455–9.
41. Bennett PR, Le Van KC, Colin Y et al. Prenatal determination of fetal RhD type by DNA amplification. *N Engl J Med* 1993; 329: 607–10.
42. Bennett PR, Warwick R, Vaughan J et al. Prenatal determination of human platelet antigen type using DNA amplification following amniocentesis. *Br J Obstet Gynaecol* 1994; 101: 246–9.
43. Mari G, Norton ME, Stone J et al. Society for maternal-fetal medicine (SMFM) clinical guideline #3: The fetus at risk for anemia—Diagnosis and management. *AJOG* 2015; 212: 697–710.
44. Weiner CP. Human fetal bilirubin levels and fetal hemolytic disease. *Am J Obstet Gynecol* 1992; 166: 1149–54.
45. Weiner CP, Williamson RA, Wenstrom KD et al. Management of fetal hemolytic disease by cordocentesis. I. Prediction of fetal anemia. *Am J Obstet Gynecol* 1991; 165: 546–53.
46. Nicolaides KH. Studies on fetal physiology and pathophysiology in rhesus disease. *Semin Perinat* 1989; 13: 328–37.
47. Nicolini U, Santolaya J, Fisk NM et al. Changes in fetal acid base during intravascular transfusion. *Arch Dis Child* 1988; 63: 710–14.
48. Moise KJ. Management of rhesus alloimmunization in pregnancy. *ACOG* 2008; 112(1): 164–76.
49. de Crespigny LC, Robinson HP, Quinn M et al. Ultrasound-guided fetal blood transfusion for severe rhesus isoimmunization. *Obstet Gynecol* 1985; 66: 529–32.
50. Moise KJ Jr, Carpenter RJ Jr, Kirshon B et al. Comparison of four types of intrauterine transfusion: Effect on fetal hematocrit. *Fetal Ther* 1989; 4: 126–37.
51. Stefos T, Cosmi E, Detti L et al. Correction of fetal anemia on the middle cerebral artery peak systolic velocity. *Obstet Gynecol* 2002; 99: 211–15.
52. Harman CR, Bowman JM, Menticoglou SM et al. Profound fetal thrombocytopenia in rhesus disease: Serious hazard at intravascular transfusion. *Lancet* 1988; 2: 741–2.
53. Segal M, Manning FA, Harman CR et al. Bleeding after intravascular transfusion: Experimental and clinical observations. *Am J Obstet Gynecol* 1991; 165: 1414–18.
54. Moise KJ. The usefulness of middle cerebral artery Doppler assessment in the treatment of the fetus at risk for anemia. *Am J Obstet Gynecol* 2008; 161: e1–4.
55. Tiblad E, Kublickas M, Ajne G et al. Procedure-related complications and perinatal outcome after intrauterine transfusions in red cell alloimmunization in Stockholm. *Fetal Diagn Ther* 2011; 30: 266–73.
56. Altunyurt S, Okyay E, Saatli B et al. Neonatal outcome of fetuses receiving intrauterine transfusion for severe hydrops complicated by Rhesus hemolytic disease. *Int J Gynaecol Obstet* 2012; 117: 153–156.
57. Pasman SA, Claes L, Lewi L et al. Intrauterine transfusion for fetal anemia due to red blood cell alloimmunization: 14 years experience in Leuven. *Facts View Vis Obgyn* 2015; 7(2): 129–136.
58. Harman CR, Biehl DR, Pollock JM et al. Intrauterine transfusion: Kinetics of absorption of donor cells in fetal lambs. *Am J Obstet Gynecol* 1983; 145: 830–6.
59. Menticoglou SM, Harman CR, Manning FA et al. Intraperitoneal fetal transfusion: Paralysis inhibits red cell absorption. *Fetal Ther* 1987; 2: 154–9.
60. Harman CR, Bowman JM. Intraperitoneal fetal transfusion. In: Chervenak FA, Isaacson GC, Campbell S (eds), *Ultrasound in Obstetrics and Gynecology*, vol. 2, pp. 1295–1313. Boston, MA: Little, Brown, 1993.
61. Harman CR, Bowman JM, Menticoglou SM et al. Current technique of intraperitoneal transfusion: Do not throw away the Renografin. *Fetal Ther* 1989; 4: 78–82.

62. Harman CR, Manning FA, Bowman JM et al. Severe Rh disease—poor outcome is not inevitable. *Am J Obstet Gynecol* 1983; 145: 823–9.
63. Harman CR, Bowman JM, Manning FA et al. Intrauterine transfusion intraperitoneal versus intravascular approach: A case control comparison. *Am J Obstet Gynecol* 1990; 162: 1053–9.
64. Garabedian C, Philippe M. Vaast P et al. Is intrauterine exchange transfusion a safe procedure for management of fetal anemia? *Eur J Obstet Gyn Reprod Biol* 2014; 179: 83–87.
65. Westgren M, Selbing A, Stangenberg M. Fetal intracardiac transfusions in patients with severe rhesus isoimmunization. *BMJ* 1988; 296: 885–6.
66. Sarno, Jr AP, Wilson RD. Fetal cardiocentesis: A review of indications, risks, applications and technique. *Fetal Diagn Ther* 2008; 23: 237–244.
67. Plapp FV, Beck ML. Transfusion support in the management of immune haemolytic disorders. *Clin Haematol* 1984; 13(1): 167–83.
68. Ruma MS, Moise KJ, Kim E et al. Combined plasmapheresis and intravenous immune globulin for the treatment of severe maternal red cell alloimmunization. *AJOG* 2007; 138: e1–e6.
69. Chitkara U, Bussel J, Alvarez M et al. High-dose intravenous gamma globulin: Does it have a role in the treatment of severe erythroblastosis fetalis? *Obstet Gynecol* 1990; 76: 703–8.
70. Margulies M, Voto LS, Mathet E, Marguelies M. High-dose intravenous IgG for the treatment of severe rhesus alloimmunization. *Vox Sang* 1991; 61: 181–9.
71. Giers G, Wenzel F, Riethmacher R et al. Repeated intrauterine IgG infusions in foetal alloimmune thrombocytopenia do not increase foetal platelet counts. *Vox Sang* 2010; 99(4): 348–53.
72. Corvaglia L, Legnani E, Galletti S et al. Intravenous immunoglobulin to treat neonatal alloimmune haemolytic disease. *J Mat Fet Neonatal Med* 2012; 25(12): 2782–2785.
73. Baschat AA, Harman CR, Alger LS et al. Fetal coronary and cerebral blood flow in acute fetomaternal hemorrhage. *Ultrasound Obstet Gynecol* 1198; 12: 128–31.
74. Senat MV, Loizeau S, Couderc S et al. The value of the middle cerebral artery peak systolic velocity in the diagnosis of fetal anemia after intrauterine death of one monochorionic twin. *Am J Obstet Gynecol* 2003; 189: 1320–4.
75. Dembinski J, Haverkamp F, Maara H et al. Neurodevelopmental outcome after intrauterine red cell transfusion for *Parvovirus B-19* induced fetal hydrops. *Br J Obstet Gynaecol* 2002; 109: 1232–4.
76. Yinon Y, Visser J, Kelly EN et al. Early intrauterine transfusion in severe red blood cell alloimmunization. *Ultrasound Obstet Gynecol* 2010; 36(5): 601–6.
77. Canlorbe G, Macé G, Cortey A et al. Management of very early fetal anemia resulting from red-cell alloimmunization before 20 weeks of gestation. *Obstet Gynecol* 2011; 118(6): 1323–9.
78. Kamping MA, Pasman SA, Bil-van den Brink CP et al. Fluid shift from intravascular compartment during fetal red blood cell transfusion. *Ultrasound Obstet Gynecol* 2013; 41(5): 550–5.
79. Klumper FJ, van Kamp IL, Vendenbussche FP et al. Benefits and risks of fetal red-cell transfusion after 32 weeks' gestation. *Eur J Obstet Gynecol Reprod Biol* 2000; 92: 91–6.
80. Sohan K, Billington M, Pamphilon et al. Normal growth and development following in utero diagnosis and treatment of homozygous alpha thalassemia. *Br J Obstet Gynaecol* 2002; 109: 1308–10.
81. Remacha AF, Badell I, Pujol-Moix N et al. Hydrops fetalis-associated congenital dyserythropoietic anemia treated with intrauterine transfusions and bone marrow transplantation. *Blood* 2002; 100: 356–8.
82. Lin SM, Chen M, Ma ESK et al. Intrauterine therapy in a fetus with congenital dyserythropoietic anaemia type I. *J Obstet Gynaecol* 2014; 34: 352–364.
83. UCSF Benioff Children's Hospital, Oakland. Thalassemia at UCSF Benioff Children's Hospital Oakland. http://thalassemia.com/services-intrauterine-therapy.aspx#gsc.tab=0. 2015. Accessed September 19, 2016.
84. Harman CR, Manning FA, Bowman JM et al. Use of intravascular transfusion to treat hydrops fetalis in a moribund fetus. *Can Med Assoc J* 1988; 138: 827–30.
85. Bussel JB. Alloimmune thrombocytopenia in the fetus and newborn. *Semin Thromb Hemost* 2001; 27: 245–52.
86. Radder CM, Brand A, Kanhai HH. A less invasive treatment strategy to prevent intracranial hemorrhage in fetal and neonatal alloimmune thrombocytopenia. *Am J Obstet Gynecol* 2001; 185: 683–8.
87. Birchall JE, Murphy MF, Kaplan C et al. European collaborative study of the antenatal management of feto-maternal alloimmune thrombocytopenia. *Br J Haematol* 2003; 122: 275–88.
88. Detti L, Oz U, Guney I et al. Doppler ultrasound velocimetry for timing the second intrauterine transfusion in fetuses with anemia from red-cell alloimmunization. *Am J Obstet Gynecol* 2001; 185: 1048–51.
89. Grubbs BH, Korst LM, Llanes A, Chmait RH. Middle cerebral artery Doppler and hemoglobin changes immediately following fetal transfusion. *J Matern Fetal Neonat Med* 2013; 26(2): 155–57.
90. Osanan GC, Silveira Reis ZN, Apocalypse IG et al. Predictive factors of perinatal mortality in transfused fetuses due to maternal alloimmunization: What really matters? *J Matern Fetal Neonatal Med* 2012; 25(8): 1333–7.
91. Weisz B, Rosenbaum O, Chayen B et al. Outcome of severely anaemic fetuses treated by intrauterine transfusions. *Arch Dis Child Fetal Neonatal Ed* 2009; 94: F201–4.

92. Sainio S, Nupponen I, Kuosmanen M et al. Diagnosis and treatment of severe hemolytic disease of the fetus and newborn: A 10-year nationwide retrospective study. *Acta Obstet Gynecol Scand* 2015; 94(4): 383–90.
93. Verduin EP, Lindenburg IT, Smits-Wintjens VE et al. Long-term follow up after intrauterine transfusion; the LOTUS study. *BMC Pregnancy Childbirth* 2010; 10: 77.
94. Dildy GA, Smith LG Jr, Moise KJ Jr et al. Porencephalic cyst: A complication of fetal intravascular transfusion. *Am J Obstet Gynecol* 1991; 165: 76–8.
95. Pessler F, Hart D. Hyporegenerative anemia associated with Rh hemolytic disease: Treatment failure of recombinant erythropoietin. *J Pediatr Hematol Oncol* 2002; 24: 689–93.

Fetal reduction and selective termination

8

MARK I. EVANS, STEPHANIE ANDRIOLE, SHARA M. EVANS, and DAVID W. BRITT

CONTENTS

INTRODUCTION

Since we first published on the subject of pregnancy management via fetal reduction (FR) a quarter century ago, the field has witnessed significant changes.[1] These changes have occurred in medical technology, outcomes, patient choices, and the large demographic and cultural shifts that are driving the pace and direction of progress and research.

FR started out as a means of managing pregnancies in which the risks to both mother and fetuses from carrying multiple embryos were unacceptably high. Selective termination (ST)—as it was called then—of some of the embryos in order to reduce the risks for morbidity and mortality for the mother and increase the viability of the remaining embryos was a desperate attempt to salvage hopeless medical situations. Like many other technological advancements, initial concerns were dominated by matters of life and death and shifted toward acceptance. Today, the indications for FR have transformed from the binary crisis of "life and death" into the broader arena of issues regarding quality of life.[2,3]

Since Louise Brown's birth in July 1978, more than 5,000,000 *in vitro* fertilization (IVF) babies have been born. The skyrocketing incidence of multiple gestations over the last 30–35 years is an undeniable side effect of infertility treatments. In the United States, the birth rate of twins has gone from the preinfertility treatment era background of 1/90 to nearly 1/30.[4,5] A woman delivering twins today has a nearly 70% chance of having conceived with the assistance of medical technology, such as IVF.

Nearly half of the babies born from IVF in the United States are products of multiple pregnancies[5] (Table 8.1). Although the incidence of higher-order multiples has somewhat plateaued, many IVF programs create as many multiples as singletons.[4,5] This assertion is supported by the U.S. Society for Assisted Reproductive Technologies (SART), which reported 37,699 singleton and 13,562 multiple pregnancies producing 65,151 infants in 2012. These numbers have remained relatively constant over the last several years.

A somewhat different picture emerges if we examine the trends of multiple births over the last 25 years.[5–7] The incidence of twin births has escalated and stayed relatively constant; however, the curves for triplets and above show a curvilinear pattern (Figure 8.1). The picture is clearest for quadruplets; there was an initial doubling and then a return to roughly the same number as in 1989, which actually may be lower, if viewed as a percentage of eligible women. The increase for higher-order multiples is an unintended result of the advancement of in vivo and IVF techniques. However, the increase in these techniques also galvanized changes in medical technology and introduced new procedures that over time have afforded greater control of the situation.

One of the key developments in controlling the number of multiples, beyond that afforded from simply moving from the use of gonadotropins to IVF, has been the codification of norms and expectations regarding single-embryo transfers (SET).[5–7] While elective single embryo transfer (eSET) can have many medical advantages, it is unlikely that eSET will ever be predominant in the United States under the current health-care system and the economics. Since IVF is associated with extremely high costs for every cycle (commonly $15,000 or more with variable insurance coverage), all parties involved—both patient and IVF provider—are under pressure to achieve a very high pregnancy rate with each cycle. As a result, SART guidelines state that under age 35, only one or two embryos should be transferred; yet, according to Centers for Disease Control (CDC) and SART data for 2014, the average number of embryos transferred is only down to 1.8 from 2.2 in 2007.[5–7] This is unlikely to change even with any further health-care reform that may ultimately emerge in the United States, either from the expansion or repealing of the Affordable Care Act. For example, 2009 SART data showed that only 7% of IVF cases in the United States

Table 8.1 Longitudinal trends in the number of multifetal pregnancies in the United States.

Year	Twins	Triplets	Quads	Quints+
2013	132,324	4,634	270	66
2011	131,269	5,137	239	41
2009	137,217	5,905	355	80
2006	137,085	6,118	355	67
2003	128,615	7,110	468	85
1996	100,750	5,298	560	81
1989	90,118	2,529	229	40
% Increase 1989–2013	46.8%	83.2%	17.9%	65.0%

Source: Martin JA et al., Births: Final data for 2013, *National Vital Statistics Reports,* Vol. 64, No. 1, January 2015, Hyattsville, MD: National Center for Health Statistics, 2015.

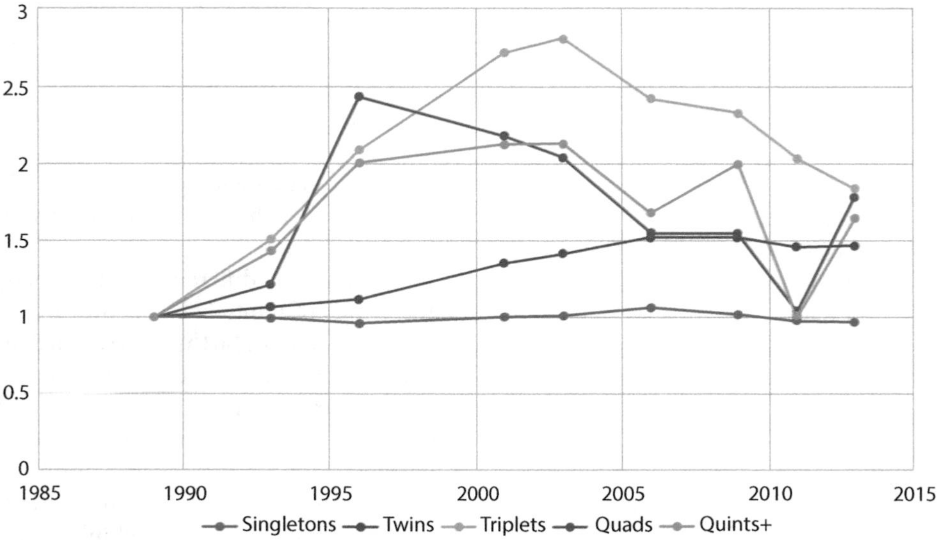

Figure 8.1 Change in ratio of multiples to singletons from 1989 to 2013: U.S. data from Centers for Disease Control (CDC). Using 1989 data set as baseline (1), ratio incidence of cases for the years are listed on the *x* axis.

in women under 35 were SET, and the numbers were much lower in older women (Table 8.2).[5–7] For 2013, the percentage of eSET for women under 35 was 22%, and for women >40 was approximately 4.5%.[5] Lawlor in 2012 using U.K. data showed that the success rate for live-borns is about 7% greater when transferring two embryos in one cycle rather than one each over two cycles.[8] It is known that the percentage of live births per transfer clearly diminishes with advancing maternal age regardless of using fresh versus frozen cycles. Thus, the impetus to be aggressive in embryo transfers is apparent but it also correlates with increased risks of multiples. Egg donors tend to be younger, so statistically they resemble the <35-year-old cohort (Table 8.3).

Due to a shift in management from ovulation induction to IVF, in which there is better control of the number of embryos transferred, the proportion of very high order multiples has diminished. Thus, the average "starting number" of patients presenting for FR procedures has slowly decreased from about 3.5 to now under 3.0 (Table 8.4).[5–8] The reduction in the number of embryos transferred is most likely attributed to tighter management control and the shifting demographics of those patients who seek FR in an effort to improve outcomes.

As the risks have become better understood and the general public has become more knowledgeable regarding the possibilities of intervention, there has been a marked shift toward skepticism, and in some cases disapproval, for multiple embryo transfers. In the 1930s, the Dionne Quintuplets were met with awe and amazement, and treated almost as a miracle, which continued with other cases for over 60 years. Similarly, "miracle" status was accorded to other high visibility instances such as the Frustasci family in the 1980s and McCoys in the 1990s. A pivotal moment in the United States was the public response to the 2009 "Octomom" in California, when the public "appreciative amazement" of the 1980s shifted noticeably to elements of shock and disgust.[9] As a result, transfer of three or more embryos significantly diminished, and many intended ovulation induction cases were converted to IVF mid-cycle, if ultrasound or hormone levels suggested a high risk of multiples.[9]

In high-order multiples, pregnancy loss is not the only deleterious outcome. For almost half a century, studies

Table 8.2 IVF management: maternal age and transfer numbers.

SART 2013	<35	35–39	40+
Mean transfer	1.7	1.7	1.8
Elective single embryo transfer	22.57%	8.0%	4.5%

Source: Lawlor DA, and Nelson SM, *Lancet*, 379: 521–27, 2012.
Abbreviations: IVF, *in vitro* fertilization; SART, Society for Assisted Reproductive Technologies.

Table 8.3 Centers for Disease Control 2013 data.

		Fresh cycles				Frozen cycles		
Nondonor egg	**Maternal age**	**Fresh cycles (*n*)**	**Mean no. of embryos transferred per cycle**	**% of live births per transfer**	**% of multiple pregnancies**	**Frozen cycles (*n*)**	**Mean no. of embryos transferred per cycle**	**% of live births per transfer**
	<305	36,958	1.8	47.7	29.2	18,801	1.7	43.9
	35–37	18,508	1.9	39.2	26.5	9,602	1.6	39.9
	38–40	16,853	23	28.5	20.9	7,116	1.7	35.4
	41–42	9,026	2.7	16.3	18.0	2,731	1.8	30.6
	42+	4,501	2.8	7.3	13.7	1,675	1.9	20.7
Donor egg		8,921	1.7	55.8	–	8,172	1.6	40.5

Source: Martin JA et al., Births: Final data for 2013, *National Vital Statistics Reports*, Vol. 64, No. 1, January 2015, Hyattsville, MD: National Center for Health Statistics, 2015.

Table 8.4 Number of embryos transferred according to maternal ages (nondonor eggs).

Year	<35	35–37	38–40	41–42	43–44	45+
1998	3.4	3.6	3.7	3.9		
2001	2.8	3.1	3.4	3.7		
2004	2.5	2.7	3.0	3.3		
2007	2.2	2.5	2.8	3.1	3.2	
2010	2.0	2.2	2.6	3.0	3.2	2.7
2013	1.8	1.9	2.3	2.7	2.8	

Source: Centers for Disease Control, *Assisted Reproductive Technology Surveillance—United States, 2013*, http://www.cdc.gov/art/reports/.

have clearly demonstrated that the incidences of prematurity and related sequelae are directly correlated with fetal number (Figure 8.2).[5–8] It should be noted that approximately 20% of fetuses born less than 750 g develop cerebral palsy.[10] In Western Australia, Petterson et al.[11] found that the rate of cerebral palsy was 4.6 times higher for twins than singletons per live births but 8.3 times higher when calculated per pregnancy. Pharoah and Cooke[12] calculated cerebral palsy rates (per 1000) at 2.3 for singletons, 12.6 for twins, and 44.8 for triplets.[13] In our experience, there is a greater sensitivity to these risks among older patients, thus leading to a corresponding increase in the utilization of prenatal diagnosis and FR.

The profound public health implications to prematurity cannot be overstated; year 2000 U.S. data showed that of $10.2 billion spent on initial newborn care with 57% of the total cost spent on the 9% of babies born at <37 weeks.[14] In 2003, more than $10 billion was spent on the 12.3% who were born preterm.[15] Data from 2005 show that there is significantly greater neurologic and developmental disability in 6-year-olds who survived birth at 26 weeks or less.[16,17] Significant cerebral palsy was present in 12%. The rates of severe, moderate, and mild disability were 22%, 24%, and 34%, respectively.[17] Hack et al.[18] also showed that in infants with birth weights less than 1000 g, the rate of cerebral palsy was 14% versus 0% for controls; asthma, poor vision, intelligence quotient (IQ) <85, and poor motor skills were also substantially higher in these very preterm infants. Advancements in neonatal intensive care have had a dramatic impact in reducing mortality, particularly at very early gestational ages, which, however, resulted in an increase in compromised, surviving infants.[19,20] As the prematurity costs rise, it is predictable that there will be corresponding changes in insurance coverage, the shaping of IVF practices, as well as a continued increase in sensitivity to these issues, especially among more at-risk patients.

History

FR was developed as a clinical procedure in the 1980s when a small group of clinicians in the United States and Europe attempted to reduce the high incidence of severe health outcomes typical of higher-order multifetal

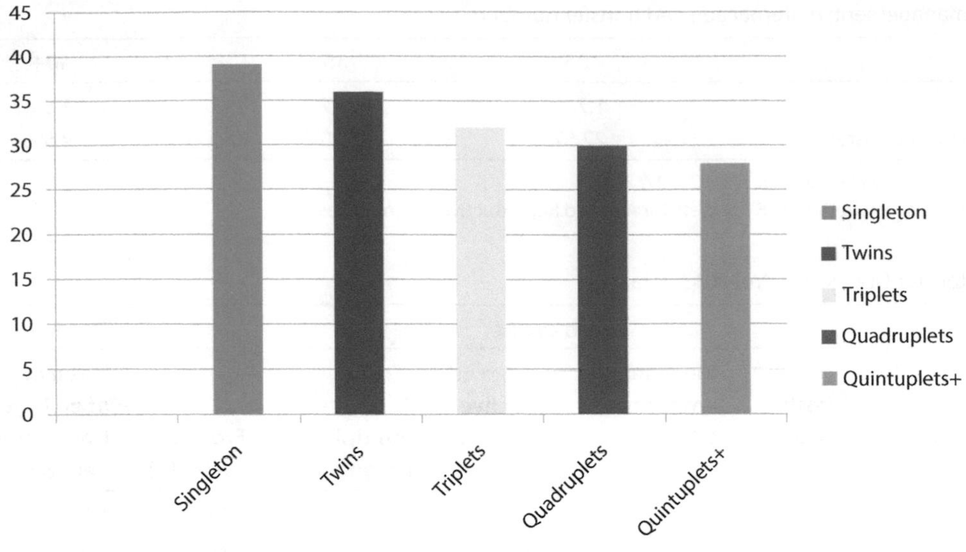

Figure 8.2 Multiples and prematurity; *y* axis depicts the average gestational age at delivery.

pregnancies by selectively terminating or reducing the number of fetuses. The first European reports by Dumez and Oury,[21] and the first American report by Evans et al.,[1] followed by a further report by Berkowitz et al.,[22] and later Wapner et al.,[23] outlined the initial surgical approaches to improve the outcome in such instances.

The surgical approach, in the mid-80s, involved transabdominally inserted needles which guided into the fetal thorax. Methods predominately involved injection of potassium chloride (KCl) but also included air embolization, electrocautery, or mechanical disruption of the fetus. Transcervical aspirations were also attempted but met with little success. Some centers also utilized transvaginal mechanical disruption or KCl; however, data suggested a significantly higher loss rate than with the transabdominal route, so this technique is less commonly utilized.[24] However, some published and unpublished data have suggested that some centers, despite considerably higher loss rates, continue to use 6- to 8-week transvaginal reduction methods. Today, the vast majority of experienced clinicians perform the procedure using ultrasound guidance with a transabdominal insertion of needles inserted into the fetal thorax.[25]

Over time, as with most surgical procedures, there has been an increased understanding of the risks, benefits, and the unique clinical nature of various approaches to FR, as well as an improvement regarding how these procedures should be best presented to patients and carried out by the clinicians. Collaboration across major centers conducting FR has resulted in significant milestones. In 1993, the first collaborative report of several centers with the greatest amount of experience showed a 16% pregnancy loss rate through 24 completed weeks.[26] Further collaborative efforts continued to highlight dramatic improvements in the overall outcomes of multifetal pregnancies (Table 8.5).

In the 1980s, the controversy surrounded the question, "At how many fetuses was it reasonable to offer FR?" Consensus was generally divided between triplets and quadruplets, although there were substantial dissimilarities in perceptions of risks by specialty and religious group beliefs.[27] In the 1990s, multiple publications showed that there was a clear improvement in reducing to twins from higher fetal numbers, including triplet pregnancies. A sizeable number of publications explored whether triplets had better outcomes when "reduced." Yaron et al.[28] compared outcomes of triplet pregnancies reduced to twins with outcomes of nonreduced twin pregnancies and expectantly managed triplet pregnancies. The results show marked improvement of outcomes for reduced twins as compared with triplets.

Antsaklis et al.[29] also showed that in triplet pregnancies, embryo reduction to twins reduced preterm delivery at ≤32 weeks (11% versus 37%) and birth weight ≤1500 g (11% versus 28%); however, this benefit was at the expense of increase in total fetal loss (15% versus 5%) in the embryo reduction group. Luke et al.[30] evaluated risk factors for adverse outcomes in spontaneous versus assisted conception twin pregnancies and found that among all twin pregnancies FR increased the risks for birth at <30 weeks, very low birth weight, and slowed mid-gestational growth. However, this analysis did not compare outcomes between nonreduced multifetal pregnancies and those reduced to twins. Kozinsky et al.[31] found that the perinatal outcomes following assisted reproductive technologies (ARTs) of singleton and twin pregnancies were similar to spontaneously conceived, matched pregnancies. McDonald et al.[32] showed in a meta-analysis that twins from IVF, even when matched to spontaneously conceived twins, had a somewhat greater risk for preterm birth, but this did not result in significant differences in low birth weight, congenital malformations, or perinatal deaths. Multiple publications over the past 15 years have echoed results showing higher risks for "unreduced" triplets versus reduced cases.[33–36] It is clear that when choosing comparison groups, extreme caution must be employed.

Table 8.5 Risks of multifetal pregnancies and improvements with FR.

Starting number of fetuses	Spontaneous loss rates	Finishing number of fetuses	Reduction of risk of pregnancy loss
6+	90%–99%	2	90%–10%
5	75%	2	50%–7%
4	25%	2	25%–4%
		1	25%–7%
3	15%	2	15%–3.5%
		1	15%–4%
2	8%	1	8%–2.5%

Data are extrapolations from various sources. When there are monozygotic twins as part of the multiple, the overall risk is increased as if there were one more as the starting number.

Abbreviation: FR, fetal reduction.

The 2001 collaborative data using late first-trimester procedures similarly demonstrated that the outcomes of triplets reduced to twins, and quadruplets reduced to twins, are very similar to those starting as twins.[37] Both pregnancy loss and prematurity rates were significantly decreased and both were correlated with the starting and finishing fetal number. Blickstein has also reported that triplets did worse than reduced twins in every perinatal category in his large database.[38] More recent data have shown continued improvements in management and overall outcomes in the hands of experienced centers (Table 8.5).

Improved clinician experience and knowledge, as well as advancements in infertility management, have also resulted in some novel clinical scenarios. As a result of increasing use of blastocyst transfers, and evolving IVF laboratory methods, the number and proportion of monozygotic (MZ) twins has increased significantly in the last 15 years.[7,9,39] Approximately 7% of our higher-order multifetal pregnancies involve a monochorionic–diamniotic twin pair.[39] In our experience, the best outcomes generally result from reduction of the MZ twins, provided the "singleton" appears healthy after evaluation by chorionic villus sampling (CVS) and ultrasound. However, if there are apparent problems with the singleton, then keeping the twins is the next best option. Other centers have reported that FR in dichorionic triplet pregnancy reduces the rate of preterm birth at the expense of a nonsignificant rate of miscarriage.[40]

In the 2001 collaborative report, the subset of patients who reduced from twins to singleton had a pregnancy loss rate similar to that of reducing triplets to twins; however, in about one-third of the patients reduced from twins to singleton had additional complicating factors, such as maternal cardiac disease, or prior twin pregnancy with severe prematurity, or uterine abnormality, which may have increased the overall risks.[37] Recently, however, the demographics have shifted, and a significant proportion of such cases are medically less complex but involve women in their forties, or even their fifties, some of whom are using donor eggs. Many of these women, for both medical and social reasons, desire a singleton pregnancy.[41–43] Our data suggest that twins reduced to a singleton have better outcomes as compared with nonreduced twins.[41,43] Therefore, it is not unexpected that more women are requesting to reduce their twins to a singleton. In a series of triplets from the late 1990s, we observed that the average age of patients reducing to twins was 37 years, and to a singleton 41 years.[28] While the reduction in risk for pregnancy loss, in the nineties, for reducing from triplets to singleton was not as great as the decrease in risk for reducing from triplets to twins (15%–7% and 15%–5%, respectively), the resulting singleton had a higher gestational age at delivery, and the incidence of births <1500 g was 10-fold higher for twins versus singletons. As a reduction to a singleton has become more common, the age difference between those women reducing to twins and those to a singleton has vanished.[39] These data have made counseling of patients far more complicated than before. Not unexpectedly, there are frequently differences in opinion among couples as to the preferability of twins versus singleton, or even as to the total number desired, which sometimes is greater than twins for one member of the couple.[43] Based on the above data, and the evolving demographics of the couples who experience infertility and elect to have reductions, we believe that reduction of twin pregnancies to a singleton is reasonable and that the practice will continue to expand.

Changing perspectives

Over the last quarter-century, we have witnessed dramatic changes in both pregnancy outcomes of multifetal pregnancies and issues surrounding FR. Outcomes have continually improved because of the following reasons: (1) improved understanding of the clinical issues involved; (2) decrease in the proportion of extremely higher-order multiples (i.e., quadruplets and above); (3) advancements in ultrasound, allowing for improved visualization, and use of CVS, thus decreasing the risk of missing, sonographically or chromosomally abnormal fetuses; and (4) cohort of highly experienced physicians currently performing the majority of cases as compared with a large number of unexperienced clinicians in the past (Table 8.5).[41–45]

There has also been a change in the context and scope of the clinical dialog between patients and physicians over the last 20–30 years. The most notable shift has been the movement from questions of mortality to questions of morbidity. This appears to be linked to an increase in the age of patients undergoing fertility treatments and a decrease in the number of presenting fetuses.[46,47] These transformations in turn appear to be changing due to advances in IVF technology and fundamental demographic changes in the age at which mothers are having their first child.[4–6] A further consequence of these shifts has been the increased utilization of donor eggs and prenatal diagnosis.[46,47] The aforementioned changes have resulted in the transformation from a salvage operation for higher-order multifetal pregnancies, to a common, and preplanned, pregnancy management strategy.

Overall, the pregnancy outcomes after FR have improved substantially over the past 25 years.[39,46,47] In the early 1990s when half of FR cases consisted of quadruplets or greater, the pregnancy loss rates (up to 24 weeks) were quite high at 13%. Preterm deliveries occurred in an additional 10% of the cases. Currently, with decreasing starting numbers, improved ultrasound visualization, enhanced understanding of zygosity, and a select cohort of experienced practitioners accounting for a high proportion of reductions performed, preterm deliveries are decreased to about 4%. However, counseling must be personalized to also take into consideration the specific starting and finishing fetal numbers (Figure 8.3; Table 8.5). Most FR procedures are still performed in one session but when reducing from higher orders (5+) to a singleton, better results may be achieved when the FR is performed in two different sessions, 5–7 days apart.

Over the past decade, the pattern of patients seeking FR has continued to evolve in response to predictable demographic and cultural shifts.[4,5] There has been a strong trend of increasing age at which women give birth to their first child (Figure 8.4) and this trend is common throughout the developed world. Actually, there are two parallel but independent trends: fewer lower- and middle-class teenage mothers delivering (and having terminations) and more women postponing childbearing for a wide variety of reasons to their thirties and forties. The latter is, of course, the group that mostly applies to our discussion here.[5] As the risks of delayed childbearing have become more widely known,[16,46] there has been a corresponding increase in the demand for donor eggs as a means of moderating the risks for older women.[46]

With the rapid expansion of the availability of donor eggs, and the increasing sensitivity and specificity of diagnostic testing, the number of "older women" seeking FR has increased dramatically. In our experience, over 10% of all patients who seek FR are now over 40 years of age, and nearly half of them are using donor eggs.[38] It would appear that as advances in care have developed of achieving pregnancies and ways of moderating, if not eliminating, the risk of older women who wish to have children, more of them are electing to do so.

As a consequence of the shift to older patients, many of whom already had previous relationships and children, there is an increased desire by these patients to have only one additional child. The number of experienced centers willing to perform FR from twins to singleton is still very limited, but we believe based upon improvement of outcomes, that it can be justified in almost all circumstances. In our center, twins currently constitute about 25% of the patients we see for FR.[39]

For patients who are "older," particularly those using their own eggs, the issue of genetic diagnosis has become progressively more salient. In 2009, about 60% of patients in the United States having ART cycles were over 35 years. If the criteria of comparable risk to that of a 35-year-old are used, then about 90% of IVF patients are at increased risk[1] (Table 8.6).

For the past decades and currently, most FR practitioners made their decisions as to which fetuses to keep or reduce by ultrasound evaluation only. In the 1980s, most of our procedures were performed between 9 and 10 weeks with decisions based principally on basic ultrasound and fetal position.[1] For those patients for whom genetic assessment was appropriate, amniocentesis was performed several weeks later[48]; subsequently, we changed our approach and performed CVS a week after FR to twins and currently we prefer to perform

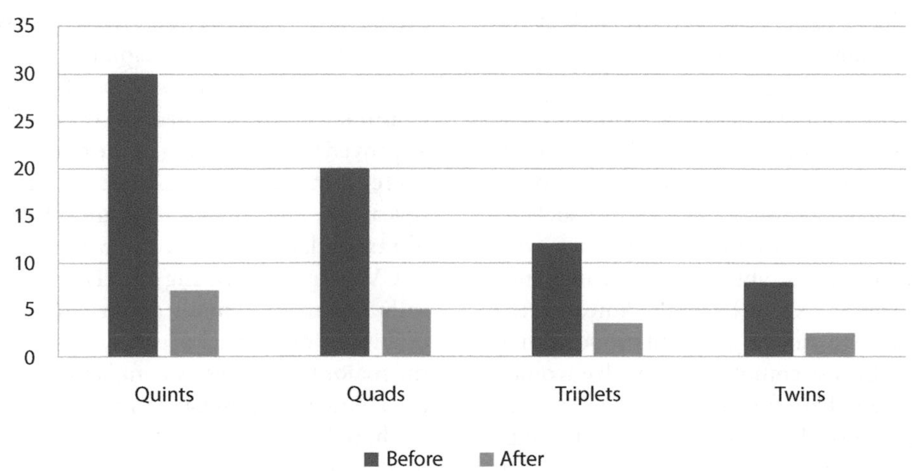

Figure 8.3 Reduction of pregnancy loss with fetal reduction (FR).

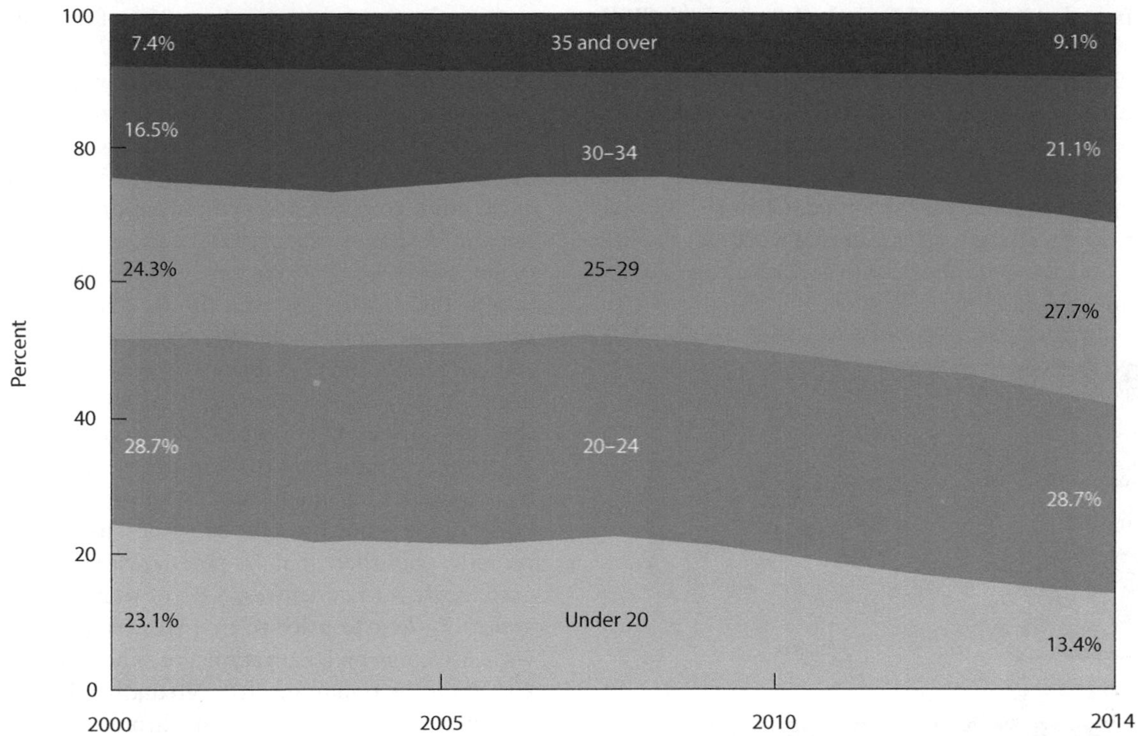

Figure 8.4 Increasing age at first birth: percentage of first births, by age of mother, U.S. 2000–2014. (Data from CDC/National Center for Health Statistics [NCHS], National Vital Statistics System, at http://www.cdc.gov/nchs/data/databriefs/db232.htm.)

Table 8.6 Fetal gender options and patient's choices.

Type of FR	Gender option (*N*, %)	Chose all M	Chose all F	Chose MF twins	*p*
3→2	79 (51%)	1 (1%)	7 (9%)	71 (90%)	<.001
3→1	20 (25%)	10 (50%)	10 (50%)	NA	NS
2→1	44 (27%)	20 (45%)	24 (55%)	NA	NS

Source: Evans MI et al., *Prenat Diagn*, 33, 935–39, 2013.
Abbreviations: NA, not applicable; NS, nonsignificant; M, male; F, female.

CVS the day before with fluorescence in situ hybridization (FISH) analysis overnight. Waiting for a full karyotype has been problematic because of the long time interval to get the results, as well as the fact that there may be a 1% error rate in matching incorrectly the karyotype results with the corresponding fetus.[49,50] Therefore, as FISH technology became reliable, we began routinely to do the FR procedures on 2 consecutive days.[45,46] Over the last 20 years, the proportion of patients having CVS before FR has steadily risen from about 20% in 2000 to about 85% currently.[39]

While there have been many studies regarding the risks of prenatal diagnosis with widely diverging statistics,[51] in our view, the net effect is in the most experienced hands is zero sum since the risks of the diagnostic procedures are counterbalanced by the reduction of risk of pregnancy loss by not allowing an abnormal fetus to continue with the pregnancy.[39]

Another distinct cohort of patients are those who consider reduction procedures for a diagnosed abnormality in one fetus of a multiple pregnancy, as opposed to the risks inherent with multiples per se.[44,45] There has been a consensus in the literature to perform FR in the first trimester for cases done for reducing the fetal number per se, and to use ST—often in the second trimester—for a diagnosed fetal anomaly. Occasionally, fetal abnormalities are found for the first time even in the third trimester, which poses medical, ethical, and legal issues.[52] We and others have likewise published large series over the past decades that have delineated the similarities and differences when there is a confirmed abnormality.[53,54] Much of this literature focuses on twins, many of which have twin to twin transfusion syndrome (TTTS) where laser therapy has become the mainstay of therapy, but ST is still sometimes necessary.[55] A complete discussion of these issues is beyond the scope of this chapter.

Modern management

Prior to FR, there should be a rigorous evaluation of fetal status, which includes more than just a nuchal translucency ultrasound measurement and position of the fetuses. Typically, we perform a 2-day procedure on most patients at approximately 12 weeks: CVS on the first day with FISH analyses overnight for chromosomes 13, 18, 21, X, and Y[39] (Figure 8.5). The results are obtained the following afternoon, and the FR is performed that day. By definition, FISH for five chromosomes cannot detect everything, but our experience and modeling suggest only about a 1/400 residual risk of a problem on karyotype.[39] This risk is lower than the risk of waiting for 2 additional weeks for the full karyotype and the potential confusion resulting from a large volume of data.[49,50]

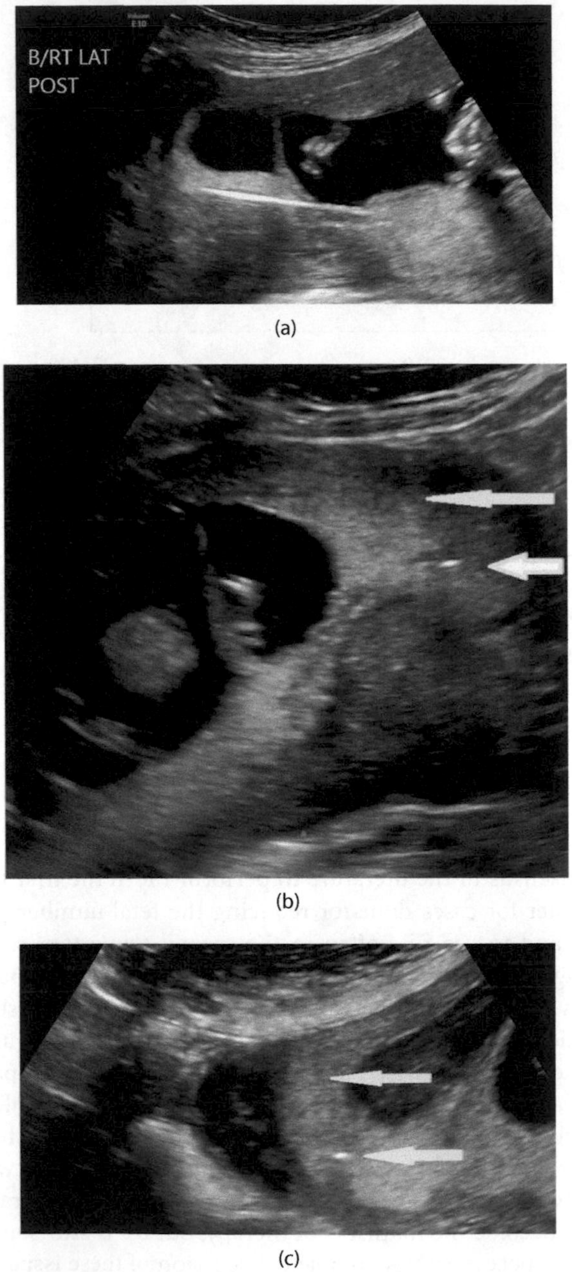

Figure 8.5 (a) Transcervical chorionic villus sampling (CVS) on triplet B; catheter with stylet in place seen as white line traversing posterior placenta. (b) Needle inserted abdominally in placenta A; arrows show tip and path of needle. (c) Needle inserted abdominally in placenta C; arrows show tip and path of needle.

Over the past few years, about 85% of our patients have combined CVS and FR procedures. We expect that the utilization of CVS prior to reduction will likely increase even further because of the increased number of "older" patients, the increased risks of chromosomal and other anomalies in patients conceiving by IVF and especially with intracytoplasmic sperm injection (ICSI), and the known 3%–6% inaccuracy rate of preimplantation genetic diagnosis (PGD).[39,45,46] We have also found that many couples in their forties, or even fifties, who are using donor eggs—whose genetic risk is the age of the egg donor—nevertheless still want CVS prior to FR because their "tolerance" for having a child with special needs is more akin to their actual ages, not the egg donor's age.

Our recent data show that our protocol of CVS followed by overnight FISH analysis with FR the second afternoon significantly improves the outcomes in such cases. We recently published that in pregnancies with ultrasonographically normal fetuses, 3.1% of women with normal-appearing fetuses prior to first-trimester FR had a fetus with an abnormal karyotype, of which FISH detected 90%.[39] Of the remaining 10%, virtually all were confined placental mosaicisms for other chromosomes or culture artifacts. Of the 350 patients with normal-appearing first-trimester fetuses, 6% had abnormal CVS on either karyotype or FISH. Those abnormal FISH and ultrasound results guided decisions at the time of the FR procedure. Ultimately, 90% of the abnormal FISH results were confirmed on final karyotype. With respect to false negatives, most were for chromosomes for which there were not FISH probes used, and most of them were actually confined placental mosaicisms. Ultimately, only 1 of the 350 cases (0.3%) had a clinically relevant false negative (sex chromosome mosaicism). On balance, we believe that the risk of a false negative is lower than the risks encountered while waiting between procedures, which increases loss rates because of the higher fetal number and the risk of making a mistake as to which fetus is which when returning for the FR procedure.

While using FISH for rapid diagnoses has worked very well, other methods have been and will become feasible over the next few years. Inexpensive methods included direct preparation CVS, which was used commonly in the 1980s but was largely abandoned because of high rates of mosaicism and aneuploidies that were not reflective of fetal status.[56] Quantitative fluorescent polymerase chain reaction (QfPCR) can also be used for rapid preparation evaluation of chromosome number.[57,58] Microarrays can provide even more detail than whole chromosomes but currently are far more expensive.[59] As the cost decreases and turn around speed increases, molecular subchromosomal techniques will clearly move into the mainstream of evaluation.[59] With the development of single nucleotide polymorphism (SNP) array technologies that are detecting copy number variants in about 1% of patients, the option of waiting for these results (nearly 3 weeks) can be considered. This may be more practical for patients reducing twins to a singleton who live locally but it may be less practical for higher-order numbers and patients traveling from too far.[39,60]

With the increasing use of PGD as part of the IVF process, many patients question if traditional CVS still has application in reduction decisions.[59] Our experience has been that over the past 5 years, there has been about a 2%–3% discordancy between PGD results and CVS results with chromosomal having higher discordant results as compared with Mendelian.[39] However, with the introduction of new PGD microarray like methods, the discordancy rate is likely to decline and in our view it may end up being approximately 1%.[61,62] Likewise, with the advent of noninvasive prenatal screening (NIPS) techniques, the same questions arise.[63] Our perspective is that both PGD and NIPS are excellent screening tests but they are not diagnostic. We have observed a number of instances in which errors have occurred resulting in babies born with conditions for which screening had been performed. Also in multiples, NIPS cannot distinguish which fetus is which, so that if an abnormality is detected, diagnostic techniques will still be required.

An increasingly common scenario in multifetal pregnancies is the combination of MZ twins with one or more singletons.[64] Changes in IVF culture techniques, including the increasing use of blastocyst transfers, have significantly increased the incidence of MZ twinning. As a result, dichorionic, triamniotic triplets, for example, have far higher rates of pregnancy loss, TTTS, and complications of prematurity.[65] We have observed that over 50% of the monochorionic (MC) twins developed TTTS, and the average gestational age at birth is about 30 weeks, which is 2 weeks less compared with trichorionic triplets.

In the vast majority of cases, the major determining factor in deciding which fetus or fetuses to reduce is based on chromosomal risk. However, the same principles can be applied to Mendelian risks. Recently, we evaluated a couple with triplets who were both cystic fibrosis carriers. Using appropriate probes, we were able to determine that two of the fetuses were carriers, and one was affected, which was subsequently reduced.

Fetal gender determination

As part of the FISH results, we also obtain gender. Historically, we perceived a significant bias among those patients who were interested and who mostly expressed a preference for males.[44,45] These requests disproportionately came from patients of cultures that classically value males over females. Because of such bias, we refused to let gender be a factor with the rare exception of genetic diseases with gender discordancy. Of course, in X-linked disorders, the males are at risk, thus making females the safer option. Over the past 15 years, however, we noticed a shift to requests coming from all ethnic groups and a perceived equalization of gender preferences. In the early 2000s, our ethics consultant, John Fletcher, PhD, encouraged us to consider, and we have adopted, the following approach.

First, a detailed ultrasound examination is performed in search for a fetus with a "potential problem." In the absence of increased nuchal translucency (>2 mm), smaller fetal size (such as more than ½ week, smaller gestational sac size), or placental concern, then and only then, gender preference is considered.

Patients are told that there will be a nongender disclosing "poker faced" discussion when the results are obtained. Then, they choose which of four "concerning gender" categories they prefer. The categories are the following: (1) those patients who want to know "everything"; (2) those who want to know "nothing"; (3) those who have no preference but want to know the identity of the gender(s) they've kept (but not the reduced); and (4) those who, all things considered, do have a preference but do not want to know the reduced fetus(es)' or gender(s).[66,67]

Recently, we have published data that show that when patients do have a gender preference, there is an equal preference for females as males. For patients reducing to twins, the overwhelming preference is for one of each; for those reducing to a singleton, it is essentially a 50/50 split (Table 8.6).[66]

We have also recently been able to use our technology to extend services to a group of patients not previously well served. In the past few years, we have seen several gay male couples, using surrogate carriers with egg donation, when both partners fertilized the eggs. The couples generally desire FR for the usual clinical reasons, but they frequently may request if possible to be left with twins—one fathered by each of them.[68] We chose to consider this request in the same vein as gender preference, i.e., only if there are no higher clinical priorities. In several cases, we have been able to assess the pregnancies with CVS and ultrasound, document normal genetic results, perform paternity testing, and discover that one man fathered two and the other one. In such cases, we may reduce one of the twins fathered by the same man.[68]

Selective termination

A separate category includes patients with mostly natural twin pregnancies but sometimes higher orders, in whom an abnormality is detected in one or more of the fetuses. We distinguish between FRs, which are procedures mostly performed in the first trimester and done for fetal number, per se, and ST, which are mostly second-trimester procedures and are performed for a diagnosed fetal abnormality. Several individual center and collaborative reports over the last 30 years have shown that the earlier the procedure is performed, the better the perinatal outcome, thus leading us to the conclusion that for all multiples, offering CVS for diagnosis is better than waiting for amniocentesis. Regardless of when the diagnosis is made, as long as it is legal in the jurisdiction, ST can be performed. In dichorionic twins, intracardiac KCl is the most effective method. Our older data suggested that after 16 weeks, the loss rate of the survivor was increased, but our experience now shows even after 20 weeks, the outcomes of the normal twin are generally improved by reduction of the abnormal twin.[69]

The situation is much more complex for the monochorionic twin pair for whom the incidence of structural fetal anomalies is actually considerably higher than for fraternal twins.[70] Unfortunate experiences from the 1970s and 1980s showed that if KCl terminations were performed because the monozygocity was unappreciated, then loss rates approached 50% with as much as 75% neurologic impairment in the survivor.[71] Even with spontaneous death of one twin, in the late second and third trimester, there is a risk of impairment to the survivor of approximately 12%, which is due to bleeding into the placenta, as opposing intravascular pressure from the other fetus ceases at death.[72] There is considerable debate on the optimal management of the abnormal twin, varying from performing immediate cesarean section, at term, to intrauterine transfusion of the surviving twin or expectant management. It is usually not possible to determine prospectively the risk of damage to the remaining twin.[71]

In the 1990s we developed the concept of umbilical cord ligation to perform ST and minimize the risk to the survivor.[73] Several approaches have been utilized, including literal cord ligation, cauterization, radio frequency ablation of the hepatic artery, and embolization. All have survival statistics of approximately 90%, but also have a 6%–10% risk of a damaged survivor.[74] As a result, we believe that an elective reduction of monochorionic twins is ill advised as the residual risk to the remaining twin is too high. Only rarely does there appear to be a complete separation of the placentas and vasculature so that FR can be considered. Even so, there always is the possibility of some vascular connection between the two.

Ethical issues

Improved outcomes, coupled with increasing availability and utilization of ART, have led to a progression in the ethical debates being considered. Nearly 30 years ago, FR seemed acceptable only in life-or-death situations.[69,70] As has been seen in numerous innovative technologies, once concepts are established, the concentration can move from "life or death" to "quality of life." Such has been the case with FR, but because of the framework of the abortion debate, FR will always be contentious. Opinions on FR, in our experience, have never followed the classic "prochoice/prolife" dichotomy.[29,47,48] We have long studied the reactions and strategies used by our patients and their families as to how to internalize and present to others their situation and choices that are made.[71,72]

It is practically impossible to isolate ethical debates from the context in which they take place particularly the number of embryos with which patients are presented for FR. In recent years, mothers presenting for FR with quadruplets and quintuplets have declined dramatically. The primary focus of research and care continues to be on the advancement of fertilization strategies and techniques that offer greater control in lowering the probabilities of such higher-order multifetal pregnancies.

Triplets are still plentiful. Even with the improved embryo-transfer control, the economics of IVF favor a modest risk of multiples, especially among women with fewer resources (for whom the cost of IVF cycles is a real consideration) and those who are over 35 (where the chances of larger transfer numbers reflect greater difficulty in getting pregnant). The serious debate is long past whether it is appropriate to offer FR to triplets but now centers on the question about whether or not it is appropriate to offer FR routinely for twins.[42,43]

Our data show that the reduction of twins to a singleton improves the outcome of the remaining fetus.[47–49] However, because of the sharp ethical divide over women's reproductive rights, no consensus on appropriateness of routine reduction from twins to singleton is ever likely to emerge.[75–77] Currently, the number of women with twins desiring FR to a singleton is small. However, in our view, the proportion of patients desiring reduction from twins to singleton will steadily increase over the next several years, and this option may be presented to all patients.

With a gradual decrease in starting fetal numbers, the emphasis has somewhat shifted to the prevention of serious morbidity, i.e., cerebral palsy from prematurity. Several studies have suggested that the rate of cerebral palsy for singletons is approximately 1/700, twins 1/100, and triplets 1/25–30.[11–13] If one's definition of success is a healthy mother and healthy family, for both morbidity and mortality, the data show conclusively with multiples, fewer is always better.

SUMMARY

Over the past 30 years, U.S. and international data have shown that by reducing the number of fetuses in multiples pregnancy outcomes are vastly improved. The efficacy of reduction for triplets or more has long been accepted by all but the most conservative of commentators. The medical data now also show that the reduction of twins to a singleton improves outcomes. The discussion then shifts to an ethical one. We understand that FR will never be universally accepted but we argue that from an autonomy and public health perspective, FR must be seen as a necessary procedure that will hopefully become increasingly rare.

REFERENCES

1. Evans MI, Fletcher JC, Zador IE et al. Selective first trimester termination in octuplet and quadruplet pregnancies: Clinical and ethical issues. *Obstet Gynecol* 1988; 71: 289–96.
2. Cohen AB, Hanft RS. *Technology in American Health Care: Policy Direction for Effective Evaluation and Management.* Ann Arbor, MI: Univ Michigan Press, 2004.
3. Evans MI, Hanft RS. The introduction of new technologies. *ACOG Clin Semin* 1997; 2(5): 1–3.
4. Centers for Disease Control. *National Survey of Family Growth.* http://www.cdc.gov/nchs/nsfg/abc_list_i.htm#infertilityservices. 2013. Accessed August 30, 2016.
5. Martin JA, Hamilton BE, Osterman MHS et al. Births: Final data for 2013. *National Vital Statistics Reports*, Vol. 64, No. 1, January 2015. Hyattsville, MD: National Center for Health Statistics.

6. Society of Assisted Reproductive Technologies. *Society of Assisted Reproductive Technologies 2013 Statistics.* https://www.sartcorsonline.com/rptCSR_PublicMultYear.aspx?ClinicPKID=0. 2013. Accessed August 30, 2016.
7. Centers for Disease Control. *Assisted Reproductive Technology Surveillance—United States, 2013.* http://www.cdc.gov/art/reports/. Accessed November 7, 2013.
8. Lawlor DA, Nelson SM. Effect of age on decisions about the number of embryos to transfer in assisted conception: A prospective study. *Lancet* 2012; 379: 521–27.
9. Evans MI, Britt DW. Medical, ethical, and legal aspects of fetal reduction. In: Schenker JL (ed), *Ethical and Legal Aspects of ART*, pp. 121–30. New York, NY, Berlin: Walter De Gruyter GmbH & Co., 2011.
10. Task Force of American College of Obstetricians and Gynecologists. Neonatal encephalopathy and cerebral palsy: Defining the pathogenesis and pathophysiology. Washington, DC: ACOG, 2003.
11. Petterson B, Nelson K, Watson L et al. Twins, triplets, and cerebral palsy in births in Western Australia in the 1980s. *BMJ* 1993; 307: 1239–43.
12. Pharoah PO, Cooke T. Cerebral palsy and multiple births. *Arch Dis Child Fetal Neonat Ed.* 1996; 75: F174–77.
13. Dimitiiou G, Pharoah PO, Nicolaides KH et al. Cerebral palsy in triplet pregnancies with and without iatrogenic reduction. *Eur J Pediatr* 2004; 163: 449–51.
14. St. John EB, Nelson KG, Oliver SP et al. Cost of neonatal care according to gestational age at birth and survival status. *Am J Obstet Gynecol* 2000; 182: 170–75.
15. Cuevas KD, Silver DR, Brooten D et al. The cost of prematurity: Hospital charges at birth and frequency of rehospitalizations and acute care visits over the first year of life: A comparison by gestational age and birth weight. *Am J Nurs* 2005; 105: 56–64.
16. Marlow N, Wolke D, Bracewell MA et al. Neurologic and developmental disability at six years of age after extremely preterm birth. *N Engl J Med* 2005; 352: 9–19.
17. Rosenbaum P, Paneth N, Leviton A et al. A report: The definition and classification of cerebral palsy April 2006. *Dev Med Child Neurol* 2007; 49: 8–14. Corrected in Rosenbaum P, Paneth N, Leviton A et al. A report: The definition and classification of cerebral palsy April 2006. *Dev Med Child Neurol Suppl* 2007; 109: 8–14.
18. Hack M, Taylor HG, Drotar D et al. Chronic conditions, functional limitations, and special health care needs of school-aged children born with extremely low birth weights in the 1990s. *JAMA* 2008; 94: 318–25.
19. Stoll BJ, Hansen NI, Bell EF et al. Neonatal outcomes of extremely preterm infants from the NICHD Neonatal Research Network. *Pediatrics* 2010; 126: 443–56.
20. Yogev Y, Melamed N, Bardin R et al. Pregnancy outcome at extremely advanced maternal age. *Am J Obstet Gynecol* 2010; 203: 558.e1–7.
21. Dumez Y, Oury JF. Method for first trimester selective abortion in multiple pregnancy. *Contrib Gynecol Obstet* 1986; 15: 50.
22. Berkowitz RL, Lynch L, Chitkara U et al. Selective reduction of multiple pregnancies in the first trimester. *N Engl J Med* 1988; 318: 1043.
23. Wapner RJ, Davis GH, Johnson A. Selective reduction of multifetal pregnancies. *Lancet* 1990; 335: 90–3.
24. Timor-Tritsch IE, Peisner DB, Monteagudo A et al. Multifetal pregnancy reduction by transvaginal puncture: Evaluation of the technique used in 134 cases. *Am J Obstet Gynecol* 1993; 168: 799–04.
25. Li R, Yang R, Chen X et al. Intracranial KCl injection—An alternative method for multifetal pregnancy reduction in the early second trimester. *Fetal Diag Ther* 2013; 34: 26–30.
26. Evans MI, Dommergues M, Wapner RJ et al. Efficacy of transabdominal multifetal pregnancy reduction: Collaborative experience among the world's largest centers. *Obstet Gynecol* 1993; 82: 61–67.
27. Evans MI, Drugan A, Fletcher JC et al. Attitudes on the ethics of abortion, sex selection & selective termination among health care professionals, ethicists & clergy likely to encounter such situations. *Am J Obstet Gynecol* 1991; 164: 1092–99.
28. Yaron Y, Bryant-Greenwood PK, Dave N et al. Multifetal pregnancy reduction (MFPR) of triplets to twins: Comparison with non-reduced triplets and twins. *Am J Obstet Gynecol* 1999; 180: 1268–71.
29. Antsaklis A, Souka AP, Daskalakis G et al. Embryo reduction versus expectant management in triplet pregnancies. *J Matern Fetal Neonatal Med* 2004; 16: 219–22.
30. Luke B, Brown MD, Nugent C et al. Risk factors for adverse outcomes in spontaneous versus assisted conception in twin pregnancies. *Fertil Steril* 2004; 81: 315–9.
31. Kozinsky Z, Zadori J, Ovros H, et al. Obstetric and neonatal risk of pregnancies after assisted reproductive technology: A matched control study. *Acta Obstet Gynecol Scand* 2003; 82: 850–6.
32. McDonald S, Murphy K, Beyene J et al. Perinatal outcomes of in vitro fertilization twins: A systematic review and meta analysis. *Am J Obstet Gynecol* 2005; 193: 141–52.
33. Leondires MP, Ernst SD, Miller BT et al. Triplets: Outcomes of expectant management versus multifetal reduction for 127 pregnancies. *Am J Obstet Gynecol* 1999; 72: 257–60.
34. Lipitz S, Shulman A, Achiron R et al. A comparative study of multifetal pregnancy reduction from triplets to twins in the first versus early second trimesters

after detailed fetal screening. *Ultrasound Obstet Gynecol* 2001; 18: 35–8.
35. Sepulveda W, Munoz H, Alcalde JL. Conjoined twins in a triplet pregnancy: Early prenatal diagnosis with three-dimensional ultrasound and review of the literature. *Ultrasound Obstet Gynecol* 2003; 22: 199–04.
36. Francois K, Sears C, Wilson R, Elliot J. Twelve year experience of triplet pregnancies at a single institution. *Am J Obstet Gynecol* 2001; 185: S112.
37. Evans MI, Berkowitz R, Wapner R et al. Multifetal pregnancy reduction (MFPR): Improved outcomes with increased experience. *Am J Obstet Gynecol* 2001; 184: 97–103.
38. Blickstein I. How and why are triplets disadvantaged compared to twins. *Best Pract Res Clin Obstet Gynecol* 2004; 18: 631–44.
39. Rosner M, Pergament E, Andriole S et al. Detection of genetic abnormalities using CVS and FISH prior to fetal reduction in sonographically normal appearing fetuses. *Prenat Diagn* 2013; 33: 940–44.
40. Chaveeva P, Kosinski P, Puglia D et al. Trichorionic and dichorionic triplet pregnancies at 10–14 weeks: Outcome after embryo reduction compared to expectant management. *Fetal Diag Ther* 2013; 34: 199–05.
41. Evans MI, Kaufman MI, Urban AJ et al. Fetal Reduction from twins to a singleton: A reasonable consideration. *Obstet Gynecol* 2004; 104: 102–09.
42. Templeton A. The multiple gestation epidemic: The role of the assisted reproductive technologies. *Am J Obstet Gynecol* 2004; 190: 894–98.
43. Kalra SK, Milad MP, Klock SC, Grobman WA. Infertility patients and their partners: Differences in the desire for twin gestations. *Obstet Gynecol* 2003; 102: 152–55.
44. Evans MI, Britt DW. Selective reduction in multifetal pregnancies. In: Paul M, Grimes, D, Stubblefield P (eds). *Management of Unintended and Abnormal Pregnancy*, pp. 312–18. London, UK: Blackwell-Wiley Publishing Co, 2009.
45. Evans MI, Britt DW. Fetal reduction: Ethical and societal issues. In: Sauer M (ed), *Semin Reprod Med* 2010; 28: 295–302.
46. Balasch J, Gratacós E. Delayed childbearing: Effects on fertility and the outcome of pregnancy. *Curr Opin Obstet Gynecol.* 2012; 24(3): 187–93.
47. Balasch J, Gratacós E. Delayed childbearing: Effects on fertility and the outcome of pregnancy. *Fetal Diagn Ther* 2011; 29: 263–73.
48. McLean LK, Evans MI, Carpenter RJ, et al. Genetic amniocentesis (AMN) following multifetal pregnancy reduction (MFPR) does not increase the risk of pregnancy loss. *Prenat Diagn* 1998; 18(2): 186–88.
49. Wapner RJ, Johnson A, Davis G, et al. Prenatal diagnosis in twin gestations: A comparison between second-trimester amniocentesis and first-trimester chorionic villus sampling. *Obstet Gynecol* 1993; 82: 49–56.
50. Brambati B, Tului L, Baldi M, Guercilena S. Genetic analysis prior to selective fetal reduction in multiple pregnancy: Technical aspects and clinical outcome. *Hum Reprod* 1995; 10: 818–25.
51. Tabor A, Alfirevic Z. Update on procedure-related risks for prenatal diagnosis techniques. *Fetal Diagn Ther* 2010; 27: 1–7.
52. Hern WM. Selective termination for fetal anomaly/genetic disorder in twin pregnancy at 32+ menstrual weeks. Report of four cases. *Fetal Diagn Ther* 2004; 19: 292–95.
53. Evans MI, Goldberg J, Horenstein J et al. Selective termination (ST) for structural (STR), chromosomal (CHR), and Mendelian (MEN) anomalies: International experience. *Am J Obstet Gynecol* 1999; 181: 893–97.
54. Eddleman KA, Stone JL, Lynch L, Berkowitz RL. Selective termination of anomalous fetuses in multiple pregnancies: Two hundred cases at a single center. *Am J Obstet Gynecol* 2002; 187: 1168–72.
55. Lu J, Ting YH, Law KM et al. Radiofrequency ablation for selective reduction in complicated monochorionic multiple pregnancies. *Fetal Diagn Ther* 2013; 34: 211–6.
56. Pergament E, Schulman JD, Copeland K et al. The risk and efficacy of chorionic villus sampling in multiple gestations. *Prenat Diagn* 1992; 12: 377–84.
57. Nicolini U, Lalatta F, Natacci F et al. The introduction of QF-PCR in prenatal diagnosis of fetal aneuploidies: Time for reconsideration. *Hum Reprod Update* November–December 2004; 10(6): 541–8.
58. Wapner RJ, Martin CL, Levy B et al. Chromosomal microarray versus karyotyping for prenatal diagnosis. *N Engl J Med* 2012; 367: 2175–84.
59. Wapner RJ, Babiarz JE, Levy B et al. Expanding the scope of noninvasive prenatal testing: Detection of fetal microdeletion syndromes. *Am J Obstet Gynecol* 2015; 212: 322.e1–9.
60. Balasch J, Gratacos E. Delayed childbearing: Effects on fertility and the outcome of pregnancy. *Curr Opin Obstet Gynecol* 2012; 24: 187–93.
61. Dreesen J, Destouni A, Kourlaba G et al. Evaluation of PCR-based preimplantation genetic diagnosis applied to monogenic disease: A collaborative ESHRE PGD consortium study. *Eur J Hum Genet* 2014; 22: 1012–8.
62. Yang Z, Liu J, Collins GS et al. Selection of single blastocysts for fresh transfer via standard morphology assessment alone and with array CGH for good prognosis IVF patients: Results from a randomized pilot study. *Mol Cytol* 2012; 5: 24–32.
63. Dondorp W, de Wert G, Bombard Y et al. Noninvasive prenatal testing for aneuploidy and beyond: Challenges of responsible innovation in prenatal screening. *Eur J Hum Genet* 2015; 57: 1–8.
64. Pantos K, Kokkali G, Petroutsou K et al. Monochorionic triplet and monoamniotic twins gestation after intracytoplasmic sperm injection and

laser-assisted hatching. *Fetal Diagn Ther* 2009; 25: 144–47.
65. Peeters SH, Evans MI, Slaghekke F et al. Pregnancy complications for di-chorionic, tri-amniotic triplets: Markedly increased over trichorionic and reduced cases. *Am J Obstet Gynecol* 2014; 210: S288–9.
66. Evans MI, Rosner M, Andriole S, et al. Evolution of gender preferences in multiple pregnancies. *Prenat Diagn* 2013; 33: 935–39.
67. Evans MI, Andriole SA, Britt DW. Fetal reduction—25 Years' experience. *Fetal Diagn Ther* 2014; 35: 69–82.
68. Evans MI, Andriole S, Pergament E et al. Paternity balancing. *Fetal Diagn Ther* 2013; 34: 135–9.
69. Evans MI, Goldberg J, Horenstein J et al. Selective termination (ST) for structural (STR), chromosomal (CHR), and Mendelian (MEN) anomalies: International experience. *Am J Obstet Gynecol* 1999; 181(4): 893–97.
70. Hack KE, Derks JB, Elias SG et al. Increased perinatal mortality and morbidity in monochorionic versus dichorionic twin pregnancies: Clinical implications of a large Dutch cohort study. *Br J Obstet Gynecol* 2008; 115: 58.
71. Evans MI, Lau TK. Making decisions when no good options exist: Delivery of the survivor after intrauterine death of the co-twin in monochorionic twin pregnancies. *Fetal Diagn Ther* 2010; 28: 191–95.
72. Quintero RA, Reich H, Puder KS et al. Brief report: Umbilical cord ligation of an acardiac twin by fetoscopy at 19 weeks of gestation. *N Engl J Med* 1994; 330: 469–71.
73. Gebb J, Rosner M, Dar P, Evans MI. Long term neurologic outcomes after fetal interventions: Meta analysis. *Am J Obstet Gynecol* 2014; 210: S115.
74. Beauchamp TL, Childress JC, *Principles of Biomedical Ethics*, 5th edition. New York, NY: Oxford University Press, 2001: 358–59.
75. Benjamin M. *Splitting the Difference. Compromise and Integrity in Ethics and Politics.* Lawrence, KA: University Press of Kansas, 1990.
76. Britt DW, Evans MI. Sometimes doing the right thing sucks: Frame combinations and multifetal pregnancy reduction decision difficulty. *Soc Sci Med* 2007; 65: 2342–56.
77. Britt DW, Evans MI. Information sharing among couples considering multifetal pregnancy reduction *Fertil Steril* 2007; 87: 490–95.

Spontaneous and indicated abortions

9

MÁRTA GÁVAI and ZOLTÁN PAPP

CONTENTS

DEFINITION AND CLINICAL PICTURE OF ABORTION

Abortion (miscarriage) is the termination of a pregnancy, induced or spontaneous, before the conceptus is sufficiently developed to survive after delivery. The precise gestational age at which the infant is able to survive is difficult to define. Spontaneous abortion is the most common complication of early pregnancy. Most authorities restrict the term "abortion" to the first 23 weeks of pregnancy; or in retrospect, to the delivery of any infant weighing less than 350 or 500 g. In the following discussion, abortion is defined as expulsion of the products of conception before gestational week 23. Abortions taking place before week 13 are termed early (first-trimester) abortions; those occurring at weeks 13–23 are called late (second-trimester, midtrimester) abortions. This subdivision into two different categories is important because of the different etiologies and types of treatment applied.

Threatened or threatening abortion

Threatened abortion (called in the past also *abortus imminens*) is characterized by vaginal bleeding, ranging from bloody vaginal discharge, or spotting to profuse, bright red bleeding. Pain may be present, either intermittent or constant, due to uterine contractions, at the loin or groin area, resembling menstrual cramps. Pelvic examination reveals the cervix intact and the os closed; the corpus uteri is soft, its size corresponding to the gestational age. This definition makes threatened abortion a common complication in early pregnancy, occurring in about one of four or five pregnancies, about one-half ending in spontaneous abortion. The bleeding and pain may be intermittent, may vary in intensity, and may persist for many days and even weeks.

Inevitable abortion

Inevitable abortion (also called in the past *abortus incipiens*) presents with bright red, often profuse, vaginal bleeding, and uterine contractions. The cervix is shortened and dilated, and parts of the conceptus may be visible in the vagina or through the os. The uterus is hard and tender during contractions. With the dilating cervix, the membranes rupture and expulsion of the conceptus, in part or in whole, will invariably follow.

Incomplete abortion

In incomplete abortion (also called in the past *abortus incompletus*), only parts of the conceptus have been expelled. The history will be that of passage of fragments of tissue together with bright red vaginal bleeding and uterine contractions. After the passage of products of conception, the bleeding will continue in varying intensity, ranging from bloody discharge, possibly accompanied by expulsion of bits of tissue, to profuse bleeding, occasionally leading to hypovolemic shock. Pain resulting from uterine contractions may be present periodically. At clinical examination, the cervix is dilated and products of conception may be seen or felt through the os. The corpus uteri is enlarged, soft, subinvoluted, and possibly tender if infection has supervened.

Complete abortion

In complete abortion (also called in the past *abortus completus*), the products of conception have been expelled completely. Its occurrence is more common in the first weeks of pregnancy due to the loose embedding of the ovum in the endometrium. After the passage of the products of conception, the hemorrhage and pain subside, but some vaginal discharge, usually bloodstained, may proceed for some days. On examination, the cervix is closed, and the corpus possibly enlarged, but firm and well involuted.

Missed abortion

Missed abortion designates the retention of the conceptus in the uterus after the conception of an anembryonic pregnancy or the death of the embryo. Before this occurs, the patient may have presented with the history of threatened abortion. The often scanty bleeding usually continues for several days or weeks, becoming a persistent brownish vaginal discharge. Pain is uncommon. With the death of the conceptus, the patient's impression of being pregnant disappears. The breasts become smaller, and the uterus fails to grow. It may even shrink in size as a result of the absorption of amniotic fluid and maceration of the fetus. With prolonged retention of the dead conceptus in the uterus, rarely disturbances in the blood coagulation mechanism may occur (e.g., hypofibrinogenemia and prolonged or uncontrolled bleeding). Prior to the widespread use of ultrasound, not infrequently the embryo or fetus was retained in utero for a prolonged period of time. In the present period of medical technology, specific criteria have been established to diagnose fetal death in utero early, and to obviate this pathologic progression.

Septic abortion

Any type of abortion may be associated with infection (also called in the past abortus septicus), but retention of the products of conception or parts of them, such as missed and incomplete abortion, are particularly predisposing. Inadequately sterilized instruments used in criminally or self-induced abortions carry a high risk of infection. The infection usually takes the course of endometritis with chills and elevated body temperature; foul-smelling, purulent vaginal discharge; and lower abdominal and pelvic tenderness. Parametritis, tubo-ovarian abscess, peritonitis—localized or generalized—or life-endangering septic shock with cardiovascular collapse and renal failure may ensue. A variety of microorganisms may cause septic abortion, but *Escherichia coli*, *Streptococcus pyogenes*, and other hemolytic streptococci, *Staphylococcus aureus* and *Bacteroides,* are the most frequently encountered. Occasionally, the potentially serious clostridial bacteria are the causative agents.

Habitual (recurrent) abortion

Habitual abortion (also called in the past *abortus habitualis*) is the occurrence of three or more consecutive spontaneous abortions. Habitual abortions take the course of one of the abovementioned types of abortion.

INCIDENCE

One of the problems in establishing the exact incidence of abortion is the various definitions used, with the lack of a definite date in pregnancy until which the expulsion of the conceptus or the death of the fetus can be called an abortion. It is generally estimated that at least 10%–15% of all pregnancies terminate in spontaneous abortion. These figures are based upon abortions recognized clinically and by means of laboratory tests and histologic examination. An unexpected delay in the menstrual period followed by excessively heavy bleeding may in many instances result from early pregnancy wastage, where the fertilized ovum never was implanted properly. The number of these early "occult" abortions cannot be accurately determined, since the evidence of pregnancy usually is missing. Hertig[1] has calculated a biologic rate of spontaneous abortion of approximately 28%, once the menstrual period was missed. Macklon et al.[2] concluded in a classic study that human pregnancy wastage occurs on such a scale that only ~30% of conceived pregnancies will progress to live birth. From various data, it appears that the real incidence of spontaneous abortion is much higher than the 10%–15% usually mentioned. The frequency of spontaneous abortion decreases with increasing gestational age. The incidence in clinically recognized pregnancies up to 20 gestational weeks is 8%–20%. The overall risk of spontaneous abortion after 15 weeks is low (about 0.6%) for chromosomally and structurally normal fetuses, but varies according to maternal age and ethnicity. Loss of unrecognized or subclinical pregnancies is even higher, occurring in 13%–26% of all pregnancies. If preimplantation losses are considered, approximately 50% of fertilized oocytes do not result in a live birth.[2,3]

ETIOLOGY

The exact causes of most spontaneous abortions are considered unknown. Spontaneous abortion is most commonly caused by chromosomal abnormalities in the embryo or exposure to teratogens. It is often difficult to determine the cause of a spontaneous abortion in an individual case. In one-third of cases occurring at 8 weeks of gestation or earlier, no embryo or yolk sac is observed in the gestational sac. In the remaining two-thirds of cases in which an embryo is identified, approximately half are abnormal, dysmorphic, stunted, or too macerated for examination.

In the early weeks of pregnancy, the expulsion of the conceptus is usually preceded by the death of the embryo. Later, the fetus frequently is expelled alive. The causes of abortion can be fetal or genetic, maternal, paternal, and combined factors.

Fetal or genetic factors

In their study of 1000 cases of spontaneous abortion, Hertig and Sheldon[4] found defects or abnormalities of the expelled conceptus in 62%. About one-half of the abortuses examined represented pathologic ova, with absent or defective embryos.[5] Embryos with localized anomalies were found in 3%, and placental abnormalities showed an incidence of 10%.

The exact causes of the anomalies are still unknown, but it has been presumed that the defective ovum resulted from "germplasm defects." Chromosome abnormalities are responsible for many early spontaneous abortions,[3,6] including cases which at histopathologic examination revealed blighted ova, placenta, and cord abnormalities (Figure 9.1).

Chromosome aberrations are present at conception in nearly 10% of zygotes. These are of reduced viability, and most of the affected embryos die and are expelled spontaneously. Chromosome aberrations are present in 60% of early abortions, 6% of midtrimester abortions, and 4%–5% of stillborn fetuses. The earlier the abortion occurs, the higher the incidence of cytogenetic defects. The prevalence of abnormal fetal karyotypes is 90% in empty sac pregnancies, 50% in abortions occurring at 8–11 weeks of gestation, and 30% in those occurring at 16–19 weeks. In cases considered normal at the cytogenetic level, single nucleotide polymorphism (SNP) chromosomal microarray analysis revealed a clinically significant copy number change or whole-genome uniparental disomy in 1%–2%. This supports the use of SNP chromosomal microarray analysis for the cytogenomic evaluation of miscarriage specimens when clinically indicated.[7]

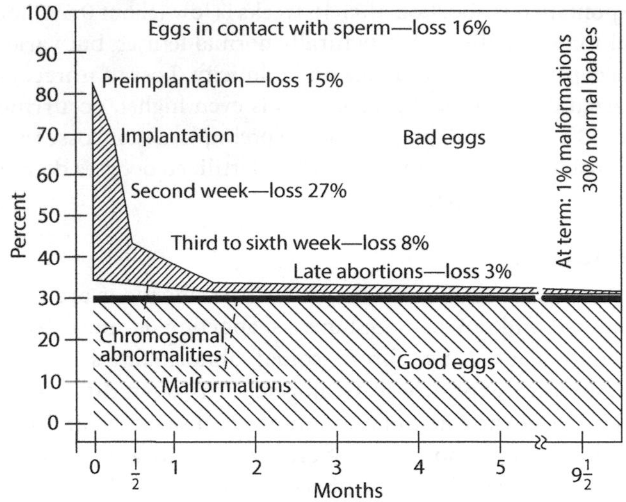

Figure 9.1 Emil Witschi's concept of the natural history of reproductive wastage. A large proportion of fertilized ova is lost soon after conception. These early losses are not apparent clinically. Many embryos and fetuses are lost because of early spontaneous abortion, others during the second trimester, and relatively few around term. Of all conceptions, only about 30% result in healthy, live-born babies.

Although there are exceptions, in general, additional chromosomal material is more compatible with life than a deficiency. In abortion material, mainly trisomies and triploidy can be found.[8] The monosomic zygotes usually die and are eliminated without any clinical signs of abortion. Among the monosomic zygotes, only those with 45, X monosomy are viable. About 2% of these survive the intrauterine period and are born with Ullrich–Turner syndrome. In samples from spontaneous abortions, trisomy for any of the chromosomes, except chromosomes 1 and 5, may be found. Trisomy 16 occurs most frequently and leads to abortion in every case. A small number of some of the other trisomies escape intrauterine selection, and their bearers may be born alive (1%–2% of trisomy 13, 5%–10% of trisomy 18, and 15%–25% of trisomy 21).[9–11] Autosomal trisomies are associated with advanced maternal age (e.g., trisomy 21), whereas monosomy X and polyploidy are not. Other mechanisms, such as the age of the gametes, virus infections, chemicals, drugs, or radiation, may possibly interfere with the chromosomal composition.

Congenital anomalies may be caused by chromosomal or other genetic abnormalities, by extrinsic factors (e.g., amniotic bands), or by exposure to teratogens. Potential teratogens include maternal disorders (e.g., diabetes mellitus with poor glycemic control), drugs (e.g., isotretinoin), physical stresses (e.g., fever), and environmental chemicals (e.g., mercury).

Maternal nonmedical factors

The preliminary condition for *implantation* of the blastocyst is a properly prepared endometrium developed under the influence of the ovarian hormones. In the cells of the endometrial glands, it is possible to detect alkaline phosphatase from early in the follicular phase. When glycogen is released into the glandular lumina after ovulation, the alkaline phosphatase breaks down glycogen into glucose and fructose, which are needed by the trophoblast during implantation. When this metabolism is adequate, the environment for nidation, and further development of the embryo is created. Factors that adversely influence the carbohydrate metabolism, and thus the nourishment of the endometrial bed, may hinder the proper development of early pregnancy.

The human blastocyst normally implants in the fundal part of the uterus. However, occasionally, the implantation takes place in abnormal locations inside the uterus (e.g., close to the internal os). With such a low implantation, spontaneous abortion frequently occurs. If the pregnancy continues, it may present as a case of placenta praevia.

Endocrine deficiencies

Endocrine deficiencies play a significant role in spontaneous abortions. The proper development of the endometrium and the maintenance of the decidua (the implantation, placentation, and embryonic development) rely on a proper hormonal function of the corpus luteum and the trophoblast. Estrogen and progesterone from the ovary stimulate and maintain the endometrium. With implantation, the trophoblast begins the production of chorionic gonadotropin, sustaining the corpus luteum of pregnancy, which in turn keeps the decidua alive and maintains the metabolic processes necessary for fetal growth. The corpus luteum and the trophoblast/early placenta are essential for further gestational development. If one of the two fails, a vicious cycle may ensue, ending in termination of the pregnancy. Inadequate progesterone production has been blamed for causing spontaneous, especially habitual, abortions. However, progestational hormone therapy seems to have a limited effect in preventing abortions. Whether deficient progesterone production is the cause or the effect of abortion is difficult to determine. The corpus luteum of pregnancy is the main site of progesterone production until gestational weeks 8–10. After this, the production in the ovary diminishes, and the placenta becomes the main source of progesterone. Bilateral oophorectomy in gestational week 10 does not interfere with the successful outcome of pregnancy.[12] Thyroid hormones are essential for the maintenance of pregnancy, and a deficiency in maternal thyroid hormones has been associated with early pregnancy losses.[13] It has been shown that thyroid hormone receptors THRα1, THRα2, THRβ1, and THRβ2 are downregulated in spontaneous and recurrent miscarriages. The majority of cells expressing the thyroid hormone receptors in the decidua are decidual stromal cells.[13]

Uterine abnormalities

These may be *congenital,* arising from anomalies of Müllerian fusion of various degree, and resulting in conditions such as uterus didelphys, uterus bicornis unicollis, uterus unicornis, or uterus subseptus. Among the *acquired* abnormalities, leiomyomas deforming the uterine cavity are especially likely to cause abortion.[14] Uterine synechiae (Asherman's syndrome), resulting from previous infection, curettage, or the scarring of the uterine wall from previous surgery, may cause abortion. Malposition of the uterus is seldom an obstacle to the proper progress of pregnancy. These uterine abnormalities, congenital, or acquired, may interfere with the blood circulation in the decidua and the nutrition of the growing embryo/fetus. On the other hand, the pregnancy may be carried to term in spite of a malformed uterus. If uterine abnormalities are suspected in connection with repeated pregnancy wastage, proper investigational procedures, including hysterosalpingography, hysterosalpingosonography, and possibly hysteroscopy, should be performed and any detected anatomic defect corrected.[15] Removal of the septum significantly increased live birth rate and was associated with a high spontaneous conception rate in infertile women.

A special entity of uterine abnormalities is cervical insufficiency. This condition is discussed in another chapter.

Infections

Viral as well as bacterial infections have been suspected of causing abortions. Syphilis is the classic example of maternal infection, spreading across the placenta and causing fetal death and abortion in the second trimester. Various other microorganisms, such as herpes simplex virus, *Toxoplasma gondii*, *Listeria monocytogenes*, parvovirus B19, rubella, cytomegalovirus, lymphocytic choriomeningitis virus, and *Mycoplasma* spp., have been associated with spontaneous abortion.[16–18]

Maternal diseases

Hypothyroidism and diabetes mellitus are conducive to the loss of early pregnancy, whereas chronic renal and cardiovascular diseases, such as nephritis and hypertension, are more likely to be associated with late fetal death or premature delivery.

Surgery during pregnancy and occupational exposure to inhalation anesthetics increases the risk of spontaneous abortion.[19] Disturbances in hemostasis, intrauterine device failures, and physical and psychic trauma, as well as occupational and other socioeconomic factors (e.g., drinking alcohol or using illicit drugs during pregnancy, smoking, and nutritional and vitamin deficiency) are also of significance in the causation of abortion.[20–22]

Considerable interest has centered in recent years on the roles of antiphospholipid antibodies and the various types of thrombophilia syndromes in pregnancy losses during both early and advanced gestations.[23–26] Since the management of these complications is a medical, rather than surgical, problem, their detailed discussion is outside of the scope of this chapter.

Paternal factors

Semen quality is influenced by factors such as radiation, certain drugs, anesthetics, occupation, and infection. The greater the frequency of abnormal sperm heads, the higher the risk of spontaneous abortion. It has been reported that the sperm concentration was significantly higher in repeated and habitual abortion groups, with a tendency to polyzoospermia (i.e., more than 200×10^6/mL sperm).[27]

Combined (maternal and paternal) factors

The frequency of structural chromosomal anomalies among aborters is higher than in the general populations (0.8% vs. 0.3%). There are also some balanced carrier translocation karyotypes among habitual aborters.[28–31]

Unexplained

The cause of abortions of chromosomally and structurally normal embryos/fetuses in apparently healthy women is unclear. As discussed above, genetic abnormalities not detected by a standard karyotype (small deletions, duplications, and point mutations) account for an undefined proportion of spontaneous abortions. In a study where embryoscopy, embryo biopsy, and karyotype were performed in more than 200 patients with missed abortion, 18% of embryos having a normal karyotype exhibited grossly abnormal developmental morphology.[32]

PATHOLOGY

Most pathologic changes are secondary to fetal death in early abortions. After this, "live abortions" become more frequent. Following fetal death, the placental function gradually deteriorates, leading to the disintegration of the decidua by hemorrhage and necrosis. The ovum acting as a foreign body stimulates the uterus, causing expulsion of the products of conception or parts of them.

In cases of spontaneous abortion after gestational weeks 6–8, some chorionic tissue usually remains adherent to the uterine wall. During months 4 and 5 of pregnancy, the placenta is divided into cotyledons. Until this has been accomplished, any spontaneous abortion should be considered as incomplete.

At histologic examination, a frequent pathologic finding is hydropic swelling or degeneration of the chorionic villi. Hydropic degeneration may resemble hydatidiform mole.

Sometimes an ovum is surrounded by extravasated blood collecting between the decidua and the chorion, where it coagulates and forms layers. This is referred to as a blood or *carneous mole*. In some cases, the appearance is nodular due to localized hematomas of varying sizes, and it is called a *tuberous mole*. In some cases of missed abortion, the amniotic fluid may be absorbed to such an extent that the fetus becomes compressed, forming a *fetus compressus*. Occasionally, this happens to such a degree that the fetal remnants resemble parchment, the so-called *fetus papyraceus*. This is not infrequently found in cases of twin pregnancy where one fetus died early in pregnancy and the other continued developing.[33]

DIAGNOSIS

When the patient presents with vaginal bleeding in early pregnancy, the fetus may have been dead for some time. If parts of the chorionic tissue are still functioning, the pregnancy test may be positive. If spontaneous termination of pregnancy is awaited, many days of unnecessary delay and anxiety will result. Only in cases where expelled products of conception can be examined or when parts of the conceptus are visible through the os can the diagnosis of irreversible abortion be made with certainty on clinical grounds alone.

A number of diagnostic tests have been applied to the evaluation of early threatened pregnancy. With the development of accurate radioimmunoassays, a variety of hormonal parameters have become diagnostic tools. Unfortunately, there are no exact hormone values, levels, or trends that permit differentiation between the doomed pregnancies and those proceeding to viability.

In the assessment of the anatomic integrity of an early pregnancy, ultrasound plays the dominant role. The gestational sac may be first demonstrated 5–6 weeks after the last menstrual period. From gestational week 7 onward, it is possible to demonstrate fetal heart movements and even fetal motion. From approximately week 12, details of the fetal body can be detected.

In a case of early pregnancy complicated by vaginal bleeding, an ultrasound examination should include the evaluation of the appearance and size of the gestational sac, the presence of embryonic echoes and life signs, the measurement of crown–rump length, and the location of the placenta.[34,35] An echo-free area between the membranes and the uterine wall represents blood indicative of threatened abortion. The size of such hematomas is predictive of the outcome of the pregnancy. The distribution of etiologic factors in spontaneous abortion differs according to whether embryonic cardiac activity is recorded.[36] In cases of anembryonic gestations, a gestational sac without echoes can be demonstrated. Absence of fetal life signs after 8 or 9 weeks' gestation is suggestive of an unsuccessful outcome for the pregnancy. The lack of growth of the embryo/gestational sac or degenerative change in the sac indicates missed abortion. A well-formed gestational sac, which on subsequent examination demonstrates fragmentation, also is evidence of a missed abortion (Table 9.1).

Ultrasonic demonstration of fetal life signifies a successful outcome for the pregnancy in 80%–90% of cases of threatened abortion.[33] In cases of incomplete abortion, it is possible to demonstrate retained conceptional products in the uterus with ultrasonography through the absence of the thin, midline echo seen in complete abortions.

The diagnosis of spontaneous abortion should be made with the help of measurement of the serum human chorionic gonadotropin (hCG). A single hCG concentration is not informative, but a baseline is useful if the ultrasound findings are nondiagnostic or if ectopic pregnancy is suspected. In the possibility of multiple gestation serum hCG must be considered because, in such cases, the serum hCG concentrations can be misleading; levels may increase or decrease, depending upon viability of the other fetuses.

TREATMENT

In cases of vaginal bleeding, thorough medical history should be taken, focusing on earlier pregnancies (abortions and deliveries), and a general physical and pelvic examination performed. If present and retrievable, an intrauterine contraceptive device should be removed. In cases of pronounced bleeding, blood should be drawn for blood indices, typing, and crossmatching. If infection is suspected, cultures should be taken from the cervical canal and the blood in order to identify any pathogens and their antibiotic sensitivity. Unless the medical history and/or pelvic examination indicates that abortion is inevitable or has taken place, adequate diagnostic procedures should be initiated to diagnose failing pregnancy. When voluntary termination of the pregnancy is a legally acceptable option, the patient is to be counseled about the prognosis of her pregnancy and the increased risk of fetal anomalies associated with threatening abortions.

Table 9.1 Ultrasonographic diagnostic and suggestive criteria of missed abortion by ACOG's Clinical Guidelines.

Diagnostic findings	Suggestive findings
CRL ≥7 mm and no heartbeat	CRL <7 mm and no heartbeat
MSD ≥25 mm and no embryo	MSD = 16–24 mm and no embryo
Absence of embryo with heartbeat 2 weeks or more after a scan that showed a gestational sac without a yolk sac	Absence of embryo with heartbeat 7–13 days after an ultrasound scan that showed a gestational sac without a yolk sac
Absence of embryo with heartbeat 11 days or more after a scan that showed a gestational sac with a yolk sac	Absence of embryo with heartbeat 7–10 days after an ultrasound scan that showed a gestational sac with a yolk sac
	Absence of embryo for 6 weeks or longer after last menstrual period
	Empty amnion (amnion seen adjacent to yolk sac, with no visible embryo)
	Enlarged yolk sac (>7 mm)
	Small gestational sac in relation to the size of the embryo (<5 mm difference between mean sac diameter and crown–rump length)

Abbreviations: ACOG, American College of Obstetricians and Gynecologists; CRL, crown–rump length; MSD, mean sac diameter.

The majority of spontaneous abortions are caused by conceptional defects; thus, therapeutic efforts rarely will prove effective. Coitus should be avoided during bleeding and for 1 or 2 weeks after its cessation.

There were attempts with progestogen therapy where progesterone deficiency has been demonstrated but a meta-analysis in 2012 was investigated the effects of early progesterone cessation on pregnancy outcomes in women undergoing *in vitro* fertilization (IVF)/intracytoplasmic sperm injection (ICSI) and concluded that progesterone supplementation beyond the first positive hCG test after IVF/ICSI might generally be unnecessary.[37]

Progestogen therapy should be restricted to the very few instances where progesterone deficiency has been demonstrated (e.g., special cases of habitual abortion).

There are no therapies available for treatment of threatened abortion which are supported by level 1 evidence. For women with recurrent pregnancy loss, a uterine study (e.g., three-dimensional [3D] sonohysterography) should be offered; parental chromosomes done; and antiphospholipid antibodies drawn. There are no other interventions supported by level 1 evidence for these women.

The frequency of miscarriage in cases of threatened abortion may approach 50%.[35] An increased incidence of premature deliveries (e.g., small-for-date infants, placental abruption and infarction, perinatal asphyxia, perinatal mortality, and congenital abnormalities) is anticipated in women whose pregnancies were complicated by vaginal bleeding during the first two trimesters.

Inevitable, incomplete, complete, habitual, and missed abortions involve hemorrhage that may require transfusion. The uncommon but serious disorders of coagulation mechanism (e.g., hypofibrinogenemia, disseminated intravascular coagulation) should be kept in mind.[38,39]

Worldwide, abortion accounts for approximately 14% of pregnancy-related deaths, and septic abortion is a major cause of the deaths from abortion. Today, septic abortion is an uncommon event in the United States. The primary critical treatment is early curettage to remove infected and devitalized tissue even in the face of continued fetal heart tones. In cases of septic abortion, bacterial cultures should be taken from the cervix and blood. Gram staining of the specimen may reveal the causative bacterial agent. Broad-spectrum antibiotics in large doses should be instituted, with therapy being individualized when bacterial sensitivity patterns are available. The central venous pressure and urinary output may need to be monitored, the fluid and electrolyte balance carefully studied, and blood-gas analyses performed for the purpose of correcting any deficits. Antibiotic administration and fluid resuscitation provide necessary secondary levels of treatment. Most young physicians have never treated septic abortion. The pathophysiology of septic abortion involves infection of the placenta, especially the maternal villous space that leads to a high frequency of bacteremia. Symptoms and signs range from mild to severe. The microbes involved are usually common vaginal bacteria, including anaerobes, but occasionally potentially very serious and lethal infection is caused by bacteria that produce toxins. Important secondary treatments are the administration of fluids and antibiotics.[40]

Once an inevitable, incomplete, or missed abortion has been diagnosed, there are several options. The first is expectant management. The second is medical abortion, using pharmacologic agents. Otherwise uterine evacuation can be elected. This is chosen also to manage pregnancy termination. Choice of technique for uterine evacuation depends on the uterine volume, the operator experience, and the cultural habits of the land. The choices include manual or electric vacuum aspiration, or dilation and evacuation (D&E) or dilation and curettage (D&C). This chapter focuses on the surgical options through uterine evacuation.

SURGICAL MANAGEMENT IN THE FIRST TRIMESTER

Nowadays surgical management is chosen for women who do not want to wait for a pregnancy to pass spontaneously or with medication evacuation and who wish to avoid the experience of pain and bleeding that accompanies the passage of the products of conception.

Before uterine aspiration cervical preparation is necessary to allow insertion of instruments and removal of the products of conception. Adequate cervical preparation can help minimize the occurrence of procedure-related complications. We strongly recommend the use of either hygroscopic dilators or prostaglandins to gradually dilate the cervix hours before a uterine evacuation, in order to avoid cervical trauma.

The selection of method for D&C should be based on the characteristics of each instrument.

Tenaculum

The employment of a single-toothed tenaculum will focus tension on a small area of the cervix, making laceration of that site more likely. The double-toothed tenaculum will lessen the effect. Some consider the bullet-type tenaculum efficient in preventing this complication. Several types of tenacula are presented in Figure 9.2. Multiple tenacula are

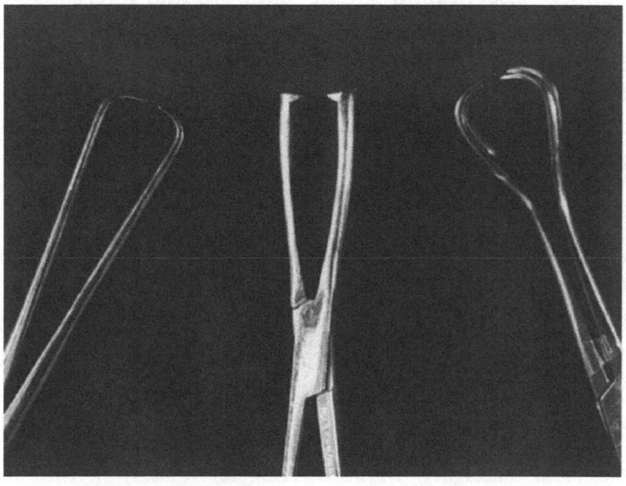

Figure 9.2 Various types of tenacula. From left to right: single-toothed, bullet type, multiple toothed.

of particular value when there is distortion of the cervix due to previous surgery or if a local lesion is present.

Dilator

A great variety of possibilities are available to dilate the cervix. The choice will vary with the condition of the cervix, the available time, and the personal preference of the surgeon. Dilation of the cervix can be performed with rigid, osmotic, balloon, and medicated dilators. If there is no medical condition (e.g., bleeding) requiring intervention, a medical rather than an instrumental approach may be considered. Injury to the cervix from dilation is positively related to the extent of dilation and inversely to the period of time over which the procedure is performed.

Hygroscopic dilators (laminaria, synthetic tents)

Removal of fluid from the cervix is primarily responsible for dilation of 0–12 mm. Hygroscopic dilators absorb water, sufficient to account for cervical dilation on the basis of volume reduction. The conventional dilator forces fluid from the cervix into the soft tissue of the lower uterine segment. Distention of tissues in this area can be detected. Dilators above 9 mm force fluid into the lower uterine segment in excess of available tissue space, resulting in displacement of the inner wall of this area of the uterus down into the path of the dilator. At higher levels of dilation, the fluid is forced farther up the uterine wall. The balloon dilator exerts uniform pressure on the entire area, not allowing movement of fluid out of the cervix and is, therefore, less effective in causing dilation.

The laminaria is prepared from seaweed (*Laminaria digitata*) which is sterilized and rolled into a small, compact, tubular structure approximately 6 cm in length. It is prepared in three diameters: small (3–5 mm), medium (6–8 mm), and large (8–10 mm). Upon exposure to a moist environment, it will increase three to four times in diameter over a 6- to 8-hour period. Its use is not associated with injury to the cervix.

Synthetic dilators (e.g., Dilapan [polyacrylonitrile], Lamicel [magnesium sulfate sponge]), and alternatively, *Laminaria japonica* are often used. These osmotic dilators serve to dilate the endocervical canal by absorbing cervical moisture. This uptake of water and the resulting expansion of the dilator produces both softening of the cervix and dilation of the endocervical canal in 4–6 hours.[41,42]

Artificial cervical dilator devices

A variety of balloon-type devices have been used to dilate the cervix.[43] The device is inserted into the cervical canal and inflated with fluid. It may be left in place up to 24 hours. A significant, immediate expulsion rate, as well as considerable pain, is associated with the instillation of the fluid.

Medical dilator

Cervical ripening in first-trimester abortion can be achieved with prostaglandins; progesterone agonists; prostaglandin analogs, such as sulprostone, gemeprost, and misoprostol; and a folic acid analog.

Prostaglandins

Prostaglandins (PG) are believed to play a critical biologic role in the control of cervical function. Various commercial PGE2 formulations are currently available for cervical ripening (intravenous solutions, intravaginal tablets, intracervical gel, intravaginal gel, intravaginal insert with retrieval system, and vaginal suppositories).[44,45]

Misoprostol is a synthetic 15-deoxy-16-hydroxy-16-methyl analog of naturally occurring PGE1. It is a viscous oil susceptible to the same types of chemical degradation as natural PGE, stable at room temperature. This means that the drug is easily stored and transported. Misoprostol exhibits a wide range of biologic activities. It is protective of the gastric mucosa, and has vasodilator, immunosuppressive, and uterotonic effects. The uterotonic features of misoprostol are of value in pregnancy termination and in the medical management of miscarriage. Vaginal misoprostol provides safe and effective preoperative dilation.[46–48] A dose of 400 μg per vaginam 2–3 hours prior to the procedure is recommended attempting to determine optimal dosing.[48,49] In a study using oral misoprostol-alone abortion regimens although most women experienced some side effects, regimens were tolerable and acceptable. Five of the seven regimens resulted in complete abortion rates of 60% or less. Only repeated doses of misoprostol resulted in efficacy exceeding 60%. Misoprostol-alone abortion regimens using oral misoprostol are too ineffective for clinical use or further investigation.[47]

The PGE1 analog *gemeprost* (1 mg per vaginam 3 hours before surgery) is commonly used, too.

Antiprogestins

Many processes in female reproductive physiology depend on progesterone. This hormone facilitates the action of estradiol in inducing the luteinizing hormone (LH) surge in the follicular cycle and supports the luteal phase. A compound action of progesterone plays an important role in the interruption of pregnancy. With the identification of the progesterone receptor came the realization that its antagonist was a potential candidate for such a compound.

Mifepristone is similar in structure to progesterone and glucocorticoids, but lacks the C19 methyl group and the two-carbon side chain at C17 of these hormones and has a conjugated C9–C10 double bond. The chemical structures of other synthetic antiprogestins are similar to that of mifepristone.[45]

The antiprogestin action of mifepristone is mediated by the PR, a ligand-activated transcription factor with domains for DNA binding, hormone binding, and transactivation. Members of this nuclear receptor superfamily include androgen, estrogen, and mineralocorticoid receptors, as well as receptors for thyroid hormones, retinoids, and vitamin D. Mifepristone binds to the progesterone and glucocorticoid receptors.

Progesterone and mifepristone produce a conformational change in the form of progesterone receptor that permits it to bind to DNA. Its activation by progesterone or mifepristone is accompanied by a loss of associated heat-shock proteins and dimerization. The activated receptor dimer binds to progesterone-response elements in the promoter region of progesterone-responsive genes. In the case of progesterone, this binding will increase the transcription rate of these genes, producing progestin effects. In contrast, a receptor–dimer complex that has been activated by mifepristone also binds to progesterone response elements, but an inhibitory function in the C-terminal region of the hormone-binding domain renders these DNA-bound receptors transcriptionally inactive. This is the basis for the progesterone-antagonistic action of mifepristone, underlying its abortifacient and contraceptive actions.[50,51]

Methotrexate is a folic acid analog that competitively inhibits dihydrofolate reductase, an enzyme necessary for the DNA synthesis. Methotrexate is approved for use in treating certain cancers, psoriasis, and rheumatoid arthritis. Treatment for ectopic pregnancy and early abortion represents off-label use of the drug.[52]

Instruments of surgical evacuation

Types of surgical instruments used to dilate the cervix

The conventional type of dilator is pressed against the external os, causing dilation of the opening. Examples of this type are the Hegar, Pratt, Hank, or Hawkin–Ambler dilators. The Hegar dilator increases in 0.5-mm increments and has a rounded tip, unlike the modified types that have tapered ends (Figure 9.3). The latter types permit more gradual dilation of the cervix and require less force during use, and therefore the potential for injury to the cervix is less.

Curette

Curettes vary in size as well as in the structure of the curetting surface. The surface may be smooth and sharp, with one continuous "cutting" surface, or serrated with teeth of varying sizes. Injury to the myometrium is more likely to occur with the latter (Figure 9.4). The zeal of the surgeon in performing the curettage can be a factor in the production of injury to the myometrium and resultant scarring. Other instruments include uterine sounds, ovum forceps, weighted speculum, right-angle retractors, and malleable probe (Figure 9.5).

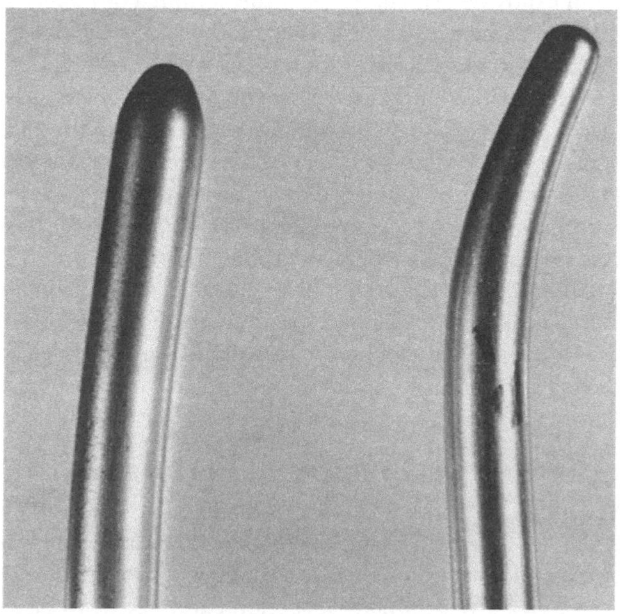

Figure 9.3 Pratt dilator (right) and Hegar dilator (left).

DILATION AND CURETTAGE FOR EVACUATION OF THE UTERUS

The procedure can be inpatient or ambulatory. Various anesthetic techniques can be used, including paracervical block or general anesthesia. Anesthetic agents that promote uterine relaxation (e.g., halothane) should be avoided. Prior to curettage, the patient should be examined under anesthesia to determine the size and position of the uterus.

After proper placement of the patient on the operating table in the lithotomy position and induction of anesthesia, the vagina and perineum are cleansed in the usual manner. No shaving or clipping of vulva/perineal hair is necessary or desirable. The urinary bladder is emptied.

A weighted speculum is placed in the vagina and a small, right-angle retractor is inserted anteriorly to expose the cervix. The cervix is grasped with a tenaculum placed on the midportion of the anterior lip. Traction is gently made downward to straighten the cervicouterine angle. While this is being done, the urethral meatus should be protected from pressure of the instrument. Any tissue present in the cervical canal can be removed with forceps.

A sound that has been shaped to conform to the position of the uterus may be passed through the cervical canal into the uterine cavity. This procedure will give confirmatory information on the uterus and the angle between the cervical canal and the uterine cavity.

The sound should pass easily due to the dilation of the cervical canal occurring with the abortion process. The fundus of the uterus will be detected by resistance to further gentle passage of the sound. The degree of resistance

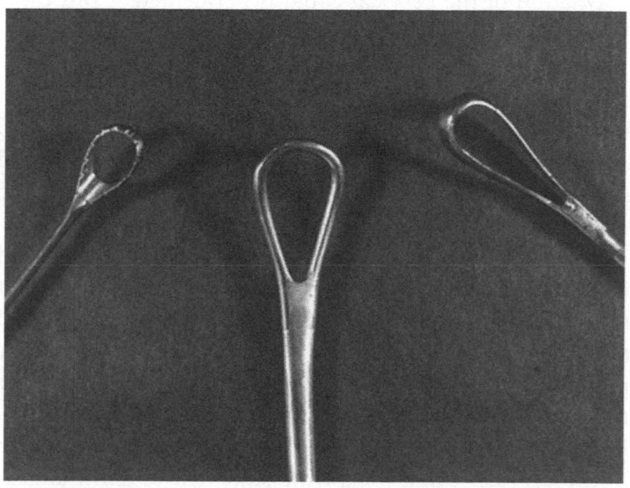

Figure 9.4 Curettes. From left to right: serrated, smooth, sharp, with one continuous cutting surface.

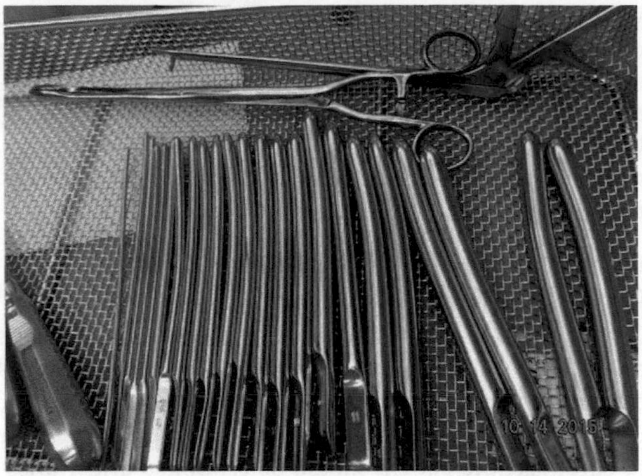

(a)

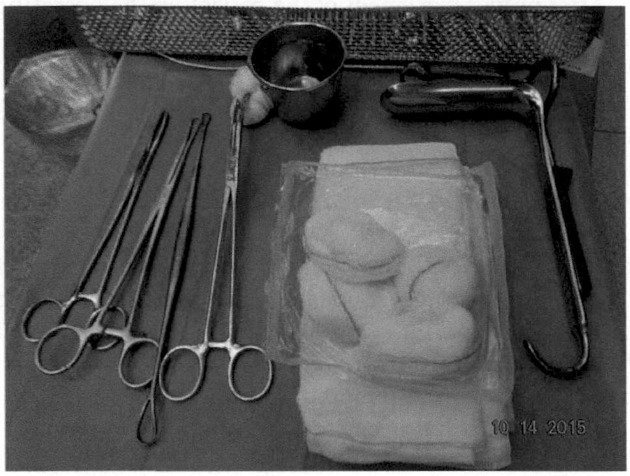

(b)

Figure 9.5 (a and b) Preparation of instruments for the operation.

will vary and may be minimal in some instances. Oxytocic agents can be administered prior to this step, but are of questionable value at the early stages of gestation.

Dilation of the cervical canal is performed at this time. Frequently, this is not required and may be harmful, especially in the young, nulliparous woman. The dilator, preferably a tapered dilator (e.g., Hanks), is gently grasped with the thumb below the instrument and the index, middle, and ring fingers above it. The little finger of the operator's hand should be supported against the perineum to minimize uncontrolled advancement of the dilator into the uterus. The tip of the dilator is inserted into the cervical canal and is advanced just beyond the internal os, using steady but minimal force. Resistance may be encountered at the level of the internal os. This can be overcome if constant, steady pressure is applied, rather than forceful thrusts. The latter maneuver can result in uncontrolled advance of the instrument and uterine perforation. Each dilator should remain in the cervical canal for a time sufficient to allow adjustment to that size before its removal. The dilator should be removed easily from the cervix before proceeding to insertion of the next larger size. Dilation should proceed to a size sufficient for curettage or evaluation to be performed. Generally, a dilator size 1 mm greater than the number of weeks of gestation is necessary. (With the use of medical dilators (e.g., misoprostol) cervix is dilated up till 7 mm in the case of primigravidae and $\geq$7 mm in multigravidae.)

In second-trimester abortions, digital exploration and evacuation of the uterus may be performed. The uterus should be positioned anteriorly. The index finger and, if possible, also the middle finger are inserted through the cervix into the uterine cavity, while the other hand is placed on the patient's abdomen to depress the fundus of the uterus. Any tissue that is felt is detached with the examining fingers and removed. The procedure is repeated until no additional tissue fragments are encountered.

A curved or straight ovum forceps (or similarly structured instrument) is introduced into the uterine cavity and the cavity systematically explored for tissue masses that can be removed. It is important that the operator introduce each instrument into the uterus with gentleness and caution.

The position of the uterus may change during the procedure. A retroverted uterus that has been repositioned anteriorly may not remain in place. The direction of the cavity must be determined during passage of the ovum forceps and also before they are opened and closed.

A standard procedure for curettage should be utilized. All areas of the uterine cavity are explored. The instrument is laid on the palmar surface of four fingers and held with the opposing thumb. The curette is introduced into the cervical canal and moved to the uterine fundus, whose resistance is gently appreciated. The curette should be pulled downward over the uterine wall while slight pressure is exerted on the inner surface of the instrument.

The curette should be removed as each area is explored to collect the tissue that has been obtained. The operator should discontinue the procedure once the yield of tissue is significantly decreased. At that time, minimal or no bleeding should be present. The uterine cavity should not be curetted too vigorously, since this can lead to removal not only of the functional layer of the endometrium, but also of the basalis. A grating sensation indicates that the curettage of the area should be discontinued. The decision of whether to proceed with currettage, if evacuation with finger exploration and ovum forceps appears to have completed the process, depends on the judgment of the surgeon.

All tissues obtained should be collected in a gauze bag placed around the weighted speculum. It should be rinsed free of blood and clots prior to submitting the tissue to pathology. The surgeon should note any intrauterine irregularities at the time of curettage.

VACUUM ASPIRATION (DILATION AND EVACUATION)

Vacuum aspiration of uterine contents seems to be preferable to sharp curettage.[53] When suction curettage was compared with conventional curettage for evacuation of the uterus, it was found that suction curettage was a faster procedure and also less painful. Can be used manual or electric vacuum aspirator.[54] Manual vacuum aspirator used at less than 10 weeks of gestation has its advantages: it may result in less pain and blood loss, it is more portable than the electric one, it is inexpensive, it does not require electricity, and it can be performed under local anesthesia. As an alternative to electric vacuum aspirations, the management of therapeutic abortion (TAB) and spontaneous abortion (SAB) supports an increasing interest in using the manual vacuum aspiration.[55]

The manual vacuum aspirator is a hand-activated syringe attached to a vacuum source. In the 50 or 60 mL syringe the vacuum is produced by retracting the plunger at the other end. The syringe is connected to a rigid or a flexible cannula. The products of conception are aspirated by rapidly withdrawing and depressing the syringe plunger 20–30 times. The cannula is moved in and out and simultaneously rotated in a 360° arc. The catheter is removed under continuous maximum negative pressure when aspiration of intrauterine contents appear to be complete. Suction will decrease when the syringe is 80% full (Figure 9.6).

Electric vacuum aspiration can be used for terminations at all gestational ages.[55]

In contrast to traditional curettage, it is the suction at the tip of the cannula, and not mechanical movement of the curette, that disrupts and separates the products of conception from their uterine attachment, facilitating removal. The relative vacuum created allows the pressure of the ambient atmosphere transmitted through the body of the mother to force the uterine contents into the collecting system. The vacuum may be considered in relative or absolute terms, depending on whether normal pressure (at sea level) is viewed as 0 or 760 mm Hg. At higher elevations, there will be an associated decrease in atmospheric pressure, with resultant reduction in available theoretical maximum vacuum from the approximate 1.0 kg/cm^2. A suction of 45 mm Hg (relative) is sufficient for completion of the procedure.

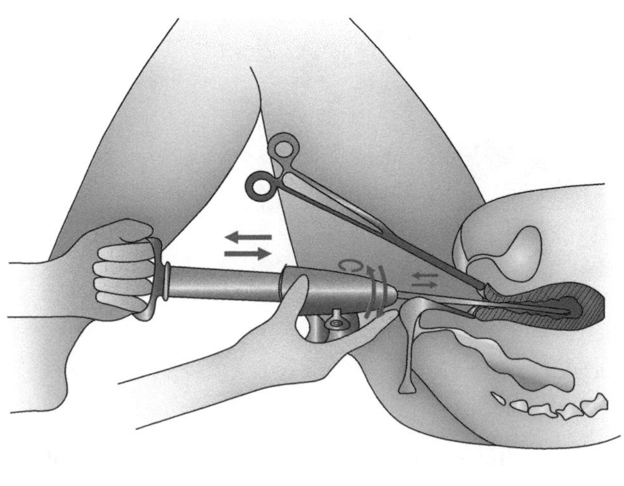

Figure 9.6 Manual vacuum aspiration: a vacuum is produced by retracting a plunger and products are aspirated by rapidly withdrawing and depressing the syringe plunger 20–30 times; simultaneously the cannula is moved in and out and rotated in a 360° arc.

Although the details of specific systems may vary, the principle is the same. A suction curette with a distal opening is placed in the uterus. The negative pressure is controlled by occluding an aperture in the proximal part of the curette. In this system, this control is provided by a sliding ring, which can be moved over the opening. The curette is connected by plastic tubing to a collection bottle, which contains a gauze trap for the tissue. There is a second collection bottle to increase the capacity of the system. The collection bottles are connected to the vacuum source.

The curettes are usually constructed of plastic and may be rigid or flexible. Generally, they have a rounded tip with one or more side openings. Selection of a cannula depends on the preference of the surgeon.

The preparation of the patient is similar to that described under conventional D&C. The patient is examined to confirm previous findings. A speculum is placed in the vagina to expose the cervix. The anterior lip of the cervix is grasped with a tenaculum, and gentle, downward traction is made. Since the suction curette is not placed into the fundus of the uterus, but just beyond the internal os of the cervix, sounding of the uterus may not be necessary. The cervical canal must be dilated sufficiently to permit insertion of the cannula.

A metal curette may be used at the end of the procedure to verify that all products of conception have been removed.

In missed abortion, there is usually sufficient time to dilate the cervix prior to suction cannula. The vacuum should not be instituted until the aperture of the cannula is just beyond the internal os of the cervix. When the cannula is withdrawn, similar precautions should be taken. Injury to the area of the internal os can occur when the suction cannula passes this area with the vacuum system operative.

The transparent tubing should be observed to ascertain the passage of the residual products of conception from the uterine cavity (Figure 9.7). The cannula should be slowly rotated to allow the aperture of the cannula to face all areas of the uterus. The cannula is not intended to "scrape" or curette the walls of the uterus. The vacuum dislodges fragments of tissue and delivers them to the suction curette. The procedure can be considered complete when the yield of tissue is greatly decreased and foamy serosanguinous fluid appears within the suction tubing.

MEDICAL TERMINATION OF PREGNANCY

Earlier the surgical evacuation was the most frequent method in the case of the evacuation of the uterus but medical methods for abortion have emerged over the past two decades as safe, effective, and feasible alternatives to surgery.[56] The choice of method depends on the gestational age, the availability and the patient's desire. Medication abortion is used to be performed up to 7–8 gestational weeks in incomplete spontaneous abort and missed abortion or socially (non-medically) indicated termination. It is less successful in the late first-trimester gestational weeks. Before the procedure, the patient must be informed of the advantages and disadvantages of both methods. Medication and surgical (cervical

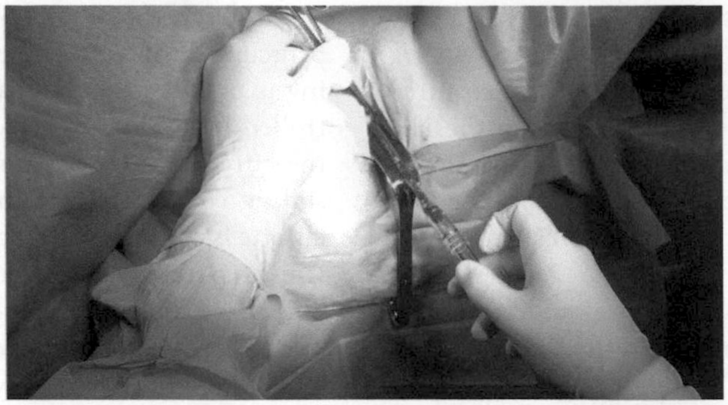

(a)

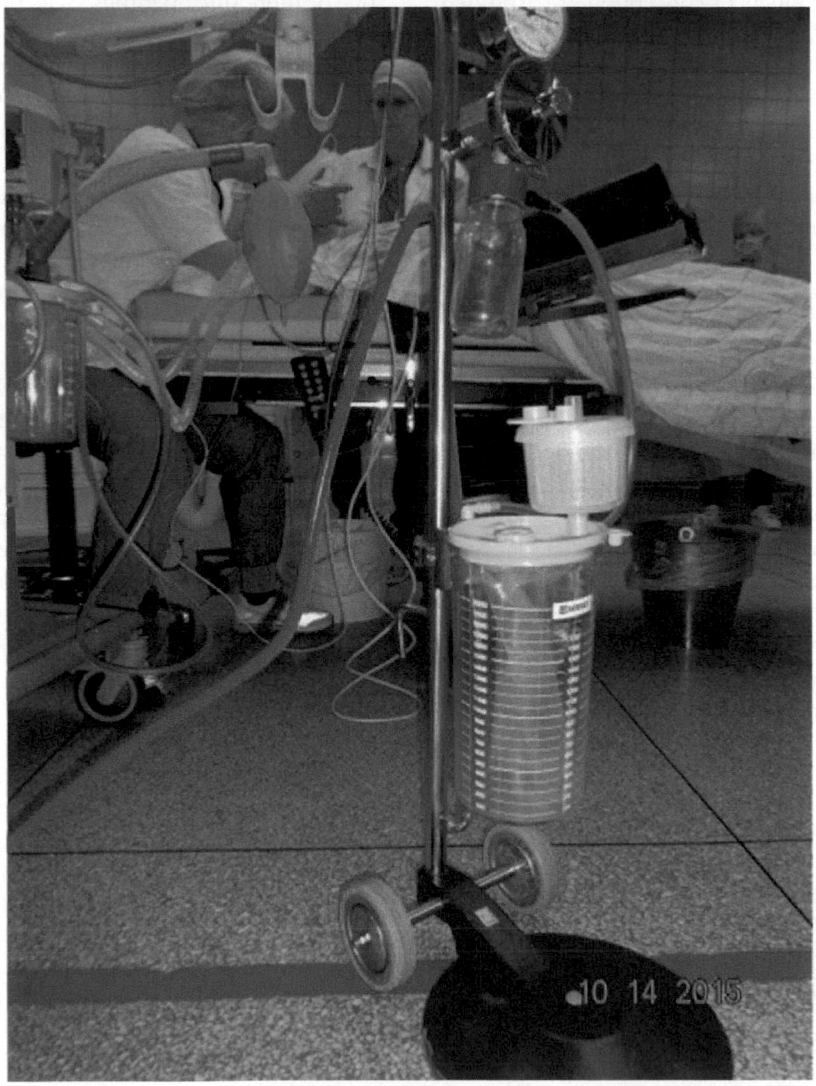

(b)

Figure 9.7 (a and b) Transparent tubing helps to visualize the products of conceptus.

D&E) abortion are both safe and effective approaches for appropriately selected patients with low complication rates.

In the management of medical evacuation there are several used regimens in clinical protocols. A time-tested method of application an oral mifepristone dose of 200 mg followed by misoprostol 400 μg vaginal after 48 hours which can be repeated (misoprostol 400 μg vaginal) after 6 and 12 hours. This is a method of the self-administration of misoprostol at home. In the case of missed abortion mifepristone can be omitted. In protocols and recommendations can be difference in the administration (self-administration, administered by a clinician), can be difference the time when misoprostol recommended to follow the mifepristone, between the route of administration (vaginal, oral, buccal, sublingual) and the dose of misoprostol.[57]

Before the procedure the ultrasound examination has an important role in the diagnosis of the gestational age and to exclude the ectopic pregnancy. After the termination, test for serum hCG can be the diagnostic procedure to exclude an ongoing pregnancy. These methods can be different following several protocols.

Many studies have compared the efficacy and complication rates of medical and surgical abortion. The efficacy of medical and surgical abortion at 9 weeks of gestation or less is extremely high and complications are infrequent. The most common complications with medical evacuation are ongoing pregnancy, unanticipated aspiration, persistent pain, bleeding, or both. The rate of serious complications was 0.1% in each groups, includes emergency department presentation, hospitalization, infection, perforation, and hemorrhage requiring transfusion.

MANAGEMENT OF MISSED ABORTION

Women with missed abortion can be managed with surgical (D&C [sharp or vacuum]) or medication (misoprostol), uterine evacuation or with expectant management.[58]

All three approaches have similar efficacy, and the choice of treatment method depends mainly on patient preference.

If medication is not available due to various reasons dilatation of the uterus cervix can be performed inter alia with laminaria.

During the first trimester and the early portion of the second one, missed abortion can be evacuated by suction curettage (Video 9.1). When the size of the uterus is considered too large for safe evacuation by D&C, medical induction should be used. Intravenous oxytocin is less effective in the second trimester than later in pregnancy in producing effective uterine contractions, but its effectiveness is improved if the cervix has undergone effacement and dilation. The preferred method of treatment is surgery through the insertion of a hygroscopic dilator into the cervical canal the evening before surgery.

The vagina and cervix should be surgically cleansed and the cervix stabilized with a tenaculum or sponge forceps. The laminaria is grasped with a sterile uterine dressing forceps and is inserted into the cervical canal until its distal tip passes the internal os. It should slide easily into the cervical canal. If the upper margin of the laminaria is not placed at the level of the internal os, it will expel itself during swelling. The proximal 5–10 mm should protrude from the external os. A folded sponge placed against the cervix will reduce the tendency for expulsion. The maximum swelling of the laminaria occurs over a 6- to 8-hour period. If further dilation is desired, it can be removed, and two small laminaria inserted in its place. It is preferable to use two small laminaria in parallel instead of a single large one.

The patient should remain recumbent after insertion to avoid vagal tone reaction and syncope. Most patients will have low abdominal cramps for a few minutes. These may recur, but are generally mild and can be relieved by analgesics. Failure of the laminaria to dilate the cervix occurs in a small percentage of patients due to its expulsion from the cervical canal. Fever and infection are infrequent complications of this procedure. Frequently, no further dilation of the cervix is required.

Follow-up

Part of the follow-up procedures after missed abortion can be the histopathological examination of the product of conception. Examinations for women, who pass the products of conception spontaneously or with the help of medication evacuation the control of the uterine cavity with ultrasound or measurements of serum human chorionic gonadotropin. Postabortion instructions, grief, and contraception counseling, information about interval to conception and future reproductive outcome may require.

Rh immunization and antibiotic prevention/treatment

Following the abortion, Rho (D) immunoglobulin (RhoGAM) should be administered to Rh-negative mothers at risk. A dose of 50 μg appears adequate to prevent sensitization in abortions occurring prior to 13 weeks' gestation. For abortions occurring at 13 weeks' gestation or later, a standard 300-μg dose is recommended.

Women with incomplete abortion may present with local and systemic evidence of infection. Generally, the infection is confined to the uterus. Antibiotic coverage should be directed to bacteria generally encountered in pelvic infection. Gram-negative aerobic and anaerobic organisms are usually present.[22] Since it is not possible to await the results of culture, treatment should be instituted on admission to the hospital. The clinical response usually is rapid once the uterus has been evacuated. Antibiotic treatment is continued during the immediate period or beyond if there is evidence of spread of the infection beyond the uterus.[59]

Complications

Complications relative to D&C of the uterus can be related to specific instrumentation. The cervix of the young nullipara, especially in early pregnancy, is resistant to dilation. This may predispose to injury of the cervix and perforation of the uterus. Signs and symptoms of the latter may not develop for several hours. Hemorrhage may be immediate or delayed. Trauma to the basal endometrium and myometrium may manifest at a later date as menstrual dysfunction or infertility (Asherman's syndrome).

Cervical laceration

The most common injury occurring during D&C is laceration of the cervix due to the tenaculum pulling free. It occurs more often with the single-toothed tenaculum. Lacerations that require repair occur in 1%–2% of procedures. Surgical repair should be performed after the completion of the D&C. In most instances, the lacerations are small and stop bleeding by the end of surgery.

Lacerations from the dilator may be more extensive, particularly in the young nullipara whose cervix is small and difficult to dilate. The amount of force exerted at the internal cervical os to produce dilation varies with stage of gestation, the type of dilator, and the extent of dilation. The cervix in the earlier stages of gestation requires greater force to produce dilation. As pregnancy progresses, less force is necessary. Age, race, and gravidity do not affect this finding. The cervix is most resistant to further dilation at 9 mm.

Only modest force is required to dilate the cervix sufficiently to accomplish evacuation. Gentle force is the least traumatic and most effective. When excessive effort is applied, the tenaculum may pull free from the cervix. If this happens, injury to the area of the internal cervical os may ensue.

False passage

When the sound or dilator is introduced without appropriate direction or control, a false cervical canal may be created. Persistence in dilation of this false passage may result in a significant laceration of the cervix, or in the formation of a canal which communicates with the vagina as a cervical fistula. Whenever there is difficulty in identifying the external cervical os (e.g., missed abortion), or if abnormal resistance is encountered during the passage of an instrument, the operator should reconfirm the position and direction of the cervical canal by gentle passage of a probe or sound.

Other cervical effects

An increased incidence of cervical pregnancy after D&C for induced abortion has been reported.[60] In rare instances, cervical or paracervical implantation of fetal tissue with subsequent symptomatology has occurred.[61]

Late effects of cervical injury may be manifest as cervical stenosis due to synechiae or reproductive failure due to cervical incompetency[62] (Figure 9.8).

Uterine hemorrhage

Bleeding during or after D&C for completion of an abortion is a frequent complication. Incomplete evacuation of the uterine contents is primarily responsible. The operative procedure should not be terminated until bleeding from the uterus is minimal and the organ is firmly contracted. Other causes of bleeding must be excluded. Generally, uterine bleeding is not associated with perforation. The cervix should be inspected carefully to determine any bleeding sites.

Since the operative procedure to empty the uterus is a "blind" one, it may not be possible to ascertain that all tissue has been removed. The symptoms caused by incomplete emptying of the uterus may be delayed, occurring after the patient has left the hospital. Bleeding and cramps, necessitate another D&C. Blood replacement should be provided as necessary. Sonography is capable of identifying retained products of conception in utero and is useful, therefore, for the diagnosis of incomplete evacuation.

In women undergoing medical termination of pregnancy vaginal bleeding is common and typically heavier than a period, but not usually excessive. The mean duration of bleeding ranges from 8 to 17 days but may be prolonged. Usually there is not necessary therapy because of the blood loss. In the case of bleeding persists for more than 1 week, unanticipated aspiration is performed, if retained products of conception is suspected.

Perforation

The quoted incidence of uterine perforation at time of D&C is derived primarily from data relating to elective termination of pregnancy. In these reports the rate of

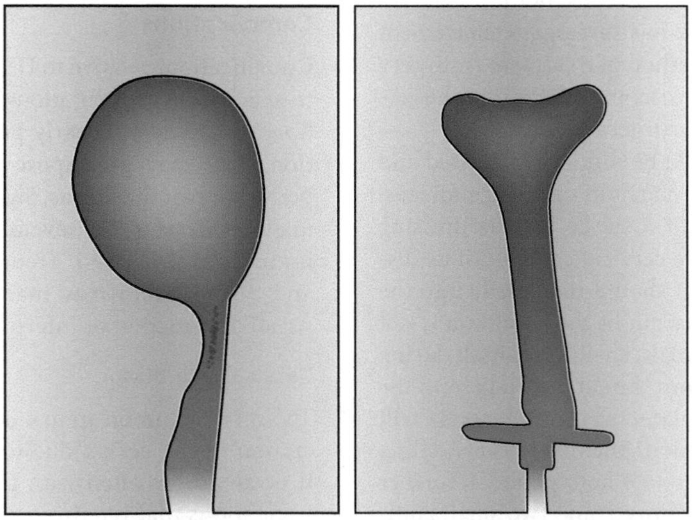

(a) (b)

Figure 9.8 Schematic representation of cervical changes in nulliparous women following first-trimester pregnancy termination. The original research rested upon cervicohysterographic studies performed immediately before (a) and 8 weeks after (b) the abortion procedures. Note the loss of the original structure of the isthmus uteri. Also note that these abortions were done prior to the introduction of the suction apparatus into gynecologic practice. (From Árvay A et al., *Rev Franc Gynec Obstet*, 62, 81–86, 1967.)

perforations varies from 0.75 to 15 per 1000 procedures. Some believe that the incidence of unrecognized perforations is many times higher. Perforation can result from any instrument, but it occurs most frequently during sounding of the uterus. For this reason many experts omit this step. Knowledge of the position of the uterus prior to instrumentation helps to avoid this complication. Not only anteroposterior uterine orientation should be determined, but lateral deviation as well. Inspection of the vaginal fornices may suggest lateral displacement when one fornix is much wider than the other. Confirmation can be obtained by observing the direction the sound or the smallest dilator takes when it is passed into the uterus. Downward traction with a tenaculum on the cervix will tend to straighten the cervicouterine angle and avoid perforation.

All instruments should be advanced slowly into the uterus. Dilators should be introduced just beyond the internal os. Suction cannulas also should be introduced to this depth and the products of conception aspirated with the cannula in this position. The cervix of early pregnancy (8 weeks or less) or of the young, nulliparous woman is most resistant to dilation. Forceful efforts must be avoided.

Perforation can be diagnosed when there is a sudden decrease in resistance to an instrument, or passage occurs to a depth greater than the measured size of the uterine cavity. This latter finding may not be reliable in lateral perforations where the structures of the intraligamentar space may limit the passage of the perforating tool. Perforation is definitely established with the recovery of obvious extrauterine tissue.

When the surgery is performed under local anesthesia, perforation may be suspected if the patient develops pain. If the perforation occurs in the midline of the uterus, she will experience severe midline pain that subsides rapidly; while with a lateral perforation, the pain is severe, persistent, and localized to the affected side.

Management will depend on circumstances, but discontinuation of the operative procedure is essential whenever perforation is suspected. The site of perforation should be noted, particularly in reference to the lateral or midline area of the uterus. The patient's vital signs must be closely monitored. A laparotomy is indicated if the perforation has resulted in removal of fat or other extrauterine tissue, if there is evidence of shock, if there has been extensive, previous abdominal surgery, if the patient is very obese, or if the urine is bloody.

If the perforation is midline and there is no urgent indication (e.g., bleeding) for completion of the evacuation, observation can be performed and the procedure completed somewhat later under laparoscopic guidance. The laparoscopist can guide the other operator away from the perforation site and observe contraction of the uterus as it is emptied. The perforation site is inspected for size, bleeding, and extrusion of the products of conception. Large lacerations with active bleeding and/or extruded products of conception require laparotomy.

When the perforation is in the lateral portion of the uterus, the uterus is empty, and there is no indication for laparotomy, ultrasound and in some instances laparoscopy should be performed. The broad ligament areas should be thoroughly inspected. If an extraperitoneal hematoma is observed, it should be watched for a change in size. An increase in size is an indication for laparotomy for control of the bleeding. The serosal surface of the bladder and bowel is inspected as completely as possible through the laparoscopy. If more than superficial injury is noted, laparotomy should be performed.

If none of the abovementioned complications exist or develop and the patient is stable, she may be discharged after 24–48 hours of observation. Sonography should be utilized to define the hematoma and to observe its resolution.

Synechiae

Curettage of the pregnant or recently pregnant uterus is the primary antecedent factor for the development of intrauterine synechiae.[63] Elective termination of a pregnancy and D&C for incomplete abortion are the most commonly associated factors. The former group is at a higher risk than the latter. The technique of sharp curettage is particularly traumatic to the endometrium. Trauma to the basal layer of the endometrium predisposes to adherence of the anterior and posterior uterine walls. Local infection also may play a role.

PREVENTION OF SPONTANEOUS ABORTIONS

After one spontaneous abortion, the risk of another in the next pregnancy is not significantly higher than in the general population. The prevention of spontaneous abortion is mainly directed toward correcting etiologic factors conducive to recurrent abortion.[39,64] A detailed history of previous abortions must be taken; careful physical and pelvic examinations performed; and andrologic, immunologic, radiologic, and other relevant laboratory tests done.[65,66]

Prior to conception, maternal disorders such as diabetes mellitus and hypothyroidism should be adequately treated. In the case of uterine abnormalities, where congenital or acquired have been demonstrated, proper operative procedure (metroplasty) should be performed. (Anomalies connected with duplication of the uterus can be documented by hysterosalpingography and/or ultrasonography.)

Overripeness of the ovum, preovulatory or postovulatory or other anomalies in the mechanism of ovulation have been associated with an increased frequency of early spontaneous abortion.[67,68] In cases of recurrent abortions where ovopathies, abnormal ovulation, or luteal phase defects are suspected, induction of ovulation may be considered.

If the second or even the third pregnancy also ends in abortion, without obvious cause, it is justifiable to search for genetic reasons— chromosome rearrangement or X-linked dominant inheritance.[11,69] Both parents should have peripheral blood cultures set up for chromosome analysis. There may be an opportunity to examine aborted products of conception. If a parent is found to carry a balanced rearrangement, and there is as yet no healthy child, the outlook is unfavorable. When a parent carries a chromosome rearrangement, options include prenatal diagnosis (chromosome analysis), artificial insemination by donor (AID), *in vitro* fertilization, or adoption. The question of X-linked dominant inheritance can be answered by clinical and genealogical examination. Also recommended are investigations for evidence of antiphospholipid and thrombophilia syndromes.[23–26]

Incarceration of the retroflexed uterus

This entity represents the only circumstance where an otherwise inevitable abortion can be prevented. On very rare occasions, a uterus in fixed retroflexion becomes trapped in the true pelvis. The patient is usually asymptomatic during the first trimester and, thus the condition remains unrecognized initially. However, around weeks 13–14 the gravida becomes symptomatic. Pelvic discomfort appears first. This is followed by urinary retention. If the condition remains unrecognized and, thus, untreated, the patient ends up in the emergency room on account of excruciating pelvic pain associated with inability to void. On account of the rarity of this complication, it may remain undiagnosed even at this point. If so, the bladder becomes immensely distended and its walls thickened due to edema. Portions of the mucous membrane may slough off and, in the same process, urinary tract infection develops and escalates into severe pyelonephritis. The distended bladder, particularly in connection with carelessly performed pelvic examination, may rupture. In the absence of timely surgical intervention, this complication can be fatal. The same is true of the alternative final outcome; development of ischemic necrosis in the uterine walls leading to pelvic and later generalized peritonitis.

For an examiner who is mindful of this clinical entity, the diagnosis is easy. The woman's excruciating pain, her inability to void, the extreme distension of the bladder, the tenderness of the lower abdomen to touch, and the associated guarding are almost diagnostic. A careful pelvic examination makes the diagnosis conclusive through the palpation of the uterus filling the posterior part of the pelvis. Not infrequently, the cervix is out of the examiner's reach as it points upward towards the ramus of the pubic bone.[70]

Whereas probably most cases of incarceration could be prevented by the use of a Hodge pessary and by the mother spending the night in the prone position, because the retroflexed uterus only rarely becomes trapped, such measures are almost never taken prophylactically. Almost invariably, the diagnosis is made when the gravida becomes symptomatic and even then, sometimes with considerable delay. By that time, the correction of the complication no longer is simple.

The removal of the uterus from its entrapped position usually requires major anesthesia. Far too often, the patient's discomfort is so extreme, that she cannot cooperate with the somewhat time-consuming process of administering a spinal anesthesia. On this account, general anesthesia is probably the most suitable for this procedure.

With the patient in the lithotomy position, after catheterization of the urinary bladder, the operator introduces two or, if possible more, fingers into the posterior fornix of the vagina. Some degree of force is needed to lift the uterus out of its entrapped position and push it into the false pelvis. The external hand takes over at this point and holds the uterus in its new position in front of the promontory of the sacrum. Later this function is taken over by an assistant, while the operator packs the fornix with gauze in order to prevent the return of the organ into its previous position. When removed 24 hours later, the gauze pack may be replaced with a pessary. With or without such measures, once lifted out from the true pelvis, the uterus seldom returns to its entrapped position. When rarely it does, the same procedure needs to be repeated. Fortunately, the growth of the uterus precludes its later entrapment as the pregnancy progresses.

This technique permits the correction of uterine entrapment in the overwhelming majority of the instances. If it fails, it can be repeated with a finger introduced into the rectum. However, if this is still unsuccessful, the complication requires immediate laparotomy. Thus, manual correction is best performed under double setup. If attempts at emptying the bladder have been unsuccessful, its overdistension must be relieved by suprapubic puncture before the abdominal incision. Once the abdomen is open, manual elevation of the pregnant uterus from the posterior pelvis seldom entails significant difficulty. If it does, allowing air to enter the space behind the organ may facilitate the procedure. If everything fails, removal of some of the amniotic fluid by uterine puncture may prove helpful. Alternatively, or in combination with the latter, the use of an obstetric vacuum extractor may be warranted.[57]

If everything fails, and particularly in those cases where necrosis of the myometrium is a threat, hysterotomy, and evacuation of the products of conception may be the ultimate solution. It has been suggested that in this eventuality antefixation of the uterus should be part of the surgical procedure.

PROCEDURES FOR MIDTRIMESTER-INDICATED TERMINATION

With the development of genetic counseling, new information has become available to affected patients and families. Prenatal diagnosis with the option of termination of pregnancy provides important reassurance for couples at risk of genetic disorders.

Conventional techniques

In patients up to 12 weeks' gestation, conventional techniques are used, including cervical dilation, either instrumental or medical, followed by vacuum aspiration or curettage. Intracervical laminaria and PG induce fetal ejection: the embryo is usually delivered whole, thus permitting pathologic examination.[11,71,72]

After week 12, generally abortion is induced medically. However, D&E also is a common technique for second-trimester pregnancy termination.[73,74] During the induction, the fetus usually is expelled completely. Nonetheless, instrumental emptying of the uterus is often required, on account of incomplete expulsion of the placenta.

Ideally, induction of abortion should not damage the fetus, and should allow full histopathologic examination, and further investigations where appropriate.[61] It is often necessary to dilate the cervix and stimulate uterine contractions for the expulsion of the products of conception. These requirements are partly met by the use of (1) PG, PG analogs, and antiprogesterones[75]; (2) intra-, and extra-amniotic abortificiant (hypertonic saline, and other solutions)[11,76]; (3) pretreatment with laminaria or synthetic dilators; and (4) concurrent intravenous oxytocin. In rare cases, abdominal hysterotomy may be considered.

Cervical ripening and induction

The role of the cervix in pregnancy has been often oversimplified. It was thought that it simply acts as a sphincter in pregnancy which relaxed during delivery. In fact, although in early pregnancy the cervix is long and tight, it begins to shorten, open, and relax by midgestation, a process termed "ripening."

In the cervical connective tissue, biochemical and biophysical changes are initiated by estrogens and PG. Cross-bridges between collagen molecules are broken, and the glycosaminoglycan and proteoglycan contents of the matrix increase. Cervical connective tissue fibroblasts synthesize PG in large amounts; these in turn stimulate collagen metabolism with diminished collagen synthesis and increased breakdown.[77]

Cervical ripening can be achieved with PG, progesteron agonits, and PG analogs. Various commercial PGE2 formulations are currently available (intravenous solutions, intravaginal tablets, intracervical gel, intravaginal gel, intravaginal insert with retrieval system, and vaginal suppositories).

PG and PG analogs

PG are naturally occurring fatty acid derivatives with a wide range of applications in obstetrics, especially relating to midtrimester pregnancy termination.[78] Intravaginal or rectal misoprostol, usually 400 μg about every 4 hours, is very safe and effective for second-trimester medical uterine evacuation, and should be the preferred technique for this clinical scenario.

Current protocols for second-trimester induction abortion typically include a PG, usually misoprostol, and may utilize mifepristone or oxytocin.[79] Oxytocin, the most commonly used induction agent at later gestational ages fails to induce labor as effectively as the other single agent therapy at midtrimester because the uterus has relatively fewer oxytocin receptors at less than 20 weeks of gestation. Oxytocin is associated with longer induction abortion intervals than newer methods, as well as higher risks of side effects such as postpartum hemorrhage and even water intoxication. Patients desiring medical abortion in the second trimester now have safer, more effective options, utilizing PG agents either alone or in combination with progesterone antagonists. Several PG agents have been used to induce abortion:

- Carboprost, a PGF2alpha analog, results in more systemic side effects than PG E analogs.[80]
- Sulprostone, a PGE2 analog, has fallen out of favor because it has been associated with myocardial infarction.[81]
- Gemeprost and misoprostol, both PGE1 analogs, are the most common medications currently used for induction abortion.[82–84]

Comparative studies have found that both misoprostol and gemeprost induce labor more effectively and with fewer side effects than other prostaglandins (e.g., carboprost, sulprostone) and than single agent oxytocin or oxytocin in combination with other types of prostaglandins.[80] Both misoprostol and gemeprost induce labor at a variety of gestational ages. The dose decreases as pregnancy advances because the uterus becomes more sensitive to PG with decreasing dose requirements as pregnancy advances.

Recently, the most used technique is misoprostol as a single agent for medical termination of pregnancy in 13–22 weeks. Route of administration in these cases, mostly is the vaginal one. Vaginal administration includes greater efficacy and fewer side effects, although there is evidence that women would prefer an oral route of administration to avoid painful vaginal examinations.

Termination of pregnancy can be successful within 48 hours in 100% of those, who receive misoprostol vaginally, that number is about 86% within 24 hours.[85,86] Protocols of dosing can be difference, a well-established possibility 400 μg per vaginam every three hours maximum five times daily.

Monitoring the patient during the procedure is necessary. The goals of monitoring are to assess treatment efficacy and assess for complications.

After expulsion of the placenta it should be examined to see whether it is complete (Figure 9.9). In the postabortion period women should be observed for at least four hours to monitor vital signs and observe for severe abdominal pain or excessive vaginal bleeding. Late complication can be fever, apart from the mentioned.

Intravenous administration of PGFa and PGE2 causes side effects—erythema, nausea, vomiting, and diarrhea—that are very troublesome. Intraamniotic injection of PG is an accepted method of termination. For this purpose, PGF2a is the most suitable. Results are somewhat better when PG are introduced extraamniotically. A blunt-tipped, flexible plastic or rubber cannula can be introduced between the uterine wall and the fetal membranes, for injection or infusion. Giving PG by this route requires a lower dosage, since the injected drug rapidly reaches the myometrium. Dosage for PGF2a would be 750 μg every 2 hours; for PGE2, 200 ng every 2 hours. Repeated injections must be given.[75,87,88]

Natural PG cannot be given intramuscularly, as they are highly irritating locally. However, PG analogs can. They have also been given in vaginal pessaries and jelly. PGF2a should not be used in active cardiac, pulmonary, renal, or hepatic disease and is relatively contraindicated for patients suffering from bronchial asthma,

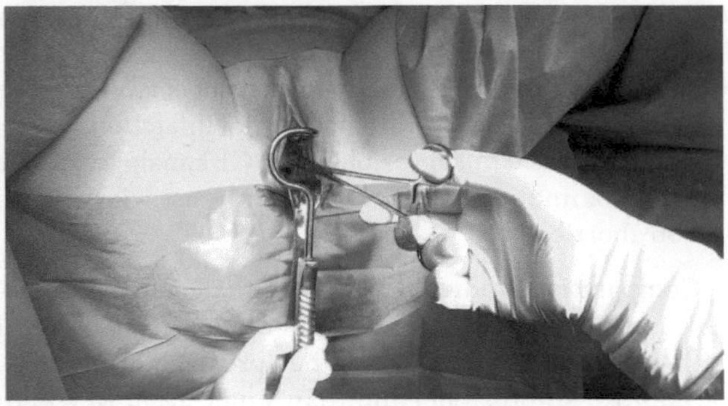

(a)

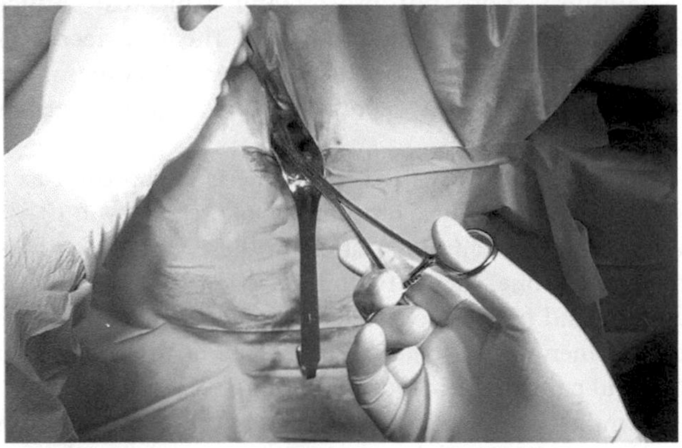

(b)

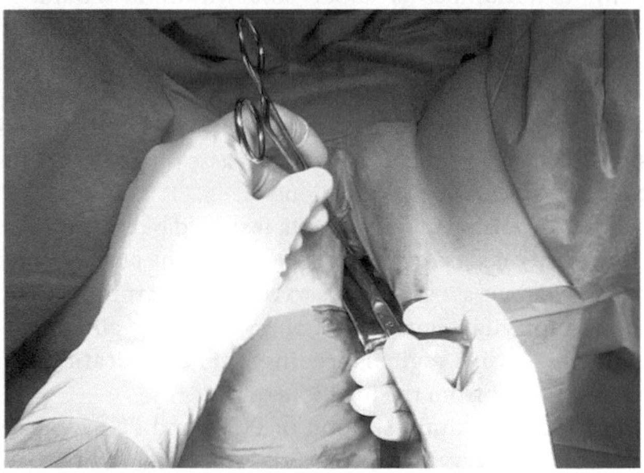

(c)

Figure 9.9 (a through c) Removal of the remnants of the conceptus after using misoprostol and mifepristone.

hypertension or sickle cell disease. PG do not damage the fetus; thus the histopathologic examination is not interfered with. However, they have undesirable side effects, and even maternal death has occasionally been reported.[89] Preference should be given to PGE2 as a local preparation for cervical ripening.

The mother's vital functions must be checked at regular intervals. The application can be repeated up to three times daily. The gel is preferable to the sponge. It rarely causes uterine hypertonus and is less likely to provoke premature rupture of the membranes. The membranes should be broken only when the internal os and the cervix appear sufficiently ripe. Oxytocin infusion can then be started, if desired.

The membranes should never be ruptured with an unripe cervix. In cases of gross hydrocephalus, or abdominal distension, with a nonviable fetus, cephalocentesis (ventriculocentesis), or abdominocentesis may be performed during labor, to preserve the birth canal and facilitate vaginal delivery.[90,91]

Rh-negative patients should be given anti-D gamma globulin at the time of any invasive procedure, or termination (200–300 μg, irrespective of gestational age).

Hypertonic saline

Intra-amniotic injection of hypertonic saline (50 mL of 20% sodium chloride) leads to abortion. Fetal death and expulsion result from dehydration. Although not without danger, this technique is still used sometimes for midtrimester termination.

Transabdominal amniocentesis is performed under local anesthesia (1% lidocaine) with a 1.2-mm diameter needle (thicker than that used in diagnostic amniocentesis). Amniotic fluid is withdrawn, approximately 10 mL for every week of gestation, and 50–100 mL of sterile 20% saline is injected. The injection must be given into the amniotic fluid. If given subcutaneously, intraperitoneally, or into the myometrium, it may cause pain and serious complications.[11]

Uterine contractions are felt immediately after injection. The uterus becomes tense and enlarges. As the injected Na and Cl ions reach the maternal circulation, the mother feels thirst.

Entry of saline into the maternal circulation provokes blushing, feeling of heat and nausea, falling blood pressure, bradycardia, and, occasionally, cardiac arrest. Saline induction must never be employed under general anesthesia or in the presence of hypertension, cardiac, or renal disease.

Late complications of hypertonic saline induction include various coagulopathies, especially drops in factor V and factor VIII levels. The platelet count may also fall, the prothrombin time increase, and fibrin degradation products appear. Such changes seldom emerge less than a few hours after injection. Most commonly, they present 10–24 hours later. Thus, women should not leave the hospital within 24 hours of the induction.

The fetal heart usually fails within 2 hours of the saline injection. Abortion occurs in about 24–36 hours. In 10% of the cases, the uterine contractions are poor and oxytocin needs to be given (5–30 IU in 500 mL 5% glucose infusion). This method has the advantage that the aborted fetus rarely shows signs of life.

As an alternative to hypertonic saline, intra-amniotic 50% glucose solution has been used. This avoids hypernatremia, but the induction is slow. Glucose is a good culture medium; thus, prophylactic antibiotics may have to be given.

Intraamniotic hypertonic urea solution has also been used, but is an inefficient way of inducing abortion. All hypertonic injection techniques have the relative disadvantage that they damage the fetus; thus, histopathologic examination is difficult or impossible, although the placenta and membranes may still be suitable for cytogenetic and biochemical examination.

DECISION MAKING REGARDING THE FATE OF PREGNANCY

Termination of pregnancy, with the aim of preventing the birth of a fetus with an incurable disorder, is a traumatic and unhappy option. However, this procedure is frequently performed. When there is a hope of treatment for a prenatally diagnosed disorder, premature induction of labor may prevent in utero progression of the disease and/or permit prompt postnatal surgery (e.g., in case of omphalocele ruptured in utero). Between these two extremes there are a great number of disorders, very variable in severity, which demand individual judgment. It seems justified to outline some general principles relating to the decision-making process in the pregnancy situation.[11,92]

- *Condition 1: correct genetic diagnosis.* The diagnosis, in affected child or adult, or in the fetus in utero, must be made with up-to-date methods and the results recorded in writing *(ethics of the clinician/the investigator; ethics of the laboratory).*
- *Condition 2: adequately informed parents.* No matter what their level of education, every couple must be informed and, as far as possible, made to understand the nature of the disease in question, its severity, its prognosis, and the possibilities of cure or treatment *(ethics of the counselor; ethics of genetic counseling).*
- *Condition 3: free decision by the parents.* The couple may choose to continue the pregnancy, or they may choose its termination (ethics of the couple/the parents; ethics of the family).
- *Condition 4: actions taken are within the law.* Society creates laws that regulate the termination of pregnancy. These and the professional codes and regulations provide a framework within which each case must be evaluated individually (*ethics of society; public health ethics*).

Medical indications for termination

Risk to the mother's life

Termination of pregnancy may be permitted at any time when serious illness threatens the mother's life (e.g., heart failure, life-threatening obstetric complications). In such cases the doctor in charge documents the illness in the notes.

Risk of genetic disorder or teratogenic damage

When the risk of genetic disorder or teratogenic damage to the fetus is high, the disorder/damage is likely to be severe, and prenatal diagnosis is not available, termination up to week 12 of pregnancy in many countries is permitted.

Risk of genetic disease or malformation

When the risk of serious genetic disease or malformation in the fetus is 50%–100%, and there is no possibility of treatment, termination may be permitted until week 20 in some countries and up to week 24 in others.

1. The theoretical probability of fetal disease is 100%: a parent carries a homologous balanced translocation (e.g., 21/21; a female fetus from a father carrying an X-linked mutant gene of a dominant trait, etc.).
2. There is 100% probability of a chromosome disorder associated with severe developmental retardation and physical defects; enzymopathies, congenital malformations, and other pathologic conditions (prenatal diagnosis).
3. The theoretical probability of a severe autosomal dominantly inherited disorder (e.g., Huntington's disease) is 50% or above.
4. A mother carrying an X-linked recessive gene is pregnant with a male fetus, and fetal hemizygosity cannot be excluded.
5. With prenatal exposure to rubella or cytomegalovirus infection, the fetal risk may reach the 50% level.

Occasionally, some serious fetal defect, likely to be fatal in the immediate postnatal period, is discovered. Such pregnancies, if continued, may be accompanied by obstetric complications threatening the mother's health (poly/oligohydramnios, placental abruption, uterine rupture, or uterine atony) and/or psychological disturbances (occasionally psychopathy).

Within the time limits permitted by the law, the mother must be given the option of pregnancy termination for a postnatally nonviable fetus, especially when her own health is endangered. Conditions considered incompatible with postnatal life include the following.[11]

1. Severe central nervous system malformations (e.g., anencephaly and/or rachischisis with or without hydrocephalus, hydranencephaly, alobar holoprosencephaly, iniencephaly).
2. Severe bilateral renal diseases (e.g., renal agenesis with Potter sequence, infantile-type polycystic kidney disease, multicystic kidney dysplasia).
3. Severe chromosome aberrations (e.g., triploidy, trisomy 13).
4. Neonatal lethal chondrodysplasia (e.g., thanatophoric dysplasia, achondrogenesis) and type II osteogenesis imperfecta.
5. Severe multiple forms of the amniotic deformity, adhesions, mutilations (ADAM) complex (e.g., craniofacial disruption, thoracoabdominal eventeration).

SELECTIVE TERMINATION IN MULTIPLE PREGNANCY

Improved ultrasound technology and invasive prenatal diagnostic procedures have facilitated the detection of fetal abnormalities in multiple gestations. Advances in assisted reproductive technologies also have led to an increased incidence of multiple gestation, particularly as result of ovulation induction.

Fetal disease or disorder in a twin pregnancy may be concordant or discordant. In the former situation both fetuses are affected, and termination may be carried out as for a single pregnancy. In a discordant twin pregnancy, when only one of the fetuses is affected, the following three outcomes are possible:

1. The couple may decide against any form of termination, and the pregnancy is continued. One should note that, in general, abnormal/affected fetuses have a much higher mortality in utero than normal ones (up to 75%–85% for trisomy 21, and up to 90 to 95% for trisomy 18, between conception and term); continuation of a discordant twin pregnancy may often result in the "natural" death of the affected twin, and survival of the healthy one.
2. The parents may decide to lose both fetuses, the affected and the healthy one.
3. Selective termination of pregnancy, bringing about the death of the affected twin while preserving the normal one, may be attempted.

Over the past 15 years, multifetal pregnancy reduction has become a well-established and integral part of infertility therapy for the sequelae of aggressive infertility management. In the mid-1980s, the risks and benefits of the procedure could only be guessed. We now have clear and precise data on the risks and benefits of the procedure and an understanding that the risks increase substantially with the starting and finishing number of fetuses in multifetal pregnancies. The collaborative loss rate numbers (i.e., 4.5% for triplets, 8% for quadruplets, 11% for quintuplets, and 15% for sextuplets or more) seem reasonable for the procedures performed by an experienced operator.[93–96] If *selective termination* is chosen, the affected fetus can be removed by hysterotomy; however, there is little experience with this technique and no real information on its safety for the second twin. Induced cardiac arrest is another mode of selective termination; air, formaldehyde, or potassium solution is injected into the circulation of the affected fetus, either into the umbilical vein under fetoscopic control, or directly into the heart, guided by ultrasound. Alternatively, or in combination with the injection method, the affected fetus may be exsanguinated.[93–96]

The following procedure is probably the least dangerous for the normal twin. A volume of 10 mL 20% NaCl solution is injected into the heart of the affected fetus. The fetus is not exsanguinated, to avoid possible bleeding from the unaffected fetus through any arteriovenous anastomoses. Presumably, the hypertonic saline acts directly on the myocardium. Within the circulation, the saline is diluted to such a degree that it will not damage the other fetus even if placental anastomoses are present.

Soon after injection, the affected fetus becomes bradycardic, and all cardiac activity ceases within a few hours. The mother is checked regularly in the clinic for several weeks, and further ultrasound examinations are made at 3- to 4-week intervals, to follow development of the surviving fetus and absorption of the other. At such times, maternal blood should also be examined for signs of diffuse intravascular coagulation. The dead fetus becomes a fetus papyraceus, but the other should develop normally.

Various technical procedures have been described, including transcervical minisuction to remove fetuses at 8–11 weeks. Another method is the transvaginal aspiration of the early embryo, usually at approximately 6–7 weeks. This technique is analogous in many respects to oocyte aspiration for *in vitro* fertilization.[97]

Disorders for which selective termination may be offered or requested can be divided into two groups. In the first one, the affected fetus might live for months or years, although severely handicapped (e.g., mental retardation), or only later develop neurologic problems (e.g., some enzymopathies). In utero development of the healthy twin would not be endangered in this situation. Intervention (selective termination) seems justifiable on grounds of the severe disorder in the affected fetus. The second group consists of congenital malformations incompatible with postnatal life. These are often associated with a progressive polyhydramnios, which may considerably disturb growth and development of the healthy twin. In this situation, intervention may be additionally justified: to ensure the development of the healthy fetus and to prevent obstetric complications. With or without intervention, the affected fetuses would not survive delivery.[11]

EMBRYOPATHOLOGY AND FETAL PATHOLOGY

As a result of recent developments in prenatal diagnosis, many diseases and disorders previously accessible only after birth can be examined in the embryo or fetus. Morphologic investigation of induced or spontaneous abortions is termed "embryopathology and fetal pathology." With an induced abortion, the aims of investigation are (1) to check the accuracy of the prenatal diagnosis and (2) to identify any abnormalities that were not detected prenatally. The aims of investigation in spontaneously aborted material are (1) to note anything suggestive of a high risk of recurrent abortion and (2) to identify any genetically significant pathology. Research into the etiology and pathology of acquired and genetic diseases and disorders is a further aim of embryo/fetopathology. To work in this field demands not only specialized embryologic and pathologic knowledge, but also experience and training in obstetrics and genetics.[11,72]

Only fresh, unfixed material can be examined. If it is necessary to transport the abortus, it should be cooled (as in melting ice). For most purposes biopsies are useless or impossible to obtain once the fetus has been exposed to formalin. Fixative, if added, also upsets the external appearances, colors the skin, and, due to its slow rate of tissue penetration, may not preserve deep viscera anyway. Before fixation, the pathologist should be convinced of the presence or absence of contractures, limb or other deformities, dermal changes, anatomic congenital malformations, and injuries.

To detect enzymopathies, samples are taken from those tissues (usually liver, kidney, heart, skeletal muscle, brain, and placenta) in which the pathologic metabolite is likely to accumulate. The skin and the fascia lata are also useful for enzyme assay; fibroblasts can be cultured *in vitro*. Samples are taken with a sterile scalpel and slices are placed in sterile serum-free culture medium or normal saline. The samples are transported to the laboratory without freezing or warming, at room temperature.

Occasionally, the prenatal diagnosis (e.g., congenital nephrosis) can be confirmed by electron microscopy. For this purpose, the electron microscope laboratory protocol must be followed at the time of sampling.

For chromosome examination, blood can be obtained from the umbilical cord or by direct cardiac puncture. The sample is collected into a sterile tube containing heparin. The blood thus obtained is suitable for serum tests. Samples for culturing bacteria, viruses, fungi, and parasites must be taken under strictly aseptic conditions. Chromosome analysis can also be performed on cultured lung, spleen, gonad, or other tissues. While dissecting dead fetuses and embryos, precautions are to be taken in handling acquired immunodeficiency syndrome (AIDS)-infected material.

After external inspection, attempts are made to separate the decidual, chorionic, amniotic, and embryonal/fetal elements. Special attention should be paid to the umbilical cord. The condition of the various tissues and membranes is noted, and any distortion, disintegration, or maceration that came about in utero is distinguished from any change or damage at the time of delivery or later. Histologic examination may help decide the exact nature and the timing of certain "injuries." The crown–rump and the crown–heel measurements are recorded.

Embryos may be sectioned sagittally, in toto, and examined microscopically. Fetuses are necropsied in detail. The face, eyes, nostrils, mouth, palate, and ears are inspected. The shape of the cranium is described and small encephaloceles are searched for. Pterygium and hygroma are looked for in the neck. The chest, the back, and the umbilical cord with its vessels are scrutinized thoroughly. One should remember that before gestational week 18 the clitoris of the female fetus is as large as the penis of the male; the labia majora develop later. The limbs, including the palms, fingers, soles, and toes, are examined. Special attention is paid to the placenta and the fetal membranes.[82]

Any detected abnormalities are described and measured carefully. The degree of maceration/autolysis is recorded. The intact embryo is photographed from the front, from the side, and from behind. Abnormalities are photographed in detail. Photographic documentation allows a retrospective review of the original findings and is useful for teaching, research, and publication.

External inspection is followed by autopsy. The organs are inspected in situ. For this purpose, scissors, forceps, a probe, and a magnifying lens are needed. The brain is fixed in toto, and later sliced, for examination. The placenta and the fetal membranes are thoroughly examined macroscopically and histologically. One should keep in mind the possibility of hydatidiform mole.

Histologic examination of lungs, liver, and kidney should be considered routine; that of other organs as appears appropriate. Buffered formalin is used as a fixative. Samples of material obtained from abortions terminated for nonmedical reasons may be used as controls.

Total body radiography is done to record skeletal disorders and to study some soft tissue disorders. Tape may be used to keep the embryo in a correct position. Anteroposterior and lateral views are taken, using 18 × 24-cm film. Skeletal abnormalities can be demonstrated convincingly with the alizarin red technique.

To obtain reliable postmortem ventriculograms, 10 mL of cerebrospinal fluid is withdrawn, and then 5 mL of buffered formalin is injected, followed by 5 mL of meglumine diatrizoate (Gastrografin). Postmortem angiography is valuable for study of vascular malformations.

POSTTERMINATION COUNSELING

It is important to follow-up women who have had termination for fetal abnormalities. They may become depressed immediately after the termination and may require support. They need to discuss what was wrong with the fetus, and the prospects for future pregnancies. It is the geneticist/obstetrician who should provide much of the support (trained nursing staff (health visitor, psychiatric social worker) attached to the genetics/obstetrics department), such as arranging for "posttermination counseling."[11]

Video 9.1 Vacuum aspiration of a missed abortion in week 8, after failed (unsuccessful) medication (misoprostol) uterine evacuation 3 days earlier (self-administration). Two hours before the procedure the patient was administered 2 tbl. vaginal misoprostol: https://goo.gl/Ez6ir2.

REFERENCES

1. Hertig AT. Implantation of the human ovum. In: Behrman SJ, Kistner RW (eds), *Progress in Infertility* (2nd edition), p. 114. Boston, MA: Little, Brown, 1975.
2. Macklon NS, Geraedts JP, Fauser BC. Conception to ongoing pregnancy: The 'black box' of early pregnancy loss. *Hum Reprod Update* 2002; 8: 333–343.
3. Boué J, Boué A, Lazar P. Retrospective and prospective epidemiological studies of 1500 karyotyped spontaneous human abortions. *Teratology* 1975; 12: 11–26.
4. Hertig AT, Sheldon WH. Minimal criteria required to prove prima facie case of traumatic abortion or miscarriage. *Ann Surg* 1943; 117: 596.
5. Shepard TH, Fantel AG, Fitzsimmons J. Congenital defect rates among spontaneous abortuses. Twenty years of monitoring. *Teratology* 1989; 39: 325–331.
6. Witschi E. Developmental causes of malformation. *Experientia (Seperatum)* 1971; 27: 1245–1247.

7. Levy B, Sigurjonsson S, Pettersen B et al. Genomic imbalance in products of conception: Single-nucleotide polymorphism chromosomal microarray analysis. *Obstet Gynecol* 2014; 124: 202–209.
8. Harris MJ, Poland BJ, Dill FJ. Triploidy in 40 human spontaneous abortuses: Assessment of phenotype in embryos. *Obstet Gynecol* 1981; 57: 600–606.
9. Canki N, Warburton D, Byrne J. Morphological characteristics of monosomy-X in spontaneous abortions. *Ann Genet* 1988; 31: 4–13.
10. Dhillon RK, Hillman SC, Morris RK et al. Additional information from chromosomal microarray analysis (CMA) over conventional karyotyping when diagnosing chromosomal abnormalities in miscarriage: A systematic review and meta-analysis. *BJOG* 2014; 121: 11–21.
11. Papp Z. *Obstetric Genetics*. Budapest, Hungary: Hungarian Academic Press, 1990.
12. Diczfalusy E, Borrell U. Influence of oophorectomy on steroid excretion in early pregnancy. *J Clin Endocrinol Metab* 1961; 21: 1119.
13. Ziegelmüller B, Vattai A, Kost B et al. Expression of thyroid hormone receptors in villous trophoblasts and decidual tissue at protein and mRNA levels is downregulated in spontaneous and recurrent miscarriages. *J Histochem Cytochem* 2015; 63: 511–523.
14. Gávai M, Berkes E, Lázár L et al. Factors affecting reproductive outcome following abdominal myomectomy. *J Assist Reprod Genet* 2007; 24: 525–531.
15. Papp Z, Mezei G, Gávai M et al. Reproductive performance after transabdominal metroplasty. A review of 157 consecutive cases. *J Reprod Med* 2006; 51: 544–552.
16. Naessens A, Foulon W, Cammu H et al. Epidemiology and pathogenesis of *Ureaplasma urealyticum* in spontaneous abortion and early preterm labor. *Acta Obstet Gynecol Scand* 1987; 66: 513–516.
17. Jamieson DJ, Kourtis AP, Bell M et al. Lymphocytic choriomeningitis virus: An emerging obstetric pathogen? *Am J Obstet Gynecol* 2006; 194: 1532–1536.
18. Crane J, Mundle W, Boucoiran I et al. Parvovirus B19 infection in pregnancy. *J Obstet Gynaecol Can* 2014; 36: 1107–1116.
19. Axelsson G, Rylander R. Exposure to anaesthetic gases and spontaneous abortion: Response bias in a postal questionnaire study. *Int J Epidemiol* 1982; 11: 250–256.
20. Csécsei K, Szeifert GT, Papp Z. Amniotic bands associated with early rupture of amnion due to an intrauterine device. *Zentralbl Gynäkol* 1987; 109: 738–741.
21. Harlap S, Shiono PH, Ramcharan S. Spontaneous foetal losses in women using different contraceptives around the time of conception. *Int J Epidemiol* 1980; 9: 49–56.
22. Kline J, Stein Z, Susser M et al. Fever during pregnancy and spontaneous abortion. *Am J Epidemiol* 1985; 121: 832–842.
23. Gharavi AE, Pierangeli SS, Levy RA et al. Mechanisms of pregnancy loss in antiphospholipid syndrome. *Clin Obstet Gynecol* 2001; 44: 11–19.
24. Kujovich JL. Thrombophilia and pregnancy complications. *Am J Obstet Gynecol* 2004; 191: 412–424.
25. Vinatier D, Duefour P, Cosson M et al. Antiphospholipid syndrome and recurrent miscarriages. *Eur J Obstet Gynecol Reprod Biol* 2001; 96: 37–50.
26. Ernest JM, Marshburn PB, Kutteh WH. Obstetric antiphospholipid syndrome: An update on pathophysiology and management. *Semin Reprod Med* 2011; 29: 522–539.
27. Homonnai ZT, Paz GF, Weiss JN et al. Relation between semen quality and fate of pregnancy. Retrospective study of 534 pregnancies. *Int J Androl* 1980; 3: 574–584.
28. Kajii T, Ferrier A. Cytogenetics of aborters and abortuses. *Am J Obstet Gynecol* 1978; 131: 33.
29. Papp Z, Gardó S, Dolhay B. Chromosome study of couples with repeated spontaneous abortions. *Fertil Steril* 1974; 25: 713–717.
30. Simpson JL, Meyers CM, Martin AO et al. Translocations are infrequent among couples having repeated spontaneous abortions but no other abnormal pregnancies. *Fertil Steril* 1989; 51: 811–814.
31. Tharapel AT, Tharapel SA, Bannerman RM. Recurrent pregnancy losses and parental chromosome abnormalities. *Br J Obstet Gynaecol* 1985; 92: 899–914.
32. Philipp T, Philipp K, Reiner A et al. Embryoscopic and cytogenetic analysis of 233 missed abortions: Factors involved in the pathogenesis of developmental defects of early failed pregnancies. *Hum Reprod* 2003; 18: 1724–1732.
33. Papp Z, Csécsei K, Tóth Z et al. Exencephaly in human fetuses. *Clin Genet* 1986; 30: 440–444.
34. Simpson JL, Mills JL, Holmes LB et al. Low fetal loss rates after ultrasound-proved viability in early pregnancy. *JAMA* 1987; 258: 2555–2557.
35. Jouppila P. Clinical and ultrasonic aspects in the diagnosis and follow-up of patients with early pregnancy failure. *Acta Obstet Gynecol Scand* 1980; 59: 405–409.
36. Liu Y, Liu Y, Zhang S et al. Etiology of spontaneous abortion before and after the demonstration of embryonic cardiac activity in women with recurrent spontaneous abortion. *Int J Gynaecol Obstet* 2015; 129: 128–132.
37. Liu XR, Mu HQ, Shi Q et al. The optimal duration of progesterone supplementation in pregnant women after IVF/ICSI: A meta-analysis. *Reprod Biol Endocrinol* 2012; 10: 107
38. Ford HB, Schust DJ. Recurrent pregnancy loss: Etiology, diagnosis, and treatment. *Rev Obstet Gynecol* 2009; 2: 76–83.
39. Diejomaoh MF. Recurrent spontaneous miscarriage is still a challenging diagnostic and therapeutic quagmire. *Med Princ Pract* 2015; 24 (Suppl. 1): 38–55.

40. Eschenbach DA. Treating spontaneous and induced septic abortions. *Obstet Gynecol* 2015; 125: 1042–1048.
41. Lindelius A, Varli IH, Hammarstrom M. A retrospective comparison between lamicel and gemeprost for cervical ripening before surgical interruption of first-trimester pregnancy. *Contraception* 2003; 67: 299–303.
42. Bartz D, Maurer R, Allen RH et al. Buccal misoprostol compared with synthetic osmotic cervical dilator before surgical abortion: A randomized controlled trial. *Obstet Gynecol* 2013; 122: 57–63.
43. Gibson KS, Mercer BM, Louis JM. Inner thigh taping vs traction for cervical ripening with a Foley catheter: A randomized controlled trial. *Am J Obstet Gynecol* 2013; 209: 272.e1.
44. Mitchell MD. Biochemistry of the prostaglandins. *Baillieres Clin Obstet Gynecol* 1992; 6: 687.
45. Robbin A, Spitz IM. Mifepristone: Clinical pharmacology. *Clin Obstet Gynecol* 1996; 39: 436–450.
46. Fong YF, Singh KP. A comparative study using two dose regimens (200 lg or 400 lg) of vaginal misoprostol for pre-operative cervical dilatation in first trimester nulliparae. *Br J Obstet Gynaecol* 1998; 105: 413–417.
47. Blanchard K, Shochet T, Coyaji K et al. Misoprostol alone for early abortion: An evaluation of seven potential regimens. *Contraception* 2005; 72: 91–97.
48. Tang OS, Ho PC. The pharmacokinetics and different regimens of misoprostol in early first-trimester medical abortion. *Contraception* 2006; 74: 26–30.
49. Marret H, Simon E, Beucher G et al. Overview and expert assessment of off-label use of misoprostol in obstetrics and gynaecology: Review and report by the Collègc national des gynécologues obstétriciens français. *Eur J Obstet Gynecol Reprod Biol* 2015; 187: 80–84.
50. Winikoff B, Dzuba IG, Creinin MD. Two distinct oral routes of misoprostol in mifepristone medical abortion: A randomized controlled trial. *Obstet Gynecol* 2008; 112: 1303.
51. Shaw KA, Shaw JG, Hugin M et al. Adjunct mifepristone for cervical preparation prior to dilation and evacuation: A randomized trial. *Contraception* 2015; 91: 313–319.
52. Creinin MD, Potter C, Holovanisin M et al. Mifepristone and misoprostol and methotrexat/misoprostol in clinical practice for abortion. *Am J Obstet Gynecol* 2003; 188: 664–669.
53. Kittiwatanakul W, Weerakiet S. Comparison of efficacy of modified electric vacuum aspiration with sharp curettage for the treatment of incomplete abortion: Randomized controlled trial. *J Obstet Gynaecol Res* 2012; 38: 681–685.
54. Dean G, Colarossi L, Porsch L et al. Manual compared with electric vacuum aspiration for abortion at less than 6 weeks of gestation: A randomized controlled trial. *Obstet Gynecol* 2015; 125: 1121–1129.
55. Wen J, Cai QY, Deng F et al. Manual versus electric vacuum aspiration for first-trimester abortion: A systematic review. *BJOG* 2008; 115: 5.
56. Ireland LD, Gatter M, Chen AY. Medical compared with surgical abortion for effective pregnancy termination in the first trimester. *Obstet Gynecol* 2015; 126: 22–28.
57. Dalenda C, Ines N, Fathia B et al. Two medical abortion regimens for late first-trimester termination of pregnancy: A prospective randomized trial. *Contraception* 2010; 81: 323–327.
58. Torre A, Huchon C, Bussieres L et al. Immediate versus delayed medical treatment for first-trimester miscarriage: A randomized trial. *Am J Obstet Gynecol* 2012; 206: 215.e1-6.
59. Larsson PG, Platz-Christensen JJ, Dalaker K et al. Treatment with 2% clindamycin vaginal cream prior to first trimester surgical abortion to reduce signs of postoperative infection: A prospective, double-blinded, placebo-controlled, multicenter study. *Acta Obstet Gynecol Scand* 2000; 79: 390–396.
60. Shinagawa S, Nagayama M. Cervical pregnancy as a possible sequela of induced abortion. Report of 19 cases. *Am J Obstet Gynecol* 1969; 105: 282–284.
61. Ayers LR, Drosman S, Saltzstein SL. Iatrogenic paracervical implantation of fetal tissue during a therapeutic abortion. *Obstet Gynecol* 1971; 37: 755–760.
62. Árvay A, Görgey M, Kapu L. La relation entre les avortements (interruptions de la grossesse) et les accouchements prématurés. *Rev Franc Gynec Obstet* 1967; 62: 81–86.
63. Taylor PJ, Cumming DC, Hill PJ. Significance of intrauterine adhesions detected hysteroscopically in eumenorrheic infertile women and role of antecedent curettage in their formation. *Am J Obstet Gynecol* 1981; 139: 239–242.
64. Houwert-de Jong MH, Eskes TKAB, Termijtelen A et al. Habitual abortion: A review. *Eur J Obstet Gynecol* 1989; 30: 39.
65. Glaser D, Wank R, Bartsch-Sandhoff M et al. Immunotherapy after recurrent abortions with a paternal chromosomal translocation. *Geburtsh Frauenheilkd* 1989; 49: 58–60.
66. Parke A, Maier D, Hakim C et al. Subclinical autoimmune disease and recurrent spontaneous abortion. *J Rheumatol* 1986; 13: 1178–1180.
67. Iffy L. Embryologic studies of time of conception in ectopic pregnancy and first trimester abortion. *Obstet Gynecol* 1965; 26: 490–498.
68. Mikamo K, Iffy L. Aging of the ovum. *Obstet Gynecol Annu* 1974; 3: 47–99.
69. Morton NE, Chiu D, Holland C et al. Chromosome anomalies as predictors of recurrence risk for spontaneous abortion. *Am J Med Genet* 1987; 28: 353–360.
70. Lancet M, Jakobovits A. Abnormalities of position, shape, and structure of the pregnant uterus. In: Iffy L, Kaminetzky HA (eds), *Principles and Practice of Obstetrics and Perinatology*, p. 1471. New York, NY: Wiley, 1981.

71. Swahn ML, Bygdeman M. Termination of early pregnancy with RU 486 (Mifepristone) in combination with a prostaglandin analogue (Sulprostone). *Acta Obstet Gynecol Scand* 1990; 68: 293–306.
72. Papp Z. (ed.). *Atlas of Fetal Diagnosis*. Amsterdam-London-New York-Tokyo: Elsevier, 1992.
73. Autry AM, Hayes EC, Jaobson GF et al. A comparison of medical induction and dilation and evacuation for second trimester abortion. *Am J Obstet Gynecol* 2002; 187: 393–397.
74. Shulman LP, Ling FW, Meyers CM et al. Dilation and evacuation is a preferable method for mid-trimester genetic termination of pregnancy. *Prenat Diagn* 1989; 9: 741–742.
75. Klinte I, Hamberger L, Wiqvist N. 2nd-trimester abortion by extra-amniotic instillation of Rivanol combined with intravenous administration of oxytocin or prostaglandin-F2-alpha. *Acta Obstet Gynecol Scand* 1983; 62: 303–306.
76. Uldbjerg N, Ekman G, Malmström A et al. Biochemical and morphologic changes of human cervix after local application of prostaglandin E2 in pregnancy. *Lancet* 1981; 1: 267–268.
77. WHO Task Force on the Use of Prostaglandins for the Regulation of Fertility. Prostaglandins and abortion. II. Single extra-amniotic administration of 0.92 mg of 15-methyl-prostaglandin F2a in Hyskon for termination of pregnancies in weeks 10 to 20 of gestation: An international multicenter study. *Am J Obstet Gynecol* 1977; 129: 593–596.
78. Hill NCW, MacKenzie IZ. 2308 second trimester terminations using extra-amniotic or intra-amniotic prostaglandin E2: An analysis of efficacy and complications. *Br J Obstet Gynaecol* 1989; 96: 1424–1431.
79. Dabash R, Vhelli H, Hajri S et al. A double-blind randomized controlled trial of mifepristone or placebo before buccal misoprostol for abortion at 14–21 weeks of pregnancy. *Int J Gynaecol Obstet* 2015; 130: 40–44.
80. Su LL, Biswas A, Choolani M et al. A prospective, randomized comparison of vaginal misoprostol versus intra-amniotic prostaglandins for midtrimester termination of pregnancy. *Am J Obstet Gynecol* 2005; 193: 1410–1414.
81. Owen J, Hauth JC. Vaginal misoprostol vs. concentrated oxytocin plus low-dose prostaglandin E2 for second trimester pregnancy termination. *J Matern Fetal Med* 1999; 8: 48.
82. Kapp N, Todd CS, Yadgarova KT et al. A randomized comparison of misoprostol to intrauterine instillation of hypertonic saline plus a prostaglandin F2alpha analogue for second-trimester induction termination in Uzbekistan. *Contraception* 2007; 76: 461.
83. Wildschut H, Both MI, Medema S et al. Medical methods for mid-trimester termination of pregnancy. *Cochrane Database Syst Rev* 2011; (1): CD005216.
84. Bartley J, Brown A, Elton R et al. Double-blind randomized trial of mifepristone in combination with vaginal gemeprost or misoprostol for induction of abortion up to 63 days gestation. *Hum Reprod* 2001; 16: 2098–2102.
85. Guest J, Chien P, Thomson M et al. Randomised controlled trial comparing efficacy of same day administration of mifepristone and misoprostol for termination of pregnancy with the standard 36 to 48 hour protocol. *BJOG* 2005; 112: 1457.
86. Bebbington MW, Kent N, Lim K et al. A randomized controlled trial comparing two protocols for the use of misoprostol in midtrimester pregnancy termination. *Am J Obstet Gynecol* 2002; 187: 853–857.
87. Schneider D, Langer R, Golan A et al. Induced early mid-trimester abortion in primigravid adolescents: Comparison between laminaria dilatation-evacuation and extra-amniotic PGFi2a infusion. *Isr J Obstet Gynecol* 1991; 2: 170.
88. WHO Task Force on Prostaglandins for Fertility Regulation, Special Programme of Research, Development and Research Training in Human Reproduction. Vaginal administration of 15-methyl-PGF2a methyl ester for preoperative cervical dilatation. *Contraception* 1981; 23: 251–259.
89. Less A, Goldberger SB, Bernheim B et al. Vaginal prostaglandin E2 and fetal amniotic fluid embolus. *JAMA* 1990; 263: 3259–3260.
90. Chervenak FA, McCullough LB. An ethically justified, clinically comprehensive management strategy for 3rd-trimester pregnancies complicated by fetal anomalies. *Obstet Gynecol* 1990; 74: 311–316.
91. Papp Z, Tóth Z, Szabó M et al. Prenatal screening for neural tube defects and other malformations by both serum AFP and ultrasound. In: Kurjak A (ed), *The Fetus as a Patient*, pp. 167–180. Amsterdam, the Netherlands: Elsevier, 1985.
92. Papp Z. Genetic counseling and termination of pregnancy in Hungary. *J Med Philos* 1989; 14: 323–333.
93. Kerenyi TD, Chitkara Y. Selective birth in twin pregnancy with discordancy for Down's syndrome. *N Engl J Med* 1981; 304: 1525–1527.
94. Itskovitz-Eldor J, Drugan A, Levron J et al. Transvaginal embryonic aspiration (TEA)—A safe method for selective reduction in multiple gestation. *Am J Obstet Gynecol* 1992; 166: 3581–3585.
95. Evans MI, Kramer RL, Yaron Y et al. What are the ethical and technical problems associated with multifetal pregnancy reduction? *Clin Obstet Gynecol* 1998; 41: 46–54.
96. Patkós P, Tóth-Pál E, Papp Z. Multiembryonic pregnancy reduction: The Hungarian experience. *Am J Obstet Gynecol* 2002; 186: 596–597.
97. Evans MI, Krivchenia EL, Gelber SE et al. Selective reduction. *Clin Perinatol* 2003; 30: 103–111.

Percutaneous intrauterine fetal shunting 10

SUNDEEP G. KESWANI, R. DOUGLAS WILSON, and MARK P. JOHNSON

CONTENTS

In utero fetal surgery continues to develop with improved diagnostic techniques, patient selection, and the use of innovative fetal therapies. The broad categories of surgical in utero fetal therapy can be separated into open uterine techniques and minimally invasive endoscopic/ultrasound-guided techniques that require only puncture of the uterus with single or multiple ports. Benefits of minimally invasive fetal intervention include diminished exposure of the mother and fetus to the traumatic nature of open fetal surgery. Minimally invasive, or "closed" techniques may result in decreased uterine irritability and a decreased incidence of preterm delivery the "Achilles' heel" of open fetal surgery. In addition, minimally invasive surgery does not subject the mother to the sequelae of a hysterotomy or commit her to cesarean delivery for subsequent pregnancies.

Fetal abnormalities involving outflow obstruction of the bladder or fluid-filled space occupying lesions in the fetal chest can result in significant morbidity or mortality. Select patients with these disorders may benefit from chronic in utero drainage of these fluid-filled lesions. This chapter aims to summarize the present status of closed in utero fetal therapy using shunts to create vesicoamniotic or thoracoamniotic decompression of the fluid-filled space.

FETAL LOWER URINARY TRACT OBSTRUCTION (LUTO)

Introduction

Congenital malformations of the renal system are present in 15% of all prenatally detected congenital anomalies and are associated with multiple system involvement in 70% of cases. Renal tract anomalies are found in greater than 300 genetic syndromes and 35% of all chromosome anomalies.[1–3] Congenital renal obstructive pathology is associated with abnormal renal development with direct effects on renal growth. Human fetuses with severe lower urinary tract obstruction during the first 30 gestational weeks may have abnormal metanephric blastema, cystic dysplasia, and apoptosis of mesenchymal and tubular cells and reduced numbers of nephrons.[2,4]

Fetal obstructive uropathies are heterogeneous and have multiple structural and pathological etiologies. Prenatally diagnosed cases with megacystis or an enlarged fetal bladder can have both obstructive and nonobstructive etiologies. LUTO is a commonly used term that encompasses the spectrum of prenatally diagnosed lower urinary tract pathologies. The most common etiology for bladder outlet obstruction in a male fetus with associated oligohydramnios includes malformations in the prostatic/urethral/bladder neck complex. In contrast, bladder outlet obstruction in a female fetus is usually due to developmental cloacal malformations. Nonobstructive megacystis cases usually have normal amniotic fluid volumes for both males and females and are due to the heterogeneous nonobstructive etiologies. Nonobstructed bladder/megacystis cases are not candidates for fetal therapy.

PATHOPHYSIOLOGY FOR FETAL BLADDER OUTLET OBSTRUCTION

Therapy for bladder outlet obstruction became a possibility with the introduction of fetal ultrasound. The rapid development of ultrasound technology in the early 1990s allowed the visualization of the fetus and identification of fetal pathology. Fetal bladder outlet obstruction was one of the first conditions to be researched with sheep models prior to translation of therapeutic treatments to humans. The variation and prevalence of congenital fetal lower urinary tract pathologies, associated with LUTO are summarized in Table 10.1.[5,6] The separation of the LUTO subtypes and associated anomalies is reported with the total number of associated LUTO cases having a prevalence of 3.34 (confidence interval [CI] 2.95–3.72) per 10,000 live births; however, these prevalence figures do not include pregnancy losses. This retrospective cohort of 284 is further categorized into complex (63) and isolated (221) groups. Only the isolated group (78%) would usually be candidates for fetal therapy. Posterior urethral valve (PUV) obstruction was the most common obstructive etiology identified with 179 cases (160 isolated cases [89%]) and the PUV etiology was 63% of the total LUTO cohort. Urethral atresia, urethral stenosis, and Prune Belly syndrome were categorized at 9.9%, 7.0%, and 2.5% of the total, respectively. The unspecified or specified as "other" subtype for LUTO was 17.6% of the total cohort. Regardless of the etiology of the bladder outlet obstruction, if obstruction is complete, the outcome would be a similar fetal "deformation" anomaly pattern/oligohydramnios sequence (Table 10.1).[5,6]

The obstructive etiology differences and outcomes are determined by urological assessment in survivors or the pathological analysis of the bladder neck or outlet obstruction and other urinary system structures in fetal/neonatal deaths. The degree of obstruction (complete—nonruptured PUV, urethral atresia; partial—ruptured PUV, urethral stenosis) will be reflected in the amniotic fluid volume ([AFI] or deepest vertical pocket; Table 10.2[3,7–18]). Complete obstruction creates a fetal megacystis with bladder smooth muscle hypertrophy and hyperplasia and subsequent impaired contractility, compliance, and elasticity. The excessive intrabladder pressure is then transmitted via the ureterovesical valves to create enlarging hydroureters and hydronephrosis as urine volume continues to expand with renal function and with secondary ureteral reflux from bladder activity. The resulting dilated renal pelvis and calyces then compress the renal parenchyma creating the type IV cystic degeneration (as visualized by ultrasound). This progressive obstructive and pressure-related process produces renal insufficiency of the fetus and neonate.

Primary fetal bladder outlet obstruction (malformation) and secondary pressure-related deformations to the bladder and kidney result in additional effects on the lung, and muscular skeletal/facial systems. These secondary effects to the lung include severe pulmonary hypoplasia, with a lack of late developing alveolar sacs and can be lethal. Amniotic fluid volume is important for allowing the hydrostatic expansion (in and out) of the developing lung airway structures as well as creating space for fetal movement and muscular development. Insufficient fluid can result in multiple sequelae; oligohydramnios sequence (Potter's syndrome) has been well described and includes the additional limb arthrogryposis and facial compression features.[19]

Table 10.1 Congenital lower urinary tract obstructive pathology (megacystis ± prenatal ultrasound visualization).

Final diagnosis	Prevalence/10,000 LB	Comment
Posterior urethral valves	2.10 (CI 1.79–2.41)	Male
Urethral atresia	0.33 (CI 0.21–0.45)	Male
Urethral stenosis	0.23 (CI 0.13–0.34)	Male
Prune belly syndrome	0.08 (CI 0.02–0.14)	Male/female (female no gonadal location issue)
Anterior urethral		Male
Valves/diverticulum		<50% bulbar; 33% penile; 33% penoscrotal junction
Congenital urethrocele		Male/female
MMIHS (lethal)		Three female/one male
Isolated megacystis		Milder variant of MMIHS/visceral myopathy
Megacystis-megaureter		Massive thin-walled bladder with UT dilatation
Associate		Large-volume repetitive urinary reflux

Abbreviations: LB, live birth; MMIHS, megacystis microcolon intestinal hypoperistalsis syndrome; UT, urinary tract.

Table 10.2 LUTO malformation: diagnosis and renal evaluation.

A. Primary ultrasound screening/diagnosis (95% sensitivity rule out false negative/80% specificity rule out false positive)

Gestational age 12–36 weeks

Megacystis (earliest 11 weeks; 1/1800 prevalence with frequent spontaneously resolution)

Definition: 10–14 weeks normal bladder <6 mm; >15–17 mm obstruction

>14 weeks large appearing bladder with no emptying after 45 minutes

Oligohydramnios: significant predictor of poor renal function postnatally

Definition: single vertical pocket <0.5–3.0 cm; amniotic fluid index (AFI) <3.0–8.0 cm

Renal appearance: hydronephrosis >4–7 mm; renal echogenicity, cystic parenchymal, abnormal renal cortical appearance best predictor for postnatal renal function

Urinary extravasation (15%): urinary ascites, perinephric urinoma, urinothorax

Associated malformations 33%

Cardiac; increased cardiothoracic ratio (21%); ventricular hypertrophy (29%); pericardial effusions (36%); bladder compresses iliac arteries, creating increased cardiac afterload

Renal volumes: for right and left kidney (5th to 95th percentile for gestational age 20–40 weeks) (Yoshizaki et al.[10])

Three-dimensional power Doppler histogram and vascular indices (Bernades et al.[11])

Four-dimensional ultrasonographic imaging (Ruano et al.[12])

B. Other imaging/MRI

Provides additional detail prenatally and as alternative to autopsy

C. Invasive analysis

Karyotype (25% risk of aneuploidy T13/18) from amniotic fluid or fetal urine

Microarray; additional copy number variant pathology 11.8% with bladder anomaly

Urinary/renal function analysis (absolute cutoffs); serial assessment x 3 q 2 days

Good prognosis screen

Sodium < 100 mmol/L (better predictor)

Chloride < 90 mmol/L

Calcium < 8 mg/dL (better predictor)

Osmolality < 200 mmol/L

Total protein < 20 mg/dL

B2-microglobulin < 6 mg/L

Amniotic fluid cell-free fetal DNA/metabolomics: limited data available

D. Diagnostic cystoscopy

Diagnostic capability for prognosis prediction is limited, but evidence-based publications using cystoscopy altered the ultrasound diagnosis in 25%–36% of cases

Abbreviations: LUTO, lower urinary tract obstruction; MRI, magnetic resonance imaging.

SCREENING AND DIAGNOSTIC EVALUATIONS FOR FETAL BLADDER OUTLET OBSTRUCTION

Table 10.2[4,7–18] summarizes the diagnostic and renal function evaluations reported and currently used for clinical decisions. The summary includes the imaging triage (ultrasound; magnetic resonance imaging [MRI]), the invasive laboratory analysis (genetic testing; renal function testing), and the diagnostic utility of fetal cystoscopy.

Noninvasive ultrasound imaging access has been evaluated by systematic review. Thirteen articles met the study criteria and a meta-analysis compared clinically similar subgroups to minimize clinical heterogeneity. The best ultrasound parameter to predict postnatal renal function in survivors was renal cortical appearance (sensitivity 0.57 [CI 0.37–0.76]; specificity 0.84 [CI 0.71–0.94] with area under the curve of 0.78).[20] Evaluation of the amniotic fluid volume (sensitivity 0.63 [CI 0.51–0.74]; specificity 0.76 [CI 0.65–0.85] with area under the curve 0.74) was also found useful. MRI[7,13] is also used for fetal imaging and the MRI technique is not dependent on amniotic fluid volume and is well-suited for fetal renal pathology evaluation, and can be used as early as 20 weeks gestation. MRI is complementary to ultrasound and should be used following ultrasound assessment (Figure 10.1).

The functional renal urinary-based values obtained by vesicocentesis (Table 10.2) have been used for many years for treatment triage decisions. Sodium, calcium, and B2 microglobulin values are considered as the better predictors of postdelivery renal function.[3,15,21] A systematic review[21] identified the predictive value of calcium at >95th percentile for gestation (likelihood ratio (LR) +6.65, 0.23–190.96; LR −0.19, 0.05–0.74) and sodium at >95th percentile for gestation (LR +4.46, 1.71–11.6; LR −0.39, 0.17–0.88) to be the most highly correlated to renal injury. B2 microglobulin was found to

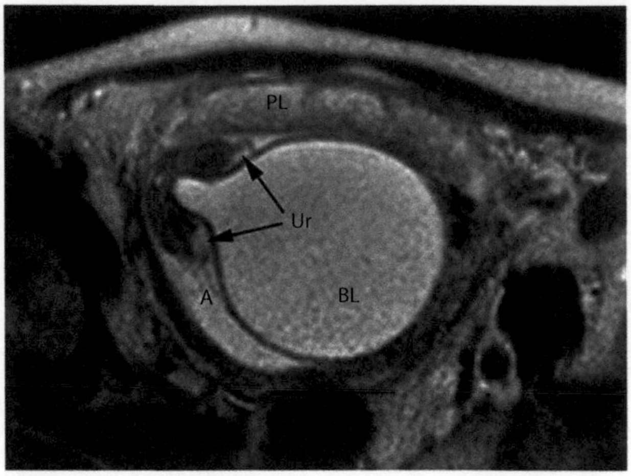

Figure 10.1 Magnetic resonance imaging (MRI) transverse image of fetal abdomen with lower urinary tract obstruction (A, ascites; BL, bladder; PL, placenta; Ur, hydroureters).

be less accurate (LR +2.92, 1.28–6.69; LR −0.53, 0.24–1.17). These urine-based predictors estimate the postnatal renal function, with sodium and calcium indicating tubular function at the time of serial evaluation. Fetal urine becomes more hypotonic with increasing gestational age, and tubular reabsorption of sodium and B2 microglobulin increases during 20–40 gestational weeks.[22] Other urinary testing for renal function using other urinary products/analysis, such as cell-free DNA or proteomics or metabolomics, has not been evaluated.

A systematic review[23] (66 manuscripts) for diagnostic cystoscopy with LUTO pathology identified 63 patients from four manuscripts. The quality of evidence, to date, for a diagnostic fetal cystoscopy with LUTO is poor. Fetal diagnostic cystoscopy in cases of LUTO should be considered, at present, to be an experimental intervention until more survival and long-term outcomes results are available.[21]

INTERVENTIONAL TECHNIQUES FOR LOWER URINARY TRACT OBSTRUCTION

The intervention techniques for LUTO must be evaluated with respect to the ethical considerations for fetal therapy and on both the fetal "benefit to risk ratio" and the maternal "risk to benefit ratio." The informed consent process may consider both the palliative survival techniques for respiratory preservation with postnatal renal evaluation and repair, or with fetal treatment techniques that try to improve the fetal renal function with decreased neonatal morbidity and possibly better childhood outcomes from pediatric medical and surgical care.[24]

Ultrasound-guided techniques, for preservation of the fetal respiratory and musculoskeletal systems, can be considered from 20 to 36 gestational weeks.[19] Serial amnio-infusions to maintain an adequate amniotic fluid volume can prevent the deformations associated with Oligohydramnios Sequence. Repeated amnio-infusion techniques introduce the risk of infection and premature rupture of membranes, with resulting preterm delivery and prematurity risks for the neonate. However, serial amnio-infusion treatments have been shown to have limited therapeutic use and value.

Vesicocentesis for fetal urinary/renal function evaluation is an ultrasound-guided needle technique similar to amniocentesis but with the fluid target being the enlarged fetal bladder.[3,21] A 22-gauge spinal needle is used for a midline lower bladder location, and color flow Doppler is used to avoid puncturing the umbilical vessels that have a bilateral bladder location. The low midline bladder location allows for a more complete aspiration of the fetal bladder. Serial vesicocentesis is recommended, with three procedures and specimen results (every 2 days) to allow optimal renal evaluation. The urine values that are consistent with a favorable prognosis for postnatal renal function are listed in Table 10.2 and can identify potential candidates for vesicoamniotic shunting (bypassing the bladder outlet obstruction).

If favorable fetal renal function is identified, with no other significant genetic/functional/organ system structural or functional anomalies are present (other than those associated with the LUTO), then counseling and informed consent can be considered or obtained for "closed" ultrasound-guided fetal vesicoamniotic shunting (VAS). Detailed descriptions of the VAS technique are published,[25,26] and the fetal VAS experience[25–30] is summarized in Table 10.3. Briefly, under ultrasound guidance, the fetal abdominal and bladder are punctured using a needle trocar through which a double pigtail catheter is passed. The distal end is deployed in the fetal bladder and the proximal end is deployed in the amniotic space created by the amnio-infusion. Following the VAS placement, ultrasound is used to determine the correct VAS location and to demonstrate flow out of the bladder through the VAS with evidence of a decompressing fetal bladder (Figure 10.2).

Complications

Counseling the patient prior to any invasive needle or shunt procedure includes discussion of risks including premature rupture of membranes, direct trauma to the fetus, placental bleeding, and possible preterm labor. Transient vesicoperitoneal fistulas occasionally occur following vescicocentesis, resulting in urinary ascites. These fistulas close spontaneously in 10–14 days with redevelopment of the megacystis. Displacement of the shunt is a fairly common complication, occurring in approximately 30%–45% of reported cases.[25] Appropriate location of the shunt in the fetus's lower abdominal region decreases the risk of shunt displacement due to bladder decompression. Repeat shunt insertions may be necessary depending on the clinical situation. There are not good estimates for the risk of loss of pregnancy as a result of the shunt procedure. In the percutaneous shunting in lower urinary tract obstruction (PLUTO) trial,[27] 4 of 16 (25%) patients had an intrauterine death rate following successful shunt placement. Vesicocentesis pregnancy loss rates are considered to be similar to amniocentesis rates at 0.5%–1.0%.

Outcome

Table 10.3 summarizes the published outcomes of vesicoamniotic shunting for LUTO. A systematic review and

Table 10.3 Review of published VAS use/outcome survival and renal evaluations.

Author	Study design	Comment
Morris et al.[25]	Systematic review (1990–2009)	Primary articles 23/statistical analysis 20 VAS improves survival (OR 3.86; 2.00–7.45) with high residual poor postnatal renal function (observational studies only)
Tonni et al.[26]	Systematic review (1987–2008)	Primary articles included 12 with treatment VAS has failed to improve the outcome and/or long-term prognosis with PUV VAS related to efficacy on renal outcome is still under debate VAS seems to ameliorate pulmonary function VAS is associated with high fetal mortality rate and limited renal function improvement
Morris et al.[27]	Randomized controlled trial	31 fetuses (16 VAS; 15 no treatment) (RCT was discontinued due to lack of enrollment) VAS was associated with higher survival, but size and direction of effect remained uncertain The chance of normal renal function is very low irrespective of VAS or conservative therapy
Ethun et al.[28]	Single center case review (2004–2012)	14 male LUTO/11 intervention VAS increases survival with significant perinatal and long-term morbidity
Diwaker et al.[29]	Secondary RCT analysis	VAS cost-effectiveness (PLUTO) VAS is more expensive than conservative care VAS is not likely to be cost-effective in the management of fetal LUTO
Ruano et al.[30]	Case review; two centers (1990–2013)	111 LUTO fetuses (VAS 16) VAS was associated with an improved 6-month survival rate, but no effect on renal function

Abbreviations: OR, odds ratio; PLUTO, percutaneous shunting in lower urinary tract obstruction; PUV, posterior urethral valve; RCT, randomized controlled trial; VAS, vesicoamniotic shunt.

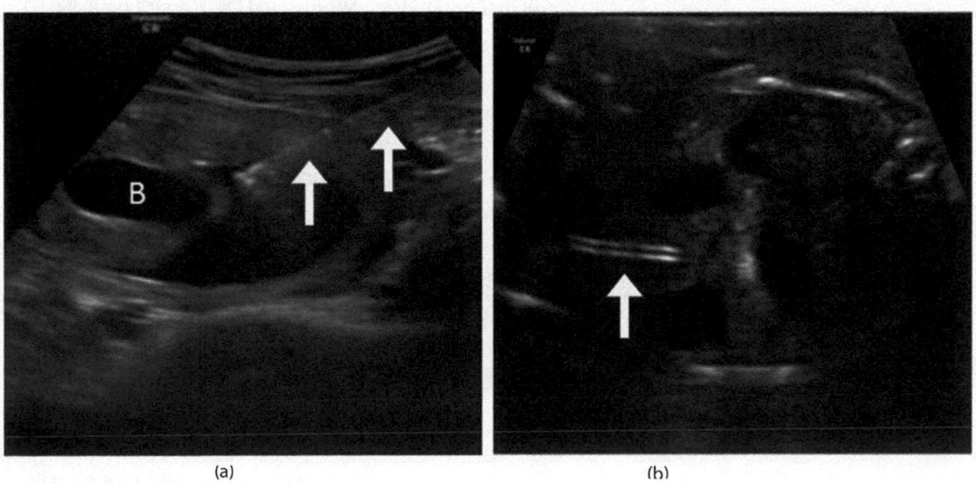

Figure 10.2 (a) A needle trocar (arrows) through the uterine wall to puncture the fetal abdominal and bladder wall; (b) shows the bladder end of the double pigtail catheter in the fetal bladder (arrow) that had been threaded through the inserted trocar.)

meta-analysis of the effectiveness of VAS for the treatment of LUTO examined 20 studies for the fetal intervention for presumed LUTO (369 fetuses), 12 studies were used for a meta-analysis for the effect of fetal intervention on perinatal survival and seven studies were used for a meta-analysis for the effect of fetal intervention on long-term renal function (although five studies had no fetal intervention).[25] In utero therapy (mainly VAS) was considered to improve perinatal outcomes compared to no treatment (odss ratio [OR] 3.86; CI 2.00–7.45). The second meta-analysis outcome demonstrated no improved long-term improvement of renal function if VAS was used over no treatment (OR 0.67; CI 0.22–2.00).

The diagnostic and therapeutic use of a fetal cystoscopy (Figure 10.3) for LUTO has been summarized in Table 10.4.[16–18,26,30,31] Ruano et al.[30] reported a case–control study and concluded from a cohort of 111 fetuses with 34 therapeutic cystoscopy procedures that fetal cystoscopy and VAS improve 6-month survival rates in cases of severe LUTO. However, only fetal cystoscopic intervention (i.e., valve ablation) may prevent impairment of renal function in fetuses with PUV. The treatment evidence provided in Tables 10.3 and 10.4 indicates that postnatal renal function is not significantly improved with placement of vesicoamniotic shunts, however, there may be a benefit to overall fetal survival by improving pulmonary function.

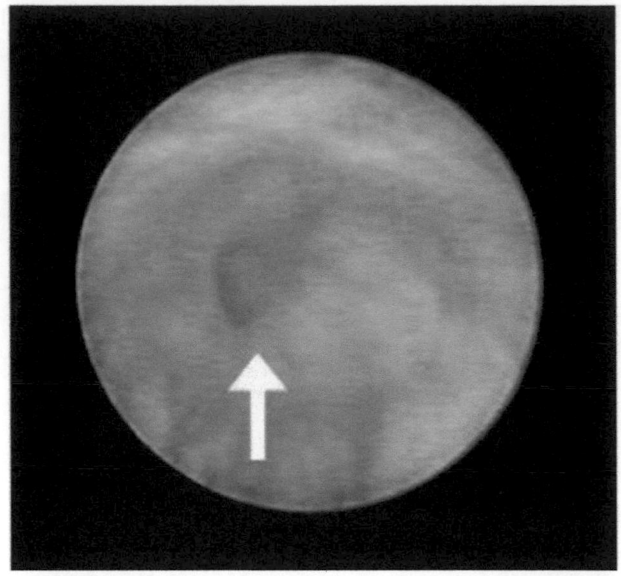

Figure 10.3 Operative image of the urethral orifice (arrow) during a diagnostic fetal cystoscopy in the management of lower urinary tract obstruction (LUTO). (Courtesy of Dr. Rodrigo Ruano.)

SUMMARY FOR LOWER URINARY TRACT OBSTRUCTION SHUNT THERAPIES

The ultrasound criteria used for the screening and identification of the fetus with fetal bladder outlet obstruction

Table 10.4 Summarized published fetal cystoscopy experience for fetal LUTO.

Author	Study design	Comment
Ruano et al.[18]	Cohort 2006–2008	Feasibility
		Seven cystoscopy with laser/PUV/four cystoscopy only (UA)
		12 expectant management only
Morris et al.[23]	Systematic review (66 papers)	Reviewed treatment for 63 patients
		Cystoscopy to no treatment: improved survival OR 20.51 (CI 3.87–108.69)
		Cystoscopy to VAS: NS survival OR 1.49 (CI 0.13–16.97)
Ruano[16]	Cohort 2008–2010	16-week gestation cysto with severe megacystis
		Seven cystoscopy (three PUV-laser; three UA; precysto demise)
		PUV two survivors/one MMIHS postnatal death/eight expectant with no survivors
Ruano[17]	Review (1995–2010)	PUV 20 cases with cystotherapy
		Laser fulguration 10/20; survival 7/10/hydroablation 4/20; survival 3/4
		Guide-wire 4/20; monopolar fulguration 1/20; urethral probe 1/20; survivors none
Tonni et al.[26]	Review (computer search)	Limited review: limited cystoscopy/LUTO use
Ruano et al.[30]	Multicenter case–control	111 fetuses(cystoscopy 34/VAS 16/no intervention 61)
		Probability of survival: cystoscopy vs. none ARR 1.86 (CI 1.01–3.42)
		VAS vs. none ARR 1.73 (CI 1.01–3.08)
		Normal renal function: cystoscopy vs. none ARR 1.73 (CI 0.97–3.08)
		VAS vs. none ARR 1.16 (CI 0.86–1.55)
		Six-month survival: cystoscopy vs. none ARR 4.10 (CI 1.75–9.62)
		VAS vs. none ARR3.76 (CI 1.42–9.97)
		Renal function: cystoscopy vs. none ARR 2.66 (CI 1.245–5.70)
		VAS vs. none ARR 1.03 (CI 0.49–2.17)
Sananes et al.[31]	Multicenter case series	40 fetal therapeutic laser cystocopies for PUV

Abbreviations: ARR, adjusted risk ratio; CI, confidence interval; UA, urethral atresia.

are well defined. These include characteristic enlargement of the bladder, pressure changes in the ureters, and alterations in the renal parenchyma associated with a decrease in amniotic fluid levels. Establishing the exact prenatal anatomic obstructive etiology requires significant skill and expertise. While still experimental, diagnostic cystoscopy may be useful in elucidating a specific etiology, if an appropriate risk–benefit ratio is established. Prenatal genetic and urinary evaluation and estimation of postnatal renal function requires amniocentesis/vescicocentesis for fetal chromosomal microarray and serial vesicocentesis. Urinary calcium, sodium, and B2 microglobulin are the most reliable predictors of postnatal renal function. In the male fetus with isolated LUTO secondary to PUVs or urethral hypoplasia, fetal/neonatal survival is improved via improvement in pulmonary development and decreased oligohydramnios can be achieved by amnio-infusion followed by VAS. The best treatment for renal preservation with isolated LUTO has not been established; however, it is generally accepted that interventional therapy for LUTO should be reserved for cases with associated oligohydramnios. Conservative management may be appropriate for a limited number of isolated LUTO presentations with incomplete bladder neck obstruction.

INTRODUCTION TO IN UTERO SHUNTING FOR THORACIC PATHOLOGIES

The fetal thoracic cavity, much like the postnatal thoracic cavity, represents a closed space which has minimal capacity to expand in response to rapid growth of masses or accumulation of fluid. Masses such as large cystic congenital pulmonary airway malformations (CPAMs) or fluid accumulation such as pleural effusions (PEs) pose a threat to the developing fetus by acting as a space-occupying lesion and result in intrathoracic compression of the developing lungs and disturbance of intrathoracic blood flow secondary to increased intrathoracic pressure and mediastinal shift of the heart and great vessels, which may lead to fetal hydrops (Figure 10.1). The risk for pulmonary hypoplasia or cardiovascular impairment is directly related to the degree of the space-occupying volume. Drainage of these lesions via in utero shunt placement or thoracentesis may lead to a decrease in volume of these space-occupying lesions with beneficial effects on fetal hemodynamics, normal lung growth, and outcome.

Pleural effusions

Fetal PE can present as part of a more generalized picture of nonimmune fetal hydrops or as an isolated sonographic finding.[32–34] They are generally divided into primary and secondary causes. Primary PE is a lymphatic malformation while secondary PE is usually due to associated anomalies such as aneuploidy, cardiac defects, anemia, or infections. Primary PE occurs in approximately 1 in 12,000 pregnancies with a 2:1 male to female ratio.[32] Gestational age at presentation is generally less than 32 weeks and the presence of hydrops is associated with high perinatal mortality ranging from 36% to 40%[33–35] (Figure 10.4). Isolated PE in the absence of fetal hydrops still poses a threat to the developing fetus by acting as a space-occupying lesion. The risk for pulmonary hypoplasia or cardiovascular impairment is directly related to the size of the space-occupying effusion volume. The laterality of the PE does not appear to influence outcome, but bilateral effusions may have more effect on pulmonary development as well as cardiac compression.[35]

Selection criteria for the treatment of fetuses with pleural effusion

Selection criteria for PE treatment by thoracoamniotic shunting (TAS) requires primary PE etiology that is not part of a more complex genetic syndrome; selection

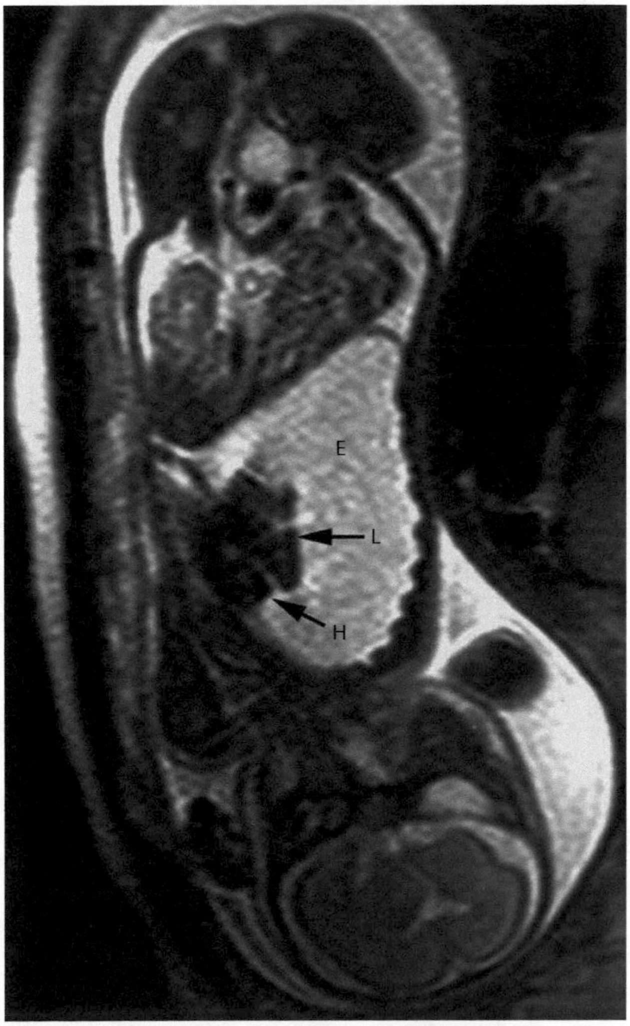

Figure 10.4 MRI image of congenital pleural effusion. Note the displacement and compression of the heart and lungs, and the presence of hydrops characterized by ascites and skin edema (E, effusion; H, heart; L, lung.)

criteria include normal karyotype, negative viral studies, normal echocardiogram, and absence of significant congenital anomalies that would affect morbidity or mortality, rapid recurrence of the effusion after thoracocentesis, and gestational age of less than 32 weeks.[32,33,36] However, a recent study advocates for shunting up to 37 weeks to improve postnatal resuscitation efforts.[37] Minimal evaluation should include confirmation of a primary lymphocytic effusion by cell count (>95% mononuclear cells) and PCR-based infectious studies for parvovirus, cytomegalovirus, herpes virus, and toxoplasmosis from the effusion fluid obtained at initial diagnostic thoracocentesis or amniocentesis.

Thoracentesis and thoracoamniotic shunting technique

Thoracocentesis utilizes a 20- to 22-gauge spinal needle under continuous ultrasound guidance with insertion into the lower lateral aspect of the fetal hemithorax in the midaxillary line. The entrance point is important as it should be the most dependent portion of the thorax into which the effusion will collect, allowing the maximum amount of fluid to be removed by aspiration. Reevaluation is performed in 24–72 hours and effusions rapidly accumulating after drainage will most likely benefit from chronic drainage by TAS (Figure 10.5). The technique for TAS is similar to that used for bladder insertion but optimal positioning of the shunt is side dependent. For right effusions, the optimal position for shunt placement is the lower third of the chest between the midclavicular and midaxillary lines. For left effusions, optimal placement is the upper third of the chest in the midaxillary line. This allows for optimal drainage as the heart returns to its normal position and the lungs expand to fill the chest. The appropriate trajectory for passage of the shunt trocar is determined by ultrasound such that the tip of the trocar ends up immediately adjacent to target location in the chest. Maternal skin is then anesthetized with 1% plain lidocaine and a small 3-mm incision is made. The trocar sheath is then passed through the maternal abdomen into the amniotic fluid space adjacent the chest. The trocar is advanced until the space between the ribs at the entrance site is located, and, using a gentle twisting action, the trocar is advanced through the chest wall until the tip lies 5–10 mm within the effusion. The sharp stylet is removed and 5–10 cc of effusion fluid aspirated. If there is suggestion of particulate matter it is beneficial to perform a lavage by alternating aspiration of 10 cc of effusion followed by infusion of 10 cc warm (37°C) normal saline until the fluid appears clear. The double-pigtail shunt is then quickly loaded into the trocar sheath so that the effusion does not drain, making catheter placement more difficult and limiting its ability to resume its original coiled shape. If necessary, it may be helpful to temporarily expand the effusion to facilitate shunt placement by infusing 10–30 cc of warm saline. Push rods (one or two push rods, depending on the manufacturer) are introduced and slowly advanced, displacing the proximal segment of the catheter into the intended cavity. The metal tip and high-density composition of the Rocket catheter optimizes visualization of its entrance into the fluid cavity. The push rod is advanced 8–9 cm to deploy the proximal pigtail into the fluid space. The sheath is then withdrawn to approximately 1 cm from the chest wall. The push rod is then held in place while

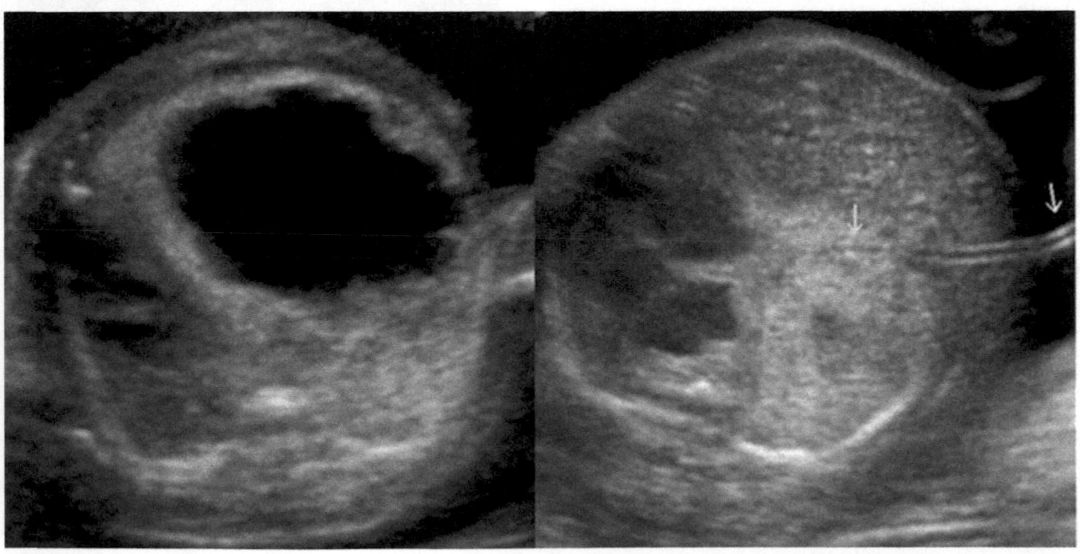

(a) (b)

Figure 10.5 Congenital pulmonary airway malformation (CPAM) with macrocyst (a) before and (b) after shunt placement. Prior fine needle drainage of the macrocyst helped to determine the optimal position to enter the fetal chest for subsequent shunt placement (arrows point at shunt within the CPAM).

the outer sheath is pulled approximately 2–3 cm backward over the push rod through the chest wall into the amniotic cavity, which deploys the central straight portion of the shunt. The shunt should then be within the amniotic cavity and while holding the pushrod in place the sheath is backed an additional 1–2 cm away from the chest wall. At this point, it is important to stop and rotate the tip of the sheath away from the insertion site without otherwise moving it and then deploy the remainder of the shunt from the sheath at an angle away from the insertion site. This is an important maneuver as it prevents the proximal pigtail from being partially deployed into the chest cavity which increases the risk of shunt migration into the chest cavity. Effusion drainage begins rapidly because of the initial increased intrathoracic pressure, but may take 12–48 hours to complete. Prophylactic single-dose intravenous (IV) antibiotic therapy is recommended. If polyhydramnios is present, amnioreduction utilizing the trocar sheath can be performed.

Complications

The most common complications of thoracic shunt procedures are related to displacement of the catheter into the amniotic cavity or less commonly into the thoracic cavity.[38] Occlusion from proteinaceous materials or thrombus may present additional complications. Pregnancy loss is estimated at approximately 5%. Thoracentesis risk for pregnancy loss is estimated at 0.5%–1.0%.

Outcome

Outcomes following TAS are dependent on correct selection of fetuses for whom treatment will provide a benefit for fetuses with hydrops or significant risk of pulmonary hypoplasia. Studies have shown that effective drainage leads to improved antenatal lung growth, hydrops resolution, and long-term survival (Table 10.5). Aubard et al.[33] identified hydrops as the only prognostic factor for outcome following multivariant analysis with survivals, with and without hydrops, of 67% and 100%, respectively, while without treatment, survival was 21%–23% in both groups. Thompson et al.[41] reviewed 17 neonatal TAS survivors with a mean gestational age of 29 weeks (range of 21–35). Twelve fetuses were hydropic at TAS. Recurrent respiratory symptoms were identified in six infants, but was not significantly different from a matched control group. Yinon et al.[37] reported on 88 fetuses with large PE, 59 (67.0%) were hydropic, 67 (76.1%) had bilateral effusions, and 36 (40.9%) had polyhydramnios. Mean age of shunt placement was 27.6 weeks (range 18–37), and delivery was 34.2 weeks (range 19–42). Seventy-four babies (84.1%) were live-born and 52 (70.3%) survived the neonatal period. In 59 hydropic fetuses, 10 (16.9%) died in utero and 18 (30.5%) died after birth for a perinatal survival of 52.5%. However, in 29 nonhydropic fetuses, neonatal survival was 72.4%. Hydrops resolved in 28 fetuses (47.5%) following shunting with 71% survival compared with 35% in 31 fetuses where hydrops persisted. In their 22 neonatal deaths, seven were due to pulmonary hypoplasia, five were due to genetic syndromes, two were due to aneuploidy, and one was due to congenital heart disease.

CONGENITAL PULMONARY AIRWAY MALFORMATION

CPAM is a benign, space-occupying tumor due to overgrowth of terminal respiratory bronchioles. CPAMs are most often unilobular (80%–95%) and can affect any lobe. They are classified prenatally by ultrasound and MRI into microcystic (50%) or macrocystic (50%) types depending on the size of the cysts.[42,43] Macrocystic CPAMs can contain a single or several large dominant macrocysts, which fill with fluid, until they formed large, space-occupying regions within the fetal lung. Large lesions can cause rapid mediastinal shift and compromise hemodynamic status with the development of hydrops. Early enlargement of lesions can result in the compression of the normal fetal lung tissue that may result in lethal pulmonary hypoplasia if it occurs at 18–24 weeks gestation during critical lung transition from canalicular to the alveolar stage. Mediastinal shift and left lung masses can also lead to compression of the fetal esophagus, decreased fetal swallowing with the development of polyhydramnios with risk of preterm delivery. CPAMs communicate with the tracheobronchial tree such that there is a risk of air trapping after birth within the macrocysts, causing rapid enlargement

Table 10.5 Pleural effusion outcomes following thoracoamniotic shunt placement.

Author	No.	LB	SB	NND	Hydrops	Survival
Nicolaides and Azar[39]	51	33 (12 HR)	2	12	18	65%
Aubard et al.[33]	80	57 (48 HR)	21	15	63	74% (O), 67% (H), 100% (NH)
Yinon et al.[37]	88	74	—	22	59	59%
Peranteau et al.[40]	37	21	3	13	21	60% (O), 50% (H), 100% (NH)
Total	**256**	**185**	**26**	**62**	**161**	**48.4% (O)**

Abbreviations: H, hydropic fetuses; HR, hydrops resolution following shunt placement; NH, nonhydropic fetuses; O, overall survival.

and compression of the newborn's lungs resulting in respiratory distress and/or pneumothorax. The greatest rate of growth of microcystic CPAM usually occurs at 20–25 weeks with a plateau in growth beginning at 26–28 weeks.[44] The natural history of CPAM with dominant macrocysts or macrocystic cluster is more unpredictable because rate of growth of the cystic and solid components can be quite different. The goal of shunt therapy is chronic drainage of the macrocysts to decrease overall volume and therefore mass effect within the fetal chest. Early therapy is directed at preventing pulmonary hypoplasia, while later interventions are done for evolving hydrops or progressive polyhydramnios.

SELECTION CRITERIA FOR SHUNT THERAPY IN FETUSES WITH CONGENITAL PULMONARY AIRWAY MALFORMATION

TAS should be considered for fetuses with secondary complications that worsen their prognosis (early-onset hydrops or progressive polyhydramnios) and have failed a course of steroid therapy, which has been shown to alter growth in primarily microcystic lesions.[45] The goal of shunting is chronic drainage of the large macrocysts that decreases mass volume and corrects the underlying physiologic disturbances (Figure 10.2). Candidates should have a macrocystic CPAM confirmed by ultrasound and/or fetal MRI; fetuses with other lesions are not likely to benefit from TAS. Initially, thoracentesis should be performed to drain the dominant macrocyst or macrocystic complex (as often there is communication between the cysts) and then reevaluate to determine how rapidly the fluid reaccumulates. Also, it is important to document "where" the macrocyst(s) drains (upward or downward in the chest cavity), which will help guide optimal shunt placement into the macrocyst(s) and decrease the risk for shunt displacement after the macrocyst(s) collapse. Polyhydramnios may require amnioreduction to decrease the risk of preterm delivery. The fetus must have a normal karyotype and negative workup for fetal hydrops, including hematologic, infectious, and cardiovascular etiologies.

THORACENTESIS AND THORACOAMNIOTIC SHUNT TECHNIQUE

The technique for thoracentesis and shunt insertion is similar to that described for PE, although there may be some minor variation related to the involved lobe of the lung on the right or left side. The point of entrance into the fetal chest for TAS must be chosen with consideration given to how the cysts shrink during the initial drainage process, so that the cyst can be completely drained, based on the original position of the shunt. Maternal single-dose IV broad-spectrum antibiotic prophylaxis is recommended.

Complications

Overall procedure complications are similar to those related to shunting for PE, although the risk of shunt malfunction due to occlusion may be increased.[45–47] Risk of rupturing a major blood vessel while traversing the pulmonary parenchyma before entering the macrocyst(s) can be minimized using color flow Doppler to visualize blood vessels that need to be avoided. Although not directly contraindicated, all efforts should be made to avoid trocar passage through the placenta. If transplacental approach is necessary, color Doppler to avoid large placental surface vessels should be employed. As in all fetal interventions, the potential of uterine irritability exist and patients should be monitored for at least 4–6 hours after these procedures, and utilize aggressive tocolytic therapy as needed.

Outcomes

A summary of published outcomes for TAS for macrocystic outcomes is presented in Table 10.6. The natural history of CPAM shows that fetal hydrops is a significant prognostic factor of fetal outcome. Review of published reports[35,41,45–47] shows that hydrops was present in only 7% (8/117) of live-born survivors but was present in 52% (22/42) that experienced perinatal loss. Laberge et al.[34] reviewed 48 cases and found that only hydrops was a significant prognostic factor for survival. We had previously reviewed our experience with TAS in large macrocystic lesions with fetal hydrops or severe polyhydramnios.[47] Ten shunts were placed at a mean gestational age of 23 weeks. Shunting resulted in a mean reduction of 50% in overall

Table 10.6 Macrocystic CPAM outcomes following thoracoamniotic shunt placement.

Author	No.	Shunts	LB	SB	NND	Survival
Bernaschek et al.[45]	4	4	3 (1 H)	—	1	75% (O,S)
Dommergues et al.[46]	33 (4 BPS)	9 (H, P)	4 BPS, 23 CCAM (5 H)	—	3 (1 H)	79% (O), 67% (S)
Baxter et al.[47]	10	10 (6 H)	7 (4 H)	1 (1 H)	2 (2 H)	70%
Wilson et al.[38]	10	13 (10 patients)	9	1	2	70%
Schrey et al.[48]	11	11	10	1	0	91% (83% H)
Peranteau et al.[40]	37	42 (37 patients, 28 H)	35 (28 H)	2 (2 H)	8 (8 H)	73% (O), 74% (H), 80% (non-H)
Total	**105**	**84 (43 H)**	**91 (38 H)**	**5 (3 H)**	**24 (10 H)**	**68.4% (O), 67.4% (S), 56% (H)**

Abbreviations: CPAM, congenital pulmonary airway malformation; BPS, bronchopulmonary sequestration; H, hydropic; non-H, non-hydropic; P, polyhydramnios; O,overall survival; S, stillbirth.

mass volume and the CPAM mass volume/head circumference ratio (CVR). The mean duration of the shunt was 10 weeks and mean age at delivery was 33 weeks with a subsequent perinatal survival of 70%, suggesting an improved outcome in this population.

Schrey et al.[48] described 11 fetuses with macrocystic CPAM that underwent TAS. Procedures were offered if fetal hydrops or signs of evolving hydrops were present or for very large lesions or rapidly enlarging lesions. If multiple cysts were present, a single shunt was used with intent to traverse several cysts. All fetuses had normal karyotype and no other anomalies. Shunts were placed at a mean gestational age of 24.6 weeks (range 17–32). Six fetuses were hydropic and of the remaining five, one had severe polyhydramnios, three had lesions rapidly increasing in size (CVR > 1.6), and one had a very large lesion at initial presentation. In total, four cases presented with severe polyhydramnios. Shunting the largest cyst always decompressed the entire lesion and hydrops and/or polyhydramnios resolved in all surviving fetuses. One severely hydropic fetus, shunted at 17 weeks, died the following day. In one case the shunt fell out and the lesion did not reaccumulate. No patient had rupture of membranes or preterm labor before 35.6 weeks. Mean gestational age at delivery was 38.2 weeks and underwent uneventful postnatal lobectomies with CPAM confirmed in all cases. Mean interval from shunting to delivery was 13.1 weeks (range 4.1–19.4). Overall survival was 10/11 (91%) and 5/6 (83%) for hydropic fetuses. All but two fetuses required respiratory support at some period after birth but prior to surgery.

In 2015, Peranteau et al.[40] reviewed their single institutional experience managing large macrocystic CPAM and PE with TAS. Ninety-seven shunts were placed in 75 fetuses who presented with macrocystic CPAM ($n = 38$) or large PE ($n = 37$) in the setting of hydrops or severe mass effect. Mean age at shunt placement was less in CPAMs (24 ± 3 weeks) than PE (26 ± 3 weeks). The CPAM volume and CVR changed by 55 ± 21% and 57 ± 21%, respectively, representing a significant decrease in mass effect of over 50% following shunting. Complete PE drainage occurred in 27% and significant, but incomplete drainage in 73%. Hydrops was present in 69% of fetuses which resolved in 83% after TAS.

Overall long-term survival was 68%, 75% for CPAM, and 60% for PE. Postnatal median NICU stay for survivors was 21 days (range 4–215). Endotracheal intubation and respiratory support beyond expected occurred in 71%. Two CPAM patients required extracorporeal membrane oxygenation (ECMO) support on day 1 for cardiorespiratory failure with only one survivor. At discharge, 27% (PE 50%, CPAM 17%) required a diuretic and/or supplemental oxygen for respiratory support. Authors concluded that survival was strongly associated with decrease in mass volume and hydrops resolution following shunt placement. No fetus survived in either group in which hydrops did not resolve. Alternatively, all fetuses that survived showed hydrops resolution, however, there were five cases each of CPAM and PE that did not survive despite hydrops resolution.

SUMMARY

TAS in appropriate selected fetuses with macrocystic CPAM or large PE has been shown to improve survival and decrease postnatal morbidity and mortality. Presence and severity of hydrops at time of TAS and resolution of hydrops following shunt placement are important prognostic factors with better outcomes in fetuses without hydrops at time of TAS and those that have resolution of hydrops following successful shunting. As such, patients with severe hydrops and/or who show limited resolution of hydrops following TAS should be counseled cautiously about the long-term prognosis.

CONCLUSIONS

Prenatal identification of renal and thoracic abnormalities is increasingly more common, and counseling regarding the in utero medical and surgical options for these lesions continues to be developed. The key to success for the in utero therapy of bladder and thoracic abnormalities is appropriate evaluation to ensure the correct diagnosis and prediction of the morbidity or mortality. The selection criteria for fetuses undergoing in utero therapy must be limited to those fetuses for whom benefit can be anticipated from the therapy. The reported data would suggest that the use of both vesicoamniotic and thoracoamniotic shunts can benefit this select group of fetuses with fluid-filled lesions of either the bladder or the chest, respectively. As the use of this therapeutic modality increases, prospective randomized trials will define the utility, efficacy, risks, and benefits of intrauterine fetal shunting for the mother and the fetus.

REFERENCES

1. Firth HV, Hurst JA. Renal tract anomalies. In: Firth HV, Hurst JA, and Hall JG (ed), *Oxford Desk Reference—Clinical Genetics*, pp. 624–626. Oxford, UK: Oxford University Press, 2005.
2. Chevalier RL. Congenital urinary tract obstruction: The long view. *Adv Kid Dis* 2015; 22(4): 312–9.
3. Johnson MP. Fetal obstructive uropathy. In: Harrison MR, Evans MI, Adzick NS, Holzgreve W (eds), *The Unborn Patient—The Art and Science of Fetal Therapy* (3rd Edition), Chapter 18, pp. 259–86. Orlando, FL: W.B. Saunders Company, 2001.
4. Chevalier RL. Fetal urinary tract obstruction: pathophysiology. In: Kilby MD, Oepkes D, Johnson A (eds), *Fetal Therapy: Scientific Basis and Critical Appraisal of Clinical Benefits*, Section 2, Chapter 14.1. pp. 238–45. Cambridge, UK: Cambridge University Press, 2013.
5. Malin G, Tonks AM, Morris RK et al. Congenital lower urinary tract obstruction: A population-based epidemiological study. *BJOG* 2012; 119: 1455–64.
6. Clayton DB, Brock III JW. Lower urinary tract obstruction in the fetus and neonate. *Clin Perinatol* 2014; 41:643–59.

7. Morris RK, Kilby MD. Congenital urinary tract obstruction. *Best Pract Res Clin Obstet Gynaecol* 2008; 22(1): 97–122.
8. Dias T, Sairam S, Kumarasiri S. Ultrasound diagnosis of fetal renal abnormalities. *Best Pract Res Clin Obstet Gynaecol* 2014; 28: 403–15.
9. Rychik J. McCann M, Tian Z et al. Fetal cardiovascular effects of lower urinary tract obstruction with giant bladder. *Ultrasound Obstet Gynecol* 2010; 36: 682–6.
10. Yoshizaki CT, Francisco RPV, Corriera de Pinho J et al. Renal volumes measured by 3-dimensional sonography in healthy fetuses from 20–40 weeks. *J Ultrasound Med* 2013; 32: 421–427.
11. Bernardes LS, Francisco RPV, Saada J et al. Quantitative analysis of renal vascularisation in fetuses with urinary tract obstruction by three-dimensional power-Doppler. *Am J Obstet Gynecol* 2011; 572: E1–7.
12. Ruano R, Pimenta EJ, Duarte S, Zugaib M. Four-dimensional ultrasonographic imaging of fetal lower urinary tract obstruction and guidance of percutaneous cystoscopy. *Ultrasound Obstet Gynecol* 2009; 33: 250–2.
13. Lefere M, Sandiate I, Hindryck A et al. Postmortem high-resolution fetal magnetic resonance imaging in three cases of lower urinary tract obstruction. *Fetal Diagn Ther* 2013; 34(3): 195–8.
14. Haeri S, Hernandez Ruano S, Farah LM et al. Prenatal cytogenetic diagnosis from fetal urine in lower urinary tract obstruction. *Congenit Anom* 2013; 53: 89–91.
15. Wu S, Johnson MP. Fetal lower urinary tract obstruction. *Clin Perinatol* 2009; 36: 377–90.
16. Ruano R, Yoshisaki CT, Salustiano EMA et al. Early fetal cystoscopy for first-trimester severe megacystis. *Ultrasound Obstet Gynecol* 2011; 37: 696–701.
17. Ruano R. Fetal surgery for severe lower urinary tract obstruction. *Prenat Diagn* 2011; 31: 667–74.
18. Ruano R, Duarte S, Bunduki V et al. Fetal cystoscopy for severe lower urinary tract obstruction—Initial experience of a single center. *Prenat Diagn* 2010; 30: 30–9.
19. Jones KL, Jones MC, Del Campo M (eds). Oligohydramnios sequence. In: *Smith's Recognizable Patterns of Human Malformation*, pp. 820–1. Philadelphia, PA: Elsevier Saunders, 2013.
20. Morris RK, Malin GL, Khan KS, Kilby MD. Antenatal ultrasound to predict postnatal renal function in congenital lower urinary tract obstruction: Systemic review of test accuracy. *BJOG* 2009; 116: 1290–9.
21. Morris RK., Quinlan-Jones E, Kilby MD, Khan KS. Systematic review of accuracy of fetal urine analysis to predict poor postnatal renal function in cases of congenital urinary tract obstruction. *Prenat Diagn* 2007; 27: 900–911.
22. Nicolini U, Spelzini F. Invasive assessment of fetal renal abnormalities: Urinalysis, fetal blood sampling and biopsy. *Prenat Diagn* 2001; 21(11): 964–9.
23. Morris RK, Ruano S, Kilby MD. Effectiveness of fetal cystoscopy as a diagnostic and therapeutic intervention for lower urinary tract obstruction: A systematic review. *Ultrasound Obstet Gynecol* 2011; 37: 629–37.
24. Clayton DB, Brock III JW. In utero intervention for urologic diseases. *Nat Rev Urol* 2012; 9: 207–217.
25. Morris RK, Malin GL, Khan KS, Kilby MD. Systematic review of the effectiveness of antenatal intervention for the treatment of congenital lower urinary tract obstruction. *BJOG* 2010; 117: 382–390.
26. Tonni G, Vito I, Ventura A, Grisolia G et al. Fetal lower urinary tract obstruction and its management. *Arch Gynecol Obstet* 2013; 287: 187–94.
27. Morris RK, Malin G, Quinlan-Jones E, Middleton KH et al. Percutaneous vesicoamniotic shunting versus conservative management of fetal lower urinary tract obstruction (PLUTO): A randomized trial. *Lancet* 2013; 382: 1496–506.
28. Ethun CG, Zamora IJ, Roth DR, Kale A et al. Outcomes of fetuses with lower urinary tract obstruction treated with vesicoamniotic shunt: A single-institution experience. *Journal Pediatr Surg* 2013; 48: 956–62.
29. Diwaker L, Morris RK, Barton P, Middleton LJ et al. Evaluation of the cost effectiveness of vesicoamniotic shunting in the management of congenital lower urinary tract obstruction (based on data from the PLUTO Trial). *PLoS One* 2013; 8(12): 1–10.
30. Ruano R, Sananess N, Sangi-Haghpeykar H, Hernandez-Ruano S et al. Fetal intervention for severe lower urinary tract obstruction: A multicenter case–control study comparing fetal cystoscopy with vesicoamniotic shunting. *Ultrasound Obstet Gynecol* 2015; 45: 452–8.
31. Sananes N, Favre R, Koh CJ, Zaloszyc A et al. Urological fistulas after fetal cystoscopic laser ablation of posterior urethral valves: Surgical technical aspects. *Ultrasound Obstet Gynecol* 2015; 45: 183–9.
32. Bianchi DW, Crombleholme TM, D'Alton ME. Hydrothorax. In: *Fetology*, pp. 313–21. New York, NY: McGraw-Hill, 2000.
33. Aubard Y, Derouineau I, Aubard V et al. Primary fetal hydrothorax: A literature review and proposed antenatal clinical strategy. *Fetal Diagn Ther* 1998; 13: 325–33.
34. Laberge JM, Crombleholme TM, Longaker M. The fetus with pleural effusions. In: Harrison MR, Golbus MS, Fily RA (eds), *The Unborn Patient*, pp. 314–9. Philadelphia, PA: WB Saunders, 1991.
35. Weber AM, Philipson EH. Reviews. Fetal pleural effusions: A review and meta-analysis for prognostic indicators. *Obstet Gynecol* 1992; 79: 281–6.
36. Johnson MP, Flake AW, Quintero RA et al. Fetal shunt procedures. In: Evans MI, Johnson MP, Moghissi KS (eds), *Invasive Outpatient Procedures in Reproductive Medicine*, pp. 61–89. Philadelphia, PA: Lippincott-Raven, 1997.

37. Yinon Y, Grisaru-Ganovsky S, Chaddha V et al. Perinatal outcome following fetal chest shunt insertion for pleural effusion. *Ultrasound Obstet Gynecol* 2010; 36: 58–64.
38. Wilson RD, Baxter JK, Johnson MP et al. Thoracoamniotic shunts: Fetal treatment of pleural effusions and congenital cystic adenomatoid malformations. *Fetal Diag Ther* 2004; 19: 413–20.
39. Nicolaides KH, Azar GB. Thoraco-amniotic shunting. *Fetal Diagn Ther* 1990; 5: 153–64.
40. Peranteau WH, Adzick NS, Boelig MM et al. Thoracoamniotic shunts for management of fetal lung lesions and pleural effusions: A single institutional review and predictors of survival in 75 cases. *J Pediatr Surg* 2015; 50: 301–5.
41. Thompson PJ, Greenough A, Nicolaides KH. Respiratory function in infancy following pleuro-amniotic shunting. *Fetal Diagn Ther* 1993; 8: 79–83.
42. Adzick NS. Fetal cystic adenomatoid malformation of the lung: Diagnosis, perinatal management and outcomes. *Semin Thorac Cardiovas Surg* 1994; 6: 247–52.
43. Stocker JT, Madewell JER, Drake RM. Congenital cystic adenomatoid malformation of the lung: Classification and morphologic spectrum. *Hum Pathol* 1977; 4: 155–71.
44. Crombleholme TM, Coleman B, Hedrick HL et al. Cystic adenomatoid malformation volume ratio predicts outcome in prenatally diagnosed cystic adenomatoid malformation of the lung. *J Pediatr Surg* 2002; 37: 331–8.
45. Bernaschek G, Deutinger J, Hansmann M et al. Feto-amniotic shunting-report of the experience of four European centres. *Prenat Diagn* 1994; 14: 821–33.
46. Dommergues M, Louis-Sylvestre C, Mandelbrot L et al. Congenital adenomatoid malformation of the lung: When is active fetal therapy indicated? *Am J Obstet Gynecol* 1997; 177: 953–8.
47. Baxter JK, Johnson MP, Wilson RD et al. Thoracoamniotic shunts: pregnancy outcome for congenital cystic adenomatoid malformation (CCM) and pleural effusion. *Am J Obstet Gynecol* 2001; 6: S245.
48. Schrey S, Kelly EN, Langer JC et al. Fetal thoracoamniotic shunting for large macrocystic congenital cystic adenomatoid malformations of the lung. *Ultrasound Obstet Gynecol* 2012; 39: 515–20.

Cordocentesis

11

CARL P. WEINER and GENE T. LEE

CONTENTS

INTRODUCTION

Fetal blood sampling was initially performed at hysterotomy.[1] The subsequent development of fetoscopy in the 1960s allowed fetal vessel puncture under direct visualization. However, fetoscopy was cumbersome and risky since the procedure-related loss rates exceeded 5%. The development of high-resolution ultrasound made it possible to clearly image the umbilical cord. Spurred by a desire to accurately diagnose fetal toxoplasmosis, Daffos performed the first intentional percutaneous umbilical blood sampling under ultrasound guidance (cordocentesis) in the early 1980s.[2] The procedure rapidly gained favor with demonstration of its safety[3–5] and directly spurred the development of fetal medicine. If necessary for technical reasons, fetal blood can also be obtained under sonographic guidance from either the fetal heart (cardiocentesis) or the intrahepatic umbilical vein (hepatocentesis).[6] A wide range of gestational appropriate fetal norms (hematological, endocrinological, immunological, biochemical, and biophysical)[7] were developed, a crucial step in the evolution of fetal medicine. While many early indications for cordocentesis have been supplanted by less invasive techniques, there remain several indications for fetal blood sampling. The most common are the assessment and treatment of red cell and platelet alloimmunization, the rapid antenatal diagnosis of inherited blood or metabolic diseases, rapid karyotyping of malformed or severely growth-restricted fetuses in some countries, and rarely the determination of fetal acid base status.[8]

METHODS

Cordocentesis is performed in the outpatient setting by a single operator with or without an assistant. There is no benefit of maternal fasting, sedation, prophylactic antibiotics, or tocolysis. Cordocentesis can be performed as early as 12 weeks gestation, though it is technically more difficult prior to 20 weeks, and the loss rate is much higher prior to 16 weeks gestation. We encourage the patient's partner to attend both the counseling session preceding the procedure and the procedure itself. The limitations and potential complications must be stated unambiguously before written informed consent is obtained, and a targeted ultrasound examination is performed.

Centers vary in their approach. There are two methods for cordocentesis: freehand and the use of a fixed needle guide. Also, there are three potential locations selected for sampling: placental cord origin, free loop of umbilical cord, or intrahepatic vein. The first few centimeters of the fetal origin of the umbilical cord are innervated and puncture in that region causes pain and bradycardia. The umbilical vein is the preferred target rather than the umbilical artery because of its lower association with complications. Like all percutaneous procedures, a "no touch" philosophy is essential. If you do not touch the shaft of the needle, you cannot contaminate it.

The selection of the site for sampling will depend on operator experience and accessibility. In general, the placental cord origin is often targeted because the location is fixed. However, the intrahepatic umbilical vein appears to be equally safe compared with cordocentesis.[9,10] In one center, the intrahepatic umbilical vein as the site for sampling was more successful and there was less streaming from the sampling site.[10]

The freehand technique typically employs a 20- to 22-gauge spinal needle 8–12 cm long.[2] The needle course is tracked by imaging the tip and shaft with the ultrasound transducer held either in the opposite hand of the operator or by the assistant. Since the needle is not fixed, the tip can move several centimeters in all axes should either the site of insertion be suboptimal or the fetus move during the procedure. Once punctured, the operator secures the needle while the assistant aspirates a series of 1-mL syringes. Larger syringes can create enough negative pressure to collapse the umbilical vein leading to the erroneous conclusion that the position has been lost. Preheparinization of the syringe is unnecessary unless a fetal blood gas is needed. The sample is immediately placed into a specimen container prepared with the appropriate preservative. The freehand technique remains the most popular method for cordocentesis because of the flexibility it allows the operator.

Cordocentesis is also performed using a fixed needle guide (Figure 11.1)[3] that is attached to the base of the ultrasound transducer. Typically, the transducer is held by the operator's assistant. The predicted course of the needle, which can travel only in the vertical plane, is displayed on the ultrasound screen. This allows the operator to select in advance a precise target for puncture. Deviation from the predicted path occurs only when there is an abrupt change in the relationship between the puncture site in the maternal abdominal wall and the uterus as the needle traverses between the two. The most common causes are abrupt patient movement and failure of the assistant to hold the transducer surface flat against the maternal abdomen. Fetal movement is rarely an issue because of the speed of the procedure. Since lateral movement of the needle is not possible, a smaller gauge needle such as a 22 or 25 is used. It is important to line up the umbilical cord longitudinally rather than in cross section. It is preferable to target the "easiest" location for a direct approach. In more than 50% of the cases, a free loop is targeted, and placental puncture is avoided if possible when the indication is alloimmunization (red blood cell [RBC] or platelet), just as the informed practitioner would do with amniocentesis. In contrast to the freehand technique where there is a larger needle gauge and movement outside the vertical axis, local anesthesia is unnecessary for diagnostic procedures when using a 22-gauge needle. A local anesthetic is placed subcutaneously, independent of the technique, when the procedure is lengthy (e.g., intravascular transfusion). Prophylactic antibiotics are not indicated for either cordocentesis or intravascular transfusion. In our experience, amnionitis complicates less than 1 in 800 diagnostic procedures when the "no touch" philosophy is rigorously adhered to and a needle guide is used (1 in 1200 procedures).

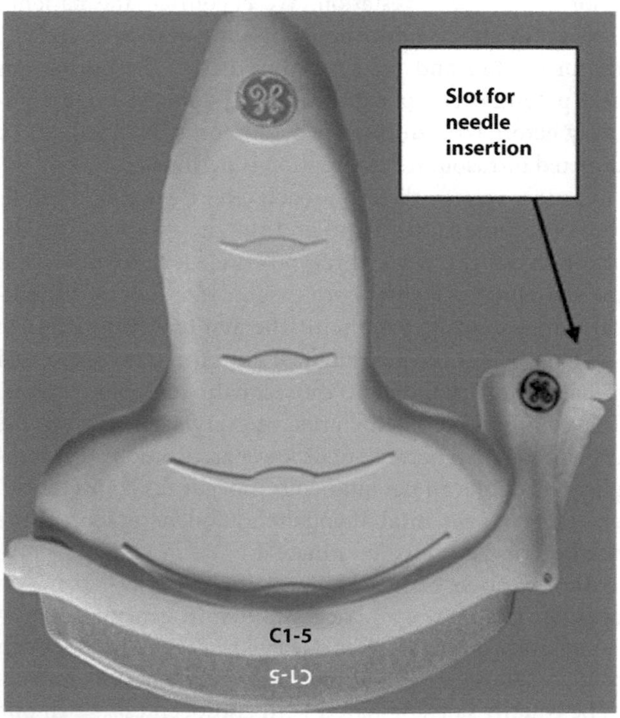

Figure 11.1 Typical example of a fixed needle guide. The one shown is made for the Voluson E10 by Civco Medical Solutions, Coralville, IA. The guideline follows the on-screen software.

Fetal movement may either prevent a successful puncture or shorten the access time available regardless of the technique used. Fetal movement while the needle is intraluminal increases the risk of umbilical cord trauma. Many operators administer a neuromuscular antagonist to eliminate the fetal movement (especially when performing a mid-loop puncture) and select either pancuronium (0.3 mg/kg estimated fetal weight), vecuronium (0.1 mg/kg EFW), or atracurium (0.4 mg/kg EFW). The agent is given either intramuscularly into the fetal buttock, or preferably, intravenously as soon as the vein is punctured. The effect is evident within seconds. Vercuronium instead of pancuronium is preferred for simple diagnostic procedures because its shorter half-life allows a more rapid return of fetal movement and heart rate variability.[11] In contrast, pancuronium is preferred for fetal transfusion because its side effect of increased fetal heart rate (FHR) helps maintain fetal cardiac output despite the volume load.[12]

The volume of blood removed depends on the gestation and indication for sampling. Five milliliters is typical and adequate for a karyotype, umbilical venous blood gas, and complete blood profile with Kleihauer–Betke testing, with 2 mL remaining for other additional tests.

MAJOR COMPLICATIONS AND RISK FACTORS FOR CORDOCENTESIS

The major complications of cordocentesis are listed in Table 11.1. They include all complications associated with amniocentesis plus fetal bradycardia, umbilical cord laceration, and thrombosis. Risk factors for cordocentesis are noted in Table 11.2.

Umbilical cord laceration and thrombosis are associated with freehand procedures. While such complications have not been formally recorded when a needle guide was used, these complications have been reported anecdotally.[13,14] Though bleeding from the umbilical puncture site is common, prolonged bleeding with sequelae is uncommon. Application of a "no touch" technique and the use

Table 11.1 Complications of cordocentesis.

1.	Bradycardia or asystole
2.	Premature rupture of membranes
3.	Premature labor
4.	Umbilical hemorrhage
5.	Placental hemorrhage
6.	Chorioamnionitis
7.	Umbilical thrombosis
8.	Fetal to maternal hemorrhage

Table 11.2 Risk factors for cordocentesis.

1.	Umbilical artery puncture (associated with bradycardia)
2.	Fetal hypoxemia (associated with bradycardia)
3.	Technique (freehand versus needle guide)
4.	Gestational age before 20 weeks (both techniques)
5.	Number of punctures (freehand technique only)
6.	Duration of procedure (freehand technique only)
7.	Inexperience

of disposable needles for a single puncture minimizes the risk of amnionitis.

Bradycardia is the major complication of cordocentesis. Virtually all emergency cesarean deliveries and most perinatal losses are associated with a fetal bradycardia. Umbilical artery puncture and hypoxia are the major risk factors for bradycardia (Figure 11.2). In the absence of profound anemia or fetal heart failure, fetal hypoxia is associated with an elevated umbilical artery resistance index and it can be used as a risk marker. The incidence of bradycardia with absent and/or reversed diastolic flow approaches 25%. Umbilical artery puncture increases the risk of fetal bradycardia 5- to 10-fold.[15] The presence of either oligohydramnios or a two-vessel cord increases the risk of arterial puncture. The observation that bradycardia may be associated with an elevated resistance index in one but not in both umbilical arteries suggests that the cause is localized vasospasm. Pancuronium use is associated with a lower prevalence of bradycardia in appropriately grown but not growth-restricted fetuses.[15] It is likely some episodes of bradycardia occur when fetal movement tugs on the umbilical cord, causing needle trauma and irritation to the underlying vascular smooth muscle. Bradycardia after umbilical vein puncture may reflect the disruption of the adjacent umbilical artery smooth muscle as the tip traverses the cord. In the event of a bradycardia, direct observation suggests that vigorous fetal stimulation by palpation is beneficial since the heart will speed up and then slow again if the manual stimulation is stopped too early. A variety of chronotropes (e.g., atropine) and bicarbonate have been given as part of a fetal resuscitation without predictable effect.

Even when performed at a mid-loop, the fetus does "react" to the cordocentesis. Umbilical artery resistance typically declines after either a diagnostic procedure or a fetal intravascular transfusion.[16] The higher the "normal" baseline resistance index, the greater the decline. The decrease is associated with prostacyclin release from

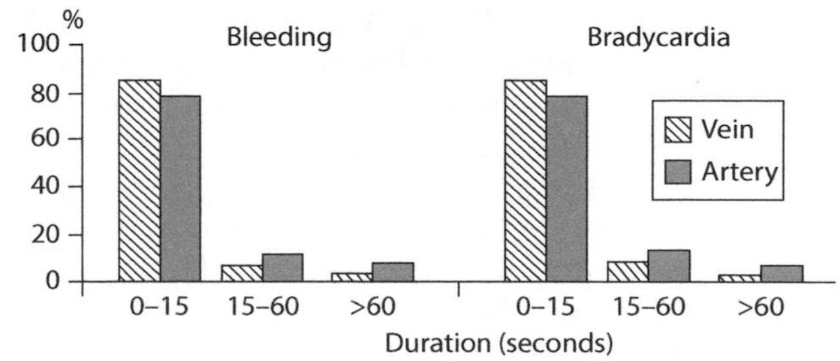

Figure 11.2 Fetal bradycardias and intra-amniotic bleeding occur more often and last longer when an umbilical cord artery rather than a vein is sampled.

the vascular endothelium.[17,18] Endothelial adaptation to hypoxia also explains why hypoxemia is a risk factor for bradycardia.[15] Rizzo et al.[19] demonstrated that endothelin is released upon umbilical vein puncture of growth-restricted but not appropriately grown fetuses. Fetuses who develop bradycardia release more endothelin, suggesting that the excess endothelin causes focal vasoconstriction at or near the puncture site.

Both techniques for cordocentesis have a learning curve. However, the learning curve may be shorter when a needle guide is used. Until recently, it was generally accepted that the technique selected was a matter of operator preference and had no impact on the outcome. However, there are a series of findings to challenge this concept.

The first line of evidence is indirect. The often stated "advantage" of the freehand technique, its flexibility, may also increase the risk. Analogous to a lever, a small movement at the hub of the needle amplifies the distance the tip moves. In association with this inescapable fact, freehand cordocentesis is produced in a significantly greater incremental increase in the maternal serum alpha-fetoprotein (MSAFP) than amniocentesis after controlling for placental puncture.[20] In contrast, the incremental change in MSAFP when a needle guide is used is similar to amniocentesis.[21] Further, the association between fetal thrombocytopenia and bleeding from the umbilical puncture site after a freehand cordocentesis is high enough to have prompted a recommendation that all fetuses at risk for alloimmune thrombocytopenia receive a prophylactic platelet transfusion at cordocentesis.[22] Yet, there is no relationship between the fetal platelet count and the bleeding time from the puncture site when a needle guide is used.[23] The latter may reflect either less lateral movement of the needle after puncture or the thinner gauge needle, or both. The loss rates reported after second-trimester amniocentesis are lower when thinner needles are used.[24] Not surprising, there are also reports which suggest that an amniocentesis performed with a needle guide is safer than one performed freehand.[25]

There is also a line of direct evidence favoring the use of a needle guide, though not a single center had an adequate volume for a randomized trial, and comparisons of loss rates sustained by groups using the freehand and needle guide techniques are problematic since it is hard to separate procedure-related losses from those secondary to the natural progression of disease. We sought to address the role of the technique by combining our experience with another fetal medicine unit which shared in common the use of a fixed needle guide for all procedures.[13] Over 25 operators with varying levels of experience performed 1260 diagnostic cordocenteses at a mean gestational age of 29 weeks. The umbilical vein (confirmed by the blood pressure reading) was punctured in 90% of the cases, demonstrating that the desired vessel can be targeted. A procedure-related loss was defined as any loss within 2 weeks of the procedure except those resulting from elective pregnancy termination. Overall, there were 12 losses (0.9%) (Table 11.3). To exclude the contribution of the underlying pathology to the loss rate, procedures should be divided into high and low risk, with the latter excluding chromosomal abnormalities, nonimmune hydrops, intrauterine growth restriction, and fetal infection. Such exclusions virtually eliminate all abnormal fetuses that might be at risk of a loss *unrelated* to the procedure. After revision, the study's procedure-related loss rate with the needle guide 0.2 (2/1021). A decade later, Liao et al.[14] reported their experience using the fixed needle guide in 1475 pregnancies. Their reported procedure loss rate was 0.8% (12/1475). Combined together, these two studies show a 0.5% (14/2496) complication rate.

The most recent studies for the freehand technique which include large sample sizes suggest that the procedure-related perinatal loss rate approaches ~1%. Donner et al.[26] reported 759 diagnostic cordocenteses *with a known outcome* using the freehand technique. After excluding 94 terminations, their loss rate is calculated at 1.1% (7/665). Tongsong et al.[27,28] reported a 1% procedure loss rate on 1320 pregnancies for cordocentesis performed between 16 and 24 weeks. This same group reported in 2011 a total perinatal loss rate of 2.2%–2.9% from 2214 cordocenteses.[29]

These findings, both indirect and direct, suggest that many of the procedure-related losses associated with cordocentesis are possibly technique dependent. Ultimately the critical issue may be the experience of the operator. While skilled operators with frequent volume may have results that approach those obtained with a needle guide, the majority of practitioners who perform only a few cordocenteses per year would benefit from using the needle guide.

INDICATIONS AND APPLICATIONS FOR CORDOCENTESIS

Antenatal diagnosis of blood disorders

The earliest indications for fetal blood sampling in the 1970s and early 1980s were the diagnosis of hemoglobinopathies and genetic defects affecting hemostasis.[1,30] The 1990s saw the application of recombinant DNA techniques to the analysis of placental biopsy material or amniocytes for the diagnosis of many of these conditions in the first trimester of pregnancy.[30,31] However, cordocentesis may still be needed for a phenotype diagnosis, in those patients requiring confirmation of normality based on a linked probe, those who lack key affected relatives, those who are not informative by any of the available probes, and those in whom DNA analysis is not feasible because of late referral.

Antenatal diagnosis of metabolic disorders

There are more than 200 inherited, metabolic conditions for which the specific enzyme deficiencies are defined, and for which accurate diagnostic biochemical assays are available. Many of these conditions have no effective therapy and result in either early childhood death or serious disability. Prenatal diagnosis of over 100 of these disorders is now possible by the analysis of amniotic fluid, placental tissue, or fetal blood. Cordocentesis may be particularly useful when a rapid diagnosis is needed. This occurs when the gestational age is close to the local limit for abortion, as with late prenatal care, or after failed chorionic villus or amniotic fluid techniques.

Red blood cell alloimmunization

Cordocentesis is not indicated in most instances of maternal RBC alloimmunization solely for fetal blood typing. The most current technology allows for detection of fetal Rhesus (Rh) antigen by polymerase chain reaction (PCR) of cell-free fetal DNA in maternal serum.[32,33] Alternatively, clinicians can obtain accurate fetal typing by applying PCR to either trophoblast or amniocytes obtained in the early second trimester when the risk of exacerbating sensitization is lower.[34,35]

During the last 50 years, several therapeutic approaches were undertaken with the aim of ameliorating the severity

Table 11.3 Frequency of major complications of cordocentesis when a needle guide is used.

Final diagnosis	GA (weeks) at cordocentesis	Percent of emergency delivery[a]	Percent of death within 2 weeks[b]
RBC alloimmunization	28 ± 4	0.2	0.2
Uteroplacental dysfunction	32 ± 4	5.0	0.9
Chromosome abnormality	29 ± 6	7.7	9.9
All others	28 ± 6	0.3	0.2

Source: Weiner CP and Okamura K, *Fetal Diagn Ther*, 11, 169–175, 1996.
Abbreviations: GA, gestational age; RBC, red blood cell.
[a] Weiner, unpublished data.
[b] From Weiner and Okamura. Thirteen fetuses with a chromosome abnormality delivered by cesarean section were delivered before the karyotype was completed.

of the condition and preventing intrauterine fetal death. Fetal blood sampling has made it possible to better understand the pathophysiology of the disease and provided an improved method for assessment and treatment of fetal anemia.[36–41] The net result of improved understanding is an improved perinatal outcome.

Previously, the severity of fetal hemolysis was estimated from (1) the history of previously affected pregnancies, (2) the level of maternal hemolytic antibodies in a first sensitized pregnancy, (3) the amniotic fluid bilirubin concentration, (4) the altered morphometry of fetus and placenta, and (5) the presence of pathological FHR patterns. However, there was a wide scatter of values around the regression lines describing the associations between the degree of fetal anemia and the data obtained from these indirect methods of assessment.[42]

Perhaps the most important advancement in the noninvasive management of RBC alloimmune disease was the recognition that most anemic fetuses have elevated peak flow velocities in the middle cerebral artery (MCA). The vast majority of fetuses with moderate or severe anemia have an elevated peak systolic velocity (PSV) in the MCA.[43,44] However, a sizable percentage of anemic fetuses have normal velocities,[45] and the relationship between velocity and the magnitude of the hemoglobin deficit varies greatly among fetuses.

The only accurate method for determining severity is blood sampling by cordocentesis with the measurement of fetal hemoglobin concentration, reticulocyte count, blood type, strength of the direct Coombs test, and total bilirubin concentration. In principle, invasive procedures should be minimized not only because of the fetal risk, but also because transplacental puncture enhances the risk of fetomaternal hemorrhage,[20,21] increases maternal antibody titer and worsens disease. The recommended approach is to avoid cordocentesis until the MCA-PSV is abnormal (>1.5 multiple of median [MoM]). Since there is a known 10%–12% false-positive rate,[44,45] some providers may choose to wait for an increasing trend in those pregnancies under 20-week gestation when cordocentesis is most difficult. In addition, since as many as half the fetuses with mild to moderate anemia have normal velocities, it is reasonable, depending on referral patterns and distances, to consider sampling all women with a history of severe disease, those with high antibody titers, and fetuses with pathological FHR patterns.

A fetal blood sample is obtained, the hemoglobin concentration measured, and an intravascular blood transfusion given as necessary (Figure 11.3).[46] The goal of the first transfusion is to correct the hemoglobin deficit completely unless there is evidence of hydrops. Immune hydrops is almost always secondary to high-output heart failure characterized by an elevated umbilical venous pressure.[47] These fetuses tolerate poorly the first intravascular transfusion and should be corrected initially to a hemoglobin level of no more than 8–9 g/dL. We routinely monitor the fetal umbilical venous pressure to avoid too much transfusion. The second transfusion

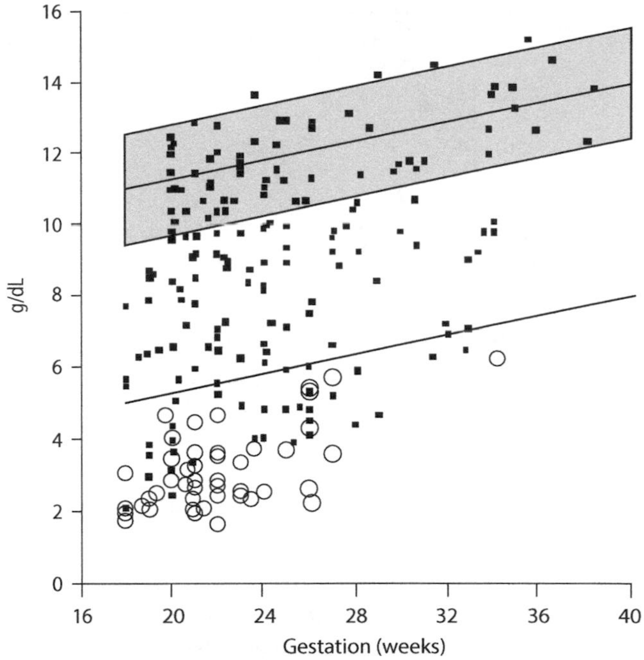

Figure 11.3 Fetal hemoglobin concentration from red cell isoimmunized pregnancies at the time of the first fetal blood sampling are plotted on the reference range (mean, 5th, and 95th centiles; shaded area) for gestation. Hydrops fetalis (O) is associated with severe anemia.

is performed a few days later at which time the target hemoglobin for this and all subsequent transfusions is 18 g/dL. Subsequent transfusions are given at 3- to 4-week intervals until 34–36 weeks' gestation, their timing based on the findings in the MCA and the knowledge that following a fetal blood transfusion the mean rate of decrease in fetal hemoglobin is approximately 0.3 g/dL/day (Figure 11.4).[46] When hydrops is not a factor for the first transfusion, investigators have found that the timing the second cordocentesis can be accurately predicted when the MoM >1.69.[48] Currently, the survival rate of red cell isoimmunized pregnancies treated with cordocentesis exceeds 90% in experienced hands, and virtually all losses are associated with immune hydrops fetalis.[47,49] Studies show that children can expect to have normal long-term neurodevelopment despite the profound anemia prior to treatment.[49,50]

Rarely, the clinician in a sensitized pregnancy will find a fetus whose PSV MCA is greater than 1.5 MoM but is not anemic (hematocrit [HCT] > 30 g/dL). In this instance, the timing of the repeat cordocentesis can be determined by the change in the peak flow velocity in the MCA and by the "hemolysis pattern" determined at the first sampling (Table 11.4).[51] This prospectively validated grading scheme is based on the reticulocyte count and the strength of the positive direct Coombs test. Most fetuses do not require a second sampling. Sensitized fetuses with no severe anemia still remain at risk for postnatal hyperbilirubinemia, which is directly correlated with their antenatal bilirubin levels (Figure 11.5).[52,53]

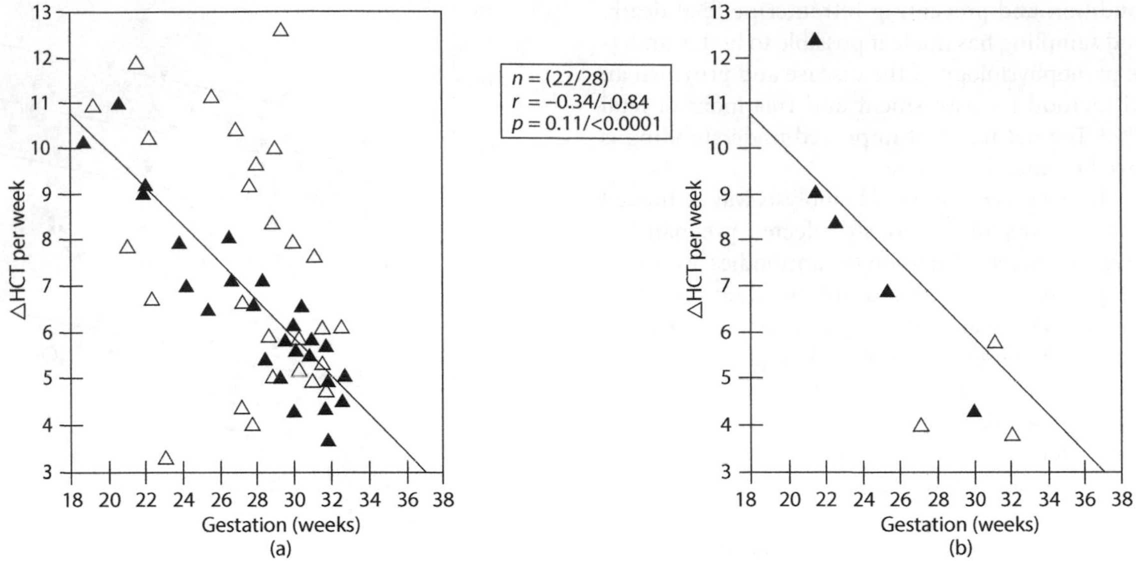

Figure 11.4 Rate of hematocrit (HCT) decline after the first and subsequent transfusions. (a) Effect of gestational age on decline in HCT after transfusion. Open triangles, decline in HCT between first and second transfusions; closed triangles, decline for all subsequent transfusions. Regression line is based on all subsequent transfusions. (b) Prospective confirmation of relationship shown (a) with new data. Open triangles, decline in HCT between first and second transfusions; closed triangles, decline for all subsequent transfusions. Regression line is from (a). (Reproduced from *American Journal of Obstetrics & Gynecology*, 165, Weiner CP et al., Management of fetal hemolytic disease by cordocentesis. II. Outcome of treatment, 1302–1307, 1991, with permission from Elsevier.)

Table 11.4 Patterns of fetal hemolysis predictive of subsequent anemia.

Pattern	Hematocrit	Reticulocytes	± Direct Coombs test results	Interval for cordocentesis (weeks)	Interval for scan (weeks)	Comments
1	Normal	Normal	−/trace	—	4	Repeat if initial maternal indirect Coombs test result <128 and twofold increase documented
2	Normal	Normal or <2.5th percentile	1+/2+	5–6	2	Do not repeat after 32 weeks if unchanged; delivery at term
3	Normal	>97.5th percentile	3+/4+	2	1	Continue through 34 weeks if hematocrit value stable; deliver at 37–38 weeks if not transfused
4	<2.5th percentile but >30%	Any	Any	1–2	1	Repeat, as long as hematocrit criteria fulfilled; deliver with pulmonary maturity if not transfused

Source: From Weiner CP et al., *Am J Obstet Gynecol*, 165, 546–553, 1991. With permission.

Maternal idiopathic thrombocytopenic purpura (ITP)

Immune thrombocytopenia (ITP) is currently not an indication for cordocentesis.[54] Severe neonatal thrombocytopenia can occur in pregnancies complicated by maternal ITP.[55,56] These newborns can require platelet transfusions, prednisone, intravenous immunoglobulin (IVIG), or combinations of these treatments. Rarely, in less than 1% of the cases, the newborns will show neonatal intracranial hemorrhage.[56,57]

Regrettably, there is no way to predict or identify the fetus at risk for severe thrombocytopenia. There is no correlation between the maternal platelet count and the infant's platelet count. There is also no study which has documented that platelet-associated immunoglobulin G (IgG) can reliably distinguish or exclude those infants who will be thrombocytopenic.

The procordocentesis argument used to be based on the assumed risk of fetal intracranial hemorrhage during labor. Modern data clearly show that this risk is lower than 1% and the stillbirth risk is even rarer.[58,59] In comparison, the risk of fetal loss due to cordocentesis

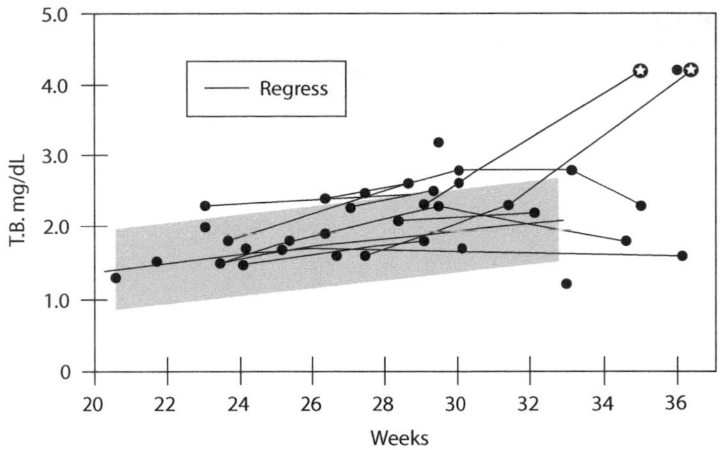

Figure 11.5 Relationship in pregnancies affected by red blood cell (RBC) alloimmunization between fetal bilirubin and postnatal hyperbilirubinemia. (Reproduced from *American Journal of Obstetrics & Gynecology*, 166, Weiner CP, Human fetal bilirubin levels and fetal hemolytic disease, 1449–4, 1992, with permission from Elsevier.)

(0.2%–3%) may equal or exceed the risk for intracranial hemorrhage. Further, there is no direct or indirect evidence that cesarean section for maternal auto-ITP improves neonatal outcome.

Neonatal alloimmune thrombocytopenia-platelet alloimmunization

Significant progress in the management of the fetus with severe alloimmune thrombocytopenia has led to clear recommendations for treatment.[60–62] It is now clear that medical therapy consisting of primarily high doses of IVIG (1–2 g/kg/week) with a prednisone rescue for suboptimal responders is an effective treatment for the majority of affected pregnancies.[63,64] Treatment is stratified by whether there was a prior affected fetus with intracranial hemorrhage, the gestational age of the hemorrhage, or severe thrombocytopenia at delivery. At-risk pregnancies begin their infusions between 10 and 20 weeks depending upon the past history. In the past decade, there is increasing consensus that fetal blood sampling should be avoided and staged acceleration of therapy should be implemented instead.[61,62] The single exception is to perform a cordocentesis at >32 weeks gestation in order to determine if a vaginal delivery can be allowed. Fetal platelet transfusion is associated with a high loss rate when used for primary therapy (up to 17%),[65] and now plays a secondary role, usually indicated for those fetuses with extremely low platelet counts or those with a count <50,000 prior to a planned vaginal delivery. There is no relationship between the fetal platelet count and bleeding from the puncture site when a needle guide is used (Figure 11.6).[23]

The characteristics of the previous sibling do not automatically predict the severity of the subsequent fetus.[66] If the father and mother are homozygous for their platelet genotype, incompatible, and the antibody is directed at the incompatible locus, then the subsequent fetus is usually more severely affected. However, if there is paternal heterozygosity, uncertainty, or unavailability, then

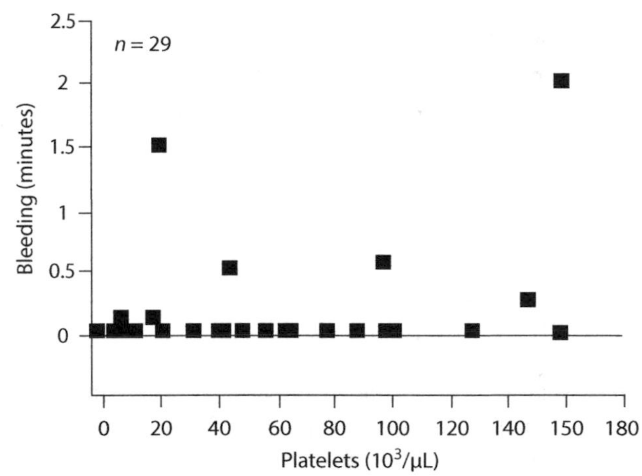

Figure 11.6 Scattergram illustrating the lack of a relationship between platelet count and the duration of bleeding from the umbilical cord puncture site in fetuses with alloimmune thrombocytopenia. (Reproduced from *Fetal Diagnosis and Therapy*, 10, Weiner CP, Fetal blood sampling and fetal thrombocytopenia, 173–177, 1995, with permission from Karger.)

amniocentesis and even fetal blood sampling would be required to determine fetal platelet type.

Rapid karyotype

The fetal lymphocytes can be stimulated to yield a rapid karyotype of high quality in less than 24 hours when the laboratory will cooperate. This is especially useful for patients referred with severe early-onset fetal growth restriction at a potentially viable gestation or those with malformations detected just prior to the legal limit for pregnancy termination (Table 11.5).

Evaluation of nonimmune hydrops fetalis

The performance of cordocentesis is essential for a complete evaluation of nonimmune hydrops since it allows

Table 11.5 Malformations and associated chromosomal abnormalities of fetuses who had antenatal karyotyping.

Defect	*n*	Incidence aneuploidy (%) Isolated	Incidence aneuploidy (%) Multiple	Common chromosomal defect
Brain				
Ventriculomegaly	185	3	27	Triploidy
Holoprosencephaly	52	<1	29	Trisomy 13
Posterior fossa cyst	45	<1	48	Trisomy 13, 18
Choroid plexus cyst	121	2	46	Trisomy 18
Face				
Cleft	64	<1	55	Trisomy 13, 18
Micrognathia	56	<1	66	Trisomy 18
Neck				
Nuchal edema	145	<1	40	Trisomy 21
Cystic hygromas	52	<1	71	Turner's syndrome
Chest				
Diaphragmatic hernia	79	<1	40	Trisomy 18
Heart defect	156	<1	65	Trisomy 13, 18, 21; Turner's syndrome
Kidneys				
Hydronephrosis				
Mild	319	2	26	Trisomy 13, 18, 21
Severe	294	3	25	Trisomy 18, 21
Gut				
Esophageal atresia	24	<1	78	Trisomy 18
Duodenal atresia	23	17	53	Trisomy 21
Abdominal wall				
Exomphalos	116	<4	47	Trisomy 13, 18
Hydrops	209	7	17	Trisomy 21

the separation of cardiac from noncardiac etiologies.[67] The umbilical venous pressure (UVP) is a surrogate for the central venous pressure. Recent studies of human fetuses[68] indicate that it is very similar to right-sided heart pressure. An elevated UVP is consistent with myocardial dysfunction whether caused by anemia (e.g., parvovirus infection, hemolytic disease), or myocarditis, or obstructed cardiac return (thoracic mass effect) (Figure 11.7a and b). Successful treatment of cardiogenic hydrops is associated with normalization of the UVP before the hydrops resolve. The UVP also predicts which fetus with a hydrothorax and hydrops whose hydrops will be cured by placement of a thoracoamniotic shunt. Hydrops that is responsive to shunting is caused by a shift of the mediastinum which then obstructs cardiac return. If the UVP is neither elevated nor normalized after draining the chest, a shunt will not help. The underlying problem lies elsewhere.

Severe early-onset growth restriction

Cordocentesis is no longer indicated solely for the measurement of the fetal acid base status, especially if the umbilical artery Doppler determined resistance is normal and labor is absent. Assuming the mother is well ventilated and the vessel punctured is correctly identified, the blood gases are less likely to be abnormal than the risk of fetal loss. In over 1200 procedures, we have yet to identify a fetus with abnormal blood gases and a normal Doppler resistance index in the absence of either hydrops or fetal sepsis. Refinements in multivessel Doppler studies allow the safe exclusion of fetal hypoxemia, and the prediction of fetal hypoxemia and acidemia with reasonable clinical accuracy.[69–71]

Miscellaneous

Not yet widely accepted but a likely valid indication for cordocentesis is the presence of maternal thyroid-stimulating antibody (TSiG) or active maternal Graves' disease.[72,73] Emerging evidence suggests even mild degrees of thyroid dysfunction may be associated with impaired long-term neurodevelopment.[74–76] While there is a relationship between the degree of maternal and fetal thyroid suppression with such agents as propylthiouracil, it is not uncommon for the fetus to be significantly over- or undertreated despite the mother being euthyroid. In the instance of fetal hyperthyroidism, the maternal antithyroid medication dose should be increased and the woman given thyroxine replacement. In the instance of fetal hypothyroidism, the fetus can be given thyroxine intra-amniotically on a weekly basis.[77] Women with a history of Graves' disease who have undergone thyroid ablation should be screened for the presence of TSiG. The fetus is at a minimal risk if the TSiG study is negative.

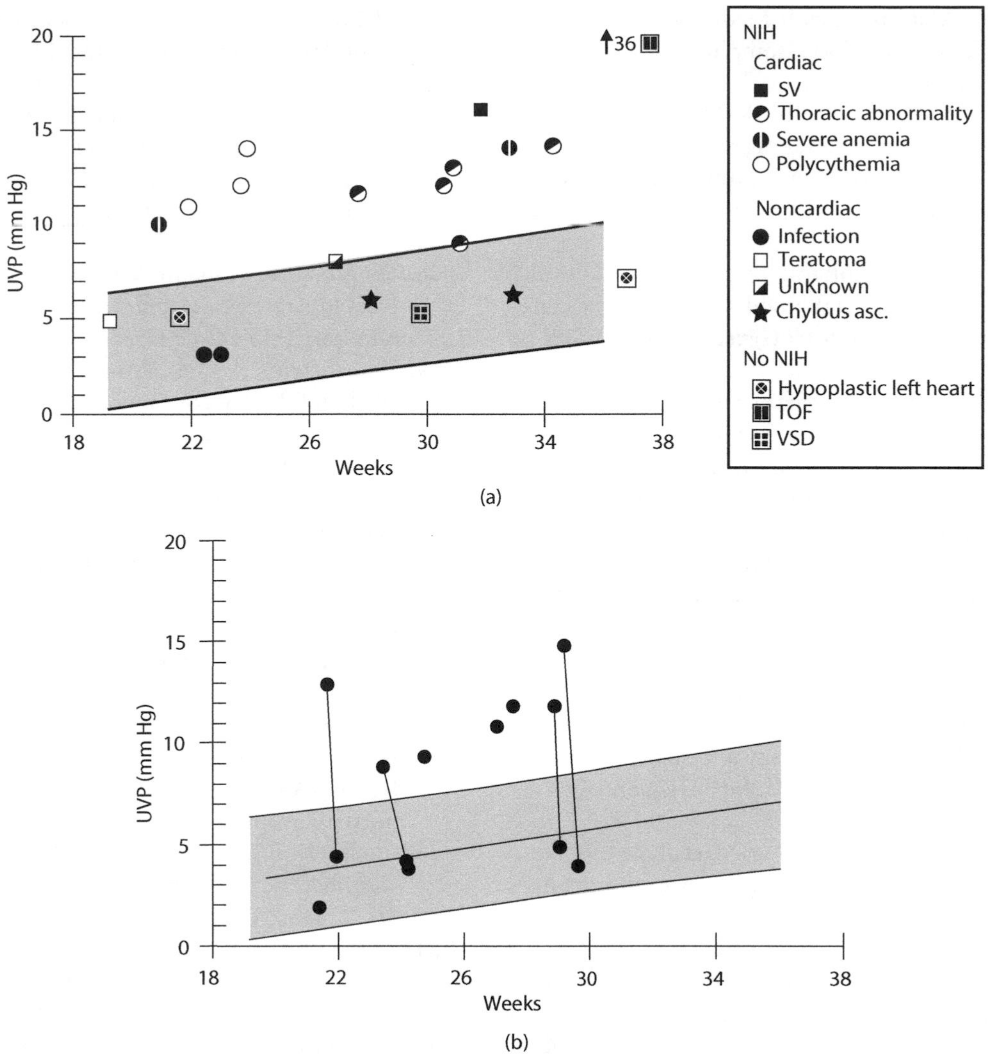

Figure 11.7 (a) Umbilical venous pressure (UVP) measurements corrected for amniotic fluid pressure of 17 untreated fetuses with nonimmune hydrops (NIH) and four nonhydropic fetuses with major cardiac structural malformations plotted against 95% confidence interval for gestational age (shaded area). Data exclude NIH fetuses in whom only umbilical artery pressure had been measured. SVT, supraventricular tachycardia; TOF, tetralogy of Fallot; VSD, ventricular septal defect; chylous asc, chylous ascites. (b) UVP measurements corrected for amniotic fluid pressure before first transfusion of eight fetuses with immune hydrops is plotted against gestational age. Umbilical venous pressure (where available) before second transfusion is shown for comparison. Seven of eight fetuses had high umbilical venous pressure. In each of these fetuses, umbilical arterial pressure returned to normal before the second transfusion and before resolution of hydrops. (Reproduced from *American Journal of Obstetrics & Gynecology*, 168, Weiner CP, Umbilical pressure measurement in the evaluation of nonimmune hydrops fetalis, 817–823, 1993, with permission from Elsevier.)

REFERENCES

1. Alter, BP. Examination of fetal blood for hemoglobinopathies. In: Alter, BP (ed) *Perinatal Hematology*, pp. 13–29. London, UK: Churchill Livingstone, 1989.
2. Daffos F, Capella-Pavlovsky M, Forestier F. A new procedure for fetal blood sampling in utero: Preliminary results of fifty-three cases. *Am J Obstet Gynecol* 1983; 146: 985–7.
3. Weiner CP. Cordocentesis for diagnostic indications: Two years' experience. *Obstet Gynecol* 1987; 70: 664–8.
4. Daffos F. Access to the other patient. *Semin Perinatol* 1989; 13: 252–9.
5. Maxwell DJ, Johnson P, Hurley P et al. Fetal blood sampling and pregnancy loss in relation to indication. *Br J Obstet Gynaecol* 1991; 98: 892–7.
6. Bang J, Bock JE, Trolle D. Ultrasound-guided fetal intravenous transfusion for severe rhesus haemolytic disease. *Br Med J Clin Res Ed* 1982; 284: 373–4.
7. Ramsay M, James D, Steer P et al. *Normal Values in Pregnancy* (3rd edition). Philadelphia, PA: WB Saunders, 2005.

8. Society for Maternal-Fetal Medicine, Berry SM, Stone J et al. Fetal blood sampling. *Am J Obstet Gynecol* 2013; 209: 170–80.
9. Somerset DA, Moore A, Whittle MJ et al. An audit of outcome in intravascular transfusions using the intrahepatic portion of the fetal umbilical vein compared to cordocentesis. *Fetal Diagn Ther* 2006; 21: 272–6.
10. Aina-Mumuney AJ, Holcroft CJ, Blakemore KJ et al. Intrahepatic vein for fetal blood sampling: One center's experience. *Am J Obstet Gynecol* 2008; 198(387): e381–6.
11. Mouw RJ, Klumper F, Hermans J et al. Effect of atracurium or pancuronium on the anemic fetus during and directly after intravascular intrauterine transfusion. A double blind randomized study. *Acta Obstet Gynecol Scand* 1999; 78: 763–7.
12. Shields LE, Brace RA. Cardiovascular responses to neuromuscular blockade in the anemic ovine fetus. *J Matern Fetal Med* 1997; 6: 195–9.
13. Weiner CP, Okamura K. Diagnostic fetal blood sampling-technique related losses. *Fetal Diagn Ther* 1996; 11: 169–75.
14. Liao C, Wei J, Li Q et al. Efficacy and safety of cordocentesis for prenatal diagnosis. *Int J Gynaecol Obstet* 2006; 93: 13–17.
15. Weiner CP, Wenstrom KD, Sipes SL et al. A. Risk factors for cordocentesis and fetal intravascular transfusion. *Am J Obstet Gynecol* 1991; 165: 1020–5.
16. Weiner CP, Anderson TL. The acute effect of cordocentesis with or without fetal curarization and of intravascular transfusion upon umbilical artery waveform indices. *Obstet Gynecol* 1989; 73: 219–24.
17. Weiner CP, Robillard JE. Effect of acute intravascular volume expansion on human fetal prostaglandin concentrations. *Am J Obstet Gynecol* 1989; 161: 1494–7.
18. Capponi A, Rizzo G, Pasquini L et al. Indomethacin modifies the fetal hemodynamic response induced by cordocentesis. *Am J Obstet Gynecol* 1997; 176: S19.
19. Rizzo G, Capponi A, Rinaldo D et al. Release of vasoactive agents during cordocentesis: Differences between normally grown and growth-restricted fetuses. *Am J Obstet Gynecol* 1996; 175: 563–70.
20. Nicolini U, Kochenour NK, Greco P et al. Consequences of fetomaternal haemorrhage after intrauterine transfusion. *BMJ* 1988; 297: 1379–81.
21. Weiner C, Grant S, Hudson J et al. Effect of diagnostic and therapeutic cordocentesis on maternal serum alpha-fetoprotein concentration. *Am J Obstet Gynecol* 1989; 161: 706–8.
22. Paidas MJ, Berkowitz RL, Lynch L et al. Alloimmune thrombocytopenia: Fetal and neonatal losses related to cordocentesis. *Am J Obstet Gynecol* 1995; 172: 475–9.
23. Weiner CP. Fetal blood sampling and fetal thrombocytopenia. *Fetal Diagn Ther* 1995; 10: 173–7.
24. Tabor A, Philip J, Bang J et al. Needle size and risk of miscarriage after amniocentesis. *Lancet* 1988; 1: 183–4.
25. Weiner C, Williamson R, Varner MW et al. Safety of second trimester amniocentesis. *Lancet* 1986; 2: 226.
26. Donner C, Simon P, Karioun A et al. Experience of a single team of operators in 891 diagnostic funipunctures. *Obstet Gynecol* 1994; 84: 827–31.
27. Tongsong T, Wanapirak C, Kunavikatikul C et al. Cordocentesis at 16–24 weeks of gestation: Experience of 1,320 cases. *Prenat Diagn* 2000; 20: 224–8.
28. Tongsong T, Wanapirak C, Kunavikatikul C et al. Fetal loss rate associated with cordocentesis at midgestation. *Am J Obstet Gynecol* 2001; 184: 719–23.
29. Tangshewinsirikul C, Wanapirak C, Piyamongkol W et al. Effect of cord puncture site in cordocentesis at mid-pregnancy on pregnancy outcomes. *Prenat Diagn* 2011; 31: 861–4.
30. Mibashan RS, Peake IR, Nicolaides K. Prenatal diagnosis of hemostatic disorders. In: Alter BP (ed), *Perinatal Hematology*, pp. 64–107. The University of Michigan, MI: Churchill Livingstone, 1989.
31. Boehm C, Kazazian HH Jr. Examination of fetal DNA for hemoglobinopathies. In: Alter BP (ed.), *Perinatal Hematology*, pp. 30–63. The University of Michigan, MI: Churchill Livingstone, 1989.
32. Bills VL, Soothill PW. Fetal blood grouping using cell free DNA—An improved service for RhD negative pregnant women. *Transfus Apher Sci* 2014; 50: 148–53.
33. Clausen FB, Damkjaer MB, Dziegiel MH. Noninvasive fetal RhD genotyping. *Transfus Apher Sci* 2014; 50: 154–62.
34. Yankowitz J, Li S, Murray JC. Polymerase chain reaction determination of RhD blood type: An evaluation of accuracy. *Obstet Gynecol* 1995; 86: 214–7.
35. Yankowitz J, Li S, Weiner CP. Polymerase chain reaction determination of RhC, Rhc, and RhE blood types: An evaluation of accuracy and clinical utility. *Am J Obstet Gynecol* 1997; 176: 1107–11.
36. Berkowitz RL, Chitkara U, Goldberg JD et al. A. Intravascular transfusion in utero: The percutaneous approach. *Am J Obstet Gynecol* 1986; 154: 622–3.
37. Grannum PA, Copel JA, Plaxe SC et al. In utero exchange transfusion by direct intravascular injection in severe erythroblastosis fetalis. *N Engl J Med* 1986; 314: 1431–4.
38. Nicolaides KH, Rodeck CH, Mibashan RS, Kemp JR. Have Liley charts outlived their usefulness? *Am J Obstet Gynecol* 1986; 155: 90–4.
39. Nicolaides KH. Studies on fetal physiology and pathophysiology in rhesus disease. *Semin Perinatol* 1989; 13: 328–37.
40. Weiner CP, Robillard JE. Atrial natriuretic factor, digoxin-like immunoreactive substance, norepinephrine, epinephrine, and plasma renin activity in human fetuses and their alteration by fetal disease. *Am J Obstet Gynecol* 1988; 159: 1353–60.
41. Soothill PW, Lestas AN, Nicolaides KH et al. 2,3-Diphosphoglycerate in normal, anaemic and transfused human fetuses. *Clin Sci (Lond)* 1988; 74: 527–30.

42. Nicolaides KH, Sadovsky G, Cetin E. Fetal heart rate patterns in red blood cell isoimmunized pregnancies. *Am J Obstet Gynecol* 1989; 161: 351–6.
43. Mari G, Moise KJ Jr, Deter RL, Carpenter RJ Jr. Flow velocity waveforms of the umbilical and cerebral arteries before and after intravascular transfusion. *Obstet Gynecol* 1990; 75: 584–9.
44. Mari G, Deter RL, Carpenter RL et al. Noninvasive diagnosis by Doppler ultrasonography of fetal anemia due to maternal red-cell alloimmunization. Collaborative Group for Doppler Assessment of the Blood Velocity in Anemic Fetuses. *N Engl J Med* 2000; 342: 9–14.
45. Pretlove SJ, Fox CE, Khan KS, Kilby MD. Noninvasive methods of detecting fetal anaemia: A systematic review and meta-analysis. *BJOG* 2009; 116: 1558–67.
46. Weiner CP, Williamson RA, Wenstrom KD et al. Management of fetal hemolytic disease by cordocentesis. II. Outcome of treatment. *Am J Obstet Gynecol* 1991; 165: 1302–7.
47. Weiner CP, Pelzer GD, Heilskov J et al. The effect of intravascular transfusion on umbilical venous pressure in anemic fetuses with and without hydrops. *Am J Obstet Gynecol* 1989; 161: 1498–1501.
48. Detti L, Oz U, Guney I et al. Doppler ultrasound velocimetry for timing the second intrauterine transfusion in fetuses with anemia from red cell alloimmunization. *Am J Obstet Gynecol* 2001; 185: 1048–1051.
49. Lindenburg IT, Smits-Wintjens VE, van Klink JM et al. Long-term neurodevelopmental outcome after intrauterine transfusion for hemolytic disease of the fetus/newborn: The LOTUS study. *Am J Obstet Gynecol* 2012; 206(141): e141–8.
50. Harper DC, Swingle HM, Weiner CP et al. Long-term neurodevelopmental outcome and brain volume after treatment for hydrops fetalis by in utero intravascular transfusion. *Am J Obstet Gynecol* 2006; 195: 192–200.
51. Weiner CP, Williamson RA, Wenstrom KD et al. Management of fetal hemolytic disease by cordocentesis. I. Prediction of fetal anemia. *Am J Obstet Gynecol* 1991; 165: 546–53.
52. Weiner CP, Wenstrom KD. Outcome of alloimmunized fetuses managed solely by cordocentesis but not requiring antenatal transfusion. *Fetal Diagn Ther* 1994; 9: 233–8.
53. Weiner CP. Human fetal bilirubin levels and fetal hemolytic disease. *Am J Obstet Gynecol* 1992; 166: 1449–4.
54. Weiner C. Why Fuss over diagnosing fetal thrombocytopenia secondary to ITP? *Contemp OB/GYN* 1995; 40: 45–50.
55. van der Lugt NM, van Kampen A, Walther FJ et al. Outcome and management in neonatal thrombocytopenia due to maternal idiopathic thrombocytopenic purpura. *Vox Sang* 2013; 105: 236–43.
56. Kelton JG. Idiopathic thrombocytopenic purpura complicating pregnancy. *Blood Rev* 2002; 16: 43–6.
57. Kutuk MS, Croisille L, Gorkem SB et al. Fetal intracranial hemorrhage related to maternal autoimmune thrombocytopenic purpura. *Childs Nerv Syst* 2014; 30: 2147–50.
58. Webert KE, Mittal R, Sigouin C et al. A retrospective 11-year analysis of obstetric patients with idiopathic thrombocytopenic purpura. *Blood* 2003; 102: 4306–11.
59. Gasim T. Immune thrombocytopenic purpura in pregnancy: A reappraisal of obstetric management and outcome. *J Reprod Med* 2011; 56: 163–8.
60. Radder CM, Brand A, Kanhai HH. Will it ever be possible to balance the risk of intracranial haemorrhage in fetal or neonatal alloimmune thrombocytopenia against the risk of treatment strategies to prevent it? *Vox Sang* 2003; 84: 318–25.
61. Bussel J. Diagnosis and management of the fetus and neonate with alloimmune thrombocytopenia. *J Thromb Haemost* 2009; 7 (Suppl 1): 253–7.
62. Pacheco LD, Berkowitz RL, Moise KJ Jr et al. Fetal and neonatal alloimmune thrombocytopenia: A management algorithm based on risk stratification. *Obstet Gynecol* 2011; 118: 1157–63.
63. Bussel JB, Berkowitz RL, Lynch L et al. Antenatal management of alloimmune thrombocytopenia with intravenous gamma-globulin: A randomized trial of the addition of low-dose steroid to intravenous gamma-globulin. *Am J Obstet Gynecol* 1996; 174: 1414–23.
64. Bussel JB, Berkowitz RL, Hung C et al. Intracranial hemorrhage in alloimmune thrombocytopenia: Stratified management to prevent recurrence in the subsequent affected fetus. *Am J Obstet Gynecol* 2010; 203(135): e131–34.
65. Overton TG, Duncan KR, Jolly M et al. Serial aggressive platelet transfusion for fetal alloimmune thrombocytopenia: Platelet dynamics and perinatal outcome. *Am J Obstet Gynecol* 2002; 186: 826–31.
66. Gaddipati S, Berkowitz RL, Lembet AA et al. Initial fetal platelet counts predict the response to intravenous gammaglobulin therapy in fetuses that are affected by PLA1 incompatibility. *Am J Obstet Gynecol* 2001; 185: 976–80.
67. Weiner CP. Umbilical pressure measurement in the evaluation of nonimmune hydrops fetalis. *Am J Obstet Gynecol* 1993; 168: 817–23.
68. Weiner Z, Efrat Z, Zimmer EZ et al. Direct measurement of central venous pressure in human fetuses. *Am J Obstet Gynecol* 1997; 176: S19.
69. Baschat AA, Weiner CP. Umbilical artery Doppler screening for detection of the small fetus in need of antepartum surveillance. *Am J Obstet Gynecol* 2000; 182: 154–8.
70. Baschat AA, Gembruch U, Gortner L et al. Relationship between arterial and venous Doppler and perinatal outcome in fetal growth restriction. *Ultrasound Obstetrics Gynecol* 2000; 16: 407–13.

71. Baschat AA, Gembruch U, Weiner CP, Harman CR. Qualitative venous Doppler waveform analysis improves prediction of critical perinatal outcomes in premature growth-restricted fetuses. *Ultrasound Obstetrics Gynecol* 2003; 22: 240–5.
72. Wenstrom KD, Weiner CP, Williamson RA, Grant SS. Prenatal diagnosis of fetal hyperthyroidism using funipuncture. *Obstet Gynecol* 1990; 76: 513–7.
73. Yankowitz J, Weiner C. Medical fetal therapy. *Baillieres Clin Obstet Gynaecol* 1995; 9: 553–70.
74. Salerno M, Militerni R, Di Maio S et al. Prognostic factors in the intellectual development at 7 years of age in children with congenital hypothyroidism. *J Endocrinol Invest* 1995; 18: 774–9.
75. Kooistra L, van der Meere JJ, Vulsma T, Kalverboer AF. Sustained attention problems in children with early treated congenital hypothyroidism. *Acta Paediatrica* 1996; 85: 425–9.
76. Weber G, Siragusa V, Rondanini GF et al. Neurophysiologic studies and cognitive function in congenital hypothyroid children. *Pediatr Res* 1995; 37: 736–40.
77. Van Loon AJ, Derksen JT, Bos AF, Rouwe CW. In utero diagnosis and treatment of fetal goitrous hypothyroidism, caused by maternal use of propylthiouracil. *Prenat Diagn* 1995; 15: 599–604.

Minimally invasive fetal surgery—The Colorado approach

12

NICHOLAS BEHRENDT and TIMOTHY M. CROMBLEHOLME

CONTENTS

INTRODUCTION

As prenatal diagnosis has become increasingly sophisticated, invasive therapies have been developed to treat an expanding number of conditions. The motivation for the development of in utero therapies springs from the realization that, with certain congenital anomalies, irreversible changes have already taken place by the time of birth, or, alternatively, may result in intrauterine fetal demise (IUFD). Several congenital anomalies have been successfully treated with open fetal surgery, but the indications for minimally invasive approaches are increasing. This chapter will review the current indications for minimally invasive fetal surgery, which have expanded significantly since the last edition of this book.

FETOSCOPIC TREATMENT FOR STRUCTURAL ANOMALIES

Lower urinary tract obstruction

The most common etiology of chronic lower urinary tract obstruction in the male fetus is posterior urethral valves (PUVs), which occur in approximately 1 in 4000 live births. In female fetuses, the most common cause of bladder outlet obstruction is urethral atresia.[1] Complications associated with fetal lower urinary tract obstruction include progressive oligohydramnios, pulmonary hypoplasia, cystic renal dysplasia, and deformations of the face and extremities. Death ensues in up to 72% of fetuses with bladder outlet obstruction if left untreated.[2] Uncorrected oligohydramnios observed in the second trimester is particularly ominous with a perinatal mortality rate of 80%–100%.

The initial approach to the fetus with suspected bladder outlet obstruction should include a detailed ultrasound examination to rule out other associated anomalies and echocardiography. Lower urinary tract obstruction must be distinguished from other pathologic causes of fetal hydronephrosis including urethral atresia, persistent cloaca, megacystis/microcolon, anterior urethral valves, bilateral ureterovesical junction obstruction, and bilateral ureteral pelvic junction obstruction. The presence of megacystis, thickened bladder wall, posterior urethral dilatation, bilateral hydronephrosis, and ureterectasis characterizes the changes associated with PUV. However, these findings are not specific to PUV alone. In addition to mechanical causes of bladder outlet obstruction, megacystis may be the presentation of "prune belly" syndrome or megacystis/microcolon hypoperistalsis syndrome (MMHS), which are both forms of functional obstruction.[3] Prune belly syndrome is characterized by diffuse dilation of the genitourinary tract. There is an intrinsic muscular deficiency which prevents the generation of increased intravesical pressures making dysplastic changes in the kidneys unusual as well as making these cases poorly responsive to vesicoamniotic shunting. In MMHS, there is an associated abnormality in the bowel which manifests as small bowel dilatation which rarely develops before 28 weeks gestation. MMHS has an extremely poor prognosis and does not respond to vesicoamniotic shunting.[4] Survivors have both severe genitourinary and gastrointestinal dysfunction with death commonly within the first year or years of life. Ureteropelvic junction obstruction, ureterovesical obstruction, and vesicoureteral reflux are more common causes of a dilated fetal urinary tract and are more commonly unilateral and do not have megacystis as a feature. A duplicated collecting system can have an ectopic ureterocele within the bladder which can enlarge and in rare cases will block the bladder outlet replicating findings of PUV or urethral atresia. Persistent cloaca in a female fetus can have functional bladder outlet obstruction related to a long common channel for drainage of the bladder, rectum, and vagina. This may present with hydrocolpos or hydrometrocolpos with debris, which may be observed to swirl in the bladder due to the rectal communication. In the setting of oligohydramnios shunting should be considered for persistent cloaca. We have experience with seven such cases which tend to have better preserved renal function postnatally compared with PUV. Since chromosomal abnormalities are found in up to 12% of fetuses with bladder outlet obstruction, fetal karyotyping is indicated.[2]

A major problem in the management of fetuses diagnosed with lower urinary tract obstruction is selecting those fetuses who are most likely to benefit from in utero intervention. Among cases of fetal urinary tract obstruction, a fetus with preserved renal function produces more hypotonic urine, whereas one with advanced renal dysfunction is a "salt waster," producing more hypertonic urine. The usefulness of assessing urine chemistry in fetal obstructive uropathy lies in the separation of fetuses into "good" or "poor" prognostic categories based on the preservation of renal function reflected by the tonicity of the fetal urine. In one study, urine samples taken from fetuses who subsequently had a good outcome revealed levels of Na less than 100 mEq/L, Cl less than 90 mEq/L, and osmolarity less than 210 mOsm/L.[5] These values were chosen because they were two standard deviations from the mean values of fetuses with a good prognosis. Fetuses with urine chemistries greater than these values had irreversible renal damage and suffered from severe oligohydramnios resulting in pulmonary hypoplasia. The efficacy of these proposed criteria was subsequently confirmed to reflect postnatal outcome and appropriately selected fetuses for intervention.

However, fetal urine electrolyte criteria were developed for use in fetuses presenting with bladder outlet obstruction after 20 weeks gestation. Today, bladder outlet obstruction is commonly diagnosed before 16 weeks gestation prior to the development of oligohydramnios. At this gestational age the amniotic fluid is primarily derived from transudation across the fetal skin. Once the barrier function of the skin develops and the fetus is reliant upon urine production for amniotic fluid, the fetus will have oligohydramnios. At gestations <20 weeks it may be developmentally appropriate to have elevated Na, Cl, osmolality, and Ca in the absence of dysplasia. If these values are below the cutoff for preserved renal function they may be informative but elevated values at this gestational age cannot be interpreted to reflect compromised renal function. This limits the utility of fetal urine electrolytes prior to 20 weeks gestation.

Johnson et al.[6] modified this approach to include three sequential vesicocenteses at 24-hour intervals. This regimen permits a comparative analysis of stagnant urine (first sample) with fresh urine (third sample). Fresh urine samples are thought to reflect fetal renal function more accurately, and this approach increases the predictive value of fetal urinary electrolytes. However, we have found that sequential taps, which may require up to three vesicocenteses, may compromise subsequent vesicoamniotic shunting due to a higher rate of premature preterm rupture of membranes (PPROM).

There are no randomized trials regarding the use of amniotic shunts for prenatal bladder drainage for obstructive uropathies. In one meta-analysis, which included nine case series (147 fetuses) and seven controlled series (195 fetuses), bladder drainage improved perinatal survival relative to no drainage in the controlled studies (odds ratio 2.5; 95% confidence interval (CI) 1.1–5.9, $p = .03$).[7]

While prenatal intervention may help the fetus survive by correcting oligohydraminos and pulmonary hypoplasia, there is a growing appreciation that the long-term outcome of children after vesicoamniotic shunting may be complicated by renal insufficiency, bladder dysfunction, and growth problems. Freedman et al.[8] reported outcomes in 14 patients who survived beyond 2 years of age after having had in utero vesicoamniotic shunt placement. Renal function was normal in only six of these patients (43%). Of the remaining eight patients, five had renal failure requiring kidney transplantation and three had chronic renal insufficiency. Three of the four whose obstructive uropathy was due to PUV required bladder augmentation. In addition, growth of these toddlers was a problem with 86% below the 25th percentile and 50% below the 5th percentile. In another study, of patients who underwent various procedures with the majority being vesicoamniotic shunts, five of eight (63%) babies born alive developed chronic renal disease.[9] Two underwent renal transplant and another was awaiting transplant at the time of report. Five of eight babies underwent urinary diversion after birth.

It has been postulated that by the time bladder outlet obstruction is diagnosed the fetal kidneys are irreversibly damaged. The Percutaneous Lower Urinary Tract Obstruction (PLUTO) trial was a randomized trial evaluating the benefits of vesicoamniotic shunting.[10] However, the trial had to be stopped early due to difficulties in enrollment. Of the patients analyzed, survival to 28 days postnatally was higher with vesicoamniotic shunting compared with observation alone, but these differences were not statistically significant.

There are two shunts commercially available and U.S. Food and Drug Administration (FDA) approved for vesicoamniotic shunting including the Harrison shunt (Cook Medical, Inc., Bloomington, IN) and the Rocket KCH or Rodeck catheter (Rocket Medical, Washington Tyne& Wear, United Kingdom). Both are double pigtail on the intravesical end and single pigtail on the external end. The Harrison catheter is softer and more easily placed while the Rodeck catheter is stiffer and more challenging to place. The Harrison shunt comes with its own introducer set, but alternatively, a Storz fetoscope can be used to place the catheter. In contrast, the Rodeck catheter is stiffer and requires a separate introducer set, which is larger than the trocar in the Harrison set. The advantage of the Rodeck catheter may be its less predisposition to dislodgement. Although the placement of a vesicoamniotic shunt seems simple, the procedure is technically challenging and carries an appreciable complication rate. Long-term shunt success is variable due in large part to shunt obstruction and displacement. Functional shunt failure has been reported to occur in 40%–50% of cases after successful placement, mostly due to displacement of the shunt into the fetal abdomen or amniotic cavity. Other reported complications of vesicoamniotic shunts include PPROM, amnionitis, and iatrogenic gastroschisis. Another report described a case in which the shunt traversed the femoral triangle and inguinal ligament in the subcutaneous tissue before entering the bladder, raising the potential of extremity injury.[11]

The postnatal problems after vesicoamniotic shunting have been a catalyst for the development of alternative fetoscopic techniques to treat obstructive uropathy in utero. An endoscopic approach is appealing because shunts can be placed under direct visualization, more accurate diagnosis can be made, and direct treatment of the urinary tract anomaly can be attempted. One approach involves cystoscopic identification of the underlying etiology and, in cases of PUVs, destruction of the membranous obstruction. Engineering and manufacturing advances have produced successive generations of smaller fiber optic endoscopes that have made fetal cystoscopy a reality. Initially, using a variety of 1.7- to 2.2-mm endoscopes, Quintero et al.[12] were able to show that in utero diagnostic fetal cystoscopy is possible and later were able to identify proximal urethral obstructions. Several attempts at laser ablation of PUVs were technical successes, but postoperative obstetric complications resulted in no long-term survivors from this early experience.[13] More recently, a 1-mm, semirigid, fiberoptic endoscopic system that allows a minimally invasive approach to diagnostic cystourethroscopy has been used. With a 1.2 × 2.4-mm, double-lumen trocar sheath, it is possible to pass guide wire probes or laser fibers to assist in diagnostic evaluation and offer the possibility of laser ablation of PUVs. Design modifications and refinements to this system have recently allowed us to visualize more reliably the source of proximal urethral obstruction and differentiate between urethral atresia and PUVs. Clifton et al.[14] have reported the use of transurethral catheters after successful laser ablation of PUV.

The hope is that, by treating the source of the obstruction in midgestation, renal function will be preserved, and the need for postnatal urologic surgery to correct secondary anatomic bladder abnormalities may be reduced or eliminated. However, despite a compelling rationale for fetal cystoscopic treatments of PUVs and advances in fetoscopic techniques, this approach has yet to be shown to be more effective treatment of lower urinary tract obstruction. It is clear that the angulation between the bladder and the posterior urethra becomes more acute after 20 weeks gestation. For this reason, visualization of the PUV may be exceedingly difficult after 20 weeks gestation and therefore, we limit this approach to cases less than 20 weeks.

Congenital diaphragmatic hernia

Congenital diaphragmatic hernia (CDH) is a defect in the diaphragm resulting from incomplete fusion of the primitive diaphragm. CDH occurs in approximately 1 in

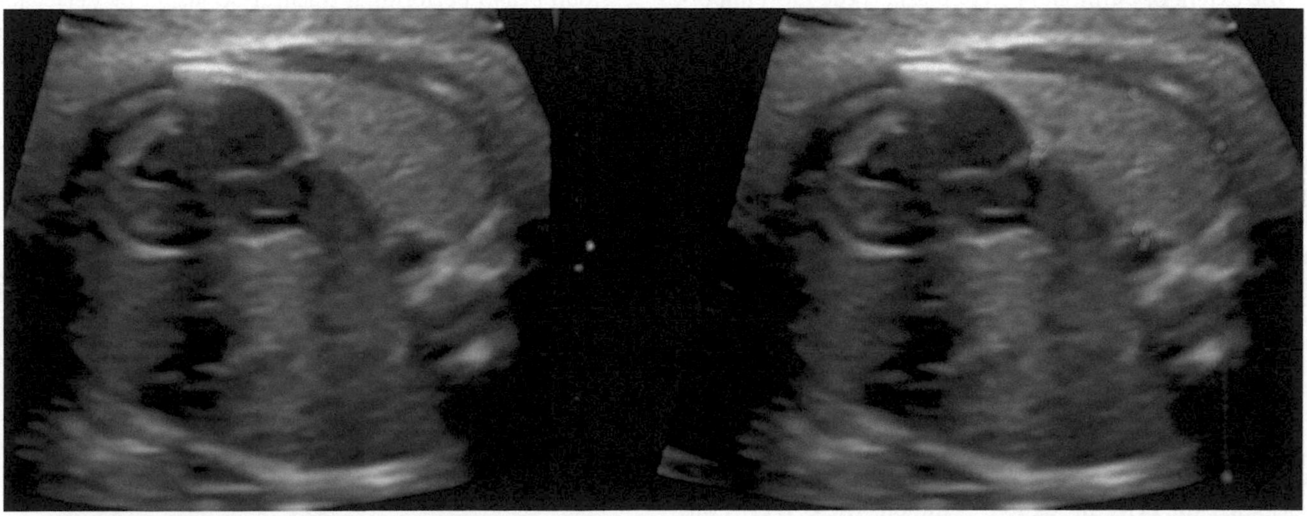

Figure 12.1 Ultrasound image demonstrating two of the techniques used to measure right lung area. The lung-to-head ratio is derived from this evaluation by dividing the lung area by the head circumference. The image on the left uses the trace method to measure the area of the right lung posterior to the displaced heart. The image on the right uses the anterior–posterior method. Both images are taken on axial images at the level of the four-chamber view of the heart.

2500–5000 live births and as frequently as 1 in 2200 on prenatal ultrasound studies. Most commonly, the CDH is on the left (85%–90%). The defect is on the right in approximately 10% of cases and may be bilateral in less than 5% of cases. Associated anomalies are seen in 25%–57% of all cases of CDH and 95% of stillborns with CDH.[15,16] Chromosomal anomalies, including trisomy 21, 18, and 13, occur in association with CDH in 10%–20% of cases that are diagnosed prenatally. The clinical spectrum of this anomaly ranges from fetuses that do very well with postnatal management to severely affected infants with profound pulmonary hypoplasia that precludes postnatal survival.

The degree of pulmonary hypoplasia is a critical determinant of survival in CDH. Herniation of viscera associated with CDH usually occurs during the pseudoglandular stage of lung development (5–17 weeks' gestation). Although the major bronchial buds are present, the number of bronchial branches is greatly reduced. If the herniation persists into later stages of lung development, the absolute number of alveoli is also reduced.[17] The pulmonary vascular bed is similarly abnormal, with both a reduction in the number of generations of vessels and an extension of muscularization to the preacinar capillary bed. These pulmonary vascular changes in preacinar capillaries are a histologic correlate of pulmonary hypertension. Although the diaphragmatic defect is easily corrected after birth, the pulmonary hypoplasia and pulmonary hypertension may not be.

General indication of severity for left-sided diaphragmatic hernia is revealed by determining whether the liver is above or below the diaphragm and also by the sonographic measurement of lung-to-head ratios (LHRs) (Figure 12.1).[18–20] Detection of liver position is enhanced by magnetic resonance imaging (MRI). One study of 38 cases of CDH reported that MRI correctly diagnosed liver position in 37 (97%), whereas ultrasound correctly diagnosed liver position in 32 (84%).[21]

The extent of pulmonary hypoplasia is the most important determinant of survival in CDH. Metkus et al.[21] reported the use of the right LHR as a sonographic predictor of survival in fetal diaphragmatic hernia. The LHR is the two-dimensional area of the right lung taken at the level of the four-chamber view of the heart. This is divided by the head circumference. In a retrospective review of 55 fetuses diagnosed with left-sided congenital diaphragmatic hernia, the LHR was found to be predictive at its extremes. At low values (i.e., small right lung), fetuses with LHRs <0.6 did not survive with postnatal therapy. However, in fetuses with LHRs >1.35, survival was 100% with conventional postnatal therapies, including extracorporeal membrane oxygenation (ECMO).[22,23]

Jani et al.[24] developed the observed-to-expected (O/E) LHR using data in 354 normal fetuses between 12 and 24 weeks to normalize the LHR throughout gestation. The O/E LHR was found to reflect postnatal survival throughout gestation but to be more accurate at 32–33 weeks than at 22–23 weeks.

Between 12 and 32 weeks' gestation, normal lung area increases four times more than head circumference.[25] For this reason, Jani et al.[25] proposed referencing LHR to gestational age by expressing the observed LHR as a ratio to the expected mean LHR for that gestational age. In a study from the CDH antenatal registry, 354 fetuses with isolated left and right CDH between 18 and 38 weeks, Jani et al. found that O/E LHR predicted postnatal survival. The O/E LHR tended to be more accurate at 32–33 weeks' than at 22–23 weeks' gestation. The O/E LHR was also found to correlate with short-term morbidity.

It was recognized long ago that occlusion of the fetal trachea results in markedly enlarged and hyperplastic lungs. This observation was applied to the problem of diaphragmatic hernia. Throughout gestation the fetal lung produces a fluid that exits the trachea during normal breathing movements. External drainage of this fluid, bypassing the glottic mechanism, results in retarded lung growth and pulmonary hypoplasia. Conversely, tracheal occlusion results in accelerated lung growth and pulmonary hyperplasia. In the fetal lamb model of diaphragmatic hernia, tracheal obstruction accelerates lung growth, pushing the viscera back into the abdomen resulting in larger lungs with significant functional improvement at birth as compared with controls. The results of experimental work were so impressive that this strategy was employed by Harrison in fetuses with herniation of the left lobe of the liver.[26]

Despite an excellent biologic response with complete tracheal occlusion, there was only one survivor in the initial series of patients treated by tracheal occlusion. The group at The Children's Hospital of Philadelphia had similar problems when the procedure was performed at 28 weeks of gestation. Survival increased to 40% in fetuses with a predicted mortality rate in excess of 90% when fetal tracheal clip application was performed at 26 weeks of gestation.[27]

Due to difficulties with open fetal surgery for tracheal clip application as well as fetoscopic tracheal clip application, the University of California at San Francisco (UCSF) group began performing tracheal occlusion by detachable endoluminal balloon placement. Figure 12.2 shows an ultrasound image of the endoluminal balloon in place within the

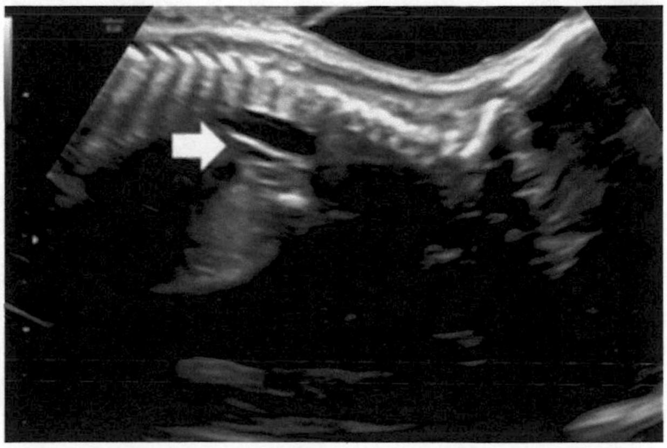

Figure 12.2 Ultrasound image of a fetal endotracheal occlusion balloon in place. The arrow points to the balloon and fluid that accumulates behind the balloon after placement.

fetal trachea. The results with fetoscopic balloon tracheal occlusion were evaluated in a National Institutes of Health (NIH)-sponsored randomized trial that compared fetoscopic tracheal occlusion (FETO) to conventional postnatal therapy in fetuses with isolated left-sided CDH with liver herniation and LHR <1.4.[28] The investigators' preliminary data suggested an anticipated survival with conventional therapy of 50% and with FETO of 75%. A crucial aspect of the trial was that patients from both arms of the trial were born and treated postnatally at UCSF. The trial was stopped after randomization of only 24 patients because of an unexpectedly high survival rate with standard postnatal care. Eight of the 11 fetuses (73%) randomized to tracheal occlusion survived and 10 of 13 fetuses (77%) randomized to standard care survived to 90 days of age. There was a significant difference in gestational age at delivery for fetal tracheal occlusion (30.8 weeks) compared with conventional therapy (37 weeks). This trial demonstrated a significant improvement in survival compared with historical controls in the same center. However, the inclusion of fetuses with LHR > 1 but < 1.4 biased the study toward the less severe end of the spectrum with insufficient power to analyze the effects in the subset of patients with LHR <1.0.

The tracheal occlusion procedure currently in use is done using maternal percutaneous access under local or regional anesthesia with a single 3.3-mm port and a detachable balloon to occlude the trachea.[29] The balloon is inserted at 27 0/7–29 6/7 weeks and removed at 34 weeks. If patients deliver prior to 34 weeks they require emergency peripartum balloon removal, which requires the availability of trained clinicians at all times. The Eurofetus group reports in their experience of over 150 cases a survival rate with tracheal occlusion of 50%–57%.[29] However, these studies have been criticized due to lack of contemporary controls. Nonetheless, no maternal complications have been reported, but iatrogenic preterm rupture of the membranes has occurred in 20% of cases. Long-term follow-up of study infants is in progress. DePrest and his Eurofetus colleagues have achieved survival of 83% with tracheal occlusion at 26–28 weeks' gestation followed by reversal of tracheal occlusion performed either by popping the balloon by an ultrasound-guided needle or by a second fetoscopic procedure.

The tracheal occlusion to accelerate lung growth trial (TOTAL trial) is a prospective randomized clinical trial that has been underway in European centers in which left-sided CDH with O/E LHR <25% is randomized to either tracheal occlusion or conventional postnatal treatment. Due to slow recruitment to the trial, North American centers were invited to join and seven formed a coalition (Colorado, Cincinnati, Children's Hospital of Philadelphia, Maryland, Toronto, UCSF, Texas Children's and Memorial Hermann Hospital) that have collaborated on getting FDA approval for an Investigational Device Exemption for the BALT balloon and the Storz fetoscope designed to insert the balloon. At the time of this writing only Colorado and CHOP had obtained both FDA and institutional review board (IRB) approvals and only Toronto and Colorado had placed balloons under this new IDE. The goal of the IDE was to qualify centers to begin randomizing subjects in the TOTAL trial once five FETO procedures had been performed at a given center.

The only other fetal surgery offered for high-risk CDH is ex utero intrapartum treatment (EXIT)-to-ECMO. In preliminary results reported by Kunisaki et al.,[30] fetuses with liver herniation and PPLV or <20% are offered EXIT-to-ECMO, with a 65% survival. We have observed similar results in a small cohort of patients with 50% survival. This therapeutic innovation remains unproven but may hold promise in these high-risk CDH cases given survival with conventional treatment is significantly lower.

Myelomeningocele (MMC)

Fetal MMC treatment has come to the forefront in the treatment of fetal conditions marked more by morbidity rather than mortality. The Management of Myelomeningocele Study (MOMS) in which fetuses with a diagnosis of MMC were randomized to either open fetal in utero treatment versus standard postnatal repair showed a decrease in the need for ventriculoperitoneal shunt by 1 year of life in patients who underwent in utero repair versus postnatal repair.[31] This has significantly increased the amount of open fetal procedures performed. Unfortunately, open fetal surgery continues to have a significant amount of morbidity for both the mother and fetus and therefore more minimally invasive approaches are being pursued.

Endoscopic MMC repair has been undertaken in animal models with promising results including improvement in Chiari malformation and improvement in neurologic function.[32,33] These results have led to the attempted development of a similar approach in humans. Bruner et al.[34] first published on this endoscopic approach to MMC with disappointing results. This seemed to lead to the further development of open fetal surgery for this approach. More recently, attempts have again taken place to take a fetoscopic approach to MMC repair. Pedreira et al.[35] recently reported a series of 10 fetuses with attempted endoscopic approach that showed this approach can be technically performed with promising outcomes; however, there was still a significant rate of complications especially preterm premature rupture of membranes. This may be due to the use of multiple endoscopic ports therefore decreasing some of the potential benefit of minimally invasive surgery.

Kohl[36] has reported a series of cases repaired using multiple large port sites but with an 84% PPROM rate, which is notably higher than observed in the MOMS trial. In contrast, Peiro et al.[37] developed both a one- and two-port technique in a sheep model and has cautiously started offering this to patients. Similarly, Belfort et al.[38] has started offering a fetoscopic approach using CO_2 insufflation and closure of the skin alone over the placode.

The safety of intra-amniotic CO_2 insufflation in humans has not been established with the concern being that the fetus lacks carbonic anhydrase, which can lead to fetal acidosis during the procedure. Clearly these approaches offer the advantage of eliminating the large hysterotomy used in open fetal surgery and eliminate the need for surgical delivery of the current and all future pregnancies. It is not clear, however, that these minimally invasive approaches can achieve the same reduction in the need for ventriculoperitoneal shunting demonstrated by open fetal surgery used in the MOMS trial. In addition, it is too early to know if these fetoscopic approaches will result in other complications such as PPROM, prematurity, or tethered cord. The current techniques for fetoscopically repairing MMC must, for now, be considered experimental and should be prospectively studied to evaluate their efficacy and complication rates compared with standard open fetal surgery.

Amniotic band syndrome (ABS)

ABS is another example of a usually nonlethal anomaly potentially treatable by fetoscopic surgery. This syndrome results from a rupture of the amnion during fetal development, which may subsequently attach to or encircle parts of the developing fetus (Figure 12.3). Constrictive bands most commonly affect the extremities but can also involve the craniofacial region, trunk, or umbilical cord. Involvement of the latter may result in fetal demise. The prenatal natural history of isolated extremity ABS is characterized by progression from distal edema owing to venous obstruction leading to in utero limb amputation secondary to vascular insufficiency. If diagnosed early enough in their course, these patients may benefit from in utero lysis of these fibrous bands.

Based on the experimental work by Crombleholme et al.[39] demonstrating the potential for functional recovery of banded extremities once released, Quintero et al.[40] performed the first fetoscopic lysis of amniotic bands in two human fetuses, using endoscissors in one fetus and yttrium aluminium garnet (YAG) laser in the other. Limb salvage was achieved, but one fetus suffered from serious facial deformities caused by ABS and the other had an incomplete release for fear of injury to the ankle. Keswani et al.[41] performed fetoscopic laser release of three extremity amniotic bands in two fetuses, both with impending limb amputation. Secondary lymphedema persisted postnatally in one fetus, while atrophy of the hand occurred in the other fetus. One lower extremity in which the band was released before irreversible damage occurred was completely normal at the time of delivery. The results of these few cases establish at least the feasibility of performing fetoscopic release of amniotic bands involving the extremities. We also have experience in cases with umbilical cord involvement; this approach has the potential of being lifesaving as acute IUFD can occur unexpectedly. Umbilical cord involvement should be suspected when a cluster of umbilical cord loops is sonographically observed to move together usually with limb movement. Predicting when a cord accident will occur is not possible so the release of amniotic bands should be considered in all cases with umbilical cord involvement.

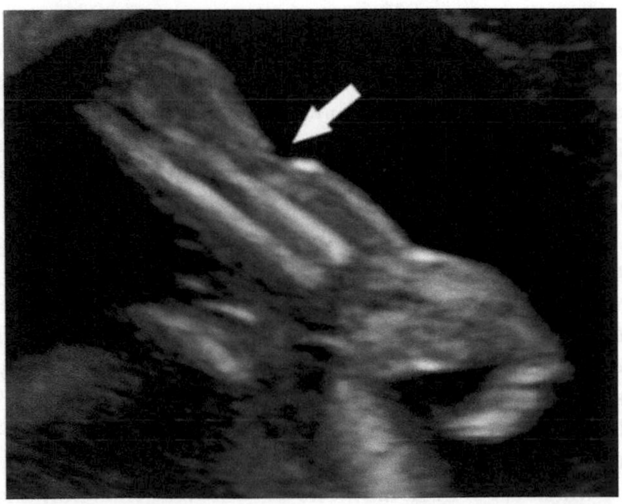

Figure 12.3 Ultrasound image of a fetus with amniotic band syndrome. The arrow points to an area of the fetal arm in which the band is constricting and an indentation can be seen.

Giant chorioangiomas

Placental chorioangiomas are thought to be abnormal proliferation of vessels arising from chorionic tissue. Chorioangiomas have an incidence of 1% and are the most common placental tumor.[42] Giant chorioangiomas defined as being >4 or 5 cm are more rare occurring in only 1 in 9,000 to 50,000 placentas.[42] Diagnosis of chorioangiomas is important because the associated complications that result in perinatal mortality as high as 18%–40%.[43,44] The high blood flow shunting through chorioangiomas may lead to polyhydramnios, preterm labor, fetal anemia, intrauterine growth restriction, high-output cardiac failure, hydrops, and death.[44,45]

Spontaneous thrombosis of giant chorioangiomas can occur so that not every case must be treated. Fetal anemia can complicate giant chorioangiomas either from hemorrhage into the tumor, or microangiopathic hemolytic anemia, as indicated by elevated middle cerebral artery peak systolic velocity (MCA PSV) indices (>1.5 multiple of median [MoM]).[46,47] Polyhydramnios may result from hyperfiltration of the shunted volume through the kidneys, or transudation from the surface of the tumor.[48] Polyhydramnios in the setting of a high cardiac output state may be temporized by amnioreduction; however, this may acutely worsen the hemodynamic state as reduced intra-amniotic pressure may allow increased blood flow through the tumor and precipitate hydrops or fetal death. The indication for fetoscopic devascularization is the presence of high-output cardiac failure or hydrops in one series.[49] In this series 5 out of 10 patients showed evidence of high-output cardiac failure necessitating intervention. Numerous techniques have been reported to treat giant chorioangiomas including embolization, ethanol, microcoils, laser photocoagulation, and bipolar coagulation. They have all been used either individually or in combination with reports showing the latter techniques having better success than embolization techniques. A common finding is that the entire flow from an umbilical artery feeds directly into the chorioangioma accounting for the high-output state observed. Control of this inflow has been achieved with bipolar electro cautery, vascular clip application, or suture ligation. In some cases, however, in the process of occlusion, the vessel ruptures which has inevitably led to immediate exsanguination. In treated cases, the collateral vessels on the surface of the chorioangioma can then be photocoagulated to prevent recurrence of the high-output state. There have been some reports of placental insufficiency following devascularization of the giant chorioangioma but in most cases the area of placenta occupied by the chorioangioma is not functional and devascularization will not worsen placental insufficiency already present.

FETOSCOPIC TREATMENT FOR COMPLICATIONS IN MONOCHORIONIC TWINS

Monochorionic twins discordant for anomaly

Fetoscopic intervention for the management of complications in monochorionic twins continues to be the area of greatest impact of minimally invasive fetal surgery. These complications include, but are not limited to anomalous cotwin with threatened fetal demise, twin-reversed arterial perfusion (TRAP) sequence, twin anemia polycythemia sequence (TAPS), and twin-to-twin transfusion syndrome (TTTS). There is also a wide range of congenital malformations that appear more commonly in twin gestations, including congenital heart defects, which are twice as prevalent in monozygotic twins when compared with dizygotic or singleton pregnancies.[50] More specific concern for the management of twins lies in the potential for harm to the nonanomalous fetus. Depending on the anomaly of one twin, there is up to a 30% risk of fetal demise in the anomalous twin.[51] The intrauterine death of one twin in a monochorionic pregnancy significantly increases the risk of cotwin demise and neurodevelopmental morbidity in the other fetus.[52] In addition, twins discordant for anomaly deliver earlier than the average twin delivery with an average age of 34 weeks.[53]

In a dichorionic pregnancy, it is possible to observe spontaneous IUFD or perform selective feticide by means of a potassium chloride injection without significant risk to the healthy cotwin. This is not the case with monochorionic pregnancies in light of the vascular connections between the twins. It is believed that these connections make for the increased morbidity and mortality in the cotwin in the case of single IUFD. Therefore, interventions have been proposed in order to attempt to decrease these complications.

The initial treatment was centered on fetoscopic cord ligation or coagulation in the abnormal fetus. Crombleholme et al.[54] reported the first use of fetoscopic cord ligation to prevent neurologic injury in a surviving twin when the death of a cotwin was imminent. This procedure is usually performed with a two-port technique in which a fetoscope and bipolar instrument can be introduced into the amniotic cavity and the cord can be coagulated and cut. In one of the larger studies performed Lanna et al.[55] showed a 71% survival overall with a low risk of neurodevelopmental morbidity in surviving twins.

More recently radiofrequency ablation (RFA) is being used on an increasing basis for the purpose of selective feticide in discordant monochorionic twin pregnancies. This technique involves the ultrasound-guided introduction of a 19-gauge RFA instrument into the anomalous twin at the level of the abdominal cord insertion. Electrical current at alternating high frequencies is then used to produce increased tissue temperatures which then cause tissue coagulation and cessation of blood flow. Varying levels of survival after RFA have been shown with most estimates in the range of 70%–88%.[56,57] The potential benefit to RFA is that it is considered less invasive and may avoid some of the complications of bipolar coagulation, the most important being preterm delivery.

However, a meta-analysis reviewing these two forms of treatment did not show a significant difference in survival or median gestational age at delivery.[58] Therefore, both of these treatments appear to be acceptable alternatives in the management of these complicated pregnancies.

Twin-reversed arterial perfusion sequence

TRAP sequence occurs only in the setting of monochorionic pregnancy. The incidence of this condition is about 1 in 35,000 births or 1% of monochorionic twin gestations. In the TRAP sequence, the acardiac/acephalic twin receives all of its blood supply from the normal or "pump" twin (Figure 12.4). The term "reversed perfusion" is used

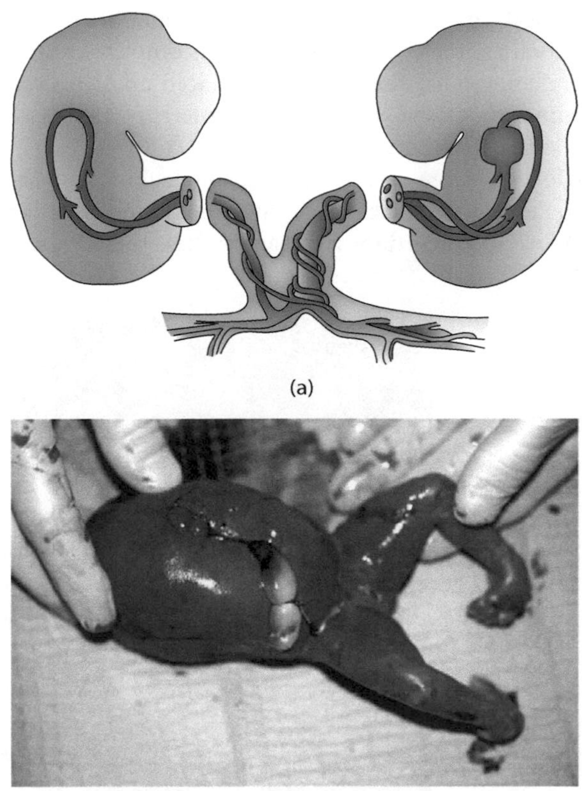

(a)

(b)

Figure 12.4 (a) Schematic illustration of pathophysiology of twin-reversed arterial perfusion (TRAP) sequence. The circulation of the acardiac twin (left) is grossly anomalous, whereby this parasitic twin is sustained by the normal "pump" twin (right). (b) Acardiac/acephalic twin delivered after cord ligation.

to describe this scenario because blood enters the acardiac/acephalic twin through its umbilical artery and exits through the umbilical vein. The grossly anomalous circulation whereby the parasitic acardiac twin is sustained by the normal pump twin places increased demand on the normal baby's heart, resulting in cardiac failure. If left untreated, the pump twin dies in up to 50%–75% of cases. In addition, there is the risk of preterm delivery, intrauterine growth restriction, and heart failure in the pump twin when significant TRAP is present. This is especially true when the acardiac/acephalic twin is greater than 50% of the size of the pump twin by estimated weight.[59] Figure 12.5 shows an example in which the TRAP fetus is significantly larger than the pump twin.

There have been multiple treatments attempted for TRAP sequence (cord embolization, cord ligation, laser, bipolar diathermy, intrafetal alcohol injection, etc.) but therapy currently focuses on either the use of cord coagulation/ligation or RFA. This treatment is aimed at interrupting the blood supply between the pump twin and the acardiac fetus. Quintero et al.[60] reported the first successful umbilical cord ligation for TRAP sequence causing cessation of blood flow communication between the fetuses. Bipolar coagulation has been shown to have a relatively high survival of the pump twin when used to interrupt the blood supply to the acardiac fetus.[61,62] Unfortunately, complication of this includes preterm premature rupture of membranes, preterm delivery, and incomplete treatment. Therefore, similar focus has been placed on using a more minimally invasive technique to interrupt the vascular communication between the fetuses.

RFA is a more minimally invasive technique that has been used with success in this population. Similar to RFA use in discordant twin anomalies, the RFA needle is sonographically guided into the area of umbilical cord vessels of the acardiac twin and the electrical current is used to interrupt the blood supply. The advantage of this approach is that it is not limited by oligohydramnios in the acardiac sac or difficulty in gaining access to the short umbilical cord of the acardius. The North American Fetal Therapy Network (NAFTNet) reported that RFA is a viable option in the case of TRAP sequence with an 80% survival of the pump twin at 30 days postdelivery.[63] Mean gestational age at delivery was 33.4 weeks overall and 36 weeks for survivors. This series shows that RFA is a reasonable treatment for cases of complicated TRAP sequence and has the potential benefits of being a less invasive technique.

We currently monitor TRAP sequence pregnancies with weekly ultrasounds evaluating the acardius/pump twin weight ratio, amniotic fluid level, hydrops, and cardiac function. If there is evidence of a large acardius (>70% of the weight of the pump twin) or heart failure in the pump twin we then offer fetal treatment. We most commonly use RFA for treatment because of its more minimally invasive approach, however, we will use bipolar coagulation in cases of monoamniotic TRAP pregnancy in which cord entanglement is potentially an issue.

TWIN-TO-TWIN TRANSFUSION SYNDROME

Treatment options in twin-to-twin transfusion syndrome

The natural history of severe TTTS is well established, with mortality approaching 100% if left untreated, especially when it presents at less than 20 weeks' gestation.[64,65] As a result, numerous treatments have been proposed, including selective feticide, cord coagulation, section parva, placental bloodletting, maternal digitalis, maternal indocin

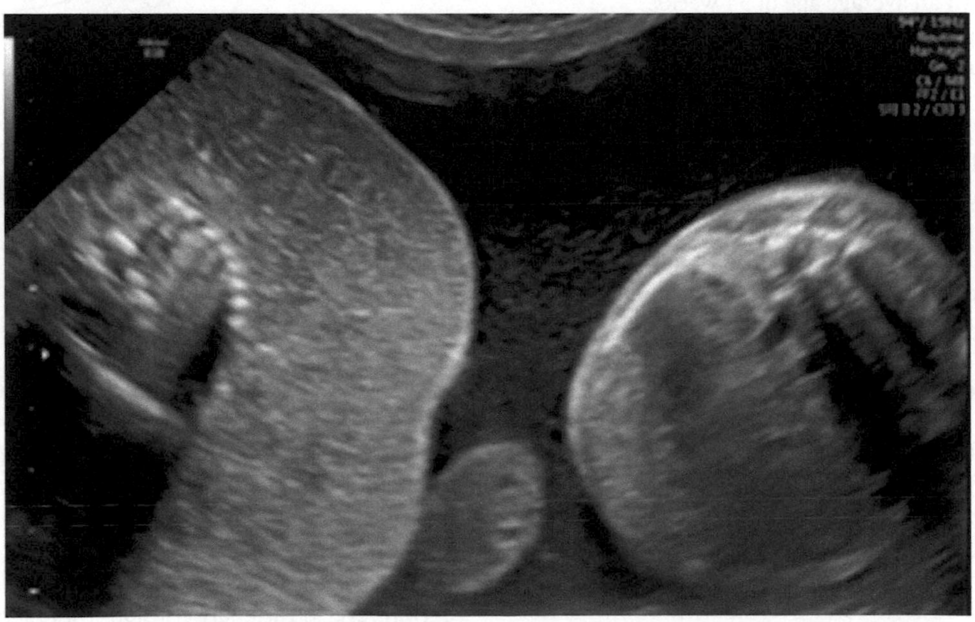

Figure 12.5 Ultrasound image of a twin pregnancy with TRAP sequence. The acardiac fetus (left) is significantly larger than the "pump" fetus (right). This increases the risks for complications for this pathologic process.

administration, serial amnioreduction, microseptostomy of the intertwine membrane, and nonselective and selective fetoscopic laser.

Traditionally, amnioreduction and intertwin membrane septostomy were the most commonly used treatments for TTTS. Initial evaluation of serial amnioreduction revealed an overall fetal survival rate of 49%.[66] Unfortunately, this survival number appeared to fluctuate based on the severity of TTTS. Mari et al.[67] found that patients presenting with advanced TTTS prior to 22 weeks' gestation and absent end diastolic flow in the recipient umbilical artery had a survival rate with aggressive amnioreduction of only 13%; with absent end diastolic flow in the donor umbilical artery, survival was 33%. The paradoxical resolution of oligohydramnios after a single amnioreduction was first suggested by Saade et al.[68] to be due to inadvertent puncture of the intertwin membrane. Although initial small studies suggested survival as high as 81% with microseptostomy a multicenter trial comparing amnioreduction and microseptostomy showed a comparable 65% survival for each modality.[69,70] The overall low survival numbers for each of these treatments are likely due to the treatments focus on relieving side effects of TTTS and not the underlying pathologic process. In cases of severe TTTS these treatments likely have little to no effect, as both fetuses still suffer the consequences of the shared placental circulation and the morbidity/mortality that comes along with it. Because of this, the goal became finding a treatment that treats the disease and interrupts the pathologic process.

Fetoscopic laser photocoagulation

The first treatment for TTTS that attempted to treat the anatomic basis of the syndrome was reported by De Lia et al.[71,72] Fetoscopic laser was used to photocoagulate vessels crossing the intertwine membrane referred to as "nonselective laser photocoagulation." The theory behind this treatment is that photocoagulating the vessels that are shared between the twins in TTTS will arrest the disease and potentially cause resolution of the effects (Figure 12.6). In the first small series, De Lia reported an overall survival of 53% in 26 patients.[72] While survival was not significantly better than previous reports with serial amnioreduction, the neurologic outcome in 96% of survivors was "normal" as assessed by head ultrasound.

Initially, nonselective laser ablation was instituted for the treatment of TTTS. A nonselective fetoscopic laser technique photocoagulates all vessels crossing the intertwin membrane regardless of where the anastomoses occur. This approach is problematic as the intertwine membrane often bears no relation to the vascular equator of the placenta. This nonselective laser photocoagulation of all vessels crossing the intertwine membrane likely sacrifices vessels not responsible for the TTTS resulting in a higher death rate of the donor twin from acute placental insufficiency.[73]

Because of this lack of significant survival advantage in nonselective laser treatment, a selective laser photocoagulation was developed.[73] In this technique the fetoscope is used to "map" the fetal placental blood vessels. Vessels that communicate between the fetuses are the only ones treated with photocoagulation. In addition, vessels that appear close (close proximity cotyledons) and unpaired arteries and veins are also treated. In theory, this approach does not necessarily favor the treatment of donor twin vessels, and therefore decreases the risk of acute placental insufficiency. Initial trials of this technique were positive and when compared with serial amnioreduction there was a 79% survival of at least one twin in the laser photocoagulation arm compared with only 60% in the amnioreduction arm.[74]

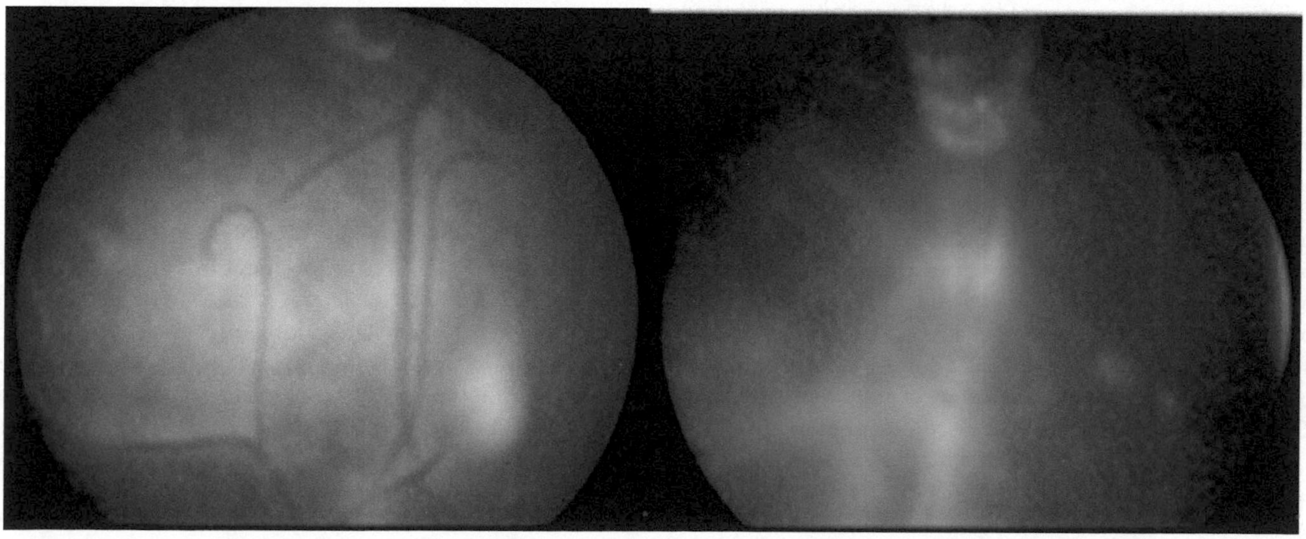

(a) (b)

Figure 12.6 (a) Fetoscopic view of the placental surface shows an example of arteriovenous connections on the placental surface. (b) The appearance of the same arteriovenous connections postlaser photocoagulation. The laser fiber can be seen at the 12 o'clock position of the picture.

The Eurofetus trial by Senat et al.[75] and the NIH-sponsored trial by Crombleholme et al. remain the two largest trials comparing laser treatment to amnioreduction.[76] The Eurofetus trial showed significant improvement in the survival of at least one twin in laser compared with amnioreduction (76% versus 56%) as well as less neurologic abnormalities on neuroimaging studies (31% versus 52%). This study showed the superiority of laser over traditional amnioreduction. The trial by Crombleholme et al. failed to show the definitive survival benefit of the Eurofetus trial but it did introduce an important adjunct diagnosis tool for TTTS. This trial showed that the Cardiovascular Profile Score was the most significant predictor of recipient mortality.

Survival in TTTS cases treated by laser photocoagulation appears to continue to improve. Habli et al.[77] reported an overall fetal survival of 77.5% with the survival of one or both twins at 88%. A recent manuscript by Mullers et al.[78] showed an overall fetal survival of 61% with the survival of one or both twins at 75%. Results in our center currently are 95% survival of one or both twins with 80% of pregnancies with dual survivorship. As the diagnosis is better understood and the treatment optimized, outcomes will hopefully continue to improve.

Additional modifications to the laser technique include the sequential laser photocoagulation and the Solomon technique.[79,80] The sequential technique describes the order of treatment of the abnormally communicating fetal vessels with the goal of minimizing feto-fetal transfusion that can occur during the laser procedure. The first vessels treated are arteriovenous communications from donor to recipient, followed by arteriovenous communications from recipient to donor, and then venous–venous and arterial–arterial connections. Initial reports suggested potential benefit to the donor twin survival using this technique compared with the center's historical control samples.

The Solomon randomized trial was recently published with promising results.[80] This was developed because of the relatively high incidence of recurrent/persistent TTTS and postlaser TAPS reported to occur in up to 14% and 13% of cases, respectively. This technique involves performing an initial selective laser photocoagulation and then proceeding with laser photocoagulation of the surface of the placenta from one edge to the other in a line. The authors of this trial found a significant decrease in the incidence of both recurrent/persistent TTTS and TAPS sequence compared with nonsolomonized placentas (5% versus 1% for TTTS and 22% versus 4% for TAPS). Although there was potentially improvement in the rate of recurrent TTTS and TAPS, there were also an increased rate of complications. Complications reported include higher rates of iatrogenic monoamnionicity, bleeding, and PPROM although none of these reached statistical significance. These complications using this technique must be weighed against the potential benefit. Despite the suggestion at improved outcomes these modifications may simply reflect improved surgical technique. Perhaps complete "mapping" of the abnormal vessel connections between fetuses prior to laser treatment can produce similar outcomes by allowing speedier treatment (to decrease volume fluctuations) and complete blood vessel treatment (to decrease recurrent/persistent TTTS and TAPS) and therefore a true selective laser photocoagulation technique may be just as beneficial.

Other improvements in the diagnosis and treatment of TTTS do not necessarily involve the use of the fetoscope but should still be mentioned. Initial description of the severity of TTTS is usually made using the staging system by Quintero.[82] This method solely relies on ultrasound evaluation of the twin pregnancy. More recent staging systems have "modified" the Quintero system by involving cardiac evaluations of the fetuses with recipient twin cardiac function being a major part of the system. There have been several systems proposed.[83–85] We use the Cincinnati modification to the Quintero staging system to describe the presence and severity of fetal cardiomyopathy.[86] This system describes the criteria for diagnosis of cardiomyopathy and then ranks as mild, moderate, or severe. There are a significant number of Quintero stage I TTTS cases that already show evidence of cardiomyopathy. A system such as ours shows the most severely affected cases of TTTS and therefore the ones that necessitate treatment. Another potential advancement in the treatment of TTTS is the use of nifedipine when complicated by cardiomyopathy. Crombleholme et al.[86] showed overall improved survival with its use compared with traditional surgical treatment alone (83% vs. 75%) and specifically improved overall recipient survival (90% vs. 82%) and in stage IIIC and IV (93% vs. 86%) with no effect on donor survival. This likely represents another treatment that focuses on stabilizing/reversing the underlying cardiac pathology specifically affecting the recipient twin.

COMPLICATIONS OF ENDOSCOPIC FETAL SURGERY

Preterm labor remains the "Achilles heel" of fetal intervention.[87] It is, to some degree, a complication of all fetal surgery. Using a fetoscopic approach should decrease this risk but does not solve the problem. The etiology of preterm labor may be related to the disease process for which the surgery is indicated (i.e., associated with polyhydramnios or specific anomalies). Preterm labor may also be related to a fetal systemic inflammatory response that is a reaction to intervention.[88] A maternal inflammatory response to uterine trauma probably also plays a role in initiating preterm contractions. Improvement in avoiding or arresting preterm labor in fetal surgery cases will allow the field to make even greater strides forward.

Preterm labor is not the only complication that occurs. Chorioamniotic separation is the most frequent complication of endoscopic fetal surgery occurring in at least 36% or cases.[89] In addition, other major complications occur at variable rates. Habli et al.[77] showed a 17.8% risk of PPROM, 3.3% risk of pregnancy loss before 24 weeks, and placental abruption rate of 8%. Each of these complications leads to increased morbidity and mortality for the pregnancies and influences the average gestational age at delivery. Decreasing these complications will also contribute to the advancement of the field.

Bleeding is not usually a major problem in endoscopic fetal surgery. It is well worth the time preoperatively to plan carefully with an ultrasound approach which allows room for manipulation of the endoscope while avoiding the placenta as well as the broad-ligament blood vessels. In the case of anterior placenta, the patient may need to lie completely on one side. In all cases it is best to tilt the patient at least slightly to avoid obstruction of the vena cava.

SUMMARY

Endoscopic fetal surgery has made great strides over the years and even since the last edition of this textbook. As the understanding of the underlying pathophysiology advances and the surgical techniques improve, better outcomes can be expected. Despite these advancements, fetal surgery should still be reserved for cases at risk for significant morbidity or mortality if left untreated.

REFERENCES

1. Reuss A, Stewart PA, Wladimiroff JW et al. Non-invasive management of fetal obstructive uropathy. *Lancet* 1988; 2: 949–51.
2. Cusick EL, Didier F, Droulle P et al. Mortality after an antenatal diagnosis of foetal uropathy. *J Pediatr Surg* 1995; 30: 463–6.
3. Ciftei AO, Cook RCM, voon Vetzen D. Megacystic microcolon enteral hypoperistaltic syndrome: Evidence of primary myocellular defect of contractile fiber synthesis. *J Pediatr Surg* 1996; 31: 1706–1711.
4. Maximel JC, Pettinato G, Reinbert Y et al. Prune Belly Syndrome: Clinicopathologic study of 29 cases. *Pediatr Pathol* 1989; 9: 691–711.
5. Glick PL, Harrison MR, Golbus MS et al. Management of the fetus with congenital hydronephrosis II. Prognostic criteria and selection for treatment. *J Pediatr Surg* 1985; 20: 376–87.
6. Johnson MP, Bukowski TP, Reitleman C et al. In utero surgical treatment of fetal obstructive uropathy: A new comprehensive approach to identify appropriate candidates for vesicoamniotic shunt therapy. *Am J Obstet Gynecol* 1994; 170: 1770–9.
7. Clark TJ, Martin WL, Divakaran TO et al. Prenatal bladder drainage in the management of fetal lower urinary tract obstruction: A systematic review and meta-analysis. *Obstet Gynecol* 2003; 102: 367–82.
8. Freedman AL, Johnson MP, Smith CA et al. Long-term outcome in children after antenatal intervention for obstructive uropathies. *Lancet* 1999; 354: 374–7.
9. Holmes N, Harrison MR, Baskin LS. Fetal surgery for posterior urethral valves: Long-term postnatal outcomes. *Pediatrics* 2001; 108: el–7.
10. Morris RK, Malin GL, Quinlan-Jones E et al. Percutaneous vesicoamniotic shunting versus conservative management for fetal lower urinary tract obstruction (PLUTO): A randomized trial. *Lancet* 2013; 382: 1496–1506.
11. Gatti JM, Kirsch AJ, Massad CA. Antenaral intervention: Jeopardizing life or limb. *Urology* 2002; 60: iii–ix.
12. Quintero RA, Johnson MP, Smith C et al. In utero percutaneous cystoscopy in the management of fetal lower obstructive uropathy. *Lancet* 1995; 346: 537–40.
13. Quintero RA, Hume R, Smith C et al. Percutaneous fetal cystoscopy and endoscopic fulguration of posterior urethral valves. *Am J Obstet Gynecol* 1995; 172: 206–9.
14. Clifton MS, Harrison MR, Ball R et al. Fetoscopic transuterine release of posterior urethral valves: A new technique. *Fetal Diag Ther* 2008; 23: 89–94.
15. Fauza DO, Wilson JM. Congenital diaphragmatic hernia and associated anomalies: Their incidence, identification, and impact on prognosis. *J Pediatr Surg* 1994; 29: 1113–7.
16. Puri P. Congenital diaphragmatic hernia. *Curr Prob Surg* 1994; 31: 787–846.
17. Albanese CT, Lopoo J, Goldstein RB et al. Fetal liver position and perinatal outcome for congenital diaphragmatic hernia. *Prenatal Diagn* 1998; 18: 1138–42.
18. Guibaud L, Filiatraut D, Gare L et al. Fetal congenital diaphragmatic hernia: Accuracy of sonography in the diagnosis and prediction of the outcome after birth. *AJR Am J Roentgenol* 1996; 166: 1195–202.
19. Lipshutz GS, Albanese CT, Feldstein VA et al. Prospective analysis of lung-to-head ratio predicts survival for patients with prenatally diagnosed congenital diaphragmatic hernia. *J Pediatr Surg* 1997; 32: 1634–6.
20. Landy JAM, Van Gucht M, Van Dooren MF et al. Congenital diaphragmatic hernia: An evaluation of the prognostic value of the lung-to-head ratio and other prenatal parameters. *Prenat Diagn* 2003; 23: 634–9.
21. Metkus AP, Filly RA, Stringer MD et al. Sonographic predictors of survival in fetal diaphragmatic hernia. *J Pediatr Surg* 1996; 31: 148–52.
22. Cannie M, Jani JC, De Keyzer F et al. Fetal body volume use at MR imaging to quantify relative lung volume in fetuses suspected of having pulmonary hypoplasia. *Radiology* 2006; 241: 847–53.
23. DePrest J, Jani J, Van Schoubroeck D et al. Current consequences of prenatal diagnosis of congenital diaphragmatic hernia. *J Pediatr Surg* 2006; 41: 423–430.
24. Jani J, Nicolaides KH, Keller RL et al. Observed to expected lung area to head circumference ratio in the prediction of survival in fetuses with isolated diaphragmatic hernia. *Ultrasound Obstet Gynecol* 2007; 30: 67–71.
25. Jani J, Nicolaides KH, Benachi A et al. Timing of lung size assessment in the prediction of survival in fetuses with diaphragmatic hernia. *Ultrasound Obstet Gynecol* 2008; 31: 37–40.

26. Harrison MR, Mychaliska GB, Albanese CT et al. Correction of congenital diaphragmatic hernia in utero. IX. Fetuses with poor prognosis (liver herniation, low lung-to-head ratio) can be saved by fetoscopic temporary tracheal occlusion. *J Pediatr Surg* 1998; 33: 1017–23.
27. Flake AW, Crombleholme TM, Johnson MP et al. Treatment of severe congenital diaphragmatic hernia by fetal tracheal occlusion: Clinical experience with fifteen cases. *Am J Obstet Gynecol* 2000; 183: 1059–66.
28. Harrison MR, Keller RL, Hagwood SB et al. A randomized trial of fetal endoscopic tracheal occlusion for severe fetal congenital diaphragmatic hernia. *N Engl J Med* 2003; 349: 1916–24.
29. Deprest J, Gratacos E, Nicolaides KH; FETO Task Group. Fetoscopic tracheal occlusion (FETO) for severe congenital diaphragmatic hernia: Evolution of a technique and preliminary results. *Ultrasound Obstet Gynecol* 2004; 24(2): 121–6.
30. Kunisaki SM, Barnewolt CE, Estroff JA et al. Ex utero intrapartum treatment with extracorporeal membrane oxygenation for severe congenital diaphragmatic hernia. *J Pediatr Surg* 2007; 41: 98–106.
31. Adzick NS, Thom EA, Spong CY et al., A randomized trial of prenatal versus postnatal repair of myelomeningocele. *N Engl J Med* 2011; 364(11): 993–1004.
32. Kohl T, Hartlage MG, Kiehitz D et al. Percutaneous fetoscopic patch coverage of experimental lumbosacral full-thickness skin lesions in sheep. *Surg Endosc* 2003; 17(8): 1218–23.
33. Fontecha CG, Peiro JL, Sevilla JJ et al. Fetoscopic coverage of experimental myelomeningocele in sheep using a patch with surgical sealant. *Eur J Obstet Gynecol Reprod Biol* 2011; 156(2): 171–6.
34. Bruner JP, Richards WO, Tulipan N et al. Endoscopic coverage of fetal myelomeningocele in utero. *Am J Obstet Gynecol* 1999; 180: 153–8.
35. Pedreira DA, Zanon N, Nishikuni K et al. Endoscopic surgery for the antenatal treatment of myelomeningocele: The CECAM trial. *Am J Obstet Gynecol* 2015; 214(1): 111.e1–111.e11.
36. Kohl T. Percutaneous minimally invasive fetoscopic surgery for spina bifida aperta. Part I: Surgical technique and perioperative outcome. *Ultrasound Obstet Gynecol* 2014; 44: 515–24.
37. Peiro JL, Fontecha CG, Ruano R et al. Single-Access Fetal Endoscopy (SAFE) for myelomeningocele in sheep model I: Amniotic carbon dioxide gas approach. *Surg Endocs* 2013; 27(10): 3835–40.
38. Belfort MA, Whitehead WE, Shamshirsaz AA et al. Fetoscopic repair of myelomeningocele. *Obstet Gynecol* 2015; 126: 881–4.
39. Crombleholme TM, Dirkes K, Whitney TM et al. Amniotic band syndrome in fetal lambs. Part I: Fetoscopic release and morphometric outcomes. *J Pediatr Surg* 1995; 30(7): 974–8.
40. Quintero RA, Morales WJ, Phillips J et al. In utero lysis of amniotic bands. *Ultrasound Obstet Gynecol* 1997; 10: 316–20.
41. Keswani SG, Johnson MP, Adzick NS et al. In utero limb salvage: Fetoscopic release of amniotic bands for threatened limb amputation. *J Pediatr Surg* 2003; 38: 848–51.
42. Fox H, Elston CW. *Pathology of the Placenta. Major Problems in Pathology*, pp. xvii, 491. Philadelphia, PA: Saunders, 1978.
43. Quintero RA, Reich H, Romero R, Johnson MP et al. In utero endoscopic devascularization of a large chorioangioma. *Ultrasound Obstet Gynecol* 1996; 8(1): 48–52.
44. Sepulveda W, Alcalde JL, Schnapp C, Bravo M. Perinatal outcome after perinatal diagnosis of placental chorioangioma. *Obstet Gynecol* 2003; 102: 1028–33.
45. Zanardini C, Papageorghiou A, Bhide A, Thilaganathan B. Giant placental chorioangioma: Natural history and pregnancy outcome. *Ultrasound Obstet Gynecol* 2010; 35: 332–6.
46. Hamill N, Rijhsinghani A, Williamson RA, Grant S. Prenatal diagnosis and management of fetal anemia secondary to a large chorioangioma. *Obstet Gynecol* 2003; 102: 1185–8.
47. Hirata GI, Masaki DI, O'Toole M et al. Color flow mapping and Doppler velocimetry in the diagnosis and management of a placental chorioangioma associated with non-immune fetal hydrops. *Obstet Gynecol* 1993; 81: 850–2.
48. Wanapirak C, Tongsong T, Sirichotiyakul S et al. Alcoholization: The choice of intrauterine treatment for chorioangioma. *J Obstet Gynaecol Res* 2002; 28: 71–5.
49. Lim FY, Coleman A, Polzin W et al. Giant chorioangiomas: Perinatal outcomes and techniques in fetoscopic devascularization. *Fetal Diagn Ther* 2015; 37: 18–23.
50. Burn J. The spectrum of genetic disorders in twins. In: Ward RH, Whittle M (eds), *Multiple Pregnancy*, pp. 74–83. London, UK: RCOG Press, 1995.
51. Kang HJ, Liao AW, Brizot ML et al. Prediction of intrauterine death and severe preterm delivery in twin pregnancies discordant for major fetal abnormality. *Eur J Obstet Gynecol Reprod Biol* 2014; 175: 115–8.
52. Ong SS, Zamora J, Khan KS, Kilby MD. Prognosis for the co-twin following single-twin death: A systematic review. *BJOG* 2006; 113(9): 992–8.
53. Malone FD, D'Alton ME. Multiple gestation: Clinical characteristics and management. In: Creasy RK, Resnik R (eds), *Maternal-Fetal Medicine* (4th edition), pp. 598–615. Philadelphia, PA: WB Saunders, 1999.
54. Crombleholme TM, Robertson F, Marx G et al. Fetoscopic cord ligation to prevent neurologic injury in monozygous twins. *Lancet* 1996; 348: 191.

55. Lanna MM, Rustico MA, Dell'Avanzo M et al. Bipolar cord coagulation for selective feticide in complicated monochorionic twin pregnancies: 118 consecutive cases at a single center. *Ultrasound Obstet Gynecol* 2012; 39(4): 407–13.
56. Bebbington MW, Danzer E, Moldenhauer J et al. Radiofrequency ablation vs bipolar umbilical cord coagulation in the management of complicated monochorionic pregnancies. *Ultrasound Obstet Gynecol* 2012; 40(3): 319–24.
57. Roman A, Papanna R, Johnson A et al. Selective reduction in complicated monochorionic pregnancies: Radiofrequency ablation vs. bipolar cord coagulation. *Ultrasound Obstet Gynecol* 2010; 36(1): 37–41.
58. Gaerty K, Greer RM, Kumar S. Systematic review and meta-analysis of perinatal outcomes after radiofrequency ablation and bipolar cord occlusion in monochorionic pregnancies. *Am J Obstet Gynecol* 2015; 213(5): 637–43.
59. Moore TR, Gale S, Benirschke K. Perinatal outcome of forty-nine pregnancies complicated by acardiac twinning. *Am J Obstet Gynecol* 1990; 163: 907–12.
60. Quintero RA, Reich H, Pruder KS et al. Brief report: Umbilical cord ligation to an acardiac twin by fetoscopy at 19 weeks gestation. *N Engl J Med* 1994; 330: 469–71.
61. Corbacioglu A, Gul A, Bakirci IT et al. Treatment of twin reversed arterial perfusion sequence with alcohol ablation or bipolar cord coagulation. *Int J Gynaecol Obstet* 2012; 117(3): 257–9.
62. Gul A, Gungorduk K, Yildirim G et al. Fetal therapy in twin reversed arterial perfusion sequence pregnancies with alcohol ablation or bipolar cord coagulation. *Arch Gynecol Obstet* 2008; 278(6): 541–5.
63. Lee H, Bebbington M, Crombleholme TM et al. The North American Fetal Therapy Network Registry data on outcomes of radiofrequency ablation for twin-reversed arterial perfusion sequence. *Fetal Diagn Ther* 2013; 33(4): 224–9.
64. Chescheir NC, Seeds JW. Polyhydramnios and oligohydramnios in twin gestations. *Obstet Gynecol* 1988; 71: 882–4.
65. Weir PE, Ratten GJ, Beischer IMA. Acute polyhydramnios—A complication of monozygous twin pregnancy. *Br J Obstet Gynaecol* 1979; 86: 849–53.
66. Moise KJ Jr. Polyhydramnios: Problems and treatment. *Semin Perinatol* 1993; 17: 197–209.
67. Mari G, Roberts A, Detti L et al. Perinatal morbidity and mortality rates in severe twin-twin transfusion syndrome: Results of the International Arnnioreduction Registry. *Am J Obstet Gynecol* 2001; 185: 708–15.
68. Saade GR, Olson G, Belfort MA et al. Amniotomy: A new approach to the 'stuck twin' syndrome. *Am J Obstet Gynecol* 1995; 172: 429–34.
69. Saade GR, Belfort MA, Berry DL et al. Amniotic septostomy for the treatment of twin oligohydramnios-polyhydramnios sequence. *Fetal Diagn Ther* 1998; 13: 86–93.
70. Saade G, Moise K, Dorman K et al. A randomized trial of septostomy versus amnioreduction in the treatment of twin oligohydramnios polyhydramnios sequence (TOPS). *Am Obstet Gynecol* (Society for Maternal-Fetal Medicine, Oral presentation, abstract 3) 2002; 187(6): S54.
71. De Lia JE, Cruikshank DP, Kaye WR. Fetoscopic neodymium–YAG laser occlusion of placental vessels in severe twin-twin transfusion syndrome. *Obstet Gynecol* 1990; 75: 1046–53.
72. De Lia JE, Kuhlmann RS, Harstad TW et al. Fetoscopic laser ablation of placental vessels in severe twin-twin transfusion syndrome. *Am J Obstet Gynecol* 1995; 172: 1202–11.
73. Quintero RA, Morales WJ, Mendoza G et al. Selective photocoagulation of placental vessels in twin-twin transfusion syndrome: Evolution of a surgical technique. *Obstet Gynecol Survey* 1998; 53: 597–603.
74. Hecher K, Plath H, Bregenzer T et al. Endoscopic laser surgery versus serial amniocenteses in the treatment of severe twin-twin transfusion syndrome. *Am J Obstet Gynecol* 1999; 180: 717–24.
75. Senat MV, Deprest J, Boulvain M et al. Endoscopic laser surgery versus serial amnioreduction for severe twin-to-twin transfusion syndrome. *N Engl J Med* 2004; 351: 136–44.
76. Crombleholme TM, Shera D, Lee H et al. A prospective, randomized, multicenter trial of amnioreduction vs selective fetoscopic laser photocoagulation for the treatment of severe twin-twin transfusion syndrome. *Am J Obstet Gynecol* 2007; 197(4): 396 el-9.
77. Habli M, Bombrys A, Lewis D et al. Incidence of complications in twin-twin transfusion syndrome after selective fetoscopic laser photocoagulation: A single-center experience. *Am J Obstet Gynecol* 2009; 201(4): 417 el-7.
78. Mullers SM, McAuliffe FM, Kent E et al. Outcome following selective fetoscopic laser ablation for twin to twin transfusion syndrome: An 8 year national collaborative experience. *Eur J Obstet Gynecol Reprod Biol* 2015; 191: 125–9.
79. Chmait RH, Kontopoulos EV, Quintero RA. Sequential laser surgery for twin-twin transfusion syndrome. *Am J Perinatol* 2014; 31 (Suppl 1): S13–8.
80. Slaghekke F, Lewi L, Middeldorp JM et al. Residual anastomoses in twin-twin transfusion syndrome after laser: The Solomon randomized trial. *Am J Obstet Gynecol* 2014; 211(3): 285 el-7.
81. Quintero RA, Morales WJ, Allen MH et al. Staging of twin-twin transfusion syndrome. *J Perinatol* 1999; 19(8 Pt 1): 550–5.

82. Stirnemann JJ, Nasr B, Proulx F et al. Evaluation of the CHOP cardiovascular score as a prognostic predictor of outcome in twin-twin transfusion syndrome after laser coagulation of placental vessels in a prospective cohort. *Ultrasound Obstet Gynecol* 2010; 36(1): 52–7.
83. Shah AD, Border WL, Crombleholme TM et al. Initial fetal cardiovascular profile score predicts recipient twin outcome in twin-twin transfusion syndrome. *J Am Soc Echocardiogr* 2008; 21(10): 1105–8.
84. Habli M, Michelfelder E, Cnota J et al. Prevalence and progression of recipient-twin cardiomyopathy in early-stage twin-twin transfusion syndrome. *Ultrasound Obstet Gynecol* 2012; 39(1): 63–8.
85. Crombleholme TM, Lim FY, Habli M et al. Improved recipient survival with maternal nifedipine in twin-twin transfusion syndrome complicated by TTTS cardiomyopathy undergoing selective fetoscopic laser photocoagulation. *Am J Obstet Gynecol* 2010; 203(4): 397 e1–9.
86. Harrison MR. Fetal surgery. *Am J Obstet Gynecol* 1996; 174: 1255–64.
87. Romero R, Gomez R, Ghezzi F et al. A fetal systemic inflammatory response is followed by the spontaneous onset of preterm parturition. *Am J Obstet Gynecol* 1998; 179: 186–93.
88. Harrison MR, Tsao K, Hirose S et al. Chorioamniotic membrane separation following fetal surgery. *Am J Obstet Gynecol* 2001; 184: SI43.

Fetal surgery—The Texas Children's Fetal Center approach

13

ALIREZA A. SHAMSHIRSAZ, MICHAEL A. BELFORT, and ROBERT H. BALL

CONTENTS

BRIEF HISTORY OF FETAL SURGERY

The availability of ultrasound imaging and screening programs has made the unborn child a true patient. Fetal surgery has evolved over the past three decades from an ambitious concept, to a familiar, regulated, and innovative field of medicine. New intraoperative techniques for open surgeries and minimally invasive image-guided percutaneous approaches for fetoscopic repairs have had a positive impact on outcomes. In addition, overall improvements in postoperative care have decreased morbidity. Advances in fetal imaging, diagnosis, anesthesia, and postoperative tocolysis have accelerated progress such that fetal interventions have now become vital for subsets of fetal patients who would otherwise endure significant lifelong morbidity and increased mortality.

The first successful direct fetal intervention was performed by Sir William Liley in 1963 when he completed a transuterine fetal intraperitoneal red blood cell transfusion for erythroblastosis fetalis. This was accomplished using fluoroscopy in a time that preceded the ultrasound era.[1] Over the subsequent decades the field rapidly developed, to a large extent fueled by the work of Dr. Michael Harrison, a pediatric surgeon and an early pioneer in fetal surgery. In 1982, one of the first organized conferences on fetal intervention occurred in the Santa Ynez Valley. Dr. Harrison summarized the conclusions of the first meeting of this group, which would later become the International Fetal Medicine and Surgery Society (IFMSS) in a seminal paper.[2] One of the key statements made in that paper established an important scientific principle to guide those involved in the nascent field, namely, "All case material, regardless of outcome, should be reported to a fetal treatment registry, so that the benefits and liabilities of fetal therapy can be established as soon as possible." This ethos is as important today as it was three decades ago. A consensus, endorsed by the IFMSS, has been reached on the criteria and indications for fetal surgery (Table 13.1).[3]

A fetal anomaly raises unique and complex issues for the pregnant woman and her family. The importance of having a multidisciplinary team involved in the prenatal evaluation, the surgical therapy, and the postnatal care cannot be over emphasized. The current ideal multidisciplinary fetal intervention team includes specialists in maternal–fetal medicine, pediatric surgery, maternal and fetal anesthesia, pediatric

Table 13.1 Criteria for fetal surgery.

1. Accurate diagnosis and staging is possible, with exclusion of associated anomalies.
2. Natural history of the disease is documented, and prognosis is established.
3. There's currently no effective postnatal therapy.
4. In utero surgery has proved feasible in animal models, reversing deleterious effects of the condition.
5. Interventions are performed in specialized multidisciplinary fetal treatment centers within strict protocols with approval of the local Ethics Committee and informed consent of the mother or parents.
6. Fetus should be a singleton with no concomitant anomalies.
7. Family should be fully counseled about risk and benefits and should be agree to treatment.

Source: Harrison MR and Adzick NS, *Ann Surg*, 213, 279–291, 1991.

neurosurgery, pediatric urology, pediatric nephrology, pediatric cardiology and interventional cardiology, neonatology and access to a bioethicist, and a social worker familiar with the issues involved.[4]

OPEN FETAL SURGERY TECHNIQUE AND COMPLICATIONS

"Open" fetal surgery refers to the creation of a hysterotomy for access to the fetus, with the intent of closing the uterine incision at the completion of the procedure, and continuing the pregnancy. Commensurate with Harrison's initial principles,[2] human experimentation in open fetal surgery was preceded by animal work which included testing the concept in a primate model.[5] This model was chosen because other gravid, large animal models, such as the sheep, have a uterus and a preterm labor profile that are much more forgiving than those seen in the human or primate. In addition, the sheep uterus is thin walled and has a multicotyledonary, epitheliochorial placenta, which is very different to the discoid, hemochorial, human placenta.

The technique used in performing open hysterotomy fetal surgery in most fetal programs in the United States is generally as follows. Preoperatively, indomethacin (as a prophylactic tocolytic) and antibiotics are given. An epidural catheter is placed preoperatively but only activated after the case for postoperative pain control. General anesthesia is initiated with propofol and moderate to high levels (1–3 Monitored Anesthesia Care) of inhalational agent (generally sevoflurane) are employed to maximize uterine relaxation. After prepping and draping, ultrasound transducers with sterile covers are used to identify fetal lie and placental location. A transverse skin incision is generally made a third of the way between the pubic symphysis and the umbilicus (lower with an anterior placenta so that the uterus can more easily be exteriorized). Occasionally, the rectus muscles need to be at least partially transected to allow appropriate exposure. Once the peritoneal cavity is entered, the ultrasound transducer is placed directly on the myometrium, and the edge of the placenta is identified and marked by cautery. The general strategy is to place the hysterotomy as far from the placenta as possible, with the direction of the incision parallel to its edge. This will minimize the risk of extension toward the placenta. The reason for this level of caution is that placental bed bleeding cannot be controlled. If necessary, the fetus is externally verted to an appropriate presentation and position for the intended procedure prior to opening the uterus. This is an important point, since once the uterus is opened there should an absolute minimum of fetal manipulation given the propensity to cardiac decompensation with such perturbation.

The hysterotomy is facilitated by the ultrasound-guided placement of two absorbable monofilament sutures parallel to the intended incision site and through the full thickness of the uterine wall. In this way, the membranes are plicated to the uterine wall to limit chorioamniotic separation. The uterus is opened between the sutures and a uterine stapler is then introduced into the cavity and fired. This device places two parallel lines of dissolving staples approximately 8 cm long and opens the uterus between them. This produces a hemostatic myometrial incision with the membranes tacked to the myometrium, minimizing the risk of separation. In some institutions hemostatic sutures are placed around the hysterotomy instead of using a stapler. Occasionally, bleeding from the myometrial edge requires placement of atraumatic clamps or a figure-of-8 stitch. When placing a staple line ultrasound should be used to confirm that no fetal part or loop of cord is pinched in the device. Bleeding between the membranes and uterine wall, leading to a subchorionic hematoma, is a potentially serious complication that can occur during hysterotomy creation, and this could potentially dissect the membranes away from the uterine wall and cause significant maternal blood loss. Recognizing this problem early allows sutures to be placed to control the bleeding.

The fetus is then partially exposed or exteriorized and monitored using ultrasound, and in some cases with pulse oximetry and direct fetal echocardiography. Prior to beginning the fetal surgery, an intramuscular dose of analgesics (fentanyl), atropine, and vecuronium is given to provide pain control to immobilize the fetus and to suppress the fetal stress response (bradycardia). A catheter for the infusion of warm saline is placed into the uterus to maintain amniotic fluid volume and prevent umbilical cord compression and fetal cooling during the procedure. After completion of the fetal portion of surgery, any exteriorized part of the fetus is gently placed inside the uterus. Warmed normal saline containing antibiotics is instilled into the amniotic cavity, and the uterus is closed in two layers with absorbable sutures. Interrupted stay sutures are placed first, but not tied, and then a continuous suture is placed to close the hysterotomy. Prior to tying the continuous suture, a catheter is used to refill the amniotic

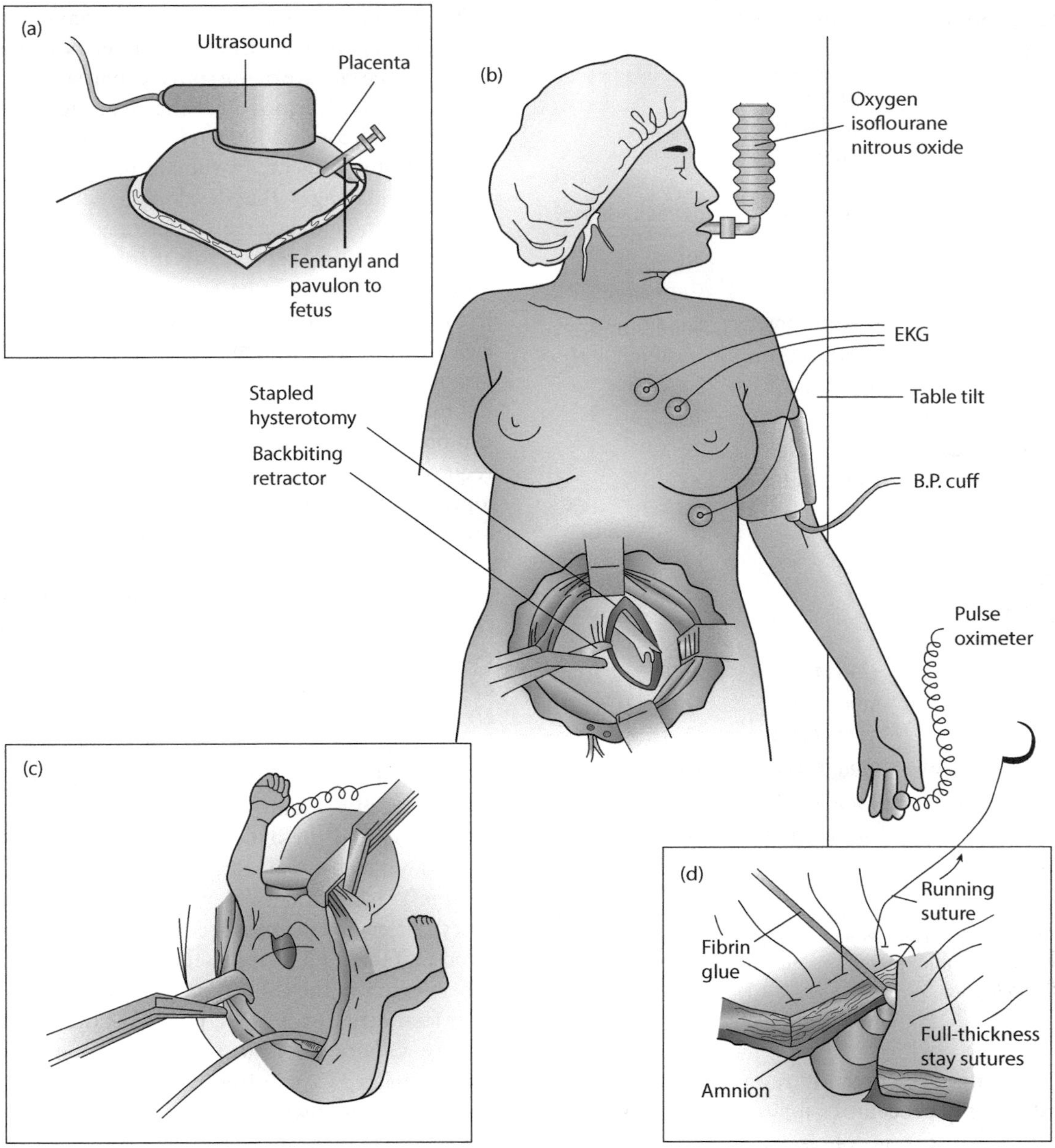

Figure 13.1 Operating room set up, and techniques for open fetal surgery.

cavity under ultrasound guidance. The fluid is replenished to a level of high normal fluid. Then, the stay sutures are tied. When it is certain that the suture line is hemostatic and watertight, the abdominal wall is closed in layers in the usual fashion. Occasionally, the hysterotomy is covered with an omental flap (Figure 13.1).

Tocolysis with intravenous magnesium sulfate is administered as the mother emerges from anesthesia. Postoperatively, the patient is treated on labor and delivery and given aggressive tocolysis with magnesium sulfate and continued indomethacin, for a total of 48 hours.

Complications of open fetal surgery include preterm contractions, maternal morbidity from tocolysis, chorioamniotic membrane separation, oligohydramnios, rupture of membranes, uterine dehiscence, and fetal decompensation. Postoperative uterine contractions are the Achilles' heel of open fetal surgery. Amniotic fluid leakage can occur through the hysterotomy site or, more commonly, vaginally because of chorioamniotic membrane separation or frank membrane rupture[6,7] (Table 13.2). Delivery by cesarean section is mandatory to avoid uterine rupture. All mothers who have had open fetal surgery with an upper segment incision subsequently require cesarean delivery and a 2-year interval between pregnancies is recommended. A potential risk in subsequent pregnancies is placenta accreta. The reason for this is that the site of a hysterotomy performed in the second trimester is highly unlikely to be in the same area as a third-trimester cesarean section entry. There is an increased risk of placenta accreta in any case where implantation is in an area

Table 13.2 Complications of open fetal surgery in repair of myelomeningocele.

	Children's Hospital of Philadelphia study (post-MOMS) trial	MOMS trial
No. of fetuses	100	78
Anesthesia	General	General
Access	Laparotomy	Laparotomy
Access diameter (mm)	Hysterectomy	Hysterotomy
Gestational age at intervention (weeks) (median and range)	23.2 (20.4–25.8)	23.6 ± 1.4
Operation time	78.5 (54–106)	n.s.
Success rate	n.s.	n.s.
Intraoperative hemorrhagic complications	n.s.	n.s.
Perioperative death rate	n.s.	2/78 (2.6%)
Chorioamnionitis	4/96 (4.1%)	2/78 (3%)
Oligohydramnios	6/96 (6.3%)	16/78 (21%)
PPROM	31/96 (32.3%)	36/78 (46%)
Delivery before 30 weeks	9/96 (9.4%)	10/78 (13%)
Delivery before 34 weeks	44/96 (45.8%)	36/78 (46%)
Gestational age at birth (weeks) (median and range)	34.3 (22.1–34.6)	34.1 ± 3.1 (n.s.)

Abbreviations: MOMS, Management of Myelomeningocele Study; PPROM, premature preterm rupture of the membranes; n.s., not significant.

of uterine scarring. We currently reserve maternal laparotomy/hysterotomy procedures for repair of neural tube defects (NTDs), resection of sacrococcygeal teratoma (SCT) and other tumors (pericardial), and for resection of congenital pulmonary airway malformations (CPAMs).

CONDITIONS TREATED WITH OPEN FETAL SURGERY

Open spina bifida

NTDs, including anencephaly, encephalocele, and myelomeningocele (MMC), are the most common human congenital structural defects. MMCs result from incomplete closure of the neural tube (which occurs on days 22–28 from conception) and are characterized by protrusion of the spinal cord and meninges through open vertebral arches. Patients with MMC are impacted by bowel and bladder dysfunction, orthopedic disabilities and lifelong paralysis, and possible learning disability.[8] The adverse effects of MMC occur both at the level of the lesion and in the brain. Before folic acid supplementation, NTDs affected 1–2 per 1000 pregnancies. The fortification of cereal and grain products in the United States has been associated with a 22.9% decrease in the incidence of NTDs.[9]

The neural damage in MMC has been explained by a "two-hit hypothesis." The first hit refers to the primary failure in the closure of the spinal canal early in embryonic life. The second hit involves the sequelae from exposure of the spinal cord and extruded nerves to direct trauma and neurotoxic agents in the amniotic fluid, which progressively damages the developing nervous system.[8] It is this secondary damage which may be ameliorated by early fetal surgical repair. This theory is supported by the observation that only half of affected fetuses have ventriculomegaly before 24 weeks of gestation, but more than 90% develop ventriculomegaly by term.[10] This theory also provides the rationale for trying to close the defect during mid-gestation. Because additional neurologic damage can occur after birth, as the result of additional surgeries required to replace a malfunctioning or infected ventriculoperitoneal shunt, any treatment that reduces the need for ventriculoperitoneal shunting would also improve outcomes.

The Management of Myelomeningocele Study (MOMS) trial was an ambitious study of prenatal compared with postnatal MMC repair, funded by the Eunice Kennedy Shriver National Institute of Child Health and Human Development and the National Institutes of Health. The study was performed in three fetal surgery units (the Children's Hospital of Philadelphia, Vanderbilt University Medical Center, and the University of California San Francisco), and the data management and analysis were carried out by the Data Study and Coordinating Center at George Washington University in Washington, DC. The entry criteria for the prospective MOMS trial are summarized in Table 13.3. Prior to the beginning of the trial, all other centers in the United States voluntarily agreed not to offer fetal surgery for MMC outside of the trial, essentially closing a "back door" to the intervention until the trial was completed. It required that all three centers develop a multispecialty team of clinicians who could evaluate all clinical and psychosocial aspects of potential patients and provide standardized prenatal, surgical, and perioperative care.[6] This was the first multicenter, prospective, randomized controlled trial (RCT) of maternal–fetal surgery for MMC, and the surgeons at all three centers had to develop and adhere to a strict protocol covering every aspect of the surgery, perioperative treatment, and maternal and fetal follow-up. Significant drawbacks were that it was not open to non-US citizens, and that the trial slowed the development of minimally invasive techniques. In 2010, the MOMS trial was stopped for efficacy by the Data Safety and Monitoring Board at a planned interim analysis of 183 out of the 200 anticipated patients.[6] Actual rates of shunt placement were 40% in the prenatal surgery group and 82% in the postnatal surgery group (relative risk [RR] 0.48, 97.7% confidence interval [CI] 0.36–0.64, $p < .001$). Prenatal surgery also resulted in an improvement in the composite score for mental development and motor function at 30 months ($p = .007$) and in improvement in several secondary outcomes, including hindbrain herniation by 12 months and ambulation by 30 months of age. However,

Table 13.3 Exclusion and entry criteria for the prospective MOMS trial.

Inclusion criteria
Pregnant women of age 18 or older
Gestational age at randomization from 19 weeks 0 days to 25 weeks 6 days
No karyotype abnormality
Lesion level no lower than S1
Established Arnold-Chiari II diagnosis on prenatal ultrasonography and MRI
Exclusion criteria
Further fetal anomaly
Pregestational insulin-dependent diabetes
Obesity (BMI $\geq$ 35 kg/m^2)
Fetal kyphosis of 30° or more
Twin, triplet, and higher-order multifetal pregnancies
Placenta previa
Short or incompetent cervix
Maternal medical condition
Previous history of spontaneous preterm labor
Maternal–fetal Rh incompatibility
Positive maternal viral serology (such as HIV, hepatitis B, or hepatitis C)
Lack of family support at the center
Uterine anomaly
Psychosocial limitations
Incompliant with travel and follow-up protocols

Abbreviations: BMI, body mass index; HIV, human immunodeficiency virus; MRI, magnetic resonance imaging.

prenatal surgery was associated with an increased risk of preterm delivery and uterine dehiscence at delivery. At 12 months of age, a significantly lower proportion of infants in the prenatal surgery group had any evidence of hindbrain herniation (64%) or moderate/severe hindbrain herniation (25%) when compared with the postnatal surgery group who had rates of 96% and 67%, respectively. In addition, the prenatal surgery group showed lower rates of brainstem kinking, abnormal fourth-ventricle location, and syringomyelia. Conversely, more children in the prenatal surgery group required surgery for tethered cord than in the postnatal surgery group (8% compared with 1%).[6]

Congenital cystic adenomatoid malformation (CCAM)

A CCAM, also known as CPAM, is a bronchopulmonary malformation usually identified on ultrasound as an intrapulmonary mass commonly localized to one lung lobe. They are classified based on the size of the cyst(s) as determined by ultrasound. Macrocystic (Stocker Type I) lesions contain at least one cyst >5 mm, whereas microcystic (Stocker Type III) lesions appear echogenic and are without visible cysts. Type II lesions are mixed.

If a fetus with a microcystic CCAM develops hydrops thought to be due to the mass effect, it is not amenable to decompression by shunting or drainage. In these cases, the use of prenatal steroids with the dosing typically given for fetal lung maturation has been associated with the resolution of the hydrops fetalis in the majority of cases (78%).[11] The mechanism is currently unknown, but it is postulated that steroids accelerate maturation or involution of the lesion. In view of this evidence, steroids seem a reasonable first-line therapy or medical adjunct in high-risk cases. To explore this issue more definitively, the same group has now embarked on a RCT (www. clinicaltrials.gov, study NCT00670956).

Rarely, some fetuses with a lung mass may benefit from open fetal surgery. We have found that fetuses with a large lung mass who develop progressive nonimmune hydrops associated with cardiac failure (as opposed to a chylothorax alone or hydrops without specific signs of cardiac failure)[12] may benefit from in utero decompression or resection of a cystic mediastinal lesion.[13] The fetuses with CCAM which have mediastinal shift with compression of developing lung tissue may benefit from the same procedure. Thoracoamniotic shunting may be performed in cases of CCAM with a large predominant cyst, while open fetal surgery is reserved for those fetuses <32 weeks gestational age (GA) with a massive multicystic, predominantly solid CCAM or bronchopulmonary sequestration. For hydropic fetuses greater than 32 weeks gestation, early delivery should be considered with resection of the lesion using an ex utero intrapartum treatment (EXIT) strategy. The reason for this is that very large CCAM lesions have airway connections to the bronchial tree and when neonatal respiration begins the lesion starts to fill with air but cannot decompress—the result is an expanding intrathoracic mass that compresses the heart and behaves like a tension pneumothorax. The optimum therapeutic option is to deliver the baby on placental support, open the fetal chest, and decompress the lung, establish an airway and begin neonatal ventilation, and then complete the delivery and transport the baby to another operating room to complete the resection. While numbers are small, results suggest benefit with this approach. Follow-up developmental testing has been normal in the majority of the survivors.[14] In an EXIT procedure, maternal laparotomy and stapled hysterotomy are performed under general endotracheal anesthesia with good uterine relaxation, and the fetal chest is exposed through the hysterotomy as described above for spina bifida repair. Our routine is to establish fetal intravenous access and to place a pulse oximeter on a fetal finger. The fetus is pretreated with intravenous atropine and volume (usually in the form of a transfusion) since sudden decompression of the fetal chest can lead to fetal bradycardia, poor ventricular filling, and a precipitous fall in cardiac output. We recommend continuous echocardiographic monitoring for all open fetal surgery cases regardless of lesion type in order to monitor fetal myocardial performance and volume status. Maternal–fetal general anesthesia is a potential fetal myocardial depressant, and we have found that having a pediatric cardiologist at the table actively managing fetal resuscitation is crucial.

For prenatal management of CCAM, minimally invasive techniques which include destruction of the lesion using thermocoagulation with laser, electrocautery and radiofrequency ablation (RFA), and the use of sclerosing agents have all been reported.[15,16]

Sacrococcygeal teratoma

Fetal SCT occurs in 1–2 per 20,000 pregnancies. The long-term outcome is excellent for SCTs diagnosed postnatally,[17] and most pregnancies with a prenatally diagnosed SCT proceed without incident. In rare cases, preterm labor develops, usually associated with polyhydramnios. Occasionally there is fetal demise from high-output cardiac failure associated with a large arteriovenous (AV) fistula.[18] Because the presence of an abnormal karyotype is rare with an isolated SCT, amniocentesis is usually not required as part of the workup.[19] Monitoring of tumor size, growth rate, and fetal cardiac function allows early identification of those fetuses at particular risk for decompensation.[20]

Large vascular fetal SCTs have uniformly dismal outcomes when associated with high-output failure and fetal hydrops before viability.[21] For this reason we believe that fetal therapy is justified in the presence of SCT with associated hydrops, and both minimally invasive and open fetal surgical approaches have been used. Minimally invasive therapies include laser ablation, RFA, interstitial laser, and vascular coil placement.[22] Open interventions have also been attempted.[23] Both types of intervention aim to decrease the impact of the mass on the fetal cardiovascular system, allowing the fetus to recover in utero. Outcomes have been mixed.

FETOSCOPIC PROCEDURES: THE TEXAS APPROACH TECHNIQUE AND COMPLICATIONS

"Closed" fetal surgeries are procedures performed by inserting a needle or a fetoscope through the uterine wall avoiding the need for a hysterotomy. In some cases the procedures are percutaneous, and in some a small incision in the maternal abdominal wall is required. Fetoscopic procedures are minimally invasive interventions.

Access to the amniotic cavity is facilitated by either thin-walled, semiflexible, disposable plastic ports, or by reusable, rigid metal cannulas; both allow a portal through which different instruments may be inserted.

Prophylactic doses of tocolytic (nifedipine 10–20 mg orally [PO] or indomethacin 50 mg PO) and antibiotics (cefazolin 2 g intravenously [IV]) are given preoperatively.

The most commonly performed fetoscopic intervention in most fetal centers today is that of laser ablation of placental anastomoses in twin-to-twin transfusion syndrome (TTTS). The technique of fetoscope insertion is described below:

The procedure is usually performed under local anesthesia, which is injected along the anticipated track of the access port. A 22-gauge needle is used to anesthetize the soft tissue down to the myometrium using ultrasound guidance. Supplemental intravenous sedation with remifentanil may also be given to sedate the mother during the procedure. After preparing and draping the abdomen, an ultrasound transducer with a sterile cover is used to identify the best place for port insertion, taking into consideration fetal lie and placental location. An 18-gauge needle is then inserted into the uterine cavity under ultrasound guidance and a guide-wire is introduced through the needle into the amniotic fluid. The needle is then removed leaving the wire in place. A Teflon cannula (Cook® Medical Inc., Bloomington, IN) loaded on a dilator is advanced over the guide wire using the Seldinger technique. The sheaths range in size from 8 to 12 Fr. Most fetoscopic surgical procedures usually involve only one uterine puncture. Current fetoscope diameters are between 1.0 and 4.0 mm with a 0–70° field of view. Occasionally, vision is obscured by blood or debris; in these cases, amnio-exchange with warmed saline (heated by a blood warmer or special amnio-irrigator) can improve visibility.

In patients with TTTS who have anterior placentation, we consider a laparoscopic-assisted fetoscopic technique. Briefly, the patient is placed in a lateral tilt opposite to the planned site of fetoscope entry. The peritoneum is exposed through an incision 2–3 cm above the fundus of the uterus. A 10-mm blunt tipped trocar is then introduced into the peritoneal cavity, and the cuff is inflated to create an airtight seal. A pneumoperitoneum is then established. A laparoscope is introduced, and under direct vision, a second trocar with a 5-mm blunt probe is inserted in the midclavicular line. Using the blunt probe, the uterus is displaced to the contralateral side exposing the uterine wall behind the broad ligament. The blunt probe is used to displace bowel or omentum that blocks access. An 18-gauge needle is then inserted into the abdominal cavity in the midaxillary line between the upper iliac crest and lower rib under laparoscopic visualization, and the needle is advanced into the uterus. A guide wire is then introduced through the needle into the amniotic fluid. The needle is then removed leaving the wire in place. Some of the intra-abdominal CO_2 is released to diminish the space between the abdominal wall and the uterus and a 12-Fr Teflon cannula loaded on a dilator is advanced over the guide-wire and into the uterus under direct laparoscopic visualization. Once the tip of the cannula is noted to be in the amniotic cavity (using ultrasound), the pneumoperitoneum is allowed to slowly escape under vision and the cannula is advanced fully into the amniotic fluid. The laparoscope is then removed leaving its access trocar in place. The fetoscope is then inserted into the amniotic cavity through the cannula and the laser ablation performed in the usual fashion.

In general, a policy should be adopted for administering fetal analgesics for any invasive procedures during which the fetus might experience pain, and certainly from 18 to 20 weeks onward. It can be given intramuscularly or IV using a 22-gauge needle under ultrasound guidance or direct vision with a fetoscope. We usually give vecuronium (0.2 mg/kg), atropine (20 μg/kg), and fentanyl (15 μg/kg) to provide analgesia, to immobilize the fetus, and to suppress the fetal stress response (bradycardia).

Despite the minimally invasive nature of fetoscopy, complications can and do occur and include preterm contractions, maternal morbidity from tocolysis, preterm premature rupture of membranes, abruption, chorioamnionitis, and fetal distress. However, unlike open fetal surgery, the risk of uterine dehiscence is not an issue, and delivery by cesarean section is not mandatory. We currently reserve fetoscopic procedures for laser photocoagulation for TTTS; percutaneous fetal endoscopic tracheal occlusion for congenital diaphragmatic hernia (CDH); and for the management of other rare cases such as chorioangioma, vasa previa, and amniotic band syndrome (ABS).

CONDITIONS TREATED WITH A FETOSCOPIC PROCEDURE

Placental laser photocoagulation for twin-to-twin transfusion syndrome

TTTS occurs in 9%–15% of monochorionic twin pregnancies and represents the most important cause of mortality in such pregnancies; it typically becomes clinically evident between 16 and 26 weeks gestation.[24,25] The pathology is usually explained by unbalanced circulatory sharing between twins. There are four types of placental vascular anastomoses: arteriovenous, venoarterial, arterio-arterial (AA), and veno-venous. AV and venoarterial anastomoses are unidirectional and result when a placental surface vessel from each twin connects to a common cotyledon. AA and veno-venous anastomoses are connections on the surface of the placenta that have the potential for either unidirectional or bidirectional blood flow. AV anastomoses allow flow in one direction only and therefore may create imbalance in interfetal circulatory shifts, potentially leading to TTTS. Bidirectional AA anastomoses are believed to protect against the development of TTTS. Although these vascular anastomoses are an anatomic prerequisite for the development of TTTS, the pathogenesis of TTTS is probably more complex than a simple transfer of red cells.

The imbalance in circulating blood volume that results from these anastomoses leads to cardiovascular responses that eventually become maladaptive. Although the donor twin usually maintains normal cardiac function, hypervolemia in the recipient twin results in increased preload, leading to right ventricular hypertrophy, and eventually hypertension and cardiomyopathy. The increased systemic pressure may also result in increased right ventricular afterload and diminished right heart output, contributing to acquired pulmonic stenosis[26] and eventually fetal death. The development of right ventricular outflow obstruction is observed in close to 10% of all recipient twins. Recipient twins who demonstrate cardiac compromise generally have poorer survival than their donor twin, while recipients with normal cardiac function may show improved survival.

In an attempt to standardize nomenclature for this condition, Quintero et al. (1999) proposed classifying TTTS into five stages based on the degree of fetal compromise (Table 13.4). The diagnosis of TTTS is based on stringent

Table 13.4 The Quintero classification system for twin-to-twin transfusion syndrome.

Stage	Classification
I	There is a discrepancy in amniotic fluid volume with oligohydramnios of a maximum vertical pocket (MVP) ≤2 cm in one sac and polyhydramnios in other sac (MVP ≥ 8 cm).[a] The bladder of the donor twin is visible, and Doppler studies are normal.
II	The bladder of the donor twin is not visible (during length of examination, usually around 1 hour), but Doppler studies are not critically abnormal.
III	Doppler studies are critically abnormal in either twin and are characterized as abnormal or reversed end-diastolic velocities in the umbilical artery, reverse flow in the ductus venosus, or pulsatile umbilical venous flow.
IV	Ascites, pericardial or pleural effusion, scalp edema, or overt hydrops present.
V	One or both babies are dead.

Source: Adapted from Quintero RA et al. *J Perinatol*, 19(8 Pt 1):550, 1999.

[a] Most European centers use a cutoff of 10 cm for gestation over 20 weeks. For presentations earlier than 18 weeks, cutoffs have not been agreed upon.

sonographic criteria of amniotic fluid and bladder filling discordance. In the donor twin, there is oliguric oligohydramnios with a deepest vertical pocket (DVP) of 2 cm or less. In contrast, the recipient twin presents with polyuric polyhydramnios and a DVP cutoff of 8 cm or greater before 20 weeks and 10 cm or greater after 20 weeks. In the United States, an 8-cm DVP cutoff throughout gestation is used. The differential diagnosis includes monoamnionicity, discordant growth, isolated polyhydramnios or oligohydramnios, and severe intertwin hemoglobin differences at the time of birth. Although the Quintero staging system predicts outcome to a certain extent, it is better to use it to reflect the more severe manifestations of disease than as an indicator of the time sequence of progressive disease.

It remains difficult to identify those monochorionic twin pregnancies that will develop TTTS. Conflicting results have been reported regarding nuchal translucency and crown–rump length discordance for predicting adverse obstetric outcomes such as TTTS.[25,27] A recent multicenter study of monochorionic diamniotic (MCDA) twin pregnancies showed that intertwin discordance in the first trimester (nuchal translucency and crown–rump length) was not predictive of adverse obstetric and neonatal outcomes.[24] However, there is some evidence to suggest that early second-trimester ultrasound examination showing abdominal circumference and estimated fetal weight discordance may be associated with an increased risk of subsequent adverse obstetric outcome.[28] Nevertheless, given that vascular anastomotic patterns and flows may change unpredictably with placental expansion, it may be impossible to predict the development of TTTS accurately. We recommend that all monochorionic twin pregnancies be monitored by ultrasound evaluation every 2 weeks from 16 weeks onward. At these examinations, relative amniotic fluid volume, bladder filling, growth, and visualization of a free-floating intertwin membrane, should be evaluated. The role of Doppler studies in early twin pregnancy evaluation, and in those unaffected by TTTS, is still debated. Patients should be informed of the symptoms of TTTS and advised to seek immediate medical advice if they notice rapidly increasing abdominal girth or premature contractions.

Fetal echocardiography is recommended in all monochorionic twins because the risk of cardiac anomalies is increased ninefold in MCDA twins. The prevalence of congenital cardiac anomalies has been reported to be 2% in otherwise uncomplicated MCDA gestations and 5% in cases of TTTS, with a higher incidence of lesions seen in recipient fetuses.[29] Functional fetal echocardiography will form an important adjunct in the management of TTTS cases, but just how it will prove to be useful is not established.

The mortality rate for untreated progressive midtrimester TTTS is approximately 90%.[30] The goal of intervention is to restore more equitable blood flow between the twins and to halt or reverse cardiac decompensation in either fetus. Even with the latest treatment modalities, the risk of adverse outcome remains significant. Following treatment the pregnancy must be monitored carefully until delivery since complications of ongoing TTTS and/or the laser therapy occur. Therefore, the option of pregnancy termination should be part of patient counseling. The treatment options for TTTS include expectant management and early delivery, selective fetal reduction, amnioreduction, amniotic septostomy, and laser photocoagulation of the surface placental anastomoses; all except selective reduction have been evaluated in randomized trials.[31–33] The Eurofetus RCT, which involved 142 enrolled patients with stages I–IV disease diagnosed between 16 and 26 weeks gestation is currently the best available data on optimal treatment for TTTS. This study showed a significantly higher likelihood of survival for at least one twin to 28 days of life (76% vs. 56%)[34] in the laser group when compared with amnioreduction. Another RCT in the United States, comparing laser coagulation with amnioreduction, was discontinued because of poor recruitment. In this small trial, the 30-day survival rate of at least one twin was 65% with laser treatment and 75% with amnioreduction.[35] Several factors may explain the lower survival rate in this RCT, including low patient numbers and relatively limited operator experience with the laser coagulation technique.

The laser photocoagulation is carried out using a diode or YAG laser and a 400 or 600-μm fiber inside a fetoscope that is introduced into the uterus via a 9-12F ported vascular catheter that is placed under ultrasound guidance. Under fetoscopic vision, the surface placental vessel anastomoses are identified and ablated.

Although a few programs offer intervention for stage I TTTS (currently being studied in an international RCT—NCT01220011), most programs consider only patients with Quintero stage II–IV TTTS or stage I with extenuating circumstances (rapidly worsening polyhydramnios, cardiac signs suggestive of impending compromise) for laser photocoagulation. The GA beyond which laser photocoagulation is typically not offered differs between programs, with some centers not offering this therapy after 24 weeks of gestation and others not offering it after 25 or 26 weeks of gestation. There has recently been a call to consider offering laser therapy before 17 weeks and after 26 weeks of gestation based on data suggesting equivalent outcomes.[36] This has, however, not been universally adopted and further research is needed.

Different surgical techniques have been proposed for performing fetoscopic laser ablation.[37,38] Initially, nonselective laser coagulation of placental vessels was performed, whereby any vessels that crossed the intertwin membranes (membranous equator) were coagulated.[37] Selective laser coagulation of placental vessels (SLCPV) was subsequently reported, in which anastomoses crossing between the twins' vascular equator were identified and coagulated.[38] Chalouhi et al.[39] proposed a SLCPV procedure with subsequent surface coagulation of the placenta between the ablated anastomotic sites in order to create a physical separation of the donor and the recipient vascular territories on the surface of the placenta. This surgical procedure is known as "Solomonization" or the "Solomon technique." In a controlled trial, 274 pregnant women with TTTS were randomized to standard laser coagulation or coagulation of the entire vascular equator. Laser coagulation of the entire vascular equator was associated with a significant reduction in twin anemia polycythemia sequence (odds ratio [OR] 0.16, 95% CI 0.05–0.49) and reduced recurrence of TTTS (OR 0.21, 95% CI 0.04–0.98), but no difference in perinatal mortality or severe neonatal morbidity.[40] The superiority of the Solomon technique has also been reported in other studies.[41]

A complete anterior placenta presents a technical challenge by limiting where the fetoscope can be inserted. A number of different techniques have been evaluated in an attempt to optimize outcomes. These include midline laparotomy and exteriorization of the uterus,[42] and the use of intracannula laser deployment.[43] Failure to adequately visualize the vascular equator (the clear area between the surface vessels fanning out from each of the two cord insertions) on the placental surface significantly impedes the ability to satisfactorily ablate all of the anastomoses that may exist. The more acute the angle of incidence of the fetoscope to the placental surface, the less effective the laser energy will be, and the more difficult the visualization becomes, because of the semirigid nature of the fiber optic fetoscopes used. In cases where there is no viable access point, our team uses a laparoscopic assisted approach, as described above. This allows the operator to view the anastomoses in a more direct fashion enabling a better opportunity for successful ablation of the anastomoses.[44]

Feto-fetal transfusion syndrome (FFTS) has been described in both dichorionic and monochorionic triplet gestations. FFTS may occur in 5% of dichorionic triplets, and in approximately 8% of monochorionic triplets.[45] Given the high risk for perinatal demise in cases of early-onset FFTS in monochorionic–triamniotic or dichorionic–triamniotic triplet pregnancies, it appears that laser photocoagulation of communicating anastomoses can lead to improved neonatal survival but is technically more challenging and potentially associated with lower success rates.[45]

Congenital diaphragmatic hernia

The incidence of CDH varies between 1 and 5 per 10,000 live-born infants, making it a rare disease.[46] The exact etiology of the condition remains unknown. Most cases are left sided, and 13% are right sided; bilateral lesions, complete agenesis, and other rarities comprise fewer than 2%. CDH can occur in association with other anomalies or as an isolated condition.

Prenatal diagnosis of CDH is based on several classic ultrasound findings, including abdominal organs (stomach, intestines, liver) seen within the thoracic cavity, displacement of the heart to the hemithorax contralateral to the defect, cardiac axis shift, and polyhydramnios. Magnetic resonance imaging (MRI) is useful to confirm the diagnosis of CDH in cases of equivocal sonographic findings.

Between 26% and 58% of fetuses with CDH have additional unrelated anomalies that may or may not be associated with a genetic syndrome. Associated anomalies include cardiac, renal, central nervous system and gastrointestinal malformations.[47] Such cases are usually not considered candidates for fetal therapy because the poor survival rate. Genetic counseling and amniocentesis are offered.

Over the past 30 years, the overall survival of neonates with isolated CDH has increased from 50% to 80%[48] and this is primarily attributable to significant advances in postnatal care with multiple modalities including the use of extracorporeal membrane oxygenation, nitric oxide, and sophisticated ventilator technology and strategies.[49]

After the diagnosis of CDH, the first goal is to exclude additional abnormalities. Karyotyping is an essential step, but the finding of normal chromosomes does not exclude other genetic conditions and syndromes. The most widely used prediction methods of CDH outcomes are based on assessment of lung size and determination of liver herniation into the thorax by ultrasound, with the so-called lung-to-head ratio (LHR). At the level of the four-chamber view, the area of the lung contralateral to the lesion is measured. The impact of pulmonary hypoplasia is estimated by calculating the lung area divided by the head circumference, measured in the standard biparietal view.

Today, the fetal therapy for severe CDH is percutaneous fetoscopic endoluminal tracheal occlusion (FETO). The procedure is believed to work because it prevents egress of lung fluid, thereby increasing airway pressure, which promotes pulmonary tissue proliferation, increases alveolar airspace, and encourages maturation of pulmonary vasculature. The balloon is inserted at 26–28 weeks gestation and then the occlusion is reversed by removal at 34 weeks. The latter intervention was included mainly because of experimental observations indicating that this would improve lung maturation.[50,51] Once the balloon has been removed delivery can occur according to obstetric principles. In the event that the patient labors before the balloon has been removed, an EXIT procedure is required to safely relieve the tracheal obstruction while on placental circulation. In rare cases, balloon removal or deflation has been achieved under emergency conditions postnatally by direct laryngoscopy or percutaneous puncture.

The European FETO (percutaneous fetal endoscopic tracheal occlusion) Task Force reported that fetal endoscopic tracheal occlusion in 201 patients[52] was complicated by premature preterm rupture of the membranes (PPROM) within 3 weeks in only 16.7%. On the basis of stratified data from the prenatal CDH registry, FETO therefore increased survival in severe cases with left-sided CDH from 24.1% to 49.1%, and in right-sided from 0 to 35.3% ($p < .001$).[50,52] In a more recent trial, patients with severe fetal CDH were randomized to fetoscopic endotracheal occlusion ($n = 20$) or standard postnatal management ($n = 21$). Fifty percent of fetuses in the fetoscopic endotracheal occlusion group survived to 6 months of age, compared with only 4.8% in the postnatal treatment group.[53] It should be noted that in this trial ECMO was unavailable for either group.

The efficacy of the FETO in utero intervention remains inconclusive, and thus it is still considered experimental and should only be performed under a monitored research protocol.

Other conditions treated with fetoscopic procedures

Amniotic band syndrome

ABS is a rare prenatal complication that occurs in 1/3000 to 1/15,000 pregnancies resulting in live birth. This syndrome can lead to fetal death from umbilical cord strangulation and/or congenital limb deformity or loss, presumed to result from ischemia caused by constriction bands that interfere with vascular perfusion.[54] The underlying causative factors and the pathophysiology of amniotic bands remain unclear. Membrane rupture, either spontaneous or iatrogenic, appears to account for the majority of cases but congenital anomalies of the amniotic membranes have also been implicated.[55]

Fetoscopic release of amniotic bands with minimally invasive surgery has been performed, and may allow preservation of life and/or limb function in cases of ABS. When possible the fetoscopic release of amniotic bands can be performed via a fetoscope using a laser or scissors in the amniotic fluid. The acceptable functional outcome in 50% of cases is reassuring, although more experience and further studies are needed to determine the selection criteria that will justify the risk of this invasive in utero therapy for ABS.[56]

Vasa previa

Vasa previa is a very rare complication in pregnancy and may be classified as either type 1 (velamentous umbilical cord with fetal blood vessels traversing the internal cervical os) or type 2 (fetal vessels crossing membranes between the two lobes of a bilobed placenta such that the vessels traverse the internal cervical os).[57] Vasa previa have been associated with a high perinatal mortality rate due to fetal exsanguination after vessel damage at the time of membrane rupture. Accurate prenatal diagnosis and appropriate timing of cesarean delivery can improve neonatal outcome.[58] Quintero et al. reported a few successful cases of intrauterine laser photocoagulation of type 2 vasa previa.[58,59]

Our team performed in utero laser photocoagulation of vasa previa vessels at 29 4/7 weeks of gestation in a pregnancy also complicated by a fetus with a large neck mass compromising the airway. The patient underwent a controlled EXIT procedure at 34 4/7 weeks of gestation following membrane rupture with good neonatal outcome.[43] We do recognize that this form of intervention has a limited scope and that the prenatal diagnosis and characterization of the type of vasa previa and proportion of placenta affected, has to be carefully assessed to ensure that an individualized plan of care is developed for each case considered.

Chorioangioma

A chorioangioma is a placental tumor that is composed of an abnormal proliferation of blood vessels. The majority of placental chorioangiomas are asymptomatic, and usually escape clinical and sonographic detection, especially those measuring less than 4 cm in diameter. In contrast, those larger than 4 cm, although rare, may be associated with adverse perinatal complications. A large chorioangioma may act as a peripheral AV shunt, leading to high-output cardiac failure, fetal disseminated intravascular coagulopathy, fetal anemia and thrombocytopenia, cardiomegaly, and ultimately nonimmune hydrops. Other complications include polyhydramnios, premature delivery, and fetal growth restriction. The overall associated perinatal mortality is 30%–40%.[60]

Several fetal therapeutic approaches have been employed to interfere with the vascular supply to the tumor and reverse fetal heart failure. Endoscopic laser ablation appears to be the most commonly used therapeutic modality, and has been associated with a favorable outcome.[61,62]

FETAL INTERVENTIONS GUIDED BY SONOGRAPHY (FIGS): TECHNIQUE AND COMPLICATIONS

The procedural approach for these procedures is identical to the fetoscopy approach described above, including fetal analgesia.

For vesicoamniotic shunt, the fetal abdominal wall and bladder are punctured using a trocar, through which the double pigtail catheter is passed (Harrison shunt or Rocket catheter). The distal end is positioned in the fetal bladder and the proximal end is deployed in the amniotic space. For thoracoamniotic shunt, we use the same double pigtail catheter. To optimize shunt placement, careful consideration needs to be given to the previously observed pattern of cyst involution during drainage. For shunt placement in the left thorax, it is important to ensure that the shunt enters the fetal chest at the superior and lateral left aspect of the macrocyst to encourage upward and lateral involution of the cyst. Placement of the shunt in the midclavicular line is not recommended because of the increased risk of displacement and potential for interfering with normal restoration of mediastinal structures.

Complications of FIGS include catheter displacement, occlusion from thrombus material, procedure-related placental abruption, premature rupture of membranes, preterm labor, preterm birth, although less common than open fetal surgery and fetoscopic procedures. We currently reserve FIGS procedures for vesicoamniotic shunt in lower urinary tract obstruction (LUTO); thoracoamniotic shunt in fetuses with pleural effusion (PE) or fluid-filled spaces occupying chest lesions; balloon valvuloplasty in critical aortic or pulmonary stenosis; and RFA or bipolar coagulation for management of anomalous multiple gestations.

CONDITIONS TREATED WITH FETAL INTERVENTIONS GUIDED BY SONOGRAPHY

Lower urinary tract obstruction

LUTO is a descriptive term for a number of heterogeneous conditions, related to the anatomical anomalies of the bladder neck The most common are posterior urethral valves (PUV) due to an obstructing membrane in the proximal male urethra, and urethral atresia in either male or female fetuses[63] Complete obstruction is associated with major consequences, including bladder dilation, hydroureteronephrosis, renal dysplasia, and, as a result of anhydramnios, pulmonary hypoplasia and skeletal deformities; Almost 45% of cases of severe obstruction end in neonatal death.[64]

LUTO is commonly diagnosed during the fetal anatomy ultrasound examination at 18–20 weeks of gestation. Sonographic findings include a dilated posterior urethra (the "keyhole sign"), an enlarged bladder (megacystis), and either unilateral or bilateral hydronephrosis with or without renal parenchymal cystic appearances (cystic kidney disease).

Because untreated LUTO can result in lethal pulmonary hypoplasia and renal failure in the neonate, careful selection of candidates for antenatal intervention is paramount to ensure that procedures to relieve LUTO are offered only to fetuses with sufficient renal function. A detailed ultrasound examination should be performed to exclude coexisting anomalies. Amnioinfusion may be helpful in some cases to improve visualization of the fetal anatomy. The fetal gender should be confirmed, as the presence of a female fetus significantly increases the likelihood of complex malformations, including urethral atresia, persistent cloaca, or megacystis microcolon intestinal hypoperistalsis syndrome. Assessment of the fetal karyotype

Table 13.5 Prognostic urine values for selection of fetuses for prenatal intervention.[a]

	Good prognosis	Poor prognosis
Sodium	<90 mmol/L	>100 mmol/L
Chloride	<80 mmol/L	>90 mmol/L
Osmolality	<180 mOsm/L	>200 mOsm/L
Calcium	<7 mg/dL	>8 mg/dL
Total protein	<20 mg/dL	>40 mg/dL
β_2-Microglobulin	<6 mg/L	>10 mg/L

Source: Muller FI et al., *Clin Chem*, 42(11), 1996.

[a] Based on the last urine specimen obtained by serial bladder drainage at 24- to 48-hour intervals between 18 and 22 weeks' gestation.

should be offered to exclude aneuploidy and in our center we perform placental biopsy or fetal blood sampling rather than vesicocentesis (anhydramnios) or amniocentesis (severe oligohydramnios) in order to ensure adequate tissue for karyotype. Usually fetal renal function cannot be determined with a single urine sample. The best prediction is obtained by two or more sequential vesicocenteses several days apart. The commonly recognized prognostic thresholds are shown in Table 13.5.[65] Examination of fetal urine samples obtained by vesicocentesis may provide some information about the degree of renal impairment, although the potential for predicting postnatal renal function using these indices was questioned in a 2007 systematic review of 23 studies.[66]

In our center, our procedure is to obtain urine for biochemical testing as part of the initial evaluation (along with karyotype, echocardiogram, and full anatomic scan). If the initial biochemistry is favorable vesicoamniotic shunting may be considered without a second specimen. If the results are unfavorable, a second specimen is obtained 48 hours later and tested. If unfavorable, shunting is not currently offered. In the future proteomic and metabolomic evaluation of fetal urine and/or blood may offer better prognostic information[67] but this is not currently the standard of care.

Ruano et al. reported on the ablation of PUVs using fetal cystoscopy combined with either mechanical or laser disruption of the valves. It is possible that this approach may prevent renal deterioration and improve postnatal outcome.[68] Because of the limitations of the currently available equipment, and the potential for fistula formation following laser fulguration, it is still too early for fetal cystoscopy to be translated into clinical practice outside of a research trial.[69]

The Percutaneous Vesicoamniotic Shunting versus Conservative Management for Lower Urinary Tract Obstruction (PLUTO) trial was performed to assess the effectiveness of vesicoamniotic shunting. Unfortunately this trial was stopped after only 31 patients because of poor recruitment and the required sample size of 150 was never reached. Despite the small sample size, the as-treated analysis showed that shunted fetuses had better survival than nonshunted fetuses (RR 3.30, 95% CI 1.02–9.62, $p = .03$). No conclusions could be made regarding the benefit (or lack thereof) of vesicoamnionic shunting on long-term renal function.[70]

Selective feticide for monochorionic, diamniotic twin pregnancies

MCDA twin pregnancies can be complicated by significant clinical problems, such as severe discordant malformations, twin-reversed arterial perfusion (TRAP) sequence, TTTS, or severe selective intrauterine growth restriction (IUGR). In many situations, selective termination of one fetus may be necessary in order to optimize the chances of survival of the normal co-twin. The presence of vascular connections leads to unacceptable risks if intrafetal injection is used as a method of selective termination.

A variety of occlusive techniques have been used to achieve selective termination in monochorionic twin pregnancies. Needle-based coagulation techniques using laser, monopolar, and radiofrequency energy involve the insertion of a 14- to 17-gauge needle into the fetal abdomen under ultrasound guidance, aiming for the intra-abdominal rather than umbilical vessels. This technique is attractive for its simplicity, the smaller membrane defect produced, and the intuitive expectation that the risk for PPROM would be less. RFA has been become more popular. It is potentially a less invasive option that utilizes an RF electrode with a 17-gauge (1.4-mm-diameter) probe and is performed solely under ultrasound guidance. Ultrasound-guided bipolar cord coagulation (BCC) has been also introduced for later GAs. There are 2.4- or 3.0- mm reusable or disposable forceps available, depending on the target cord diameter. Under ultrasound guidance, a portion of the umbilical cord is grasped, and coagulated. Bebbington et al. published a retrospective review of 58 cases of RFA compared with 88 cases of BCC. Despite the smaller-caliber instrument for RFA, there appeared to be no advantages in terms of obstetric outcomes.[71]

Thoracoamniotic shunting

Fetuses with PE or fluid-filled spaces occupying chest lesions may be candidates for shunt placement. The most commonly diagnosed lung lesions include CCAMs, bronchopulmonary sequestrations (BPS), and hybrid lesions.[72] A small number of fetuses will present with a lung lesion or PE large enough to cause mediastinal shift and compression of the heart and lungs bilaterally. These fetuses are at an increased risk of developing pulmonary hypoplasia and/or hydrops fetalis. Hydrops, in itself, may be a predictor of impending fetal demise.[73] Additionally, even in the absence of hydrops, pulmonary hypoplasia is associated with significant morbidity and mortality in the perinatal period.[74] Thus, fetuses with congenital lung lesions or primary PEs resulting in a significant intrathoracic mass effect and risk for pulmonary hypoplasia and/or hydrops without other anatomical or chromosomal abnormalities may be candidates for fetal intervention. The mode of intervention is dependent on the type of lesion (microcystic vs. macrocystic vs. PE) as well as the GA of the fetus. For hydropic fetuses after 32 week's gestation, delivery is typically recommended. However, it has been proposed that intervention be considered up to 37 weeks, with a rationale of potentially improving hydrops while the fetus remains on placental support, allowing further lung maturation[75,76] and recovery without the stress of the hemodynamic changes associated with the neonatal period.

Severe PEs and space-occupying fluid-filled chest lesions may increase hydrostatic pressure within the fetal thorax causing pulmonary hypoplasia or compression of the fetal heart, leading to cardiac decompensation and nonimmune hydrops. A detailed evaluation of the fetal anatomy and a fetal echocardiogram are essential. Karyotyping of the fetus is recommended because of the association of aneuploidy with PE.[77] Maternal blood type, antibody status, Kleihauer–Betke testing, virology testing, including toxoplasmosis, rubella, cytomegalovirus, herpes simplex virus, and parvovirus B19 are also recommended in the evaluation.

The National Institute for Health and Clinical Excellence Guidelines state that invasive fetal therapy for fetal hydrothorax should be restricted to fetuses with primary or isolated effusions resulting in hydrops.[78] Some experienced clinicians have suggested that criteria for intervention should include the following: fetal hydrops with the PE as the likely etiology, isolated PE without hydrops occupying more than 50% of the thoracic cavity, a shift in mediastinum, rapid increase in lesion size, polyhydramnios, or isolated effusion without associated anomalies.[79]

Thoracocentesis under ultrasound guidance is generally the first approach with removal of as much pleural fluid as possible. The fluid should be assessed for lymphocyte count to determine if it is a chylothorax (accumulation of lymph). A high lymphocyte count (usually greater than 80%) will confirm a chylothorax. After fluid drainage the fetus can be assessed for the degree of lung re-expansion, and the lungs can be evaluated to rule out underlying abnormalities. Fetuses in whom the effusion rapidly reaccumulates may benefit from placement of a thoracoamniotic shunt.

Another congenital abnormality that may benefit from thoracoamniotic shunting is CCAMs.[80] The CCAM volume ratio (CVR) has been proposed as a prognostic measure for the development of hydrops. The CCAM volume (in milliliters) is sonographically measured by using the formula for an ellipse: CCAM volume = length × height × width × 0.52, CVR = CCAM volume/head circumference. When the CVR is greater than 1.6, an 80% risk for fetal hydrops is predicted.[81] Our protocol for sonographic follow-up, based on the CVR, is weekly for CVR <1.2, twice weekly for CVR 1.2–1.6, and even more often for a CVR >1.6. For fetuses with macrocystic CCAMs who develop hydrops, fetal intervention to protect residual lung tissue should be considered because of the poor prognosis of expectant management. In a review by Knox et al.[82] in utero therapy was associated with significantly improved survival in hydropic fetuses.

Fetal pulmonary lesions should be evaluated using color Doppler to differentiate CCAMs from bronchopulmonary sequestration (a lesion that is associated with systemic blood supply from an anomalous aortic vessel). MRI is a useful tool for imaging fetal chest masses, and can aid in distinguishing CCAMs from other intrathoracic lesions, localizing the lesion to a specific lobe, and for visualizing the compressed normal lung. An echocardiogram is suggested to rule out cardiac anomalies and to evaluate cardiac function in cases of evolving or fulminant hydrops. A karyotype is not indicated for CCAMs unless associated anomalies are present. At present, the benefit and safety of thoracoamniotic shunting in fetuses with macrocystic lesions and no hydrops has yet to be determined. Our group has noted that even once a fetus with a chest mass has developed hydrops, unless the hydrops is associated with cardiac decompensation, intervention may be unnecessary.[83]

Congenital heart defects

Severe aortic stenosis usually presents in midgestation with severe left ventricular (LV) dysfunction and an enlarged left ventricle. There is subsequent progressive LV dysfunction evolving to hypoplastic left heart syndrome (HLHS). Despite improvement in neonatal care this cardiac anomaly is still associated with poor outcomes. This cardiac malformation has become the chief indication for antenatal intervention. Despite initially disappointing attempts with prenatal balloon valvuloplasty for aortic stenosis, researchers in Linz, Austria, and in Boston, MA, pursued the idea of prenatal intervention for severe cases. There is a window of time during which fetal aortic valvuloplasty may be successful in preserving LV function and preventing single ventricle physiology and this has been shown to reduce short-term and long-term morbidity and mortality.[84] The group at Boston Children's Hospital reported promising results with 43% of all live-born patients (n = 100) achieving a biventricular circulation.[85]

Fetal cardiac interventions may be performed under general or regional anesthesia. For HLHS, once the fetus is motionless a needle (17–19 gauge depending on the procedure and fetal size) is inserted into the fetal left ventricle at the level of the apex and in alignment with the left ventricular outflow tract. A guide wire and a catheter with a coronary dilation balloon are advanced through the aortic valve, which is dilated to 120% of the annulus. There are no specifically designed, commercially available intracardiac devices for fetal interventions,. Needles chosen for the procedure should be as small as possible and must allow convenient insertion of the balloon system of choice. Similar percutaneous cardiac balloon procedures have been proposed for HLHS with a highly restrictive foramen ovale (atrial septostomy) and for pulmonary atresia with an intact ventricular septum.[86]

After a successful procedure, the needle and balloon catheter are withdrawn from the fetal heart and maternal abdomen. In most cases a fetal pericardial effusion will occur and if this causes bradycardia, or appears to be rapidly expanding, it needs to be drained using a 22- or 20-gauge needle. Fetal bradycardia is quite common following these procedures, and resuscitation drugs including epinephrine, atropine, calcium, and bicarbonate should be available for intracardiac administration.

EX UTERO INTRAPARTUM TREATMENT

The principles of the EXIT procedure were first developed for reversing tracheal occlusion performed in fetuses with severe CDH. The EXIT procedure offers the advantage of ensuring uteroplacental gas exchange while on placental support, and delaying the need for a patent airway or ventilation. To permit optimal uteroplacental perfusion and hence ample time to perform a potentially complex fetal airway procedure, EXIT is done under maximal uterine relaxation, typically provided by deep inhalational general anesthesia. The maternal anesthetic protocol typically involves rapid sequence induction with propofol, rocuronium bromide, and remifentanil, followed by intubation and maintenance of anesthesia by propofol, remifentanil, and minimum alveolar concentration of sevoflurane in oxygen. Sevoflurane is preferred to isoflurane because of its faster onset of action and faster elimination to reverse uterine relaxation after cord clamping. In this procedure, a hysterotomy is created with a stapling device using absorbable staples (identical to the one used for hysterotomies for fetal surgeries, described above), and the fetal head and shoulders are delivered through the incision. While the placenta is still providing gas exchange, fetal intubation by laryngoscopy or rigid bronchoscopy, tracheostomy, or even tumor resection can be performed to establish an airway. Bleeding from the uterus is controlled by the staples on the edge of the hysterotomy incision. Coordination between the surgeon and anesthesiologist regarding the timing of decreasing the inhaled anesthetic and the administration of oxytocin will adjust the balance of uterine relaxation and increased tone. To avoid the collapse of the uterine cavity and possible triggering of placental separation as well as umbilical cord compression, warm saline can be infused into the uterus. In addition umbilical arterial and venous catheters allow for adequate vascular access for perinatal resuscitation.

The range of indications for the EXIT procedure has expanded and currently includes giant fetal neck masses, lung or mediastinal tumors, EXIT to extracorporeal membrane oxygenation (ECMO) and fetuses with congenital high airway obstruction syndrome (the absence or blockage of the larynx or trachea).[87,88] In one review of 52 cases, the average operating time available while remaining on the placental circulation was 45 + 25 minutes and the average blood loss was 970 ± 510 mL.[89] However, this review also noted that successful completion of the EXIT procedure without fetal or maternal complications has been reported for as long as 150 minutes on placental circulation.

Placental histopathology has identified coagulopathy changes in cases undergoing EXIT. Thrombotic complications are not usually considered among the risks for EXIT procedures, however this has now been documented, leading to the potential for adverse short-term and long-term outcomes. Thus, the possibility of residual neonatal coagulopathy should be considered in the management of fetuses and neonates delivered by EXIT.[90]

THE FUTURE OF FETAL SURGERY

It is quite possible that some recent advances in fetoscopic surgery may revolutionize the field. The authors and others[90–96] believe that with appropriate maternal anesthetic management and careful surgical technique to protect the fetal membranes, CO_2 gas may be introduced into the human uterus at or beyond 22 weeks to allow the development of a new surgical space in which fetal surgical procedures can be performed. These include fetal neural tube repair, amniotic band dissection and extirpation, and removal of shunts.[91–98] Our current method involves a maternal laparotomy to expose the uterus, allowing positioning of the fetus and the affected area of the body under the access point. Two or three vascular access ports (7F–16F in size) can then be placed through the uterine wall, and a variety of endoscopic instruments and cameras can be used. While there is a theoretical risk of CO_2 causing fetal acidosis, fetal sheep experiments have suggested that maternal hyperventilation can reduce the risk of this[95] and we have yet to see evidence of severe acidosis during a fetoscopic case that is attributable to CO_2 toxicity. Others have attempted percutaneous fetoscopy in gas to repair fetal NTDs, but currently that approach has been hampered by excessive rates of preterm premature rupture of the membranes and preterm delivery.[93,96] This may be due to technical issues related to less protection of the membranes using a percutaneous technique than can be directed using an open abdomen technique. Clearly, the percutaneous technique is less invasive.[96] Going forward the risk of maternal laparotomy to enable a delivery after 35 weeks of gestation without PPROM versus a percutaneous approach without laparotomy but which results in a delivery closer to 34 weeks with an increased risk of PPROM must be settled.

Fetoscopy in CO_2 gas is clearly an experimental area and should only be attempted under appropriate institutional review board (IRB) and Food and Drug Administration (FDA) oversight by experienced teams at high-volume fetal centers. We believe that going forward, as more and more purpose-built instruments are developed, and more and more sophisticated technology is introduced, that fetoscopic surgery may replace open fetal surgery. The use of an upper segment hysterotomy has such a long-lasting and deleterious effect on the mother's reproductive health that striving for a less invasive option is a worthy cause.

REFERENCES

1. Liley AW. Intrauterine transfusion of foetus in haemolytic disease. *Br Med J* 1963; 2: 1107.
2. Harrison MR, Filly RA, Golbus MS et al. Fetal treatment. *N Engl J Med* 1982; 307: 1651.

3. Harrison MR, Adzick NS. The fetus as a patient. Surgical considerations. *Ann Surg* 1991; 213(4): 279–91.
4. Bliton MJ. Ethics: "Life before birth" and moral complexity in maternal–fetal surgery for spina bifida. *Clin Perinatol* 2003; 30: 449.
5. Adzick NS, Harrison MR, Glick PL et al. Fetal surgery in the primate. III. Maternal outcome after fetal surgery. *J Pediatr Surg* 1986; 21: 477–80.
6. Adzick NS, Thom EA, Spong CY et al. A randomized trial of prenatal versus postnatal repair of myelomeningocele. *N Engl J Med* 2011; 364: 993.
7. Moldenhauer JS, Soni S, Rintoul NE et al. Fetal myelomeningocele repair: The post-MOMS experience at the Children's Hospital of Philadelphia. *Fetal Diagn Ther* 2015; 37: 235–40.
8. Meuli M, Meuli-Simmen C, Hutchins GM et al. The spinal cord lesion in human fetuses with myelomeningocele: Implications for fetal surgery. *J Pediatr Surg* 1997; 32: 448.
9. Centers for Disease Control and Prevention (CDC). Racial/ethnic differences in the birth prevalence of spina bifida—United States, 1995–2005. *MMWR Morb Mortal Wkly Rep* 2009; 57(53): 1409.
10. Babcook CJ, Goldstein RB, Barth RA et al. Prevalence of ventriculomegaly in association with myelomeningocele: Correlation with gestational age and severity of posterior fossa deformity. *Radiology* 1994; 190: 703.
11. Curran PF1, Jelin EB, Rand L et al. Prenatal steroids for microcystic congenital cystic adenomatoid malformations. *J Pediatr Surg* 2011; 45: 145–50.
12. Cass DL, Olutoye OO, Cassady CI et al. Prenatal diagnosis and outcome of fetal lung masses. *J Pediatr Surg* 2011; 46: 292.
13. Adzick NS. Open fetal surgery for life-threatening fetal anomalies. *Semin Fetal Neonatal Med* 2010; 15: 1.
14. Adzick NS. Management of fetal lung lesions. *Clin Perinatol* 2009; 36(2): 363.
15. Ruano R, da Silva MM, Salustiano EM et al. Percutaneous laser ablation under ultrasound guidance for fetal hyperechogenic microcystic lung lesions with hydrops: A single center cohort and a literature review. *Prenat Diagn* 2012; 32: 1127–32.
16. Lee FL1, Said N, Grikscheit TC et al. Treatment of congenital pulmonary airway malformation induced hydrops fetalis via percutaneous sclerotherapy. *Fetal Diagn Ther* 2012; 31: 264–8.
17. Swamy R, Embleton N, Hale J et al. Sacrococcygeal teratoma over two decades: Birth prevalence, prenatal diagnosis and clinical outcomes. *Prenat Diagn* 2008; 28: 1048.
18. Bond SJ, Harrison MR, Schmidt KG et al. Death due to high-output cardiac failure in fetal sacrococcygeal teratoma. *J Pediatr Surg* 1990; 25: 1287–91.
19. Batukan C, Ozgun MT, Basbug M et al. Sacrococcygeal teratoma in a fetus with prenatally diagnosed partial trisomy 10q (10q24.3→qter) and partial monosomy 17p (p13.3→pter). *Prenat Diagn* 2007; 27: 365–8.
20. Westerburg B, Feldstein VA, Sandberg PL et al. Sonographic prognostic factors in fetuses with sacrococcygeal teratoma. *J Pediatr Surg* 2000; 35: 322; discussion 325.
21. Benachi A, Durin L, Maurer SV et al. Prenatally diagnosed sacrococcygeal teratoma: A prognostic classification. *J Pediatr Surg* 2006; 41: 1517.
22. Van Mieghem T, Al-Ibrahim A, Deprest J et al. Minimally invasive therapy for fetal sacrococcygeal teratoma: Case series and systematic review of the literature. *Ultrasound Obstet Gynecol* 2014; 43: 611.
23. Hedrick HL, Flake AW, Crombleholme TM et al. Sacrococcygeal teratoma: Prenatal assessment, fetal intervention, and outcome. *J Pediatr Surg* 2004; 39(3): 430.
24. Allaf MB, Vintzileos AM, Chavez MR et al. First-trimester sonographic prediction of obstetric and neonatal outcomes in monochorionic diamniotic twin pregnancies. *J Ultrasound Med* 2014; 33: 135.
25. Lewi L, Jani J, Boes AS et al. The natural history of monochorionic twins and the role of prenatal ultrasound scan. *Ultrasound Obstet Gynecol* 2007; 30: 401.
26. Simpson LL, Marx GR, Elkadry EA et al. Cardiac dysfunction in twin-twin transfusion syndrome: A prospective longitudinal study. *Obstet Gynecol* 1998; 92: 557.
27. Kagan KO, Gazzoni A, Sepulveda-Gonzalez G et al. Discordance in nuchal translucency thickness in the prediction of severe twin-to-twin transfusion syndrome. *Ultrasound Obstet Gynecol* 2007; 29: 527.
28. Allaf MB, Campbell WA, Vintzileos AM et al. Does early second-trimester sonography predict adverse perinatal outcomes in monochorionic diamniotic twin pregnancies? *J Ultrasound Med* 2014; 33(9): 1573.
29. Bahtiyar MO, Dulay AT, Weeks BP et al. Prevalence of congenital heart defects in monochorionic/diamniotic twin gestations: A systematic literature review. *J Ultrasound Med* 2007; 26: 1491.
30. Simpson LL for the Society of Maternal-Fetal Medicine (SMFM). Twin–twin transfusion syndrome. *Am J Obstet Gynecol* 2013; 208: 3.
31. Saade GR, Belfort MA, Berry DL et al. Amniotic septostomy for the treatment of twin oligohydramnios-polyhydramnios sequence. *Fetal Diagn Ther* 1998; 13(2): 86.
32. Moise KJ Jr, Dorman K, Lamvu G et al. A randomized trial of amnioreduction versus septostomy in the treatment of twin-twin transfusion syndrome. *Am J Obstet Gynecol* 2005; 193(3 Pt 1): 701, Erratum in: *Am J Obstet Gynecol* 2005; 193(6): 2183.

33. Moise KJ Jr, Dorman K, Lamvu G et al. A randomized trial of amnioreduction versus septostomy in the treatment of twin-twin transfusion syndrome. *Am J Obstet Gynecol* 2005; 193(3 Pt 1): 701, Erratum in: *Am J Obstet Gynecol* 2005; 193(6): 2183.
34. Senat MV, Deprest J, Boulvain M et al. Endoscopic laser surgery versus serial amnioreduction for severe twin-twin transfusion syndrome. *N Engl J Med* 2004; 351: 136.
35. Crombleholme TM, Shera D, Lee H et al. A prospective, randomized, multicenter trial of amnioreduction vs selective fetoscopic laser photocoagulation for the treatment of severe twin-twin transfusion syndrome. *Am J Obstet Gynecol* 2007; 197(4): 396.e1.
36. Baud D, Windrim R, Keunen J et al. Fetoscopic laser therapy for twin-twin transfusion syndrome before 17 and after 26 weeks' gestation. *Am J Obstet Gynecol* 2013; 208(3): 197.e1.
37. De Lia JE, Cruikshank DP, Keye WR Jr. Fetoscopic neodymium: YAG laser occlusion of placental vessels in severe twin–twin transfusion syndrome. *Obstet Gynecol* 1990; 75: 1046.
38. Ville Y, Hyett J, Hecher K et al. Preliminary experience with endoscopic laser surgery for severe twin–twin transfusion syndrome. *N Engl J Med* 1995, 332: 224.
39. Chalouhi GE, Essaoui M, Stirnemann J et al. Laser therapy for twin-to-twin transfusion syndrome (TTTS). *Prenat Diagn* 2011; 31: 637.
40. Slaghekke F, Lopriore E, Lewi L et al. Fetoscopic laser coagulation of the vascular equator versus selective coagulation for twin-to twin transfusion syndrome: An open-label randomized trial. *Lancet* 2014; 383: 2144.
41. Ruano R, Rodo C, Peiro JL et al. Fetoscopic laser ablation of placental anastomoses in twin–twin transfusion syndrome using 'Solomon technique'. *Ultrasound Obstet Gynecol* 2013; 42: 434.
42. Deprest JA, Van Schoubroeck D, Van Ballaer PP et al. Alternative technique for Nd: YAG laser coagulation in twin-to-twin transfusion syndrome with anterior placenta. *Ultrasound Obstet Gynecol* 1998; 11: 347.
43. Quintero RA, Chmait RH, Bornick PW et al. Trocar-assisted selective laser photocoagulation of communicating vessels: A technique for the laser treatment of patients with twin-twin transfusion syndrome with inaccessible anterior placentas. *J Matern Fetal Neonatal Med* 2010; 23(4): 330.
44. Shamshirsaz AA, Javadian P, Ruano R et al. Comparison between laparoscopically assisted and standard fetoscopic laser ablation in patients with anterior and posterior placentation in twin-twin transfusion syndrome: A single center study. *Prenat Diagn* 2015; 35(4): 376.
45. Blumenfeld YJ, Shamshirsaz AA, Belfort MA et al. Fetofetal transfusion syndrome in monochorionic-triamniotic triplets treated with fetoscopic laser ablation: Report of two cases and a systematic review. *Am J Perinatol* 2015; 5(2): 153.
46. Torfs CP, Curry CJ, Bateson TF. A population based study of congenital diaphragmatic hernia. *Teratology* 1992; 46: 555.
47. Holder AM, Klaassens M, Tibboel D et al. Genetic factors in congenital diaphragmatic hernia. *Am J Hum Genet* 2007; 80: 825.
48. Skari H, Bjornland K, Haugen G et al. Congenital diaphragmatic hernia: A meta-analysis of mortality factors. *J Pediatr Surg* 2000; 35: 1187.
49. Downward CD, Jaksic T, Garza JJ et al. Analysis of an improved survival rate for congenital diaphragmatic hernia. *J Pediatr Surg* 2003; 38: 729.
50. Jani J, Keller RL, Benachi A et al. Prenatal prediction of survival in isolated left-sided diaphragmatic hernia. *Ultrasound Obstet Gynecol* 2006; 27: 18.
51. Deprest J, Nicolaides K, Done E et al. Technical aspects of fetal endoscopic tracheal occlusion for congenital diaphragmatic hernia. *J Pediatr Surg* 2011; 46: 22.
52. Jani JC, Nicolaides KH, Gratacos E et al. Severe diaphragmatic hernia treated by fetal endoscopic tracheal occlusion. *Ultrasound Obstet Gynecol* 2009; 34: 304.
53. Ruano R, Yoshizaki CT, Da Silva MM et al. A randomized controlled trial of fetal endoscopic occlusion versus postnatal management of severe isolated congenital diaphragmatic hernia. *Ultrasound Obstet Gynecol* 2012; 39: 20.
54. Garza A, Cordero JF, Mulinare J et al. Epidemiology of the early amnion rupture spectrum of defects. *Am J Dis Child* 1988; 142: 541.
55. Sentilhes L, Verspyck E, Eurin D et al. Favorable outcome of a tight constriction band secondary to amniotic band syndrome. *Prenat Diagn* 2004; 24: 198.
56. Javadian P, Shamshirsaz AA, Haeri S et al. Perinatal outcome after fetoscopic release of amniotic bands: A single-center experience and review of the literature. *Ultrasound Obstet Gynecol* 2013; 42(4): 449.
57. Catanzarite V, Maida C, Thomas W et al. Prenatal sonographic diagnosis of vasa previa: Ultrasound findings and obstetric outcome in ten cases. *Ultrasound Obstet Gynecol* 2001; 18(2): 109.
58. Lee W, Kirk JS, Comstock CH et al. Vasa previa: Prenatal detection by three-dimensional ultrasonography. *Ultrasound Obstet Gynecol* 2000; 16(4): 384.
59. Chmait RH, Chavira E, Kontopoulos EV et al. Third trimester fetoscopic laser ablation of type II vasa previa. *J Matern Fetal Neonatal Med* 2010; 23(5): 459.
60. Hosseinzadeh P, Shamshirsaz AA, Cass DL et al. Fetoscopic laser ablation of vasa previa for a fetus with a giant cervical lymphatic malformation. *Ultrasound Obstet Gynecol* 2015; 46(4): 507.
61. Amer HZ, Heller DS. Chorangioma and related vascular lesions of the placenta—A review. *Fetal Pediatr Pathol* 2010; 29(4): 199.
62. Hosseinzadeh P, Shamshirsaz AA, Javadian P et al. Prenatal therapy of large placental chorioangiomas: Case report and review of the literature. *Am J Perinatol* 2015; 5(2): 196.

63. Gunn TR, Mora JD, Pease P. Antenatal diagnosis of urinary tract abnormalities by ultrasonography after 28 weeks gestation: Incidence and outcome. *Am J Obstet Gynecol* 1995; 172: 479.
64. Makayama DK, Harrison MR, deLorimer AA. Prognosis of posterior urethral valves presenting at birth. *J Pediatr Surg* 1986; 21: 43.
65. Muller FI, Dommergues M, Bussières L et al. Development of human renal function: Reference intervals for 10 biochemical markers in fetal urine. *Clin Chem* 1996; 42(11): 1855.
66. Morris RK, Quinlan-Jones E, Kilby M et al. Systematic review of accuracy of fetal urine analysis to predict poor postnatal renal function in case of congenital urinary tract obstruction. *Prenat Diagn* 2007; 27: 900.
67. Klein J; Lacroix C, Caubet C et al. Fetal urinary peptides to predict postnatal outcome of renal disease in fetuses with posterior urethral valves (PUV). *Sci Transl Med* 2013; 5(198): 14.
68. Ruano R, Sananes N, Sangi-Haghpeykar H et al. Fetal intervention for severe lower urinary tract obstruction: A multicenter case-control study comparing fetal cystoscopy with vesicoamniotic shunting. *Ultrasound Obstet Gynecol* 2014; 45(4): 452.
69. Sananes N, Favre R, Koh CJ et al. Urological fistulas after fetal cystoscopic laser ablation of posterior urethral valves: Surgical technical aspects. *Ultrasound Obstet Gynecol* 2015; 45(2): 183.
70. Morris RK, Malin GL, Quinlan-Jones E et al. Percutaneous vesicoamniotic shunting versus conservative management for lower urinary tract obstruction (PLUTO): A randomised trial. *Lancet* 2013; 382: 1496.
71. Bebbington MW, Danzer E, Moldenhauer J et al. Radiofrequency ablation vs bipolar umbilical cord coagulation in the management of complicated monochorionic pregnancies. *Ultrasound Obstet Gynecol* 2012; 40: 319.
72. Khalek N, Johnson MP. Management of prenatally diagnosed lung lesions. *Semin Pediatr Surg* 2013; 22: 24.
73. Wilson RD, Baxter JK, Johnson MP et al. Thoracoamniotic shunts: Fetal treatment of pleural effusions and congenital cystic adenomatoid malformations. *Fetal Diagn Ther* 2004; 19: 413.
74. Laberge JM, Flageole H, Pugash D et al. Outcome of prenatally diagnosed congenital cystic adenomatoid lung malformations: A Canadian experience. *Fetal Diagn Ther* 2001; 16: 178
75. Peranteau WH, Adzick NS, Boelig MM et al. Thoracoamniotic shunts for the management of fetal lung lesions and pleural effusions: A single-institution review and predictors of survival in 75 cases. *J Pediatr Surg* 2015; 50(2): 301.
76. Yinon Y, Kelly E, Ryan G. Fetal pleural effusions. *Best Pract Res Clin Obstet Gynaecol* 2008; 22(1): 77.
77. Achiron R, Weissman A, Lipitz SA et al. Fetal pleural effusion: The risk of fetal trisomy. *Gynecol Obstet Invest* 1995; 39: 153.
78. NICE Guideline IPG 190. *Insertion of Pleuro-Amniotic Shunt for Fetal Pleural Effusion.* London, UK: National Institute for Health and Clinical Excellence, 2006.
79. Yinon Y, Grisaru-Granovsky S, Chadda V et al. Perinatal outcome following fetal chest shunt insertion for pleural effusion. *Ultrasound Obstet Gynecol* 2010; 36: 58.
80. Stocker JT, Madewell JE, Drake RM. Congenital cystic adenomatoid malformation of the lung. Classification and morphologic spectrum. *Hum Pathol* 1997; 8: 155.
81. Crombleholme TM, Coleman B, Hedrick H et al. Cystic adenomatoid malformation volume ratio predicts outcome in prenatally diagnosed cystic adenomatoid malformation of the lung. *J Pediatr Surg* 2002; 37: 331.
82. Knox EM, Kilby MD, Martin WL et al. In-utero pulmonary drainage in the management of primary hydrothorax and congenital cystic lung lesion: A systematic review. *Ultrasound Obstet Gynecol* 2006; 28: 726.
83. Cass DL, Olutoye OO, Ayres NA et al. Defining hydrops and indications for open fetal surgery for fetuses with lung masses and vascular tumors. *J Pediatr Surg* 2012; 47(1): 40.
84. Donofrio MT, Moon-Grady AJ, Hornberger LK et al. Diagnosis and treatment of fetal cardiac disease: A scientific statement from the American Heart Association. *Circulation* 2014; 129: 2183.
85. McElhinney DB, Marshall AC, Wilkins-Haug LE et al. Predictors of technical success and postnatal biventricular outcome after in utero aortic valvuloplasty for aortic stenosis with evolving hypoplastic left heart syndrome. *Circulation* 2009; 120: 1482.
86. Tulzer G, Arzt W, Franklin RCG et al. Fetal pulmonary valvuloplasty for critical pulmonary stenosis or atresia with intact septum. *Lancet* 2002; 360: 1567.
87. Laje P, Peranteau WH, Hedrick HL, et al. Ex utero intrapartum treatment (EXIT) in the management of cervical lymphatic malformation. *J Pediatr Surg* 2015; 50(2): 311.
88. Cass DL, Olutoye OO, Cassady CI et al. EXIT-to-resection for fetuses with large lung masses and persistent mediastinal compression near birth. *J Pediatr Surg* 2013; 48: 138.
89. Hirose S, Farmer DL, Lee H et al. The ex utero intrapartum treatment procedure: Looking back at the EXIT. *J Pediatr Surg* 2004; 39: 375.
90. Stanek J, Sheridan RM, Le LD et al. Placental fetal thrombotic vasculopathy in severe congenital anomalies prompting EXIT procedure. *Placenta* 2011; 32(5): 373.

91. Belfort MA, Shamshirsaz AA, Whitehead WE et al. Unusual pleuro-amniotic shunt complication managed using a 2-port in-CO2 fetoscopic technique: Technical and ethical considerations. *Ultrasound Obstet Gynecol* 2015; 47(1): 123–4.
92. Belfort MA, Whitehead WE, Shamshirsaz AA et al. Fetoscopic repair of meningomyelocele. *Obstet Gynecol.* 2015; 126(4): 881–4.
93. Kohl T. Percutaneous minimally invasive fetoscopic surgery for spina bifida aperta. Part I: Surgical technique and perioperative outcome. *Ultrasound Obstet Gynecol* 2014; 44(5): 515–24.
94. Degenhardt J, Schürg R, Winarno A et al. Percutaneous minimal-access fetoscopic surgery for spina bifida aperta. Part II: Maternal management and outcome. *Ultrasound Obstet Gynecol* 2014; 44(5): 525–31.
95. Saiki Y, Litwin DE, Bigras JL et al. Reducing the deleterious effects of intrauterine CO_2 during fetoscopic surgery. *J Surg Res* 1997; 69: 51–4.
96. Pedreira DA, Zanon N, Nishikuni K et al. Endoscopic surgery for the antenatal treatment of myelomeningocele: The CECAM trial. *Am J Obstet Gynecol* 2015; pii: S0002-9378(15)01104-7. [Epub ahead of print]
97. Bevilacqua NS, Pedreira DA. Fetoscopy for meningomyelocele repair: Past, present and future. *Einstein (Sao Paulo)* 2015; 13(2): 283–9.
98. Whitehead WE, Ball R, Silver R et al. Fetoscopic amniotic band release in a case of chorioamniotic separation: An innovative new technique. *AJP Rep* 2016; 6(2): e222-5.

Cervical insufficiency

14

RUPSA BOELIG and VINCENZO BERGHELLA

CONTENTS

DEFINITION OF CERVICAL INSUFFICIENCY (CI)

The concept of the cervix being "so slack that it cannot rightly … keep in the seed" was first hypothesized in the 1658 text *Practice of Physick* by Rivière et al.[1] In the 1940s and 1950s, the term "cervical incompetence" came into vogue, and surgical interventions were described to treat the "weak" cervix. Only recently have properly controlled scientific studies on the subject been performed.

CI, formerly known as cervical incompetence, represents a subgroup of preterm birth (PTB). Its definition has been controversial but the most accepted one is painless dilation leading to recurrent second-trimester losses.[2] The gestational age when these second-trimester losses (preceded by painless dilation) occur is usually 16–28 weeks. This definition implies that the PTB is caused by a cervical problem: the cervix is too weak to retain the pregnancy. Historically, cervical "sufficiency" was viewed as a dichotomous variable: the cervix either is sufficient to retain the pregnancy to term, or it is not, leading to painless dilation and second-trimester loss. Recently, Iams et al.[3] have convincingly shown that cervical sufficiency (or competence) is a continuous variable. Cervical shortening, in the absence of labor or other symptoms, can also be considered CI in certain conditions. Specifically, in women with a prior spontaneous PTB (sPTB), a cervical length (CL) <25 mm between 16 and 24 weeks is on the spectrum of CI and may be treated as such. This new concept has opened the way for new therapeutic approaches, in particular ultrasound-indicated cerclage, to attempt to alter cervical shortening in progress before it leads to PTB. In theory, this approach would obviate the clinical limitation of having to wait for two or more losses or PTB before therapeutic approaches are offered.

INCIDENCE

Given the difficulties with diagnosis, the incidence of CI is difficult to ascertain. CI represents only a portion of all PTB under 32 weeks, which is 2% in the United States and 1% in other developed (e.g., European) nations. The best estimation of the incidence of CI is obtained by reviewing the incidence of cervical cerclage, the most commonly employed surgical intervention for CI. The best estimates report a range of 0.3%–0.4%[4] for the incidence of cerclage in the United States. It should be noted that women with a prior second-trimester loss have a 70%–90% chance of delivering at term in the subsequent pregnancy, even without undergoing a cerclage.[5]

ANATOMY AND PHYSIOLOGY OF THE HUMAN CERVIX

The uterine cervix is derived from the fusion of the distal Müllerian ducts and subsequent central atrophy. The cervix consists primarily (>70%) of fibrous connective tissue, mostly collagen types I and III, with most of the remainder consisting of smooth muscle. The percentage of smooth muscle is more prominent in the upper (29%) than in the lower (6%) parts of the cervix.[6] Only about 1% of cervical tissue is made of elastin. The upper limit of the cervix is difficult to distinguish from the uterine corpus in the nonpregnant woman. In pregnancy, the muscular lower segment of the corpus, or isthmus, distends and elongates, making its inferior border with the mostly fibrous cervix the functional internal cervical os. This sphincter-like region, not easy to discern to the millimeter histologically, helps keep the pregnancy in utero.

The strength of the cervix derives mostly from the connective tissue. The amount of connective tissue in the cervix is directly proportional to its strength, while the amount of smooth muscle tissue is inversely proportional to its strength.[6]

During pregnancy, the collagen bundles of the cervix become more dissociated, with fewer cross-links, and more soluble collagen fragments, with less hydroxyproline. Elastin is decreased in women with CI. Relaxin causes connective tissue remodeling and may play a role in CI. Elevated second-trimester serum relaxin has been related to decreased CL.

ASSOCIATIONS AND POSSIBLE CAUSES

A higher incidence of CI has been postulated in women exposed to diethylstilbestrol (DES) in utero[7] and those with Ehlers–Danlos syndrome or other connective tissue disorders. It is very rare for a woman to have a congenital cause of CI, and such associations have never been proven. Several historical factors have been associated with CI, as described in Table 14.1. The overwhelming majority of CI cases are associated with acquired factors. Most of the acquired factors involve surgery or trauma to the cervix and can be considered iatrogenic. Ablation of cervical intraepithelial neoplasia by cold-knife or laser cone biopsy or loop electrosurgical excision procedure (LEEP) could lead to CI based upon the amount of cervical tissue removed. Dilation and curettage (D&C) or diethylstilbestroldilation and evacuation (D&E) procedures, especially when more than one, for voluntary terminations, and even for spontaneous abortions, have been associated with CI. Gentle dilation of the cervix with laminaria before the D&C or D&E is recommended,[8] but seldom used in clinical practice except in the second trimester. Data definitively linking obstetric cervical lacerations with CI are not available.

Table 14.1 Conditions associated with insufficiency.

Congenital
Ehlers–Danlos syndrome Müllerian anomaly
DES exposure
Acquired (usually traumatic and iatrogenic) cone biopsy
Cold-knife laser LEEP
Multiple D&E[a]
Obstetric cervical laceration

Abbreviations: DES, diethylstilbestrol; D&E, dilation and evacuation; LEEP, loop electrosurgical excision procedure.

[a] For either spontaneous or voluntary terminations.

More than just anatomic cervical defects, functional cervical deficiencies may play an important role. CI may represent a final common pathway of many causes of midtrimester pregnancy loss at the severe end of the spectrum of PTB. The main pathways leading to PTB include infectious, inflammatory, immunologic, uterine distention, or structural factors (Müllerian, DES, fibroids, etc.) and fetal abnormalities (genetic or structural/syndromic).

DIAGNOSTIC APPROACHES

Obstetrical history

A history of painless dilation leading to recurrent second-trimester losses is the most accepted definition of CI. Unfortunately, the requirement for recurrent second-trimester losses implies that a woman must lose at least two fetuses before a diagnosis is made and preventive measures need to be implemented. Clinical characteristics of the second-trimester loss (whether the patient was symptomatic of painful contractions and/or bleeding, or not) do not seem to predict which women will have a recurrent second-trimester loss.[8]

CI should be diagnosed with caution when second-trimester loss occurs in a multiple-gestation pregnancy. We have shown that the incidence of recurrent PTB at <24 weeks after the early loss (mean 23 weeks) of a twin gestation when subsequently carrying a singleton gestation is 12%, with 88% delivering at ≥35 weeks.[9]

These limitations of diagnostic approaches based on obstetric history alone have prompted exploration of prepregnancy tests and diagnostic approaches during pregnancy in an attempt to diagnose CI before multiple losses occur.

Nonpregnant testing

Evaluation of the cervix in the nonpregnant state has been employed extensively in the past for the evaluation of CI. Several screening tests have been proposed, including the ease of passage of a no. 8 Hegar dilator, catheter traction tests using Foley catheters, ease of leakage of fluid during hysteroscopy or hysterosalpingogram, measurement of the width of the upper cervical canal (by radiography or hysterography), and others. While most of these reports associate abnormalities of testing with *prior* pregnancy outcome, almost none of the studies report prediction of *future* pregnancy outcome. Based on a combination of these tests, cervical compliance scores have been proposed,[10] but do not appear to be very predictive or clinically useful. The prediction of CI in a future pregnancy based on pre- or interpregnancy tests is therefore very poor according to current evidence. This might be because the functionality of cervical tissues may be different in the nonpregnant from the pregnant state in the same woman. More research is needed in the area of nonpregnant testing before it can be of practical clinical use.

Testing during pregnancy

Transvaginal ultrasound CL

CI or early PTB is usually preceded by cervical opening, which begins to occur first at the internal os. This progressive opening of the cervix "from the inside out" results in shorter functional length of the cervix and is not detectable by manual/digital evaluation of the cervix. Measurements of CL by transvaginal ultrasound (TVU) have been shown to be safe, well accepted by women, reproducible, and predictive of PTB. A recent review summarizes a large literature on this subject.[11] TVU is the reference standard for assessment of the cervix in pregnancy for prediction of PTB. No clinical decisions should be based on transabdominal (TA) ultrasound of the cervix alone, given its shortcomings.[11] TVU of the cervix has better predictive accuracy than manual/digital evaluation of the cervix.[12] Shortening and opening of the cervix starts at the internal os, and about three-fourths of women with asymptomatic short cervix on ultrasound have no appreciable changes by manual examination.[13] Screening of cervical changes in pregnancy to predict PTB or CI should be done with TVU and *not* with manual examination or a different ultrasound technique. The technique of TVU has been well described (Figures 14.1–14.3).[11,14] While different parameters can be measured, CL is the most reproducible, with low (<10%) inter- and intraobserver variability. Other variables, such as funneling, do not add significantly to the prediction of PTB based on CL alone (Figures 14.2 and 14.3).[15] The shortest best multiple CL measurements after spontaneous or transfundal-pressure changes should be used for PTB prediction. A CL of 25–50 mm is normal at 14–24 weeks in all pregnant women. In low-risk women, CL is a continuous variable, with a mean of 35–40 mm at 14–30 weeks, with the lower 10th percentile being 25 mm and the upper 10th (90th percentile) 50 mm.[16] Rarely do women have a short cervix under 25 mm before 14 weeks, and only those with a prior cone biopsy or second-trimester loss.[17] Early detection of short CL before 20 weeks can predict second-trimester losses and CI. Many women who will have PTB have a short cervix first around 18–22 weeks.[11,14] The earlier the short CL is detected by TVU, and the shorter the CL, the higher the risk of PTB. A cervix under 25 mm has a positive predictive value (PPV) of 70% for PTB under 35 weeks when detected at 14–18 weeks and of 40% when detected at 18–22 weeks in high-risk women.[12] Therefore, it may be that patients at the highest risk of PTB (e.g., patients with possible CI, early PTB, or cone biopsies) may benefit from early (i.e., 14–18 weeks) ultrasound examination to determine their need for intervention.

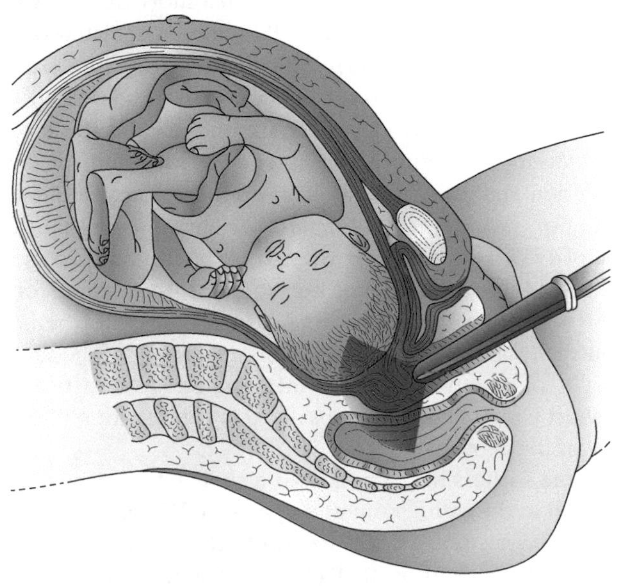

Figure 14.1 The endovaginal ultrasound probe is placed into the anterior fornix of the vagina to obtain the corresponding ultrasound image of the cervix.

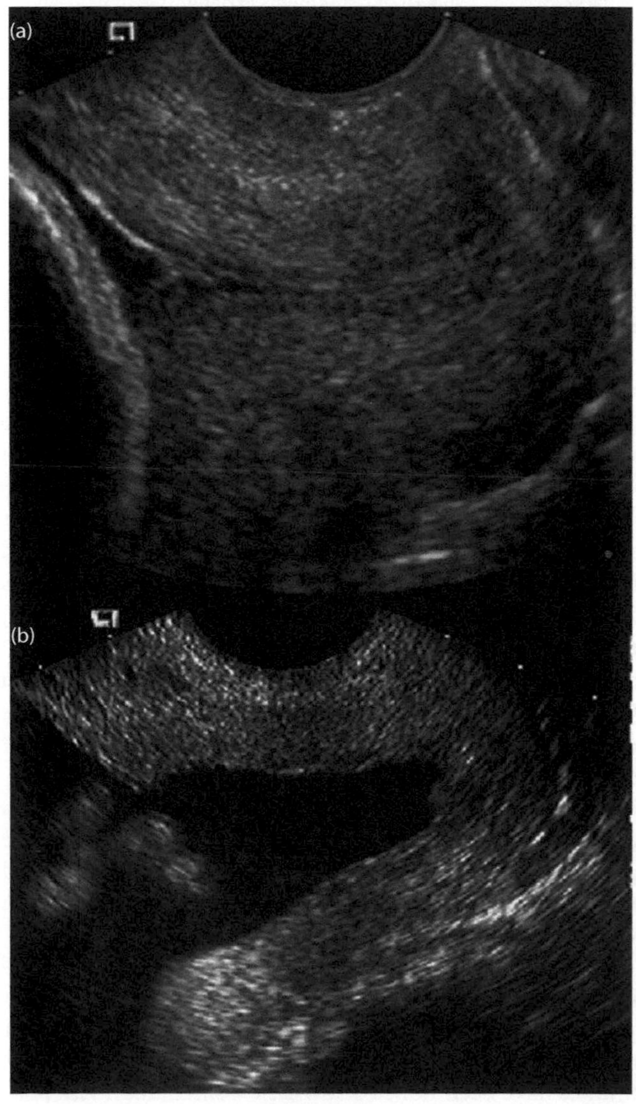

Figure 14.2 Transvaginal ultrasonography (TVU) of (a) closed normal cervix and (b) a short cervix with significant funneling.

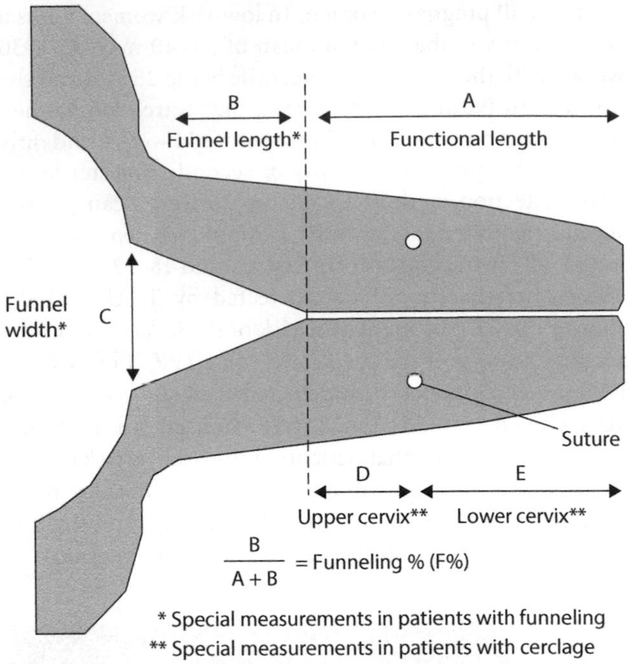

Figure 14.3 Schematic illustration of TVU cervical measurements.

TVU CL screening is recommended for women with a singleton pregnancy and a history of a prior sPTB. A large randomized trial and meta-analysis have demonstrated the efficacy of cerclage in reducing the risk of PTB <35 weeks and in perinatal morbidity for women with a prior sPTB and CL <25 mm detected prior to 24 weeks.[18,19] The current recommendation is for women with a prior sPTB to have biweekly TVU CL screening from 16 0/7 to 23 6/7 weeks, increased to weekly for a CL 25–30 mm, with the recommendation of an ultrasound-indicated cerclage for a CL <25 mm.

For low-risk women (i.e., singletons without a prior sPTB), universal TVU-CL screening can be considered (American College of Obstetricians and Gynecologists [ACOG], Society for Maternal-Fetal Medicine [SMFM] refs). These women may be screened once between 18 0/7 and 23 6/7 weeks, with vaginal progesterone started for a CL ≤20 mm, as this has been demonstrated to reduce the risk of sPTB by ~40%.[11,20,21] Even though the incidence of short cervix (≤20 mm) in this population is low, ~1% studies have demonstrated that CL screening is a cost-effective measure and is something we practice in our unit for the prevention of PTB.[22,23] A meta-analysis has demonstrated that this intervention may even be beneficial to women with CL 21–25 mm.[24]

Many different populations have been screened, including asymptomatic women with singleton, twin, and triplet pregnancies and symptomatic women with preterm labor or premature preterm rupture of the membranes (PPROM). Studies have been done on low-risk women, high-risk populations, and women with a cerclage in place. The actual population screened has a tremendous effect on the significance of the TVU CL results. In low-risk women carrying singleton gestations without prior sPTB, the sensitivity for PTB under 35 weeks of TVU CL under 25 mm at 22–24 weeks was only 37%, with a PPV of only 18%.[16] This means that 82% of these low-risk women who were found to have a short CL under 25 mm at 24 weeks delivered at ≥35 weeks. In women carrying singleton gestations but with a prior sPTB under 32 weeks, the sensitivity of TVU CL under 25 mm at 16–24 weeks increased to 69%, with a PPV of 55%.[15]

In twin gestations, TVU CL under 25 mm in the second trimester has a sensitivity of 30% and a PPV of 60%.[25] The low sensitivity may be due to the fact that multiple gestations have PTB not because of CI, but because of uterine overdistention. Furthermore, although some studies may demonstrate a benefit with vaginal progesterone, results are mixed, and there is insufficient evidence to recommend any intervention (progesterone, pessary, or cerclage) for twins with an asymptomatic short, but not dilated CL.[24,26–30]

The cervix may shorten in the second trimester, too early in pregnancy, for a variety of reasons. A short CL is a common final pathway, eventually leading to PTB. While some rare women can develop an early short CL because of an intrinsic weakness of the cervix due to a congenital disorder or a connective tissue disease, CI is more commonly due to prior traumatic or surgical damage. Other mechanisms leading to a short cervix include inflammatory, infectious, or immunologic processes, as well as simply contractions. Women with normal CL have mechanical and immunologic protection against the ascent of lower vaginal microorganisms. Once shortened by these processes, the CL can provide easier access of potentially pathologic vaginal microorganisms to the intrauterine environment, leading to prolonged subclinical chorioamnionitis and subsequent CI or PTB. There is a strong association between a short CL on TVU and infection. High amniotic fluid interleukin (IL)-6, later development of chorioamnionitis, and acute inflammatory lesions of the placenta have all been associated with a short CL on TVU. A short CL leading to CI or PTB is often associated with PPROM instead of preterm labor(PTL), providing additional evidence for the role of infection in these women.

Usually, the cause and effect are unclear: did the short CL develop first and allow ascending infection, or did infection and inflammation develop first and cause shortening of the cervix?[31] Recent studies have shown that the majority of asymptomatic women with CL under 25 mm before 24 weeks have some contractions, more than controls with a normal cervix.[32,33] Again, it is unclear whether contractions cause the short CL or are a result of the short cervix, or whether these two factors work synergistically. A short CL probably develops due to a combination of several of the above factors.

Some authors have considered a short CL in pregnancy by itself as the pathognomonic sign of CI. We do not believe this to be accurate, since the short CL is just a common final pathway leading to PTB. For example, twin gestations that contract from overdistention develop a short CL, which in this case is a secondary and not a primary process. We postulate that a short CL might be confirmatory of CI only in women with prior second-trimester losses who asymptomatically develop a short CL early in the second trimester (<24 weeks) in the following pregnancy.

MANAGEMENT

Avoidance of intervention *(primum non nocere)*

The negative predictive value of a CL of ≥25 mm in predicting PTB is relatively high if this length is obtained at 14–24 weeks in different populations. It is about 88%–96% even in women at high risk of PTB such as those with a prior PTB or carrying twins. This information has been used by clinicians to avoid cerclage and other interventions in women in whom the obstetric history is poor but not clearly consistent with CI.

In fact, about 60% of these high-risk women maintain a normal CL until after 24 weeks and deliver at term and can be spared any intervention. Only about 40% develop a short CL, are at true risk of PTB, and should be offered intervention. A meta-analysis of four randomized controlled trials[34–37] including 466 women demonstrated that CL screening with ultrasound-indicated cerclage as appropriate had similar incidences of PTB prior to 37 weeks and 34 weeks, as well as similar perinatal mortality compared with history-indicated or prophylactic cerclage (Table 14.2).[38]

Nonsurgical interventions

Bed rest or modified activity

Bed rest is commonly recommended for women with clear, possible, or even signs of CI. Unfortunately, no trials have been done to demonstrate its efficacy or detriment. Up to 1.5% incidence of thromboembolism has been reported in association with prolonged bed rest.[39] A recent review found little benefit of activity restriction in PTB prevention.[40] Furthermore, bed rest may actually increase the risk of PTB. A recent study found an increased rate of PTB among nulliparous women with a short CL placed on activity restrictions compared with those without any restrictions.[41]

Medical

Administering 17-hydroxy progesterone 250 mg once a week intramuscularly (IM) from 16 to 20 weeks until 36 weeks has been shown to decrease PTB by about 33% in women with a prior PTB that occurred at 20–36 weeks.[42] The benefit is slightly higher for women with a prior PTB under 28 weeks and possible CI. In view of results from a prior meta-analysis[43] and another recent trial,[44] obstetricians should consider offering progesterone prophylaxis to all women with a prior PTB, including those with CI.[45] For women without a prior sPTB but with a current asymptomatic CL ≤20 mm, vaginal progesterone may be offered to reduce the risk of sPTB by ~40%.[20,21,45]

Indomethacin, antibiotics, omega-3 fatty acids, and other medical interventions have been postulated to be helpful in the management of women with CI or early PTB, but no evidence is available to demonstrate clear benefit. More research is needed.[45]

Pessary

Minimal research has been done on the efficacy of a pessary to prevent CI or PTB. One retrospective study on women with cervical dilation and exposed membranes between 15 and 24 weeks compared pessary with cerclage and expectant management found that examination-indicated cerclage significantly improved perinatal outcomes and prolonged pregnancy while pessary did not provide any additional benefit compared with expectant management.[46] One small study found that pessary as an adjunct to examination-indicated cerclage in the second trimester may improve outcomes as well.[47] Trials on the benefit of pessary in low-risk singletons with a short CL have had mixed results.[48,49] One large randomized controlled trial on pessary use in twins found no benefit while another did find a benefit only for the subgroup of women with a CL less than the 25th percentile.[26,50] At this point there is insufficient evidence to recommend pessary for the treatment of CI.

Surgical intervention: cerclage

Cervical cerclage has been the traditional treatment for the diagnosis of CI. This intervention was originally devised by Lash and Lash,[51] and then refined by Shirodkar[52] and McDonald.[53] In their studies, cerclage was used for women with both a history of PTB or CI *and* recurrent manual cervical dilation. Over 35 different procedures for the treatment of CI have been reported in the world's literature.[54] Table 14.3 summarizes guidelines for perioperative management of a cerclage,[55] which are discussed in further detail below under "Medical and technical considerations for cerclage."

Table 14.2 Randomized trials of ultrasound-indicated versus prophylactic cerclage in high-risk populations.

			PTB, *n*(%)		
	n	PTB (weeks)	HC	TVU	Risk ratio
Althuisius et al.[34]	67	<34	3/23 (13)	6/44 (14)	NS
Kassanos et al.[35]	55	<37	11/27 (41)	11/28 (39)	NS
Beigi et al.[36]	97	<37s	9/45 (20)	13/52 (25)	NS
Simcox et al.[37]	247	<37	44/125 (35)	39/122 (32)	NS
Total	466	<37 or 34	67/220 (30)	69/246 (28)	1.08 (0.82, 1.44)
Total	399	<37	64/197 (32)	63/202 (31)	0.97 (0.73, 1.29)

Source: Berghella V and Mackeen AD, *Obstet Gynecol*, 118(1), 148–155, 2011.
Abbreviations: NS, nonsignificant; PTB, preterm birth; HC, history indicated cerclage; TVU, ultrasound indicated cerclage.

Table 14.3 Perioperative management strategies for cerclage.

Variable	History indicated	Ultrasound indicated	Examination indicated
Preoperative			
Fetal ultrasound	Yes	Yes	Yes
Amniocentesis	No	No	Consider
Perioperative antibiotics	No	No	Consider
Perioperative indocin	No	Consider	Consider
Intraoperative			
Anesthesia	Spinal	Spinal	Spinal
Cerclage type	McDonald	McDonald	McDonald
Suture	Operator preference	Operator preference	Operator preference
Needle	Operator preference	Operator preference	Operator preference
Cerclage height	As high as possible	As high as possible	As high as possible
Number of stitches	One	One	One
Management of membrane prolapse	Operator preference	Operator preference	Operator preference
Postoperative			
Hospitalization vs. outpatient	Outpatient	Outpatient	Outpatient
Activity restriction	No	No	No
Repeat cerclage if failure	No	No	No

Source: Berghella V et al., *Am J Obstet Gynecol*, 209(3), 181–192, 2013.

Indications for cerclage

History indicated

Definition. A cerclage placed solely on the basis of prior obstetric or gynecologic history is often called a prophylactic or elective cerclage. The term "elective" we believe to be misleading, since there is nothing elective about the procedure, which should be performed for specific indications only.

Indications. The only indication that has been confirmed by evidenced-based data is a singleton pregnancy with a history of three or more second-trimester losses or PTBs.[56] The other clinical indication might include CI (again defined as prior painless cervical dilation leading to recurrent second-trimester losses). Other indications such as prior cone biopsy, Müllerian anomaly, DES exposure, prior PTB not associated with CI, and Ehlers–Danlos syndrome have occasionally been used clinically, but have not been confirmed as indications that benefit from history-indicated cerclage.

Performed. History-indicated cerclage is usually performed at 12–15 weeks' gestation. This allows time to perform an early ultrasound to confirm viability and normal early anatomy (e.g., nuchal translucency) after the first-trimester spontaneous loss period has passed.

Efficacy. Prevention of PTB has been proven only for three or more prior second-trimester losses or PTBs[56] (Table 14.4). Trials on women at a lower risk of PTB based on prior obstetric history have not shown benefit from history-indicated cerclage.[56,58,59] There are limited randomized data showing that history-indicated cerclage is not beneficial in other populations at high risk of PTB such as twins.[57] Unfortunately, there are very limited nonrandomized data showing that history-indicated cerclage is not beneficial in other populations at high risk of PTB such as patients with prior cone biopsy, Müllerian anomaly, DES exposure, prior PTB not associated with CI, and Ehlers–Danlos syndrome. Given the paucity of data showing benefit from history-indicated cerclage, alternative management has recently moved to screening of high-risk pregnancies with TVU of the cervix to determine during pregnancy the risk of PTB, since the majority of women at high risk of PTB deliver at term even without intervention.[11]

Ultrasound indicated

Definition. Ultrasound-indicated cerclage is defined as cerclage performed because a short cervix has been detected on TVU during pregnancy, usually in the second trimester, without cervical dilation. This cerclage has also been called therapeutic, salvage, or rescue cerclage. These terms cause confusion with emergency cerclage (defined below), and so the term "ultrasound-indicated cerclage" seems the most appropriate.

Indications. As discussed previously, a short CL on TVU in the second trimester significantly increases the risk of PTB in all populations studied. Women with three or more second-trimester losses or PTBs should receive a history-indicated cerclage. Singleton gestations with a prior sPTB are candidates for ultrasound-indicated cerclage if the cervix shortens <25 mm on TVU between 16 0/7 and 23 6/7 weeks.[2,45,60]

Performed. As a short CL is usually not detected on TVU before 14 weeks, ultrasound-indicated cerclage is usually performed when the short CL is detected, usually at 14–24 weeks. Ultrasound-indicated cerclage is usually not offered at or after 24 weeks. This is because viability usually is possible at this gestational age, and the uterus is more sensitive

Table 14.4 Randomized trials of prophylactic cerclage.

		PTB <37 weeks		
	n	**Cerclage (%)**	**No cerclage (%)**	***p***
Dor et al.[57]	50	45	48	NS
Lazar et al.[58]	506	7	6	NS
Rush et al.[59]	194	34	32	NS
MRC/RCOG[56]	1292	26	31	NS
2:3STL/PTB[56]	45	32	53	a

Abbreviations: CI, confidence interval; MRC, Medical Research Council; RCOG, Royal College of Obstetricians and Gynaecologists; RR, risk ratio; STL, second trimester losses.

[a] RR = 0.6, 95%CI = 0.37–0.95.

Table 14.5 Randomized trials for ultrasound indicated cerclage in women with prior PTB.

Author	**Group**	***n***	**GA studied (weeks)**	**CL cutoff (mm)**	**PTB <35 weeks, *n* (%)**	**Risk ratio**
Althuisius et al.[60]	Cerclage	14	16–27	<25	0 (0)	
	Control	12	16–27	<25	6 (50)	
Rust et al.[62]	Cerclage	53	16–24	<25	13 (25)	
	Control	49	16–24	<25	16 (32)	
To et al.[61]	Cerclage	21	22–24	<15	5 (24)	
	Control	23	22–24	<15	8 (35)	
Berghella et al.[63]	Cerclage	14	14–24	<25	5 (36)	
	Control	17	14–24	<25	11 (65)	
Owen et al.[18]	Cerclage	148	16–21	<25	48 (32)	
	Control	153			64 (42)	
Total	Cerclage	250			71 (28)	0.70 (0.55, 0.89)
	Control	254			105 (41)	

Source: Berghella V et al., *Obstet Gynecol*, 117(3), 663–671, 2011.
Abbreviations: CL, cervical length; GA, gestational age.

to a foreign body, such as cerclage, at this gestational age. SomeAUthors, especially in Europe, continue to offer ultrasound-indicated cerclage up to 27–28 weeks.[60,61]

Efficacy. Five randomized trials[18,60–63] (Table 14.5) have been done examining the efficacy of an ultrasound-indicated cerclage in women with singleton gestations and a history of prior sPTB. A meta-analysis of these trials has demonstrated that there is a significant 30% reduction in the rate of PTB <35 weeks as well as an improvement in perinatal mortality and morbidity with the use of ultrasound-indicated cerclage versus expectant management.[38] Notably, in twins, an ultrasound-indicated cerclage was associated with an increase in PTB, and a recent meta-analysis found that cerclage was associated with greater neonatal morbidity and thus should not be offered for this indication for multiple gestations.[28,64]

Physical Examination Indicated

Definition. Examination-indicated cerclage (i.e., emergency or urgent) is a cerclage placed because of cervical dilation detected by physical examination.

Indications. Examination-indicated cerclage is performed for singleton or twin pregnancies with cervical dilation prior to 24 weeks' gestation.

Performed. Like ultrasound-indicated cerclage, examination-indicated cerclage is usually performed at 14–23 6/7 weeks. Bulging membranes, at or beyond the external os, are often encountered and Trendelenburg position, retrograde bladder filling, Foley catheter, sponge-on-a-stick, and/or amniocentesis may be necessary to reduce the membrane prolapse before adequate suture placement is possible.

Efficacy. Over 50% of women with cervical dilation of ≥2 cm have microbial invasion of the amniotic cavity.[65] Therefore, amniocentesis should be considered before offering examination-indicated cerclage. Given the high incidence of infection and inflammation, the prognosis is usually guarded, with or without intervention.

Only one trial has evaluated the efficacy of examination-indicated cerclage.[66] Twenty-three women (seven with twins) with membranes at or beyond the external os at around 20–24 weeks were randomized to cerclage and indomethacin or usual care. All women received bed rest, thrombosis prophylaxis, and antibiotics. The 13 women in the cerclage group gained more days (54 vs. 20 days [$p < .05$]) and delivered 4 weeks later than the control women (30 vs. 26 weeks). The major limitations of this study are the small sample size and the inclusion of twins.

A recent meta-analysis on the efficacy of examination-indicated cerclage, which included the randomized trial as well as nine other cohort studies, found that examination-indicated cerclage is associated with improved neonatal survival, increased pregnancy latency, decreased incidence of PTB, and specifically, early PTB.[67]

Transabdominal

Definition. As the word implies, *transabdominal* (TA) cerclage is a cerclage placed around the cervix from an abdominal incision, and therefore "from above," in contrast with transvaginal cerclage, which is placed from a vaginal approach, and therefore "from below."

Indications. TA cerclage has been performed for two main indications; that is, a prior failed history-indicated TV cerclage, or a cervix with no intravaginal portion (i.e., due to prior cervical surgery/excision). By "prior failed cerclage," authors have usually meant that the woman had a history suggestive of CI, for which she received a history-indicated cerclage that failed to prevent another early PTB. The indication of "prior failed transvaginal cerclage" is supported by controlled data for TA cerclage.[68] Women with no or minimal intravaginal cervix usually have a history of large cone biopsies, surgical trauma, or cerclage complications, and also a history suggestive of CI.

Performed. TA cerclage is usually performed prophylactically at around 10–12 weeks. As with history-indicated cerclages, an early TVU at 10–12 weeks should be performed to exclude gross fetal anomalies. Given the difficulty of operating around the pregnant uterus, TA cerclage should be performed by 12 weeks. If the woman presents after 12 weeks, TA cerclage can still be performed up to 18–20 weeks, but is increasingly technically difficult with each gestational week. About half of the case series have reported TA cerclage performed before pregnancy. The benefits of this approach are that technical difficulties with the pregnant uterus are avoided. The shortcomings of preconceptional TA cerclage placement are that spontaneous miscarriages and anomalous fetuses may necessitate more involved operating room procedures for management.

Efficacy. Over 22 observational case series have been published on the outcome of TA cerclage pregnancies. Almost all report excellent term delivery rates, usually over 80%, whether it was placed pre- or postconceptionally.[69] Unfortunately, almost all of these studies did not have controls for adequate comparison of less invasive management. The only adequately controlled study of TA cerclage compared women with a similar history of a failed (PTB under 33 weeks) transvaginal cerclage who received either a TA cerclage or another transvaginal cerclage (both at 10–15 weeks). The women who received TA cerclage had a better outcome than controls with transvaginal cerclage (PTB under 35 weeks, 18% vs. 42%; $p = .04$; gestational age at delivery 36.3 vs. 32.8 weeks, $p = .03$, respectively).[68] It should be noted that in this trial antibiotics and progesterone were uniformly given to the TA women. There is limited data on the effectiveness of laparoscopic and robotic cerclage, as almost all series on these procedures have no controls. All data in the literature so far have been on TA cerclage performed on women with a singleton pregnancy for historical risk factors for PTB. There are no specific data on TA cerclage performed for cervical (examination or TVU) changes.

Surgical techniques for cerclage

Transvaginal cerclage

After adequate analgesia (typically with spinal anesthesia), the patient is placed in the dorsal lithotomy position, and surgical prep of the perineum and vagina is performed (gently in the vagina if the membranes are protruding from the cervix). Wc utilize a weighted speculum and right-angle retractors, as well as two or three sponge forceps (or DeLee cervical tenacula) on the cervix to optimize visualization of the surgical field (Figure 14.4). The vast majority of cerclages performed today are modifications of the techniques described by Shirodkar and McDonald.

Shirodkar cerclage. First presented at a film festival in Paris in 1950, Shirodkar's procedure for the treatment of CI used human fascia lata as the suture material. After transverse incision of the cervicovaginal epithelium on both the anterior (at the reflection of the bladder) and posterior aspects of the cervix, the vesicovaginal and rectovaginal fascia is reflected cephalad to the level of the internal os, as when beginning a vaginal hysterectomy (Figure 14.5). Long Allis clamps are placed laterally with the jaws in the anterior and posterior incisions as high on the cervix as possible to maximize the cephalad dissection. The Allis

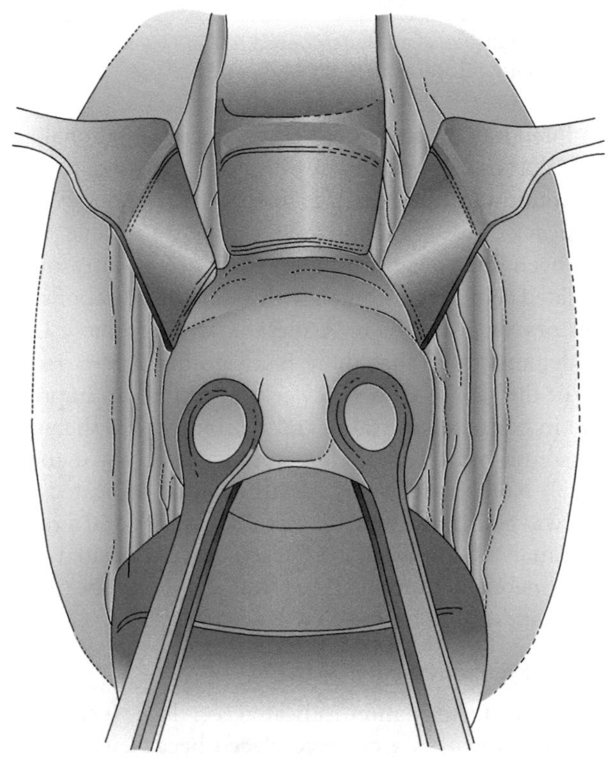

Figure 14.4 Transvaginal cerclage. A weighted speculum, right-angle retractors, and two or three sponge forceps on the cervix are used to optimize visualization of the surgical field.

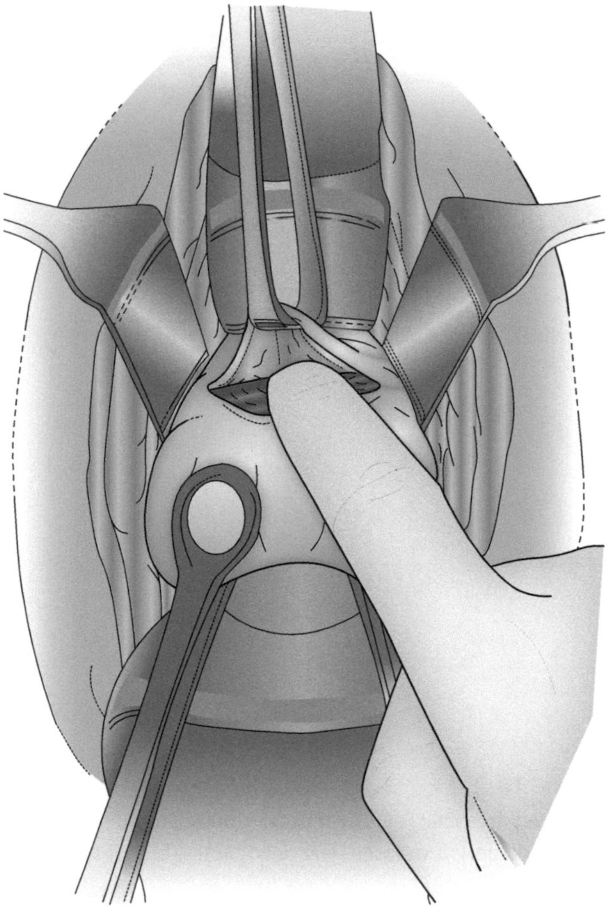

Figure 14.5 Modified Shirodkar cerclage. The initial transverse incision is made in the anterior cervicovaginal epithelium at the reflection of the bladder, and the vesicovaginal fascia is reflected cephalad to the level of the internal os, similarly to when beginning a vaginal hysterectomy.

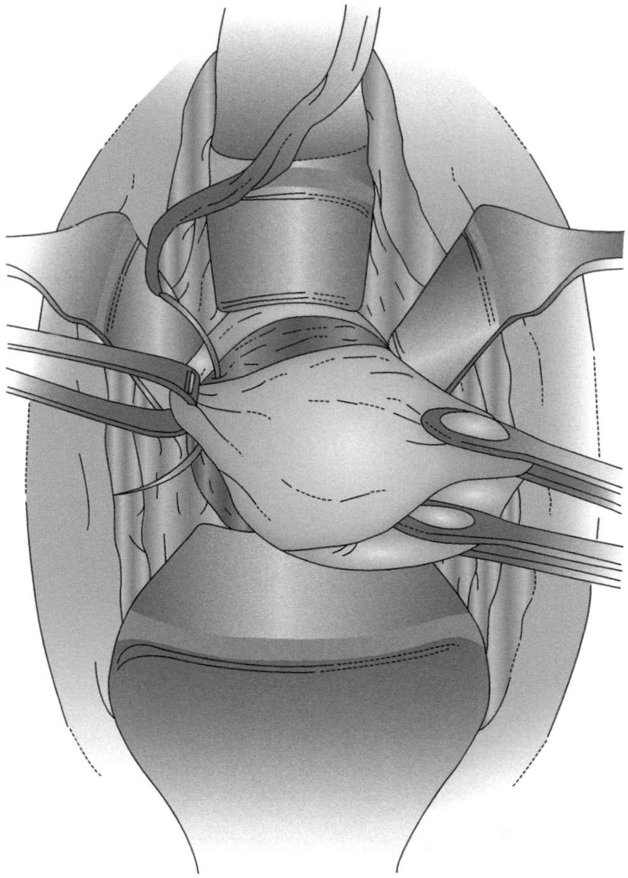

Figure 14.6 Modified Shirodkar cerclage. An Allis clamp is placed laterally with the jaws in the anterior and posterior incisions as high on the cervix as possible to maximize the cephalad dissection. Lateral traction is placed on the submucosal tissue to avoid the uterine vasculature.

clamps are used to place lateral traction on the submucosal tissue so that the cerclage can be effectively placed close to the medially located cervix while avoiding the laterally displaced uterine vessels (Figure 14.6). The suture is driven by two successive passes with an atraumatic needle on each side (from posterior to anterior or vice versa) just distal to the Allis clamp above the insertion of the cardinal ligaments (Figure 14.7). After ensuring that the suture tape lies flat posteriorly, the suture is tied anteriorly, tight enough as to admit a fingertip at the external os, but closed at the internal os (Figure 14.8). Successive knots are placed to facilitate identification and later removal. The mucosal incisions are closed over (with the cerclage suture passing through) only if active bleeding is noted (Figure 14.9).

McDonald cerclage. In 1957, McDonald described a cerclage technique that requires no submucosal dissection. Just distal to the vesicocervical reflection (at the junction of the ectocervix and the anterior rugated vagina), a purse-string suture is placed in four to six passes circumferentially around the cervix (Figure 14.10). Each pass should be deep enough to contain sufficient cervic stroma to avoid "pulling-through" but not so deep as to enter the endocervical canal (and risk rupture of the membrane). The uterine vessels should be avoided laterally (Figure 14.11). The suture should be placed high on the posterior aspect of the cervix, as this is the most likely site of suture displacement. The suture is tied anteriorly, successive knots are placed, and the ends are left long enough (2–3 cm) to facilitate later removal (Figure 14.12). As with the Shirodkar technique, the suture is tight enough to ensure the internal os is closed.

Transabdominal cerclage

Several techniques have been described to place the cerclage higher, closer to the internal os, including the TA cervicoisthmic cerclage. In our center, where over 100 of these procedures have been performed, a simple atraumatic technique under spinal anesthesia with a Pfannesteil incision is employed. After digital displacement of the uterine vessels bilaterally, a 5-mm Mersilene band is guided through the broad ligament at the level of the internal os by blunt perforation with a right-angle clamp (Figure 14.13).[68] The suture is tied anteriorly and left in place at the time of the necessary cesarean delivery at 38–39 weeks.

Laparoscopic/robotic-assisted laparoscopic cerclage. A laparoscopic approach has been described[70,71] as an

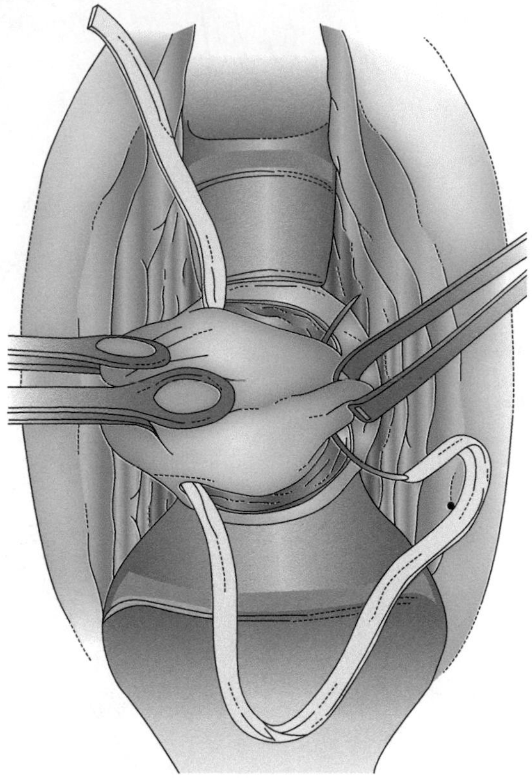

Figure 14.7 Modified Shirodkar cerclage. The suture is driven by successive passes with an atraumatic needle on each side just distal to the Allis clamp above the insertion of the cardinal ligaments.

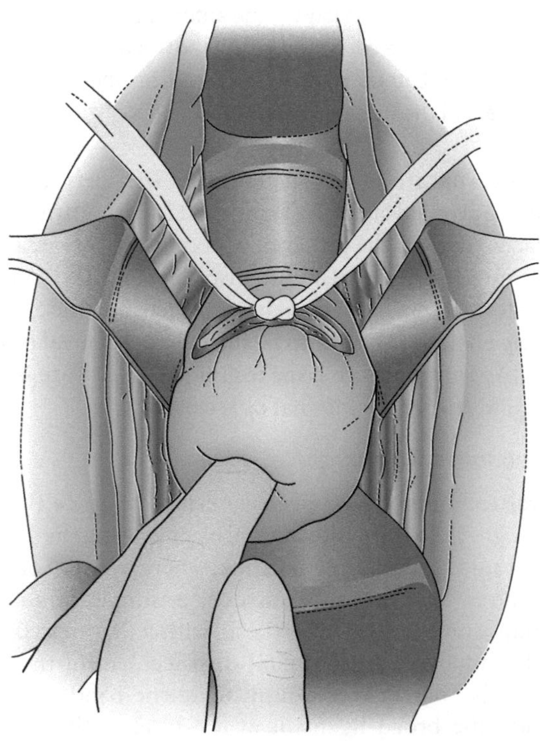

Figure 14.8 Modified Shirodkar cerclage. After ensuring that the suture tape lies flat posteriorly, the suture is tied anteriorly, tight enough as to admit a fingertip at the external os, but closed at the internal os.

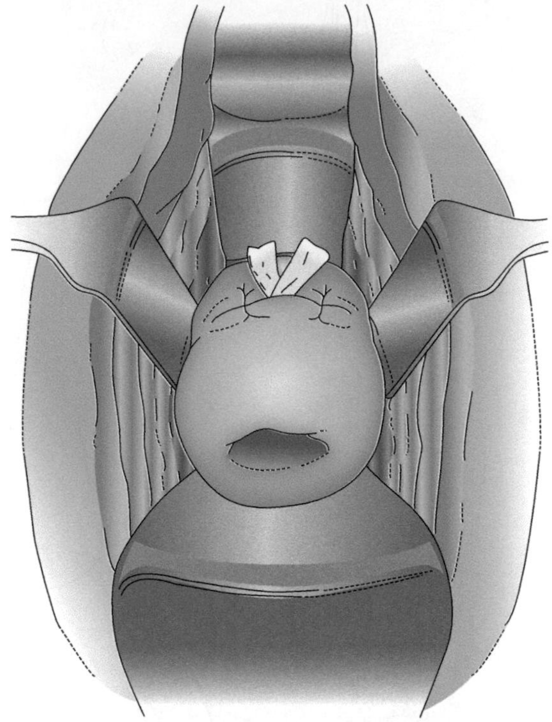

Figure 14.9 Modified Shirodkar cerclage. Successive knots are placed to facilitate identification and later removal. The mucosal incisions are closed over only if active bleeding is noted.

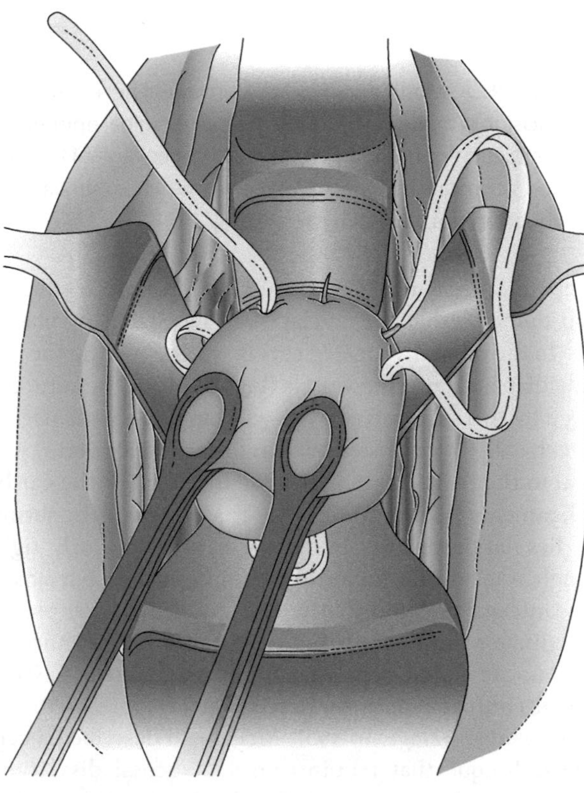

Figure 14.10 McDonald cerclage. Just distal to the vesicocervical reflection a purse-string suture is placed in four to six passes circumferentially around the cervix. The suture should be placed high on the posterior aspect of the cervix, as this is the most likely site of suture displacement.

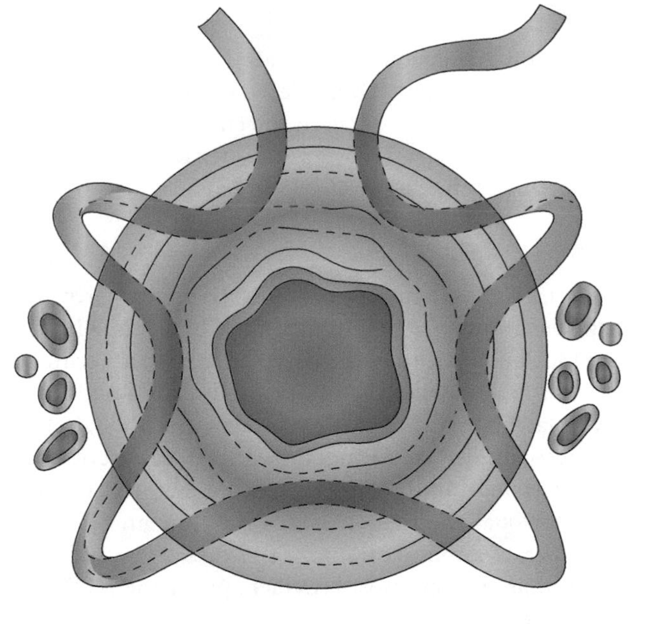

Figure 14.11 McDonald cerclage coronal section. Each pass should be deep enough to contain sufficient cervic stroma to avoid "pulling-through," but not so deep as to enter the endocervical canal. The uterine vessels should be avoided laterally.

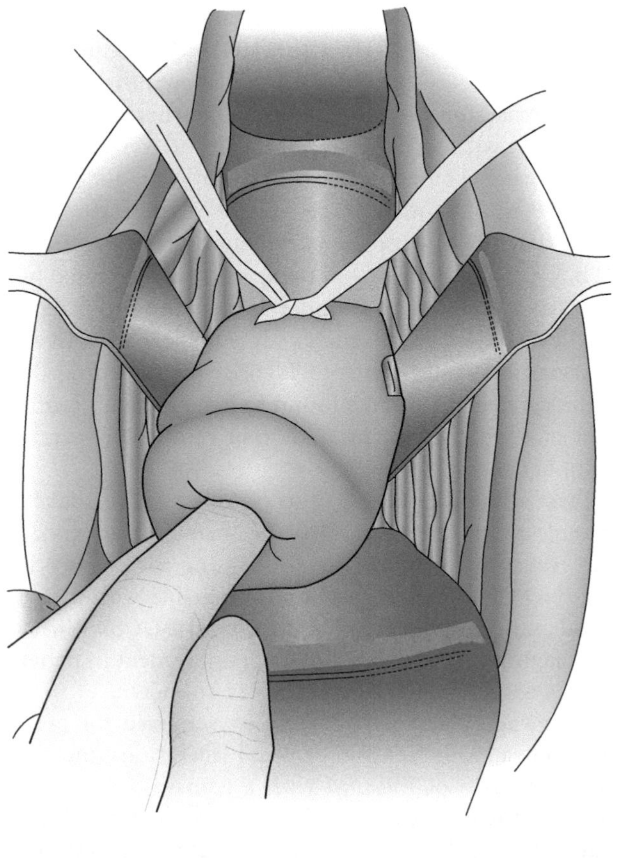

Figure 14.12 McDonald cerclage. The suture is tied anteriorly, tight enough to admit a fingertip at the external os, but closed at the internal os. Successive knots are placed, and the ends are left long enough to facilitate later removal.

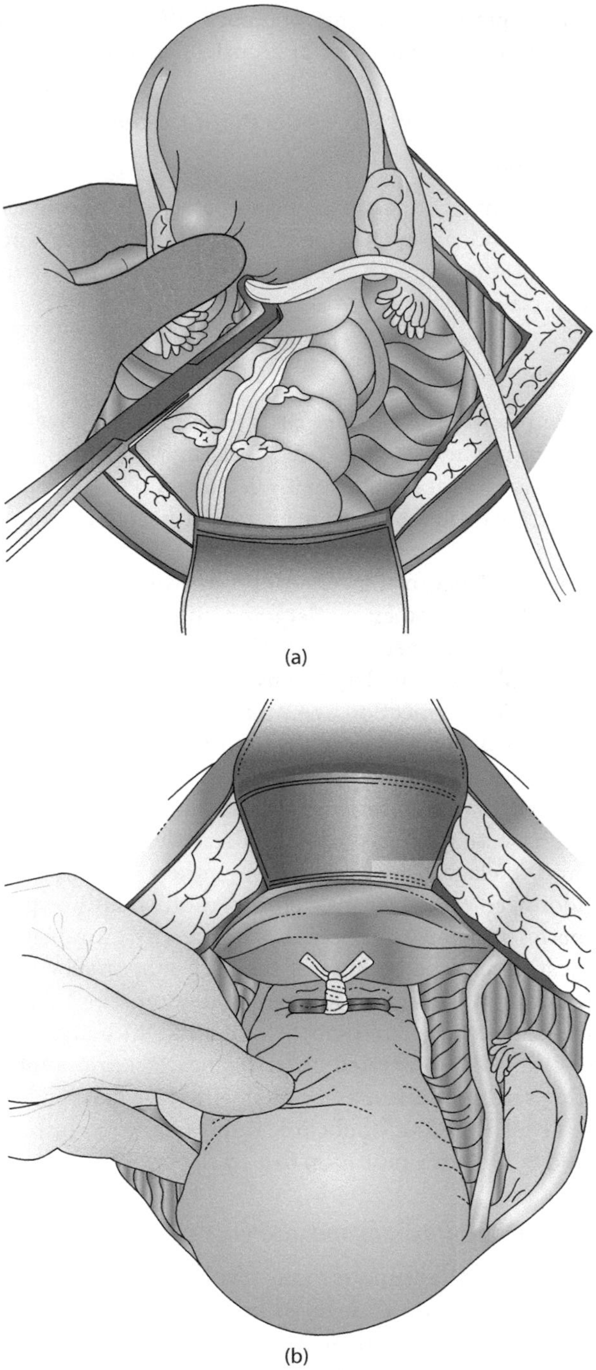

(a)

(b)

Figure 14.13 (a and b) Transabdominal cerclage. After the digital displacement of the uterine vessels bilaterally, a 5-mm Mersilene band is guided through the broad ligament at the level of the internal os by blunt perforation with a right-angle clamp. The suture is tied anteriorly.

interval procedure, but should not be attempted without appropriate laparoscopic suturing experience. Recent reviews found that outcomes of a laparoscopic cerclage were comparable to a laparotomy with no increase in complications, although this has not been studied in a randomized controlled fashion; a recent prospective cohort study confirmed this finding.[69,72,73] More recently, centers have published their experience with robotic-assisted laparoscopic cerclage; this approach also appears to be safe, again, at a center with appropriate experience.[74]

Medical and technical considerations for cerclage

Ultrasound

Before placing the cerclage, it is imperative to ensure fetal viability, and, as much as possible by gestational age, normal fetal anatomy. This is particularly important before TA cerclage.

Screening for infection

Before placing the cerclage, it is important to screen for infections when appropriate. Although bacterial vaginosis may be associated with recurrent PTB,[75] routine preoperative vaginal cultures have not been shown to be beneficial.[55]

The incidence of intraamniotic microbial infection is under 2% in women undergoing ultrasound-indicated cerclage,[62] and over 50% in those undergoing examination-indicated cerclage.[65] Given the low incidence of intraamniotic infection, routine amniocentesis in the setting of a history or ultrasound-indicated cerclage is not recommended. However, cohort studies have demonstrated that an amniocentesis evaluating for intraamniotic infection selects for candidates that would benefit from a cerclage. Therefore, although there has not been a randomized study, strong consideration should be given to performing an amniocentesis before any examination-indicated cerclage because of the high rate of subclinical intraamniotic infection in this population.[55,76–78] Overall these patients are at a high risk for PPROM or PTL, and one study demonstrated that diagnostic amniocentesis in this setting was not associated with a higher incidence of PTB or PPROM.[79] Subclinical intraamniotic infection would be a contraindication to a cerclage.[55]

Prophylactic antibiotics and tocolytics

"Prophylactic" antibiotics and tocolytics are commonly used at the time of cerclage, without any evidence of their benefit. Given the high success rate and early timing of history-indicated cerclage, when infection, inflammation, and contractions are rare, it is very doubtful that these adjunctive therapies would be shown to add benefit. For ultrasound-indicated cerclage, indomethacin might contribute to the benefit of cerclage in the one positive trial, but another retrospective cohort study found no benefit of tocolytics.[60,80,81] Since subclinical infection, inflammation, and uterine activity are more common at the time of examination-indicated cerclage, antibiotics and indomethacin therapy may be beneficial in this setting. One randomized trial demonstrated increased rate of latency >28 days in women who received both perioperative indocin and antibiotics (cefazolin × three doses) compared with women who received no perioperative medications.[82]

Sutures

Several different suture materials have been employed for cerclage. The only controlled data on this subject do not show a difference between the efficacies of Mersilene, Tevdek, and Prolene. Tevdek was associated with a nonsignificant higher incidence of PPROM.[83]

Cerclage technique

There are no randomized controlled trials comparing cerclage techniques. The main difference between Shirodkar and McDonald techniques is that the Shirodkar technique requires dissection of the bladder and rectum off the cervix to facilitate higher suture placement. Although it has not been studied in a randomized trial, case series have demonstrated similar efficacy of the two techniques.[55] The McDonald technique avoids the time and potential intraoperative complications of this dissection, and given the similar efficacy, most providers prefer the McDonald technique.

Management once cerclage is placed

TVU of the cervix has been evaluated for the follow-up of women with history-indicated, ultrasound-indicated, or physical examination-indicated cerclage in place. Most studies have shown that transvaginal cerclage is placed in the middle part of the cervix in the majority of cases, except for TA cerclage, always placed higher near the internal os (Figure 14.14).[84–86] Evaluation of pre- and postcerclage TVU CL has shown that CL usually increases postcerclage, and that an increase in CL is associated with a higher rate of term delivery.[87] Several studies have evaluated the accuracy of TVU for predicting PTB in patients with cerclage.[84–86] These studies all show that TVU cervical parameters are predictive of PTB. CL under 25 mm and upper cervix (the closed portion above the cerclage) under 10 mm are probably the two best predictive parameters. It is unclear what (if any) intervention would prevent PTB once the screening TVU of the cerclaged cervix is found to be abnormal. Limited data show that performing another reinforcing cerclage is not beneficial.[88]

Three-dimensional (3D) ultrasound (3DUS) makes it possible to obtain an axial plane through the cervix at the level of the cerclage, demonstrating the entire stitch (Figure 14.14). This view is not obtainable with conventional two-dimensional (2D) ultrasound (2DUS). Whether 3D imaging will improve clinical management in patients with or without a cerclage in place is unknown.

Transvaginal cerclage should be removed for persistent contractions to avoid cervical lacerations and evulsions. In cases of PPROM with a transvaginal cerclage in place, the cerclage should usually be removed immediately to avoid the high rates of ensuing infection for both the mother and fetus/neonate. Before 28 weeks, it might be discussed to consider removing the cerclage after steroids for fetal maturity have been administered.[89]

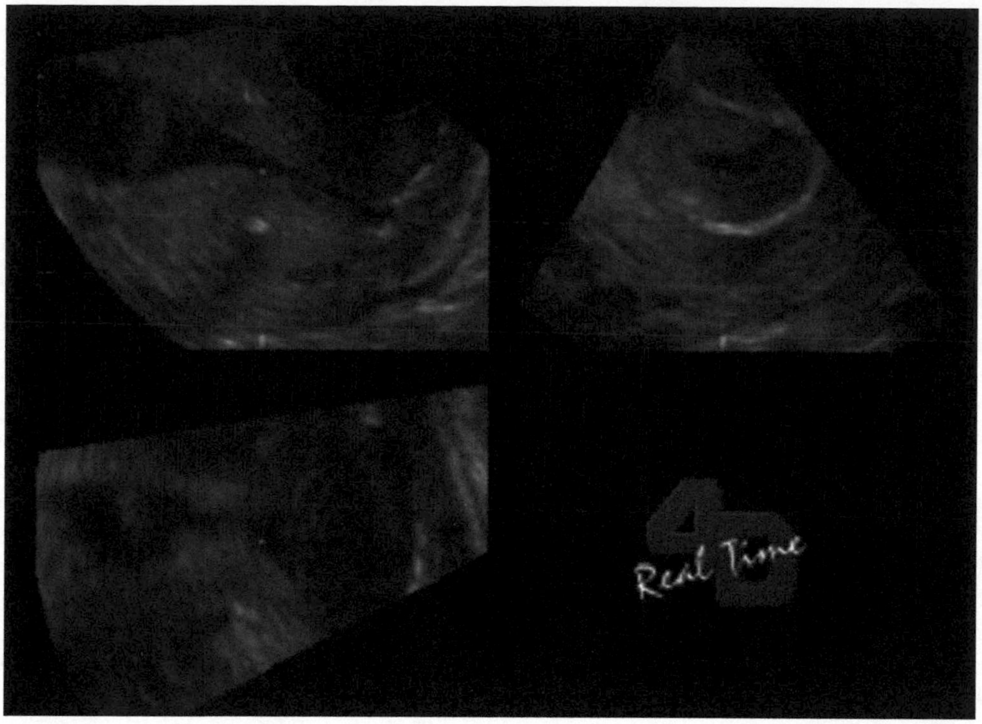

Figure 14.14 Ultrasound images of a transabdominal cerclage in two and three dimensions. Three-dimensional multiplanar display of a cervix with a cerclage in place. In two-dimensional ultrasound (2DUS), we normally see just two bright dots representing the suture. In three-dimensional ultrasound (3DUS) in the axial plane, we can see the suture in its entirety. This view enables a complete assessment of the cerclage and its relationship with the cervical canal, which is "fishmouth"-shaped in the axial plane.

Transvaginal cerclage should always be removed around 36 weeks to avoid complications from term contractions. A meta-analysis of six retrospective studies found a 30% (11.4% vs. 6.4%) nonsignificant reduction in the incidence of cervical lacerations of cerclages that were a planned removal versus a removal in labor. Although not significant, given the risk of Type 2 error, we still recommend planned removal at 36 weeks.[90]

Removal of McDonald cerclage is usually straightforward as long as enough length has been left on the cut knot to be identified. Removal can almost always (94% of cases) be done in the office without anesthesia with just a speculum, a pair of ring forceps, and long suture scissors. Occasionally (less than 10% of cases), a knot which is buried in tissue or a woman with low discomfort tolerance might necessitate removal in the operating room under regional anesthesia. Once it is removed, many women and their doctors anticipate cervical dilation, labor, and delivery to follow very soon. In fact, the mean interval between cerclage removal and spontaneous delivery is 16 days, with only 3% of women delivering within 48 hours of cerclage removal.[91] For women who have had a cerclage in their prior pregnancy for unclear indications, performing a cerclage in their next pregnancy has not been shown to be beneficial compared with close observation only.[92,93] Therefore, the saying, "once a cerclage, always a cerclage," is misleading. This reinforces the importance of performing the initial cerclage only when appropriate.

Contraindications

Contraindications to cerclage placement include the presence of a lethal fetal abnormality, evidence of intrauterine infection (chorioamnionitis), active bleeding, preterm labor, and ruptured membranes. If resolved, prior bleeding and preterm labor can become relative contraindications. The minimum gestational age of fetal viability should serve as the maximum upper gestational age of cerclage placement. In developed countries this is 23–24 weeks' gestation, while it may be as high as 26–28 weeks in areas of the world with limited neonatal care capabilities. The increased sensitivity of the uterus and cervix to this surgical manipulation later in gestation should also limit later cerclage placement.

Complications

The most common major morbidities associated with cerclage placement are rupture of membranes, chorioamnionitis, and suture displacement.[2] The presence of the cerclage can lead to preterm contractions or labor and cervical lacerations. Intrapartum fever and endometritis occur more frequently in women with cerclage.[94] Cervical bleeding and contractions during and immediately after cerclage placement are common but not well studied. Some clinicians use indomethacin either prophylactically or therapeutically for the cramps and contractions that often occur after cerclage placement. Ultrasound-indicated and examination-indicated cerclages are associated with a higher incidence of morbidity than history-indicated cerclage, probably due to the already ongoing inflammation/infectious labor process.

Bladder or urethra injuries at the time of cerclage placement have been reported[95,96]; they are extremely rare but increasing theoretical risks with attempts at "higher" suture placement. Whether intraoperative ultrasound can minimize this theoretical risk has not been determined.

TA cerclage is associated not only with the increased risks of a laparotomy or laparoscopy at the time of cerclage placement, but also with the increased risk of hemorrhage from inadvertent uterine vessel laceration. Furthermore, an additional laparotomy is necessitated for delivery of the fetus, whether this be (ideally) at term or in the second trimester soon after cerclage placement if membrane rupture or labor ensues. Laparoscopically placed TA cerclage holds the promise of decreasing this laparotomy-associated morbidity. Uterine rupture and maternal septicemia are extremely rare but life-threatening complications that have been reported in association with all types of cerclage.

CONCLUSIONS

CI, that is, painless dilation leading to recurrent second-trimester losses, occurs in <0.5% of pregnancies and probably represents the most extreme cases of the continuum of PTB. Diagnostic criteria are based not only on this history but also currently on a asymptomatic TVU CL ≤25 mm before 24 weeks in a woman with a prior sPTB or ≤20 mm in a singleton gestation without prior sPTB. Prepregnancy tests are unreliable, while TVU of the cervix during pregnancy may unmask a risk of recurrent PTB in women with a prior unclear CI or early PTB history by revealing a short CL in the second trimester.

Medical management is limited but progesterone use starting at 16–20 weeks is beneficial in preventing recurrent PTB in women with a prior PTB. Operative management involves cerclage, with modifications of the technique described by McDonald most commonly used today. Since no trials compare the efficacy of different techniques, and since almost all RCTs on cerclage used the McDonald technique, McDonald cerclage remains more popular, also given its simplicity in placement and removal. Randomized trials show evidence of benefit for history-indicated cerclage in women with three or more second-trimester losses or PTB. Women with unclear CI, such as those with just one or two PTBs or just one second-trimester loss, can be followed with TVU of the cervix. In about 40% of these women who develop a TVU CL ≤25 mm, ultrasound-indicated cerclage should be performed. A small trial showed the benefit of physical examination-indicated cerclage. In women who had a prior PTB under 33 weeks even with an early history-indicated transvaginal cerclage, TA cerclage decreases recurrent PTB compared with repeating a transvaginal cerclage.

REFERENCES

1. Rivieère L, Culpeper N, Cole A et al. *Practice of Physick*. London, UK: Peter Cole, 1658.
2. American College of Obstetricians and Gynecologists. ACOG practice bulletin no. 142: Cerclage for the management of cervical insufficiency. *Obstet Gynecol* 2014; 123(2 Pt 1): 372–9.
3. Iams JD, Johnson FF, Sonek J et al. Cervical competence as a continuum: A study of ultrasonographic cervical length and obstetric performance. *Am J Obstet Gynecol* 1995; 172(4 Pt 1): 1097–103; discussion 1104–6.
4. Friedman AM, Ananth CV, Siddiq Z et al. Trends and predictors of cerclage use in the United States from 2005 to 2012. *Obstet Gynecol* 2015; 126(2): 243–9.
5. Berghella V, Haas S, Chervoneva I, Hyslop T. Patients with prior second-trimester loss: Prophylactic cerclage or serial transvaginal sonograms? *Am J Obstet Gynecol* 2002; 187(3): 747–51.
6. Danforth DN. The fibrous nature of the human cervix, and its relation to the isthmic segment in gravid and nongravid uteri. *Am J Obstet Gynecol* 1947; 53(4): 541–60.
7. Ludmir J, Landon MB, Gabbe SG et al. Management of the diethylstilbestrol-exposed pregnant patient: A prospective study. *Am J Obstet Gynecol* 1987; 157(3): 665–9.
8. Harlap S, Shiono PH, Ramcharan S et al. A prospective study of spontaneous fetal losses after induced abortions. *N Engl J Med* 1979; 301(13): 677–81.
9. Pelham J, Arvon R, Berghella V. Prior preterm birth of twins: Risk of preterm birth in a subsequent singleton pregnancy. *Am J Obstet Gynecol* 2003; 101: 78S.
10. Zlatnik FJ, Burmeister LF. Interval evaluation of the cervix for predicting pregnancy outcome and diagnosing cervical incompetence. *J Reprod Med* 1993; 38(5): 365–9.
11. Berghella V. Universal cervical length screening for prediction and prevention of preterm birth. *Obstet Gynecol Surv* 2012; 67(10): 653–8.
12. Berghella V, Tolosa JE, Kuhlman K et al. Cervical ultrasonography compared with manual examination as a predictor of preterm delivery. *Am J Obstet Gynecol* 1997; 177(4): 723–30.
13. Berghella V, Kuhlman K, Weiner S et al. Cervical funneling: Sonographic criteria predictive of preterm delivery. *Ultrasound Obstet Gynecol* 1997; 10(3): 161–6.
14. Berghella V, Bega G, Tolosa JE, Berghella M. Ultrasound assessment of the cervix. *Clin Obstet Gynecol* 2003; 46(4): 947–62.
15. Owen J, Yost N, Berghella V et al. Mid-trimester endovaginal sonography in women at high risk for spontaneous preterm birth. *JAMA* 2001; 286(11): 1340–8.
16. Iams JD, Goldenberg RL, Meis PJ et al. The length of the cervix and the risk of spontaneous premature delivery. National Institute of Child Health and Human Development Maternal Fetal Medicine Unit Network. *N Engl J Med* 1996; 334(9): 567–72.

17. Berghella V, Talucci M, Desai A. Does transvaginal sonographic measurement of cervical length before 14 weeks predict preterm delivery in high-risk pregnancies? *Ultrasound Obstet Gynecol* 2003; 21(2): 140–4.
18. Owen J, Hankins G, Iams JD et al. Multicenter randomized trial of cerclage for preterm birth prevention in high-risk women with shortened midtrimester cervical length. *Am J Obstet Gynecol* 2009; 201(4): e1–8.
19. Berghella V, Rafael TJ, Szychowski JM et al. Cerclage for short cervix on ultrasonography in women with singleton gestations and previous preterm birth: A meta-analysis. *Obstet Gynecol* 2011; 117(3): 663–71.
20. Fonseca EB, Celik E, Parra M et al. Fetal Medicine Foundation Second Trimester Screening Group. Progesterone and the risk of preterm birth among women with a short cervix. *N Engl J Med* 2007; 357(5): 462–9.
21. Hassan SS, Romero R, Vidyadhari D et al. Vaginal progesterone reduces the rate of preterm birth in women with a sonographic short cervix: A multicenter, randomized, double-blind, placebo-controlled trial. *Ultrasound Obstet Gynecol.* 2011; 38(1): 18–31.
22. Orzechowski KM, Boelig RC, Baxter JK, Berghella V. A universal transvaginal cervical length screening program for preterm birth prevention. *Obstet Gynecol.* 2014; 124(3): 520–5.
23. Werner EF, Hamel MS, Orzechowski K et al. Cost-effectiveness of transvaginal ultrasound cervical length screening in singletons without a prior preterm birth: An update. *Am J Obstet Gynecol* 2015; 213(4): 554.e1–554.e6.
24. Romero R, Nicolaides K, Conde-Agudelo A et al. Vaginal progesterone in women with an asymptomatic sonographic short cervix in the midtrimester decreases preterm delivery and neonatal morbidity: A systematic review and metaanalysis of individual patient data. *Am J Obstet Gynecol* 2012; 206(2): 124.e1–124.19.
25. Goldenberg RL, Iams JD, Miodovnik M et al. The preterm prediction study: Risk factors in twin gestations. national institute of child health and human development maternal-fetal medicine units network. *Am J Obstet Gynecol* 1996; 175(4 Pt 1): 1047–53.
26. Nicolaides KH, Syngelaki A, Poon LC et al. Cervical pessary placement for prevention of preterm birth in unselected twin pregnancies: A randomized controlled trial. *Am J Obstet Gynecol* 2016; 214(1): 3.e1–3.e9.
27. Rafael TJ, Berghella V, Alfirevic Z. Cervical stitch (cerclage) for preventing preterm birth in multiple pregnancy. *Cochrane Database Syst Rev* 2014; 9: CD009166.
28. Saccone G, Rust O, Althuisius S et al. Cerclage for short cervix in twin pregnancies: Systematic review and meta-analysis of randomized trials using individual patient-level data. *Acta Obstet Gynecol Scand* 2015; 94(4): 352–8.
29. Brubaker SG, Pessel C, Zork N, et al. Vaginal progesterone in women with twin gestations complicated by short cervix: A retrospective cohort study. *BJOG* 2015; 122(5): 712–8.
30. Senat MV, Porcher R, Winer N et al. Prevention of preterm delivery by 17 alpha-hydroxyprogesterone caproate in asymptomatic twin pregnancies with a short cervix: A randomized controlled trial. *Am J Obstet Gynecol* 2013; 208(3): 194.e1–194.e8.
31. Odibo AO, Talucci M, Berghella V. Prediction of preterm premature rupture of membranes by transvaginal ultrasound features and risk factors in a high-risk population. *Ultrasound Obstet Gynecol.* 2002; 20(3): 245–51.
32. Berghella V. Frequency of uterine contractions in asymptomatic pregnant women with or without a short cervix on transvaginal ultrasound. *Am J Obstet Gynecol* 2003; 187: S127.
33. Lewis D, Pelham J, Sawhney H et al. Most asymptomatic pregnant women with a short cervix on ultrasound are having uterine contractions. *Am J Obstet Gynecol* 2001; 185: S144.
34. Althuisius SM, Dekker GA, van Geijn HP et al. Cervical incompetence prevention randomized cerclage trial (CIPRACT): Study design and preliminary results. *Am J Obstet Gynecol* 2000; 183(4): 823–9.
35. Kassanos D, Salamalekis E, Vitoratos N et al. The value of transvaginal ultrasonography in diagnosis and management of cervical incompetence. *Clin Exp Obstet Gynecol* 2001; 28: 266–8.
36. Beigi A, Zarrinkous F. Elective versus ultrasound-indicated cervical cerclage in women at risk for cervical incompetence. *Med J Islamic Rep Iran* 2005; 19: 103–7.
37. Simcox R, Seed PT, Bennett P et al. A randomized controlled trial of cervical scanning vs history to determine cerclage in women at high risk of preterm birth (CIRCLE trial). *Am J Obstet Gynecol* 2009; 200: 623–9.
38. Berghella V, Mackeen AD. Cervical length screening with ultrasound-indicated cerclage compared with history-indicated cerclage for prevention of preterm birth: A meta-analysis. *Obstet Gynecol* 2011; 118(1): 148–55.
39. Kovacevich GJ, Gaich SA, Lavin JP et al. The prevalence of thromboembolic events among women with extended bed rest prescribed as part of the treatment for premature labor or preterm premature rupture of membranes. *Am J Obstet Gynecol* 2000; 182(5): 1089–92.
40. Sciscione AC. Maternal activity restriction and the prevention of preterm birth. *Am J Obstet Gynecol* 2010; 202(3): 232.e1-232.e5.
41. Grobman WA, Gilbert SA, Iams JD et al. Activity restriction among women with a short cervix. *Obstet Gynecol* 2013; 121(6): 1181–6.
42. Meis PJ, Klebanoff M, Thom E et al. Prevention of recurrent preterm delivery by 17 alpha-hydroxyprogesterone caproate. *N Engl J Med* 2003; 348(24): 2379–85.

43. Keirse MJ. Progestogen administration in pregnancy may prevent preterm delivery. *Br J Obstet Gynaecol* 1990; 97(2): 149–54.
44. da Fonseca EB, Bittar RE, Carvalho MH, Zugaib M. Prophylactic administration of progesterone by vaginal suppository to reduce the incidence of spontaneous preterm birth in women at increased risk: A randomized placebo-controlled double-blind study. *Am J Obstet Gynecol* 2003; 188(2): 419–24.
45. Committee on Practice Bulletins-Obstetrics, The American College of Obstetricians and Gynecologists. Practice bulletin no. 130: Prediction and prevention of preterm birth. *Obstet Gynecol* 2012; 120(4): 964–73.
46. Gimovsky AC, Suhag A, Roman A et al. Pessary versus cerclage versus expectant management for cervical dilation with visible membranes in the second trimester. *J Matern Fetal Neonatal Med* 2016: 29: 1363–6.
47. Kosinska-Kaczynska K, Bomba-Opon D, Zygula A et al. Adjunctive pessary therapy after emergency cervical cerclage for cervical insufficiency with protruding fetal membranes in the second trimester of pregnancy: A novel modification of treatment. *Biomed Res Int* 2015; 2015: 185371.
48. Goya M, Pratcorona L, Merced C et al. Cervical pessary in pregnant women with a short cervix (PECEP): An open-label randomised controlled trial. *Lancet* 2012; 379(9828): 1800–6.
49. Hui SY, Chor CM, Lau TK et al. Cerclage pessary for preventing preterm birth in women with a singleton pregnancy and a short cervix at 20 to 24 weeks: A randomized controlled trial. *Am J Perinatol* 2013; 30(4): 283–8.
50. Liem S, Schuit E, Hegeman M et al. Cervical pessaries for prevention of preterm birth in women with a multiple pregnancy (ProTWIN): A multicentre, open-label randomised controlled trial. *Lancet* 2013; 382(9901): 1341–9.
51. Lash AF. The incompetent internal os of the cervix: Diagnosis and treatment. *Am J Obstet Gynecol* 1960; 79: 552–6.
52. Shirodkar VN. A new method of operative treatment for habitual abortions in the second trimester of pregnancy. *Antiseptic* 1955; 52: 299–300.
53. McDonald IA. Suture of the cervix for inevitable miscarriage. *J Obstet Gynaecol Br Emp* 1957; 64(3): 346–50.
54. Shortle B, Jewelewicz R. *Clinical Aspects of Cervical Incompetence.* Chicago, IL: Yearbook Medical Publishers, 1989.
55. Berghella V, Ludmir J, Simonazzi G, Owen J. Transvaginal cervical cerclage: Evidence for perioperative management strategies. *Am J Obstet Gynecol* 2013; 209(3): 181–92.
56. Final report of the Medical Research Council/Royal College of Obstetricians and Gynaecologists multicentre randomised trial of cervical cerclage. MRC/RCOG working party on cervical cerclage. *Br J Obstet Gynaecol* 1993; 100(6): 516–23.
57. Dor J, Shalev J, Mashiach S et al. Elective cervical suture of twin pregnancies diagnosed ultrasonically in the first trimester following induced ovulation. *Gynecol Obstet Invest* 1982; 13(1): 55–60.
58. Lazar P, Gueguen S, Dreyfus J et al. Multicentred controlled trial of cervical cerclage in women at moderate risk of preterm delivery. *Br J Obstet Gynaecol* 1984; 91(8): 731–5.
59. Rush RW, Isaacs S, McPherson K et al. A randomized controlled trial of cervical cerclage in women at high risk of spontaneous preterm delivery. *Br J Obstet Gynaecol* 1984; 91(8): 724–30.
60. Althuisius SM, Dekker GA, Hummel P et al. Final results of the cervical incompetence prevention randomized cerclage trial (CIPRACT): Therapeutic cerclage with bed rest versus bed rest alone. *Am J Obstet Gynecol* 2001; 185(5): 1106–12.
61. To MS, Alfirevic Z, Heath VC et al. Cervical cerclage for prevention of preterm delivery in women with short cervix: Randomised controlled trial. *Lancet* 2004; 363(9424): 1849–53.
62. Rust OA, Atlas RO, Reed J et al. Revisiting the short cervix detected by transvaginal ultrasound in the second trimester: Why cerclage therapy may not help. *Am J Obstet Gynecol* 2001;185(5): 1098–105.
63. Berghella V, Odibo AO, Tolosa JE. Cerclage for prevention of preterm birth in women with a short cervix found on transvaginal ultrasound examination: A randomized trial. *Am J Obstet Gynecol* 2004; 191(4): 1311–17.
64. Berghella V, Odibo AO, To MS et al. Cerclage for short cervix on ultrasonography: Meta-analysis of trials using individual patient-level data. *Obstet Gynecol* 2005; 106(1): 181–9.
65. Romero R, Gonzalez R, Sepulveda W et al. Infection and labor. VIII. Microbial invasion of the amniotic cavity in patients with suspected cervical incompetence: Prevalence and clinical significance. *Am J Obstet Gynecol* 1992; 167(4 Pt 1): 1086–91.
66. Althuisius SM, Dekker GA, Hummel P, van Geijn HP. Cervical incompetence prevention randomized cerclage trial. Cervical incompetence prevention randomized cerclage trial: Emergency cerclage with bed rest versus bed rest alone. *Am J Obstet Gynecol* 2003; 189(4): 907–10.
67. Ehsanipoor RM, Seligman NS, Saccone G et al. Physical examination-indicated cerclage: A systematic review and meta-analysis. *Obstet Gynecol.* 2015; 126(1): 125–35.
68. Davis G, Berghella V, Talucci M, Wapner RJ. Patients with a prior failed transvaginal cerclage: A comparison of obstetric outcomes with either transabdominal or transvaginal cerclage. *Am J Obstet Gynecol* 2000; 183(4): 836–9.
69. Tulandi T, Alghanaim N, Hakeem G, Tan X. Pre and post-conceptional abdominal cerclage by laparoscopy or laparotomy. *J Minim Invasive Gynecol* 2014; 21(6): 987–93.

70. Scibetta JJ, Sanko SR, Phipps WR. Laparoscopic transabdominal cervicoisthmic cerclage. *Fertil Steril* 1998; 69(1): 161–3.
71. Gallot D, Savary D, Laurichesse H et al. Experience with three cases of laparoscopic transabdominal cervico-isthmic cerclage and two subsequent pregnancies. *BJOG* 2003; 110(7): 696–700.
72. Ades A, Dobromilsky KC, Cheung KT, Umstad MP. Transabdominal cervical cerclage: Laparoscopy versus laparotomy. *J Minim Invasive Gynecol* 2015; 22(6): 968–73.
73. Burger NB, Brolmann HA, Einarsson JI et al. Effectiveness of abdominal cerclage placed via laparotomy or laparoscopy: Systematic review. *J Minim Invasive Gynecol* 2011; 18(6): 696–704.
74. Foster TL, Addleman RN, Moore ES, Sumners JE. Robotic-assisted prophylactic transabdominal cervical cerclage in singleton pregnancies. *J Obstet Gynaecol* 2013; 33(8): 821–2.
75. McDonald H, Brocklehurst P, Parsons J. Antibiotics for treating bacterial vaginosis in pregnancy. *Cochrane Database Syst Rev* 2005; (1): CD000262.
76. Diago Almela VJ, Martinez-Varea A, Perales-Puchalt A et al. Good prognosis of cerclage in cases of cervical insufficiency when intra-amniotic inflammation/infection is ruled out. *J Matern Fetal Neonatal Med* 2015; 28(13): 1563–8.
77. Mays JK, Figueroa R, Shah J et al. Amniocentesis for selection before rescue cerclage. *Obstet Gynecol* 2000; 95(5): 652–5.
78. Suhag A, Berghella V. Cervical cerclage. *Clin Obstet Gynecol* 2014; 57(3): 557–67.
79. Airoldi J, Pereira L, Cotter A et al. Amniocentesis prior to physical exam-indicated cerclage in women with midtrimester cervical dilation: Results from the expectant management compared to physical exam-indicated cerclage international cohort study. *Am J Perinatol* 2009; 26(1): 63–8.
80. Visintine J, Airoldi J, Berghella V. Indomethacin administration at the time of ultrasound-indicated cerclage: Is there an association with a reduction in spontaneous preterm birth? *Am J Obstet Gynecol* 2008; 198(6): 643.e1-643.e3.
81. Smith J, DeFranco EA. Tocolytics used as adjunctive therapy at the time of cerclage placement: A systematic review. *J Perinatol* 2015; 35(8): 561–5.
82. Miller ES, Grobman WA, Fonseca L, Robinson BK. Indomethacin and antibiotics in examination-indicated cerclage: A randomized controlled trial. *Obstet Gynecol* 2014; 123(6): 1311–6.
83. Pereira L, Llevy C, Lewis D et al. Effect of suture material on the outcome of emergent cerclage. *Am J Obstet Gynecol* 2004; 103:S35.
84. Andersen HF, Karimi A, Sakala EP, Kalugdan R. Prediction of cervical cerclage outcome by endovaginal ultrasonography. *Am J Obstet Gynecol* 1994; 171(4): 1102–6.
85. Berghella V, Davis G, Wapner RJ. Transvaginal ultrasound of the cervix in pregnancies with prophylactic cerclage. *Am J Obstet Gynecol* 1999; 180: S173.
86. Guzman ER, Houlihan C, Vintzileos A et al. The significance of transvaginal ultrasonographic evaluation of the cervix in women treated with emergency cerclage. *Am J Obstet Gynecol* 1996; 175(2): 471–6.
87. Althuisius SM, Dekker GA, van Geijn HP, Hummel P. The effect of therapeutic McDonald cerclage on cervical length as assessed by transvaginal ultrasonography. *Am J Obstet Gynecol* 1999; 180(2 Pt 1): 366–9.
88. Baxter JK, Airoldi J, Berghella V. Short cervical length after history-indicated cerclage: Is a reinforcing cerclage beneficial? *Am J Obstet Gynecol* 2005; 193(3 Pt 2): 1204–7.
89. Jenkins TM, Berghella V, Shlossman PA et al. Timing of cerclage removal after preterm premature rupture of membranes: Maternal and neonatal outcomes. *Am J Obstet Gynecol* 2000; 183(4): 847–52.
90. Simonazzi G, Curti A, Bisulli M et al. Cervical lacerations in planned versus labor cerclage removal: A systematic review. *Eur J Obstet Gynecol Reprod Biol* 2015; 193: 19–22.
91. Arvon R, Berghella V, Farrell C, Sawnhey H. Interval to spontaneous delivery after elective removal of cerclage. *Am J Obstet Gynecol* 2002; 187: S119.
92. Fejgin MD, Gabai B, Goldberger S et al. Once a cerclage, not always a cerclage. *J Reprod Med* 1994; 39(11): 880–2.
93. Pelham J, Lewis D, Farrell C, Berghella V. Prior cerclage: To repeat or not to repeat, that is the question. *Am J Obstet Gynecol* 2002; 187: S115.
94. Drakeley AJ, Roberts D, Alfirevic Z. Cervical stitch (cerclage) for preventing pregnancy loss in women. *Cochrane Database Syst Rev* 2003; (1): CD003253.
95. Ben-Baruch G, Rabinovitch O, Madjar I et al. Ureterovaginal fistula—A rare complication of cervical cerclage. *Isr J Med Sci* 1980; 16(5): 400–1.
96. Bates JL, Cropley T. Complication of cervical cerclage. *Lancet* 1977; 2: 1035.

Advanced extrauterine pregnancy

15

DAVID KULAK, GERSON WEISS, and SARA S. MORELLI

CONTENTS

An advanced extrauterine pregnancy (AEP) is defined as one that has implanted outside the endometrial cavity on any of the surrounding reproductive organs, intra-abdominal organs, and/or peritoneum, and has survived to 20 weeks of gestation or more. Advanced extrauterine pregnancies are a rare complication and are highly associated with maternal and fetal morbidity and mortality. Ectopic pregnancies at any gestational age account for 9% of pregnancy related deaths,[1] and the risk of maternal death increases with gestational age. Typically, AEP is classified by two factors: (1) the location of the gestation, and (2) whether the site of implantation is primary or secondary. The latter most commonly occurs in the case of a tubal pregnancy that ruptures or extrudes through the fimbriated end and implants on the surrounding tissue, leaving evidence of a damaged tube and a concurrent pregnancy in a different location.[2,3] The common sites for AEP are abdominal, ovarian, intraligamentary and rudimentary uterine horn.

The first description of an extrauterine gestation was given by Albucasis (AD 936–1013), an Arab physician, in his treatise *At-Tasrif liman 'Ajiza 'an at-Ta'lif (The Method of Medicine)*,[4] and since then, reports have abounded on the subject. The first operative delivery of an abdominal pregnancy was done by Jacob Nufer in the 1500s, wherein both the mother and the fetus survived.[5] A lithopedion, or "petrified embryo," in the city of Sens (France) was reported by Cordaeus in the sixteenth century. In the eighteenth century, John Bard, surgeon to George Washington, reported the first successful operation of an ectopic pregnancy in the United States. Then, in 1903, Sir Edwin Craig championed the cause for early surgical intervention as a means of decreasing maternal mortality.[6]

During those early times, the only means of estimating gestational age was by the duration of amenorrhea. Clinical signs such as Chadwick's sign (blue-purple hue of the cervix and congestion of the vaginal mucosa) and Hegar's sign (softening of the isthmus)[7] in the first trimester and the eventual onset of fetal movements in the second trimester were presumptive evidence of pregnancy.

Today, refinements in sensitive human chorionic gonadotropin (b-hCG) assays and the increased resolution of ultrasonography and magnetic resonance imaging (MRI) allow a more accurate estimation of the gestational age of the pregnancy and its location, making timely diagnosis possible. Further, these advances facilitate a better understanding of the natural evolution of AEP. For example, we now know that the progression of AEP past 20 weeks is dependent on specific characteristics inherent to the site of implantation, such as vascularity and distensibility to accommodate the growing gestation. While in the past the chance of survival for the fetus was essentially null, with increased access to advanced imaging and surgical techniques in conjunction with modern methods of neonatal resuscitation, there have now been a number of reports of viable deliveries.

ABDOMINAL PREGNANCY

Abdominal pregnancy is a rare form of ectopic pregnancy, with a worldwide incidence ranging from 1:10,000 to 1:30,000 deliveries[8] and accounts for 1%–4% of all ectopic gestations.[9] Maternal and perinatal mortality rates of 0.5%–18% and 40%–95%,[9,10] respectively, have been reported in the literature. Rarely do these progress to advanced gestation; moreover, expectant management until viability is seldom an option. Several recently published case reports describe advanced abdominal pregnancies culminating in the delivery of a liveborn infant at term.[11,12] Even in those cases in which the fetus survives, advanced abdominal pregnancies are often complicated by massive hemorrhage at delivery and an approximate 20% risk of fetal anomalies.[11,13]

Although the most commonly reported sites of abdominal pregnancy are the Pouch of Douglas and the posterior uterine wall, other sites include the uterine fundus, as well as extrapelvic sites such as the liver, spleen, lesser sac, and diaphragm.[14] In 1942, Studdiford[2] suggested four diagnostic criteria to distinguish a primary from a secondary peritoneal pregnancy: (1) normal tubes and ovaries without evidence of injury; (2) no evidence of uteroperitoneal fistula; (3) pregnancy related exclusively to the peritoneal surface; and (4) pregnancy at an early enough stage of gestation to exclude the possibility of a secondary implantation, eliminating primary tubal nidation. Secondary implantation occurs more commonly, however, since both primary and secondary AEP is managed in the same manner, the origin has little clinical impact.

Prior to the use of MRI or ultrasound technology, diagnosis was often difficult and the clinician had to rely on certain signs and symptoms, such as abdominal pain, gastrointestinal symptoms, painful fetal movements, abnormal presentations, an uneffaced and displaced cervix, vaginal bleeding, and palpation of a pelvic mass distinct from the uterus. Failure to induce uterine contractions during oxytocin infusion was also a well-established diagnostic technique.[15] Today imaging techniques can corroborate any clinical suspicion and precisely locate the site of implantation and vascular sources galvanizing timely therapeutic planning. However, despite advances in imaging techniques, as many as 40% of cases worldwide may go undiagnosed until delivery.[13]

Treatment usually requires surgical management with evacuation of all products of conception by laparotomy. However, in instances in which a patient refuses surgical treatment due to religious, moral, or personal beliefs, a more conservative approach may be possible. These cases mandate hospitalization and continuous supervision of both fetal and maternal well-being. Patients must be informed of the 20%–40% risk of malformation in living infants attributed to oligohydramnios and compression, such as facial asymmetry, torticollis, pulmonary hypoplasia, and joint deformities (Figure 15.1).[4] Decisions regarding timing, method, and management of delivery are discussed later in this chapter.

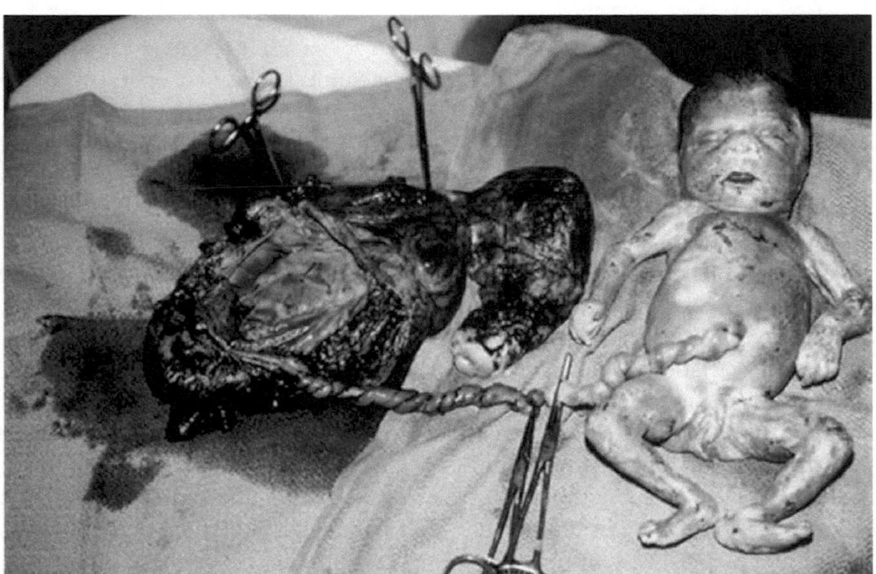

Figure 15.1 Advanced abdominal pregnancy. Fetal demise at 28 weeks' gestation with placental attachment to the right cornual region and to the broad ligament. Abdominal hysterectomy was performed without significant blood loss, and no postoperative complications were reported. (Courtesy of Dr. JJ Apuzzio.)

TUBAL PREGNANCY

The ampullary region of the fallopian tube is by far the most common of all extrauterine sites for ectopic gestations. Early tubal pregnancies may end as tubal abortions, with extrusion of the pregnancy from the fimbriated end. Tubal pregnancies usually do not progress past 12–14 weeks. After this point in time, tubal rupture occurs, sometimes with catastrophic effects, and these pregnancies therefore do not become AEP. Further discussion of this topic is beyond the scope of this chapter and is usually reserved for general gynecology texts.

CERVICAL PREGNANCY

Cervical pregnancy occurs when the implantation of placental tissue is established below the internal cervical os. Prior to the use of transvaginal sonography (TVUS), the diagnosis was made in only 18% of cases preoperatively, and usually not until the time of dilation and curettage for a presumed incomplete abortion, with subsequently severe hemorrhagic complications. Today, a correct diagnosis is made 87.5%[16] of the time when b-hCG, ultrasound, and MRI are used together.

While estimates differ as to the true incidence of cervical ectopic pregnancies in the United States, it is clear that it is an extremely rare occurrence. The incidence in the United States ranges in the literature from 1:2,500 to 1:12,422 deliveries.[16–18] The typical presenting symptom is painless, first-trimester, vaginal (uterine) bleeding. On speculum examination, the cervix is hyperemic and considerably enlarged, creating the "hourglass" (softened and significantly enlarged cervix equal to or larger than the uterine corpus) appearance on an abdominal ultrasound.

Cervical ectopic pregnancies with fetal cardiac activity at 10 or more weeks' gestation may be successfully managed with ultrasound-guided intrafetal injection of feticidal agents, but this form of ectopic pregnancy never reaches an advanced gestational age before the onset of symptoms, and thus further discussion is beyond the scope of this chapter.

OVARIAN PREGNANCY

First reported in 1682 by Saint Maurice de Périgod, ovarian ectopic pregnancy constitutes only 0.5%–3% of all ectopic pregnancies, and the incidence is only 1 out of every 7,000–40,000 deliveries.[19,20] The existing literature regarding ovarian AEP is limited to case reports, most of which are from outside the United States. Approximately 75% of ovarian pregnancies are terminated in the first trimester, 12% in the second trimester, and 12% in the third trimester.[21] Fertilization of the ovum inside the ovary and reverse migration of the embryo from the fallopian tube and implantation on the ovary are the accepted theories for its pathogenesis. Factors such as pelvic inflammatory disease or intrauterine disease (IUD) use have not been associated with ovarian pregnancy. Several investigators have indicated that patients with ovarian pregnancies are younger, have higher parity, and have fewer fertility problems than the typical tubal pregnancy patients. Lehfeldt et al.[22] demonstrated that the IUD is effective in preventing intrauterine pregnancy in 99.5% of subjects and tubal pregnancy in 95% of subjects, but it has little effect on preventing ovarian pregnancy. Shibahara et al.[23] postulate that blastocyst-stage embryo transfers may also be associated with ectopic implantation of embryos on the ovaries, but the mechanism underlying this needs further elucidation.

The diagnosis of ovarian ectopic pregnancy is often made intraoperatively since the preoperative findings are similar to those of a tubal pregnancy. Imaging such as transvaginal ultrasound may arouse suspicion; however, a definitive diagnosis is reached only by laparoscopy or laparotomy. Ultrasonographic signs specific for unruptured intrafollicular ovarian pregnancy are a thickened, uniformly echogenic wall of the sac, surrounded by ovarian stroma, and in a primary ovarian ectopic the absence of a preexisting corpora lutea on either ovary, since the fetus grows within its confines.

In 1873, Spiegelberg[24] established the following four criteria for a primary ovarian pregnancy: (1) the oviduct on the affected side must be intact; (2) the amniotic sac must occupy the position of the ovary; (3) the amniotic sac must be connected to the uterus by the ovarian ligament; (4) ovarian tissue must be present in the wall of the amniotic sac, with concomitant histologic confirmation postoperatively. Histology alone confirms the diagnosis. It can distinguish four distinct forms: intrafollicular, juxtafollicular, juxtacortical, and interstitial.

Conservative surgeries such as ovarian cystectomy or wedge resection may be done in order to remove the products of conception when the diagnosis is made early or for those who may desire future childbearing. Definitive management is unilateral salpingo-oophorectomy. Hemorrhage may occur in advanced cases, as in abdominal pregnancy. Use of the folic acid antagonist methotrexate (MTX) is indicated as an adjunct only for organ-preserving operations with an incomplete resection or persistence of trophoblastic tissue.

Although rare, an ovarian ectopic pregnancy can advance well into the second trimester if an adequate blood supply is maintained. In a recent case report, a live ovarian ectopic pregnancy was diagnosed at 16 weeks' gestation by ultrasound after the patient complained of vague abdominal pain.[25] A subsequent pelvic MRI revealed robust parasitized vasculature from the internal iliac and periuterine vessels. After transfer to a higher acuity level facility, the patient underwent an exploratory laparotomy. Ureterolysis and a right salpingo-oophorectomy were performed and the fetus and placenta were able to be completely removed without complication.

INTRALIGAMENTARY PREGNANCY

While some prefer to group this type of pregnancy within the broader category of abdominal pregnancies, an intraligamentary pregnancy is a retroperitoneal pregnancy that occurs due to rupture of the fallopian tube with a subsequent implantation between the two leaves of the broad ligament. The similarities to an abdominal pregnancy include risk factors and clinical presentation. The reported incidence ranges between 1:75 and 1:613 of all extrauterine pregnancies.[26] It is often not diagnosed before surgery because of the proximity to the uterine cavity and the rarity with which it occurs. MRI has proven to be very effective in confirming whether the pregnancy is retroperitoneal or intrauterine and is used when ultrasound findings suggest a gestational sac separate from the uterus. Although rupture of the gestational sac can entail some bleeding, massive hemorrhage is not likely to occur due to the tamponade-like effect provided by the adjacent leaves of the broad ligament.[27] In fact, the broad ligament can expand to accommodate a pregnancy to viability. If diagnosed early, it can be treated laparoscopically, although laparotomy is usually warranted. There are no reports of the use of MTX in pregnancies confined to the broad ligament.

RUDIMENTARY HORN PREGNANCY

The rudimentary horn of a uterus is the incompletely developed remnant of the contralateral Müllerian duct of a unicornuate uterus. Pregnancy in this location is very rare with an incidence of 1/76,000–150,000 births.[28] However, since the rudimentary horn does have greater distensability and vasculature than other ectopic locations, only about half of rudimentary horn pregnancies will present with rupture.[29]

Pregnancy can occur in the rudimentary horn even if there is no gross evidence of communication with the cervix. Two theories of how such a paradoxical pregnancy occurs are transperitoneal sperm migration[30] or microscopic communication with the cervix, which is sometimes found on pathological examination after surgical removal.[31]

As mentioned earlier, approximately half of rudimentary horn pregnancies are discovered after rupture. These cases generally present with severe abdominal pain and often in the setting of what was thought to be a normal intrauterine pregnancy. In these cases the actual location may be determined by imaging studies such as an MRI during the work-up for the etiology of the pain.[32] Occasionally, the pregnancy location is only discovered at the time of surgery. A 2002 case report from Japan described a viable fetus delivered at 26 weeks' gestation from a rudimentary horn during an exploratory laparotomy for what was thought to be an intrauterine pregnancy with intra-abdominal hemorrhage due to a ruptured ovarian cyst.[31]

A pregnancy that is initially established in a rudimentary horn can subsequently rupture and then reimplant in a secondary location, similar to a tubal ectopic. A recent case report described a ruptured rudimentary horn pregnancy that secondarily implanted in the abdomen. Delivery of a live infant and excision of the rudimentary uterine horn via laparotomy was performed at 30 weeks, prompted only by the sonographic finding of anhydramnios.[33]

Although a rudimentary uterine horn may contain normal endometrial tissue, pregnancies within a rudimentary horn are associated with an increased risk of placental anomalies including placenta accreta, percreta, or increta.[32] Therefore, when pregnancy does occur in this location, complete surgical removal of the horn and ipsilateral fallopian tube should be performed prior to viability.[34] In cases where a viable fetus is delivered, the rudimentary uterine horn should be removed after the delivery. When a unicornuate uterus with a rudimentary horn is discovered in a nonpregnant patient, the prophylactic removal of the rudimentary horn should be performed to avoid the risk of ectopic pregnancy and/or endometriosis from retrograde menstruation arising from the noncommunicating horn.[35,36]

DIAGNOSTIC EVALUATION

Once an ectopic pregnancy has reached a viable gestational age, rarely are serum hormones or markers necessary to evaluate AEP. Nevertheless, a thorough understanding of their use within this clinical context is of the utmost importance so that an appropriate plan of care can be undertaken at an earlier gestational age when maternal morbidity is significantly reduced.

Hormonal assessment

Human chorionic gonadotropin

Quantitative b-hCG measurements continue to be an important tool in the evaluation of extrauterine pregnancies. Measurements of b-hCG are used to make a diagnosis of an ectopic pregnancy in the setting of an empty uterine cavity or abnormal doubling of the hCG and to assess the efficacy of either medical or surgical therapy with serial measurements.[16]

Under normal conditions, serum concentrations of hCG double approximately every 48–84 hours, in a curvilinear fashion, until reaching its maximum level, usually 100,000 mIU/mL, where it begins to plateau at around weeks 8–12 of gestation. Because the increase in hCG is essentially linear in early pregnancy, the rate of increase can be used to assess the viability of the pregnancy.[37,38] Using a cutoff of less than 53% rise in serum b-hCG levels over 48 hours will yield a 91% sensitivity, but only a 66% specificity, in establishing the diagnosis of ectopic pregnancy.[39] There is no agreement as to what level of b-hCG is diagnostic of ectopic pregnancy.[40,41] In the past, using hCG cutoff values of 1500 mIU/mL or 2000 mIU/mL were recommended as the "discriminatory zone" for visualization of an intrauterine pregnancy. More recently, however, Connolly et al.[42] demonstrated that using these discriminatory levels would not predict seeing a gestational sac in a viable pregnancy in 20% and 10% of cases, respectively. As progression of the extrauterine pregnancy continues, b-hCG titers will peak at approximately 100,000 mIU/mL after 20 weeks, similar to the plateau seen in an intrauterine pregnancy gestation and then subsequently declines.

Serum progesterone

Several investigators have attempted to study the use of progesterone levels as a way to distinguish a viable from a nonviable pregnancy. However, a meta-analysis showed that the use of serum progesterone levels alone is insufficient to diagnose ectopic pregnancy.[43] Although levels of at least 25 ng/mL are generally indicative of normal gestation, serum progesterone levels less than 5 ng/mL are rarely associated with viability. The concomitant finding of low serum progesterone together with a rising hCG level raises the level of suspicion for the presence of extrauterine pregnancy. Values of 5–25 ng/mL fall within the diagnostic "gray zone" and cannot be used to reliably distinguish an intrauterine from an extrauterine gestation. Unfortunately, the routine use of progesterone alone in this clinical setting has not proven to be the panacea investigators had hoped for.

Serum markers

Vascular endothelial growth factor (VEGF)

A well-known angiogenic factor, VEGF, has been implicated in the mechanisms involved in implantation and early pregnancy. It is also believed that this permeability factor is a critical regulator of amniotic fluid transport in the fetal membranes. Several investigators have reported that VEGF expression in the endometrium and corpus luteum is regulated by ovarian steroids and hCG. A positive correlation has been made between elevated levels of VEGF during the first trimester of normal intrauterine pregnancy and gestational age, b-hCG, estradiol, and progesterone levels. Abnormal implantation further enhances the production of VEGF locally. Daniel et al. postulate that because VEGF production is dependent on hypoxia and because implantation outside the endometrial cavity presents a hostile environment for the trophoblast, VEGF production must be elevated. To test their hypothesis, they compared serum levels in three groups: group I (normal intrauterine pregnancy), group II (abnormal intrauterine pregnancy), and group III (ectopic pregnancy). Each group was matched for gestational age as assessed by last menstrual period and ultrasound measurements.

The serum level of VEGF was significantly higher in women with ectopic pregnancy (median, 226.8 pg/mL; range, 19.4–561.7 pg/mL) than in women with normal intrauterine pregnancy (median, 24.4 pg/mL; range, 2.7–196.8 pg/mL). Serum levels of VEGF in women with ectopic pregnancy were significantly higher than in women with abnormal intrauterine pregnancy (median, 59.4 pg/mL; range, 12.1–334.1 pg/mL), though this was not statistically significant. Serum VEGF level of over 200 ng/mL can distinguish an intrauterine from an extrauterine pregnancy with a specificity of 90% and a positive predictive value (PPV) of 86%, and abnormal intrauterine from extrauterine pregnancy with a specificity of 80% and a PPV of 86%. In addition, combining progesterone levels with VEGF produces better results than using either marker alone—a reflection of their different sources. A serum VEGF level of over 200 pg/mL associated with a serum progesterone level of under 18 ng/mL can distinguish intrauterine from extrauterine pregnancy with a specificity of 95% and a PPV of 92%. It is even more significant that it can distinguish ectopic from abnormal intrauterine pregnancy with a specificity of 95% and a PPV of 92%, which is better than either marker alone.[44,45]

Serum creatine kinase (CK)

Because CK is an enzyme present in muscle cells, it has been hypothesized that injury to these cells would cause an increase in its levels. Several prospective studies have found that it is not specific for tubal muscle cells and therefore is not useful as a serum marker in this setting.[46]

Radiologic assessment

Radiography

With the advances made in ultrasonography in the last 20 years, the routine use of radiographic films in the evaluation of AEP has been relegated to medical anecdotes. In the past, it was used predominantly for both suspected abdominal and saccular (within a uterine horn, such as in uterus didelphys) pregnancies,[15] with the pathognomonic finding on lateral films of an overlapping of the maternal spine by fetal parts.[46] Similarly associated findings are (1) a persistent and unusual position of the fetus; (2) a transverse lie with the back up and high in the abdomen; (3) the position of the fetal head oddly placed in relation to the trunk; (4) the maternal gas pattern overlying the fetus; (5) an unusually clearly appearing fetus, due to the absence of an intervening uterine wall or "uterine shadow"; and (6) in 2% of cases, after fetal death, the presence of calcifications, resulting in the formation of a lithopedion. In most cases, lithopedion is an incidental finding at autopsy, surgery, or imaging studies of the abdomen or pelvis, but it can also present with an acute abdomen secondary to a cecal volvulus or intestinal obstruction, a fistula, or even a pelvic abscess.

Ultrasonography

Since its inception, ultrasonography has revolutionized the management of ectopic pregnancy, and the combination of ultrasound and hCG levels is the diagnostic factor mainly responsible for the significant decrease in maternal morbidity and mortality rates in the last 25 years.[44] Current protocols utilize a serum hCG concentration of 3000 mIU/mL as the minimum level necessary to visualize intrauterine gestation on TVUS. This level in the absence of intrauterine pregnancy predicts ectopic pregnancy with a sensitivity and specificity of 100% and 99%, respectively.[44] Since ectopic pregnancies are generally associated with lower b-hCG levels than intrauterine pregnancies at similar lengths of gestation, they can often be visualized with TVUS at far lower levels of hCG. By transabdominal ultrasound, the threshold of detection of extrauterine pregnancy is set higher at 6000–6500 mIU/mL. Kadar et al.[47] reported that, regardless of singleton or multiple gestation, a sac can be seen sonographically beyond 38 days from the last menstrual period.

Undoubtedly, ultrasound has become extremely important in the diagnosis and management of AEP. Rarely is this more apparent than in the setting of abdominal pregnancy. Signs of abdominal pregnancy are a fetus separate from the uterus and extrauterine placenta (Figure 15.2). Interestingly, many of the same radiologic signs found on

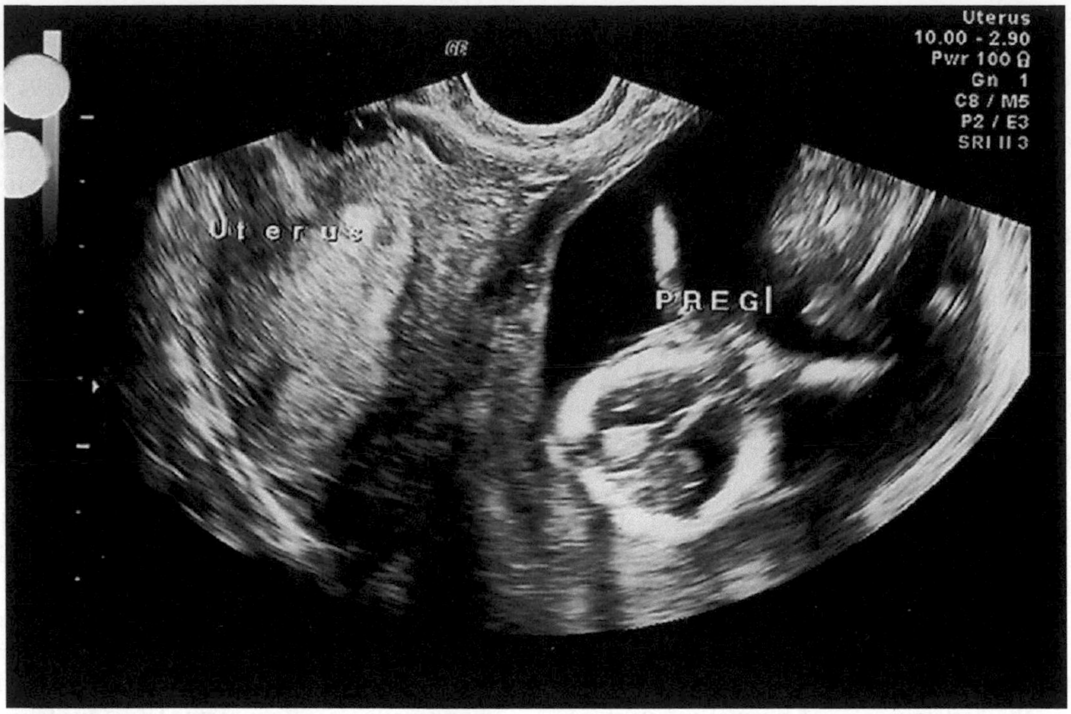

Figure 15.2 Ultrasound at 14 weeks of abdominal pregnancy. Note that uterus is adjacent to but not surrounding the fetus. (From Dahab AA et al., *J Med Case Rep*, 5, 531, 2011, published under open access.)

plain film (anteroposterior/lateral views) are those that are seen on abdominal ultrasound, albeit with far superior resolution and clarity. For example, the close approximation of the fetal parts to the abdominal wall, malpresentation of the fetus found high in the abdomen, and fetal parts overlying the maternal spine on a lateral scan, as well as the absence of the uterine wall between the maternal bladder and fetus, are all signs of abdominal pregnancy.[48]

Improvements have also been made in the diagnostic capabilities of ultrasonography in the evaluation of cervical pregnancy. The most important one has been in differentiating cervical pregnancy from various forms of abortion.[16] For the diagnosis of ovarian or intraligamentary pregnancy, ultrasonographic assessment is not as reliable. Ultrasound echoes do not delineate clearly the site of implantation; therefore, MRI or direct visualization is necessary in these situations. Color and pulsed Doppler, which can be used to assess blood flow, have been a useful adjunct to standard ultrasonography for the initial evaluation of all forms of extrauterine pregnancy. Color Doppler is used primarily to assess the enhanced blood flow surrounding a pregnancy sac, sometimes called the chorionic ring or "ring of fire" in light of its red appearance on color Doppler ultrasound. Studies utilizing color Doppler to quantify the difference in blood flow between the two sides of the adnexae have found a 20% increase in blood flow in the presence of ectopic pregnancy when compared with only an 8% increase in intrauterine pregnancies.[49] When color Doppler is added to standard ultrasonography, the sensitivity for diagnosing an ectopic pregnancy increases from 71% to 95%.[49]

Magnetic resonance imaging

MRI is not a first-line method of radiologic evaluation of pregnancy location, growth, or evaluation of abdominal pain. It is expensive and impractical for use in an emergency situation. However, it can aid in difficult cases when the resolution by TVUS is insufficient. For instance, hemorrhagic ascites is often hypointense to water on T2-weighted images, and a gestational sac with hematoma shows heterogeneous signal intensity displaying areas of low signal.[50] In the late second and third trimester it becomes progressively more difficult to assess the relationship of a fetus to adjacent myometrium or to distinguish myometrium from other intra-abdominal tissue using ultrasound alone. By producing images in multiple planes, MRI clearly demarcates the area of implantation. Thus, using MRI, a pregnancy in the broad ligament can easily be distinguished from intrauterine pregnancy.

MRI angiography and computer reconstruction may be utilized for preoperative planning to assess the location of placental tissue and to establish a complete map of the placental vasculature and its sources. MRI is useful in accurate localization of the placenta and its level and depth of adherence to surrounding tissue and detection of arterial and feeding vessels.[51] Blood vessels supporting the placenta may arise from various sources, including the infundibulopelvic ligaments, uterine arteries, mesenteric vessels, or other large vessels.[52] Therefore, a preoperative determination of the relationship between the placenta and surrounding organs can aid in the decision of whether or not to remove the placenta, and which other surgical teams (i.e., urology, vascular, or general surgery) should be present at the time of surgery. MRI can also be employed to monitor the precise location, as well as the involution of remaining placental tissue during postoperative treatment with MTX. MRI is safe for both the mother and the fetus because it does not use ionizing radiation. This holds true even in the first trimester of gestation.[7]

Fluoroscopic visualization for vascular mapping is also possible. Smrtka et al. utilized fluoroscopy to fully map the vascular supply of a bilobed placenta in a third trimester live abdominal pregnancy. As was done in that case, the catheters are generally left in situ after the angiography for use during surgery if embolization of the placental bed is necessary due to intraoperative hemorrhage.[53]

MANAGEMENT

Management, whether medical or surgical, is dependent on the gestational age and the site of implantation. Continuation of the pregnancy carries the possibility of fetal demise from inadequate perfusion at the placental site.[54] Occasionally, a patient desires conservative management despite the serious risks to both mother and fetus of continuing the pregnancy, and this situation requires immediate hospitalization and close monitoring of maternal and fetal well-being. Weekly ultrasound monitoring of fetal growth and, after the fetus reaches viability, nonstress tests twice per week are indicated in these situations. Shiu and Langer[5] reported the delivery of two surviving infants at, respectively, 28.5 and 33 weeks' gestation. Fetal assessment should begin in the second trimester after fetal viability if the mother refuses surgical intervention.

Medical management

The use of MTX has changed our approach to the treatment of early extrauterine pregnancies, and in selected cases of very early extrauterine pregnancy, is as effective as laparoscopy. MTX has a limited role, however, in the management of AEP. In the early 1980s, Tanaka and Miyazaki pioneered its use in the treatment of ectopic pregnancy, based on Li's work some 30 years before, when using the same antimetabolite in the treatment of choriocarcinoma.[55–57] While this is primarily indicated for cases of early unruptured tubal pregnancy in a hemodynamically stable patient, MTX can serve as an adjunct to surgical management or embolization in the treatment of AEP, since it can be used to facilitate the involution of placental tissue left in situ at the time of laparotomy. MTX interacts with actively proliferating trophoblasts, as well as other cells with a high mitotic index,[58,59] by functioning as a folic acid analog that disrupts the synthesis and repair of DNA, and the multiplication of cells by inhibiting dihydrofolate reductase.[60] Initially, most cases were treated with MTX protocols similar to those used in gestational trophoblastic disease with intramuscular (IM) MTX 1 mg/kg on days 1, 3, 5, and 7 and folinic acid (leucovorin rescue) 0.1 mg/kg on days 2, 4, 6, and 8.[61]

Today, the conversion to a single (50 mg/m^2 body surface area or approximately 1 mg/kg body weight) IM dose is most commonly used due to the efficacy and rare side effects compared with multidose regimens. The most common side effects associated with the administration of MTX are stomatitis, bone marrow depression, anorexia, and gastrointestinal disturbances, which, thanks to the modification in dosing regimens and addition of leucovorin to most extended protocols, are rarely reported today.[62]

There are no reports of the successful resolution of any gestation greater than 13 weeks treated with MTX alone. Lipscomb et al.[37] found that a high serum hCG (6500 mIU/mL) level is the most important factor associated with treatment failure and because advanced gestations are usually associated with levels well above this threshold for eligibility, MTX is usually reserved only for the treatment of trophoblastic tissue left in situ.

Surgical management

AEP carries a maternal mortality rate eight times higher than that of early extrauterine pregnancy.[63] Surgical management is generally similar for AEP cases, independent of the exact extrauterine location in the second and third trimester. However, there are some important considerations that must not be forgotten for optimal management.

In ovarian pregnancies, laparoscopy allows for diagnosis at an early gestational age and removal of the pregnancy tissue while attempting to conserve as much ovarian tissue as possible by wedge resection. In cases of advanced gestation, there is no alternative to the removal of the ovary and other adjacent structures.[64]

When a pregnancy is in the abdominal cavity or confined to the broad ligament, the ureter is an important consideration. Preoperative placement of a ureteral stent on the ipsilateral side, or bilaterally if necessary, may be useful for optimal visualization as the ureter courses under the uterine artery or more proximally along the pelvic brim. Proper localization of the ureter is effective at reducing and recognizing injury.[65]

Once delivery of the fetus is complete, the placenta may either be removed or left in situ and allowed to resorb after ligation of the umbilical cord. The residual placental tissue may be treated with MTX to accelerate absorption. If the placenta is left in situ, whether MTX is used or not, sepsis, intra-abdominal or pelvic abscess, delayed hemorrhage, adhesions, fistula formation, and urinary or gastrointestinal obstruction are all complications that should be anticipated and prevented, if possible.

In rudimentary horn pregnancies, the entire horn and ipsilateral fallopian tube should be removed. In these cases, the placental tissue can invade beyond the uterine decidua but generally not into the surrounding pelvic tissue, and can thus be removed intact at the primary surgery.[34]

Before proceeding with an operative intervention, it is essential to localize the placenta and identify its blood supply by MRI or arteriography.[66] Adequate preoperative preparation is essential in anticipation of massive blood loss from placental detachment and inability to ligate the vascular supply to the placental bed.

Cell saver, an autologous blood salvage system used intraoperatively, has proven to be an important tool to avoid or reduce the need for transfusion with donor blood. In women who are Rh negative, extra care needs to be taken to assess for contamination of maternal blood with fetal red cells. A Kleihauer–Betke test should be performed after an autologous transfusion is completed and the Rh-negative patient should be treated accordingly with anti-Rh(D) immune globulin as needed.[67]

Adjunctive use of arterial embolization

Initially developed for use in the gastrointestinal tract, arterial embolization is now applied to various other areas of the body for the control of hemorrhage. With regards to AEP management, arterial embolization is primarily reserved for abdominal and cervical pregnancy and is extremely effective in reducing the risk of hemorrhagic complications at the time of surgery for AEP. Rahaman et al. reported a 29-year-old primigravida who had a 21-week abdominal pregnancy treated with preoperative arterial embolization before laparoscopically assisted fetal delivery. Postoperatively, four cycles of MTX were administered at 50 mg/m^2 IM every 3 weeks for the retained abdominal placenta. Blood transfusion was not required and serial ultrasound and b-hCG measurements demonstrated complete involution 13 weeks after the last dose of MTX. Two years later, in a subsequent pregnancy the patient delivered a full-term infant.[68] In a similar case report, a 33-year old woman with an abdominal pregnancy presented at 33 weeks' gestation with fetal death. Preoperatively, the placental vasculature was embolized and after operative delivery of the fetus, the placenta was left in situ in an effort to preserve fertility given its implantation on the reproductive organs. The patient suffered prolonged postoperative ileus but otherwise recovered well. Placental function ceased after 2 months.[69] Cardosi et al.[69] recommend removing the placenta if possible even after embolization due to the risks of fibrosis and incomplete resorption.

In general, preoperative embolization of the placental bed has proven to be an effective method for reducing blood loss at the time of surgery for AEP and promotes the involution of trophoblastic tissue when the placenta is left in situ. Stents may be placed in the arterial vasculature supplying the placenta for preoperative embolization and may be utilized perioperatively as needed, allowing for expedited treatment. In cases of a planned delivery of a viable fetus, preoperatively placed stents can be utilized after delivery of the fetus. Whether or not embolization is employed, the delivery should be performed by experienced obstetrical surgeons, with extreme caution to avoid unexpected or premature separation of trophoblastic tissue that may hemorrhage.[70]

Intraoperative decision making: fate of the placenta

When dealing with abdominal pregnancy, after extraction of the fetus, the vexatious dilemma commonly encountered is whether to leave or remove the placenta, which may be adherent to vital abdominal structures including the bowel (Figure 15.3), iliac vessels, pelvic ligaments, hepatic portal vasculature, or spleen.[71] Separating the placenta may therefore lead to uncontrollable hemorrhage, but leaving it in situ may predispose the patient to abscess formation, pelvic ascites, or fibrosis.[72,73]

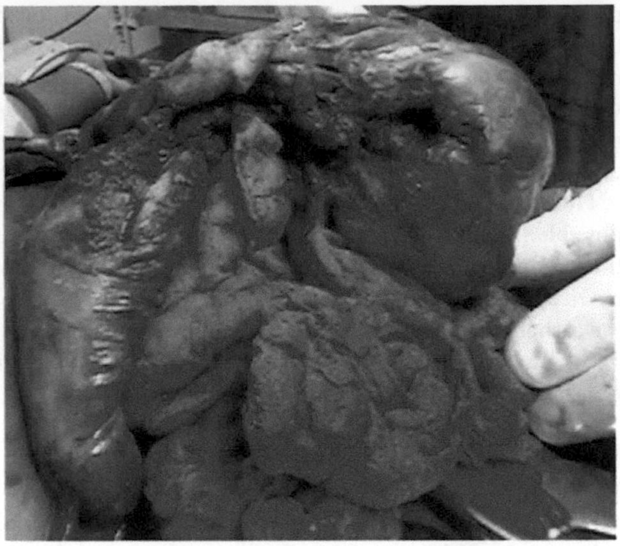

Figure 15.3 Placenta and membranes adherent to loop of bowel were left in situ after delivery of a full-term abdominal pregnancy. (From Masukume G et al., *J Med Case Rep*, 7, 10, 2013, published under open access.)

If the decision is made to remove the placenta, there should be adequate resources available for hemodynamic resuscitation should a hemorrhage occur. A multidisciplinary team including interventional radiology and other appropriate surgical subspecialties should be present or immediately available. Interventional radiologic techniques can often be utilized intraoperatively now due to the advent of hybrid operating suites. These suites combine full surgical and interventional radiology capabilities, and there has been an effort to utilize angiography for diagnostic and therapeutic purposes both preoperatively and intraoperatively, especially in cases of viable ectopic pregnancies.

If the decision is made to leave the placenta in situ due to the risk of hemorrhage or trauma to the surrounding tissue, extreme care must be taken. Using a very gentle technique so as not to dislodge the placenta, the cord should be cut close to its attachment on the placenta and excess membranes should be trimmed away. Most placentas left in situ will gradually undergo involution[42] and be absorbed uneventfully.[74] Valenzano et al. described the natural course of placental involution without the use of MTX in one abdominal pregnancy culminating in the delivery of a live infant at 30 weeks' gestation, at which time physicians elected to leave the placenta in situ. Placental involution was documented by serial b-hCG and color and pulsed Doppler sonography. The b-hCG value was negative 47 days postdelivery, and regression of placental volume over time coincided with a reduction in vascularization. At 11 months, placental volume had decreased by 82%, and after 5 years, the placenta was still present and appeared as a small residual echogenic mass with no vascularity.[74] When MTX is used as an adjunct to surgery, complete placental involution takes an average of 4–6 months. Huang et al. (2014) reported a case in which a patient was treated with oral mifepristone (50 mg twice daily [BID] for 12 days) postsurgically to cause slow degeneration and fibrosis of the placenta, followed by IM MTX (75 mg). By 3 months after surgery, the b-hCG was negative.[71]

Unfortunately, uncomplicated placental involution is not always the case. After surgery, rapid necrosis can lead to acute separation and hemorrhage. Abdominal pelvic abscess can be a very serious complication of retained placenta.[75] A second surgery to remove fibrotic residual tissue may be necessary if infection or other sequelae occur.[13]

CONCLUSION

In the last century, advances in medicine and technology have emerged to help propel us into an era of significant decreases in maternal mortality. Nowhere is this more apparent than in the setting of AEP. Developments in bioassays such as those for measuring hCG and imaging techniques such as ultrasonography, MRI, and angiography help clarify the pathogenesis and evolution of AEP by affording us the ability to deliver prompt and effective care without untoward consequences to the mother. Overall, there has been a significant advancement in the treatment of AEP and the importance of using a combined approach applying several therapeutic modalities cannot be overstated. Programs that promote early prenatal care make early intervention possible and significantly reduce morbidity.

ACKNOWLEDGMENT

The authors of this chapter acknowledge Armando E. Hernandez-Rey, who was an author of this chapter in the previous edition.

REFERENCES

1. Centers for Disease Control. Ectopic pregnancy—United States, 1988–1989. *MMWR Morb Mortal Wkly Rep* 1992; 41(32): 591–4.
2. Studdiford WE. Primary peritoneal pregnancy. *Am J Obstet Gynecol* 1942; 44: 487–91.
3. Friedrich EG Jr, Rankin CA Jr. Primary pelvic peritoneal pregnancy. *Obstet Gynecol* 1968; 31(5): 649–53.
4. Costa SD, Presley J, Bastert G. Advanced abdominal pregnancy. *Obstet Gynecol Surv* 1991; 46: 515–24.
5. Shiu AT, Langer A. Advanced extrauterine pregnancy. In: Iffy L, Apuzzio JJ, Vintzileos AM (eds), *Operative Obstetrics* (2nd edition), pp. 144–53. New York, NY: McGraw-Hill, 1992.
6. King G. Advanced extrauterine pregnancy. *Am J Obstet Gynecol* 1954; 67: 712–40.
7. Pritchard JA, MacDonald PC, Gant NF (eds). *Williams' Obstetrics* (17th edition), pp. 85–89. Norwalk, CT: Appleton-Century-Crofts, 1985.
8. Badria L, Amarin Z, Jaradat A et al. Full-term viable abdominal pregnancy: A case report and review. *Arch Gynecol Obstet* 2003; 268(4): 340–2.
9. Atrash HK, Friede A, Hogue CJR. Abdominal pregnancy in the United States: Frequency and maternal mortality. *Obstet Gynecol* 1987; 84: 1257–68.
10. Foster HW, Moore DT. Abdominal pregnancy. Report of 12 cases. *Obstet Gynecol* 1967; 30: 249–57.
11. Dahab AA, Aburass R, Shawkat W et al. Full-term extrauterine abdominal pregnancy: A case report. *J Med Case Rep* 2011; 5: 531.
12. Mengistu Z, Getachew A, Adefris M. Term abdominal pregnancy: A case report. *J Med Case Rep* 2015; 9: 168.
13. Masukume G, Sengurayi E, Muchara A et al. Full-term abdominal extrauterine pregnancy complicated by post-operative ascites with successful outcome: A case report. *J Med Case Rep* 2013; 7: 10.
14. Martin JN, Sessums K, Martin RW et al. Abdominal pregnancy: Current concepts of management. *Obstet Gynecol* 1988; 71: 549–56.
15. Beacham WD, Hernquist WC, Beacham DW et al. Abdominal pregnancy at Charity Hospital in New Orleans. *Am J Obstet Gynecol* 1962; 84: 1257–72.
16. Ushakov FB, Elchalal U, Aceman PJ et al. Cervical pregnancy: Past and future. *Obstet Gynecol Surv* 1997; 52: 45–59.
17. Parente JT, Ou CS, Levy J, Legatt E. Cervical pregnancy analysis: A review and report of five cases. *Obstet Gynecol* 1983; 62(1): 79–82.
18. Dicker D, Feldberg D, Samuel N, Goldman JA. Etiology of cervical pregnancy. Association with abortion, pelvic pathology, IUDs and Asherman's syndrome. *J Reprod Med* 1985; 30(1): 25–7.
19. Gaudoin MR, Coulter KL, Robins AM et al. Is the incidence of ovarian ectopic pregnancy increasing? *Eur J Obstet Gynecol Reprod Biol* 1996; 70(2): 141–3.
20. Raziel A, Golan A, Pansky M et al. Ovarian pregnancy: A report of twenty cases in one institution. *Am J Obstet Gynecol* 1990; 163(4 Pt 1): 1182–5.
21. Sandberg EC. Ovarian pregnancy. In: Langer A, Iffy L (eds), *Extrauterine Pregnancy*, pp. 245–53. Littleton, MA: PSG Publishing, 1986.
22. Lehfeldt H, Tietze C, Gorstein F. Ovarian pregnancy and the intrauterine device. *Am J Obstet Gynecol* 1970; 108: 1005–9.
23. Shibahara H, Funabiki M, Shiotani T et al. A case of primary ovarian pregnancy after in vitro fertilization and embryo transfer. *J Assist Reprod Genetic* 1997; 14: 63–4.
24. Spiegelberg O. Zur Casuistik der Ovarialschwangerschaft. *Arch fur Gynakol* 1873; 13: 73.
25. Elwell KE, Sailors JL, Denson PK et al. Unruptured second-trimester ovarian pregnancy. *J Obstet Gynaecol Res* 2015; 41(9): 1483–86.
26. Vorapong P, Ruangsak L, Surang T et al. Pregnancy in the broad ligament. *Arch Gynecol Obstet* 2003; 268: 233–5.

27. Dorfman SF. Deaths from ectopic pregnancy, United States, 1979–1980. *Obstet Gynecol* 1983; 62: 344–8.
28. Nahum GG. Rudimentary uterine horn pregnancy. The 20th-century worldwide experience of 588 cases. *J Reprod Med* 2002; 47(2): 151–63.
29. Lewis AD, Levine D. Pregnancy complications in women with uterine duplication abnormalities. *Ultrasound Q* 2010; 26(4): 193–200.
30. Nahum GG, Stanislaw H, McMahon C. Preventing ectopic pregnancies: How often does transperitoneal transmigration of sperm occur in effecting human pregnancy? *BJOG* 2004; 111(7): 706–14.
31. Nishi H, Funayama H, Fukumine N et al. Rupture of pregnant noncommunicating rudimentary uterine horn with fetal salvage: A case report. *Arch Gynecol Obstet* 2003; 268(3): 224–6.
32. Pillai SA, Mathew M, Ishrat N et al. Ruptured rudimentary horn pregnancy diagnosed by preoperative magnetic resonance imaging resulting in fetal salvage. *Sultan Qaboos Univ Med J* 2015; 15(3): e429–32.
33. Fekih M, Memmi A, Nouri S et al. Asymptomatic horn rudimentary pregnant uterine rupture with a viable fetus. *Tunis Med* 2009; 87(9): 633–6.
34. Reichman D, Laufer MR, Robinson BK. Pregnancy outcomes in unicornuate uteri: A review. *Fertil Steril* 2009; 91(5): 1886–94.
35. Canis M, Wattiez A, Pouly JL et al. Laparoscopic management of unicornuate uterus with rudimentary horn and unilateral extensive endometriosis: Case report. *Hum Reprod* 1990; 5(7): 819–20.
36. Nezhat F, Nezhat C, Bess O, Nezhat CH. Laparoscopic amputation of a noncommunicating rudimentary horn after a hysteroscopic diagnosis: A case study. *Surg Laparosc Endosc* 1994; 4(2): 155–6.
37. Lipscomb GH, Stovall TG, Ling FW. Nonsurgical treatment of ectopic pregnancy. *N Engl J Med* 2000; 343: 1325–9.
38. Braunstein GD, Rasor J, Adler D et al. Serum human chorionic gonadotropin levels throughout normal pregnancy. *Am J Obstet Gynecol* 1976; 152: 299–303.
39. Barnhart K, Sammel MD, Chung K et al. Decline of serum human chorionic gonadotropin and spontaneous complete abortion: Defining the normal curve. *Obstet Gynecol* 2004; 104(5 Pt 1): 975–81.
40. Tay JI, Moore J, Walker JJ. Ectopic pregnancy. *BMJ* 2000; 320: 916–19.
41. Mol BWJ, Hajenius PJ, Engelsbel S et al. Serum human chorionic gonadotropin measurement in the diagnosis of ectopic pregnancy when transvaginal sonography is inconclusive. *Fertil Steril* 1998; 70: 972–81.
42. Connolly A, Ryan DH, Stuebe AM, Wolfe HM. Reevaluation of discriminatory and threshold levels for serum beta-hCG in early pregnancy. *Obstet Gynecol* 2013; 121(1): 65–70.
43. McCord ML, Muram D, Buster JE et al. Single serum progesterone as a screen for ectopic pregnancy: Exchanging specificity and sensitivity to obtain optimal test performance. *Fertil Steril* 1996; 66: 513–16.
44. Lemus JF. Ectopic pregnancy: An update. *Curr Opin Obstet Gynecol* 2000; 12: 369–75.
45. Daniel Y, Geva E, Lerner-Geva L et al. Levels of vascular endothelial growth factor are elevated in patients with ectopic pregnancy: Is this a novel marker? *Fertil Steril* 1999; 72: 1013–17.
46. Borlum KG, Blorn R. Primary hepatic pregnancy. *Int J Gynecol Obstet* 1988; 27: 427–43.
47. Kadar N, Bohrer M, Kemmann E et al. The discriminatory human chorionic gonadotropin zone for endovaginal sonography: A prospective, randomized study. *Fertil Steril* 1994; 61: 1016–21.
48. Ombelet W, Vandermerve JV, Van Assche FA et al. Advanced extrauterine pregnancy: Description of 38 cases with literature survey. *Obstet Gynecol Surv* 1988; 43: 386–92.
49. Stenchever MA, Droegmuller W, Herbst AL, Mishell DR (eds). *Comprehensive Gynecology* (4th edition), pp. 443–78. Norwalk, CT: Mosby, 2001.
50. Nishino M, Hayakawa K, Iwasaku K et al. Magnetic resonance imaging findings in gynecologic emergencies. *J Comput Assist Tomogr* 2003; 27: 564–70.
51. Kao LY, Scheinfeld MH, Chernyak V et al. Beyond ultrasound: CT and MRI of ectopic pregnancy. *AJR Am J Roentgenol* 2014; 202(4): 904–11.
52. Malian V, Lee JH. MR imaging and MR angiography of an abdominal pregnancy with placental infarction. *AJR Am J Roentgenol* 2001; 177(6): 1305–6.
53. Smrtka MP, Gunatilake R, Miller MJ et al. Improving the management of an advanced extrauterine pregnancy using pelvic arteriography in a hybrid operating suite. *AJP Rep* 2012; 2(1): 63–6.
54. Gilbert W, Moore J, Resnick R. Angiographic embolization in the management of hemorrhagic complications of pregnancy. *Am J Obstet Gynecol* 1992; 116: 43–9.
55. Li MC, Hertz A, Spencer DB. Effect of methotrexate therapy on choriocarcinoma and chorioadenoma. *Proc Soc Exp Biol Med* 1956; 93: 361–6.
56. Tanaka T, Hayashi H, Kutsuzawa T et al. Treatment of interstitial ectopic pregnancy with methotrexate: Report of a successful case. *Fertil Steril* 1982; 37: 851–2.
57. Miyazaki Y, Shrina Y, Wake N et al. Studies on nonsurgical therapy of tubal pregnancy. *Acta Obstet Gynaecol Jpn* 1983; 35: 489.
58. Berkowitz RS, Goldstein DP, Bernstein MR. Ten years' experience with methotrexate and folinic acid as primary therapy for gestational trophoblastic disease. *Gynecol Oncol* 1986; 23: 111–18.
59. Gabbe SG, Niebyl JR, Simpson JL (eds). *Obstetrics: Normal and Problem Pregnancies* (4th edition), pp. 745–6. London, UK: Churchill Livingstone, 2002.
60. Takimoto CH. Antifolates in clinical development. *Semin Oncol* 1997; 24 (5 Suppl 18): S18–40–51.
61. Yankowitz J, Leake J, Hugguns G et al. Cervical ectopic pregnancy: Review of the literature and report of a case treated by single-dose methotrexate therapy. *Obstet Gynecol Surv* 1990; 45: 405–14.

62. Maymon R, Shulman A, Maymon BBS et al. Ectopic pregnancy, the new gynecological epidemic disease: Review of the modern work-up and the nonsurgical treatment option. *Int J Fertil* 1992; 37: 146–64.
63. Atrash HK, Friede A, Hogue CJ. Abdominal pregnancy in the United States: Frequency and maternal mortality. *Obstet Gynecol* 1987; 69(3 Pt 1): 333–7.
64. Tulandi T, Saleh A. Surgical management of ectopic pregnancy. *Clin Obstet Gynecol* 1999; 42: 31–8.
65. Tanaka Y, Asada H, Kuji N, Yoshimura Y. Ureteral catheter placement for prevention of ureteral injury during laparoscopic hysterectomy. *J Obstet Gynaecol Res* 2008; 34(1): 67–72.
66. Tulandi T, Sammour A. Evidenced-based management of ectopic pregnancy. *Curr Opin Obstet Gynecol* 2000; 12: 289–92.
67. Sullivan I, Faulds J, Ralph C. Contamination of salvaged maternal blood by amniotic fluid and fetal red cells during elective Caesarean section. *Br J Anaesth* 2008; 101(2): 225–9.
68. Rahaman J, Berkowitz R, Mitty H et al. Minimally invasive management of an advanced abdominal pregnancy. *Obstet Gynecol* 2004; 103: 1064–8.
69. Cardosi RJ, Nackley AC, Londono J et al. Embolization for advanced abdominal pregnancy with a retained placenta: A case report. *J Reprod Med* 2002; 47: 861–3.
70. Strafford JC, Ragan WD. Abdominal pregnancy: Review of current management. *Obstet Gynecol* 1977; 50: 548–58.
71. Huang K, Song L, Wang L et al. Advanced abdominal pregnancy: An increasingly challenging clinical concern for obstetricians. *Int J Clin Exp Pathol* 2014; 7(9): 5461–72.
72. Cagnazzi A, Landi S, Volpe A. Rhythmic variation in the rate of ectopic pregnancy throughout the year. *Am J Obstet Gynecol* 1999; 180: 67–71.
73. Babic D, Colic G, Mrden D. Complications after surgery for abdominal pregnancy due to retained placenta. *Ginekol Obstet* 1983; 23: 93–4.
74. Cetinkaya MB, Kokcu A, Alper T. Follow up of the regression of the placenta left in situ in an advanced abdominal pregnancy using the Cavalieri method. *J Obstet Gynaecol Res* 2005; 31(1): 22–6.
75. Worley KC, Hnat MD, Cunningham FG. Advanced extrauterine pregnancy: Diagnostic and therapeutic challenges. *Am J Obstet Gynecol* 2008; 198(3): 297. e1–7.

The role of cesarean delivery in the management of fetal malformations

16

NADIA B. KUNZIER, TRACY ADAMS, MARTIN R. CHAVEZ, and ANTHONY M. VINTZILEOS

CONTENTS

INTRODUCTION

Human development is an intricate and continuous process determined by genetics and environment. Major structural anomalies are recognized at birth in approximately 3% of all neonates.[1] Ultrasound resolution and accuracy continue to improve, thus allowing for early prenatal diagnosis. Utilization of this technology allows for maximization of management options for the patient and her caregivers. The first step with any prenatally diagnosed fetal malformation is to determine its prognosis. In general, invasive diagnostic testing should be offered as the risk of aneuploidy increases in the presence of congenital malformations. Early diagnosis and understanding of prognosis allow for discussions of in utero treatments, which may be available in certain centers, and also for condition-specific subspecialists to become involved in the patient's care throughout gestation.

This chapter will discuss the role of cesarean delivery for fetal malformations. We will review the indications for cesarean delivery for both lethal and nonlethal malformations and also outline the fundamental concepts that should guide intrapartum management decisions.

LETHAL MALFORMATIONS

Congenital malformations, deformations, and chromosomal abnormalities are the leading causes of infant death in the United States.[2] Prenatal ultrasound is an effective tool for the identification of fetal malformations with reported detection rates of up to 80% for major fetal anomalies.[3] This means that many women who seek prenatal care will know about a fetal malformation prior to birth and have the opportunity to decide upon the course of their pregnancy. When a lethal malformation is identified, a woman may choose discontinuation of pregnancy; however, there are many circumstances in which the pregnancy will be continued. There is debate surrounding the use of the term "lethal" when referring to fetal malformations.[4] However, for the purpose of this article, the term "lethal malformation" is used to describe fetal anomalies in which the overwhelming majority of affected fetuses are stillborn or die within the first year of birth. Some examples of lethal malformations are shown in Table 16.1 and Figures 16.1 and 16.2. The decision to continue affected pregnancies can be due to maternal choice, religious, or fundamental beliefs, socioeconomic concerns or due to state legal regulations with regards to gestational age limits for termination of pregnancy. It is noteworthy that many women (40%–85%) may choose to continue a pregnancy affected by a lethal malformation to term when they are offered a perinatal hospice program.[5–7] Perinatal hospice is described as a multidisciplinary approach incorporating prenatal diagnosis, grief management, and hospice care to address the needs of women with a fetal diagnosis of a lethal malformation.[8]

Vaginal delivery is the preferred route for fetuses with lethal fetal anomalies in order to avoid the added morbidities of cesarean delivery including hemorrhage, thromboembolism, infection, and risk to future reproductive health. However, cesarean delivery may be necessary for reasons of *maternal safety*, *maternal request*, or *dystocia*.

Table 16.1 Commonly detected fetal malformations.

Lethal	Nonlethal
Acrania	Spina bifida and hydrocephalus
Exencephaly	Facial and cervical masses
Iniencephaly	Omphalocele
Alobar holoprosencephaly	Nonsolid masses
Hydranencephaly	Sacrococcygeal teratoma
Trisomy 13[a]	
Trisomy 18[a]	
Renal agenesis	
Obstructive uropathy with long-standing anhydramnios	
Lethal skeletal dysplasias:	
Thanatophoric dysplasia	
Short rib polydactyly syndromes	
Campomelic dysplasia	
Osteogenesis imperfecta type 2	
Hypophosphatasia congenital	
Meckel–Gruber syndrome	

[a] Excluding mosaicism.

Maternal safety

Maternal safety must be considered first when deciding on the route of delivery. In cases of abnormal placentation (placenta previa or suspected placenta accreta) cesarean delivery should be performed to avoid maternal hemorrhage. If the patient has obstetrical factors predisposing to uterine rupture, such as prior classical cesarean delivery, prior uterine rupture, myomectomy, or more than two previous cesarean deliveries, the risk of uterine rupture must be weighed against the risk of cesarean delivery. One should keep in mind that during labor a nonreassuring heart rate tracing is often one of the first signs of uterine rupture.[9] If there is a considerable maternal risk from vaginal delivery, due to hemorrhage or uterine rupture, then cesarean delivery should be offered regardless of fetal prognosis.

Maternal request

For many women who choose to continue a pregnancy affected by a lethal fetal malformation, their only desire may be to see their infant alive. Their desire could be to hold a live infant or have a religious ceremony performed prior to death. If this is the desire of the patient and her family, a discussion regarding intrapartum fetal monitoring and the possibility of cesarean delivery for fetal indications should be raised. In such cases, as long as the patient expresses an understanding of the severity of the fetal condition and the increased risks associated with cesarean delivery, the patient's wishes should be upheld.[8–10]

Dystocia

Due to the physical characteristics of some of the lethal malformations, cesarean delivery may be indicated due to dystocia reasons. Important characteristics to evaluate sonographically prior to deciding the route of delivery include fetal biometry, fetal positioning, and the fetal head circumference to abdominal circumference ratio. In disorders such as *hydranencephaly* or *alobar holoprosencephaly with hydrocephalus present*, the fetal head may be too large to pass through the maternal pelvis. This will most likely lead to labor dystocia and the need for subsequent cesarean delivery. There are reports of cepahlocentesis to decreased fetal head size and allow for vaginal delivery[11]; however, it is important that the patient understands that the procedure itself can lead to fetal death and not all cases result in progression to vaginal delivery. An example of a lethal fetal malformation which can lead to labor dystocia due to abnormal fetal positioning is *iniencephaly*. Iniencephaly is a rare neural tube defect in which there is a dysraphism of the cervical spine with a fixed retroflexed fetal head and lordosis of the spine.[12] If carried to term, labor dystocia is common and cesarean delivery is often indicated. One report from Chile, where elective termination is not legal, recommends offering preterm induction of labor to decrease the risk of cephalopelvic disproportion.[12] Another fetal anomaly with the potential for dystocia is *Meckel–Gruber syndrome*, since these fetuses at term have a significantly larger abdominal circumference when compared with head circumference. Meckel–Gruber syndrome is classically described as a triad of encephalocele, bilateral multicystic kidneys, and postaxial polydactyly. The increased abdominal circumference is due to enlarged kidneys and at term this can lead to cephalopelvic disproportion and need for cesarean delivery.

Although several other fetal syndromes may lead to labor dystocia, the aforementioned fetal malformations are the most common examples which highlight the importance of fetal evaluation of fetal biometry and proportions, as well as fetal positioning, when contemplating the delivery mode of a patient with a known fetal lethal anomaly.

NONLETHAL MALFORMATIONS

Similarly to lethal malformations, decisions regarding mode of delivery in cases of nonlethal malformations should be taken in a multistep-wise approach. Sonographic imaging and invasive testing are crucial in establishing accurate diagnosis and prognosis, thus facilitating patient counseling. In some cases, a fetal diagnosis may be made after a single sonographic evaluation, and if the long-term prognosis is known, it can be communicated with the parents at that point. However, often times, serial ultrasound examinations may be necessary to reach the correct diagnosis or to understand the progression of disease. This may be followed by offering additional invasive diagnostic testing to determine etiology, arrange prenatal subspecialty consultation, and guide further treatments. A nurse navigator can be very helpful in scheduling all necessary appointments with the appropriate pediatric subspecialty consultants. The

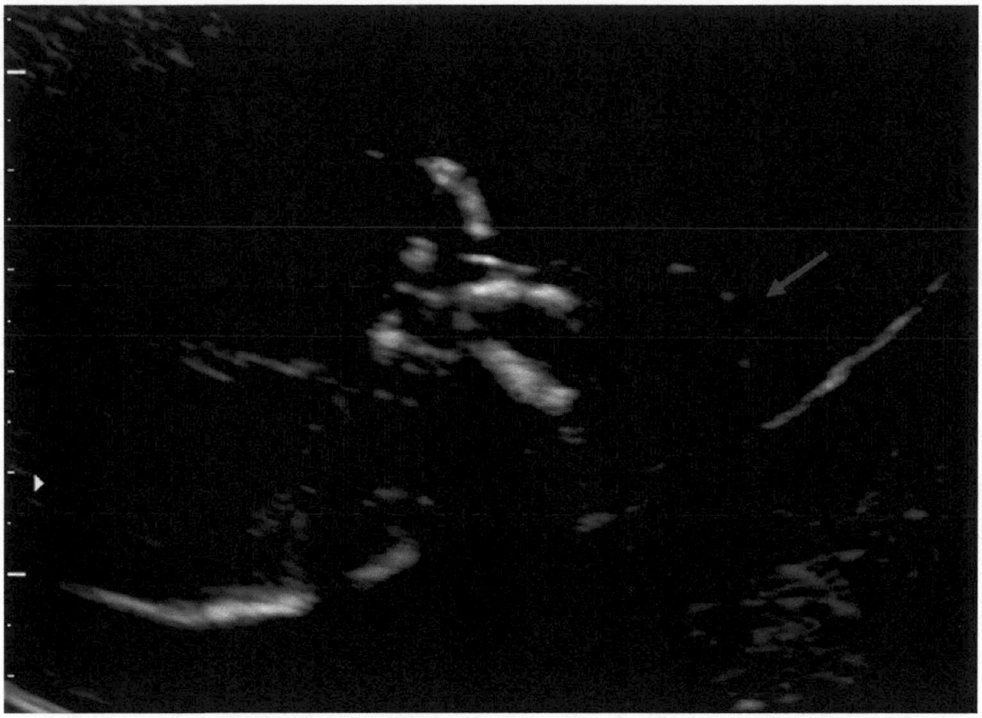

Figure 16.1 Sagittal view of anencephalic fetus at 16 weeks' gestation with arrow demonstrating free-floating brain and absence of calvaria.

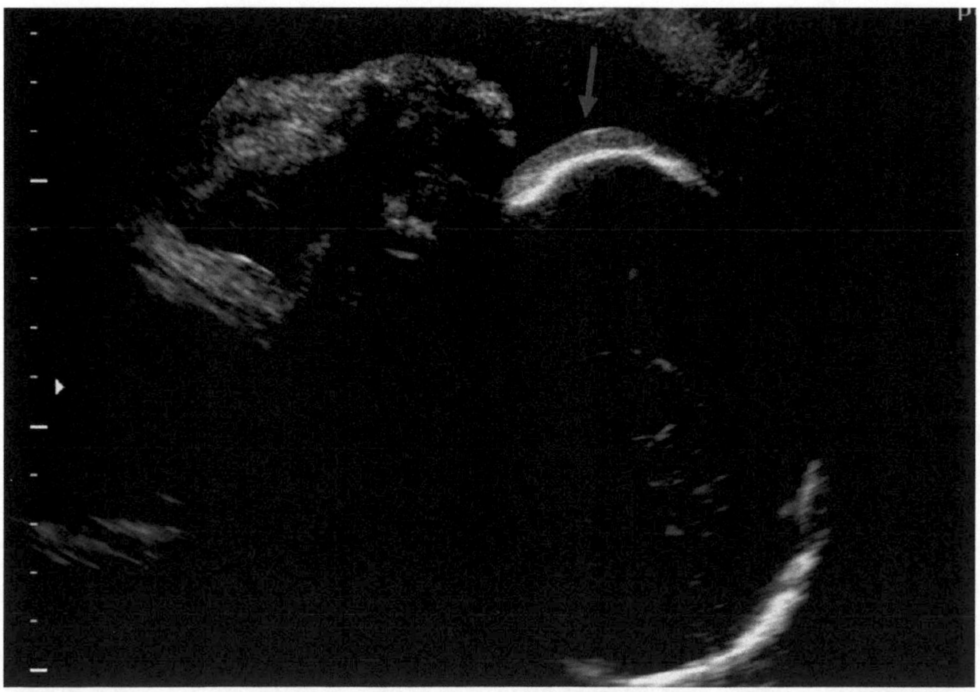

Figure 16.2 Sagittal scan of a fetus affected with thanatophoric skeletal dysplasia with arrow demonstrating an increased fetal head anteroposterior (AP) diameter and prefrontal thickening at 32 weeks' gestation.

mode of delivery is often determined in consultation with the pediatric consultants who may need to be available at birth. However, in some cases, especially those which evolve throughout gestation, it is impossible to determine the optimal delivery mode until late in the third trimester.

It is important to counsel patients that not all congenital malformations have shown to benefit from cesarean delivery. There is a significant maternal morbidity associated with nonindicated cesarean delivery and the choice of this delivery option should optimize both maternal safety and neonatal outcomes, keeping in mind the same principles as previously described in cases of lethal malformations. In these cases, however, the decision for cesarean delivery should be made if there is increased likelihood for neonatal morbidity from a vaginal birth. Fetal malformations which may lead to cephalopelvic disproportion or dystocia will benefit from cesarean delivery, thus reducing the risk for maternal tissue trauma and/or uterine rupture. Likewise, there may be some specific fetal conditions that require immediate medical or surgical intervention. Such cases may benefit from a timed cesarean delivery when all necessary pediatric subspecialists are available. Below are described some of the most common prenatally diagnosed fetal malformations requiring cesarean delivery.

Spina bifida and hydrocephalus

Neural tube defects are a heterogeneous group of congenital structural anomalies of the spinal column and brain which occur in isolation (80%) or in association with genetic syndromes.[13] The etiology and severity of the deformity will often guide consultation and management strategies. The subgroup of neural tube defects which are nonlethal carry a wide spectrum of neonatal prognosis and often pose a challenge to the managing perinatal team. Prenatal diagnosis relies on a thorough ultrasound examination with precise description of cranial and spinal findings, as well as any other associated anomalies.

Spinal bifida (Figures 16.3 and 16.4) is one of the most common nonlethal congenital anomalies of the central nervous system with myelomeningocele being the most frequent form.[14] Meningoceles typically have relatively benign neurologic sequelae, whereas myelomeningoceles are most frequently associated with various degrees of neurological impairment. Prognosis is dependent on the level of the spinal segment abnormality, the extent of the lesion, etiology, and presence of associated anomalies[15]; invasive diagnostic testing should be offered to these patients as there is an increased risk of chromosomal abnormalities especially in the presence of associated anomalies.[16] Prognosis is poor when spina bifida is associated with chromosomal abnormalities or genetic syndromes. In isolation, the extent of the defect and the affected location will determine the neurologic disability. However, the severity of the neonatal deficit depends not only on the malformation itself but also on the in utero duration of the exposure of the neural tissues to the amniotic fluid.[17] Based on this theory, intrauterine fetal surgical repair of the anatomical defect has been attempted in order to minimize exposure of the neural elements to amniotic fluid, thus improving neonatal and long-term outcomes. Since the maternal and fetal risks associated with these procedures, especially when done via open fetal surgery, are considerable a fetoscopic approach has been recently advocated.[18] Once the diagnosis and extent of disease is determined, management options, including fetal surgery, should be tailored according to prognosis and after taking into consideration the patient's wishes.[14]

Historically, most authors have advocated that cesarean delivery is superior to vaginal birth in cases of myelomeningocele. The hypothesis was that cesarean delivery prevented mechanical forces of labor which would further damage the already compromised and exposed neural tissue.[19] However, more recent data suggest that elective cesarean delivery, when compared with vaginal birth, is not associated with improved long-term outcomes or

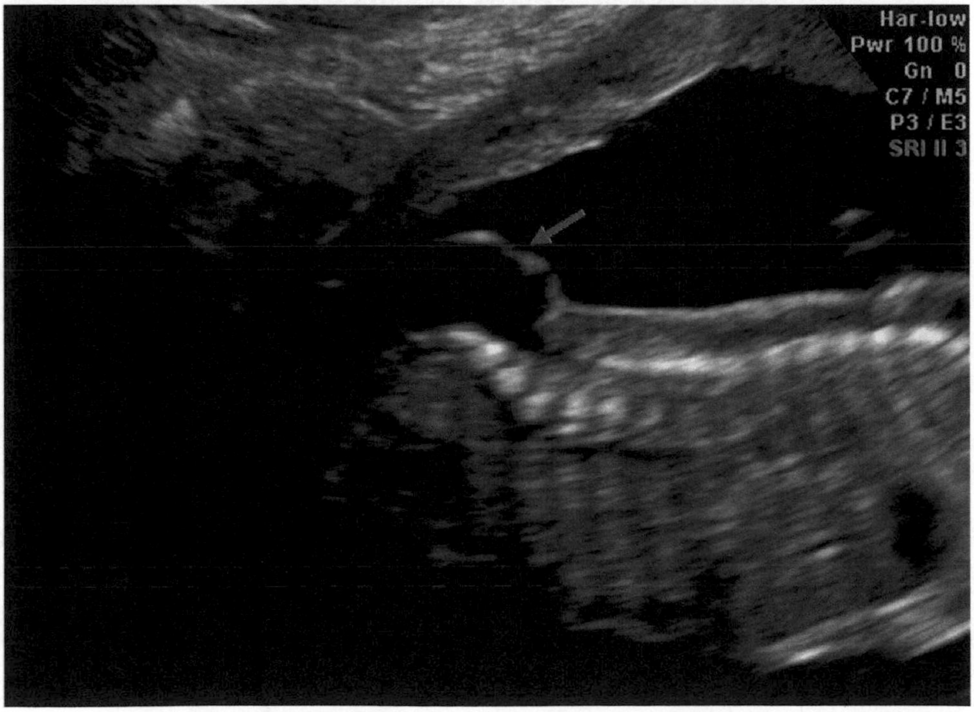

Figure 16.3 Fetal spine with spina bifida at 18 weeks' gestation with arrow indicating level of spinal defect.

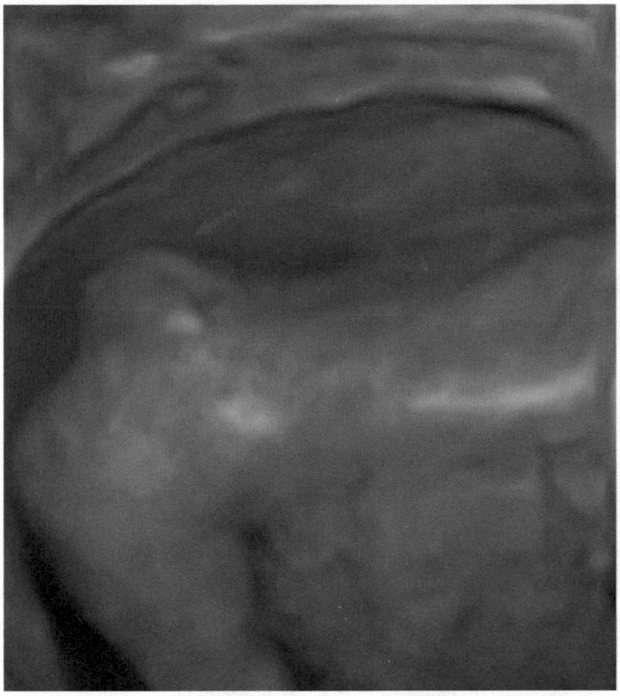

Figure 16.4 Three-dimensional image of the fetal spine demonstrating accuracy of diagnosing levels affected with spina bifida at 18 weeks' gestation with arrow indicating spinal defect.

decreased neurological impairment over vaginal delivery, regardless of anatomical location of the lesion.[20,21] Therefore, at the present time it seems reasonable to consider a trial of labor, especially in the presence of small flat defects or skin-covered defects. However, for large defects (>5 cm) cesarean delivery may be justified to reduce the risk of sac disruption and dystocia. Additionally, consideration should be given to other factors such as geographical area of practice and availability of neonatal specialists to evaluate and or treat the neonate immediately after birth. A timed delivery may be appropriate in cases where urgent neonatal care is expected by subspecialists.

Isolated hydrocephalus (Figure 16.5) or hydrocephalus associated with neural tube defects is considered as a nonlethal fetal malformation where cesarean delivery is most often necessary. When assessing for appropriate mode of delivery, fetal biometry should be monitored, especially in the third trimester. Cases of significant hydrocephalus in a fetus with a hopeful prognosis should be delivered by cesarean delivery to decrease perinatal mortality and morbidity. Vaginal delivery in these cases may lead to cephalopelvic disproportion, dystocia, and increased risk of maternal hemorrhage, secondary to protracted labor, and uterine rupture.

Fetal facial and cervical masses

Cystic hygromas (Figure 16.6) are typically diagnosed in the first trimester and are generally located in the posteriolateral aspect of the fetal neck. Large hygromas, however, can become very broad and extend beyond this region into the fetal face and thorax. More than half of all prenatally diagnosed cystic hygromas are associated with chromosomal anomalies and 30% of those with a normal karyotype have associated anomalies.[22] Large cystic hygromas and those persisting beyond 14 weeks are at an even higher risk of aneuploidy.[22] Fetal hydrops in combination with cystic hygroma is uniformly lethal. Invasive diagnostic testing should be offered to determine prognosis. In patients with normal chromosomal analysis, serial ultrasound examinations and fetal echocardiography are recommended. Cyst aspiration throughout gestation has not been associated with decreased neonatal morbidity or deformity. However, there may be a role for aspiration around the time of delivery to decompress the cyst and attempt vaginal birth by allowing the cardinal movements of labor to occur. This decompression may also help in securing an airway for the neonate. In certain circumstances with an isolated large cervical mass, the fetus may benefit from cesarean delivery at a tertiary care center with pediatric surgeons and maternal–fetal medicine specialists who can perform an ex utero intrapartum treatment (EXIT procedure), which allows for an endotracheal tube to be placed while the blood supply to the neonate remains placental in origin.[23] EXIT procedures are generally performed at or near term in fetuses that meet certain criterion for eligibility based on sonographic imaging (deviation/compression/obstruction of the airway and involvement of the floor of the mouth) which place them at a very high risk of airway obstruction and difficult intubation at the time of delivery.

Other facial and cervical occupying masses (facial and cervical teratomas) follow the same principle for delivery management. Although the majority of facial teratomas are benign, they often carry a very poor prognosis as they arise from the oral cavity and have the potential to completely replace cranial contents. Cervical teratomas are also typically benign tumors in nature, although they do have malignant potential, but have the added possible complication of pulmonary hypoplasia secondary to in utero compression on the fetal thorax. Invasive diagnostic testing to access for aneuploidy is recommended, especially when additional malformations are present. In cases, where a solid, or partially solid, mass creates a nonmobile, hyperextended fetal neck, vaginal birth may be unachievable as the fetus presents with a mechanical blockade to the cardinal movements of labor. Therefore, cesarean delivery at or near term is recommended with possible implementation of an EXIT procedure in carefully selected cases.

Omphalocele

By approximately 12 weeks, gestation, after completion of the physiologic inward rotation of the midgut, the diagnosis of omphalocele can be made (Figure 16.7). Omphaloceles are midline defects of the anterior abdominal wall with herniation of the abdominal contents covered by a two-layer membrane composed of amnion and peritoneum. A detailed anatomical survey at this time can help to

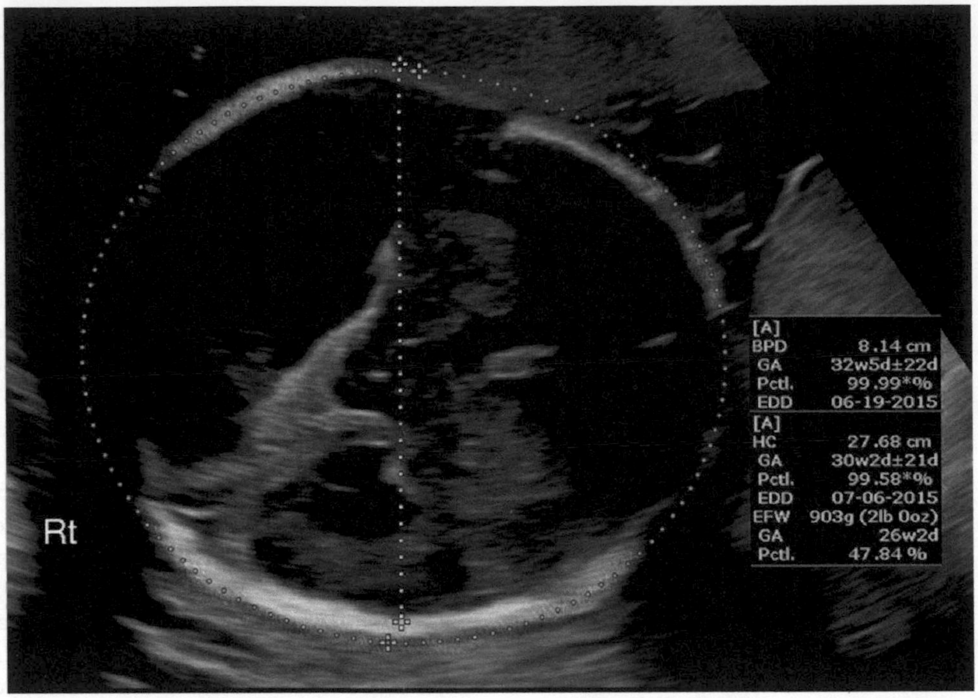

Figure 16.5 Coronal image demonstrating hydrocephalus at 26 weeks' gestation.

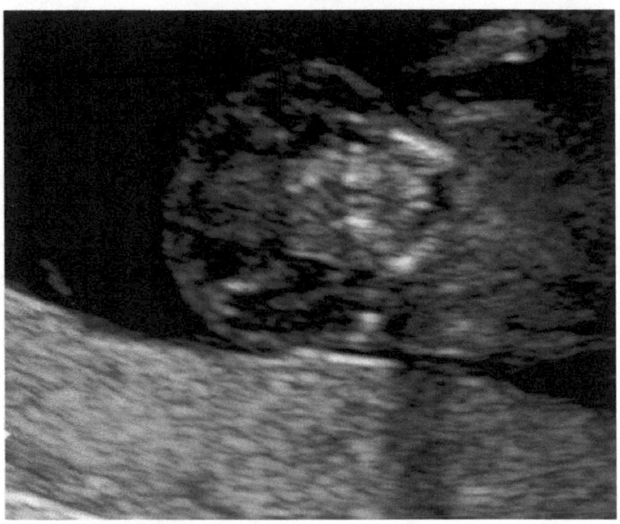

Figure 16.6 Large septated cystic hygroma at 13 weeks' gestation with arrow pointing to posteriolateral neck mass.

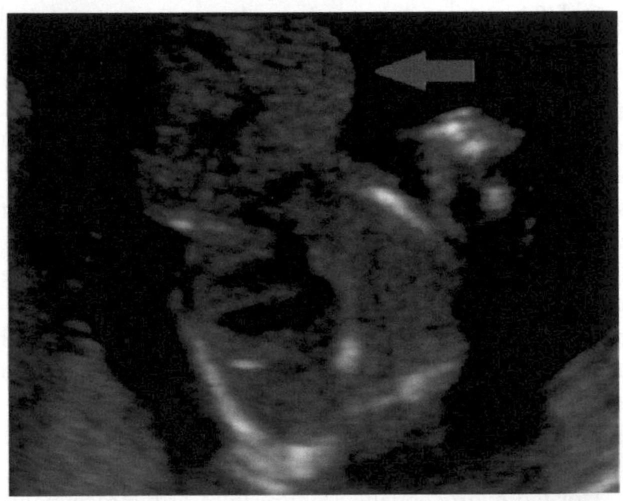

Figure 16.7 Tranverse abdominal view of fetus with omphalocele at 18 weeks' gestation with arrow pointing to the herniated abdominal organs.

determine the etiology and associated malformations present. Invasive diagnostic testing should be offered to determine prognosis and guide management. Omphaloceles are classified and managed according to the presence or absence of other associated anomalies, as well as the size and contents of the herniated sac. Omphaloceles are typically considered small if they are less than 5 cm and contain bowel and stomach but no liver. Omphaloceles greater than 5 cm containing bowel, stomach, and liver are classified as large or giant. It is possible for the omphaloceal sac to rupture resulting in free-floating abdominal organs in the amniotic cavity.[24] The size of the defect and presence of extracorporeal liver have been associated with a greater likelihood of associated anomalies and genetic syndromes. Omphaloceles with extracorporeal liver have an increased risk of associated cardiac, limb, and renal malformations, whereas small omphaloceles have an increased risk of associated gastrointestinal and central nervous system (CNS) anomalies.[25] The vast majority of omphaloceles have associated anomalies with only approximately 30% being isolated. The remaining 70% are associated with chromosomal anomalies, single gene disorders, and genetic syndromes.[25] Fetal echocardiography should be performed as approximately 50% of cases have associated cardiac defects.[26]

Intrapartum management in nonlethal cases should be based on omphalocele classification. Trial of labor should be offered in cases of small omphaloceles as cesarean delivery is not associated with improved maternal or neonatal outcomes. However, in giant omphaloceles with extracorporeal liver, cesarean delivery should be offered at or near term (in the absence of indications for earlier delivery) to prevent labor dystocia, sac rupture, and trauma to abdominal viscera.[24] Ideally, these fetuses should be delivered in a tertiary care center where experienced medical and surgical pediatric subspecialists are available to care for these neonates.

Nonsolid masses

Virtually any organ system or potential peritoneal space can be the location of fluid collection forming a nonsolid fetal mass. Diagnosis and etiology can often times be made by ultrasound alone. However, in some cases sampling of the fluid may be necessary in order to provide clues regarding the origin of the collection (i.e., urine ascites or urinoma), kidney function (distended fetal bladder) (Figure 16.8), or etiology (i.e., pleural effusion for diagnosing fetal chylothorax). Once a specific diagnosis is made, the pregnancy is monitored closely with ultrasound surveillance and often times with repeat fluid sampling or drainage to preserve organ function (i.e., bladder outlet obstruction to preserve renal function). Timing and mode of delivery should be case specific. Fetal biometry should be assessed prior to delivery to determine risks of labor dystocia as these patients may have increased abdominal circumference. The majority of the patients should be allowed trial of labor. In some cases consideration may be given to draining the fluid around the delivery time in order to reduce the neonatal effects of increased diaphragmatic pressure and respiratory compromise, and possibly decrease the fetal abdominal circumference, thus reducing the need for cesarean delivery secondary to dystocia.

Sacrococcygeal teratoma

Sacrococcygeal teratomas (Figure 16.9) are exophytic tumors consisting of cystic and solid components arising from the fetal coccyx. Fetal hydrops and intrauterine demise secondary to high output cardiac failure can occur in large, highly vascularized tumors. Intrauterine fetal interventions including amnioreduction, tumor resection, and, most recently, minimally invasive percutaneous fetal surgery with vascular laser ablation have been implemented in order to improve perinatal outcomes.[27] Vaginal delivery should be reserved for small, less-vascularized tumors as the risk of labor trauma causing fetal hemorrhage is high. Intrapartum cyst aspiration may be attempted to allow for a trial of labor, if this can be safely accomplished, in the nonvascular lesion. Cesarean delivery is the safest and preferred delivery method for the great majority of these tumors with availability of an experienced pediatric surgical team to provide immediate care to the neonate.[28]

OTHER CONSIDERATIONS

In general, cesarean delivery may be considered in every prenatally diagnosed fetal malformation that requires a planned, timed delivery due to the need for urgent care by neonatal and pediatric subspecialists. An example is critical congenital heart disease where the intrapartum management and mode of delivery may be dictated by the immediate availability (or nonavailability) of pediatric cardiologists and surgeons. In cases where availability is

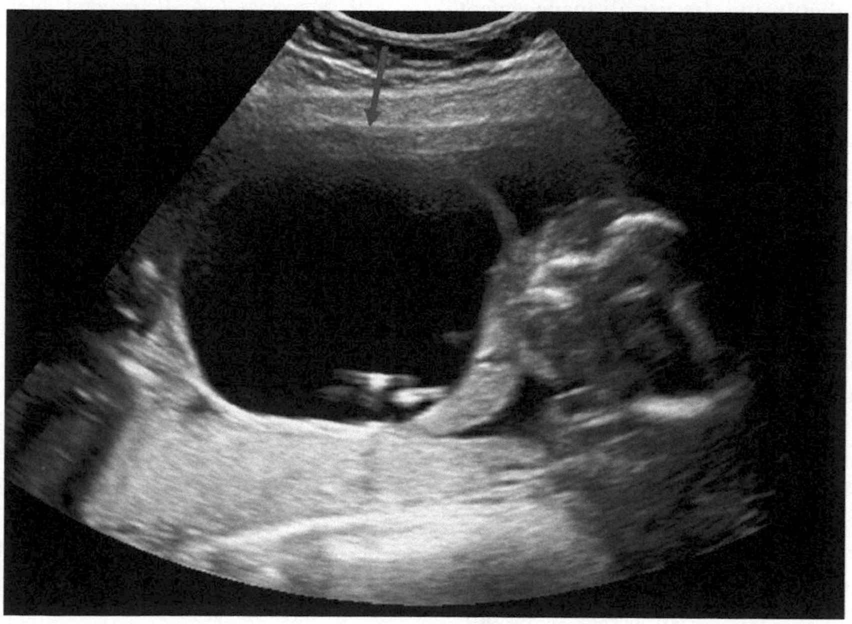

Figure 16.8 Sagittal image with arrow demonstrating an enlarged fetal bladder secondary to bladder outlet obstruction at 28 weeks' gestation.

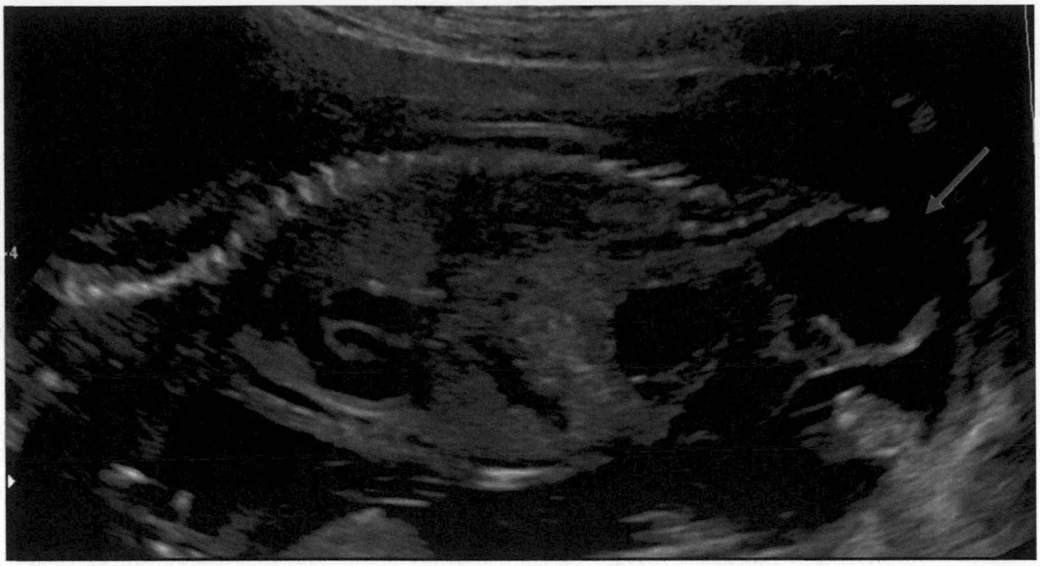

Figure 16.9 Spinal image demonstrating cystic sacrococcygeal teratoma at 21 weeks' gestation with arrow pointing to lesion in the sacrococcygeal region on the fetal spine.

determined by time of day or is limited by other logistical issues, patients should either be transferred to a tertiary care center with full-time subspecialist coverage allowing for spontaneous labor or undergo a timed cesarean section to optimize neonatal outcomes.

SUMMARY

Accurate and thorough prenatal diagnosis with ultrasound and invasive diagnostic testing can help to navigate the difficult management decisions when faced with prenatally diagnosed fetal malformations. Health care providers should provide consultation for the condition-specific prognosis with their patients and discuss all management options available. A nurse navigator may facilitate the patient's appointments with pediatric subspecialists and neonatologists. Decisions regarding mode of delivery for both lethal and nonlethal malformations should be guided by the principles of maternal safety, fetal and neonatal prognosis, and availability of condition-specific specialists. Cesarean delivery should be reserved for cases which will decrease maternal and neonatal morbidity and mortality.

REFERENCES

1. Martin J, Hamilton B, Osterman M et al. Births: Final data for 2013. *Natl Vital Stat Rep* 2014; 64(1): 1–68.
2. Heron M. Deaths: Leading causes for 2011. *Natl Vital Stat Rep* 2015; 64 (7): 76–9.
3. American College of Obstetricians and Gynecologists. *ACOG Practice Bulletin 101.* Ultrasound in pregnancy. February 2009.
4. Wiliknson D, de Crespigny L, Xafis V. Ethical language and decision-making for prenatally diagnosed lethal malformations. *Semin Fetal Neonatal Med* 2014; 19(5): 306–11.
5. Almeida M, Hume R, Lathrop A et al. Perinatal hospice: Family-centered care of the fetus with a lethal condition. *J Am Phys Surg* 2006; 11(2): 52–5.
6. Calhoun BC, Napolitano P, Terry M et al. Perinatal hospice: Comprehensive care for the family of the fetus with a lethal condition. *J Reprod Med* 2003; 48(5): 343–8.
7. Leuthner S, Jones EL. Fetal concerns program: A model for perinatal palliative care. *MCN An J Matern Child Nurs* 2007; 32: 272–8.
8. Hoeldtke NJ, Calhoun BC. Perinatal hospice. *Am J Obstet Gynecol* 2001; 185(3): 525–9.
9. Macones GA, Peirpert J, Nelson D et al. Maternal complications with vaginal birth after cesarean delivery: A multicenter study. *Am J Obstet Gynecol* 2005; 193(5): 1656–62.
10. Spinnato J, Cook V, Cook C, Voss D. Aggressive intrapartum management of lethal fetal anomalies: Beyond beneficence. *Obstet Gynecol* 1995; 85(1): 89–92.
11. Chasen ST, Chervenak FA, McCullough LB. The role of cephalocentesis in modern obstetrics. *Am J Obstet Gynecol* 2001; 185(3): 734–6.
12. Sahid S, Sepulveda W, Dezerega V et al. Iniencephaly: Prenatal diagnosis and management. *Prenatal Diagnosis* 2000; 20: 202–5.
13. Parker SE, Yazdy MM, Mitchell AA et al. Description of spina bifida cases and co-occurring malformations, 1976–2011. *Am J Med Genet A* 2014; 164A(2): 432–40.
14. Adzick NS, Thom EA, Spong CY et al. MOMS investigators. A randomized trial of prenatal versus postnatal repair of myelomeningocele. *N Engl J Med* 2011; 364: 993–4.
15. Bowmen RM, McLone DG, Grant JA et al. Spina bifida outcome: A 25 year prospective. *Pediatr Neurosurg* 2001; 34: 114–20.

16. Goetzinger KR, Stamilio DM, Dicke JM et al. Evaluating the incidence and likelihood ratios for chromosomal abnormalities in fetuses with common central nervous system malformations. *Am J Obstet Gynecol* 2008; 199(3): 285.el.
17. Sival DA, Beeger JH, Staal-Schreine-machers AL et al. Perinatal motor behavior and neurolical outcome in spina bifida aperta. *Early Hum Dev* 1997; 50: 27–37.
18. Kohl T, Tchatcheva K, Merz W et al. Percutaneous fetoscopic patch closure of human spina bifida aperta: Advances in fetal surgical closure techniques may obviate the need for early postnatal neurosurgical intervention. *Surg Endosc* 2009; 23: 890–5.
19. Chervenak FA, Ducan C, Ment LR et al. Perinatal management of myelomeningocele. *Obstet Gynecol* 1894; 63: 376–80.
20. Lewin D, Tolosa JE, Kaufmann M et al. Elective cesarean delivery and long-term motor function or ambulation status in infants with meningomyelocele. *Obstet Gynecol* 2004; 103(3): 469–73.
21. Preis K, Swiatkowska-Freund M, Janczewska I. Spina bifida—A follow-up study of neonates born from 1991 to 2001. *J Perinatal Med* 2005; 33(4): 353–6.
22. Scholl J, Durfee SM, Russell MA et al. First-trimester cystic hygroma: Relationship of nuchal translucency thickness and outcomes. *Obstet Gynecol* 2012; 120(3): 551–9.
23. Laje P, Peranteau WH, Hedrick HL et al. Ex utero intrapartum treatment (EXIT) in the management of cervical lymphatic malformation. *J Pediatr Surg* 2015; 50(2): 311–4.
24. Mann S, Blinman TA, Wilson RD. Prenatal and postnatal management of omphalocele. *Prenat Diagn* 2008; 28: 626–32.
25. Boyd PA, Bhattacharjee A, Gould S. Outcome of prenatally diagnosed anterior abdominal wall defects. *Arch Dis Child Fetal Neonatal Ed* 1998; 78(3): F209–13.
26. Gibbin C, Touch S, Broth RE. Abdominal wall defects and associated congenital heart disease. *Ultrasound Obstet Gynecol* 2003; 21(4): 334–7.
27. Sananes N, Javadian P, Britto IS et al. Technical aspects and effectiveness of percutaneous fetal therapies for large sacrococcygeal teratomas: Cohort study and a literature review. *Ultrasound Obstet Gynecol* 2015; 47(6): 712–9.
28. Anteby E, Yagel S. Route of delivery of fetuses with structural anomalies. *Eur J Obstet Gynecol Reprod Biol* 2003; 106(1): 5–9.

Evaluation and management of stillbirth

17

SEVAN A. VAHANIAN, WENDY L. KINZLER, and ANTHONY M. VINTZILEOS

CONTENTS

Stillbirth is a devastating and difficult experience for parents as well as healthcare providers. A systematic, yet empathetic approach to the diagnosis, evaluation, and management, regardless of gestational age, is crucial. The World Health Organization (WHO) defines fetal death as "death prior to the complete expulsion or extraction from its mother of a product of conception, irrespective of the duration of pregnancy; the death is indicated by the fact that after such separation the fetus does not breathe or show any other evidence of life, such as a beating heart, pulsation of the umbilical cord, or definite movement of voluntary muscles."[1] Stillbirths are classified as early if they occur at less than 20 weeks' gestation, intermediate if they occur at 20–27 weeks' gestation, and late if they occur at 28 weeks' gestation or greater. In the United States, stillbirth affects 1 in 160 pregnancies, resulting in 26,000 stillbirths annually.[2]

Although attempts have been under way to standardize criteria for reporting fetal death and to improve the quality of the National Center for Health Statistics (NCHS) fetal death data file, even within the United States there is underreporting and inconsistencies.[3] NCHS defines fetal death as the spontaneous intrauterine death of a fetus at any time during pregnancy. Most states report fetal deaths at 20 weeks or greater if gestational age is known or a birth weight greater than or equal to 350 g if the gestational age is unknown. Based on NCHS statistics, the fetal mortality rate after 20 weeks' gestation has remained stable from 2006 to 2012, with an overall fetal mortality rate of 6.05 (per 1000 live births plus fetal deaths). However, racial disparity is evident, with the fetal mortality rate in non-Hispanic white women being 4.9 per 1000 compared with 5.33 per 1000 in Hispanic women and 10.67 per 1000 in non-Hispanic black women.[4] The Stillbirth Collaborative Research Network (SCRN) was initiated in order to address and better understand these racial/ethnic and geographic disparities in causes of death among stillbirths.[5]

DIANOSIS OF STILLBIRTH

With the widespread availability of real-time ultrasound equipment, the diagnosis of stillbirth is simple and reliable, with 100% sensitivity and specificity. Fetal heart motion can be detected by 7–8 weeks' gestation by abdominal ultrasound and as early as 5½–6 weeks' gestation by high-frequency transvaginal probes.[6] Failure to detect cardiac activity is diagnostic of stillbirth. Other sonographic signs include absent fetal motion, abnormal head shape due to overlapping skull bones, and reduced or absent amniotic fluid. Prior to obtaining ultrasound confirmation, stillbirth may be suspected from a variety of clinical signs and symptoms. These include decreased or absent fetal movements, decreased fundal height, vaginal bleeding, inability to auscultate the fetal heart by transabdominal Doppler, and possibly elevated maternal serum α-fetoprotein.

Stillbirth is usually quickly evident to the person performing the ultrasound. There is a "stillness" within the uterine cavity, with no motion other than the pulsation of the maternal aorta. After confirming the absence of cardiac activity, it is important that the mother be included in confirming the diagnosis of stillbirth. She should be allowed to visualize the screen after localizing the fetal heart with the ultrasound transducer kept still so as not to create motion artificially.

After several seconds, she, too, will be able to confirm the diagnosis. This helps to eliminate the doubt surrounding the diagnosis and to reduce subsequent denial. Often, women are immediately asked when the last time fetal movement was experienced. This question is likely to elicit strong feelings of guilt that she did not seek medical attention in a timely fashion and does little to assist the medical team in making a diagnosis; it should be avoided, if possible.

EVALUATION OF STILLBIRTH

There are many conditions associated with stillbirth (Table 17.1).[7] In general, the earlier the gestational age at which death occurs, the more likely there is a chromosomal abnormality (Table 17.2).[8] Identification of the cause of stillbirth, whenever possible, is important for several reasons. First, it aids the parents in understanding what led to the demise of their fetus, and in doing so often alleviates self-imposed guilt. Second, if the cause of death is found, the parents may be counseled appropriately as to the recurrence risks of the specific condition. Third, for conditions which may recur, subsequent pregnancies may be managed with closer fetal surveillance and possible therapeutic interventions. Because the causes of stillbirth are many, a systematic diagnostic approach addressing potential maternal, fetal, and placental factors is most beneficial (Table 17.3 is on next page). A research tool entitled Initial Causes of Fetal Death (INCODE) was developed by the SCRN to assign cause of death in stillbirths. This tool spanned six categories, including maternal medical conditions; obstetric complications; maternal or fetal hematologic conditions; fetal genetic, structural, and karyotypic abnormalities; placental infection, fetal infection, or both; and placental pathological findings. The purpose of this was to identify conditions of interest that might be a potential cause of stillbirth. These conditions can then be further classified into "probable cause of death" or "possible cause of death."[7] This tool was used in a multicenter,

Table 17.2 Percentage of fetal losses associated with chromosomal abnormalities by gestational age.

Gestational age (weeks)	With chromosomal abnormalities (%)
8–11	53.5
12–15	47.9
16–19	23.8
20–23	11.9
24–27	13.2
≥28	6.0

Source: Warburton D, *Clin Obstet Gynecol,* 30, 268, 1987.

Table 17.1 Conditions associated with fetal death.

Maternal medical conditions	Red cell isoimmunization
Hypertensive disorders	Platelet alloimmunization
Diabetes	
Obesity	**Fetal genetic, structural, or karyotypic abnormalities**
Autoimmune disease (SLE)	Chromosomal
Intrahepatic cholestasis of pregnancy	Autosomal recessive disorders
Thyroid disease	X-linked dominant disorders in males
Renal disease	Structural anomalies
Substance abuse	Fetal metabolic disorders
Maternal infection	
Seizure disorder	**Placental and/or fetal infection**
	Fetal infection involving brain, heart, lung, and liver (listeriosis, ascending polymicrobial)
Obstetric complications	Fetal infection causing congenital anomaly (CMV, rubella, parvovirus, toxoplasmosis, varicella)
Fetomaternal hemorrhage	Placental infection (syphilis)
Cervical insufficiency	
Preterm labor	**Placental pathologic findings**
Preterm premature rupture of membranes	Implantation abnormalities (previa, accrete)
Chorioamnionitis	Placental membranes (velamentous cord insertion, amnion rupture sequence)
Intrapartum asphyxia	Umbilical cord (vasa previa, cord accident, entanglement, true knots, strictures)
Placental abruption	Fetal membrane infection
Multiple gestation	Circulatory disorders
Uterine rupture	
Maternal trauma	**Other**
Uteroplacental insufficiency	
Maternal or fetal hematologic conditions	
Inherited thrombophilia	
Acquired thrombophilia (antiphospholipid syndrome)	

Source: Dudley DJ et al., *Obstet Gynecol,* 116, 254–260, 2010.
Abbreviations: CMV, cytomegalovirus; SLE, systemic lupus erythematosus.

Table 17.3 Diagnostic approach to the evaluation of stillbirth.[5]

Maternal	Fetal
History and physical examination	***Ultrasound evaluation***
Underlying medical conditions	Assess gestational age (long bones)
Obstetric history	If multiple gestation, check chorionicity, signs of twin-to-twin transfusion syndrome
Current pregnancy history	Congenital anomalies
Medication or substance use	Placental location
Infectious exposures	Evidence of placental abruption
Trauma	Evidence of infection or erythroblastosis fetalis
Family history	Amniotic fluid volume
Laboratory evaluation	***Fetal testing***
Complete blood count	Amniocentesis (karyotype, microarray, cultures)
Indirect Coombs	Placental block below umbilical cord insertion site, segment of umbilical cord, or fetal tissue (costochondral junction or patella)
Kleihauer–Betke	Imaging (photographs, radiographs, magnetic resonance imaging [MRI])
Toxicology screen	Autopsy
Syphilis serology	**Placental**
Parvovirus B-19 IgG and IgM	Cultures
Inherited thrombophilia testing (selected cases)	Pathology
Acquired thrombophilia testing (selected cases)	
TORCH titers (uncertain utility)	
Thyroid-stimulating hormone (uncertain utility)	
Glycosylated hemoglobin A1c (uncertain utility)	

population-based, case–control study conducted by the SCRN that evaluated 663 women with stillbirth between 2006 and 2008 in the United States. In their sample, a probable cause of death was identified in 60.9% of cases, with the most common causes being obstetric complications (29.3%), placental abnormalities (23.6%), fetal genetic or structural abnormalities (13.7%), infection (12.9%), umbilical cord abnormalities (10.4%), hypertensive disorders (9.2%), and other maternal medical conditions (7.8%).[5] While there can be many conditions of interest that are present, an in-depth evaluation is required to determine causality. For example, the presence of histologic chorioamnionitis alone is not a possible cause of death unless there is documented funisitis.

Maternal

A careful maternal history and physical examination is part of the diagnostic evaluation of fetal death. Women should be asked about underlying medical conditions, obstetric history, current pregnancy history, medication or substance use, potentially infectious exposures, trauma, and family history. It is extremely important to question the mother carefully so as not to induce blame. Laboratory evaluation includes complete blood count, screening for the presence of fetal cells or evidence of fetomaternal hemorrhage (Kleihauer–Betke test), indirect Coombs test, toxicology screen, syphilis serology, and parvovirus B-19 immunoglobulin G (IgG) and immunoglobulin M (IgM) serology. Testing for antiphospholipid syndrome (lupus anticoagulant, IgG and IgM anticardiolipin and anti-β2-glycoprotein antibodies) and inherited thrombophilias (factor V Leiden mutation; prothrombin G20210A mutation; protein C, protein S, and antithrombin III deficiencies) can be useful in selected cases, such as in the setting of fetal growth restriction or pre-eclampsia, recurrent fetal loss, or personal or family history of thrombosis.[9] Other tests such as infectious serology screening for TORCH (toxoplasmosis, rubella, cytomegalovirus [CMV], herpes simplex virus [HSV]), thyroid-stimulating hormone, and serum glycosylated hemoglobin (HbA1c) are of uncertain utility.[10]

Fetal

Ultrasound plays a key role in the evaluation of potential fetal and placental factors contributing to stillbirth. The approximate gestational age at which death occurred can be estimated by fetal long bone (e.g., femur, humerus) measurements, assuming that there is no early fetal growth restriction. While the calvarium and intracranial anatomy are assessed, the biparietal diameter is not used to date the age at death, since soon after death the head becomes quite compressible, resulting in underestimation of the gestational age. The long bones, on the other hand, will remain relatively unchanged for several weeks. Congenital anomalies and the presence of hydrops should be sought in all cases of stillbirth. However, care should be exercised not to confuse postmortem ultrasound findings (e.g., skin and scalp edema) with fetal congenital malformations.

Since chromosomal abnormalities are significant causes of stillbirth at all gestational ages, chromosomal analysis with karyotype and microarray is indicated. This information is best obtained by amniocentesis or chorionic villus sampling at the time of diagnosis. Autolysis of fetal tissues occurs soon after death. For this reason, viable tissue may not be available at birth for cytogenetic analysis. On the other hand, fetal cells floating in the amniotic fluid may survive for days after fetal death,[11] making amniocentesis the preferred method of obtaining a specimen for cytogenetic analysis. If amniocentesis is not performed, other acceptable specimens for cytogenetic analysis include a placental block from below the umbilical cord insertion site, a segment of umbilical cord, or internal fetal tissue (costochondral junction or patella). Recently, the role of fetal cell-free DNA has been investigated in the evaluation of 50 pregnancies with intrauterine fetal demise or miscarriage.[12] Overall, adequate fetal fractions, and therefore results, were obtained in 76% of the patients; the yield was better for pregnancies of 8 weeks or greater (88%) compared with pregnancies less than 8 weeks (53%). The results revealed fetal euploidy (76%), trisomy (21%), and microdeletion (3%).[12] This practice, however, at least at the time of the writing of this chapter, may miss many cases of monosomy X, which constitutes approximately 25% of the aneuploidies in fetal losses. At the present time, the use of cell-free DNA in the evaluation of stillbirths or miscarriages may be advisable only when amniocentesis or postmortem karyotype with microarray are not feasible. In the future, cell-free DNA may become a routine test for investigating the cause of fetal death and miscarriage.

If the fetus is delivered intact, photographs and radiographs should be taken and kept on file, particularly if unusual or dysmorphic features are found. Consultation with a geneticist may also be helpful. Parents should be urged to consent to autopsy in all cases of fetal death. Once the benefits of such an examination are pointed out to them, consent can usually be obtained. Eighty-one percent of women surveyed in a study by Rankin et al.[13] agreed to a postmortem examination, and 14% of those that declined regretted that decision. Even when a fetal anomaly has been identified by ultrasound, autopsy has been shown to add information affecting the risk of recurrence in 27% of cases.[14] This examination should ideally be performed by a pathologist who has experience and/or special interest in perinatal pathology. Postmortem fetal magnetic resonance imaging is also a feasible adjunct in cases of maternal refusal to conventional autopsy, particularly in diagnosing intracranial anomalies.[15,16]

Placental

Placental and umbilical cord abnormalities may offer many clues as to the cause of fetal death. The placenta may be abnormally thickened in cases of erythroblastosis fetalis and certain infections (e.g., syphilis, Parvovirus B19). A retroplacental clot, increased placental thickness, subchorionic hematoma, or intra-amniotic blood may be visualized in cases of abruption. After delivery, placental cultures for aerobic and anaerobic bacteria, *Listeria monocytogenes*, and ureaplasma and mycoplasma may be sent. The placenta should always be examined histologically for evidence of thrombi, infarcts, inflammation, villitis, parasitic infestation, etc. Gross examination of the umbilical cord and placenta can identify circumvallate placentation, velamentous cord insertions, abnormal twisting, and/or thrombosis of the umbilical cord. Pathologic findings should correlate with the cause of death. For example, the presence of a nuchal cord alone is not a probable cause of stillbirth unless there is evidence of umbilical cord occlusion or fetal hypoxia.

Stillbirth in multiple gestations

Death of one fetus in a multiple gestation deserves special attention. Although the exact incidence of this event is unknown, it complicates approximately 0.5%–6.8% of twin gestations.[17] Demise of both twins is less likely. Outcome is influenced by gestational age at the time of the demise and by chorionicity. First-trimester fetal demise does not appear to adversely affect the outcome of the surviving twin.[18] During the second and third trimesters, both dichorionic and monochorionic twins are at risk of prematurity. In addition, monochorionic gestations are at risk of multiorgan ischemic damage, multicystic encephalomalacia, and neurologic sequelae in the surviving co-twin. Injury to the remaining twin is estimated to occur in 5%–40% of monochorionic demises. Since the timing of this insult is most likely at the time of the demise, immediate delivery has not been shown to alter outcomes. [19,20]

Ultrasound assessment plays a key role in evaluating stillbirth in multifetal gestations. Attempts should be made to determine chorionicity, as this determines the risk to the surviving fetus. The presence of a dividing membrane and signs of twin–twin transfusion syndrome should also be evaluated if a monochorionic gestation is confirmed. Both twins should be examined for the presence of structural abnormalities, and karyotyping of both fetuses by amniocentesis should be considered. At previable gestations, both expectant management and pregnancy termination are options. At term, delivery is recommended. At 24–34 weeks, close surveillance of the pregnancy, monitoring the surviving fetus for growth and well-being, and watching for signs and symptoms of preterm labor, is recommended. The risk of maternal consumptive coagulopathy in a multiple gestation where one fetus has died is rare. Baseline hematologic studies are recommended, including prothrombin time, partial thromboplastin time, fibrinogen, and platelet count, and should be followed periodically as the pregnancy continues.

MANAGEMENT OF STILLBIRTH

Once confronted with stillbirth, the parents and healthcare provider must decide upon subsequent management. Options include expectant management while awaiting spontaneous uterine evacuation, medical management, or surgical intervention. Variables to take into consideration in making these choices include gestational age, uterine size at diagnosis, preexisting medical, and obstetric conditions including previous uterine scars, provider experience, and the emotional aspects involved.

Expectant

Expectant management in the second half of pregnancy is a feasible option, particularly if the patient is not mentally prepared to proceed with intervention. A disadvantage is the potential risk of hypofibrinogenemia. Fortunately, coagulation abnormalities in association with fetal demise are uncommon. In the absence of placental abruption or uterine perforation, this risk is estimated at 3%.[21] In addition, most patients will deliver within two weeks of fetal death,[22] minimizing the risk of a coagulopathy developing with prolonged retention in utero.[23] Baseline fibrinogen levels followed by weekly assessment has been recommended if expectant management is chosen. If a coagulation defect is identified, steps should be taken to correct the coagulopathy with the appropriate blood products and promptly evacuate the uterus of the retained products of conception.

Surgical techniques

Dilation and evacuation

It is of paramount importance before deciding to perform dilatation and evacuation that cesarean scar pregnancy is ruled out by careful ultrasound examination in *all patients with previous cesarean delivery and anterior low-lying placenta or placenta previa* because in such cases dilatation and evacuation may result in a catastrophic hemorrhage. The treatment options for cesarean scar pregnancies are described in Chapter 32.

In the absence of cesarean scar pregnancy, in the second trimester, surgical emptying of the uterus by dilation and evacuation (D&E) involves dilation of the cervix followed by evacuation of the products of conception by a combination of suction aspiration, sharp curettage, and forceps as needed. Preoperative preparation with either prostaglandins (PG) or laminaria tents may be considered. Hackett et al.[24] reported greater preoperative cervical dilation when the balloon of a 14F Foley catheter inserted into the cervical canal was inflated with 25 mL of water compared with 3 mg PGE_2 inserted into the posterior fornix.

The most serious and significant complications of D&E are cervical lacerations, uterine perforation, hemorrhage, retained products of conception, infection, and intrauterine adhesion formation. These complication rates increase with advancing gestational age and are greatest after 20 weeks' gestation.[25] While the death/case ratio is 3/100,000 procedures at 13–15 weeks' gestation, it increases fourfold when performed at 21 weeks' gestation.[26]

Although D&E is generally very effective, occasional difficulty is encountered in completely evacuating the uterus, especially at more advanced gestational ages (>16 weeks). In particular, the fetal calvarium and thorax are most often retained. Inspection of fetal tissue at the time of the procedure should help to confirm that all the major fetal parts have been removed. If one recognizes that the evacuation is incomplete, the procedure can be completed under ultrasonic guidance. An alternative approach is to administer an intravenous oxytocin infusion for several hours before returning the patient to the operating room. By that time the retained fetal parts will usually be visible at the internal cervical os, where they can be grasped and removed. Either approach is preferable to blind attempts at locating or removing the retained tissue; such efforts are more likely to result in uterine perforation and hemorrhage. Some have even advocated performing all D&E procedures under continuous direct ultrasound guidance, which is associated with lower complication rates (3.7% vs. 15.9%) and less operative time.[27]

Surgical management, in addition to being safe and effective, avoids the unpredictable and longer experience of expectant or medical management. However, pathologic evaluation of a fragmented D&E specimen may not provide the same information as an intact fetus and placenta. It is also impossible for the parents to see and/or hold the object of their profound grief when the fetus is not intact. Parents should be counseled about both the advantages and disadvantages of this option.

Hysterotomy, hysterectomy, and laparotomy

Hysterotomy and hysterectomy are rarely required or indicated in the management of stillbirth unless there is advanced cesarean scar pregnancy (placenta accreta). Although the mother often states that she wants the baby removed from her uterus immediately, the physician must resist the temptation to accommodate her. Performing a nonindicated hysterotomy in such cases subjects the mother to significant morbidity, increased chance of mortality, and a much longer recuperative period. Moreover, pregnancies after hysterotomies are frequently associated with thin scars,[28] thus increasing the likelihood of uterine rupture; for this reason, most subsequent pregnancies are delivered by elective cesarean section.

Under unusual circumstances, hysterotomy or hysterectomy may be the preferred method of uterine evacuation. If a coexisting condition requires laparotomy, such as abdominal trauma, suspected ovarian cancer, or invasive cervical cancer, hysterotomy or hysterectomy may be performed. Other potential indications include suspected placenta accreta, obstructed labor, abdominal pregnancy, or maternal hemorrhage. If hysterotomy is performed, the techniques employed should be those used in cesarean section, except that the uterine incision should be only as large as necessary to remove all products of conception. If the uterus is to be preserved for subsequent pregnancies, the uterine incision should avoid the fundus, and a careful multilayered closure should be performed. Failed induction of labor should raise the suspicion of a possible abdominal, cesarean scar, or cervical pregnancy. When abdominal pregnancy is diagnosed, laparotomy, and removal of the fetus is indicated. The cord should be tied close to the placental insertion and the placenta should be left in situ, where gradual resorption will occur. Attempts at removal are associated with a significant risk of hemorrhage and should be avoided.

Medical management

PGE_1 (misoprostol) is a safe and effective way to facilitate uterine evacuation. It is inexpensive and well tolerated, does not require special storage techniques, and can be administered in similar dosing by the oral, sublingual, vaginal, or rectal routes. The most common side effects include transient pyrexia, nausea, and diarrhea, the last of which can be reduced with vaginal rather than oral dosing.[29] Premedication with antipyretics, antiemetics, and antidiarrheals will further minimize these side effects. Sublingual misoprostol has been found to have higher bioavailability with higher peak serum concentrations than oral and vaginal routes.[30] In addition, it avoids first-pass metabolism through the liver and minimizes vaginal examinations. Therefore, it should be considered as a reasonable alternative, along with the rectal route, particularly for patients experiencing bleeding that may interfere with vaginal absorption.

Prior to 28 weeks' gestation, typical misoprostol doses include 200–400 μg vaginally or orally/sublingually every 4 hours. After 28 weeks' gestation, induction is managed according to usual third-trimester obstetric protocols such as misoprostol 25–50 μg vaginally or orally/sublinqually every 4 hours; or PGE_2 (dinoprostone) suppositories every 12 hours. Alternatively, oxytocin administration per usual hospital infusion protocol is safe and effective. Uterine activity should be monitored and uterine hyperstimulation avoided. If the cervix is unfavorable, pretreatment with laminaria tents, intracervical Foley catheter, or low-dose PG preparations may shorten the induction-to-delivery time. Oxytocin should not be administered if contraindications to labor exist, such as previous classical uterine scar, transverse lie near term, cephalopelvic disproportion, or placenta previa.

Because of the increased rate of cesarean delivery, it is not uncommon to be faced with the challenge of managing a woman with a stillbirth and a previously scarred uterus. Multiple studies have shown that induction of labor with PGs in the second trimester appears to be safe and effective. Misoprostol at doses of 600–800 μg[31]or, less commonly used, extra-amniotic PGE_2[32,33] leads to delivery in 11–15 hours with no cases of uterine rupture reported in a total of 122 women. Although uterine rupture has been reported at 23 weeks after one 200 μg dose of misoprostol, this patient had two prior low-transverse cesarean sections, preterm premature rupture of membranes, and chorioamnionitis.[34] Therefore, prior to 28 weeks' gestation, recommended induction of labor with a history of a uterine scar follows the same protocol as for an unscarred uterus: misoprostol 200–400 μg vaginally, orally, or sublingually every 4 hours. After 28 weeks' gestation, oxytocin infusion is recommended, with transcervical Foley balloon for ripening in patients with an unfavorable cervical examination.

EMOTIONAL ASPECTS OF FETAL DEMISE

Fetal death is not the expected outcome of pregnancy. It is now well understood that the emotional reactions a couple experiences after a fetal demise are similar to those after the death of any loved one. These emotional responses occur not only after late fetal death, but also after early miscarriage,[35] loss of one twin,[36] and midtrimester termination of pregnancy because of fetal anomalies.[37] Although the grief response is complex, there are fairly consistent and characteristic phases that can be recognized.[38] There is considerable variation, however, in how each individual moves through and copes with these reactions. It is imperative that any healthcare provider assisting a couple at the time of a fetal loss be familiar with these emotional responses. Only then can the need for appropriate support be recognized and provided.

Most women will first experience an intense, immediate emotional response.[39] The initial phase is characterized by shock, which may last from several hours to 2 weeks, and is often accompanied by denial. Some of this denial may be lessened by involving the mother in confirmation of the diagnosis by showing her the absent cardiac activity on ultrasound. This is followed by the feelings of grief, dysphoria, guilt, and anxiety. It is particularly important at this time to avoid questions and comments that may be misinterpreted and add to the self-blame which invariably exists. Minimizing feelings of guilt is important, as they are predictors of grief intensity, coping difficulties, and progression to depression.[39] From these first few moments, the situation should be handled in a compassionate, sensitive, and sincere manner. The next phase of the grief process is characterized by a longer period of disorganization, often interrupted by feelings of grief.[38] By 3–4 months, resolution and reorganization should have occurred. The intensity and duration of these emotional reactions, however, may be heightened if there has been a history of pregnancy losses, if there are no living children, if the loss occurred late in the pregnancy, particularly in the absence of warning signs, and if there is a history of poor coping, depression, or lack of social support.[39] All couples should be provided with referrals to support groups, bereavement teams, social workers, and/or psychologists with special interest and experience in perinatal loss.

It is important to have an increased awareness of the emotional impact of perinatal loss on both the mother and the father. The outward response of the father may be quite different from that of the mother. Men often suppress their feelings of sadness and anger in their attempts to focus and support their partner. As a result of this restricted expression of grief, they tend to receive less support, feel very isolated, and are at increased risk of developing a chronic grief response.[40,41] These differences in grief reactions can subsequently strain a couple's relationship. Therefore, being supportive and communicating with both parents is essential.

By providing ongoing psychological support to parents experiencing a perinatal loss, significantly fewer depressive symptoms have been reported.[42] Supportive interventions for these couples exist on a variety of levels. As previously discussed, minimizing the feelings of denial and guilt occur at the time of diagnosis. It is important that options of pregnancy management be discussed, but that the couple not be rushed into making decisions, as long as immediate hospitalization is not required for medical necessity. At the time of delivery, encouraging the parents to see and hold the baby and collect mementos (photographs, locks of hair, footprints, and identification bracelets) can aid in grief resolution. Kellner et al.[43] found that 92% of parents chose to see their baby and 54% chose to hold their baby after perinatal death. This decision is not based on physical appearance, and even in severely macerated or anomalous fetuses, parents will benefit from this interaction. While those who see their baby never regret their choice, those who do not, often regret the decision. In addition, naming the baby helps in affirming his/her existence and should be encouraged.[44] Regarding disposal of the body, all options available to the patient should be discussed. These may include hospital disposal, private burial, and private cremation. In cases of cremation, the ashes can be offered to the parents. While hospital disposal may be most convenient to the parents, a privately arranged memorial service or funeral has several benefits. Such a service offers closure to the fetal death, allowing progression of the normal grieving process. It also offers family and friends the opportunity to express their sorrow, and many find comfort in knowing where their baby is buried.[45]

Although parents should be given adequate privacy, they should not be isolated and abandoned. An expression of our own feelings and a discussion of potential reactions from family and friends will be of assistance. Under no circumstances, regardless of gestational age at time of death, should comments be made such as, "You are young; you can have another," or "you already have a healthy child—you should be grateful for that." It has been estimated that over 50% of women experiencing a perinatal loss felt that healthcare providers were insensitive and failed to provide the opportunity to talk about the loss, and these women sensed a lack of caring and sympathy. As a result, anger is fostered and women often seek the care of new providers in subsequent pregnancies.

Follow-up outpatient visits should address both the physical and emotional needs of the mother. The loss should be discussed openly and available information regarding etiology disclosed. The healthcare provider should not only be familiar with the signs of normal grieving, but should also be able to recognize signs of pathologic grief reactions, including the development of depression, anxiety, neuroses, psychosomatic reactions, or suicidal ideation. If these states are suspected, immediate psychiatric referral is warranted. More than half of women become pregnant within 1–2 years after a perinatal loss.[46] Although some studies have reported that patients who become pregnant within 6 months are more likely to suffer from a prolonged grief reaction,[45,47] other studies have not confirmed this.[48] Recommendations should be based on the individual couple's emotional functioning. Regardless of the time of delivery, a subsequent pregnancy is often marked by strong anxiety, which becomes most intense near the gestational age at which the previous loss occurred.[48]

CONCLUSION

Stillbirth is a devastating event in the lives of parents and distressful for healthcare workers as well. The obstetrician must deal with the physical aspects of death—confirmation of the diagnosis, diagnostic evaluation, and management—as well as the emotional needs of the parents. Physicians and parents may choose to await the spontaneous onset of labor or actively to effect uterine evacuation. The latter can be achieved by both medical and surgical methods. The method of choice as well as the timing of delivery is determined by the gestational age, the experience of the physician, and the medical and emotional needs of the patient. A thorough sonographic and pathologic evaluation of the fetus and placenta is indicated and can assist in explaining the present loss, assessing recurrence risks, and determining the need for special interventions during subsequent pregnancies. Compassion, sensitivity, and openness are essential and help both parents and healthcare providers through these difficult times.

REFERENCES

1. World Health Organization. *Manual of the International Classification of Diseases, Injuries and Causes of Death* (9th revision, volume 1), p. 763. Geneva, Switzerland: WHO, 1977.
2. MacDorman MF, Kirmeyer Se, Wilson EC. Fetal and Perinatal Mortality, United States, 2006. *Natl Vital Stat Rep* 2012; 60(8): 1–22.
3. Goldhaber MK. Fetal death ratios in a prospective study compared to state fetal death certificate reporting. *Am J Public Health* 1989; 79: 1268–70.
4. Gregory ECW, MacDorman MF, Martin JA. *Trends in Fetal and Perinatal Mortality in the United States, 2006–2012*. NCHS Data Brief No. 169. Hyattsville, MD: National Center for Health Statistics, 2014.
5. Stillbirth Collaborative Research Network Writing Group. Causes of death among stillbirths. *JAMA* 2011; 306(22): 2459–68.
6. Goldstein SR, Timor-Tritsch IE. *Ultrasound in Gynecology*, p. 150. New York, NY: Churchill Livingstone, 1995.
7. Dudley DJ, Goldenberg R, Conway D, et al. A new system for determining the causes of stillbirth. *Obstet Gynecol* 2010; 116: 254–60.
8. Warburton D. Chromosomal causes of fetal death. *Clin Obstet Gynecol* 1987; 30: 268.
9. Arkel YS, Ku DH. Thrombophilia and pregnancy: Review of the literature and some original data. *Clin Appl Thromb Hemost* 2001; 7: 259–68.
10. Silver RM, Varner MW, Reddy U et al. Work-up of stillbirth: A review of the evidence. *Am J Obstet Gynecol* 2007; 196(5): 433–44.
11. Saal HM, Rodis JF, Weinbaum PJ et al. Cytogenetic evaluation of fetal death: The role of amniocentesis. *Obstet Gynecol* 1987; 70: 601.
12. Clark-Ganheart CA, Fries MH, Leifheit KM et al. Use of cell-free DNA in the investigation of intrauterine fetal demise and miscarriage. *Obstet Gynecol* 2015; 125: 1321–9.
13. Rankin J, Wright C, Lind T. Cross sectional survey of parents' experience and views of the postmortem examination. *BMJ* 2002; 324: 816–8.
14. Boyd PA, Tondi F, Hicks NR et al. Autopsy after termination of pregnancy for fetal anomaly: Retrospective cohort study. *BMJ* 2004; 328: 137–40.

15. Woodward PJ, Sohaey R, Harris DP et al. Postmortem fetal MR imaging: Comparison with findings at autopsy. *AJR Am J Roentgenol* 1997; 168(1): 41–6.
16. Cannie M, Votino C, Moerman P et al. Acceptance, reliability and confidence of a diagnosis of fetal and neonatal virtuopsy compared with conventional autopsy: A prospective study. *Ultrasound Obstet Gynecol* 2012; 39(6): 659–65.
17. Cleary-Goldman J, D'Alton M. Management of single fetal demise in a multiple gestation. *Obstet Gynecol Survey* 2004; 59: 285–98.
18. Pompler HJ, Madjar H, Klosa W et al. Twin pregnancies with single fetal death. *Acta Obstet Gynecol Scand* 1994; 73: 205–8.
19. D'Alton ME, Newton ER, Cetrulo CL. Intrauterine fetal demise in multiple gestation. *Acta Genet Med Gemellol* 1984; 33: 43–9.
20. Fusi L, Gordon H. Twin pregnancy complicated by single intrauterine death. Problems and outcomes with conservative management. *Br J Obstet Gynaecol* 1990; 97: 511–6.
21. Maslow AD, Breen TW, Sarna MC et al. Prevalence of coagulation abnormalities associated with intrauterine fetal death. *Can J Anaesth* 1996; 43: 1237–43.
22. Tricomi V, Kohl SG. Fetal death in utero. *Am J Obstet Gynecol* 1957; 74: 1092.
23. Prichard JA. Fetal death in utero. *Obstet Gynecol* 1959; 14: 573.
24. Hackett GA, Reginald P, Paintin DB. Comparison of the foley catheter and dinoprostone pessary for cervical preparation before second trimester abortion. *Br J Obstet Gynaecol* 1989; 96: 1432–4.
25. Peterson WF, Berry FN, Grace MR et al. Second trimester abortion by dilation and evacuation: An analysis of 11,747 cases. *Obstet Gynecol* 1983; 62: 185.
26. Grimes DA, Schulz KF. Morbidity and mortality from second trimester abortions. *J Reprod Med* 1985; 30: 505.
27. Acharya G, Morgan H, Paramanantham L et al. A randomized controlled trial comparing surgical termination of pregnancy with and without continuous ultrasound guidance. *Eur J Obstet Gynecol Reprod Biol* 2004; 114: 69–74.
28. Clow WM, Crompton AC. The wounded uterus: Pregnancy after hysterotomy. *BMJ* 1973; 1: 321.
29. Pang MW, Lee TS, Chung TKH. Incomplete miscarriage: A randomized controlled trial comparing oral with vaginal misoprostol for medical evacuation. *Hum Reprod* 2001; 16: 2283–7.
30. Zeiman M, Fong S, Benowitz N et al. Absorption kinetics of misoprostol with oral or vaginal administration. *Obstet Gynecol* 1997; 90: 88–92.
31. Herabutya Y, Chanarachakul B, Punyavachira P. Induction of labor with vaginal misoprostol for second trimester termination of pregnancy in the scarred uterus. *Int J Gynecol Obstet* 2003; 83: 293–7.
32. Debby A, Golan A, Sagiv R et al. Midtrimester abortion in patients with a previous uterine scar. *Eur J Obstet Gynecol Reprod Biol* 2003; 109: 177–80.
33. Shapira S, Goldberger S, Beyth Y et al. Induced second trimester abortion by extra-amniotic prostaglandin infusion in patients with a cesarean scar: Is it safe? *Acta Obstet Gynecol Scand* 1999; 78: 511–4.
34. Chen M, Shih JC, Chiu WT et al. Separation of cesarean scar during second-trimester intravaginal misoprostol abortion. *Obstet Gynecol* 1999; 94: 840.
35. Peppers LG, Knapp RJ. Maternal reactions to involuntary fetal/infant death. *Psychiatry* 1980; 43: 155.
36. Wilson AL, Fenton LJ, Stevens DC et al. The death of a newborn twin: An analysis of parental bereavement. *Pediatrics* 1982; 70: 587.
37. Adler B, Kushnick T. Genetic counseling in prenatally diagnosed trisomy 18 and 21: Psychosocial aspects. *Pediatrics* 1982; 69: 94.
38. Parkes CM. Bereavement. *Br J Psychiatry* 1985; 146: 11.
39. Brier N. Understanding and managing the emotional reactions to a miscarriage. *Obstet Gynecol* 1999; 93: 151–5.
40. Murphy FA. The experience of early miscarriage from a male perspective. *J Clin Nurs* 1998; 7: 325–32.
41. Samuelsson M, Radestad I, Segesten K. A waste of life: Fathers' experience of losing a child before birth. *Birth* 2001; 28: 124–30.
42. Carrera L, Diez-Domingo J, Montanana Vetal. Depression in women suffering perinatal loss. *Int J Gynecol Obstet* 1998; 62: 149–53.
43. Kellner KR, Donnelly WH, Gould SD. Parental behavior after perinatal death: Lack of predictive demographic and obstetrical variables. *Obstet Gynecol* 1984; 63: 809.
44. Peppers LG, Knapp RJ. *Motherhood and Mourning. Perinatal Death*, p. 125. New York, NY: Praeger, 1980.
45. LaRoche C, Lalinee-Michaud M, Engelsmann F et al. Grief reactions to perinatal death—A follow-up study. *Can J Psychiatry* 1984; 29: 14.
46. Cuisinier M, Janssen H, de Graauw C et al. Pregnancy following miscarriage: Course of grief and some determining factors. *J Psychosom Obstet Gynaecol* 1996; 17: 168–74.
47. Hughes PM, Turton P, Evans CDH. Stillbirth as risk factor for depression and anxiety in the subsequent pregnancy: Cohort study. *BMJ* 1999; 318: 1721–4.
48. Cote-Arsenault D, Nomvuyo M. Impact of perinatal loss on the subsequent pregnancy and self: Women's experiences. *J Obstet Gynecol Neonat Nurs* 1999; 28: 274–82.

Antepartum hemorrhage

18

SHAUNA F. WILLIAMS

CONTENTS

Antepartum hemorrhage (APH) is a common complication of pregnancy and occurs in about 15% of all pregnancies. It is defined as bleeding from the genital tract between week 20 of the pregnancy and the onset of labor. Obstetric hemorrhage is a significant threat to the fetus and to the mother. Premature delivery and perinatal mortality rates are increased several-fold in connection with second- and third-trimester bleeding episodes. The most frequent causes of APH are abruptio placentae and placenta previa. Other causes include cervical lesions, genital infections, trauma, and rarely vasa previa, vulvovaginal varicosities, and genital tumors. Nongynecologic causes such as hematuria and rectal bleeding also should be considered. Because of the increased risks and high morbidity and mortality rates that are associated with APH, careful clinical evaluation and management is of critical importance.

ABRUPTIO PLACENTAE

Etiology and epidemiology

Separation of a normal implanted placenta is a potentially dangerous obstetric complication for both the mother and the fetus, with a perinatal mortality rate significantly higher than the general obstetric population.[1] The clinical picture ranges from mild, and thus innocuous, to severe and potentially fatal forms.

Rates of placental abruption have been reported to range from 0.6% to 1% of births.[1,2] Interestingly, some have reported an increase in the incidence of abruption, while other reports have shown a decrease over the past several decades.[2,3] In the 1930s, a maternal mortality rate of 1.7% was reported from the New York Lying-In Hospital in connection with APH presenting with external bleeding. However, by the 1970s maternal death from obstetric hemorrhage had become exceedingly rare.[4] In contrast, abruption of the placenta still entails high fetal and neonatal mortality rates. Even in recent years, about one out of nine cases of abruption of the placenta was associated with perinatal mortality.[5] Other adverse neonatal outcomes include complications of prematurity, anemia, growth restriction, intraventricular hemorrhage, and periventricular leukomalacia.[6,7]

Placental abruption occurs when bleeding occurs between the decidua and the myometrium with subsequent compression of the placenta. In a typical case, acute retroplacental separation probably derives from the rupture of maternal small vessels. The cause of this may be due to vasospasm of the maternal vessels or could be due to thrombosis and subsequent necrosis. It is generally assumed that the rupture of spiral arteries results in high-pressure bleeding that eventually expands and separates the placenta from the implantation site. The bleeding could continue and ultimately lead to a total abruption. Abruption could also be an acute process such as after an abdominal trauma or rapid decompression of the uterus.

Several factors increase a patient's risk for abruption. History of abruption in a prior pregnancy significantly increases the risk in the next pregnancy. It appears that the greater the severity of the first abruption, the higher the risk of recurrence. Recurrence risk may range from less than 2%–24% in patients with two previously affected pregnancies.[8]

Gestational hypertension, preeclampsia, and chronic hypertension have all been associated with abruption. In women with chronic hypertension, the risk of placental abruption is increased threefold over patients without preexisting hypertensive disease.[9,10] Younger age may be a predisposing factor.[11] Parity may be a factor, although studies that have investigated this association have reported conflicting results.[11,12]

Maternal tobacco use, both before and during pregnancy, has been linked to placental abruption with an increase in risk seen with more use.[13,14] Cocaine use has also been shown to be independently associated with placental abruption.[15] This increased risk with smoking and cocaine use should be discussed with the patient and smoking and cocaine use should be discouraged during pregnancy.

Abdominal trauma and motor vehicle accidents could result in a force sufficient to shear the placenta from its attachment to the uterine wall. Placental abruption is a risk of prenatal procedures such as external cephalic version and cordocentesis. Sudden decompression could also result in an abruption, as in the case of a multifetal pregnancy after the delivery of the first twin. Similarly, the decompression that accompanies spontaneous or artificial rupture of the membranes, particularly in patients with polyhydramnios, may also lead to abruption.

Leiomyomas and first-trimester bleeding are additional risk factors.[16] Abnormal serum screening results have also been associated with abruption, specifically high mid-pregnancy levels of maternal serum alpha-fetoprotein (AFP) and low pregnancy-associated plasma protein A (PAPP-A).[17,18] Other associations with abruption have been described, such as with hyperhomocystinemia and dysfibrinogenemia.[19] Retrospective data suggest a relationship with thrombophilias, although this has not been confirmed in all studies.[20,21]

When preterm premature rupture of membranes (PROM) complicates a pregnancy, there is an increased risk of abruption, estimated to be more than three times higher than in patients without preterm PROM. When infection is present in the setting of ruptured membranes, the risk increases more than ninefold.[22,23] Interestingly in patients with abruption, pathologic examination confirms that even in patients without overt clinical infection, there is an increase in histologic chorioamnionitis.[24]

Clinical presentation and diagnosis

The clinical presentation of placental abruption can vary widely, from a small amount of vaginal bleeding to massive hemorrhage. Commonly associated signs and symptoms are back pain, vaginal bleeding, fetal compromise evidenced by nonreassuring fetal heart rate tracings, and abdominal pain from tetanic uterine contractions. Syncope, shock, diffuse intravascular coagulation (DIC), and fetal demise may occur.

Traditionally, the vaginal bleeding associated with placenta previa was described as painless, whereas that deriving from abruption of the placenta was characterized as painful. Although this differentiation may have been helpful in the past, contemporary obstetricians seldom need to rely only on this distinction, as ultrasound can, in most instances, quickly rule out the presence of a placenta previa.

Abruption of the placenta is to be suspected in the presence of the following signs:

- Vaginal bleeding after 20 weeks' gestation
- Uterine irritability manifesting in frequent uterine contractions (more than five contractions in 10 minutes) or uterine hypertonus
- Uterine tenderness or backache
- Evidence of fetal compromise on electronic fetal monitoring: late decelerations, variable decelerations, minimal or absent variability, bradycardia or sinusoidal pattern

Placental detachment is categorized as retroplacental or marginal (Figure 18.1). However, the magnitude of bleeding may not correlate with the degree of fetal or maternal compromise because of the location of the separation. In 10%–20% of the cases, placental abruption entails little or no vaginal bleeding, known as concealed abruption. This can also have devastating consequences as the reliance upon the magnitude of visible bleeding may lead to serious underestimation of the actual blood loss. It should be remembered in patients who present with abdominal pain without bleeding, other causes for the pain should be considered including nonobstetric causes of abdominal pain such as appendicitis, urinary tract infection, ovarian torsion, and degenerating fibroids.

A conclusive prenatal diagnosis of abruption of the placenta is often difficult prior to delivery. Although an ultrasound examination is critical for ruling out abnormalities of placenta location, it is not a sensitive tool for diagnosing abruption. Since ultrasound examination may not reveal evidence of a retroplacental bleed, the differential diagnosis essentially rests upon sonographic exclusion of low implantation of the placenta and placenta previa. It is important to recognize that if changes are not seen by ultrasound, this does not exclude abruption. The sensitivity of the ultrasound examination may be as low as 24%, with a negative predictive value of 53%. On the other hand, specificity and positive predictive value are 96% and 88%, respectively.[25] Ultrasound findings of early abruption may be hyperechoic or isoechoic. Over time the area becomes hypoechoic. The presence of retroplacental hematoma is suggested by the finding on ultrasound examination of a thickened, heterogeneous placenta with rounded margins and intraplacental sonolucencies. The placenta may appear as much as 9 cm in thickness, compared with the normal 4–5 cm.[26]

There are few other tools available for diagnosis. Initial laboratory studies may show anemia, coagulopathy, or a low fibrinogen. Occasionally a Kleihauer–Betke test is ordered. However, it is not diagnostic and not helpful in guiding management, except for calculating dose of Rh-immune globulin required in a Rhesus-negative patient. A comparison of low-risk patients with those who experienced an abdominal trauma showed no difference in rate of positive tests. The trauma patients with the positive tests did not have any clinical evidence of

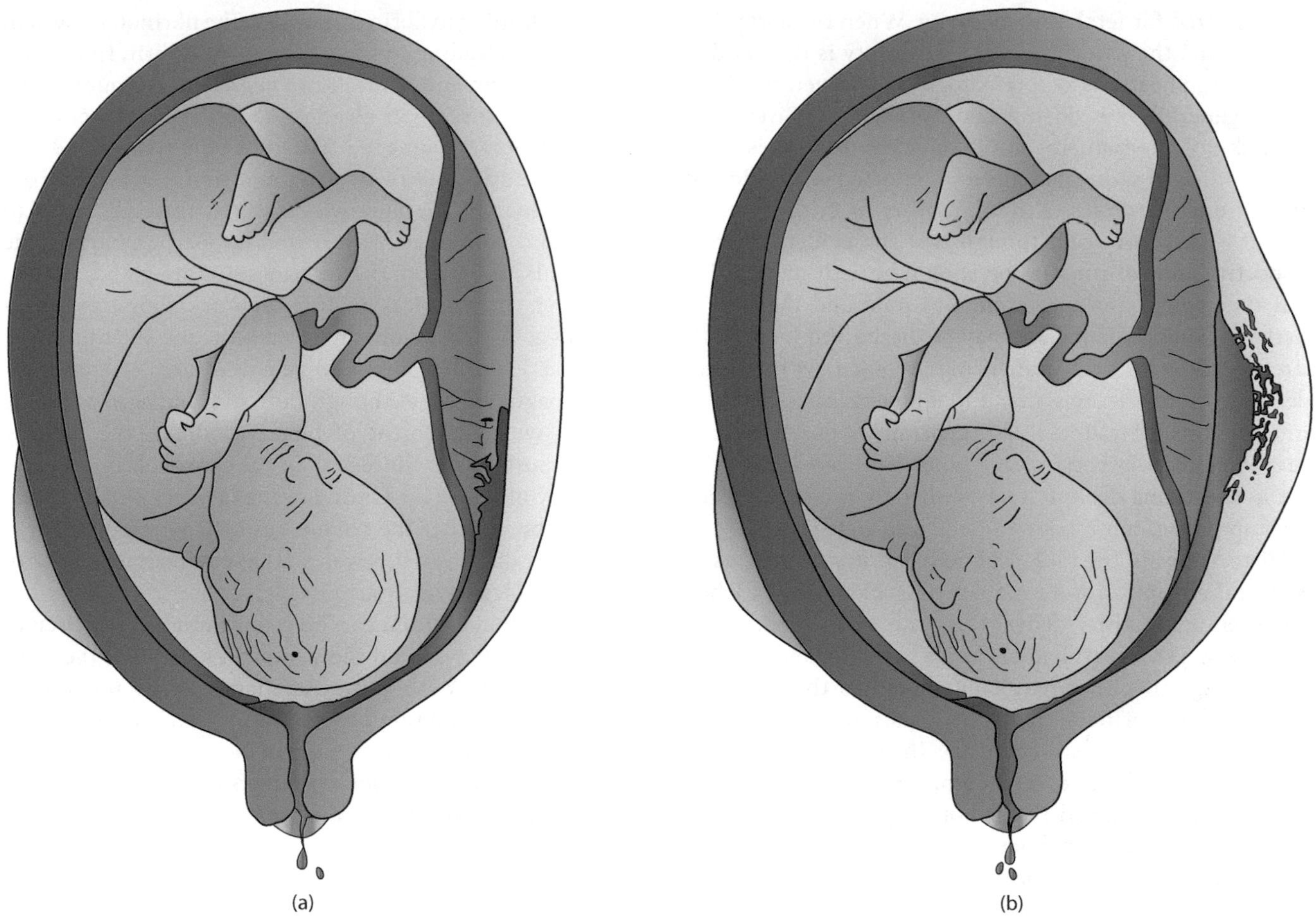

Figure 18.1 The two main types of placental separation: (a) marginal and (b) retroplacental. (This illustration was contributed to the first edition by Drs. Kjell Haram, Per Bergsjo, and Magnar Ulstein. ©2006 Leslie Iffy.)

abruption.[27] Other imaging modalities such as computed tomography (CT) and magnetic resonance imaging (MRI) have been used and may aid in diagnosis.[28,29] When MRI was compared with ultrasound in patient who ultimately were diagnosed with abruption, MRI identified all cases compared with ultrasound which picked up 52% (10 out of 19).[29]

After delivery, careful examination of the placenta may display signs of detachment as well as infarction. Small impressions are covered by firm clots, the extent of which provides a clue to the severity of the abruption. Pathologic examination shows clot on the maternal surface and may show compression of the tissue. Chronic abruptions may be brown with fibrinous strands.[30]

Management

The management of antepartum bleeding in early pregnancy requires good medical judgment and depends upon the severity of the bleeding, the duration of gestation, and the clinical condition of the mother and fetus. The viability of the fetus at a given gestational age must be measured against the likely impact of the bleeding upon maternal and fetal well-being and the long-range outlook for the pregnancy in case expectant management is an option. Delays in diagnosis can be catastrophic and changes in fetal status can occur rapidly. Patients with evidence of placenta abruption must be hospitalized and evaluated. Careful monitoring of maternal vital signs, urine output, electrolytes and acid–base status, coagulation studies including fibrinogen are standard. In selected cases, central venous pressures may need to be monitored. Serial laboratory testing is done until the patient is stable. Large bore intravenous (IV) access should be placed upon presentation and type and crossmatch should be performed as hemodynamic status could change rapidly. A Foley catheter should be utilized for close monitoring of urine output. Adequate kidney function is indicated by a urine output of 30 mL/hour or 0.5 mL/kg/hour or more. Continuous fetal monitoring is initially required until the patient is deemed stable. Neonatology and anesthesia consultation is appropriate should delivery need to occur.

The gestational age and the stability of the patient guide management. When greater than 34 weeks gestation, patients with abruption should be delivered. Prior to 34 weeks gestation, expectant management is an option if the clinical condition of the patient is stable and bleeding has significantly decreased. Corticosteroids should be administered for fetal lung maturity. When the abruption is moderate, the associated fetal morbidity is usually due to the complications of prematurity. However, tocolytic use is generally considered contraindicated. Given that the risks of prematurity are significant, tocolytics have been studied in stable patients and reported results do not suggest untoward effects to the mother or to the fetus. It should be kept in mind though that the evidence is retrospective and administration should be with caution.[31,32]

If the vaginal bleeding event was mild and there is no further bleeding the patient may be discharged home with careful follow-up and monitoring. Women with vaginal bleeding or contractions after a motor vehicle accident or a direct abdominal trauma should generally be observed for at least 24 hours. Discharge after 6 hours has been found to be safe in the setting of blunt trauma when there is no evidence of compromise, contractions or fetal heart rate changes.[33]

Historically, in the mid-twentieth century most cases of placental abruption were managed by induction of labor and eventual vaginal delivery. By the 1980s, abdominal delivery was the treatment of choice in the United States.[34] This change in philosophy contributed to the dramatic reduction of perinatal mortality rates during the last decades of the twentieth century.[35] In case of mild abruption with no evidence of fetal compromise, a trial of labor is acceptable, provided that labor progresses and is well tolerated by the maternal–fetal pair. When the outlook for vaginal delivery is favorable and a trial of labor is decided upon, amniotomy may hasten delivery. After the abruption of the placenta, spontaneous onset of labor frequently ensues. In such cases, the progress of the labor tends to be rapid. If otherwise, uterine stimulation with oxytocin is required.

The time interval between the occurrence of the abruption and delivery has considerable bearing upon the prospect of neonatal survival. It should be kept in mind that the time between the first appearance of fetal distress and in utero fetal demise may be short. Continuous electronic fetal heart rate monitoring is critically important. Recurrent hemorrhage or sign of deterioration in the fetal condition requires delivery without delay as prolonged intervals to delivery are associated with poor outcomes.[36] Renal failure and clotting defects due to hemorrhage do not represent a contraindication to abdominal delivery. However, vigorous blood replacement is important when prompt surgical intervention is deemed necessary.

In case of in utero fetal death, amniotomy can be performed followed by oxytocin stimulation. Hysterotomy may be still necessary, however, when the attempt is unsuccessful, insofar as both placental abruption and the presence of a dead fetus predispose to coagulation defects. When hemorrhage extends into the myometrium, termed the Couvelaire uterus, hysterectomy may be required in rare cases.

When it occurs against the background of obstetric hemorrhage, disseminated intravascular coagulation (DIC) originates from the release of tissue factor into the maternal circulation. This release activates the coagulation process leading to fibrin formation. The fibrinolytic system is activated leading to the production of fibrin split products. As fibrin and platelets are degraded, a coagulopathy results. Microvascular bleeding can arise from areas subject to trauma. Damage occurs not only from blood loss but also as a result of hypoxia and tissue ischemia from fibrin plugs in the microvasculature. This can result in renal and pulmonary failure and in Sheehan's syndrome (avascular necrosis of the anterior pituitary gland).

When the clinical picture and/or laboratory studies suggest a coagulopathy is present, the inciting event may be due to DIC or could be a dilutional or consumptive coagulopathy. Although both are managed with the aggressive replacement of blood products, the inciting event must also be addressed. In the case of abruption, it is delivery of the fetus. Timing of the delivery will be determined by whether the patient can deliver vaginally or if blood products can be given so that cesarean delivery can be performed as safely as possible.

Crystalloid solution can be given initially. The circulation parameters should show improvement after the infusion of 1–2 L. With administration of large amounts of crystalloids, a dilution coagulopathy could result, as well as third spacing and worsening of kidney injury, so in this setting transfusion of blood products should be considered early in the management and there is no reason for delaying resuscitation. The transfusion of packed red blood cells (PRBC) is ideal for increasing the oxygen-carrying capacity of the patient's blood. Fresh frozen plasma (FFP) should be administered in the face of liver disease, coagulation defects, thrombotic and thrombocytopenic purpura. It should be given when the prothrombin time and/or activated partial thromboplastin time values are more than 1.5 times normal. In the setting of severe obstetric hemorrhage, administration of FFP should not be delayed. From the trauma literature, higher ratios of FFP to PRBC have shown improved mortality, so it has been recommended to give it in a 1:1 ratio.[37] Another approach is to administer 2 units of FFP for 3 units of PRBCs, then after the first 6 units of PRBC have been given, to continue with a 1:1 ratio.[38] Further study is needed to determine the optimal protocol in obstetrics. With DIC, large amounts of products may be necessary to stabilize the patient. Institutional massive transfusion protocols allow for rapid preparation and administration of large volume of products and should be developed in collaboration with blood bank staff, anesthesiologists, and obstetricians.

Thrombocytopenia is also likely to result when 1.5–2 times the woman's blood volume has been transfused, or in the case of consumptive or dilutional coagulopathy. Platelet transfusion is indicated if the platelet count falls below 20,000, if operative intervention is planned and the platelet count is 50,000, or with massive hemorrhage. Cryoprecipitate is often given in case of declining fibrinogen levels out of proportion to other coagulation factors.

Postpartum hemorrhage frequently follows delivery in connection with abruption of the placenta as a result of a clotting defect or uterine atony. On this account, routine infusion of oxytocin during the third stage of labor is advisable. It is to be remembered that, once delivery has been effected and all products of conception have been removed from the uterus, spontaneous correction of the bleeding and clotting defects can be anticipated within hours.

Prevention

Prevention of placenta abruption includes discontinuation or reduction of smoking and avoidance of illicit drugs. Appropriate treatment of chronic hypertension and timely delivery in case of preeclampsia also reduce the risk of placental separation. Proper use of automobile safety belts protects against abruption. It is important to use both shoulder and lap belts, with the latter applied low at the level of the pelvic bones.

Although prior history of abruption increases the risk of this complication, no preventive intervention is currently recommended. Ultrasound examinations for fetal growth can be considered, but fetal surveillance is generally not warranted.

PLACENTA PREVIA

After abruption, placenta previa is the most frequent cause of APH. Previously, previas have been categorized as central, partial, marginal, or low lying. With the use of transvaginal ultrasonography, the location of the placenta can be determined more accurately and so is called a previa if the placenta covers the internal os, and low lying, if the edge lies within 2 cm of the os.

The placenta appears implanted over the lower segment with relative frequency on ultrasound examinations performed during the early second trimester. However, in about 90% of the instances, this is not demonstrated on follow-up ultrasound examinations. The apparent change in location is thought to be due to placental growth toward the area with greater blood supply. Additionally, as the uterus grows in size, the distance between the lower edge of the placenta and cervix also lengthens. Because of this, it is recommended to repeat the ultrasound examination in the early part of the third trimester (28–32 weeks) to reevaluate for placental location.

A history of previous placenta previa, prior cesarean delivery or other prior uterine surgery, advanced maternal age, previous infertility, multiparity, smoking and history of a variety of reproductive abnormalities, as well as previous occurrence of low implantation, predispose to the occurrence of placenta previa.[39,40]

It has previously been reported that the incidence of fetal growth restriction is increased in connection with placenta previa,[41] but recent reports have not confirmed this or that of an association with stillbirth. Whereas the major neonatal risks associated with placenta previa are associated with prematurity.[42]

Signs and symptoms

The typical manifestation of placenta previa is painless vaginal bleeding during the second half of the gestation. In the past, on rare occasions, patients with placenta previa remained asymptomatic and thus undiagnosed, until the onset of labor at or near term. This is now rare with the widespread use of ultrasound. Placenta previa is to be included in the differential diagnosis whenever vaginal bleeding occurs during the second half of the pregnancy. On external examination, the uterus is usually found to be soft and nontender. If ultrasonography has not previously been performed and ruled out a placenta previa, this should be done before a pelvic examination is performed. Transabdominal sonography may quickly rule out a previa, as the site of the implantation of an anteriorly implanted placenta is easy to detect with ultrasound. But if the placenta appears close to the cervical os, transvaginal sonography should then be performed by an experienced sonographer, as this is more accurate. The exact localization of the posteriorly implanted placenta may also be difficult. Maternal obesity, distended bladder, and uterine activity may hinder the diagnosis in these cases. The visualization of the internal cervical os is facilitated by transvaginal sonography. In expert hands, such examination can be performed with relative ease without eliciting bleeding and has been found to be safe.[43,44] Digital vaginal examination in suspected placenta previa is absolutely contraindicated. The initial examination in APH must be limited to speculum examination.

Management

As late as the mid-nineteenth century, the maternal mortality rate from placenta previa was about 25%. Irrespective of the method of delivery, the fetal mortality rate was almost 100% until the introduction of cesarean section into obstetric practice. By the turn of the twentieth century, cesarean section could be performed with relative safety by obstetric surgeons. Soon it became the standard method of delivery in cases of placenta previa. As a result, the maternal mortality rate fell to 5% by the early 1900s, and the majority of babies could be delivered alive. By the 1920s, cesarean section was used liberally for the management of placenta previa. At that time, the maternal mortality rate was as low as 2%, despite the fact that blood transfusion and antibiotics were still more than a decade away.[45] Before and during World War II, the perinatal mortality was still 25% in New York City. By the 1980s, the reported perinatal mortality rate was reported as high as 81 per 1000 and maternal mortality rates were 0.03%.[46,47]

The general principles governing the management of bleeding from placenta previa in the late second and early third trimesters resemble those previously outlined in connection with abruption of the placenta, including laboratory investigations, fetal surveillance, and stabilization of the maternal circulatory status. The diagnosis having been established, the management decision rests upon the length of the gestation, the degree of the bleeding, and the fetal condition. Recurrent and severe bleeding episodes often necessitate delivery before term. The high incidence of premature delivery still translates into a relatively high rate of perinatal morbidity from complications of prematurity. Neonatal anemia necessitating blood transfusion is a frequent complication.

The idea of delaying cervical dilation and, thus the occurrence of bleeding from placenta previa, by cerclage has been debated over the past decades. However review of outcomes after cerclage placement does not convincingly support its routine use.[48] If tocolysis is considered, magnesium sulfate has fewer adverse cardiovascular side effects, may have neonatal neuroprotective benefit, and may be given when APH is associated with preeclampsia.

Anti-D immunoglobulin in Rh-negative, nonimmunized mothers should be administered.

If delivery is not immediately indicated, corticosteroids should be administered for fetal lung maturity if gestation is less than 34 weeks. When continued expectant management is feasible, liberal hospitalization of the patient is warranted. If the patient is anemic, iron supplementation should be given. Patients with placenta previa may be kept in the hospital from the time of the first episode of bleeding until delivery, since the magnitude of the hemorrhage is not predictable and 1 or 2 hours' delay may make the difference between fetal, and occasionally even maternal, life and death. Patients who are asymptomatic can be managed on an outpatient basis.[49,50] If this management is elected, the patient must rest at home and under circumstances that permit her immediate transfer to the hospital when the next bleeding episode occurs. Limited activity and pelvic rest are usually advised, whereas strict bed rest cannot be recommended as there is no data to support its benefit and risks have been described.

If the patient remains stable then delivery should ideally take place in a nonemergent fashion and so can be performed at the end of the 36th week or beginning of the 37th week[51] to decrease the risks associated with prematurity. Regional anesthesia can be considered in these cases and may be associated with less blood loss compared with general anesthesia.[52] Close cooperation between the obstetric and anesthesia teams is critical.

Cesarean section for placenta previa can prove to be challenging as the most commonly encountered problem is hemorrhage. The site of the uterine incision should be chosen cautiously in order to avoid, if possible, the necessity of cutting through the placenta before the delivery of the fetus. An ultrasound examination can be performed prior to surgery in order to determine the site of the uterine incision. The surgical difficulties depend largely upon the site of the placental implantation. When the placental implantation is anterior, it may be necessary to cut through the placenta in order to reach the fetus in utero. If there is significant delay in delivery of the fetus, this may lead to fetal compromise. In order to minimize these risks, some surgeons prefer a classical cesarean section instead of the lower-segment transverse approach in connection with placenta previa. This approach may be particularly useful when the lower uterine segment is poorly developed (less than 34 weeks' gestation). With this approach, the time between the uterine incision and the removal of the fetus can be shortened.

As a rule of thumb, anterior implantation hinders the entry into the uterus but, in the absence of invasion of the myometrium by the placenta, facilitates the surgical control of the bleeding that inevitably occurs. In contrast, when the implantation is posterior, entry into the uterine cavity and removal of the fetus entail little difficulty. However, since the posterior aspect of the lower segment of the uterus may not contract well, control of the hemorrhage arising from the implantation site may create difficulties. Whatever is done, it should be done quickly and efficiently in order to minimize blood loss.

For a variety of reasons, the degree of intraoperative hemorrhage is unpredictable. Therefore, the preparation for cesarean section in connection with placenta previa must be thorough and farsighted. The surgical team must be prepared to handle extreme difficulties that require exceptional measures. These may include uterine artery ligation, hypogastric artery ligation, B-Lynch suture, oversewing the area of bleeding, or cesarean hysterectomy. Because the lower uterine segment cannot contract efficiently, the degree of hemorrhage is dependent, to a great extent, upon the site of the implantation of the placenta. When the previa is central and thus covers the internal cervical os, profuse bleeding should be anticipated. The blood replacement must keep pace with the blood loss in such instances. Thus, close cooperation among the members of the team is essential.

When the placenta is more than 2 cm from the internal cervical os, the patient can attempt labor with cesarean delivery reserved for usual obstetric indications. With the placenta within 2 cm, attempt at vaginal delivery can be done with caution and careful monitoring. One report provides reassuring information, with a vaginal delivery rate of 76.5% when the placenta was 1–2 cm from the os. For those less than 1 cm, the group was small, and most patients were delivered by cesarean delivery prior to labor.[53] Because of the risk of hemorrhage, most patients are delivered by cesarean delivery if the placenta is less than 1 cm from the os. Repeat ultrasound close to the time of the delivery should be considered though to prevent cesarean sections in patients with placentas that may no longer be low lying.

PLACENTA ACCRETA, INCRETA, AND PERCRETA

Placenta accreta occurs when there is abnormal placental attachment and invasion into the uterine wall. Deficient development of the endometrial decidua predisposes to deep penetration of the uterine wall by the chorionic villi. The invasion can be extensive enough to allow the placenta to burrow through the wall of the lower uterine segment and to invade the urinary bladder. Placental invasion into the myometrium is termed *placenta increta*, and *placenta percreta* is when there is invasion beyond the uterine serosa. The rate of placenta accreta has increased over the past several decades, parallel to the rise in cesarean deliveries.[54] A previous cesarean section increases the risks of both placenta previa and placenta accreta. In a large prospective observational cohort, the risk of placenta accreta without a previa is 0.2%, 0.1%, 0.8%, and 0.8% with 1, 2, 3, and 4 prior cesarean deliveries, respectively. With a previa, the risk of accreta was 11%,40%, 61%, and 67% with 1, 2, 3, and 4 prior cesarean deliveries, respectively.[55] Other risk factors include advanced maternal age, multiparity, previous myomectomy, other prior uterine surgery or submucus fibroids.[56]

Since placenta accreta is asymptomatic throughout pregnancy, its early diagnosis requires a high level of suspicion and awareness of the predisposing factors. One should determine the location of the placenta and search for venous lakes penetrating the myometrium. The ultrasound findings suggestive of placental invasion include thinning of the myometrium, abnormalities in the interface between the uterus and the bladder, and extension of the placental tissue beyond the uterine serosa and lacunar spaces or "Swiss cheese" appearance in the placental parenchyma. These lacunar spaces, when present in the second trimester, may be most predictive, with a sensitivity of 79% and positive predictive value of 92%.[57] Sensitivity ranges from 77% to 93%, and specificity ranges from 71% to 91%.[58] Interestingly, a study looking at blinded reviews of ultrasound images from patients with known placenta accreta compared with controls reported a sensitivity of 53.5%, demonstrating the importance of knowing a patient's history when performing these ultrasounds.[59]

Supplemental use of Doppler studies, including three-dimensional power Doppler, may aid in making the diagnosis, with up to 100% sensitivity.[60,61] MRI can be helpful if the diagnosis is unclear, the placenta is posterior, or there is a suspicion for percreta with reported sensitivity of 75%–100% and specificity of 65%–100%.[58,62]

Placenta percreta is the complete penetration of the entire thickness of the uterus and is a life-threatening obstetric complication. In this clinical entity, the placenta may invade the bladder as well as other pelvic structures. Predisposing factors include previous cesarean section, dilation and curettage or myomectomy, advanced maternal age, retained products of conception, previous endometritis, and past trophoblastic disease. Anticipation of this diagnosis preoperatively can allow for a multidisciplinary approach and appropriate preparations in the operating room.

Management

The optimal timing of delivery in patients with previa and accretas would minimize risks of prematurity without increasing the chance of an emergent delivery. A decision analysis compared scheduled delivery from 34 to 39 weeks and concluded that delivery at 34 weeks was preferred, although there were some circumstances where waiting until term, or 37 weeks' could be considered.[63] Extensive preparations for any surgical procedure involving placenta previa after a previous cesarean section is of great importance as placenta accreta or placenta percreta may be encountered. These preparations should include the placement of two intravenous lines as well as the availability of several units of cross-matched blood. It needs to be remembered that adhesions caused by the preceding surgery may hinder the performance of an emergency hysterectomy. When this occurs, it is necessary, therefore, to release all adhesions that may hinder quick removal of the uterus in an emergency situation Delivery at a tertiary center/specialized center with a multidisciplinary approach has been shown to decrease the amount of blood loss[64] and criteria for centers specializing in care of these patients have been developed, which include experienced surgeons, urologist, general surgeon, interventional radiologist, neonatologist, blood bank, and intensive care facilities.[65]

Management options for this entity include elective cesarean hysterectomy and abdominal delivery with conservative management and retention of the placenta.[66] Cesarean hysterectomy has been long regarded as the management of choice. However, it carries a high maternal morbidity rate, including both physical and psychological consequences, as well as the loss of fertility.[67] Conservative management leaving the placenta in situ is an alternative, which frequently permits the avoidance of massive intraoperative hemorrhage as well as the loss of the uterus, but this is not without risk of serious complications.

At the time of the procedure, the patient may be placed in a modified dorsal lithotomy position with placement of pneumatic compression devices and a three-way foley. A vertical incision with vertical fundal incision on the uterus is generally performed. After the delivery of the infant, the surgeon may wait for spontaneous placental separation. If it does not separate, then the uterus should be quickly closed prior to doing the hysterectomy. In order to minimize additional blood loss, if all clamps can be placed first, then transection of the vessels can be done. Prophylactic antibiotics are given prior to the procedure, with a repeat dose given after 2–3 hours or 1500 mL blood loss.

Placement of ureteral stents has been suggested as a way to decrease ureteral injury.[68] Placement of uterine artery balloons or catheters have been investigated as a way to decrease blood loss, but studies reviewing their use have reported conflicting results. A review of cases from 1990 to 2011 showed a lower estimated blood loss with uterine artery balloon catheters.[69] However, another retrospective case–control study comparing patients with intravascular balloon catheters with a control group without catheters showed no difference in blood loss or number of blood products administered. These authors also reported three complications in the 19 subjects (15.8%), including internal iliac artery thrombosis, groin hematoma, femoral artery thrombosis, and an internal iliac artery dissection.[70] A randomized control trial of 27 women also did not show a difference in blood loss or number of PRBC units transfused.[71]

Conservative management leaving the placenta in situ is an uncommon but alternate management strategy. The technique involves ligation of the umbilical cord close to its insertion site. Although this method does not have the same potential for intraoperative morbidity, there is an increased risk for complications such as delayed hemorrhage, sepsis, fistula, and emergent hysterectomy.[72] Reports of methotrexate use has not shown consistently positive results and complications include sepsis, peritonitis, and DIC.[73,74]

VASA PREVIA AND VELAMENTOUS CORD INSERTION

Vasa previa is present when fetal vessels, unsupported by placenta or umbilical cord, traverse the membranes on their way to a velamentous umbilical cord. A less frequent type of vasa previa involves the passage of vessels between lobes of the placenta (placenta bilobata and placenta succenturiata). Rupture of the membranes, whether spontaneous or artificial, may cause rupture of some of the vessels passing over the membranes, leading to rapid fetal exsanguination.[75] Velamentous insertion of the umbilical cord, which is a prerequisite for vasa previa, occurs in about 1% of singleton and 10% of multiple gestations. On rare occasions, even in the absence of bleeding, compression of aberrant vessels may cause hypoxia and even fetal demise. Apart from artificial rupture of the membranes, bleeding from an aberrant vessel has been described in connection with the placement of a fetal scalp electrode.

Traditionally, the diagnosis of bleeding from an aberrant vessel rested upon the following triad:

1. Spontaneous or artificial rupture of the membranes
2. Occurrence of bleeding shortly after the rupture of the membranes
3. Evidence of fetal distress on electronic monitoring within seconds or minutes after events (1) and (2)

It is intuitive that prevention of perinatal mortality would depend on prenatal diagnosis of this condition and abdominal delivery before rupture of the membranes occurs. For this reason, standard obstetric ultrasound protocols should include evaluation of the placenta location and the placental cord insertion site when possible.[76] In women at increased risk (second-trimester, low-lying placenta pregnancies resulting from *in vitro* fertilization, and those with accessory placental lobes), a routine transvaginal color Doppler sonography of the region over the cervix, if vasa previa cannot be excluded by transabdominal sonography, could facilitate the diagnosis. Sonographic prenatal diagnosis has the potential to prevent fatal outcomes deriving from vasa previa.

EXTRACHORIAL PLACENTA

This anomaly describes a condition where the chorionic plate of the placenta is smaller than its basal plate. Thus, the villous tissue projects beyond the borders of the chorionic plate. When the placenta is "circummarginata," the border between the villous and membranous chorion is provided by a flat ring of membrane. When the placenta is "circumvallata," this marginal ring has raised edges. Between the extrachorial placenta and the fetal membranes, there is a decidual layer. The placenta is extrachorial in about 30% of all cases. The incidence of circumvallata is in the range 0.5%–6.9%.[77] The diagnosis rests upon careful inspection of the placenta after delivery. The clinical importance of placenta circummarginata is negligible. On the other hand, 25%–50% of all patients with placenta circumvallata suffer APH secondary to separation of the placenta from the implantation site and bleeding from its margin. This hemorrhage often resembles the clinical manifestations of placenta previa. Although the bleeding is modest in most instances, it may occasionally result in second-trimester abortion, preterm delivery, and significant APH.

ACKNOWLEDGMENT

The author of this chapter acknowledges Gabor Nemeth, Gerard Hansen and Gyorgy Bartfai, who were the authors of this chapter in the previous edition.

REFERENCES

1. Salihu HM, Bekan B, Aliyu MH, Rouse DJ et al. Perinatal mortality associated with abruptio placenta in singletons and multiples. *Am J Obstet Gynecol* 2005; 193(1): 198–203.
2. Ananth CV, Oyelese Y, Yeo L, Pradhan A et al. Placental abruption in the United States, 1979 through 2001: Temporal trends and potential determinants. *Am J Obstet Gynecol* 2005; 192: 191–8.
3. Cunningham F, Leveno KJ, Bloom SL et al. Obstetrical hemorrhage. In: Cunningham F, Leveno KJ, Bloom SL et al. (eds), *Williams Obstetrics* (24th edition). New York, NY: McGraw-Hill, 2013. http://accessmedicine.mhmedical.com.proxy.libraries.rutgers.edu/content.aspx?bookid=1057&Sectionid=59789185. Accessed October 20, 2015.
4. Kaunitz AM, Hughes JM, Grimes DA et al. Causes of maternal mortality in the United States. *Obstet Gynecol* 1985; 65: 605–12.
5. Ananth CV, Wilcox AJ. Placental abruption and perinatal mortality in the United States. *Am J Epidemiol* 2001; 153: 332–7.
6. Ananth CV, Berkowitz GS, Savitz DA, Lapinski RH. Placental abruption and adverse perinatal outcomes. *JAMA* 1999, 3; 282(17): 1646–51.
7. Gibbs JM, Weindling AM. Neonatal intracranial lesions following placental abruption. *Eur J Pediatr* 1994; 153: 195–7.
8. Rasmussen S, Irgens LM. Occurrence of placental abruption in relatives. *BJOG* 2009; 116: 693–9.
9. Ananth CV, Savitz DA, Williams MA. Placental abruption and its association with hypertension and prolonged rupture of membranes: A methodologic review and meta-analysis. *Obstet Gynecol* 1996; 88(2): 309–18.
10. Boisramé T, Sananès N, Fritz G et al. Placental abruption: Risk factors, management and maternal-fetal prognosis. Cohort study over 10 years. *Eur J Obstet Gynecol Reprod Biol* 2014; 179: 100–4.
11. Ananth CV, Wilcox AJ, Savitz DA et al. Effect of maternal age and parity on the risk of uteroplacental bleeding disorders in pregnancy. *Obstet Gynecol* 1996; 88(4 Pt 1): 511–6.
12. Toohey JS, Keegan KA Jr, Morgan MA et al. The "dangerous multipara": Fact or fiction? *Am J Obstet Gynecol* 1995; 172(2 Pt 1): 683–6.
13. Ananth CV, Savitz DA, Luther ER. Maternal cigarette smoking as a risk factor for placental abruption, placenta previa, and uterine bleeding in pregnancy. *Am J Epidemiol* 1996; 144: 881–9.

14. Tikkanen M, Surcel HM, Bloigu A et al. Self-reported smoking habits and serum cotinine levels in women with placental abruption. *Acta Obstet Gynecol Scand* 2010; 89(12): 1538–44.
15. Addis A, Moretti ME, Ahmed Syed F et al. Fetal effects of cocaine: An updated meta-analysis. *Reprod Toxicol* 2001; 15(4): 341–69.
16. Stout MJ, Odibo AO, Graseck AS et al. Leiomyomas at routine second-trimester ultrasound examination and adverse obstetric outcomes. *Obstet Gynecol* 2010; 116(5): 1056–63.
17. Tikkanen M, Hämäläinen E, Nuutila M et al. Elevated maternal second-trimester serum alpha-fetoprotein as a risk factor for placental abruption. *Prenat Diagn* 2007; 27: 240–3.
18. Dugoff L, Hobbins JC, Malone FD et al. First-trimester maternal serum PAPP-A and free-beta subunit human chorionic gonadotropin concentrations and nuchal translucency are associated with obstetric complications: A population-based screening study (the FASTER Trial). *Am J Obstet Gynecol* 2004; 191(4): 1446–51.
19. Edwards RZ, Rijhsinghani A. Dysfibrinogenemia and placental abruption. *Obstet Gynecol* 2000; 95(6 Pt 2): 1043.
20. Kupferminc MJ, Eldor A, Steinman N et al. Increased frequency of genetic thrombophilia in women with complications of pregnancy. *N Engl J Med* 1999; 340(1): 9–13.
21. Procházka M, Happach C, Marsál K et al. Factor V Leiden in pregnancies complicated by placental abruption. *BJOG* 2003; 110(5): 462–6.
22. Ananth CV, Oyelese Y, Srinivas N, et al. Preterm premature rupture of membranes, intrauterine infection, and oligohydramnios: Risk factors for placental abruption. *Obstet Gynecol* 2004; 104(1): 71–7.
23. Gonen R, Hannah ME, Milligan JE. Does prolonged preterm rupture of the membranes predispose to abruptio placentae? *Obstet Gynecol* 1989; 73: 347–50.
24. Darby MJ, Caritis SN, Shen-Schwarz S. Placental abruption in preterm gestation: An association with chorioamnionitis. *Obstet Gynecol* 1989; 74: 88–92.
25. Glantz C, Purnell L. Clinical utility of sonography in the diagnosis and treatment of placental abruption. *J Ultrasound Med* 2002; 21: 837–40.
26. Nyberg DA, Finberg HJ. The placenta, placental membranes and umbilical cord. In: Nyberg DA, Mahony BS, Pretorius DH (eds), *Diagnostic Ultrasound of Fetal Anomalies.* Text and Atlas, p. 623. Chicago, IL: YearBook Medical Publishers, 1990.
27. Dhanraj D, Lambers D. The incidences of positive Kleihauer-Betke test in low-risk pregnancies and maternal trauma patients. *Am J Obstet Gynecol* 2004; 190: 1461–3.
28. Kopelman TR, Berardoni NE, Manriquez M et al. The ability of computed tomography to diagnose placental abruption in the trauma patient. *J Trauma Acute Care Surg* 2013; 74(1): 236–41.
29. Masselli G, Brunelli R, Di Tola M et al. MR imaging in the evaluation of placental abruption: Correlation with sonographic findings. *Radiology* 2011; 259(1): 222–30.
30. Benirschke K, Burton GJ, Baergen RN. *Pathology of the Human Placenta* (6th edition), Berlin Heidelberg: Springer-Verlag 2012.
31. Saller DN Jr, Nagey DA, Pupkin MJ, Crenshaw MC Jr. Tocolysis in the management of third trimester bleeding. *J Perintaol* 1990; 10(2): 125–8.
32. Combs CA, Nyberg DA, Mack LA et al. Expectant management after sonographic diagnosis of placental abruption. *Am J Perinatol* 1992; 9(3): 170–4.
33. Towery R, English TP, Wisner D. Evaluation of pregnant women after blunt injury. *J Trauma* 1993; 35(5): 731–5.
34. Hurd WW, Miodovnik M, Hertzberg V et al. Selective management of abruptio placentae: A prospective study. *Obstet Gynecol* 1983; 61: 467–73.
35. Nimmo RA, Murphy GA, Adhate A et al. Factors affecting perinatal mortality in an urban center. *Natl Med Assoc J* 1991; 83: 147–52.
36. Kayani SI, Walkinshaw SA, Preston C. Pregnancy outcome in severe placental abruption. *BJOG* 2003; 110: 679–83.
37. Wafaisade A, Maegele M, Lefering R et al. High plasma to red blood cell ratios are associated with lower mortality rates in patients receiving multiple transfusion (4 ≤ red blood cell units < 10) during acute trauma resuscitation. *J Trauma* 2011; 70(1): 81–8.
38. Shields LE, Wiesner S, Fulton J, Pelletreau B. Comprehensive maternal hemorrhage protocols reduce the use of blood products and improve patient safety. *Am J Obstet Gynecol* 2015; 212(3): 272–80.
39. Silver RM. Abnormal placentation: Placenta previa, vasa previa, and placenta accreta. *Obstet Gynecol* 2015; 126(3): 654–68.
40. Handler AS, Mason ED, Rosenberg DL, Davis FG. The relationship between exposure during pregnancy to cigarette smoking and cocaine use and placenta previa. *Am J Obstet Gynecol* 1994; 170(3): 884–9.
41. Gabert HA. Placenta previa and fetal growth. *Obstet Gynecol* 1971; 38: 403–6.
42. Yeniel AO, Ergenoglu AM, Itil IM et al. Effect of placenta previa on fetal growth restriction and stillbirth. *Arch Gynecol Obstet* 2012; 286(2): 295–8.
43. Timor-Tritsch IE, Yunis RA. Confirming the safety of transvaginal sonography in patients suspected of placenta previa. *Obstet Gynecol* 1993; 81(5 Pt 1): 742–4.
44. Leerentveld RA, Gilberts EC, Arnold MJ, Wladimiroff JW. Accuracy and safety of transvaginal sonographic placental localization. *Obstet Gynecol* 1990; 76(5 Pt 1): 759–62.
45. Bill AH. The treatment of placenta previa by prophylactic blood transfusion and cesarean section. *Am J Obstet Gynecol* 1927; 14: 523.
46. McShane PM, Heyl PS, Epstein ME. Maternal and perinatal morbidity resulting from placenta previa. *Obstet Gynecol* 1985; 65: 176–82.

47. Iyasu S, Saftlas AK, Rowley DL et al. The epidemiology of placenta previa in the United States, 1979 through 1987. *Am J Obstet Gynecol* 1993; 168: 1424–9.
48. Neilson JP. Interventions for suspected placenta praevia. *Cochrane Database Syst Rev* 2003; (2): CD001998.
49. Mouer JR. Placenta previa: Antepartum conservative management, inpatient versus outpatient. *Am J Obstet Gynecol* 1994; 170: 1683–5.
50. Wing DA, Paul RH, Millar LK. Management of the symptomatic placenta previa: A randomized, controlled trial of inpatient versus outpatient expectant management. *Am J Obstet Gynecol* 1996; 175(4 Pt 1): 806–11.
51. Spong CY, Mercer BM, D'Alton M et al. Timing of indicated late-preterm and early-term birth. *Obstet Gyncol* 2011; 118: 323–33.
52. Hong JY, Jee YS, Yoon HJ, Kim SM. Comparison of general and epidural anesthesia in elective cesarean section for placenta previa totalis: Maternal hemodynamics, blood loss and neonatal outcome. *Int J Obstet Anesth* 2003; 12: 12–6.
53. Bronsteen R, Valice R, Lee W et al. Effect of a low-lying placenta on delivery outcome. *Ultrasound Obstet Gynecol* 2009; 33: 204–8.
54. Wu S, Kocherginsky M, Hibbard JU. Abnormal placentation: Twenty-year analysis. *Am Obstet Gynecol* 2005; 192: 1458–61.
55. Silver RM, Landon MB, Rouse DJ et al. Maternal morbidity associated with multiple repeat cesarean deliveries. *Obstet Gynecol* 2006; 107(6): 1226–32.
56. Committee on Obstetric Practice. Committee opinion no. 529: Placenta accreta. *Obstet Gynecol* 2012; 120(1): 207–11.
57. Comstock CH, Love JJ, Bronsteen RA et al. Sonographic detection of placenta accreta in the second and third trimesters of pregnancy. *Am J Obstet Gynecol* 2004; 190: 1135–40.
58. Warshak CR, Eskander R, Hull AD et al. Accuracy of ultrasonography and magnetic resonance imaging in the diagnosis of placenta accreta. *Obstet Gynecol* 2006; 108(3): 573–81.
59. Bowman ZS, Eller AG, Kennedy AM et al. Accuracy of ultrasound for the prediction of placenta accreta. *Am J Obstet Gynecol* 2014; 211(2): 177.e1–7.
60. Shih JC, Palacios Jaraquemada JM, Su YN et al. Role of three-dimensional power Doppler in the antenatal diagnosis of placenta accreta: Comparison with gray-scale and color Doppler techniques. *Ultrasound Obstet Gynecol* 2009; 33(2): 193–203.
61. Collins SL, Stevenson GN, Al-Khan A et al. Three-dimensional power doppler ultrasonography for diagnosing abnormally invasive placenta and quantifying the risk. *Obstet Gynecol* 2015; 126(3): 645–53.
62. Rahaim NS, Whitby EH. The MRI features of placental adhesion disorder and their diagnostic significance: Systematic review. *Clin Radiol* 2015; 70(9): 917–25.
63. Robinson BK, Grobman WA. Effectiveness of timing strategies for delivery of individuals with placenta previa and accreta. *Obstet Gynecol* 2010; 116(4): 835–42.
64. Shamshirsaz AA, Fox KA, Salmanian B et al. Maternal morbidity in patients with morbidly adherent placenta treated with and without a standardized multidisciplinary approach. *Am J Obstet Gynecol* 2015; 212: 218.e1–9.
65. Silver RM, Fox KA, Barton JR et al. Center of excellence for placenta accreta. *Am J Obstet Gynecol* 2015; 212(5): 561–8.
66. O'Brien JM, Barton JR, Donaldson ES. The management of placenta percreta: Conservative and operative strategies. *Am J Obstet Gynecol* 1996; 175: 1632–8.
67. Bennett MJ, Sen RC. 'Conservative' management of placenta previa percreta: Report of two cases and discussion of current management options. *Aust NZ J Obstet Gynaecol* 2003; 43: 249–51.
68. Tam Tam KB, Dozier J, Martin JN Jr. Approaches to reduce urinary tract injury during management of placenta accreta, increta, and percreta: A systematic review. *J Matern Fetal Neonatal Med* 2012; 25(4): 329–34.
69. Ballas J, Hull AD, Saenz C, et al. Preoperative intravascular balloon catheters and surgical outcomes in pregnancies complicated by placenta accreta: A management paradox. *Am J Obstet Gynecol* 2012; 207(3): 216.e1–5.
70. Shrivastava V, Nageotte M, Major C et al. Case-control comparison of cesarean hysterectomy with and without prophylactic placement of intravascular balloon catheters for placenta accreta. *Am J Obstet Gynecol* 2007; 197: 402.e1–5.
71. Salim R, Chulski A, Romano S et al. Precesarean prophylactic balloon catheters for suspected placenta accreta. *Obstet Gynecol* 2015; 126(5): 1022–8.
72. Pather S, Strockyj S, Richards A et al. Maternal outcome after conservative management of placenta percreta at caesarean section: A report of three cases and a review of the literature. *Aust N Z J Obstet Gynaecol* 2014; 54(1): 84–7.
73. Mussalli GM, Shah J, Berck DJ et al. Placenta accreta and methotrexate therapy: Three case reports. *J Perinatol* 2000; 20(5): 331–4.
74. Sentilhes L, Ambroselli C, Kayem G et al. Maternal outcome after conservative treatment of placenta accreta. *Obstet Gynecol* 2010; 115(3): 526–34.
75. Oyelese Y, Catanzarite V, Prefumo F et al. Vasa previa: The impact of prenatal diagnosis on outcomes. *Obstet Gynecol* 2004; 103: 937–42.
76. Society of Maternal–Fetal (SMFM) Publications Committee, Sinkey RG, Odibo AO, Dashe JS. Diagnosis and management of vasa previa. *Am J Obstet Gynecol* 2015; 213(5): 615–9.
77. Fox H. *Pathology of the Placenta*, p. 107. Philadelphia, PA: WB Saunders, 1978.

Intrapartum fetal monitoring

19

MARIA ANDRIKOPOULOU, YINKA OYELESE, and ANTHONY M. VINTZILEOS

CONTENTS

BACKGROUND

Until the mid-twentieth century, most intrapartum interventions were aimed at preserving the maternal, rather than the fetal, well-being. The reason was that it was rarely possible to safely intervene on behalf of the fetus because procedures such as cesarean delivery were largely unsafe. It was the advent of surgical asepsis, intravenous transfusions, and safe anesthesia that made intrapartum interventions on behalf of the fetus possible. These advances made possible the expectation that the mother would survive the cesarean delivery without life-threatening complications. Yet, until the mid-1900s, no reliable methods existed for intrapartum fetal assessment.

While auscultation of the fetal heart rate (FHR) was first reported in 1818 by the Geneva surgeon Francois Mayor, who distinguished it from the maternal pulse, it was Kegadarac, in 1822, who first described the FHR, and asked, "Will it not be possible to judge the state of health or disease of the fetus from the variations that occur in the beat of the fetal heart?"[1] Today, the modern era of intrapartum fetal assessment is due to the introduction of continuous electronic fetal heart rate monitoring (EFM) by Ed Hon[2] at Yale in the late 1950s. Later, in the early 1960s, Saling[3] introduced fetal scalp sampling for assessing fetal pH and oxygenation status of the fetus. By 2002, over 85% of labors in the United States were monitored continuously using EFM.[4]

The main objectives of intrapartum FHR monitoring are to prevent stillbirth and, potentially, fetal brain damage resulting from oxygen deprivation during labor.

PATHOPHYSIOLOGY

Labor exposes the fetus to considerable stress. During contractions, the pressure in the myometrium exceeds that in the uterine vessels. As a consequence, uterine blood flow supplying the placenta and fetus is interrupted during each contraction. Normally, the fetus has sufficient oxygen reserve to cope with the temporary isolation from its oxygen supply that occurs during uterine contractions. If there is no break between uterine contractions (or contractions are more frequent than five in 10 minutes) or if there is inadequate fetal oxygen reserve, the fetus may lose its ability to cope with the stress of labor, even in the presence of normal uterine activity. The effects of physiologic interruption of fetal blood flow are more pronounced in fetuses with preexisting compromise such as intrauterine growth restriction. These fetuses may be unable to cope with normal uterine contractions.

An interruption of fetal blood supply or oxygenation may also occur from umbilical cord compression (i.e., prolapsed cord, cord knot, oligohydramnios, or tight cord loop around the fetal neck or body part), placental abruption, or rupture of fetal vessels.

Intrapartum fetal assessment aims primarily at early detection of inadequate fetal oxygenation, thus allowing for a timely intervention in order to avoid asphyxia-related fetal or neonatal death and hopefully irreparable neurological injury.

INTERMITTENT FETAL HEART RATE MONITORING

Intermittent FHR auscultation is considered acceptable by some authorities for fetal evaluation during labor in low-risk patients. However, in the presence of high-risk factors, the American College of Obstetricians and Gynecologists (ACOG) recommends continuous EFM for all patients.[5] After palpation of the patient's abdomen to identify fetal lie and position, a fetal stethoscope or hand-held Doppler device is used to listen to the fetal heart tones over the fetal back at the level of the fetal chest. In low-risk pregnancies, the FHR should be monitored and recorded every 15 minutes in the first stage and every 5 minutes in the second stage.[5] It is important that the examiner simultaneously takes the maternal pulse so as not to record it as the FHR in error. The examiner should also palpate the uterus regularly for contractions and listen to the heart rate for at least 1 minute after each contraction. The FHR and the timing, duration, and intensity of contractions should be recorded in the patient's medical record on each occasion. Studies that have demonstrated good outcomes with intermittent FHR monitoring have usually had one-on-one continuous care of the patient by a nurse or midwife throughout labor. Needless to say, the demands on personnel and time make this impractical in most modern obstetric settings in the United States. Importantly, some catastrophic intrapartum events that may have been picked up earlier by continuous monitoring may occur between periods of auscultation leading to adverse outcomes. These events include cord accidents, placental abruption, and uterine rupture. Nonetheless, carefully selected cases may have intermittent monitoring provided the patient is aware of its limitations and that one-on-one obstetrical care is available.

CONTINUOUS ELECTRONIC FETAL HEART RATE MONITORING

Continuous EFM, also known in Europe as cardiotocography (CTG), is almost universally used in the United States, with over 80% of births assessed with EFM.[4] In EFM, the FHR is monitored continuously, typically using a Doppler ultrasound transducer strapped on the mother's abdomen. The transducer is placed so that it overlies the fetal back at the level of the fetal chest. Doppler ultrasound detects the Doppler shift that occurs with movement of the fetal atrioventricular heart valves; this is then translated into a heart rate by a microprocessor. Because the particular valve movement used to calculate the heart rate varies from one beat to the next, errors may result in the rate counting of these monitors. Therefore, autocorrelation is used to attempt to improve the accuracy of heart rate counting. A separate monitor, the tocodynamometer, attached by another strap records uterine contractions. The tocodynamometer provides quantitative data on the frequency of contractions, semiquantitative data on the duration of contractions, and nonquantitative data on the amplitude or strength of contractions. The tocodynamometer is a strain gauge and may respond to other activities that increase abdominal pressure such as movement or coughing. Thus, both FHR and uterine activity are recorded simultaneously, usually on a computer monitor and/or continuous paper roll. The recording of both the FHR and contractions should be of adequate quality for visual interpretation. The paper speed in the United States is 3 cm/minute, while in Europe the speed is frequently 1 cm/minute. On the upper vertical scale, the FHR in beats per minute (bpm) is recorded, while on the lower scale uterine contractions are recorded.

In some situations, invasive fetal monitoring may be required. In a number of labors, it may be difficult to obtain an adequate FHR tracing. This is often the result of maternal obesity, excessive fetal or maternal movement, or descent of the fetus in the birth canal in the second stage of labor. In these circumstances, a small spiral electrode may be passed through the cervix and attached to the fetal scalp or buttocks, in the event of a planned vaginal breech delivery. In order to attach the electrode, the membranes must be ruptured and there must be sufficient cervical dilation to permit the placement of the electrode on the fetal scalp or buttocks. The electrocardiographic signal from the fetus is calculated by the R–R interval; this is recorded each time the fetal heartbeats. Besides allowing more accurate assessment of the FHR, signal loss, a not uncommon problem with external monitoring, is overcome in most circumstances when internal monitoring is used. Complications are infrequent. However, adverse events such as fetal scalp abscess, cranial osteomyelitis, penetrating ocular injury, and leakage of cerebrospinal fluid have been reported in association with fetal scalp electrode placement.[6–9] Thus, a scalp electrode should be used only when it is indicated. In addition, transmission of the maternal pulse via a fetal scalp electrode in a situation where there is a dead fetus has been described.[10]

Intrauterine pressure catheters (IUPCs) may be used to monitor the force of uterine contractions as well as their frequency in an objective manner. IUPCs are soft, pliable silicone or plastic catheters. Quantitative data relating to the duration, frequency, and amplitude of contractions are displayed continuously. This may be helpful in situations where there is failure of progress despite oxytocin augmentation, or when monitoring of uterine contractions is considered essential and cannot be achieved externally due to maternal obesity or fetal movement. The IUPC may also be used to infuse saline into the uterine cavity for the relief of variable decelerations. Most modern IUPCs have a clear channel through which the color of the amniotic fluid may be observed. Complications are rare, but include placental abruption, injury to the umbilical cord, and, very rarely, uterine perforation or rupture. Contraindications to invasive monitoring include active genital herpes, human immunodeficiency virus infection, and maternal hepatitis B infection.

GUIDELINES FOR ELECTRONIC FETAL HEART RATE MONITORING INTERPRETATION

Despite wide acceptance and utilization of EFM, there remains considerable variation in the interpretation and management of different FHR patterns. Studies have shown that the inter- and intraobserver differences in interpreting the same FHR patterns are substantial.[11] In an attempt to standardize EFM interpretation, a National Institute of Child Health and Human Development (NICHD) Research Planning Workshop convened in 1997 and reported on standardized definitions for FHR patterns.[12] Subsequently, in 2008, the Eunice Kennedy Shriver NICHD, the American College of Obstetricians, and the Society for Maternal–Fetal Medicine held another workshop of experts in EFM to revisit nomenclature, interpretation, and research recommendations for EFM.[13] The workshop recommended standard definitions for the components of EFM (Table 19.1) and also proposed a new three-tier classification system for interpretation of FHR patterns. The key features for FHR pattern classification in Categories I, II, or III are shown in Table 19.2.

In this classification, the features of FHR patterns are categorized as baseline, periodic, or episodic.[13] Periodic patterns are those associated with uterine contractions, while episodic patterns are not associated with contractions. Periodic patterns are defined as "abrupt" or "gradual" depending on waveform shape. Accelerations are increases from the baseline and decelerations are

Table 19.1 Definitions of components of electronic fetal heart rate monitoring patterns.

Pattern	Definition

Baseline	• The mean FHR rounded to increments of 5 bpm during a 10-minute segment, excluding the following:
	  • Periodic or episodic changes.
	  • Periods of marked FHR variability.
	  • Segments of baseline that differ by more than 25 bpm.
	• The baseline must be for a minimum of 2 minutes in any 10-minute segment, or the baseline for that time period is indeterminate. In this case, one may refer to the prior 10-minute window for determination of baseline.
	• Normal FHR baseline: 110–160 bpm.
	• Tachycardia: FHR baseline is greater than 160 bpm.
	• Bradycardia: FHR baseline is less than 110 bpm.

Baseline variability	• Fluctuations in the baseline FHR that are irregular in amplitude and frequency.
	• Variability is visually quantitated as the amplitude of peak-to-trough in beats per minute.
	  • Absent—amplitude range undetectable.
	  • Minimal—amplitude range detectable but 5 bpm or fewer.
	  • Moderate (normal)—amplitude range 6–25 bpm.
	  • Marked—amplitude range greater than 25 bpm.

Acceleration	• A visually apparent abrupt increase (onset to peak in less than 30 seconds) in the FHR. • At 32 weeks of gestation and beyond, an acceleration has a peak of 15 bpm or more above baseline, with a duration of 15 seconds or more but less than 2 minutes from onset to return. • Before 32 weeks of gestation, an acceleration has a peak of 10 bpm or more above baseline, with a duration of 10 seconds or more but less than 2 minutes from onset to return. • Prolonged acceleration lasts 2 minutes or more but less than 10 minutes in duration. • If an acceleration lasts 10 minutes or longer, it is a baseline change.
Early deceleration	• Visually apparent, usually symmetrical, gradual decrease and return of the FHR associated with a uterine contraction. • A gradual FHR decrease is defined as from the onset to the FHR nadir of 30 seconds or more. • The decrease in FHR is calculated from the onset to the nadir of the deceleration. • The nadir of the deceleration occurs at the same time as the peak of the contraction. • In most cases the onset, nadir, and recovery of the deceleration are coincident with the beginning, peak, and ending of the contraction, respectively.

(Continued)

Table 19.1 (*Continued*) Definitions of components of electronic fetal heart rate monitoring patterns.

Late deceleration	• Visually apparent, usually symmetrical, gradual decrease and return of the FHR associated with a uterine contraction. • A gradual FHR decrease is defined as from the onset to the FHR nadir of 30 seconds or more. • The decrease in FHR is calculated from the onset to the nadir of the deceleration. • The deceleration is delayed in timing, with the nadir of the deceleration occurring after the peak of the contraction. • In most cases, the onset, nadir, and recovery of the deceleration occur after the beginning, peak, and ending of the contraction, respectively.
Variable deceleration	• Visually apparent abrupt decrease in FHR. • An abrupt FHR decrease is defined as from the onset of the deceleration to the beginning of the FHR nadir of less than 30 seconds. • The decrease in FHR is calculated from the onset to the nadir of the deceleration. • The decrease in FHR is 15 bpm or greater, lasting 15 seconds or greater, and less than 2 minutes in duration. • When variable decelerations are associated with uterine contractions, their onset, depth, and duration commonly vary with successive uterine contractions.
Prolonged deceleration	• Visually apparent decrease in the FHR below the baseline. • Decrease in FHR from the baseline that is 15 bpm or more, lasting 2 minutes or more but less than 10 minutes in duration. • If a deceleration lasts 10 minutes or longer, it is a baseline change.
Sinusoidal pattern	• Visually apparent, smooth, sine wave–like undulating pattern in FHR baseline with a cycle frequency of 3–5 per minute, which persists for 20 minutes or more.

Source: Macones GA et al., *Obstet Gynecol*, 212, 661–666, 2008. With permission.
Abbreviations: bpm, beats per minute; FHR, fetal heart rate.

Table 19.2 Categories of FHR patterns according to the 2008 NICHD classification.

Category I (normal)
It should include *all* of the following:
Baseline rate: 110–160 bpm
Variability: Moderate
Accelerations: Present or absent
Decelerations: No late, variable or prolonged decelerations
Category II (indeterminate)
Includes all FHR patterns not classified as Category I or Category III
Category III (abnormal)
Absent variability with any of the following:
Recurrent late decelerations
Recurrent variable decelerations
Bradycardia
or
Sinusoidal pattern

Abbreviation: NICHD, National Institute of Child Health and Human Development.

decreases in FHR from the baseline FHR. Definitions of baseline heart rate, baseline FHR variability, accelerations, and decelerations are given in Table 19.1. The interpretation of FHR is visual and a full description of an EFM tracing includes descriptions of all of the following: the baseline FHR, baseline FHR variability, presence of accelerations, contractions, presence of periodic or episodic decelerations, and changes of FHR patterns over time.

SIGNIFICANCE OF DIFFERENT COMPONENTS OF THE FETAL HEART RATE PATTERN

Baseline rate

A normal baseline rate is 110–160 bpm.[13] Fetal tachycardia may occur with maternal fever; intra-amniotic infection; fetal thyrotoxicosis; fetal anemia; fetal tachyarrhythmia; fetal oxygen deprivation; and maternal administration of certain drugs, including beta-sympathomimetic tocolytics and parasympatholytic agents such as atropine or scopolamine. An uncomplicated tachycardia (i.e., one without loss of variability or decelerations) is generally associated with good outcomes.[14] Bradycardia may occur due to cord compression; medications such as maternal beta-blockers; oxygen deprivation; and fetal heart block, typically due to damage to the fetal conduction system from transplacental transfer of maternal antibodies, as may be seen in maternal systemic lupus erythematosus.

Baseline variability

This refers to the variation of the heart rate from the baseline. Normal variability is highly predictive of a nonacidemic fetus.[13] FHR variability represents as an interplay between the cardioaccelerator and cardioinhibitor centers in the fetal brain stem and is regulated by the autonomic nervous system.[5] Physiologically, there is a variability on a beat-by-beat basis of 3–8 bpm around the average. When no baseline amplitude changes are detectable, variability is said to be absent.[13] A persistent loss of variability may be one of the most ominous characteristics of an FHR tracing. However, an absence of variability does not necessarily imply fetal acidemia.[13] Short periods of reduced variability (30–45 minutes or less) may be associated with fetal sleep. Administration of narcotics or sedatives in labor may also reduce variability.[5]

Accelerations

FHR accelerations often occur with fetal movements. The presence of FHR accelerations, whether spontaneous or stimulated, reliably rules out fetal metabolic acidemia.[5,13,15,16] This is because fetal accelerations are controlled by a center in the brain (posterior hypothalamus and medulla) that is extremely sensitive to pH changes. Thus, the presence of accelerations implies that this central nervous system (CNS) center is intact and functional and therefore not hypoxemic. Importantly, though, the converse cannot be assumed; i.e., the absence of FHR accelerations could be due to a sleeping cycle and it does not necessarily imply fetal acidemia.[13]

Variable decelerations

Variable decelerations generally imply cord compression.[17] They vary in timing, shape, depth, and duration. The deceleration is mediated by the vagus nerve, and the degree of fall in heart rate is dependent on the degree of cord compression. Variable decelerations are frequently observed in breech presentations, with oligohydramnios, and when there is a nuchal cord, or the cord is around some other part of the fetus. As the umbilical cord is occluded the fetal peripheral resistance increases, the fetal pO falls, and the pCO_2 rises. Through the baroreceptors and chemoreceptors, a reflex release of acetylcholine at the sinoatrial node causes an almost instantaneous and somewhat erratic drop in FHR. Variable decelerations occur frequently during labor. Often, they can be corrected by changing the maternal position or by amnioinfusion.[5]

Variable decelerations may lead to a reduction in umbilical blood flow resulting in fetal respiratory acidosis. With repetitive or prolonged variable decelerations, fetal metabolic acidosis may be superimposed resulting in mixed fetal acidemia. As oxygen deprivation worsens, a delayed recovery in the FHR to the baseline level may develop. On occasion the FHR may fall below 60 bpm. Severe or deep variable decelerations should lead to a vaginal examination to rule out a cord prolapse or vasa previa.[18] Moreover, in patients undergoing a trial of labor after prior cesarean, variable decelerations may be the first sign of uterine rupture.[19] Finally, severe intrapartum variable decelerations may be a sign of intra-amniotic infection, especially in the premature fetus.[20]

Late decelerations

Late decelerations are thought to represent uteroplacental insufficiency and decreased intervillous exchange between the fetus and the mother.[21–23] Initially, they may represent a vagally mediated reflex response with normal heart rate variability. However, late decelerations may be associated with fetal hypoxemia and acidemia, especially when there is an associated absence of FHR variability.[21–24] They may occur with placental abruption, excessive uterine activity (whether spontaneous or oxytocin induced), maternal hypotension, anemia, or ketoacidosis. Even shallow repetitive late decelerations of only 5–10 bpm may indicate a sufficient degree of fetal oxygen deprivation to result in acidosis and brain damage. Persistent late decelerations may indicate fetal myocardial depression.

Early decelerations

Early decelerations are generally considered benign and are thought be caused by pressure on the fetal head during its descent down the birth canal in the active phase of labor, with a resultant reflex slowing of the heart rate mediated by the vagus nerve.

Sinusoidal fetal heart rate pattern

A sinusoidal fetal heart tracing is an abnormal FHR pattern that should be regarded as an ominous sign of fetal compromise, associated with a significant risk of fetal mortality or severe morbidity (Figure 19.1).[25] Sinusoidal FHR

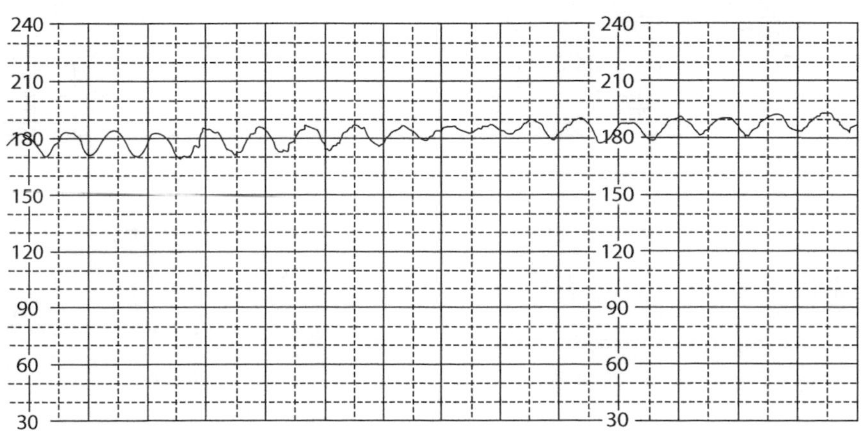

Figure 19.1 Sinusoidal fetal heart rate (FHR) pattern showing stable baseline with smooth oscillations, 3–5 per minute, amplitude 5–15 beats per minute (bpm).

pattern is defined as one with a stable baseline, oscillations of the heart rate above and below the baseline with a frequency of three to five cycles per minute and amplitude of 5–15 bpm and absent short-term variability lasting 20 minutes or more.[13,26] These FHR patterns demand immediate evaluation and intervention because they have been associated with severe fetal anemia resulting from alloimmunization, ruptured vasa previa, fetomaternal hemorrhage, placental abruption, uterine rupture, twin-to-twin transfusion, fetal hypoxia, fetal cardiac malformations, or maternal cardiopulmonary bypass.[18] Similar patterns, termed pseudosinusoidal, may result from the administration of opiates in labor.[27] While pseudosinusoidal patterns are most often associated with normal neonatal outcome, careful fetal assessment is indicated when such FHR patterns are detected.

Sawtooth fetal heart rate pattern

This FHR pattern, which may resemble sinusoidal, has been previously confused with pseudo-sinusoidal or benign salutatory pattern. Although this specific FHR pattern was not described in the 2008 NICHD FHR pattern classification, this rare FHR pattern has been recently reported to be associated with fetal CNS injury in utero of ischemic or hemorrhagic etiology.[28] This FHR pattern has *unstable* or *indeterminate* baseline, periods of *sawtooth-like oscillations* with a *frequency of 3–5 per minute* and *amplitude greater than 20 bpm*. This FHR pattern should be differentiated from a true sinusoidal pattern, usually linked to fetal anemia, which also has three to five cycles per minute but the oscillations are smooth with smaller amplitude (10–15 bpm) and with a stable baseline (Figure 19.2). We have observed three cases of sawtooth FHR pattern associated with evidence of in utero fetal CNS injury.[28] Hence, we suggest that when such an FHR pattern is observed, it be considered a Category III, rather than Category II, FHR pattern.

FETAL HEART RATE PATTERN CATEGORIES AND THEIR INTERPRETATION AND MANAGEMENT

A Category I FHR tracing generally implies that the fetus has normal fetal acid–base status.[5,13] Perhaps the most important finding in a Category I FHR tracing is the presence of accelerations, whether spontaneous or provoked. This reliably predicts the absence of fetal metabolic acidemia.[5,13] Similarly, the presence of moderate FHR variability reliably excludes metabolic acidemia.[5,13] Thus, when the FHR tracing is a Category I pattern, it is considered normal and generally no further intervention is needed.[5,13] It can be managed with intermittent monitoring every 30 minutes at the first stage of labor and then every 15 minutes in the second stage or with continuous fetal monitoring.

Conversely, a Category III FHR tracing is considered abnormal and predictive of abnormal fetal acid–base status.[5,13] The hallmark of a Category III FHR pattern is *absent FHR variability* associated with recurrent late or variable decelerations or fetal bradycardia.[5,13] Sinusoidal FHR patterns are also considered Category III.[5,13] In these situations, fetal well-being cannot be guaranteed, and there is a significant likelihood of fetal compromise with strong possibility for adverse outcomes. Hence, when there is a Category III FHR tracing, prompt evaluation and efforts to resolve the FHR pattern or expeditious delivery are indicated. In some cases, resuscitative efforts may be attempted in preparation for delivery—such as discontinuation of labor stimulation, uterine relaxants, maternal repositioning, oxygen therapy, or intravenous hydration.[5,13]

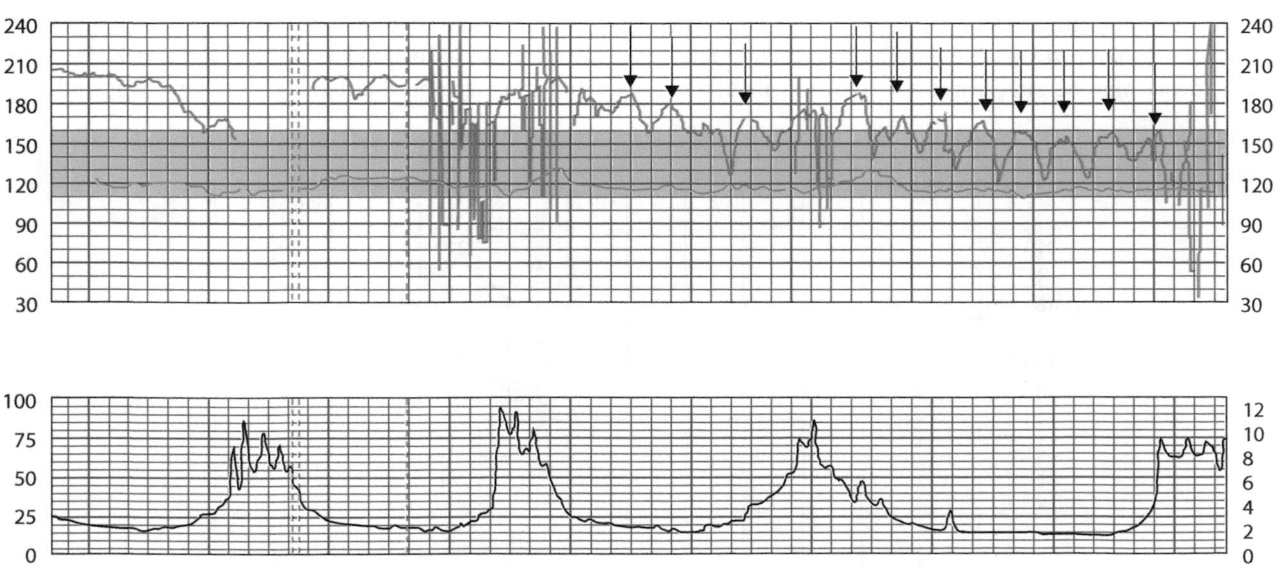

Figure 19.2 Sawtooth FHR pattern showing the unstable baseline with arrows pointing to the periods of sawtooth-like oscillations, 3–5 per minute, amplitude >20 bpm. (Modified from Andrikopoulou M and Vintzileos AM, *Am J Obstet Gynecol*, 214, 403.e1–4, 2016.)

A Category II FHR is one that does not fit into Category I or III.[5,13] Essentially, a Category II FHR pattern implies that the FHR is not completely reassuring, but is not necessarily indicative of abnormal fetal acid–base status. The overwhelming majority of FHR patterns in labor are Category II. Since Category II FHR patterns have enormous variations with respect to their clinical significance and management, these FHR patterns have been the subject of great controversy.

THE MANAGEMENT OF CATEGORY II FETAL HEART RATE PATTERNS

While the interpretation and management in the presence of Category I or III FHR patterns are fairly clear, there remains great controversy regarding the significance and management of a Category II FHR.[5,13] Unfortunately, neither the NICHD workshop guidelines nor the ACOG Practice Bulletin have given clear guidelines for the management of Category II FHR patterns despite the fact that over 80% of intrapartum FHR patterns will be Category II at some point during the labor.[5,29,30] Unfortunately, oftentimes in clinical practice, it is difficult to differentiate between Category II and Category III FHR patterns, thus resulting in unnecessary interventions or intervention delays due to misclassification. The two most important reasons for misclassifying the severity of the FHR pattern, thus leading to inappropriate management are (1) human inability to distinguish between *absent* and *minimal* variability and (2) the *severity* of FHR decelerations were not taken into consideration in the 2008 NICHD classification. In order to circumvent the aforementioned shortcomings of the three-tier categorization, Parer et al.[31] proposed a five-tier system to improve on the management of these FHR patterns. More recently, Clark et al.[29] argued that it was time for standardization of management of Category II FHR patterns and proposed an algorithm for their evaluation and management (Figure 19.3). This algorithm does not rely in the differentiation between *absent* from *minimal* variability; instead it considers as main criteria: (1) whether there are *accelerations* or *moderate variability*, both features suggesting a nonacidemic fetus; (2) presence or absence of *significant* decelerations with >50% of contractions; and (3) the stage, as well as progress, of labor. The definition of significant decelerations is shown in Table 19.3. Essentially, if a Category II FHR pattern has moderate variability and/or accelerations and labor is progressing normally, observation is warranted, even in the presence of decelerations. If there are recurrent decelerations for >30 minutes with no accelerations or moderate variability, delivery by cesarean or operative vaginal delivery may be indicated.[29] Since many of the fetuses, who are born acidemic, do not present with Category III FHR patterns, the clinical application of the Clark et al. algorithm becomes extremely important not only for the timely identification of these fetuses but also for avoiding progression to Category III FHR pattern which could be preterminal.

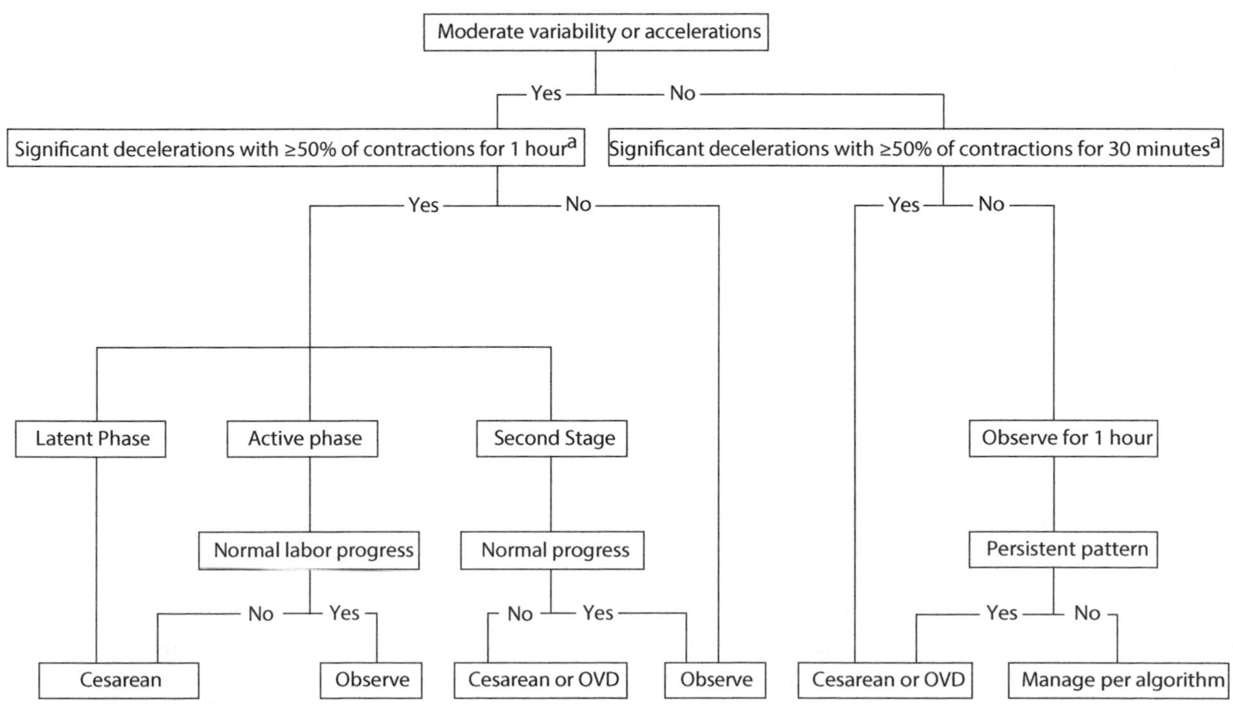

OVD, operative vaginal delivery.

[a]That have not resolved with appropriate conservative corrective measures, which may include supplemental oxygen, maternal position changes, intravenous fluid administration, correction of hypotension, reduction or discontinuation of uterine stimulation, administration of uterine relaxant, amnioinfusion, and/or changes in second stage breathing and pushing techniques.

Figure 19.3 Algorithm for managing Category II FHR patterns in labor. (From Clark SL et al., *Am J Obstet Gynecol*, 209, 89, 2013. With permission.)

Table 19.3 Definition of "significant" FHR decelerations.

- Variable decelerations lasting longer than 60 seconds and reaching a nadir more than 60 bpm below baseline.
- Variable decelerations lasting longer than 60 seconds and reaching a nadir less than 60 bpm regardless of the baseline.
- Late decelerations of any depth.
- Any prolonged deceleration (>2 to <10 minutes).
- Any decelerations that are accompanied by compensatory fetal tachycardia.

Table 19.4 Correlation between duration of second stage bradycardia and fetal academia.[a]

FHR (bpm)	Duration (minutes)
80	25
70	13
60	8
50	6
40	5

Source: Tranquilli AL et al., *J Matern Fetal Neonatal Med*, 26, 1425–1429, 2013.

[a] Cord artery pH < 7.10.

INTRAPARTUM EVOLUTION OF FETAL HEART RATE PATTERNS

In assessing the FHR tracing, it is important to realize that FHR patterns and categories are dynamic processes and that changes of both patterns and categories may evolve over time sometimes rapidly during labor.[5,13] Not infrequently, an FHR pattern may change from one category to another. Hence, any interpretation of FHR pattern is valid only for the time at which the FHR pattern is read.[5,13] Such factors as gestational age, maternal position, stage of labor, medications administered, including oxytocin, uterine relaxants and epidurals, and the presence of fever, may have a significant impact on FHR patterns. It is important that the FHR tracing be interpreted in the context of the clinical situation, such as stage in labor or labor progress, if there is a cord prolapse or the presence or absence of vaginal bleeding. The transitional changes from one FHR pattern category to another depend on the nature of the insult, its severity and its duration. Thus, not all transitions from category to category are similar.

A Category I FHR tracing can abruptly change to a Category III pattern following catastrophic event such as an umbilical cord prolapse, placental abruption, uterine rupture, ruptured vasa previa, acute cord compression, or during the second stage of labor, especially in occiput posterior presentations. All these entities should be included in the differential diagnosis when interpreting a sudden change of the Category I FHR tracing. For instance, a sudden bradycardia in a patient undergoing a trial of labor after cesarean should lead to consideration of a diagnosis of uterine rupture or placental abruption. When a Category I FHR suddenly becomes a Category III pattern with a sinusoidal pattern or bradycardia, the possibility of a ruptured vasa previa must be entertained, especially when there is bleeding or when this FHR pattern change follows rupture of the membranes. Finally, a category I FHR pattern, indicating normal fetal reserve, can suddenly become Category II or III during the second stage of labor. In such cases, there is a correlation between the severity and duration of the second stage bradycardia and fetal acidemia[32] (Table 19.4).

As seen in Figure 19.4a through c, a Category I FHR tracing may gradually progress during labor to a Category III due to primary uteroplacental insufficiency or uteroplacental insufficiency secondary to tachysystole or excessive uterine activity. Typically, this is a gradual change, with the FHR pattern first becoming Category II after the development of a *significant* variable or late decelerations followed by fetal *tachycardia* and *minimal variability.* It is important to diagnose the aforementioned sequential FHR changes (Figure 19.5) because these changes signal the end of Category II FHR and intervention should be implemented to avoid transitioning to Category III, which is characterized by possibly preterminal changes such as *absent* variability with prolonged decelerations and finally bradycardia. If not accurately interpreted and acted on, the above sequence of events has the potential to lead to intrapartum stillbirth or irreparable fetal CNS injury. At this point, it should be emphasized that some fetuses may become acidemic while still exhibiting Category II FHR pattern and transition to Category III is not a prerequisite for developing academia.

Rarely, following amelioration of the inciting circumstances (such as treatment of diabetic ketoacidosis, treatment of tachysystole, therapies to raise blood pressure following hypotension with an epidural), a Category III heart rate tracing may revert to a Category I tracing. However, in the majority of situations, resuscitative efforts for a Category III pattern are unlikely to be successful, and should be done only in preparation for delivery. The physician should be familiar with the circumstances and the gradual FHR changes so as to recognize them in a timely manner and to intervene before a preterminal or terminal FHR tracing.

FETAL INFECTION AND FETAL HEART RATE PATTERNS

Although the initial aim of EFM was to identify the hypoxic and/or acidemic fetus due to uteroplacental insufficiency, after its wide clinical application, it became apparent that fetal compromise in the presence of intra-amniotic infection can also cause abnormal fetal behavior and FHR patterns—even in the absence of fetal academia—in mothers with or without clinical signs of infection[33,34] (Figure 19.6). The mechanism by which fetal infection can cause FHR abnormalities in the absence of acidemia is not known but it is possible that infection increases metabolism and fetal oxygen demands, thus resulting in tissue hypoxia and malfunction of the central nervous system centers that control FHR patterns. Another possibility for the frequently observed decelerations is increased sensitivity

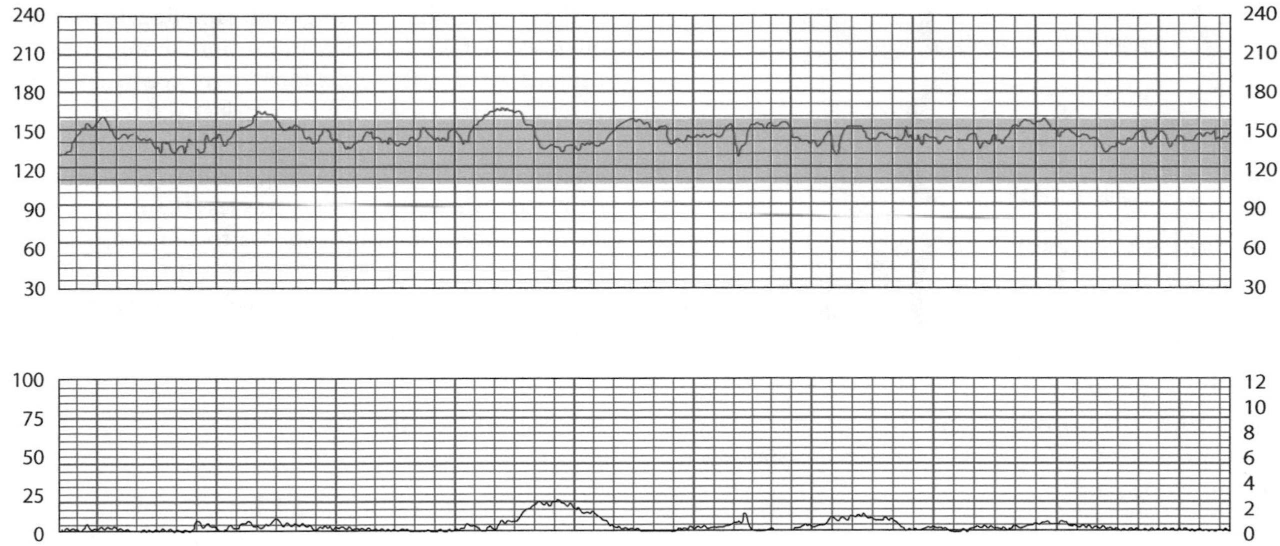

(a)

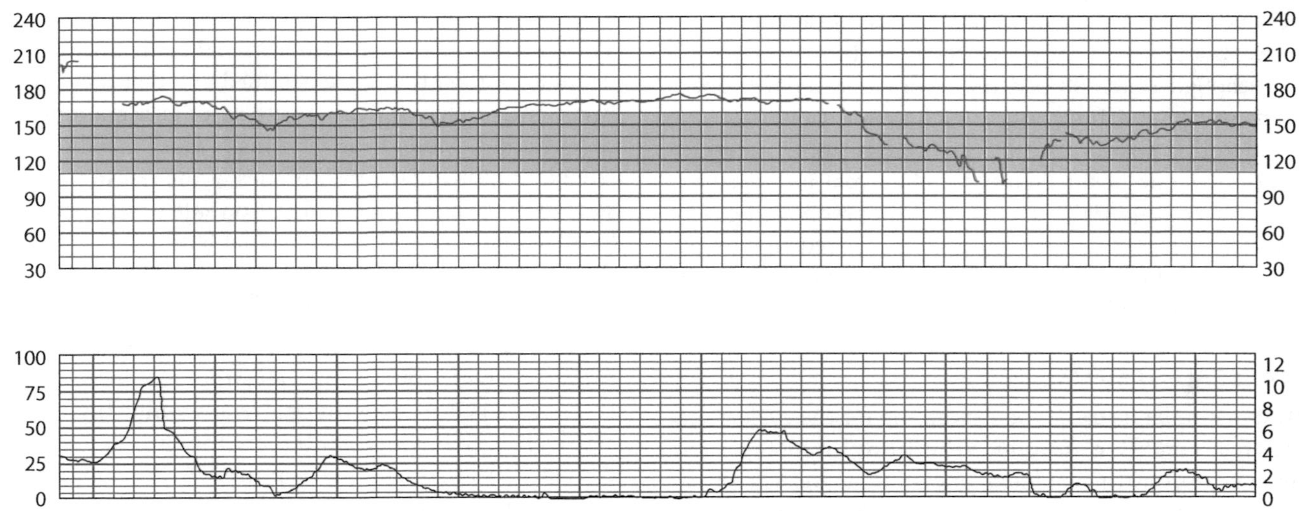

(b)

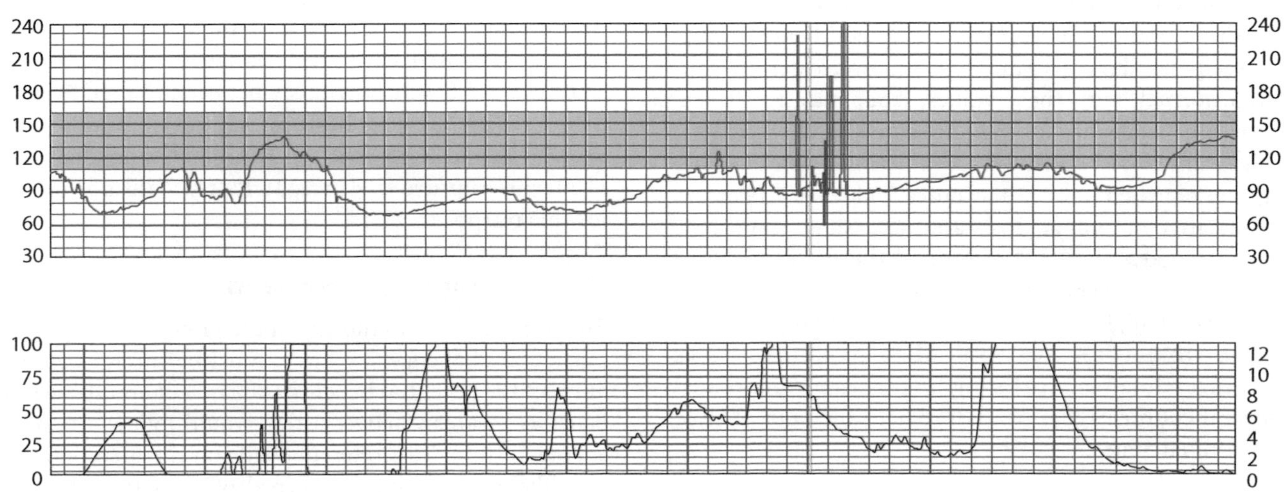

(c)

Figure 19.4 Transition from Category I (a) to Category II (b) to Category III (c) FHR pattern due to excessive uterine activity from uterotonic agents.

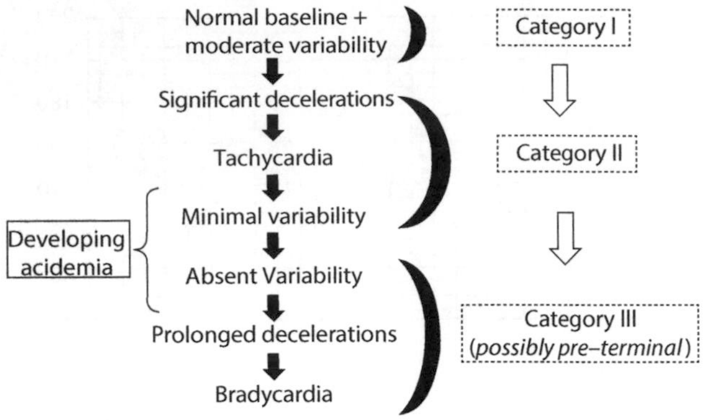

Figure 19.5 Gradual progression of Category I to Category III FHR pattern due to primary uteroplacental insufficiency or excessive uterine activity.

and vasoconstriction of the umbilical and chorionic placental vessels in the presence of intra-amniotic infection. These newborns are usually born depressed (low APGAR scores), but the cord pH is invariably within normal limits. Although the 2008 NICHD Workshop report[13] does not mention fetal infection, the clinician should always consider the possibility of fetal and/or intra-amniotic infection as one of the causes for abnormal intrapartum FHR patterns especially in patients with predisposing factors such as preterm, premature, or prolonged rupture of membranes—but also in the absence of any predisposing factors or maternal clinical signs of infection.

FETAL SCALP SAMPLING

Intrapartum fetal scalp blood sampling for the evaluation of the fetal condition, introduced by Saling[3] in 1960, gives a fairly accurate estimate of fetal oxygenation and acid–base status. However, it provides only a snapshot of fetal status at the time of the sampling. Thus, repeated scalp sampling is necessary until delivery occurs. The main indication for scalp sampling is a nonreassuring fetal heart tracing. Fetal scalp capillary pH values of 7.25 or greater are considered normal; with these values, labor may be allowed to proceed. Values of 7.20–7.24 are considered preacidotic and warrant close continued reevaluation, with the scalp sampling repeated in 20–30 minutes. Values of 7.19 or less are indicative of fetal acidosis and necessitate immediate delivery. Goodwin et al.[35] examined the pattern of fetal scalp sampling over 7 years at their institution, where an average of 16,330 births took place annually. The rate dropped from 1.76% to 0.03%. More recent experience shows that while scalp pH sampling is widely performed in several countries, the procedure has fallen out of favor in the United States.

FETAL SCALP STIMULATION

Perhaps two main factors have contributed to the demise of fetal scalp sampling in the United States. First, the inconvenience and complexity of repeatedly performing scalp sampling during labor, and secondly, the observation that in the process of performing scalp sampling, fetuses would often exhibit FHR accelerations and those fetuses that demonstrated such accelerations were consistently found to have pH values above 7.2.[16] Clark et al.[16] retrospectively analyzed 200 fetal heart tracings where the fetuses had undergone fetal scalp sampling for pH. They found that in no case where the fetal pH was less than 7.20 was there an FHR acceleration in response to the scalp sampling. However, 142 of 144 fetuses with a scalp pH greater than 7.28 responded with heart rate acceleration. Consequently, scalp stimulation with a positive acceleration response has been used as a marker for a nonacidemic fetus.

SPECIAL SITUATIONS

Twins

The monitoring of twins in labor presents a particular diagnostic dilemma. Bakker et al.[36] examined 172 twin pregnancies in labor and found that the FHR signal was suboptimal in 26%–33% of twins in the first stage and 41%–63% of twins in the second stage. It is important, when monitoring twins in labor, to make sure that two different fetal heart traces are obtained and that they do not persistently follow the same pattern of accelerations and decelerations. Monitoring of twins in labor may be facilitated by rupturing the membranes of the leading twin as soon as cervical dilation and station safely allow this and by attaching a scalp electrode to that fetus.

Trial of labor after cesarean (TOLAC)

Labor after cesarean is associated with a risk of uterine rupture, which could have catastrophic consequences. In cases of TOLAC, continuous fetal monitoring is indicated since FHR abnormalities are the earliest and most consistent sign of uterine rupture.[37,38] Repetitive variable or late decelerations and bradycardia are the most frequently observed FHR abnormalities in uterine rupture in patients undergoing TOLAC.[36,37] Hence, variable decelerations, often treated as benign in normal labors, must be assessed early and managed appropriately in TOLACs.[37,38] It was previously believed that IUPCs may help predict uterine rupture. However, studies have shown that no IUPC pattern is predictive or diagnostic of uterine rupture.[39] Hence, IUPCs should not be used for this purpose.

Monitoring of the preterm fetus

The intrapartum monitoring of the preterm fetus presents particular challenges.[5,40] There must be careful consideration of the potential benefits and risks of an intervention (such as cesarean delivery) that would follow a nonreassuring FHR.[5,40] This often depends on the gestational age and likelihood of intact survival of the fetus. This decision should involve the patient, neonatologist, and obstetrician.[5,40] Prematurity, independent of mode of delivery, is a strong risk factor for neurologic handicap. The FHR responses of the preterm fetus may be different from the term fetus. For instance, in preterm fetuses, FHR

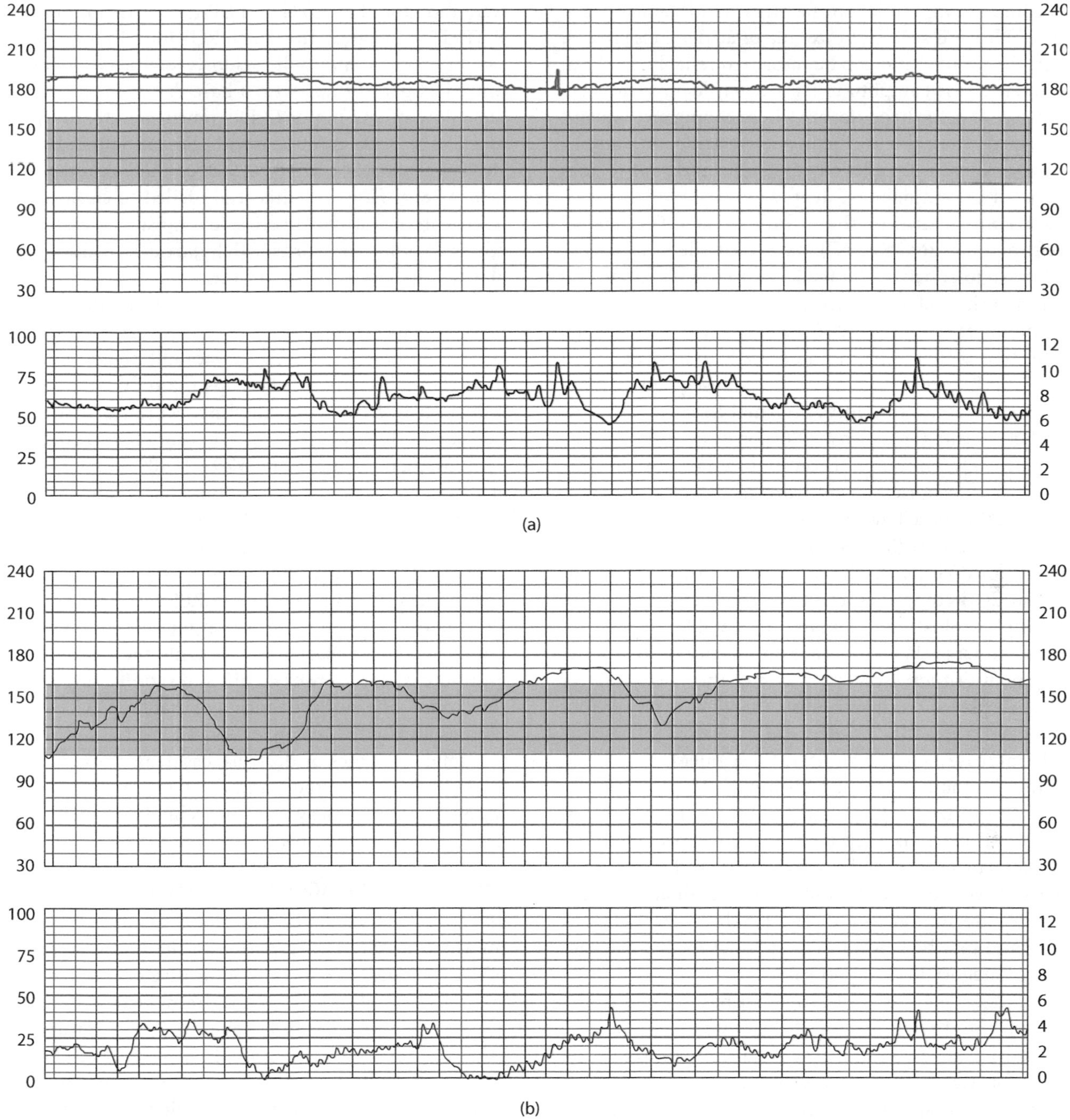

Figure 19.6 Category III FHR pattern on admission (a) and before delivery (b) of a woman at term admitted because of back pain and reduced fetal movement. At cesarean delivery, the amniotic fluid was foul-smelling, the Apgar scores 1 and 6 at 1 and 5 minutes, respectively, and the cord pH values were 7.21 (vein) and 7.18 (artery); the blood cultures of the neonate were positive for *Listeria monocytogenes*.

accelerations may not be present. Preterm fetuses, especially when there intrauterine growth restriction, malpresentation, preeclampsia, or oligohydramnios may be less likely to cope with abnormalities of FHR that would be tolerated by a term fetus. Nonreassuring FHR patterns occur in 60% of preterm labors. Furthermore, variable decelerations occur in 55%–70% of preterm labors compared with 20%–30% of term labors.[5,40] Hence, a preterm fetus is more likely to be delivered by cesarean for a Category II or III FHR tracing.

NEWER TECHNOLOGIES: ST SEGMENT ANALYSIS OF THE FETAL ELECTROCARDIOGRAM

Over the past decade, much attention has been directed at using the fetal electrocardiogram (ECG) for intrapartum monitoring of the fetus.[41–43] Data from animal experiments have indicated that the ST segment pattern of the fetal ECG reflects the ability of the myocardium to respond to hypoxia. Fetal acidemia results in a catecholamine surge, beta-adrenergic activation, myocardial glycogenolysis, elevation of the ST segment, and increased amplitude of the T-wave.[44] The

QRS complex amplitude, on the other hand, remains relatively stable until severe hypoxemia or acidemia is present. Hence, the T/QRS ratio can be measured reliably. ST elevation and increased amplitude T-wave may identify the fetus that is experiencing hypoxia, but whose coping mechanisms are adequate to deal with the insult. As acidemia worsens, the myocardium is unable to compensate and cardiac ischemia occurs, resulting in ST depression.

As a consequence of these findings, a CTG plus ST waveform analyzer (STAN®) have been developed. The STAN system consists of a fetal scalp ECG electrode and a maternal skin reference electrode, and a microprocessor that compares fetal ST and T wave changes with a baseline for that patient. The monitor needs to have an initial normal FHR pattern against which subsequent changes may be compared. This initial normal heart rate pattern must be present for at least 500 consecutive heartbeats (approximately 5 minutes of continuous monitoring). This monitor uses proprietary software to detect when there is ST elevation or a T wave with increased amplitude and issues a visual alert (ST event). Baseline T/QRS ratios are different for each fetus. The monitor records 30 consecutive fetal ECG complexes and from these creates an average complex. Most fetuses maintain a stable T/QRS ratio throughout labor. When there is an increased slope of the ST segment or increased amplitude of the T-wave, an ST event is displayed on the monitor. There are three types of ST events: (1) episodic T/QRS ratio increases, (2) baseline T/QRS increases, and (3) biphasic ST segment.

Using a combination of STAN and EFM, the FHR pattern is categorized into green, yellow, or red categories. Green zone patterns may be managed expectantly, red zone patterns need expeditious delivery and yellow zone patterns need close observation and reevaluation. These categories are similar to the NICHD three-tier EFM categories and may be helpful as an adjunct for the management of Category II FHR patterns.

STAN is widely used in Europe but has not had acceptance in the United States. STAN was conditionally approved by the Food and Drug Administration (FDA) in 2005 for use as an adjunct to conventional EFM. There have been several randomized controlled trials (RCT) comparing traditional intrapartum fetal monitoring using CTG alone with CTG and ST analysis of the fetal ECG.[41–47] The first of these, the Plymouth trial, demonstrated a 46% reduction in the rate of operative deliveries for "fetal distress" when compared with traditional FHR monitoring alone.[45] Following this, the Swedish multicenter trial, which included 4966 women, showed a 61% reduction in umbilical artery metabolic acidosis (defined as a pH under 7.05 and base deficit over 12.0 mmol/L) at birth in the group monitored by CTG and ST analysis compared with CTG alone.[46] In that study, there was also a 28% lower rate of operative delivery for abnormal FHR patterns in the STAN group. Subsequently, the Finnish RCT and the French RCT failed to find any differences in neonatal outcomes and operative delivery rates between women monitored by conventional monitoring (CTG) and those who were monitored by CTG and STAN.[41,42] In a more recent RCT of 5681 women, the Dutch RCT found a slightly lower rate of neonatal metabolic acidosis (defined as an arterial umbilical pH of <7.05 with a base deficit in the extracellular fluid of >12 mmol/L) in women monitored by CTG and STAN (0.7%) compared with those monitored by CTG (1.1%) (relative risk [RR] 0.70; 95% confidence interval [CI] 0.38–1.28).[47] However, this study failed to show any difference in operative deliveries, low Apgar scores, neonatal admissions and newborns with hypoxic–ischemic encephalopathy between the two groups.

Several meta-analyses have found no difference in neonatal outcomes and operative delivery rates between labors monitored by CTG alone and those monitored by CTG and STAN.[48–50] Perhaps the only difference is a reduction in fetal scalp sampling. More recently, a multicenter RCT was carried out by the NICHD Maternal–Fetal Medicine Units Network of 11,108 women in labor at >36 weeks of gestation, randomizing women to "open" or "masked" monitoring with fetal ST segment analysis.[43] The primary outcome was a composite of intrapartum fetal death, neonatal death, Apgar score of <4 at 5 minutes, an umbilical artery blood gas of <7.05 with a base deficit of 12 mmol/L or greater, intubation for ventilation at delivery or neonatal encephalopathy. Only the frequency of a 5-minute Apgar score of <4 differed significantly between the groups. The authors concluded that fetal ECG analysis used as an adjunct to conventional EFM did not improve perinatal outcomes or decrease cesarean delivery rates.[43] As a result of this study, and the meta-analyses evaluating STAN, it is unlikely that this technology will be widely used in the United States at this time.

UMBILICAL CORD ACID–BASE STATUS

The umbilical cord pH and blood gases give objective information about oxygenation in the infant at the time of delivery and therefore are indicative of whether or not labor has resulted in hypoxia. Immediately after delivery, a segment of the cord should be double clamped and put aside. Ideally, samples should be taken from both the artery and the vein. The samples are drawn in heparinized syringes. The ACOG has recommended that cord gases be obtained only in cases where labor and delivery or the pregnancy have been complicated[51] or when the 5-minute Apgar score is 5 or less.[52] However, some authorities recommend obtaining cord blood gases at all deliveries.[53] The argument for this is that less than 10% of all cases of cerebral palsy result from intrapartum events, and several of these cases occur in vigorous newborns. These authorities argue that cord gases may determine, in an objective manner, whether the brain damage was the consequence of an intrapartum hypoxic insult. The ACOG task force, in 2003, reported that *severe* intrapartum fetal acidemia (umbilical artery blood pH less than 7 and base deficit 12 mmol/L or more) should be included as one of the four criteria linking intrapartum asphyxia to ischemic neonatal encephalopathy.[54] Therefore, routine cord pH determinations may be advisable from a medicolegal standpoint,

Table 19.5 Abnormal cutoff cord blood gas values for defining type of acidemia at birth and taking into consideration the presence or absence of labor.

	No labor	Labor
Artery		
Acidemia	pH < 7.20	pH < 7.15
Metabolic	BE < −10 mmol/L and $pCO_2 \le 60$ mm Hg	BE < −11 mmol/L and $pCO_2 \le 65$ mmHg
Respiratory	BE ≥ −10 mmol/L and $pCO_2 > 60$ mm Hg	BE ≥ −11 mmol/L and $pCO_2 > 65$ mmHg
Mixed	BE < −10 mmol/L and $pCO_2 > 60$ mm Hg	BE ≥ −11 mmol/L and $pCO_2 > 65$ mmHg
Vein		
Acidemia	pH < 7.26	pH < 7.20
Metabolic	BE < −6 mmol/L and $pCO_2 \le 50$ mmHg	BE < −8 mmol/L and $pCO_2 \le 55$ mmHg
Respiratory	BE ≥ −6 mmol/L and $pCO_2 > 50$ mmHg	BE ≥ −8 mmol/L and $pCO_2 > 55$ mmHg
Mixed	BE < −6 mmol/L and $pCO_2 > 50$ mmHg	BE < −8 mmol/L and $pCO_2 > 55$ mmHg

Source: Vintzileos AM et al., *J Matern Fetal Med*, 1, 7–13, 1992.
Abbreviation: BE, base excess.

and would also help understand the pathophysiology of the brain damage, since most depressed neonates will not have such a severe fetal acidemia at birth. Certainly, there is consensus that cord gases should be obtained in all high-risk and complicated pregnancies, and when neonatal depression occurs. Both Helwig et al.[55] and Vintzileos et al.[56] have established normal ranges for umbilical blood gas values. In addition, Vintzileos et al. found no differences in cord blood gases and acid–base measurements between preterm and term infants. However, there were differences depending on the presence or absence of labor with labor being associated with lower pH values. In the presence of labor, fetal acidemia was defined as a cord artery pH < 7.15 or cord vein pH < 7.20, whereas in the absence of labor, these cut-offs were higher, i.e., cord artery <7.20 or cord vein pH < 7.26.[56] The abnormal cutoff cord blood gas values for defining the type of acidemia at birth after taking into consideration the presence or absence of labor are depicted in Table 19.5.[56]

THE IMPACT OF CONTINUOUS ELECTRONIC FETAL HEART RATE MONITORING ON OUTCOMES

Despite initial enthusiasm that the advent of intrapartum EFM would lead to the disappearance of stillbirth and cerebral palsy, experience indicates that this has not been the case. Rather, cesareans done for "fetal distress" have skyrocketed with no overall improvement in change in the rate of cerebral palsy.[5,57] Early reports, including a review of nearly 47,656 electronically monitored patients, noted a substantial reduction in the rates of intrapartum and neonatal deaths.[58] Years later, however, it has become apparent that these initial lofty expectations were unduly optimistic.[5,29] Several randomized controlled studies failed to show any reduction in intrapartum stillbirths in women who had continuous EFM when compared with those monitored by intermittent fetal auscultation.[59–64] The best known of these, the Dublin trial, was a randomized controlled study of 12,964 women in whom continuous EFM was compared with intermittent auscultation.[62] Stillbirths, neonatal deaths, cesarean and forceps delivery rates, Apgar scores, and neonatal intensive care admissions were similar in both groups. While there were twice as many seizures in the intermittently auscultated group as in the EFM group, both 1-year and 4-year follow-up failed to show any differences in the rate of cerebral palsy or neurological outcomes between the two groups.[65]

In a study that differed from the others, Vintzileos et al.[66] carried out a RCT of 1428 pregnant women, comparing intrapartum EFM with intermittent auscultation. They demonstrated a significant reduction in intrapartum deaths due to asphyxia in women who had continuous intrapartum electronic fetal surveillance (0/746 in the EFM group versus 6/682 in the intermittent auscultation group (p = .03). However, there was a higher rate of interventions (cesarean, forceps, and vacuum deliveries) in that group (11.2% versus 4.8% in the intermittent auscultation group; p = .04). These authors carried out a further analysis of the same study, with the primary outcome measure being the prediction of fetal acidemia at birth (defined as an umbilical arterial pH <7.15).[67] The sensitivity of EFM for acidemia was 97% compared with 34% for auscultation (p < .001). While this study was at variance with previous studies, it was the only study at the time that had used strict criteria for defining normal and abnormal FHR patterns. Subsequently, a meta-analysis by Vintzileos et al.[68] examining nine randomized controlled studies indicated that the perinatal mortality due to fetal hypoxia was reduced by EFM when compared with intermittent auscultation (odds ratio [OR] 0.41). However, in the EFM group, there was an increased rate of cesarean (OR 2.55), forceps, and vacuum deliveries (OR 2.50) for fetal distress. A year later, another meta-analysis by Thacker et al.[69] examined 12 RCTs and found that EFM was associated with fewer neonatal seizures (RR 0.5) and fewer neonates with a 1-minute Apgar score less than 4 (RR 0.82), again at the cost of an increased cesarean delivery rate (RR 1.33).

Importantly, no studies have compared EFM with no monitoring at all. It is likely that with no monitoring, there would be a great number of intrapartum deaths and asphyxiated fetuses. Clearly, EFM has led to an overall increase in cesarean delivery rates for abnormal FHR (RR 1.63, 95% CI 1.29–2.07) when compared with intermittent auscultation.[70] In addition, the use of EFM increased the risks for forceps and vacuum deliveries.[70]

It is not clear why EFM has failed to make an impact on the rates of cerebral palsy. Parer and King[71] offered a number of explanations. First, probably only 10% or less of cases of cerebral palsy can be attributed to intrapartum asphyxia. Therefore, intrapartum fetal monitoring could not be expected to prevent the other 90% of cases of cerebral palsy. Second, some episodes of fetal asphyxia are so rapid and catastrophic that even prompt delivery may not prevent fetal brain damage. Finally, there is considerable variability in the interpretation of FHR patterns, and in the responses of physicians to these patterns.[72] More recently, Clark et al.[29] have argued that the failure to demonstrate a benefit of EFM may be largely due to nonstandardization of EFM patterns and a lack of standardized protocols for the management and intervention of abnormal patterns. Interestingly, perhaps the only randomized study that showed a benefit from EFM, by Vintzileos et al.,[66] defined abnormal heart rate patterns and used a well-defined algorithm for the management of these abnormal FHR patterns.

Clark et al.[72] carried out a prospective study of 14,398 women undergoing oxytocin induction of labor. In this study, a decrease in the rate of oxytocin administration when a Category II FHR pattern occurred was associated with improved perinatal outcomes (admissions to the neonatal intensive care unit and Apgar scores of <7 at 1 and 5 minutes). These authors concluded that EFM improves neonatal outcomes when unambiguous definitions are coupled with specific interventions.

Hence it is likely that the failure to observe a benefit of EFM has been to some extent the result of nonstandardized definitions of FHR patterns and a lack of standardized responses to abnormal FHR patterns. Hopefully, the new definitions, if coupled with standardized responses, will help to improve neonatal outcomes while reducing the cesarean rates.

REFERENCES

1. Baskett TF. *On the Shoulders of Giants; Eponyms and Names in Obstetrics and Gynaecology.* London, UK: RCOG Press, 1988.
2. Hon E. The electronic evaluation of the fetal heart rate: Preliminary report. *Am J Obstet Gynecol* 1958; 77: 1084–99.
3. Saling E. Neues vorgehen zur untersuchung des kindes unter der gebrut: Einführung, technik, und grundlagen. [New technique for examining the fetus during labor: Introduction, technique and basics]. *Arch Gynakol* 1962; 197: 108–22.
4. Martin JA, Hamilton BE, Sutton PD et al. Births: Final data for 2002. *Natl Vital Stat Rep 2003*; 52(10): 1–113.
5. American College of Obstetricians and Gynecologists. ACOG Practice Bulletin No. 106: Intrapartum fetal heart rate monitoring: Nomenclature, interpretation, and general management principles. *Obstet Gynecol* 2009; 114: 192–202.
6. Cordero L, Anderson CW, Zuspan FP. Scalp abscess: A benign and infrequent complication of fetal monitoring. *Am J Obstet Gynecol* 1983; 146: 126–30.
7. McGregor JA, McFarren T. Neonatal cranial osteomyelitis: A complication of fetal monitoring. *Obstet Gynecol* 1989; 73(3 Pt 2): 490–2.
8. Nieburg P, Gross SJ. Cerebrospinal fluid leak in a neonate associated with fetal scalp electrode monitoring. *Am J Obstet Gynecol* 1983; 147: 839–40.
9. Miyashiro MJ, Mintz-Hittner HA. Penetrating ocular injury with a fetal scalp monitoring spiral electrode. *Am J Ophthalmol* 1999; 128: 526–8.
10. Ramsey PS, Johnston BW, Welter VE et al. Artifactual fetal electrocardiographic detection using internal monitoring following intrapartum fetal demise during VBAC trial. *J Matern Fetal Med* 2000; 9: 360–1.
11. Nielsen PV, Stigsby B, Nickelsen C, Nim J. Intra- and inter-observer variability in the assessment of intrapartum cardiotocograms. *Acta Obstet Gynecol Scand* 1987; 66: 421–4.
12. American College of Obstetricians and Gynecologists. Electronic fetal heart rate monitoring: Research guidelines for interpretation. National Institute of Child Health and Human Development Research Planning Workshop. *Am J Obstet Gynecol* 1997; 177: 1385–90.
13. Macones GA, Hankins GD, Spong CY et al. The 2008 National Institute of Child Health and Human Development workshop report on electronic fetal monitoring: Update on definitions, interpretation, and research guidelines. *Obstet Gynecol* 2008; 212: 661–6.
14. Sherer DM, Onyeije CI, Binder D et al. Uncomplicated baseline fetal tachycardia or bradycardia in postterm pregnancies and perinatal outcome. *Am J Perinatol* 1998; 15: 335–8.
15. Parer JT, King T, Flanders S et al. Fetal acidemia and electronic fetal heart rate patterns: Is there evidence of an association? *J Matern Fetal Neonatal Med* 2006; 19: 289–94.
16. Clark SL, Gimovsky ML, Miller FC. Fetal heart rate response to scalp blood sampling. *Am J Obstet Gynecol* 1982; 144: 706–8.
17. Ball RH, Parer JT. The physiologic mechanisms of variable decelerations. *Am J Obstet Gynecol* 1992; 166: 1683–8.
18. Cordero DR, Helfgott AW, Landy HJ et al. A nonhemorrhagic manifestation of vasa previa: A clinicopathologic case report. *Obstet Gynecol* 1993; 82: 698–700.
19. Sheiner E, Levy A, Ofir K et al. Changes in fetal heart rate and uterine patterns associated with uterine rupture. *J Reprod Med* 2004; 49: 373–8.

20. Salafia CM, Ghidini A, Sherer DM et al. Abnormalities of the fetal heart rate in preterm deliveries are associated with acute intra-amniotic infection. *J Soc Gynecol Invest* 1998; 5: 188–91.
21. Low JA, Victory R, Derrick EJ. Predictive value of electronic fetal monitoring for intrapartum fetal asphyxia with metabolic acidosis. *Obstet Gynecol* 1999; 93: 285–91.
22. Murata Y, Martin CB Jr, Ikenoue T et al. Fetal heart rate accelerations and late decelerations during the course of intrauterine death in chronically catheterized rhesus monkeys. *Am J Obstet Gynecol* 1982; 144: 218–23.
23. Martin CB, de Haan J, van der Wildt B et al. Mechanisms of late decelerations in the fetal heart rate. A study with autonomic blocking agents in fetal lambs. *Eur J Obstet Gynecol Reprod Biol* 1979; 9: 361–73.
24. Williams KP, Galerneau F. Intrapartum fetal heart rate patterns in the prediction of neonatal acidemia. *Am J Obstet Gynecol* 2003; 188: 820–3.
25. Manseau P, Vaquier J, Chavinie J et al. Sinusoidal fetal cardiac rhythm. An aspect evocative of fetal distress during pregnancy. *J Gynecol Obstet Biol Reprod (Paris)* 1972; 1: 343–52.
26. Modanlou HD, Murata Y. Sinusoidal heart rate pattern: Reappraisal of its definition and significance. *J Obstet Gynaecol Res* 2004; 30: 169–80.
27. Hofmeyr GJ, Sonnendecker EW. The prevalence, aetiology and clinical significance of pseudosinusoidal fetal heart rate patterns in labour. *Br J Obstet Gynaecol* 1992; 99: 528–9.
28. Andrikopoulou M, Vintzileos AM. Sawtooth fetal heart rate pattern due to in-utero fetal central nervous system injury. *Am J Obstet Gynecol* 2016; 214: 403.e1–4.
29. Clark SL, Nageotte MP, Garite TJ, et al. Intrapartum management of category II fetal heart rate tracings: Toward standardization of care. *Am J Obstet Gynecol* 2013; 209: 89.
30. Jackson M, Holmgren CM, Esplin ES, et al. Frequency of fetal heart rate categories and short-term neonatal outcome. *Obstet Gynecol* 2011; 118: 803–8.
31. Parer TJ, Ikeda T, King TL. The 2008 National Institute of Child Health and Human Development report on fetal heart rate monitoring. *Obstet Gynecol* 2009; 114: 136–8.
32. Tranquilli AL, Biagini A, Greco P et al. The correlation between fetal bradycardia area in the second stage of labor and acidemia at birth. *J Matern Fetal Neonatal Med* 2013; 26: 1425–9.
33. Vintzileos AM, Campbell WA, Nochimson DJ et al. The fetal biophysical profile in patients with premature rupture of the membranes—An early predictor of fetal infection. *Am J Obstet Gynecol* 1985; 152: 510–6.
34. Vintzileos AM, Campbell WA, Nochimson DJ, Weinbaum PJ. The use of the nonstress test in patients with premature rupture of the membranes. *Am J Obstet Gynecol* 1986; 155: 149–53.
35. Goodwin TM, Milner-Masterson L, Paul RH. Elimination of fetal scalp blood sampling on a large clinical service. *Obstet Gynecol* 1994; 83: 971–4.
36. Bakker PCAM, Colenbrander GJ, Vestraeten AA, et al. Quality of intrapartum cardiotocography in twin deliveries. *Am J Obstet Gynecol* 2004; 191: 2114–9.
37. Ridgeway JJ, Weyrich DL, Benedetty TJ. Fetal heart rate changes associated with uterine rupture. *Obstet Gynecol* 2004; 103: 506–12.
38. Sheiner E, Levy A, Ofir K et al. Changes in fetal heart rate and uterine patterns associated with uterine rupture. *J Reprod Med* 2004; 49: 373–8.
39. Rodriguez MH, Masaki DI, Phelan JP, et al. Uterine rupture: Are intrauterine pressure catheters useful in the diagnosis? *Am J Obstet Gynecol* 1989; 161: 666–9.
40. Ecker JL, Kaimal A, Mercer BM et al. American College of Obstetricians and Gynecologists and the Society for Maternal–Fetal Medicine: Periviable birth. *Am J Obstet Gynecol* 2015; 213: 604–14.
41. Ojala K, Vaarasmaki M, Makikallio K et al. A comparison of intrapartum automated electrocardiography and conventional cardiotocography—A randomised controlled study. *BJOG* 2006; 113: 4189–423.
42. Strachan BK, van Wijngaarden WJ, Sahota D et al. Cardiotocography only versus cardiotocography plus PR-interval analysis in intrapartum surveillance: A randomised, multicentre trial. FECG Study Group. *Lancet* 2000; 355: 456–9.
43. Belfort MA, Saade GR, Thom E et al. A randomized trial of intrapartum fetal ECG ST-segment analysis. *N Eng J Med* 2015; 373: 632–41.
44. Belfort MA, Saade GR. ST segment analysis as an adjunct to electronic fetal monitoring, Part 1: Background, physiology, and interpretation. *Clin Perinatol* 2011; 38: 143–57.
45. Westgate J, Harris M, Curnow JS et al. Plymouth randomized trial of cardiotocogram only versus ST waveform plus cardiotocogram for intrapartum monitoring in 2400 cases. *Am J Obstet Gynecol* 1993; 169: 1151–60.
46. Amer-Wahlin I, Hellsten C, Noren H et al. Cardiotocography only versus cardiotocography plus ST analysis of fetal electrocardiogram for intrapartum fetal monitoring: A Swedish randomised controlled trial. *Lancet* 2001; 358: 534–8.
47. Westerhuis ME, Visser GH, Moons KG et al. Cardiotocography plus ST analysis of fetal electrocardiogram compared with cardiotocography only for intrapartum monitoring: A randomized controlled trial. *Obstet Gynecol* 2010; 115: 1173–80.
48. Steer PJ, Hvidman LE. Scientific and clinical evidence for the use of fetal ECG ST segment analysis (STAN). *Acta Obstet Gynecol Scand* 2014; 93: 533–8.
49. Potti S, Berghella V. ST waveform analysis versus cardiotocography alone for intrapartum fetal monitoring: A meta-analysis of randomized trials. *Am J Perinatol* 2012; 29: 657–64.

50. Salmelin A, Wiklund I, Bottinga R et al. Fetal monitoring with computerized ST analysis during labor: A systematic review and meta-analysis. *Acta Obstet Gynecol Scand* 2013; 92: 28–39.
51. American College of Obstetricians and Gynecologists. *Umbilical Artery Blood Acid-Base Analysis.* Technical Bulletin No. 216. Washington, DC, ACOG, November 1995.
52. American College of Obstetricians and Gynecologists. The Apgar score. ACOG Committee Opinion Number 644, October 2015. *Obstet Gynecol* 2015; 126: e52–5.
53. Thorp JA, Rushing RS. Umbilical cord blood gas analysis. *Obstet Gynecol Clin North Am* 1999; 26: 695–709.
54. Hankins GD, Speer M. Defining the pathogenesis and pathophysiology of neonatal encephalopathy and cerebral palsy. *Obstet Gynecol* 2003; 102: 628–36.
55. Helwig JT, Parer JT, Kilpatrick SJ et al. Umbilical cord blood acid-base state: What is normal? *Am J Obstet Gynecol* 1996; 174: 1807–12.
56. Vintzileos AM, Egan JFX, Campbell WA et al. Asphyxia at birth as determined by cord blood pH measurements in preterm and term gestations: Correlation with neonatal outcome. *J Matern Fetal Med* 1992; 1: 7–13.
57. Freeman R. Intrapartum fetal monitoring: A disappointing story. *N Eng J Med* 1990; 322: 624–6.
58. Yeh SY, Diaz F, Paul RH. Ten-year experience of intrapartum fetal monitoring in Los Angeles County/University of Southern California Medical Center. *Am J Obstet Gynecol* 1982; 143: 496–500.
59. Haverkamp AD, Orleans M, Langendoerfer S et al. A controlled trial of the differential effects of intrapartum fetal monitoring. *Am J Obstet Gynecol* 1979; 134: 399–412.
60. Luthy DA, Shy KK, van Belle G et al. A randomized trial of electronic fetal monitoring in preterm labor. *Obstet Gynecol* 1987; 69: 687–95.
61. Kelso IM, Parsons RJ, Lawrence GF et al. An assessment of continuous fetal heart rate monitoring in labor. A randomized trial. *Am J Obstet Gynecol* 1978; 131: 526–32.
62. MacDonald D, Grant A, Sheridan-Pereira M et al. The Dublin randomized controlled trial of intrapartum fetal heart rate monitoring. *Am J Obstet Gynecol* 1985; 152: 524–39.
63. Shy KK, Luthy DA, Bennett FC et al. Effects of electronic fetal heart-rate monitoring, as compared with periodic auscultation, on the neurologic development of premature infants. *N Engl J Med* 1990; 322: 588–93.
64. Herbst A, Ingemarsson I. Intermittent versus continuous electronic monitoring in labour: A randomised study. *Br J Obstet Gynaecol* 1994; 101: 663–8.
65. Grant A, O'Brien N, Joy MT et al. Cerebral palsy among children born during the Dublin randomised trial of intrapartum monitoring. *Lancet* 1989; 2(8674): 1233–6.
66. Vintzileos AM, Antsaklis A, Varvarigos I et al. A randomized trial of intrapartum electronic fetal heart rate monitoring versus intermittent auscultation. *Obstet Gynecol* 1993; 81: 899–907.
67. Vintzileos AM, Nochimson DJ, Antsaklis A et al. Comparison of intrapartum electronic fetal heart rate monitoring versus intermittent auscultation in detecting fetal acidemia at birth. *Am J Obstet Gynecol* 1995; 173: 1021–4.
68. Vintzileos AM, Nochimson DJ, Guzman ER et al. Intrapartum electronic fetal heart rate monitoring versus intermittent auscultation: A meta-analysis. *Obstet Gynecol* 1995; 85: 149–155.
69. Thacker SB, Stroup DF, Peterson HB. Efficacy and safety of intra-partum electronic fetal monitoring: An update. *Obstet Gynecol* 199; 86: 613–620.
70. Alfirevic Z, Devane D, Gyte GM. Continuous cardiotocography (CTG) as a form of electronic fetal monitoring (EFM) for fetal assessment during labour. *Cochrane Database Syst Rev* 2013; (5): CD006066.
71. Parer JT, King T. Fetal heart rate monitoring: Is it salvageable? *Am J Obstet Gynecol* 2000; 182: 982–7.
72. Clark SL, Meyers JA, Frye DK et al. Recognition and response to electronic fetal heart rate patterns: Impact on newborn outcomes and primary cesarean delivery rate in women undergoing induction of labor. *Am J Obstet Gynecol* 2015; 212: 494.

Normal vaginal delivery

20

LISA N. GITTENS-WILLIAMS

CONTENTS

The role of the operator conducting delivery is to guide the fetus through the lower portion of the birth canal without injury to the mother or infant. To achieve this goal, the attendant must have an understanding of the preceding events. He or she must have the ability to perform interventions that either facilitate delivery or prevent unwanted complications.

Most modern obstetric suites provide labor delivery recovery rooms (LDRs) for the patient who is ready to deliver. This setting allows family-centered care and immediate infant bonding. In this setting spontaneous and instrumental vaginal deliveries can take place as allowed.[1] Maternal delivery positions may include the dorsal lithotomy position, maternal squatting, and the mother on side or knee to chest position. If instrumental delivery is not anticipated, the mother may remain in any position she feels comfortable. Neither maternal nor fetal outcomes have been demonstrated to change when various positions in the second stage of labor have been compared.[2] Stirrups can be used but are not required,[3,4] but legs should never be fixed into position as they may need to be released in the event that shoulder dystocia occurs. Care should be taken to avoid injury to maternal nerves. Draping of the perineum serves to protect both the mother and the operator from infection.

DELIVERY OF THE HEAD

After the fetal head descends, flexes, and rotates to the occiput anterior position, the labia minora will distend, and crowning will occur. At this time, an opening of approximately 3–4 cm will be seen at the introitus. Routine episiotomy, which refers to the performance of a surgical incision of the maternal perineum to increase the diameter of the pelvic outlet, should be avoided.[5] Restrictive use of episiotomy is described below.

As the occiput passes under the pubic arch, the operator should be facing the perineum with a towel draped over the dominant hand. Numerous approaches to the delivery of the fetal head have been described. As the fetal head delivers by extension, the birth attendant may use the techniques of no-touch, passive perineal support, the Ritgin maneuver, or perineal massage. The Ritgin maneuver is accomplished by palpating the fetal chin, applying traction in the anterior–inferior direction, which will reduce the perineal body over the fetal head and chin (Figure 20.1). Whereas manual perineal support has not been demonstrated to reduce obstetrical anal sphincter injuries, a hands-on technique is advised to avoid rapid expulsion of the fetus.[6,7]

If one hand provides perineal support, the opposite hand is placed flat with fingers extended and partially separated over the vertex. As the vertex delivers under

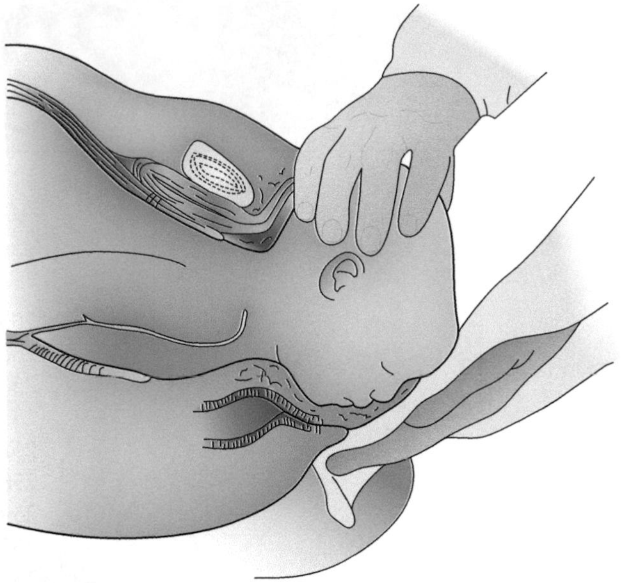

Figure 20.1 Demonstration of modified Ritgen's maneuver.

the symphysis, the lower hand guides the head over the perineum, while the upper one ensures that sudden expulsion and rapid extension do not occur with maternal pushing or uterine contractions. The operator should have a direct view of the perineum, so as to observe for and prevent tearing or extension of an episiotomy.

As soon as the head is delivered, the operator should discard the towel as it may be contaminated with fecal material. The head will restitute to its previous position (left occiput anterior [LOA], left occiput anterior [ROA], etc.). The infant face may be wiped with a towel to clear the mucus. Routine suctioning in infants without obvious obstructed breathing is not advised.[8–12] Wiping the mouth and nose at birth has been demonstrated to be equal efficacy in neonates who are 35 weeks and above.[13] Infants who appear to have respiratory difficulty can undergo suction of the mouth and nares with attention to avoid the posterior pharynx, which may result in vagal reaction and bradycardia followed by apnea.[14]

The current delivery management of infant with meconium stained fluid suggests that routine oropharyngeal or nasopharyngeal suctioning is not advised and has not been shown to decrease the rate of meconium aspiration syndrome.[14]

After wiping the fetal mouth and nasopharynx, the operator should inspect and palpate the fetal neck for the presence of a nuchal cord. Any identified nuchal cord should be reduced, if possible, by gently slipping it over the infant's head. Management of the tight nuchal cord, which cannot easily be reduced, is controversial. Many textbooks suggest that such a nuchal cord should be doubly clamped and cut. However, such a practice may be unwise and should be avoided unless absolutely necessary because if the operator encounters difficulty with the extraction of the body, irreversible damage to the fetus can result. Several such cases were reported by Iffy et al.[15] who concluded that the practice of severing the cord prior to full delivery of the baby can be dangerous.

DELIVERY OF THE BODY

After restitution of the fetal head, the operator should place his or her hands on either side of the fetal head along the parietal bones with the fingers pointing toward the occiput. The operator should avoid placing hands on the fetal neck, as this may result in nerve injury. In many cases, spontaneous delivery of the fetal shoulders will immediately follow the delivery of the fetal head; however, frequently, a delay occurs. A 2- to 4-minute pause before the rotation and passage of the shoulder through the pelvis at the peak of the next contraction is a natural physiologic process, which allows for rotation of the fetal shoulders.[16] In the absence of complications, such as cord prolapse or abruptio placentae, this delay creates no risk. If the shoulders are not spontaneously delivered, the operator should wait for the next contraction, and then encourage the mother to push.[16] The application of continuous gentle downward traction on the fetal head, directed toward the floor, should result in the delivery of the anterior shoulder at this time (Figure 20.2a). The operator should then visualize the perineum and next lift the body upward to deliver the posterior shoulder (Figure 20.2b). Once both shoulders are delivered, the accoucheur guides the body along his or her arm (Figure 20.3). Once the baby is delivered, it is held at or below the level of the placenta until cord clamping is completed or placed directly on the maternal abdomen (see Section Management of the Infant).

CUTTING OF THE CORD

Optimal timing of cord clamping has been a source of controversy and debate.[17,18] Proponents of immediate clamping believe that infusing additional volume into the fetus may result in excessive red cell destruction or hypervolemia. The opposite argument states that the fetus may benefit from the extra volume contained in the placenta. Randomized controlled trials in both term and preterm infants have evaluated the benefits of delayed cord clamping versus immediate cord clamping, however, an ideal timing for cord clamping has not been established. Several studies support a delay of 30–60 seconds with the infant held at or below the level of the placenta. Benefits include increased infant blood volume, decreased need for transfusion, decreased intracranial hemorrhage in preterm infants, and lower frequency of iron deficiency anemia at 4–6 months in term infants. The major benefit of delayed cord clamping is that a 50% reduction in the intraventricular hemorrhage is seen in the preterm infants.[19–21] A technique of cord milking compared with delayed clamping showed no difference in neonatal hemoglobin 1 hour after birth in preterm infants less than 33 weeks.[22–25]

The umbilical cord should be cut between two clamps and placed approximately 4–5 cm from the fetal abdomen. To manage the neonate, a plastic cord clamp is

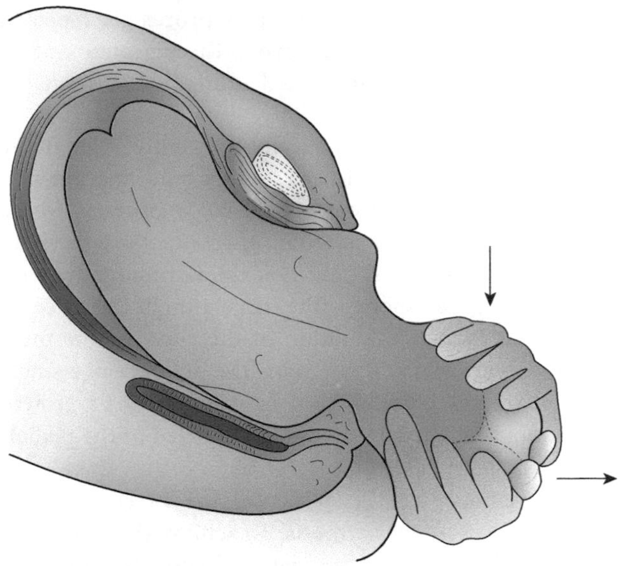

(a)

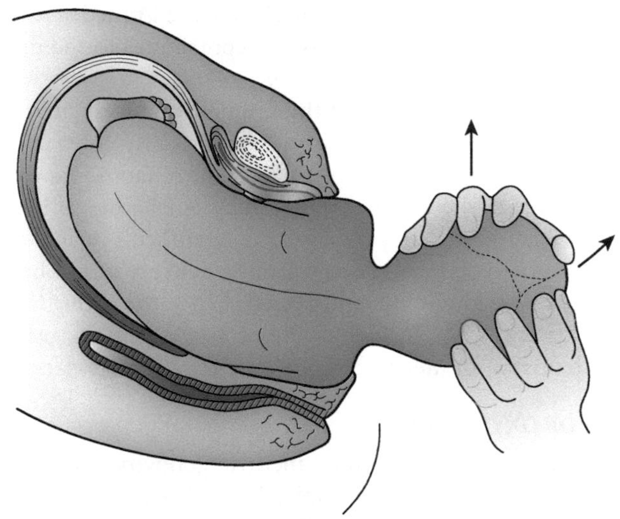

(b)

Figure 20.2 Delivery of shoulders. (a) Anterior and (b) posterior.

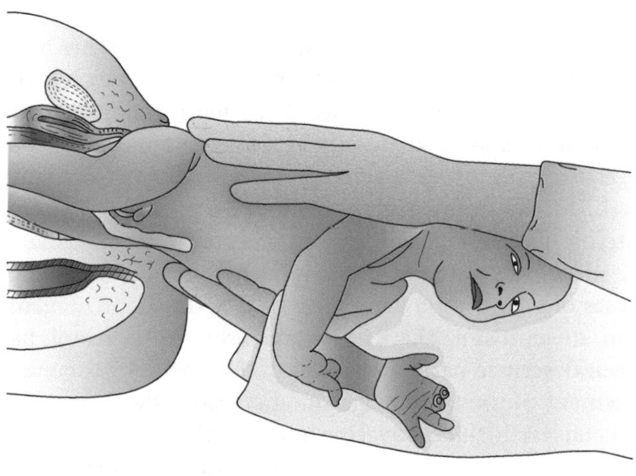

Figure 20.3 Delivery of body.

placed later 1–2 cm from the fetal abdomen and the cord is cut again. If assessment of cord pH is indicated, a segment of the remaining cord is clamped, cut, and set aside for blood gas analysis, prior to collecting blood samples for newborn testing.

Management of the infant

An infant who does not require further assistance can be immediately handed to the mother, implementing the skin-to-skin technique. The infant is placed on the maternal chest, skin to skin with the mother and the fetus can be further dried for improved thermoregulation.[25] Early skin-to-skin contact has been demonstrated to improve breastfeeding outcomes and early infant–mother attachment.[26] In a multicentered trial, a delivery technique of placing the term infant on the maternal abdomen prior to cord clamping did not affect the volume of placental blood transfusion, hence when early infant skin-to-skin placement is a priority, cord clamping can be done with infant on maternal abdomen.[27]

DELIVERY OF THE PLACENTA

The third stage of labor is commonly managed actively by the administration of oxytocics after infant delivery and with assisted placental separation, followed by uterine massage. This process has been shown to reduce blood loss.[28–30] Signs of placental separation include elongation of the cord, a palpable globular mass on the maternal abdomen, and a sudden gush of blood with protrusion of the placenta through the cervix into the vagina.

The average duration of the third stage of labor is 8 minutes. Placental separation occurs within 30 minutes after the delivery of the fetus in 97% of parturients, and a longer third stage of labor is seen with decreasing gestational age.[31,32] Because there is no increase in hemorrhage the third stage of labor is less than 30 minutes, it is recommended that manual placental removal should not be considered until at least 30 minutes have elapsed without signs of placental separation.

Once signs of separation are noted, the attendant may assist in the delivery of the placenta. This is achieved by placing the extended fingers of one hand on the maternal abdomen, just above the symphysis pubis, and then moving the fingers over the uterine fundus. With the opposite hand the attendant may apply gentle traction on the cord (Brant–Andrews maneuver) (Figure 20.4a and b).[33] The mother may then be asked to bear down.

In delivering the placenta, the operator must not force placental separation. The practice of holding the fundus with the abdominal hand may be continued until the placenta is delivered. This can reduce risks of cord avulsion or uterine inversion.[34] An alternative method, Credé's maneuver, in which the cord is fixed with the lower hand while the uterine fundus is gently compressed by the abdominal hand, may also be used. Controlled cord traction has been compared with hands-off approach of placental delivery with data supporting that controlled cord

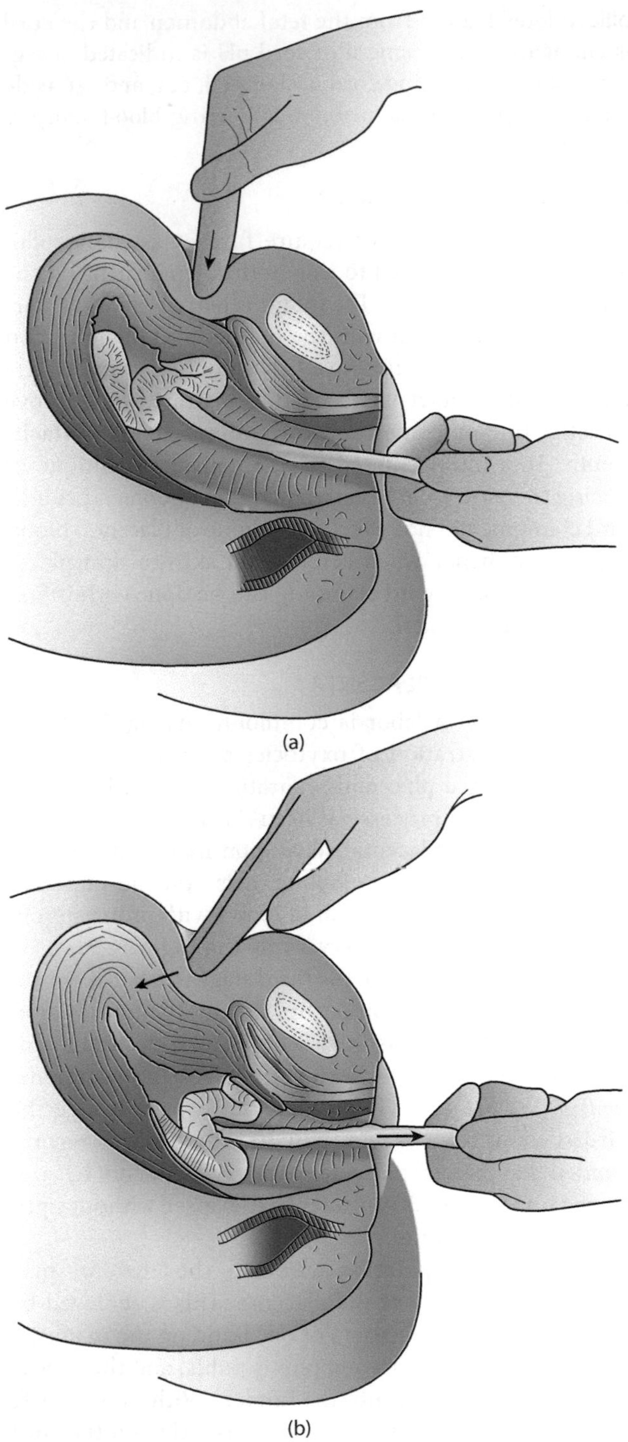

Figure 20.4 Brandt–Andrews maneuver for delivery of placenta. (a) Positioning of abdominal hand; (b) performance of the maneuver.

traction results in a decreased risk of postpartum hemorrhage; however, the use of oxytotics is the most important aspect of this process.

Occasionally, the placenta delivers but the membranes do not rapidly separate and remain, extending up into the uterus. Such membranes may be grasped with ring forceps and twisted to achieve removal. The trailing membranes may be grasped with another ring forceps placed higher up on the membranes. This process is repeated until all membranes are removed. The placenta and its membranes should be inspected immediately to ensure that they are intact.

A succenturiate placenta may inadvertently be left in the uterus. A ruptured vessel near the placental margin or a jagged edge to the placenta may alert the operator to the possibility of retained cotyledon. If retained products are suspected, the uterus should be explored manually with or without a gauze sponge. The inspection of the placenta should also include evaluation of the cord for the presence of two arteries and one vein. The presence of a single artery increases possibility of fetal anomaly or growth restriction. This finding should be reported to the pediatric attendant.

After removal of the placenta, the uterine fundus should be assessed for firmness. To achieve this, the operator places his hand on the maternal abdomen and gently massages the fundus while oxytocin is administered. Although commonly performed, there are limited studies that support that uterine massage contributes to the prevent postpartum hemorrhage.[35]

The habit of palpation of the fundus and assessment of uterine size can alert the operator to a poorly contractile and atonic uterus. In an obese patient, it should be recognized that the uterine fundus may not be palpable or easily felt and uterine massage may be difficult to achieve secondary to obesity. When planning delivery of an obese gravida, this should be considered, hence the immediate availability of pharmacological uterotonic agents or other mechanisms for uterine compression may be necessary.

USE OF OXYTOCICS

Oxytocin (Pitocin) and methylergonovine maleate (Methergine) and misoprostol (Cytotec) are widely used to control blood loss after delivery.[36,37] Oxytocin has been shown to be superior to placebo or no prophylaxis. Uterine contractions are critical in the control of blood loss. The contractions close the vessels in the uterine wall. Oxytocin causes rhythmic uterine contractions that affect primarily the fundal portion. It has little or no secondary effect on blood pressure when administered as a continuous infusion. Methergine can cause uterine spasm that involves the lower uterine segment and has a hypertensive effect in many women. It is associated with increases in femoral arterial pressure, pulmonary, arterial pressure, and wedge pressure.

15-Methyl-F-prostaglandin (Prostin 15 M) is a potent uterotonic agent which can be injected intramuscularly or directly into the myometrium. It is used primarily in cases of postpartum hemorrhage, as is the E1 prostaglandin, misoprostol. The E1 prostaglandin, misoprostol, has been described as an alternative to oxytocin for the management of the third stage of labor. Side effects are dose related and include shivering and fever.[38] This agent is recommended for reduction of postpartum hemorrhage in resource-poor areas.[39]

Trials comparing oxytocin to ergot alkaloids for the management of the third stage show that ergot alkaloids often causes nausea vomiting and raised blood pressure.[38] Most experts agree that the management of the third stage of labor should include the routine administration of oxytocin to reduce maternal blood loss, however, the dosing regimens vary among institutions.

MANAGEMENT OF THE RETAINED PLACENTA

Retained placenta affects 0.5%–3% of women after delivery. Dynamic visualization of the uterus during the third stage of labor by radiography and ultrasound has shown that placental separation depends upon contraction of the myometrium and subsequent detachment and expulsion. The risk of retained placenta and hemorrhage is increased in gestations less than 26 weeks and when the duration of the third stage is prolonged.[40]

Regardless of gestational age, the frequency of hemorrhage peaks 40 minutes after the delivery. About 90% of placentas at term will be delivered by 15 minutes and only 2%–3% will still be undelivered at 30 minutes.[41] If the placenta is not expelled after 30 minutes, it may be abnormally adherent or may be entrapped by the contracted cervix. Under such circumstances, manual placental removal is indicated because there is evidence of increase in hemorrhage when more than 30 minutes have elapsed without placental delivery. The incidence of postpartum hemorrhage, transfusion, and uterine curettage all increases after the placenta is retained more than 30 minutes.[41]

The prerequisites for manual removal include the following: Placement of an intravenous line and fluids administration as necessary. A tube of maternal blood should be sent for type and screen or crossmatch or same confirmed. The necessity for the procedure should be explained to the patient and her consent obtained. Adequate anesthesia, regional, general, or intravenous (IV) sedation should be given.

The operator should wear fresh sterile gloves. A sterile sleeve should be placed over the dominant arm if available. The field should be redraped. The operator then holds the umbilical cord with the assisting hand and introduces the dominant hand into the uterine cavity. The outside hand is then placed on the uterine fundus. The operator uses his fingers to locate the plane between the uterine wall and the placenta. When this plane is identified, gentle motion of the fingertips is used to separate the placenta from the uterine wall (Figure 20.5). The operator should resist the urge to exert undue traction on the cord, as this may tear the placenta or cord and result in retained fragments. The operator should also resist the urge to scoop out fragments of the placenta in pieces. Generally, separation occurs with ease. The process should be continued until the placenta is completely detached. The opposite hand assists in the placental delivery by lifting the fundus toward the examining hand and giving counterpressure. Once the placenta is removed, with or without a sterile piece of gauze placed over the operator's hand, manual curettage is performed. The goal is to remove an intact placenta.

After the placenta has been removed, it should be inspected for completeness. If it does not appear intact or if it has been removed in fragments, the operator should re-explore the uterus and remove the remaining fragments and membranes. Exceptionally, if remaining placental fragments cannot be removed manually, a large blunt curette may be introduced to remove them. Sharp curettage should be avoided. Routine use of antibiotics for manual exploration is not proven to beneficial.[42] Manual removal of the placenta may be challenging in the obese patent where the uterine fundus cannot be felt. If curettage is necessary, ultrasonographic guidance may be of assistance.

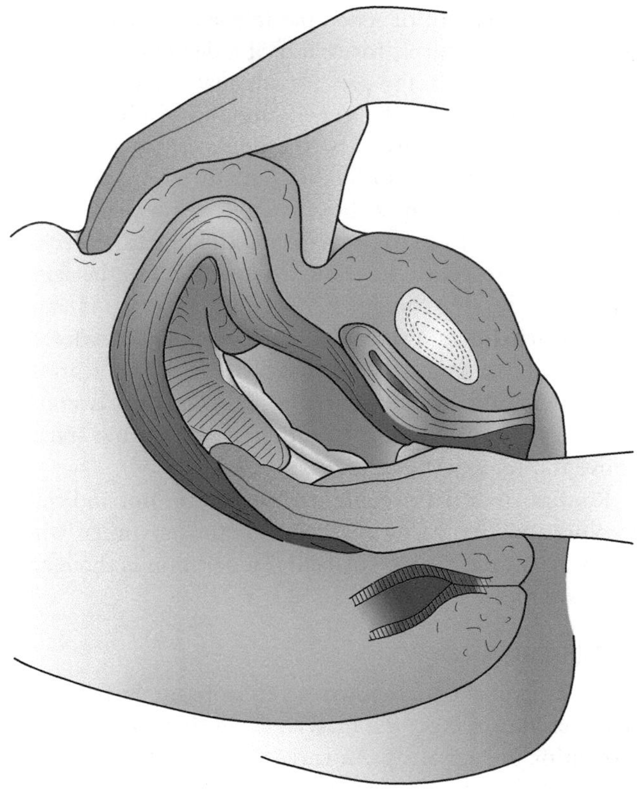

Figure 20.5 Demonstration of maneuver to remove placenta from uterus manually.

MANAGEMENT OF THE FOURTH STAGE OF LABOR

The fourth stage of labor includes the time when inspection of the birth canal and repair of lacerations and episiotomy take place. During this immediate postpartum period, the mother is observed for stability and postpartum hemorrhage.

Inspection of the birth canal involves a systematic evaluation of lacerations and bleeding. The first step is to inspect the perineum for laceration and assess the episiotomy site if one has been performed and determine whether extension has occurred or other perineal damage exists. Blood loss related to episiotomy should be noted. If excessive, it may require immediate intervention. The vagina is then inspected for lacerations. The operator should place one hand into the vagina and inspect its deep areas using a ring forceps with a large sponge. Lacerations of the vagina should be noted and repair performed with

2-0 chromic catgut or a comparable synthetic absorbable suture. In some cases, for repair of a deep vaginal laceration, an assistant has to provide adequate pelvic exposure.

After the vagina, the cervix should be checked. The cervix may be visualized by the operator placing a hand onto the pelvic floor to facilitate its direct inspection. If the entire cervix cannot be seen, a useful technique is to place ring forceps onto the anterior and posterior cervical lips, and, with gentle traction, lift and observe the cervix. Alternatively, ring forceps may be used to grasp the anterior cervical lip, and the cervix may be grasped with a second forceps in a circumferential fashion, to "walk around the cervix" until all areas are visualized. Any laceration noted on the cervix must be repaired with suture starting above the apex of the laceration.

Routine manual uterine exploration is not indicated. Exploration should be reserved for those women where bleeding is excessive, or placental separation is thought to be incomplete.

USE OF EPISIOTOMY

A relaxing incision, known as episiotomy, is frequently performed to protect the maternal soft tissue from unduly stretching or lacerating. A decrease in episiotomy rates has been noted between 1985 and 2004 in the United States and a survey of 510 hospitals reported an episiotomy rate of 12% in 2012.[43,44] Although there is no evidence to support use of routine episiotomy, some common clinical indication for selective use of episiotomy includes performance to hasten delivery in cases of fetal compromise, when instrumental delivery is planned, or when the likelihood of spontaneous laceration is high, such as in the case of a short perineal body. Episiotomy has not been associated with improvement in neonatal outcome or perineal support or improved outcomes of operative delivery.[45]

Two types of episiotomy may be performed. A median (midline) episiotomy refers to a vertical incision made from the posterior fourchette toward the rectum.[45] This incision in the midline severs the skin, the subcutaneous tissue, and the central junction of the paired bulbocavernosus, ischiocavernosus, and superficial transverse perineal muscles: the area known as the perineal body.

A mediolateral episiotomy may reduce the risk of third and fourth degree laceration.

Since the mediolateral incision protects against posterior perineal trauma, it has long been recommended as the preferred incision for women with inflammatory bowel disease, prior rectovaginal fistula, or prior posterior perineal repair, where protection of the rectum is critical.

TECHNIQUE OF EPISIOTOMY

A midline episiotomy should be made when the fetal head is crowning and has distended the vulva to 2–3 cm. If a regional block is in place, no additional anesthesia may be required; alternatively, local anesthesia should be given. The operator should place his or her fingers inside the perineum to protect the fetal head. Using a straight scissors, a downward incision is made from the midpoint of the posterior fourchette, toward the rectum, through approximately half of the perineal body. The incision can be extended further vertically, up the vaginal mucosa for a length of approximately 2–3 cm.

A mediolateral episiotomy is made by cutting from the midpoint of the posterior fourchette through the vaginal mucosa at a 45° angle. The incision may be made to the right or to the left. The direction usually depends upon the operator's dominant hand. The length of the median incision should be adequate to allow delivery of the head.

COMPLICATIONS OF EPISIOTOMY

In addition to increased incidence of third- and fourth-degree lacerations, episiotomy can be associated with excessive blood loss, particularly if the incision is made before the fetal head distends the vulva. Midline episiotomy is associated with more perineal and pelvic floor damage than no episiotomy or spontaneous lacerations. Those episiotomies that are complicated by extension to third- and fourth-degree lacerations may be associated with anal sphincter incontinence, pelvic floor injury, rectovaginal fistula, and pelvic prolapse.[45]

The mediolateral incision is associated more commonly with poorer cosmetic results and greater blood loss. There is, however, no evidence to indicate that the mediolateral episiotomy is associated with more pain than the midline incision. Both types of episiotomy can be complicated by infection, hematoma, and dehiscence.[45]

REPAIR OF EPISIOTOMY

Repair of episiotomy is generally delayed until after delivery of the placenta. This practice avoids the disruption of the repair should the placenta be retained and manual exploration of the uterus be required. Midline episiotomy is generally repaired with 2-0 or 3-0 chromic catgut or a comparable synthetic absorbable suture in a continuous fashion.[46]

Repair of the episiotomy begins with the identification of the apex of the incision. The first suture is placed above the apex and tied. Suturing should progress in a continuous running fashion to approximate the vaginal mucosa. The first stitch should be locked to aid in hemostasis at the apex, but not the remainder of them unless the edges of the incision are bleeding. Locking the sutures in this region may invert the vaginal mucosa and lead to inclusion cysts. When the vaginal suture reaches the hymenal ring, it should be brought inside the vaginal mucosa and completed by the placement of a deep suture, which approximates the two bulbocavernous muscles in the midline. The suture is then tied and the knot buried (Figure 20.6a). Next, two to three interrupted sutures are placed to approximate the deep layers of the perineum (Figure 20.6b). Lastly, a continuous subcutaneous suture is begun at the vaginal edge of the perineum, leaving the end tied for later use. This end may be held temporarily by a hemostat. The subcutaneous sutures are placed in a continuous running fashion to the lower perineal edge of the wound (Figure 20.6c), and then returned in a subcuticular

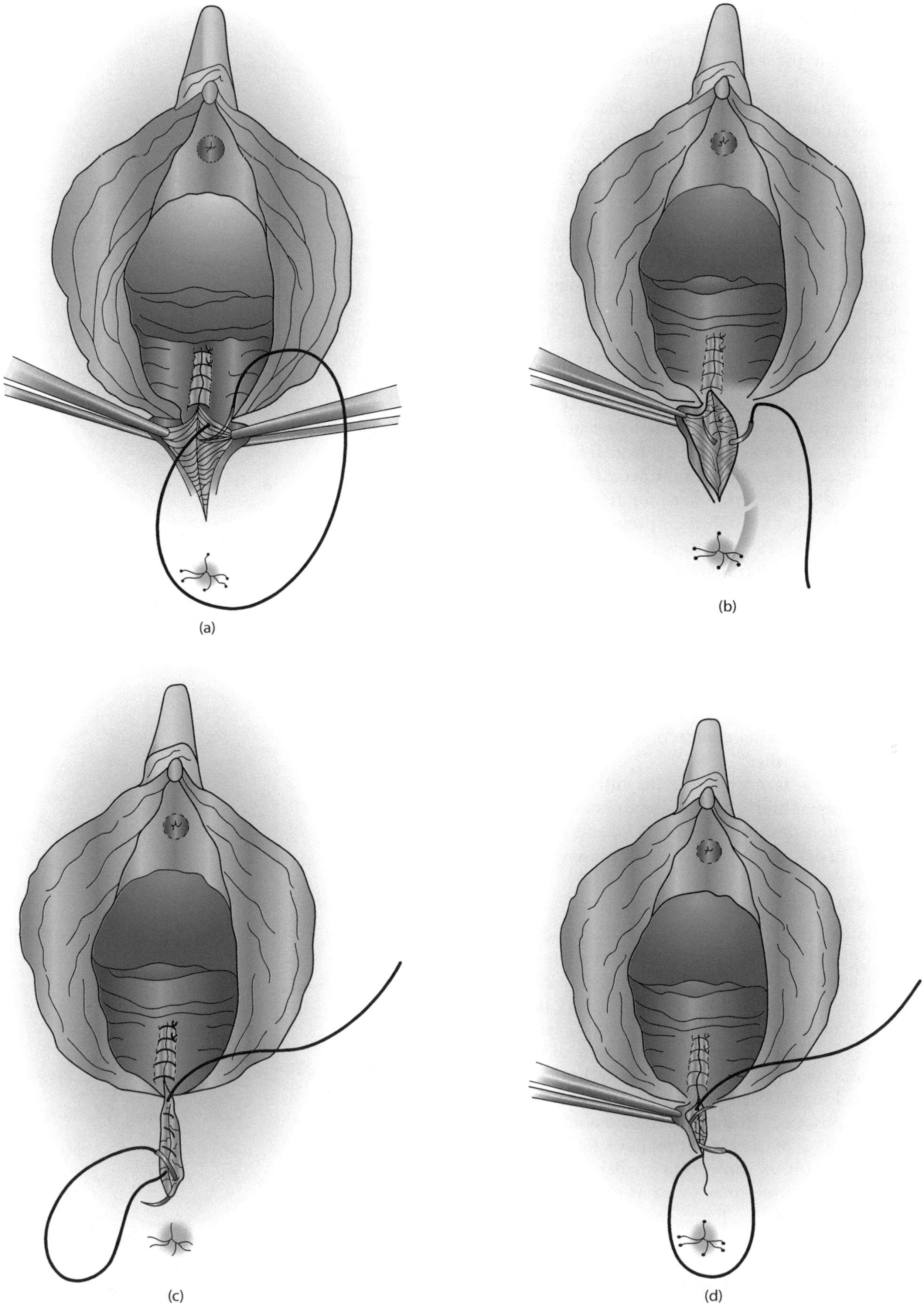

Figure 20.6 Repair of median episiotomy. (a) Closure of vaginal and bulbocavernosal muscles, (b) closure of deep layers, (c) subcutaneous closure, and (d) subcuticular closure.

pattern back to the vaginal perineal margin (Figure 20.6d). The suture is then tied to the original hemostat end. This allows for burying of the final knot so that no suture will remain exposed.

Postepisiotomy pain and swelling can be managed with ice packs and oral or topical analgesia.

DELIVERY OF THE MALPRESENTING FETAL HEAD

Face presentation

The incidence of face presentation is 0.1%–0.3% of all vertex deliveries and infants weighing more than 4000 g have a 2.9-fold increased risk for this malpresentation.[47,48] Cesarean delivery is indicated for cases of suspected cephalopelvic disproportion, large infants, desultory labor, or labor arrest. If the mentum is persistently posterior, cesarean section should be performed, since this position does not allow for natural expulsion of the fetus.

Overall, there is a 50% cesarean rate associated with face presentation. In a review of 50,300 deliveries, 40 cases of face presentation were examined. Thirty percent of the operative deliveries were for fetal distress; the rest were performed for failure to progress in labor. Vaginal delivery occurred in 88% with mentum anterior, 45% with the mentum transverse, and 2.5% of those with mentum posterior rotations. Twenty-seven percent of mentum posterior spontaneously rotated to mentum anterior. Fetal stress was particularly common in the mentum posterior presentation. Appropriate management of face presentation is to allow spontaneous labor unless indications for abdominal delivery are present. If the pelvis and the uterine contractions are adequate, vaginal delivery may ensue.[49]

After descent, as the face appears at the vulva, the chin will be under the symphysis and the operator can deliver the head by assisted flexion (Figures 20.7a and b). The shoulders are then delivered as in a cephalic presentation.

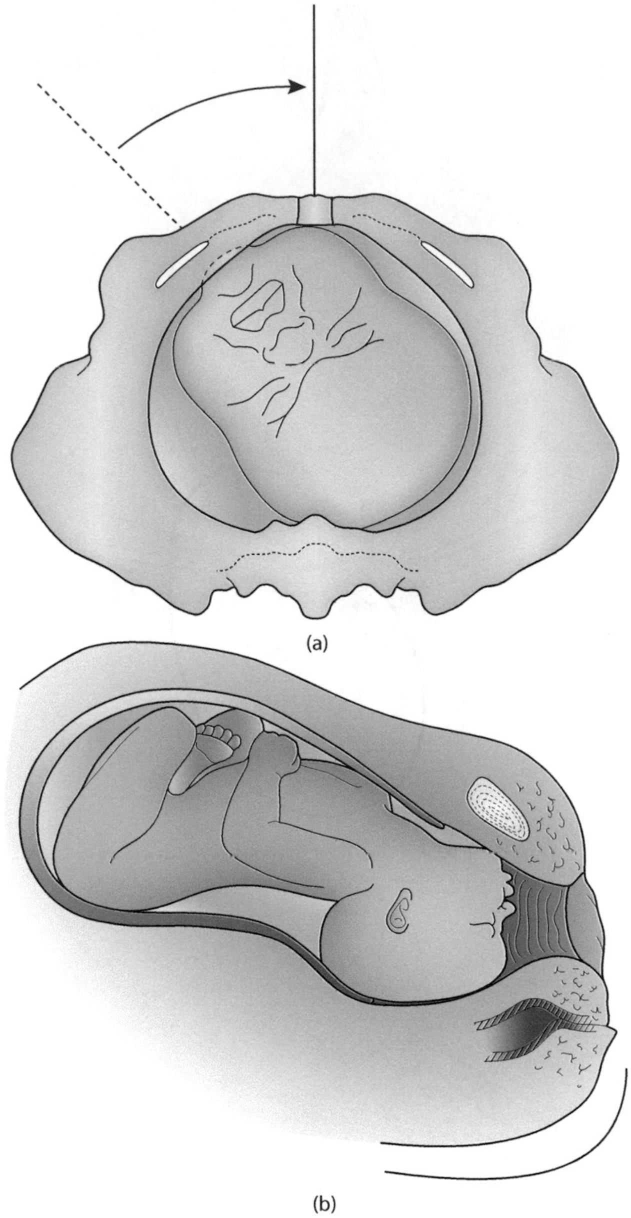

Figure 20.7 (a and b) Face presentation with the mentum anterior.

BROW PRESENTATION

Brow presentation represents a fetal position midway between the full flexion of the occiput presentation and the full extension of the face presentation (Figure 20.8). Except in the case of a very small fetus or a very large pelvis, engagement of the fetal head in the brow presentation is impossible. Since there is cephalopelvic disproportion and because a great deal of molding has taken place, thereby locking the head into a fixed position, cesarean delivery is indicated. If during the course of labor, the brow presentation persists, the prognosis for vaginal delivery is poor. If the brow converts to smaller presenting fetal head diameter, delivery may occur as in the occiput presentation. Manual rotation has been reported with no untoward outcomes reported.[50]

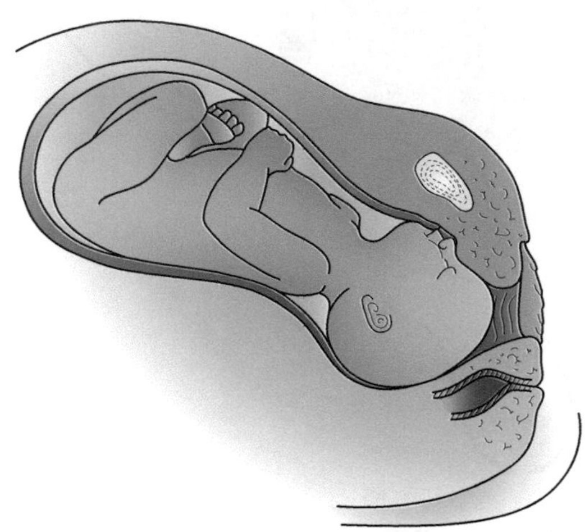

Figure 20.8 Brow presentation.

MALROTATIONS OF THE FETAL HEAD

Occiput posterior rotation has been reported in 10%–25% of the cases in the early stage of labor and in 10%–15% in the active phase. Persistent fetal occiput posterior position occurs in approximately 5% of all deliveries. The incidence is higher in primiparas than in multiparas.[49] Persistent occiput posterior rotation is associated with prolonged labor, and need for induction, oxytocin augmentation, and epidural use. Persistent occiput posterior rotation is associated with short maternal stature and prior cesarean delivery.

VAGINAL DELIVERY OF THE PREMATURE INFANT

The majority of occiput posterior positions change to anterior during labor even at full cervical dilation. With good flexion of the head, its presenting diameter is minimized; with less flexion, the large occipitofronatal diameter is presenting. In either case, the head is delivered by further flexion. The face should be expelled to the chin before one attempts to deliver the rest of the head.[49]

A variety of maneuvers, including positioning the mother in the knee-to-chest position and pelvic rocking, have been described to facilitate rotation of the fetus. These efforts have not proven to be effective. Occiput posterior rotation is also associated with high rates of third- and fourth-degree perineal lacerations, excessive blood loss, and postpartum infections when compared with delivery in the occiput anterior position.

VAGINAL DELIVERY OF THE PREMATURE INFANT

Delivery of the premature infant presenting by the vertex is a variation of normal vaginal birth. Because of the small fetal size relative to the maternal pelvis, malpresentation, asynclitism, and compound presentations and rapid delivery are relatively common. These are managed in the same way as for the term fetus. The operator must be vigilant in observing for a loop of cord or other fetal part that may present alongside the fetal head. If a hand or arm accompanies the head into the pelvis, watching and waiting is the best approach. If the compound presentation persists, gentle maneuvering of the arm or hand toward the pelvis may be attempted.

If the fetus is small relative to the pelvis, even in compound presentation it may be delivered without difficulty. Most studies have shown that for the low-birth-weight fetus without signs of fetal compromise, vaginal delivery is preferable. Reducing trauma to the premature fetus at delivery and optimizing neonatal care are paramount in the management. Personnel for the resuscitation of the infant should be immediately available. Often a bulging bag of water is presenting as the cervix dilates. The operator must remember that the cervical dilation may prove incomplete, once the membranes are ruptured. A portion of cord or a small fetal part may be in advance of the vertex. Use of ultrasound may be helpful to clarify this situation. Artificial rupture of the membranes in these circumstances must be approached judiciously, and should be attempted only when the cervix is approaching full dilation. The membranes may then be needled, allowing slow decompression of the amniotic sac and safe descent of the vertex into the pelvis. Spontaneous delivery can then be allowed with focus on controlling the delivery of the head to prevent rapid expulsion.

ACKNOWLEDGMENT

The author acknowledges that this chapter contains material from the previous edition chapter coauthored by Morten A. Stenchever.

REFERENCES

1. Hawkins J, Gibbs C, Orleans M et al. Use of labor-delivery-recovery rooms. *Anesthesiology* 1998; 88(1): 283.
2. Gupta JK, Hofmeyr GJ, Shehmar M. Position in the second stage of labour for women without epidural anaesthesia. *Cochrane Database Syst Rev* 2012; 5: CD002006.
3. Corton MM, Lankford JC, Ames R et al. A randomized trial of birthing with and without stirrups. *Am J Obstet Gynecol* 2012; 207: 133.el–5.
4. Kemp E, Kingswood CJ, Kibuka M et al. Position in the second stage of labour for women with epidural anaesthesia. *Cochrane Database Syst Rev* 2013; 1: CD008070.
5. Argentine Episiotomy Trial Collaborative. Routine vs selective episiotomy: A randomised controlled trial. *The Lancet* 1993; 342(8886): 1517–8.
6. Bulchandani S, Watts E, Sucharitha A et al. Manual perineal support at the time of childbirth: A systematic review and meta-analysis. *BJOG: An International Journal of Obstetrics & Gynaecology* 2015; 122(9): 1157–65.
7. McCandlish R, Bowler U, van Asten H et al. A randomised controlled trial of care of the perineum during second stage of normal labour. *Br J Obstet Gynaecol* 1998; 105: 1262.
8. Carrasco M, Martell M, Esotl PC. Oronasopharyngeal suction at birth: Effects on arterial oxygen saturation. *J Pediatr* 1997; 130: 832.
9. Waltman PA, Brewer JM, Rogers BP, May WL. Building evidence for practice: A pilot study of newborn bulb suctioning at birth. *J Midwifery Women's Health* 2004; 49: 32.
10. Estol PC, Piriz H, Basalo S et al. Oro-naso-pharyngeal suction at birth: Effects on respiratory adaptation of normal term vaginally born infants. *J Perinat Med* 1992; 20(4): 297–305.
11. Gungor S, Teksoz E, Ceyhan T et al. Oronasopharyngeal suction versus no suction in normal, term and vaginally born infants: A prospective randomised controlled trial. *Aust N Z J Obstet Gynaecol* 2005; 45: 453–6.
12. Gungor S, Kurt E, Ceyhan T et al. Oronasopharyngeal suction versus no suction in normal and term infants delievered by elective cesarean section: A prospective randomized controlled trial. *Gynecol Obstet Invest* 2006; 61: 69.

13. Kelleher J, Bhat R, Salas AA et al. Oronasopharyngeal suction versus wiping of the mouth and nose at birth: A randomised equivalency trial. *Lancet* 2013; 382: 326.
14. American Heart Association. 2005 American Heart Association (AHA) guidelines for cardiopulmonary resuscitation (CPR) and emergency cardiovascular care (ECC) of pediatric and neonatal patients: Pediatric basic life support. *Pediatrics* 2006; 117: e989.
15. Iffy L, Varadi V, Papp E. Untoward neonatal sequelae deriving from cutting of the umbilical cord before delivery. *Med Law* 2001; 20: 627–34.
16. Gittens Williams L. Contemporary management of shoulder dystocia. *Women's Health* 2010; 6: 861–869.
17. Laines VB, Bergel AE, Cafferrate Thompson ML et al. [Early or late cord clamping. A systematic review of the literature]. *An Pediatr (Barc)* 2005; 63: 14.
18. Andersson O, Lindquist B, Lindgren M et al. Effect of delayed cord clamping on neurodevelopment at 4 years of age: A randomized clinical trial. *JAMA Pediatr* 2015; 169: 631.
19. Committee on Obstetric Practice, American College of Obstetricians and Gynecologists. Committee Opinion No. 543. Timing of umbilical cord clamping after birth. *Obstet Gynecol* 2012; 120: 1522.
20. McDonald SJ, Middleton P, Dowswell T et al. Effect of timing of umbilical cord clamping of term infants on maternal an neonatal outcomes. *Cochrane Database Syst Rev* 2013; (7): CD004074.
21. Duley L, Dorling J, Gyte G. When should the umbilical cord be clamped? *BMJ* 2015; 351: h4206.
22. Rabe H, Jewison A, Alvarez RF et al. Milking compared with delayed cord clamping to increase placental transfusion in preterm neonates: A randomized controlled trial. *Obstet Gynecol* 2011; 117: 205.
23. Hosono S, Mugishima H, Fujita H et al. Umbilical cord milking reduces the need for red cell transfusions and improves neonatal adaptation in infants born at less than 29 weeks' gestation: A randomised controlled trial. *Arch Dis Child Fetal Neonatal Ed* 2008; 93: F14.
24. Al-Wassia H, Shah PS. Efficacy and safety of umbilical cord milking at birth: A systematic review and meta-analysis. *JAMA Pediatr* 2015; 169: 118.
25. Van Den Bosch CA, Bullough CH. Effect of early sucking on term neonates' core temperature. *Ann Trop Paediatr* 1990; 10: 347–53.
26. Moore ER, Anderson GC, Bergman N, Dowswell T. Early skin-to-skin contact for mothers and their healthy newborn infants. *Cochrane Database Syst Rev* 2007; (5): CD003519.
27. Vain NE, Satragno DS, Gorenstein AN et al. Effect of gravity on volume of placental transfusion: A multicentre, randomised, non-inferiority trial. *Lancet* 2014; 384: 235.
28. Gülmezoglu AM, Lumbiganon P, Landoulsi S et al. Active management of the third stage of labour with and without controlled cord traction: A randomised, controlled, non-inferiority trial. *Lancet* 2012; 379: 1721.
29. Du Y, Ye M, Zheng F. Active management of the third stage of labor with and without controlled cord traction: A systematic review and meta-analysis of randomized controlled trials. *Acta Obstet Gynecol Scand* 2014; 93: 626.
30. Hofmeyr GJ, Abdel-Aleem H, Abdel-Aleem MA. Uterine massage for preventing postpartum haemorrhage. *Cochrane Database Syst Rev* 2013; (7): CD006431.
31. Dombrowski MP, Bottoms SF, Saleh AA et al. Third stage of labor: Analysis of duration and clinical practice. *Am J Obstet Gynecol* 1995; 172: 1279.
32. Combs CA, Laros RK Jr. Prolonged third stage of labor: Morbidity and risk factors. *Obstet Gynecol* 1991; 77: 863.
33. Brandt ML. The mechanism and management of the third stage of labour. *Am J Obstet Gynecol* 1933; 25: 662–7.
34. Prendiville WJ, Harding JE, Elbourne DR et al. The Bristol third state trial: Active versus physiological management of third stage of labour. *BMJ* 1988; 297: 1295–300.
35. Chen M, Chang Q, Duan T et al. Uterine massage to reduce blood loss after vaginal delivery: A randomized controlled trial. *Obstet Gynecol* 2013; 122: 290.
36. Saito K, Hakuri A, Ishikawa H et al. Prospective study of intramuscular ergometrine compared with intramuscular oxytocin for prevention of post partum hemorrhage. *J Obstet Gynaecol Res* 2007; 33(3): 254–8.
37. Tuncalp O, Hofmeyer GJ, Gulmezoglu AM. Prostaglandins for preventing postpartum hemorrhage. *Cochrane Database Syst Rev* 2012; (8): CD 000494.
38. Tang J, Kapp N, Dragoman M et al. WHO Recommendations for misoprostol use for obstetric and gynecological indications. *Int J Gynaecol Obstet* 2013; 121(2): 186.
39. Liabsuetrakul T, Choobun T, Peeyananjarassi K et al. Prophylactic use of ergot alkaloids in the third stage of labour. *Cochrane Database Syst Rev* 2007; (2): CD005456.
40. Romero R, Hsu YC Athanassiadis AP et al. Preterm delivery: A risk factor for retained placenta. *Am J Obstet Gyncol* 1990: 1936: 823.
41. Combs CA, Laros RK Jr. Prolonged third stage of labor: Morbidity and risk factors. *Obstet Gynecol* 1991; 77: 863.
42. Chongsomchai C, Lumbiganon P, Laopaiboon M. Prophylactic antibodies for manual removal of retained placenta in vaginal birth. *Cochrane Database Syst Rev* 2014; (10): CD004904.
43. Goldberg J, Holtz D, Hyslop T et al. Has the use of routine episiotomy decreased? Examination of episiotomy rates from 1983 to 2000. *Obstet Gynecol* 2002; 99: 395–400.
44. Friedman AM, Ananth CV, Prendergast E et al. Variation in and factors associated with use of episiotomy. *JAMA* 2015; 313: 197.

45. American College of Obstetricians Gynecologist. ACOG Practice Bulletin No. 71: Episiotomy. *Obstet Gynecol* 2006; 107: 957.
46. Kettle C, Dowswell T, Ismail K. Continuous and interrupted suturing techniques for repair or episiotomy or second degree tears. *Cochrane Database Syst Rev* 2012; (11): CD000947.
47. Shaffer BL, Cheung YW, Vargas JE et al. Face presentation: Predictors and delivery route. *Am J Obstet Gynecol* 2006; 194: 10.
48. Tapisiz OL, Aytan H, Kiykae Altinbas S et al. Face presentation at term: A forgotten issue. *J Obset Gynaecol Res* 2014; 40: 1573–7.
49. Ponkey SE, Cohen AP, Heffner LJ et al. Persistent fetal occiput posterior position: Obstetric outcomes. *Obstet Gynecol* 2003; 101: 915–20.
50. Verspyck E, Bisson, V, Gromez A et al. Prophylactic attempt at manual rotation in brow presentation at full dilation. *Acta Obstet Gynecol Scand* 2012; 91: 1342–5.

Shoulder dystocia

21

JOHN P. KEATS

CONTENTS

Based upon my experience as an obstetric hospitalist, I can recall my share of unusual cases and emergencies during the management of laboring women. One such case from a number of years ago comes to mind as a way to introduce the important topic of shoulder dystocia (SD) in this chapter.

It was late at night and I had been following a primiparous patient in labor all day. She had a long latent phase but her active phase of labor proceeded smoothly along the Friedman curve as modified by Zhang et al.[1] She was a gestational diabetic and her blood sugars were well controlled on dietary management alone. Although she had been pushing for nearly 3 hours, she tolerated the longer second stage because she had an epidural for analgesia. She had been at plus three station for over 30 minutes with little further advancement of the fetal head. She began to complain of exhaustion and I had decided then that this should be an easy vacuum delivery. I could see the head when I separated the labia during a push, although the head did seem to recede a bit between contractions. I applied the vacuum extractor and with the second contraction the fetal chin emerged over the perineum and rotated counterclockwise. As I removed the vacuum device I realized that the head had retracted back tightly against the perineum. I began to apply gentle downward traction on the fetal head with my hands as my patient pushed again. The fetus did not budge. I realized immediately that I was dealing with a SD!

DEFINITION

There are few obstetric complications that can cause as much sudden concern and morbidity as an unexpected severe SD during delivery. Obstetricians are responsible for the safety of two patients (mother and child) and the unexpected retraction of the fetal head, when the end of a normal second stage of labor is anticipated, can be hazardous to both patients and is a challenging complication for the obstetrician to manage.

SD has been defined as the difficult delivery of the fetal shoulder requiring the use of special maneuvers in addition to gentle downward traction on the fetal head or a prolongation of the head-to-body delivery interval to more than 60 seconds.[2,3] The complication is more common when the size of the maternal pelvis is small in relation to the size of the fetus. The immediate cause is the impaction of the fetal shoulder on the pubic symphysis anteriorly or the sacral promontory posteriorly.

INCIDENCE

The incidence of SD ranges from less than 1% to nearly 2%.[4,5] This large reported range may reflect a lack of agreement on the diagnosis of SD or may be due to differences in patient characteristics in the studied populations. Interestingly, the reported incidence of this complication has not declined in recent years even though the rate of cesarean delivery has increased 5- to 10-fold.[6,7] The brachial plexus injuries that the fetus may sustain as a result of a significant SD make up a large proportion of obstetric medical malpractice claims. The legal liability can be significant.[8,9]

CONTRIBUTING FACTORS

Risk factors for SD (Box 21.1) include fetal macrosomia[10–12] defined as >4500 g or >4000 g in patients with diabetes—frank or gestational diabetes mellitus (GDM), obesity, post-term gestation, multiparity, short maternal stature, and previous history of macrosomic birth or SD. Other contributing factors include the use of oxytocin for induction of labor, epidural analgesia, prolonged labor, and the use of operative vaginal delivery (OVD).

Box 21.1 Recommended order for the application of maneuvers.

- McRobert's maneuver is typically performed first as it can be quickly applied and is often successful.
- Suprapubic (not fundal) pressure with careful attention being paid to its correct application is attempted when McRobert's fails.
- Delivery of the posterior fetal arm should be attempted next as being most likely to accomplish delivery.
- Rotational maneuvers applied in rapid succession.
- Gaskin maneuver (see Figure 21.4).
- Attempt at clavicular fracture (rarely successful).
- Abdominal delivery preferably without the Zavanelli maneuver.

One important additional risk factor associated particularly with unexpected SD is a lack of adequate assessment of fetal and maternal size along with other historical risk factors so as to be *prepared* for the possibility of a difficult SD. Although it is widely reported that the initial SD is usually not expected,[13] adequate prenatal assessment could lead to prediction and prevention or mitigation of the complication. Patient safety initiatives are now focused on methods to predict and prepare for SD along with trained medical team management of the complication once it occurs.[14,15]

PREDICTION AND PREVENTION

Efforts to predict the likelihood of SD based upon known risk factors are intended to create a state of preparedness for the complication. There have been attempts made to develop algorithms to predict which laboring patients will develop a SD at the time of delivery with cesarean *required* for all patients who meet the criteria. None of these has been shown to have sufficient predictive value to be useful. Some feel that the number of elective cesarean deliveries required to prevent one episode of SD would be excessive and not justified.[16,17] This would apply even more to attempts to predict and prevent permanent brachial plexus palsy, many of which occur even in the absence of a clinical SD.[8] However, the presence of certain specific risk factors has been shown to be *associated* with a high enough risk of SD that a scheduled cesarean birth should be offered to the patient as an option. Recently, some have suggested that even with a small risk of recurrence—given the significant adverse consequences of a severe SD, that cesarean delivery should be *indicated* with a history of previous SD. These authors point out that similarly low but significant risks for uterine rupture in women with previous uterine scars can justify elective cesarean delivery.[18] There should be careful documentation of the discussion of risks and complications of either course of action, cesarean versus vaginal birth, in these circumstances (see Section Documentation and Debriefing below).

The specific antepartum risk factors because of which cesarean birth should be offered are (1) macrosomia[14] based on an estimated fetal weight (preferably by ultrasound measurement using multiple views) of >5000 g in nonobese and nondiabetic patients and >4500 g in obese and diabetic patients[4] and (2) a history of previous severe SD with any fetal injury. It may seem counterintuitive that there is a lower weight limit for obese and diabetic or GDM patients in this management guideline. The reason is that due to the effects of maternal insulin resistance and glucose metabolism, the fetuses in diabetic (including GDM) and obese patients tend to have proportionately larger bodies relative to their head size. This creates the situation where greater fetal body mass, particularly a larger bisacromial diameter, increases the risk that the fetal head may fit through the bony pelvis but the larger after-coming shoulders will then impact on the pubic symphysis or sacral promontory. Both diabetic (including GDM) and maternal obesity alone or in combination are independently associated with adverse pregnancy outcomes including SD.[19–22]

Intrapartum risk factors should also be taken into account in an attempt to lessen the incidence of SD.[23,24] Primary in this is the principle that when electing to perform an OVD, such as forceps or vacuum, for slow or arrested descent, one should give consideration to the possibility that one will accomplish safe delivery of the fetal head over the perineum only to discover that the shoulders are now stuck. This principle does not always refer to emergency OVD done for fetal bradycardia at a low station, but rather elective OVD for "maternal exhaustion" or a prolonged second stage. Questions to ask (and be prepared to document) are as follows: (1) How long has the second stage been? Longer second stages are associated with higher SD). (2) What is the station and position of the presenting part, and is it vertex or caput? Mid-pelvis OVD has a higher association with SD. (3) Is the patient diabetic (including GDM), obese, or of short stature? (4) What is the estimated fetal weight? If multiparous, what was the weight of previous fetuses, and were there any difficulties with those deliveries?

When there is concern that one or more of these risk factors is present, it is prudent to brief the entire delivery team of your concern prior to initiating OVD. It may also be appropriate to have an extra nurse in the room, particularly one who is experienced in the treatment of SD and the correct application of suprapubic pressure (see Section Primary Maneuvers below). One might even consider alerting the neonatal intensive care unit (NICU) staff or pediatrician on call to have them attend the birth and to alert the anesthesia department should they be needed on short notice. Most of the time they will not be needed but when a difficult SD occurs this will save precious minutes. Importantly, whether one is using forceps or vacuum as their preferred modality for OVD, one should always approach this procedure as a "trial" of OVD. In other words, one should always have a plan for when to declare the attempt at OVD a failed trial—defined as the inability to achieve significant descent of the head, too many pop-offs of the vacuum, or the expiration of a preset time limit.

Lastly, one should never declare one comparable method of OVD as a failure and then switch to a trial of the other modality (e.g., failed forceps followed by a trial of vacuum). This carries too high a risk of fetal and/or maternal injury, including SD. The appropriate response to failure to accomplish delivery with one attempt at OVD is to move expeditiously to cesarean delivery.[25,26]

MANAGEMENT

The key to a successful and safe delivery when SD occurs is to have a plan of management firmly in mind with every vaginal delivery. Because SD is largely unpredictable and has been described in fetuses of widely varying sizes,[27] it is important to always be prepared to begin your management plan when SD is recognized. Recognition of SD can begin with what is described as the "turtle sign"—a tight withdrawal of the rotated fetal head against the maternal perineum immediately upon delivery of the head.[28] This alone is not necessarily sufficient to make the diagnosis of SD, neither is it seen in every case. The more definitive way to make the diagnosis is to experience failure of the anterior fetal shoulder to emerge under the pubic symphysis with maternal pushing efforts combined with gentle downward traction on the fetal head. When this occurs with the first attempt at maternal pushing after delivery of the head, it is best to desist with further downward traction in the face of an impacted shoulder, as it is exactly this lateral deviation of the fetal head relative to the anterior shoulder[29–31] that can cause fetal nerve damage as described below.

Once there is a failure of the anterior shoulder to clear the pubic symphysis, an SD management plan should be activated. When the fetal head delivers and the body is in the pelvis, blood flow in the umbilical cord will be compromised while the fetus is unable to gasp.[32,33] Therefore, time is of the essence to effectively complete the delivery, because fetal acidemia and acidosis will progressively worsen until the SD is resolved.[34,35] Any management plan for SD, therefore, must begin with the delivering provider announcing loudly and clearly that a SD is occurring. This can be thought of as the first step in a virtual checklist of steps that every obstetric provider should have in their head. This announcement then triggers a cascade of events, which the entire obstetric team has rehearsed through drills and simulations as described below.

After announcing the problem, the next item on the virtual checklist is the summoning of additional help. This should include one or more extra nurses, an additional obstetrician or other obstetric provider, a neonatal resuscitation team or pediatrician, and an anesthesia provider. Preliminary preparations to open an operating room should also be made at this time. One of the nurses should be assigned the role of time and record keeper. S/he should note the time of delivery of the fetal head and its position so as to identify which shoulder is anterior. S/he would then record the sequence and timing of whatever maneuvers are employed. It is extremely helpful to call out the amount of time elapsed after delivery of the fetal head in 30-second increments. Time perception may be distorted and inaccurate during management of a SD and calling out time intervals is helpful to prevent spending too much time on a maneuver that is not working before moving onto the next one in the preferred sequence. Once delivery of the fetal body is accomplished, the timekeeper notes the total time elapsed between delivery of the head and body of the fetus.

After additional help has been summoned, the delivering provider can then embark on a sequence of maneuvers described below to resolve the SD and deliver the fetal body. Once this is done, it is important to secure a section of umbilical cord so that fetal blood gases and pH can be determined from both the umbilical artery and vein. This information can be helpful to the pediatrician or neonatologist in the event of fetal compromise. In addition, it can be important medicolegally to document the absence of fetal acidemia/acidosis when Appearance, Pulse, Grimace, Activity, Respiration (APGAR) scores are low. From the medicolegal perspective it is always best to obtain both well-marked venous and arterial cord blood samples. This not only allows for comparison but also eliminates the possibility that a plaintiff's attorney will claim that a single set of values is a venous sample when it was in fact arterial.[36]

Last on the virtual checklist should be a debrief for everyone involved in the SD as soon as possible after the event. This should be done even if the outcome was a timely delivery of a healthy newborn. Reviewing how the care was rendered will allow for continual improvement in performance on the labor and delivery unit for the inevitable next SD. The debrief is also a good opportunity to review timing and sequence of maneuvers so that the documentation of the event recorded by the obstetric provider matches that produced by the nursing personnel. This not only represents an important feature of good patient care but it is also important from a medicolegal perspective should the case result in a malpractice suit.[37]

PRIMARY MANEUVERS

There are several maneuvers that are classically described in the management of SD to allow the anterior shoulder that is impacted against the pubic symphysis to emerge under it. First, all of the individual maneuvers will be described followed by comments on their application.

1. McRobert's maneuver: This is accomplished by having the mother hyperflex her hips as far as possible, so that her knees are pressed against her chest and upper abdomen.[38] Although some women can accomplish this themselves by placing their hands behind their knees (Figure 21.1) and pulling them in, this is often best achieved by having one nurse or other attendant on each leg, assisting the flexion. This has the effect of rotating the pelvic girdle so that the distance between the pubic symphysis and sacral promontory is increased. This is frequently all that is required to allow maternal pushing efforts combined with gentle traction on the fetal head to resolve the SD.

2. Suprapubic pressure: SD occurs when the anterior fetal shoulder becomes lodged behind the maternal pubic symphysis in a direct anterior–posterior orientation. The key to dislodging the shoulder, allowing it to slip under the symphysis, is to deflect it off of a plane that is "straight up and down." One of the most effective ways to do this is by the application of suprapubic pressure (Figure 21.2). This

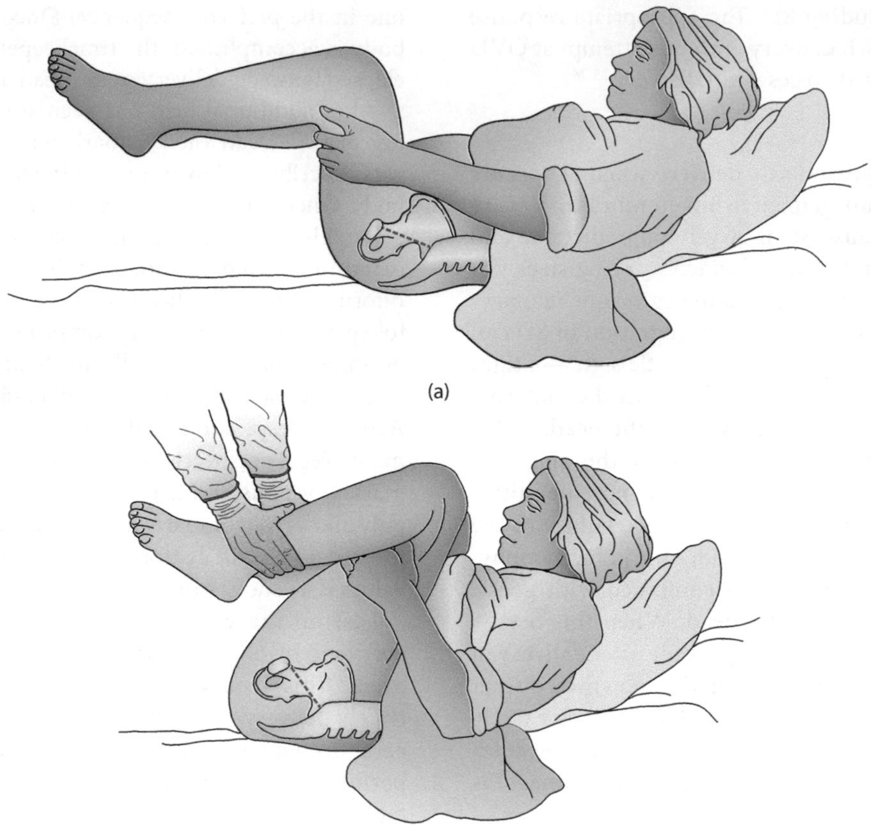

(a)

(b)

Figure 21.1 Self-implemented hyperflexion of the legs by the laboring patient: For the management of shoulder dystocia (SD), the legs should be supported and flexed by an obstetric assistant on each leg. (a) The diameter before assisted flexion. (b) The larger pubosacral diameter for allowing passage of a trapped shoulder after assisted flexion.

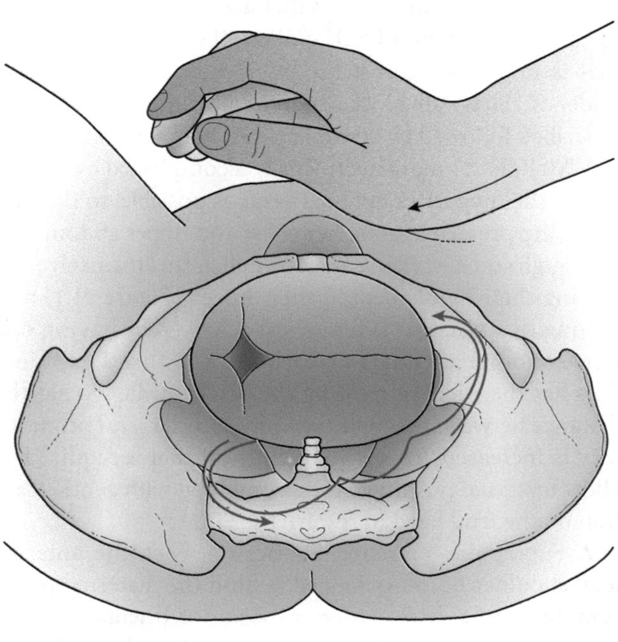

Figure 21.2 Proper application of suprapubic pressure for SD. Pressure applied higher (uterine fundus) could make the clinical situation worse.

should not be confused with fundal pressure, which in the setting of SD is not only counterproductive but potentially harmful.[39] Fundal pressure (applied higher at the level of the uterine fundus) will more tightly impact the shoulder against the symphysis, making it even harder to ultimately dislodge. In addition, vigorous application of fundal pressure can cause catastrophic uterine rupture and should always be avoided. On the other hand, suprapubic pressure is the application of force with the fist or heel of an assistant's hand to the maternal lower abdomen just above the pubic symphysis. The object of this maneuver is to move the fetal shoulder off the direct vertical by applying force to the back of the anterior shoulder and getting the shoulder to rotate in the direction of the fetal chest. Therefore, it is critical that the operator attempting delivery indicates to the assistant which fetal shoulder is anterior and what direction force should be applied. The assistant places his or her hand slightly to the side of midline over the fetal back and pushes down and toward the opposite side. So, for example, if the right fetal shoulder is anterior, the assistant would place his or her hand suprapubically to the maternal left of midline and direct the force down and to the right. The ability of the assistant to do this maneuver properly is sometimes aided by use of a stepstool to elevate the assistant over the patient. When performed properly in conjunction with McRobert's maneuver above, the operator will feel the fetal shoulder release as it moves off the vertical and emerges under the symphysis. Delivery can then be completed in the usual manner.

3. Rotational maneuvers: As stated above, the goal of the initial maneuvers to relieve SD is to get the anterior shoulder to rotate off the vertical plane. Another way to accomplish this is by applying rotational maneuvers, where the operator's hand is used to rotate the fetus.[40] Two rotational maneuvers have been described: Woods Corkscrew (Figure 21.3) and Rubin's maneuver.[41,42]

In the former, pressure is applied by the operator's fingers and hand to the anterior surface of the posterior fetal shoulder in an attempt to rotate the fetal body. In the latter, pressure is applied to the posterior surface of whichever shoulder is most accessible, again with the goal of rotating the fetal body to the point that the anterior shoulder is no longer directly vertical and can emerge under the symphysis. Either maneuver can be accomplished in less than a minute so both can be attempted in sequence if the first rotational maneuver is not successful.

4. Delivery of the posterior arm: This maneuver involves the operator placing their hand into the posterior vagina and grasping the posterior fetal hand.[43] To accomplish this one has to introduce the entire hand into the vaginal canal by sliding it over the perineum and below the fetal body. To do this one has to bring all the fingertips together, including the thumb, before passing the hand over the perineum. A common mistake by inexperienced operators is to leave the thumb external to the vagina. This will make it almost impossible to reach the posterior fetal hand in most cases. As a "rule of thumb" the operator should choose to introduce the entire hand that will be on the side of the fetal chest—the right hand if the left fetal shoulder is anterior and the left hand if the right fetal shoulder is anterior. Once in the vagina, the fetal hand should be readily palpable if the fetal arm is flexed. The hand should then be grasped and drawn across the fetal chest as the operator's hand is withdrawn, causing the fetal hand to emerge alongside the impacted anterior shoulder. To try to bring the fetal hand out otherwise risks fracturing the humerus of the posterior arm.[44] If the fetal hand is not readily palpable because the fetal arm is extended, the operator's hand should be advanced along the fetal arm until the antecubital fossa is reached. Pressure here should readily cause the fetal arm to flex and make it possible to grasp the hand. Then the arm is withdrawn as just described. Once the posterior arm is delivered, the anterior shoulder usually readily slides under the symphysis and the delivery can be completed. In the case of a very large fetus, sometimes it will be necessary to rotate the fetus 180° once the arm is delivered so that the posterior arm is now anterior. The previously impacted shoulder can now be delivered over the perineum.

5. Gaskin maneuver: This technique, also called the "all fours maneuver," was named for the midwife, Ida May Gaskin, who first described it.[45] The patient is placed on all fours (Figure 21.4), and then maternal pushing efforts are combined with gentle downward traction on the fetal head in its new position. It is theorized that the effect of gravity creates more room in the posterior vagina, with the result that in this position the posterior shoulder and arm can be delivered readily. Then upward traction will deliver the shoulder that was behind the symphysis with the fetal body quickly following. Similarly to the description of delivery of the posterior arm above, if the other shoulder does not deliver easily the fetal body can then be rotated without difficulty to allow delivery of the other shoulder over the perineum.

7. Additional extreme (and riskier) measures: When the use of these initial basic maneuvers described above is

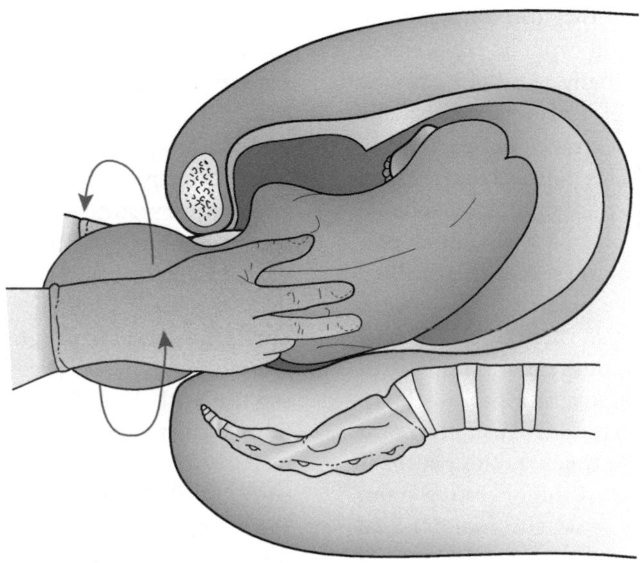

Figure 21.3 The corkscrew maneuver. The fetal shoulders are rotated by applying pressure on the scapula and the clavicle. The fetal head should be stabilized and not separately rotated.

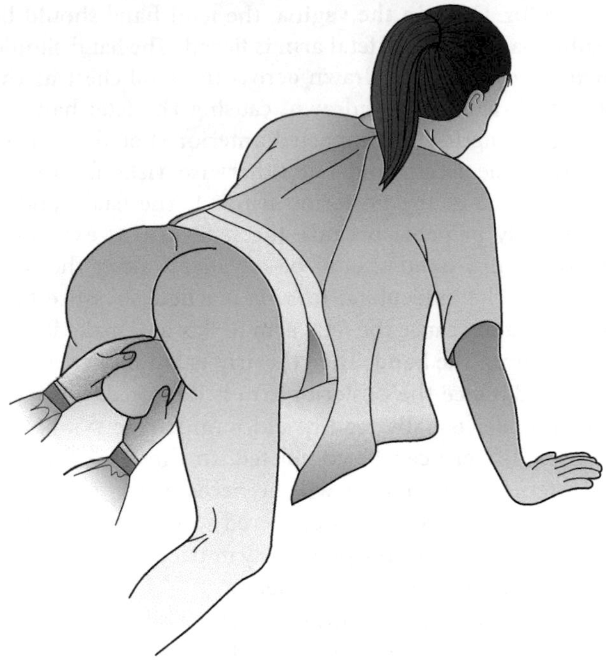

Figure 21.4 The Gaskin maneuver. The patient is placed on all fours, which facilitates the creation of a larger pubosacral diameter for passage of the fetus. This position also allows for greater gravitational force.

unsuccessful in accomplishing delivery, there are additional maneuvers that can be attempted but are rarely used today. Purposeful fracture of the anterior fetal clavicle is thought to allow collapse of the shoulder in an anterior direction.[46] This in effect rotates the anterior shoulder out from under the symphysis, but this is surprisingly difficult to accomplish using just the operator's fingers. Some have suggested pressing against the clavicle with a hemostat or other small metal instrument, but this too is difficult and is not suggested. If all else fails the patient can be taken to the operating room for a hysterotomy with either direct rotation of the anterior shoulder or assistance in cephalic replacement and delivery of the fetus abdominally. Another extreme measure is the Zavanelli maneuver,[47] also called cephalic replacement. This maneuver is presented mainly for historical purposes because most experts now feel that the fetal and maternal risks of this maneuver are significant and that abdominal delivery can be accomplished without first performing it. The technique calls for reversing the cardinal movements of the fetus during the normal birth process. The operator rotates the fetal head so that the chin is posterior. The fetal head is then flexed to the maximum extent possible until the chin slides back up over the perineal body. Once this is accomplished, the fetal head will usually retreat back up into the birth canal quite quickly. The patient is then moved as rapidly as possible to the operating room for an emergent cesarean birth. It is wise to monitor fetal heart tones during this transfer and if the tracing is consistent with good oxygenation of the fetus then a short time can be taken to allow intrauterine fetal resuscitation while more orderly preparations are made for surgery. Last, if the fetus has succumbed and is still trapped in the pelvis, surgical symphysectomy will allow the shoulder of the demised fetus to be delivered.[48–50]

HOW TO APPLY THE PRIMARY MANEUVERS

For many years it was stated that there was insufficient evidence to recommend the order in which the primary maneuvers should be applied for SD. More recently, evidence is accumulating to suggest a preferred order of application of the above maneuvers for SD.[51–54] The recommended order for the application of the maneuvers is contained in Box 21.1. To be noted in the sequence listed in Box 21.1 is the absence of cutting a generous episiotomy. Although once thought to be an important initial step in the management of SD, it is now recognized that routine episiotomy itself does not aid in release of the impacted anterior shoulder.[55] However, it is reasonable to perform or extend an episiotomy at any point in the recommended sequence if doing so will allow the operator to perform the next step. For example, many find it useful to perform an episiotomy to allow more room for delivery of the posterior arm. Lastly, it is important that one not persist too long in attempting any of the above maneuvers that is not working. To reiterate, that is the importance of appointing a timekeeper. When 30–60 seconds have elapsed with a failed maneuver to correct for SD it is time to move onto the next step.

TRAINING: SIMULATION AND DRILLS

SD is a true obstetric emergency requiring rapid action by a trained team working together toward the goal of a safe delivery. This is best accomplished by practicing for this emergent event using drills and simulations. Drilling for this emergency has been shown to improve both physician and team performance and to improve neonatal outcomes.[56,57] Although an in-depth discussion is beyond the scope of this chapter, there are many options for organizing SD drills and simulations in almost any care setting. These can be performed in a simulation laboratory with sophisticated mannequins, some of which will register the amount of force applied by the operator. Simulations often involve teams with representatives of different disciplines, and video taping of the drills to assist in debriefing afterward. Effective drills can also be performed in the labor and delivery suite using simpler mannequins and less special equipment. The goal of these rehearsal drills is to develop a team-based response to SD in the local labor and delivery unit.[58]

It is important to assign in advance who will perform the critical roles, such as timekeeper or assistant operator, during the drill. As in few other situations in obstetrics, with SD "failing to plan" is tantamount to "planning to fail."

COMPLICATIONS

With appropriate training, preparation and teamwork, most cases of SD can be successfully resolved without injury to mother or fetus.[59] However, it is important to be aware of some of the adverse effects that an episode of SD can have on both. Patients are at risk for soft tissue injury to the vagina and perineum from the manipulative maneuvers that require insertion of the operator's fingers or hand into the vagina. This can include third and fourth degree extensions of an episiotomy if one is performed, as well as possible vaginal wall lacerations. Patients with SD are at higher risk for postpartum hemorrhage, so close observation for this after delivery is required.[60] Last, it is important to recognize that any difficult birth can put the mother at risk for posttraumatic stress disorder. Evaluation by a mental health professional may be advisable if the patient shows signs of insomnia, hyperarousal, or inability to perform normal daily activities in the postpartum period.[61,62]

For the fetus, the greatest risk is damage to the brachial plexus of the anterior arm.[63] This can be due simply to the uterine expulsive forces attempting to push the fetal body past the entrapped shoulder, causing stretching of the nerves in the fetal neck that supply the ipsilateral arm. This may occur without any operator intervention. However, this stretching can be exacerbated by excessive traction on the fetal head and neck during attempts at delivery, especially if that traction is exerted while deflecting the fetal head toward the floor and away from the entrapped shoulder. This puts the nerves of the brachial plexus on maximal stretch and risks damaging them, so traction in this direction needs to be avoided if at all possible. Two major forms of brachial plexus palsy are recognized, Erb's Palsy and Klumpke's Palsy.[64–66] The former is more common and involves damage to the roots of cervical nerves C-5 and C-6. The muscles of the upper arm are most affected, with the arm held in the so-called waiter's tip position with the upper arm flaccid and adducted and the wrist flexed with the finger tips pointing backwards. The latter is due to damage to nerve roots C-8 and T-1 causing weakness of the hand and forearm muscles.

Additionally, the fetus is at risk for fractures. Most common sites of fracture are the clavicle and humerus, usually associated with delivery of the posterior arm as the method by which the SD is resolved.[67] Fortunately, these will heal without permanent sequelae in almost all cases. Last, the fetus is at risk for hypoxia and even death if the time to accomplish delivery is prolonged. There have been conflicting studies published over the years as to what time interval between diagnosis of SD and delivery puts the fetus at risk for hypoxic encephalopathy. Although no clear consensus exists, these studies in total seem to indicate that the risk of severe brain injury to the fetus is low if delivery is accomplished within 4–5 minutes of diagnosis, and begins to increase somewhere between 6 and 10 minutes of diagnosis if a SD is still unresolved.[35,68]

DOCUMENTATION AND DEBRIEFING

Appropriate documentation of SD sometimes begins in the antepartum period. If a patient has a significant risk factor for SD, as described above, such as excessive estimated fetal weight or history of previous SD with fetal injury, a thorough discussion of possible risks and complications of vaginal delivery should be held during the pregnancy. This should be carefully documented in the antenatal record, along with the recommendation for cesarean birth. If the patient refuses, then this documentation of her informed refusal will become very important should an SD occur at birth.

In the case of an unanticipated SD, once delivery has been successfully accomplished, it is important to carefully document all critical elements related to the event. An important first step is to debrief the entire team to include every staff member present in the delivery room, as soon after the delivery as is possible. This will bring to light any possible areas for improvement in the response to SD on the labor and delivery unit. Importantly, however, it will also foster agreement as to what just transpired so that physician and nursing documentation will coincide. As noted previously, this will be important medicolegally should there be a permanent fetal injury that results in a malpractice suit.

Proper documentation is important also for the completeness of the medical record in terms of future care of the patient postpartum or in subsequent pregnancies and as an aid to analysis of the care provided should that prove necessary in retrospect for quality improvement or peer review purposes. There are certain critical elements that should be included in all documentation of an episode of SD. These include identifying all participants present in the delivery room; the presence of antepartum risk factors; the use of OVD instruments; the timing of events such as onset of labor and onset of second stage; recognition of the SD; initiation of various maneuvers; and time of delivery of the body; which shoulder was anterior; maneuvers utilized and neonatal outcome measures such as APGAR scores, weight, and evidence of injury. It is also good to note communications that occurred with family, pediatrics, or NICU personnel, and plans for postpartum care.

There are a considerable number of elements that should be included for proper documentation of SD.[69] It is helpful to use a standardized form for documentation that can be either paper or electronic.[70] One example of such a form was published by the American College of Obstetricians and Gynecologists (ACOG) in 2012.[71] Poor documentation of SD events is unfortunately common and can have undesired repercussions in the event of a malpractice suit.[72]

SUMMARY

SD is one of only a few obstetric emergencies where prompt recognition, initiation of a well-thought-out plan and reliable, rehearsed teamwork can make the difference between a healthy mother and baby and a disastrous outcome with permanent injury to the fetus. The chance of a successful outcome is increased significantly by offering cesarean birth to selected patients at very high risk for SD. Additional keys to appropriate management of SD are adequate preparation for this complication when risk factors are present and avoiding OVD in those situations. Once a SD occurs, having drilled on the standard maneuvers has been shown to improve both individual and team performance and reduction in fetal injury. Full documentation of a SD is important for patient care, quality improvement, and risk management efforts. Attention to all of these important aspects of SD management reduces the anxiety felt by many birth attendants faced with this uncommon but inevitable complication of the birth process.

Guidance about ways to reduce the risk of brachial plexus birth injuries with and without SD is presented in Box 21.2.

Box 21.2 ACOG recommendations for avoiding neonatal brachial plexus palsy

1. Axial traction (keeping the skull in line with the fetal spine) preferable to lateral deviation of the fetal head but may still put strain on the brachial plexus
2. Prioritization of posterior arm delivery
3. Team training
4. Simulation
5. Appropriate documentation

Source: American College of Obstetricians and Gynecologists, *Obstet Gynecol;* 123(4): 902–4, 2014.

REFERENCES

1. Zhang J, Landy HG, Branch DW et al. Contemporary patterns of spontaneous labor with normal neonatal outcomes. *Obstet Gynecol* 2010; 116: 1281–7.
2. Hobel C. Uterine contractility and dystocia. In: *Essentials of Obstetrics and Gynecology*, Chapter 11 (6th edition). Philadelphia, PA: Saunders-Elsevier, 2016.
3. Beall MH, Spong C, McKay J, Ross MG. Objective definition of shoulder dystocia: A prospective evaluation. *Am J Obstet Gynecol* 1998; 179: 934–7.
4. American College of Obstetricians and Gynecologists. ACOG Practice Bulletin No. 40. Shoulder dystocia. *Obstet Gynecol* 2002; 100: 1045–50.
5. Lanni SM, Seeds JW. Malpresentations. In: Gabbe SG, Niebyl JR, Simpson JL (eds), *Obstetrics* (4th edition), p. 473. New York, NY: Churchill Livingston, 2002.
6. Hankins GD, Clark SM, Munn MB. Cesarean section on request at 39 weeks: Impact on shoulder dystocia, fetal trauma, neonatal encephalopathy, and intra-uterine fetal demise. *Semin Perinatol* 2006; 30: 276–87.
7. Towner D, Castro MA, Eby-Wilkens E et al. Effect of mode of delivery in nulliparous women on neonatal intracranial injury. *N Engl J Med* 1999; 341: 1709–14.
8. American College of Obstetricians and Gynecologists. Executive Summary: Neonatal brachial plexus palsy. Report of the American College of Obstetricians and Gynecologists' Task Force on Neonatal Brachial Plexus Palsy. *Obstet Gynecol.* 2014; 123(4): 902–4.
9. Mavroforou A, Koumantakis E, Michalodimitrakis E. Physicians' liability in obstetric and gynecology practice. *Med Law* 2005; 24: 1–9.
10. Benedetti TJ, Gabbe SG. Shoulder dystocia. A complication of fetal macrosomia and prolonged second stage of labor with mid-pelvic delivery. *Obstet Gynecol* 1978; 52: 526.
11. Modanlou HD, Dorchester WY, Phorosian A et al. Macrosomia—Maternal, fetal and neonatal implications. *Obstet Gynecol* 1980: 55: 420–4.
12. Nesbitt TS, Gilbert WM, Herrchen B. Shoulder dystocia and associated risk factors with macrocosmic infants born in California. *Am J Obstet Gynecol* 1998; 179: 476–80.
13. Gherman RB, Chauhan S, Ouzounian JG et al. Shoulder dystocia: The unpreventable obstetric emergency with empiric management guidelines. *Am J Obstet Gynecol* 2006; 195: 657–72.
14. Draycott TJ, Crofts JF, Ash JP et al. Improving neonatal outcome through practical shoulder dystocia training. *Obstet Gynecol* 2008; 112:14–20.
15. Crofts JR, Fox R, Ellis D et al. Observations from 450 shoulder dystocia simulations: Lessons for skills training. *Obstet Gynecol* 2008; 112: 906–12.
16. Rouse DJ, Owen J, Goldenberg RL et al. The effectiveness and costs of elective cesarean delivery for fetal macrosomia by ultrasound. *JAMA* 1966; 276: 14.
17. Langer O, Berkus MD, Huff RW et al. Shoulder dystocia: Should the fetus weighing >4,000 gm be delivered by cesarean section. *Am J Obstet Gynecol* 1991; 165: 831–7.
18. Jaspan D, Cohen AW. First person: Our shoulder dystocia policy. *Contem Obstet Gynecol* August 13, 2015.
19. Iffy L, Djordjevic MM, Apussio JJ et al. Diabetes, hypertension and birth injuries: A complex interrelationship. *Bull Isr Soc Obstet Gynecol* 2004; 2: 36.
20. Robinson H, Katch S, Mayes DC et al. Is maternal obesity a predictor of shoulder dystocia? *Obstet Gynecol* 2003; 101: 24–7.
21. Klebanoff MA, Mills JL, Berendes HW. Mother's birthweight as a predictor of macrosomia. *Am J Obstet Gynecol* 1985; 153: 353–7.
22. Catalano PM, McIntyre HD, Cruickshank JK et al. The hyperglycemia and adverse pregnancy outcomes study. Associations of GDM and obesity with pregnancy outcomes. *Diabetes Care* 2012; 35: 780–6.
23. Hassaan AA. Shoulder dystocia: Risk factors and prevention. *Aust N Z J Obstet Gynaecol* 1988; 28: 107–9.
24. El Madany AA, Jallad KB, Radi FA et al. Shoulder dystocia: Anticipation and outcome. *Int J Gynaecol Obstet* 1990; 34: 7–12.
25. American College of Obstetricians and Gynecologists. Practice Bulletin No. 154. Operative vaginal delivery. *Obstet Gynecol* 2015; 126: e56–65.
26. Bofill JA, Rust OA, Devidas M et al. Shoulder dystocia and operative vaginal delivery. *J Matern Fetal Med* 1997; 6: 220–224.
27. Bryant DR, Leonardi MR, Landwehr JB, Bottoms SF. Limited usefulness of fetal weight in predicting neonatal brachial plexus injury. *Am J Obstet Gynecol* 1998; 179: 686–9.

28. Baxley EG, Gobbo RW. Shoulder dystocia. *Am Fam Physician* 2004; 69: 1701–14.
29. Gonik B, Zhang N, Grimm NG. Prediction of brachial plexus stretching during shoulder dystocia using a computer simulation model. *Am J Obstet Gynecol* 2003; 189: 1168–72.
30. Ouzounian LG, Korst LM, Phelan JP. Permanent Erb's palsy: A traction related injury? *Obstet Gynecol* 1997; 89: 139–41.
31. Deering SH, Weeks L, Benedetti TJ. Evaluation of force applied during deliveries complicated by shoulder dystocia using simulation. *Am J Obstet Gynecol* 2011; 204: 234.e1–5.
32. Iffy L, Gittens-Williams LN. Shoulder dystocia and nuchal cord. *Acta Obstet Gynecol Scand* 2007; 86: 253.
33. Cunningham FG, MacDonald PC, Grant NF et al. *Williams Obstetrics* (20th edition). Norwalk, CT: Appleton & Lange, 1997.
34. Stallings SP, Edwards RK, Johnson JWC. Correlation of head-to-body delivery intervals in shoulder dystocia and umbilical artery acidosis. *Am J Obstet Gynecol* 2001; 185: 268–74.
35. Leung TY, Stuart O, Sahota DS et al. Head-to-body delivery interval and risk of fetal acidosis and hypoxic ischaemic encephalopathy in shoulder dystocia: A retrospective review. *BJOG* 2011; 118: 474–9.
36. Gottlieb AG, Galan HL. Shoulder dystocia: An update. *Obstet Gynecol Clin N Am* 2007; 34: 501–31.
37. Gurewitsch ED, Johnson TL, Narayan AK et al. Subjective debriefing following shoulder dystocia: How good is it? *Reprod Sci* 2009; 16: 308A.
38. McRoberts WA. Maneuvers for shoulder dystocia. *Contemp Obstet Gynecol* 1984: 24: 17.
39. Focus Group Shoulder Dystocia. In: *Confidential Enquiries into Stillbirths and Deaths in Infancy. Fifth Annual Report*, pp. 73–9. London, UK: Maternal and Child Health Research Consortium, 1998.
40. Gurewitsch ED. Optimizing shoulder dystocia management to prevent birth injury. *Clin Obstet Gynecol* 2007; 50: 592–606.
41. Woods CE. A principle of physics as applicable to shoulder delivery. *Am J Obstet Gynecol* 1943; 45: 796–804.
42. Rubin A. Management of shoulder dystocia. *JAMA* 1964; 189: 835–7.
43. Barnum CG. Dystocia due to the shoulders. *Am J Obstet Gynecol* 1945; 50: 439–42.
44. Gherman RB, Ouzounian JG, Goodwin TM. Obstetric maneuvers for shoulder dystocia and associated fetal morbidity. *Am J Obstet Gynecol* 1998; 178: 1126–30.
45. Bruner JP, Drummond SB, Meenan AL, Gaskin IM. All-fours maneuver for reducing shoulder dystocia during labor. *J Reprod Med* 43: 439–43.
46. Bankoski BR, Allen RH, Nagey DA et al. Measuring clavicle strength and modeling birth: Towards understanding birth injury. In: Vossoughi J (ed), *Proceedings of the 13th Southern Biomedical Engineering Conference*, April 1994. Washington, DC. pp. 586–9.
47. Sandberg EC. The Zavanelli maneuver: A potentially revolutionary method for the resolution of shoulder dystocia. *Am J Obstet Gynecol* 1985; 152: 479–84.
48. Van Roosmalen J. Shoulder dystocia and symphysiotomy. *Eur J Obstet Gynecol Reprod Biol* 1995; 59: 115–6.
49. Hartfield VJ. Symphysiotomy for shoulder dystocia. *Am J Obstet Gynecol* 1986; 155: 228.
50. Goodwin TM, Banks E, Millar LK, Phelan JP. Catastrophic shoulder dystocia and emergency symphysiotomy. *Am J Obstet Gynecol* 1997; 177: 463–4.
51. Royal College of Obstetricians and Gynecologists. RCOG Green-top Guideline No. 42, Shoulder dystocia. *R Coll Obstet Gynecol* 2012; 6–9.
52. Leung TY, Stuart O, Suen SS et al. Comparison of perinatal outcomes of shoulder dystocia alleviated by different type and sequence of manoeuvres: A retrospective review. *BJOG* 2011; 118: 985–90.
53. Hoffman MK, Bailit JL, Branch DW et al. A comparison of obstetric maneuvers for the acute management of shoulder dystocia. *Obstet Gynecol* 2011; 117: 1272–8.
54. Poggi SH, Spong CY, Allen RH. Prioritizing posterior arm delivery during severe shoulder dystocia. *Obstet Gynecol* 2003; 101: 1068–72.
55. Gurewitsch ED, Donithan M, Stallings SP et al. Episiotomy versus fetal manipulation in managing severe shoulder dystocia: A comparison of outcomes. *Am J Obstet Gynecol* 2005; 192: 153–7.
56. Crofts JF, Lenguerrand E, Bentham GL et al. Prevention of brachial plexus injury—12 years of shoulder dystocia training: An interrupted time-series study. *BJOG* 2016; 123: 111–8. doi:10.1111/1471–0528. 13302.
57. Inglis SR, Feier N, Chetiyaar JB et al. Effects of shoulder dystocia training on the incidence of brachial plexus injury. *Am J Obstet Gynecol* 2011; 204: 322. e1–6.
58. Grobman WA, Miller D, Burke C et al. Outcomes associated with introduction of a shoulder dystocia protocol. *Am J Obstet Gynecol* 2011; 205: 513–7.
59. Gurewitsch ED, Allen RH. Reducing the risk of shoulder dystocia and associated brachial plexus injury. *Obstet Gynecol Clin North Am* 2011; 38: 247–69, x. doi: 10.1016/j.ogc.2011.02.015.
60. Mazouni C, Menard JP, Porcu G et al. Maternal morbidity associated with obstetrical maneuvers in shoulder dystocia. *Eur J Obstet Gynecol Reprod Biol* 2006; 129: 15–8.
61. Menage J. Post-traumatic stress disorder in women who have undergone obstetric and/or gynaecological procedures. *J Reprod Infant Psychol* 1993; 11: 221–8.
62. Beck, CT. Post-traumatic stress disorder due to childbirth: The aftermath. *Nurs Res* 2004; 53: 216–24.
63. Donelly V, Foran A, Murphy J et al. Neonatal brachial plexus palsy—An unpredictable injury. *Am J Obstet Gynecol* 2002; 187: 1209–12.

64. McFarland LV, Raskin M, Daling JR et al. Erb/Duchenne's palsy: A consequence of fetal macrosomia and method of delivery. *Obstet Gynecol* 1986; 68: 784–8.
65. Gilbert WM, Newbitt TS, Danielsen B. Associated factors in 1611 cases of brachial plexus injury. *Obstet Gynecol* 1999; 93: 536–40.
66. Jennett RJ, Tarby TJ. Brachial plexus palsy: An old problem revisited again. *Am J Obstet Gynecol* 1997; 176: 1354–7.
67. Nocon JJ, McKenzie DK, Thomas LJ, Hansell RS. Shoulder dystocia: An analysis of risks and obstetric maneuvers. *Am J Obstet Gynecol* 1993; 168: 1732–9.
68. Leung T, Stuart O, Sahota D et al. Head-to-body delivery interval and risk of fetal acidosis and hypoxic ischaemic encephalopathy in shoulder dystocia: A retrospective review. *BJOG* 2011; 118(4): 474–9. doi: 10.1111/j.1471-0528.2010.02834.x.
69. Crofts JF, Bartlett C, Ellis D et al. Documentation of simulated shoulder dystocia: Accurate and complete? *BJOG* 2008; 115: 1303–8.
70. Deering SH, Tobler K, Cypher R. Improvement in documentation using an electronic checklist for shoulder dystocia deliveries. *Obstet Gynecol* 2010; 116: 63–6.
71. American College of Obstetricians and Gynecologists. Patient Safety Checklist No. 6. Documenting shoulder dystocia. *Obstet Gynecol* 2012; 120: 430–1.
72. Gross TL, Sokol RJ, Williams T et al. Shoulder dystocia: A fetal-physician risk. *Am J Obstet Gynecol* 1987; 156; 1408–18.

Postpartum hemorrhage

22

HAYWOOD L. BROWN, JAMES EDWARDS, and MARIA SMALL

CONTENTS

DEFINITION AND CLASSIFICATION

Traditionally, postpartum hemorrhage (PPH) is defined as blood loss in excess of 500 mL after a vaginal delivery and greater than 1000 mL following a cesarean delivery. Severe hemorrhage is the most common cause of maternal death worldwide accounting for approximately 25% of all maternal deaths.[1] More than one half of these deaths due to severe hemorrhage occur within 24 hours of delivery. In Africa and Asia, hemorrhage accounts for 30.8% and 33.9% of all direct obstetric mortality.[1] This amounts to approximately 140,000 deaths annually worldwide or one death every 4 minutes.[2] In the United States hemorrhage is among the top three causes for pregnancy-related death along with hypertensive disorders and embolism.[3]

PPH is implicated in 2.9% of all deliveries and is associated with 19.1% of all in-hospital deaths after delivery.[4] PPH is classified as immediate or primary if it occurs within 24 hours after the completion of the third stage; and as delayed or secondary if it occurs between 24 hours and within 6–12 weeks of the puerperium. PPH is also a significant cause for maternal morbidity or near miss mortality including coagulopathy, shock and adult respiratory distress syndrome, and peripartum intensive care unit admission.[4,5]

The definition of blood loss in excess of 500 mL as abnormal is arbitrary. Another definition for PPH that has been proposed is a postpartum decline in hematocrit concentration level of 10%. However, there are concerns with this definition because the physiological changes of pregnancy with rapid blood loss may trigger a significant hypotensive cardiovascular response before a measurable decline in hematocrit concentration is demonstrated. The Royal College of Obstetricians and Gynecologists defines PPH as minor (500–1000 mL) or major (>1000 mL). There are further subdivisions of major hemorrhage: moderate (1000–2000 mL) or severe (>2000 mL).[6]

An international expert panel defined PPH as "active bleeding >1000 mL within the 24 hours following birth that continues despite the use of initial measures, including first-line uterotonic agents and uterine massage."[7] In cases of twin gestation, the postpartum blood loss exceeds 500 mL in 38.2% and 1000 mL in 6.6% of the cases. The zygocity and gender of the twins have no identifiable effect upon the amount of the bleeding.[8]

According to data from France, 58% of all obstetric bleeding develops after delivery. Of these, 51% follow instrumental vaginal deliveries, 19% spontaneous vaginal births, and 30% cesarean sections. The authors found that in cases of severe bleeding, patients had often received inadequate care due to late recognition of the severity of the hemorrhage. They considered 90% of the maternal deaths preventable.[9–11]

Depending on the definition of PPH the incidence varies from 1% to 5% of deliveries.[12] Data accumulated from the United States National Inpatient Sample suggested an incidence between 2% and 3% during the years 1994–2006.[13]

The difficulty in estimating blood loss accurately makes the diagnosis of PPH imprecise.[14] Methods to quantitate blood loss are cumbersome, time-consuming, and require complicated laboratory analysis; they are, therefore, seldom employed. For the most part, clinical estimation of blood loss is subjective. This explains the wide range in reported incidence.[15] A drop in hematocrit from the intrapartum to postpartum period of more than 5% reflects blood loss in excess of 500 mL and may be a useful guide, provided the determination is made on the third day postpartum and there has been no significant late bleeding. The shifts in fluids and diuresis that occur in the first few days postpartum make the drop in hematocrit less reliable during the first 24 hours after delivery, when the calculation of blood loss is most crucial. From a practical stand point, because of the increase in blood volume during pregnancy and the hemodynamic changes that occur in the postpartum period, most patients can tolerate hemorrhage up to 1500 mL, if not severely anemic prior to delivery.[16]

RISK FACTORS AND PREVENTION

Studies from Canada and Australia demonstrate an increase in the incidence of PPH during the past decade.[17,18] Advanced maternal age, parity, and previous PPH are historical risk factors. In the United States, change in obstetric practice over the last few decades including an increase in the rate of cesarean delivery[19] and multiple gestations births[20] have likely contributed to the increased risk for PPH. Existing complications during pregnancy, such as hypertensive disorders, diabetes, anemia, blood disorders, uterine anomalies and leiomyomas, third-trimester bleeding, and overdistended uterus, predispose to hemorrhage. Oxytocin is widely used in developed countries for induction or augmentation of labor and is an independent risk factor for severe PPH.[21] Other risk factors for PPH during labor include chorioamnionitis, the use of tocolytic agents such as magnesium sulfate, precipitous or prolonged labor, cephalopelvic disproportion, and prolonged second stage. Finally, improper delivery of the placenta significantly increases the risk of PPH (Table 22.1).[22]

When risk factors are present, preventive measures should be instituted. These include correction of anemia before the onset of labor, the placing of a large-caliber intravenous (IV) access to permit rapid infusion of fluids; typed, crossmatched blood being readily available; replacement of coagulation factors with bleeding disorders; and the prophylactic use of oxytocic agents after

Table 22.1 Risk factors for postpartum hemorrhage.

Historical	Antepartum	Intrapartum	Miscellaneous
Advanced maternal age	Overdistended uterus	Rapid labor	Preeclampsia
Multiparity	Macrosomia	Prolonged labor	Hypertension
Previous postpartum hemorrhage	Multiple gestation	Oxytocin use	Saline abortion
Previous uterine rupture	Hydramnios	General anesthesia	Sepsis
Previous uterine surgery	Placenta previa	Instrument delivery	Fetal demise
Previous placenta accreta	Abruption placentae	Forceps	Thromboembolic disease
Previous placenta previa	Amnionitis	Podalic version	
Known uterine malformation	Magnesium sulfate	Duhrssen's incision	
Leyomyomata/adenomyosis	Drugs	Genital tract trauma	
Coagulation disorders	Aspirin, NSAID	Lacerations	
ITP	Antibiotics	Hematomas	
TTP	Thiazide diuretics	Ruptured uterus	
Hemophilia	Sedatives	Placenta accreta	
von Willebrand's disease	Tranquilizers		

Abbreviations: ITP, immune thrombocytopenic purpura; NSAID, nonsteroidal anti-inflammatory drugs; TTP, thrombotic thrombocytopenic purpura.

delivery. A full bladder hinders postpartum uterine involution, which can be overcome by catheterization.

DIAGNOSIS

Massive blood loss is readily apparent, especially during the first hour after the completion of the third stage of labor. Immediately after the delivery of the placenta, there is heavy and continuous vaginal blood flow from the introitus. Within a short period after rapid blood loss, the patient may demonstrate signs and symptoms of cardiovascular compromise that include pallor, tachycardia, tachypnea, and hypotension, and if blood loss has exceeded critical levels, then the patient may demonstrate shock and cardiovascular collapse. The diagnosis may be less obvious if the bleeding is intermittent or protracted, mild to moderate, and the vital signs remain stable. Under these circumstances, it may be a few days before the magnitude of blood loss is recognized, when the patient feels weak and dizzy upon ambulation, appears pallid and tachycardic, and a significant drop in hematocrit is observed.

It is practical to classify PPH according to the pathophysiologic mechanism involved (Table 22.2). The major causes of immediate PPH include uterine atony, genital tract trauma, and retained placental tissue. The major causes of delayed PPH include subinvolution of the placental site, retained placental fragments, and chronic endometritis.

GENERAL PRINCIPLES OF MANAGEMENT

Severe hemorrhage can be dramatic and immediately life threatening. Excessive blood loss can rapidly lead to coagulopathy that further complicates the resuscitation and contributes to significant complications and sequela. These include hypovolemic shock, renal injury, hypopituitarism (Sheehan's syndrome), postpartum amenorrhea (Asherman's syndrome), and rarely transfusion-related complications. However, the outcome in most women with PPH is favorable with prompt recognition of its development, correct identification of its cause, and aggressive and prompt transfusion therapy of appropriate blood products.

A systematic sequence of therapeutic measures to control the bleeding must be followed. These include aggressive treatment of causative factors, maintenance of effective circulating intravascular volume by adequate replacement of blood and crystalloids, and prompt recognition and correction of coagulopathy. Coagulopathy is a secondary to consumption of clotting factors and hemodilution of with aggressive fluid resuscitation and leads to further bleeding.

Table 22.2 Causes of postpartum hemorrhage.

Immediate	Delayed
Uterine atony	Subinvolution
Retained products	Retained placental tissue
Genital tract trauma	Chronic endometritis
Uterine inversion	Placental polyp
Coagulation disorders	

Blood should be transfused as quickly as possible to minimize the further loss of clotting factors necessary to control the hemorrhage. Many institutions have adopted emergency hemorrhage or massive transfusion protocols to guide transfusion management in PPH. These protocols utilize a combination of packed red blood cells (pRBCs), type-specific plasma, thawed plasma, cryoprecipitate, and apheresis platelets. If typed and crossmatched blood is not available, group O Rh-negative blood may be used. The use of equipment to warm and infuse under pressure expedites rapid transfusion. More than one IV line should be placed and large-bore IV catheters are preferred, although central venous catheter may be placed. A transuretheral Foley catheter may be useful to monitor fluid therapy. The transfusion protocol further lays out the algorithm for obtaining laboratory studies including hemoglobin/hematocrit and platelets, dissemination intravascular coagulation (DIC) panel, arterial blood gases, and electrolytes (potassium, calcium, and glucose). Adequate crystalloids, such as Ringer's lactate or saline, are integral to resuscitation. Recent evidence places resuscitation using semisynthetic colloid solutions, such as hydroxyethyl starch, into question based on alterations in coagulation, specifically viscoelastic measurements and fibrinolysis.[23] A quick and easy test for coagulopathy is to draw an extra tube of blood (in a tube without anticoagulant/plain red tube), tape it to the bed or wall, and observe for clot formation 5–7 minutes after it is drawn.

Timely blood transfusion in obstetric emergencies can be lifesaving. However, transfusion is not without risk. Excessive/massive blood transfusion can lead to pulmonary edema and transfusion-related acute lung injury (TRALI) necessitating ventilator support. Transfusion-related acute circulatory overload (TACO) is manifest as hypertension, dyspnea, and pulmonary edema. Differentiation can be difficult but is essential to appropriate therapy.[24–26] Other potential dangers include isoimmunization, hemolytic reactions, homologous serum jaundice, allergic and anaphylactic reactions, febrile reactions, citric acid intoxication, and cardiac arrest.[27] Modern screening of blood donors for infectious diseases such as human immunodeficiency virus (HIV) and hepatitis has reduced the risk of its transmission to an extremely low level.

Successful management of PPH depends on a team approach. Nurses, obstetricians, anesthesiologists, and blood bank and laboratory personnel must work in concert to effect the systematic and orderly implementation of therapeutic measures.

MANAGEMENT OF THE THIRD STAGE OF LABOR

The conduct of the third stage of labor has a major influence on the development of PPH. Placental separation usually occurs within a few minutes after the delivery of the fetus and is thought to result from the shearing mechanical force of the ensuing uterine contractions.

The signs of placental separation include a gush of fresh vaginal bleeding, descent of the umbilical cord, and a change in the shape and position of the uterine fundus. However, these may be signs of placental descent, so that the clinical differentiation between separation and expulsion is difficult. In traditional expectant management of the third stage, uterotonic medications are not administered until after delivery of the placenta and placental separation occurs without intervention. Data from Fleigner[28] and Hibbard[29] showed that when minimal manipulation of the fundus and cord was performed, and the placenta was expressed only after signs of descent were evident, 90% of the placentas were delivered within 15 minutes and only 2–3% were retained after 30 minutes.

There is a broad spectrum of opinion and practice regarding the routine management of the third stage of labor. In active management (1) a uterotonic medication is administered within 1 minute after delivery of the fetus, (2) controlled umbilical cord traction and countertraction to support the uterus is performed until separation and delivery of the placenta, and (3) uterine massage is carried out after the delivery of the placenta. Early administration of oxytocic drugs at the delivery of the shoulders enhances uterine contractility and expedites placental separation.[30,31] In one published series, expression of the placenta by a combination of traction of the umbilical cord with the Brandt maneuver reduced the frequency of PPH from about 5% to 2%.[32]

After the cord has been clamped and cut and an uterotonic administered controlled cord traction is applied with countertraction on the fundus. Slight tension is maintained on the cord while awaiting strong uterine contractions. Once the contraction occurs a gentle downward pull on the cord facilitates placenta delivery. If the placenta fails to deliver within 30–40 seconds of controlled cord traction it is best to avoid further pulling on the cord until the uterine is well contracted again. It is important not to massage the fundus until after the delivery of the placenta.

A past issue of concern was that administering an uterotonic medication prior to delivery of the placenta would increase the incidence of trapped placenta requiring manual removal. A Cochrane systematic review identified five randomized controlled trials comparing active and expectant management that included more than 6400 women. Compared to expectant management, active management was associated with a shorter third stage of labor, a reduced risk for PPH and severe hemorrhage, a reduced risk of postpartum anemia, a decreased need for blood transfusion, and a decreased need for additional uterotonic medication. Furthermore, there was no increase in the risk of manual removal of the placenta with active management and no increased risk for uterine inversion or cord separation.[33]

Oxytocin remains the first choice medication for the prevention of PPH. It is more effective than ergot alkaloids or prostaglandins and has fewer side effects. While routine administration of oxytocic agents after the placenta is delivered has been a universal practice in the United States for several decades, the increased rate of PPH indicates that active management should become the routine management of choice for women delivering vaginally. During cesarean, oxytocin is routinely given after cord clamping to assist in expression of the placenta with less blood loss. Routine active management is superior to expectant management in the prevention of PPH and serious morbidity from hemorrhage. There is no international consensus on the selection of oxytocic agent after delivery. Many agents and doses are appropriate depending on local customs and presence of electricity. Oxytocin is administered by adding 10–40 IU to 1000 mL IV fluid and running it at 150 mL/hour. Alternately, oxytocin may be given as a bolus of 5–10 IU slowly over 1–2 minutes or 10 IU intramuscular (IM).[34] When given intravenously or intramuscularly, it has little or no adverse side effect. Some data indicate that a single dose of carbetocin 100 µg IM may be superior to oxytocin 5 IU IM.[35] Ergonovine maleate (Ergotrate) and methylergonovine (Methergine), although equally effective, may lead to acute pulmonary edema, cerebrovascular accident, and retinal detachment because of their vasopressor activity.[36] In an overview of 27 controlled trials on the effects of routine oxytocic administration in the management of the third stage of labor, a 40% reduction in the risk of PPH was calculated for the study group.[37]

It is standard practice to examine the placenta and confirm that it is intact. Routine postpartum digital exploration of the uterine cavity had been advocated, but several studies have refuted its utility.[38]

UTERINE ATONY

The most common cause for PPH is uterine atony. Uterine atony results when the myometrium fails to contract or stay contracted after the expulsion of the placenta, thereby allowing blood loss to continue at the implantation site. The rate of PPH has increased by 27.5% from 1995 to 2004 due to the increasing incidence of uterine atony.[4] Uterine atony complicates 1 in 20 births and contributes to nearly 80% of all cases of PPH.[39–41] If any predisposing factor is present, the potential for excessive blood loss should be anticipated, a large-bore IV catheter should be placed and blood should be readily available. The anesthesiologist should also be aware of the potential problem and consulted regarding the need to avoid deep anesthesia and uterine-relaxant drugs.

The diagnosis of uterine atony is suggested by the presence on abdominal examination of a large, boggy uterus that rises above the umbilicus. On this basis, a stepwise sequence of maneuvers designed to reverse uterine atony should be implemented (Table 22.3). The first step is the firm abdominal massage of the uterine fundus with one hand. As uterine massage is performed, 20 U of oxytocin diluted in 1 L of normal saline or Ringer's lactate should be infused at a rate of 500–1000 mL/h. IV bolus

Table 22.3 Steps to control uterine atony.

Abdominal uterine massage
Oxytocin 20-40 units IM or 20-40 units/L IV
Prostaglandins 15-methyl analog $PGF_{2\alpha}$, 0.25 mg IM, IV, MYOM
Uterine tamponade
Uterine cavity exploration/curettage
Uterine packing
Angiographic embolization
Hypogastric/uterine artery ligation
Hysterectomy

Abbreviations: IM, intramuscularly; IV, intravenously; MYOM, intramyometrially; PGF2a, prostaglandin F2 alpha.

administration of oxytocin should be avoided because it can lead to sudden and profound hypotension, hypertension cardiac compromise,[42] and even death.[43]

Bleeding that has failed to respond to uterine massage and uterotonic therapy calls for exploration of the birth canal. With the patient under adequate anesthesia, the lower genital tract should be carefully examined to rule out lacerations of the vulva, vagina, and cervix. The uterine cavity should be explored next with a hand and any retained cotyledon be removed.

If bleeding continues and the uterus is still atonic, the administration of prostaglandins (PG) has been shown to be successful in 60–80% of patients unresponsive to standard oxytocic therapy. The use of PG of the F2a and E series is integral to the treatment of PPH.[44] A 0.25-mg dose of the 15-methylated analog prostaglandin F2 alpha (PGF2a) is more potent and has a longer duration of action than its parent compound.[45] This can be injected intramuscularly, intravenously, or intramyometrially with equal effectiveness. Peak blood levels occur 15–60 minutes after intramuscular injection. Depending on the clinical situation, repeated injections can be made at 15- to 90-minute intervals. Most patients respond to one or two doses. The total dose should not exceed 1–1.5 mg. Side effects of PG therapy include gastrointestinal symptoms, such as diarrhea and vomiting, which occur in 10–25%, and fever, which occurs in 5% of the cases. Although blood-pressure elevation occurs rarely, the drug is contraindicated in women with cardiovascular and pulmonary disease because of its potential hypertensive and bronchoconstrictive effects.[46] Cardiovascular collapse with pulmonary edema after an overdose of intramyometrially injected PGF2a has also been reported.[47]

Balloon therapy has essentially replaced intrauterine packing as a tamponade technique in PPH management. Uterine packing with gauze is seldom used in modern obstetric practice and its effectiveness remains a controversial issue. The use of balloon tamponade deserves an attempt before resorting to surgical or angiographic modalities. Before the procedure is carried out, it is essential to ensure that there is no retained placental tissue, uterine rupture or inversion, genital tract trauma, or untreated coagulopathy. The tamponade balloon is inflated to fill the uterine cavity and pressure is applied against the uterine walls from inside. Meanwhile, its catheter tip drains any blood accumulating in the dead space above it. The Bakri tamponade balloon is specifically designed for tamponade within the uterine cavity in cases of PPH secondary to atony.[48] Approximately 300–500 mL of saline is instilled into the balloon to obliterate the cavity and produce the tamponade effect. Other balloons that have been used to tamponade the uterus include the gastric Sengstaken–Blakemore tube and the urological Rusch balloon. In low-resource countries Foley catheter or condoms have been used to create a tamponade effect to stop the bleeding.[49] If successful, it may temporarily control the bleeding and offer time for preparations for surgery and blood replacement. Effective hemostasis should be observed soon after balloon insertion and inflation. Rarely should the balloon be left in for more than 24 hours. If bleeding continues or recurs the patient should be taken for embolization or surgical management. The use of prophylactic antibiotics while the packing or balloon is in place may be beneficial in controlling infectious morbidity.

In cases of severe postpartum bleeding, the following course of action has been recommended[50]:

1. Detailed documentation.
2. Asking for help.
3. Activation of a massive transfusion protocol.
4. Placement of large bore IV access.
5. Placement of a Foley catheter.
6. Fluid replacement with crystalloids and colloids until blood becomes available.
7. Attention to signs of developing hemorrhagic coagulopathy.
8. Consult hematologist.
9. Initiate central venous pressure monitoring.
10. Give O Rh-negative blood if fully compatible blood is not available.
11. Warm the blood if it needs to be infused rapidly.
12. Implement treatment in the environment of the intensive care unit.

RETAINED PLACENTA

The incidence of retained secundines is 4–8% of all deliveries.[38,51] The spectrum varies from complete retention of a separated or still attached placenta to retention of placental fragments, cotyledons, or membranes. A retained placenta that is partially or completely separated is characteristically associated with early PPH, whereas retained placental fragments relatively commonly lead to late postpartum bleeding. Retained fragments of membranes are rather common and do not cause PPH.

Failure of the placenta to be delivered may be due to entrapment by a contracted lower uterine segment; failure of separation; or placenta accreta, increta, or percreta. In addition, the injudicious conduct of the third stage of labor may result in cord avulsion, or retention of a succenturiate lobe or fragmented placental pieces. Entrapment of a separated placenta is common. Independent risk factors for retained placenta include previous retained placenta, preterm delivery, preeclampsia and greater than two miscarriages. A study by Endler et al.[52] suggests that prolonged oxytocin use is also an independent risk factor with an odds of 2.00 when oxytocin use is between 195 and 415 minutes and an odds of 6.55 when oxytocin used for labor exceeded 415 minutes. Furthermore, the chance of blood loss requiring transfusion was significantly increased.

MANUAL REMOVAL

Manual removal is indicated if the placenta is still retained 30 minutes after the delivery of the fetus or if significant bleeding mandates earlier intervention. The procedure should be carried out under appropriate anesthesia to minimize patient discomfort. A uterine relaxant such as nitroglycerin given intravenously or sublingually may be administered to provide rapid and effective relaxation of the uterus in order to facilitate manual removal. The dose of nitroglycerin is 50 μg and can be repeated as tolerated by the patient in order to achieve results.[53–55] While the uterine fundus is held firm by one hand placed abdominally (Figure 22.1), the other hand is introduced into the uterine cavity along the cord until the placenta is reached and its margin is identified. A cleavage plane between the placenta and the uterine wall is then developed by deliberate digital separation.

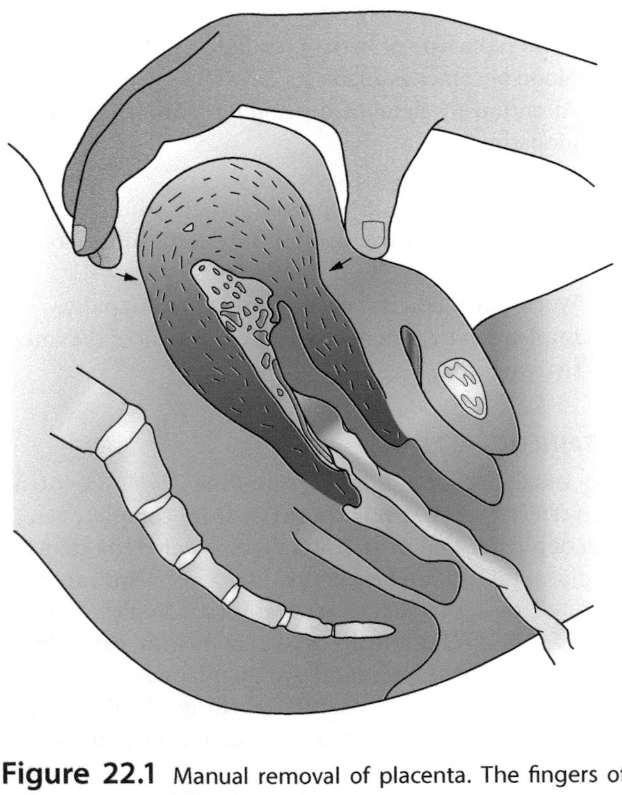

Figure 22.1 Manual removal of placenta. The fingers of the vaginal hand will dissect the cleavage plane between the uterine wall and placental margin until the placenta is completely detached.

If a cleavage plane cannot be developed, undue force should not be used. Pulling on the body of the placenta prior to digital separation is not advisable. Forceful attempts at removal can result in retention of placental fragments, uterine inversion, colporrhexis, or uterine rupture. Once the placenta has been removed, it should be carefully examined for the site of cord insertion, margins, abruptly terminating vessels, missing cotyledons, or retention of succenturiate lobes. When incomplete removal is apparent, the uterine cavity should be explored and any remaining placental tissue removed by gentle digital manipulation. Throughout these procedures, the external hand holds the fundus in a firm grasp and serves as a guide for the internal hand. Rarely, gentle and careful curettage using a large banjo-type curette may need to be employed to remove any remaining placental fragments. There is currently insufficient evidence to argue for or against the use of prophylactic antibiotics in these situations.[56]

Failure of these measures to effect complete delivery of the placenta or to control bleeding calls for immediate additional measures. These include uterine packing, vessel ligation, and hysterectomy. Oxytocic drugs are administered to ensure that the uterus remains contracted. If the placenta cannot be separated, placenta accreta should be suspected and further attempts to remove the placenta should be abandoned. Instead, immediate preparation for laparotomy must be initiated.

PLACENTA ACCRETA, INCRETA, AND PERCRETA

Placental invasive abnormalities have become a more common cause for PPH. Mhyre et al.[57] reported that the most common risk factors associated with the need for massive transfusion during hospitalization for delivery are abnormal placentation (1.6/10,000 deliveries, adjusted odds ratio [OR] 18.5, 95% confidence interval [CI] 14.7–23.3), placental abruption (1.0/10,000, adjusted OR 14.6, 95% CI 11.2–19.0), severe preeclampsia (0.8/10,000, adjusted OR 10.4, 95% CI 7.7–14.2), and intrauterine fetal demise (0.7/10,000, adjusted OR 5.5, 95% CI 3.9–7.8). This abnormal invasion of the myometrium may involve the whole (total) or part (partial/focal) of the placenta (accreta). The depth of penetration may be deep myometrial (increta) or may extend through the entire musculature to the serosa (percreta) (Figure 22.2). Various degrees of placenta accreta occur in connection with 1/500 to 1/70,000 deliveries.[58] Predisposing factors include cesarean delivery, multiparity, advanced maternal age, implantation on a submucous myoma, and endometrial scarring from previous curettage, myomectomy, or Asherman's syndrome.

Of particular note is the association with placenta previa when the latter occurs overlying a previous uterine incision. The relationship between placenta previa and

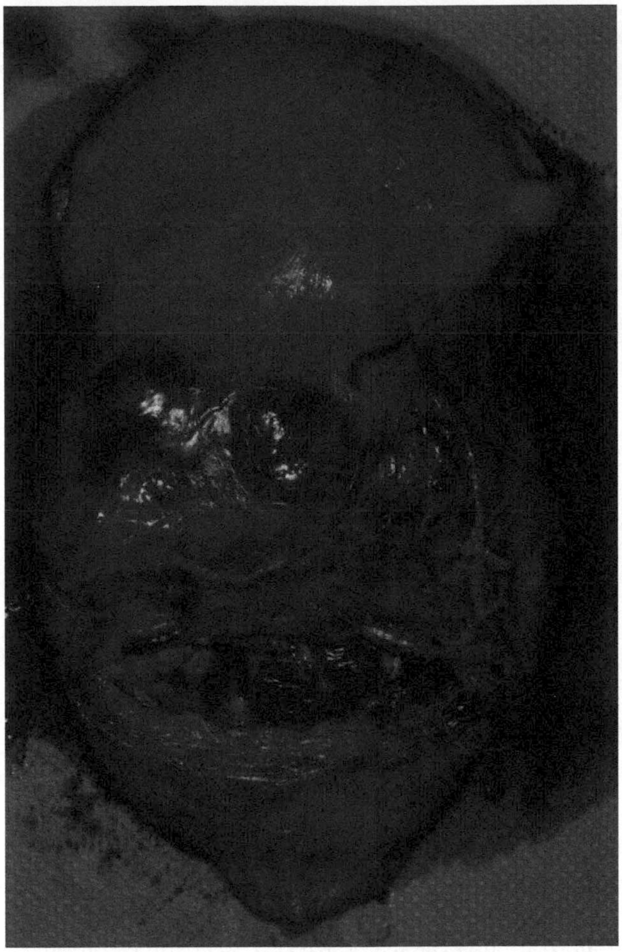

Figure 22.2 Gross hysterectomy specimen of placenta left in situ with serosa survey of vasculature of placenta percreta.

placental invasive abnormalities and the number of previous cesareans was demonstrated by Clark et al.[59] The risk for placenta previa was 0.26% with an unscarred uterus compared to 10% in women with four or more previous cesareans. In a series of 109 placenta percreta cases, a maternal mortality rate of 7% was observed.[60] Maternal morbidity and mortality are greatly improved if abnormal placentation is detected by antenatal ultrasound prior to delivery. Color Doppler ultrasound is helpful in detecting abnormal extension of placental vessels into adjoining structures such as the bladder (Figure 22.3).[61] Magnetic resonance imaging (MRI) can be useful in confirmed suspected cases of placenta percreta.[62]

Placenta previa in patients with two or more previous cesarean sections raises the risk for placenta accreta to 40–60%. Ultrasound remains the primary screening modality and can help detect placenta accreta in 50–80% of cases.[63,64] The presence of lacunae and an abnormal color Doppler imaging pattern are the most helpful findings in making the diagnosis of placental invasion (Figure 22.4). Subplacental clear space and myometrial thickness are less helpful and should be used in conjunction with other findings as evidence for placenta accreta. MRI is most clearly

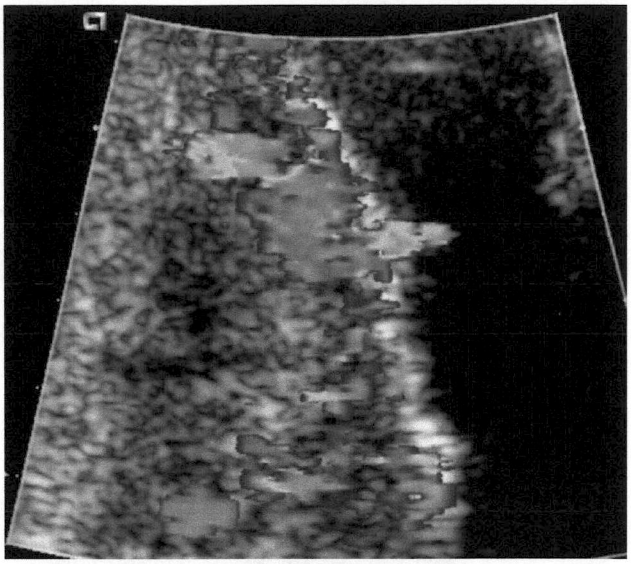

Figure 22.3 Doppler ultrasound of placental percreta with vasculature into the maternal bladder.

indicated when ultrasound findings are ambiguous or there is a posterior placenta. The most reliable MR findings are uterine bulging, heterogeneous placenta, and placental bands. Focal interruptions in the hypointense myometrial border can also be seen at sites of placental invasion during MRI.[65]

Elective planned cesarean delivery with primary or delayed hysterectomy has played a major role in lowering morbidity and mortality for placental invasion disorders.[66] Perioperative management with maternal preparation that includes a multidisciplinary operative team of obstetrician, maternal fetal medicine subspecialist, and surgical specialists (gynecologic oncologist, vascular surgeon, and urologist) and planned elective delivery around 35 weeks in a setting capable of managing potential hemorrhage is critical to decreasing maternal morbidity and mortality from placental percreta.[39] Performing the procedure in a hybrid operative suite where the capability of placing intravascular catheters for balloon occlusion and selective arterial embolization can be lifesaving if serious bleeding is encountered at the time of surgery.

MISCELLANEOUS ETIOLOGIES

Uterine rupture or dehiscence of a uterine scar is a major cause of obstetric hemorrhage. The risk of rupture is eight times higher after a preceding abdominal delivery than when the uterus is intact. Transverse incision placed at a relatively high level of the lower uterine segment is more prone to antepartum rupture than one at a low level. Other risk factors are multiparity, twin pregnancy, and instrumental deliveries.[14,67,68]

Retroperitoneal hematoma is an infrequent but dangerous form of postpartum bleeding. It is concealed and thus difficult to diagnose. The blood loss can be severe enough to cause hemorrhagic shock. The source of the bleeding may be

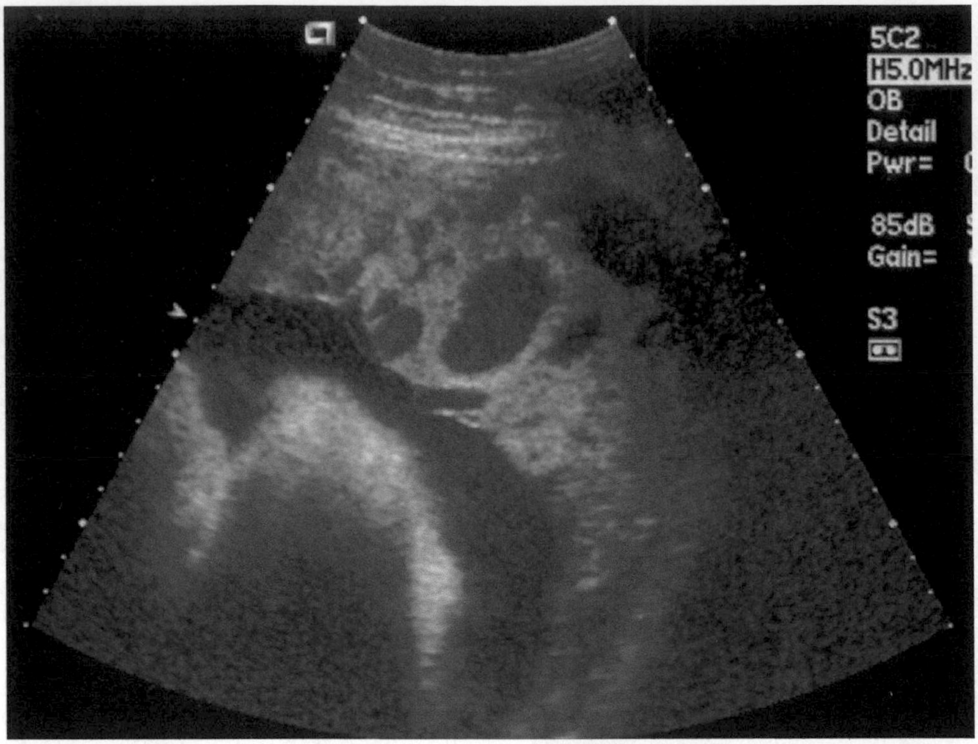

Figure 22.4 Ultrasound of placenta accreta showing multiple vascular lacunae (arrows) within the placenta.

difficult to find; thus, the involvement of a vascular or oncologic surgeon is desirable. When the bleeding vessel escapes detection, hypogastric artery ligation may be helpful.

ANGIOGRAPHIC EMBOLIZATION

Uterine artery embolization was introduced as a treatment for PPH in 1979.[69] Selective angiography to locate the bleeding site and angiographic embolization have been shown to be efficacious in controlling bleeding when other measures have failed.[70] The procedure has been shown to be associated with high technical success rates and good clinical outcomes for the treatment of primary and secondary PPH.[71,72]

The decision to perform uterine artery embolization should be made on the basis of persistent bleeding despite maximization of medical and obstetrical measures to control the bleeding or in cases of PPH not amenable to surgical therapy, such as a deep vaginal hematoma.[73] It should also be resorted to in cases where bleeding has not been adequately controlled by surgical means, such as hysterectomy or selective artery ligations.

Only skilled and experienced personnel in facilities where proper equipment is available should carry out this procedure. The technique involves the passage under fluoroscopic guidance of an intravascular catheter through the femoral artery, and advancing the catheter cephalad while performing an arteriogram of the bleeding site. Knowledge of the pelvic collateral vessels is important during angiography in order to identify all possible bleeding sites. The catheter should be advanced to a level just below the renal arteries in order to identify all collateral vessels. After embolization, aortography should be done to confirm cessation of bleeding. If bleeding continues after embolization of the major artery, repeat embolization can be performed and collateral branches can be individually identified and occluded.

Various embolic and vasoconstrictive agents for the above have been used. These currently include Gelfoam or gelatin sponge, a dissolvable sponge like material and polyvinyl alcohol particles which is ground from blocs of foam into two sizes (355–500 μm and 500–710 μm). Each micron is one thousandth of a meter, or the size of a grain of sand. Embosphere microspheres are clear acrylic microspheres approved by the Food and Drug Administration (FDA) in 2000 for uterine embolization. A variety of vasoconstrictors such as vasopressin, dopamine, and norepinephrine have a historic mention. The use of vasoconstrictors (e.g., vasopressin) has the advantage of reducing the risk of ischemic complications. With regional vasoconstriction, bleeding from collateral reconstitution is also reduced. However, because the dose of these drugs needs to be tapered over 24 hours, it requires leaving the catheter in situ for an extended period of time. This requires intensive physician and nursing care to monitor the infusion.

A major potential complication of pelvic embolization is ischemia, resulting in nerve injury or infarction of the areas affected by the vascular supply. Embolization of both the anterior and posterior branches of the internal iliac artery can obstruct the vascular supply of the sciatic and femoral nerves, resulting in paresis of the lower limbs.[74] This complication is more likely to occur with the smaller particles of Gelfoam powder and if central surgical ligation had preceded embolization of the collateral vessels. Short-lived emboli such as blood clot can also be used; however, Gelfoam may be easier to prepare and its particle size easier to control. Arterial recanalization with subsequent pregnancy has been reported.[75]

AORTIC COMPRESSION

Aortic compression is often overlooked, yet it is a simple adjuvant method in the management of PPH while other surgical or medical therapies are being prepared. The maneuver consists of compressing the aorta by pushing on the abdominal wall with a closed fist at the level of the lumbosacral junction, which is just above the bifurcation and below the level of the renal arteries. The postpartum patient is an ideal candidate for this maneuver, since the abdominal wall is lax and the rectus muscle diastasis. If the abdomen is opened, direct aortic compression can be an effective initial step in controlling the bleeding until uterine or hypogastric artery ligation is done or the bleeding site identified. If compression is needed for an extended period of time, an aortic compression device such as the Harris instrument can be utilized.[76]

ANTISHOCK TROUSERS

The antishock trousers or military anti-shock trouser (MAST) suit evolved primarily from military applications.[77,78] Although the MAST suit has a variety of medical applications, its primary use is in patients with severe intra-abdominal bleeding either preoperatively or postoperatively when surgical intervention has failed to control bleeding.[79] In the latter circumstances, the use of the MAST suit has successfully allowed stabilization of vital signs and control of bleeding and has obviated the need for surgery.[78] The reported uses in obstetrics has been to manage uncontrollable PPH due to ischiorectal hematoma and disseminated intravascular coagulation.

The device is made of one piece of double-layered polyvinyl fabric and resembles a pair of wraparound trousers. It encloses the body from the lower margin of the ribs to the ankles. There are three separate chambers for inflation — one abdominal and two leg compartments. When inflated, it is capable of sustaining an internal air pressure up to 104 mmHg indefinitely. With foot pumps, the legs are inflated first, followed by the abdominal compartments. The pressure is measured by a manometer or gauge placed in the circuit. Beginning as low as 10 mmHg, it is increased by 5- to 10-mmHg increments until the vital signs are stabilized and adequate perfusion is established. Pressures of 40–60 mmHg halt most venous bleeding. Pressures up to 100 mmHg have been applied in patients with arterial bleeding, but such high pressures should not be maintained for long periods of time. The suit should remain inflated at moderate pressures for a period of 12–24 hours after the bleeding has stopped. Deflation should be done gradually with decrements of 5 mmHg. The abdominal compartment is to be deflated before the legs.[78] When successful, the blood pressure is increased rapidly and blood loss is decreased. Increased peripheral resistance secondary to the direct pressure effect on the vessels improves blood pressure, shunting of blood flow from the lower body to the more vital upper body, improving venous return to the central circulation, and increasing cardiac output. Bleeding is reduced because the pressure applied to the exterior of the vessels results in a significant reduction of both the venous and arterial diameters. The MAST suit is also useful in decreasing the IV crystalloid requirements and it allows valuable time for safe and complete cross-matching of blood for transfusion.

Potential adverse effects include hypoventilation, hypercarbia, and hypoxia, especially if the increased intra-abdominal pressure is so high as to compromise diaphragmatic excursion. If the inflation pressure is greater than the systolic pressure, reduction of blood flow to the lower extremities can result in lactic acid production and hyperkalemia. Decreased urinary output, skin breakdown, and deepening of cardiogenic shock are additional dangers. Most potential adverse effects are preventable if the trousers are positioned correctly and if only moderate pressures are used for not more than 48 hours. Initial concern about air embolism, prompted by a case of postpartum bleeding without placental separation, has not been confirmed subsequently.[80]

SURGICAL TREATMENT

In the face of uncontrollable bleeding, such as from a ruptured uterus, one must proceed directly to surgical exploration. If the patient is desirous of future childbearing and is hemodynamically stable, elective or therapeutic pelvic vessel ligation or suturing of the identified bleeding site may be attempted first.

The choice of uterine artery ligation versus hypogastric artery and/or ovarian artery ligation depends upon the site and cause of bleeding and the surgeon's expertise with each procedure. The higher success rate with uterine artery ligation would make this the initial procedure of choice.[81] However, if proper criteria are not met, pelvic vessel ligation should not be attempted and hysterectomy should be promptly performed.

UTERINE ARTERY LIGATION

In most cases of intractable PPH especially with cesarean delivery, uterine vessel ligations should be among the first surgical steps taken as it can be performed quickly. The uterine artery originates as a branch from the anterior hypogastric artery. After coursing along the lateral wall of the pelvis, it arches over the ureter about 2 cm lateral from the uterus as the ureter runs beneath the cardinal ligament in its fascial tunnel. At this point, it gives off a descending branch to the cervix, which anastomoses with vaginal branches and the more important ascending branch. The ascending branch runs along the medial aspect of the broad ligament upward to anastomose with the ovarian vessels at the upper inner angle of the broad ligament. During pregnancy, the uterine artery elongates, hypertrophies, and carries 90% of uterine blood flow. The uterine veins and the hypertrophied ovarian veins provide the majority of return flow.

Uterine artery ligation is a simple technique, whereby bilateral ligation of the ascending branch of the uterine artery is performed. Waters first suggested this technique as a method to manage PPH when more conservative methods failed in 1952.[82] O'Leary found the procedure effective 95% of the time, with a 1% complication rate.[81]

The technique entails mass ligation or individual ligation of the uterine artery. The early descriptions stressed the importance of dissecting the uterine artery and vein, and ligating only the artery.[82] Recently, mass ligation of both the artery and vein has been advocated as a simple, effective, and more rapidly performed procedure.[81] The fingers of one hand compress the leaves of the broad ligament and run down to the level of the internal os or, in cases of cesarean section, just below the standard transverse uterine incision. Without dissecting the broad ligament, the pulsations of the ascending branch of the left uterine artery are palpated. Then, a no. 0 polyglycolic suture or other delayed absorbable suture on a large needle is passed at this level into and through the myometrium from anterior to posterior, 2–3 cm medial to the uterine vessel. Once the needle is extracted from the posterior myometrium, it is redirected from posterior to anterior through an avascular area in the broad ligament lateral to where the uterine vessel is palpated and the suture is then securely tied (Figure 22.5). This procedure is facilitated by placement of a malleable retractor posteriorly to protect the retroperitoneum and bowel. A figure-of-8 suture may be placed, particularly if there is a large uterine artery laceration or the hysterotomy is inadvertently extended into the broad ligament. Alternatively, this stitch may be run in a locking fashion superiorly to close this type of defect. It is important to include a significant amount of myometrium in the suture and to obliterate intramyometrial ascending arterial branches because the degree of uterine ischemia is directly related to the amount of myometrium in the suture. Even if the uterus remains atonic, bleeding usually comes under control. Higher failure rates have been reported in cases of placenta previa/accreta, especially if the implantation of the placenta was over the scar of a previous lower segment cesarean section; in cases where the source of bleeding is from vessels supplied by the vaginal artery; and in those due to a clotting defect.

Complications of uterine artery ligation are rare. Vein damage from multiple passages with the needle can result in broad-ligament hematoma. Arteriovenous sinus formation has also been reported, but this complication can be prevented by using absorbable suture material, avoiding figure-of-8 sutures, and including a substantial amount of myometrium in the ligature.[83] No long-term adverse effects of bilateral uterine artery ligation have been reported. Recanalization uniformly occurs with resumption of normal menstrual flow and subsequent pregnancies.[84]

HYPOGASTRIC ARTERY LIGATION

Hypogastric artery ligation will control blood loss by reducing arterial pulse pressure and decreasing distal blood flow by converting the pelvic arterial circulation into a venous system. The procedure is technically challenging

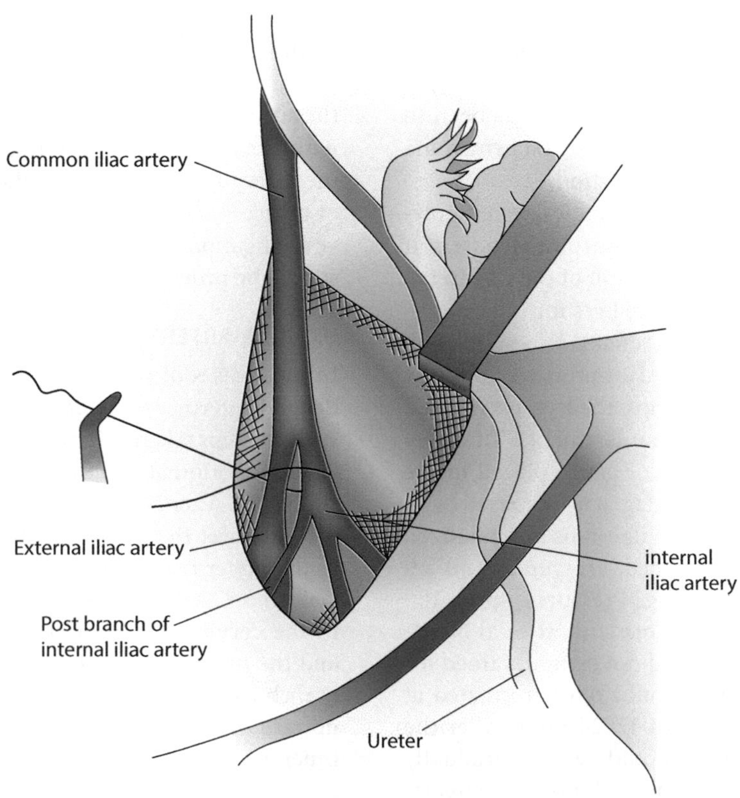

Figure 22.5 Technique of uterine artery ligation. Sutures are placed to encompass the ascending uterine arteries, as well as anastomotic branches from the ovarian arteries. (Courtesy CA Apuzzio)

and requires the skills of an experienced pelvic surgeon. Hypogastric artery ligation may confer a greater risk than hysterectomy in controlling severe hemorrhage and is only successful in controlling severe hemorrhage in 42% of cases.[85]

Knowledge of the anatomic location and relationship to neighboring structures facilitates their identification, dissection, and ligation. The aorta bifurcates at the level of the fourth lumbar vertebra into the common iliac arteries. These in turn bifurcate at the level of the sacral promontory into the external iliac artery, which courses laterally to the leg, where it becomes the femoral artery, and into the hypogastric artery, which descends medio-inferiorly along the border of the psoas muscle into the pelvis. The ureter is retroperitoneal and crosses the hypogastric artery from a lateral to medial direction at its origin. The external iliac vein and the obturator nerve are located posterolaterally and the internal ileac posteromedially. Lateral to the hypogastric artery are the major and minor psoas muscles. The hypogastric artery divides into anterior and posterior branches. The anterior branches supply blood to the pelvic viscera. The posterior division supplies blood to the fascia, buttocks, and medial surfaces of the thigh. An extensive network of anastomoses occurs in each hemipelvis vertically, ipsilaterally, and horizontally across the midline. This abundant collateral blood supply ensures that reproductive function is preserved and term pregnancies can follow even the ligations of both hypogastric and ovarian arteries.[86]

Since the hypogastric artery is a retroperitoneal structure, the first step is to enter this space. This can be done by an extraperitoneal or transperitoneal approach, depending on the source of the bleeding, the skill of the surgeon, and the condition of the patient. If there is any question on whether intra-abdominal bleeding is present, the transperitoneal route should be utilized. Initially, the uterus is pulled forward over the symphysis pubis. The intestines are packed away from the operative field into the upper abdomen. The round and infundibulopelvic ligaments are visualized. The peritoneum between the two ligaments is tented with tissue forceps and incised parallel to the infundibulopelvic ligament. Only after identification of the ureter, infundibulopelvic ligament, common iliac artery, hypogastric artery, and external iliac artery is the ligation performed. Once the hypogastric is identified, a right-angle clamp is passed below the hypogastric artery. Next, a suture is placed in the tip of the clamp and passed under the hypogastric artery, usually from the medial to the lateral side, to avoid the junction of right and left common iliac veins forming the inferior vena cava. The suture must be placed at the bifurcation of the common iliac artery to prevent thrombus formation proximal to the tie. An absorbable suture is preferred, and the artery is not transected (Figure 22.6a). This procedure may then be repeated for the contralateral vessel. The use of absorbable sutures will allow for subsequent canalization of vessels, although ultimate uterine blood flow is not compromised if permanent suture material is used.[87]

The incidence of serious complications associated with hypogastric artery ligation is low if proper identification and careful dissection of landmark structures are carried out. Unfortunately, the skill level of surgeons performing this procedure have significantly diminished over the last couple of decades due to it rarely being performed for the modern management of massive obstetric hemorrhage. Complications include misidentification and accidental ligation of the external iliac artery, laceration of the internal and external iliac veins, ureter injury, retroperitoneal hematoma, and ischemic sequelae.[88]

Accidental ligation of the external iliac artery, if unrecognized, can lead to loss of vascular supply to the ipsilateral leg. Laceration of the thin walled iliac vein occurs when too vigorous dissection of areolar tissue surrounding the artery is carried out or when the right angle clamp is improperly passed beneath the hypogastric artery. Such laceration results in severe hemorrhage and is difficult to repair. Elevation of the artery with a Babcock clamp and passing the tip from lateral to medial may avoid injury to the iliac vein.

Properly identifying the ureter and retracting it manually out of the field before dissecting the areolar tissue surrounding the hypogastric artery decreases the risk of ureteral injury. Retroperitoneal hematoma is prevented by meticulous hemostasis in the retroperitoneal space. Ischemic sequelas are rare because of the extensive collateral circulation, but can result in central pelvic ischemia, breakdown of the perineal skin and episiotomy site, and paresis of the lower extremities from lower motor neuron damage.

OVARIAN ARTERY LIGATION

Bilateral ovarian artery ligation can be a valuable adjunct to hypogastric or uterine artery ligation.[89] The ovarian artery is a retroperitoneal branch of the aorta that travels in the infundibulopelvic ligament. It enters the mesovarium at the fimbriated end of the fallopian tube, where it courses above the ovary, giving off numerous branches to the fallopian tube. During pregnancy, it contributes 5–10% of the blood supply to the uterus. Due to the enlargement of all vessels, the ovarian vessels are easy to palpate and visualize in the mesovarium.

The area for ligation should be at the junction of the utero-ovarian ligament and the ovary, which is where the ovarian artery anastomoses with the uterine artery (Figure 22.7). Ligation at this site will allow maintenance of adequate blood flow to the ovary and the fallopian tube. At this point in the mesovarium, an avascular area above the artery should be identified and a no. 0 polyglycolic suture or other delayed absorbable suture passed directly or through a window formed by a Kelly clamp. The ligature is then similarly passed through an avascular area below the artery and tied. Two simple ligatures can be used and there is no need to divide the vessel.

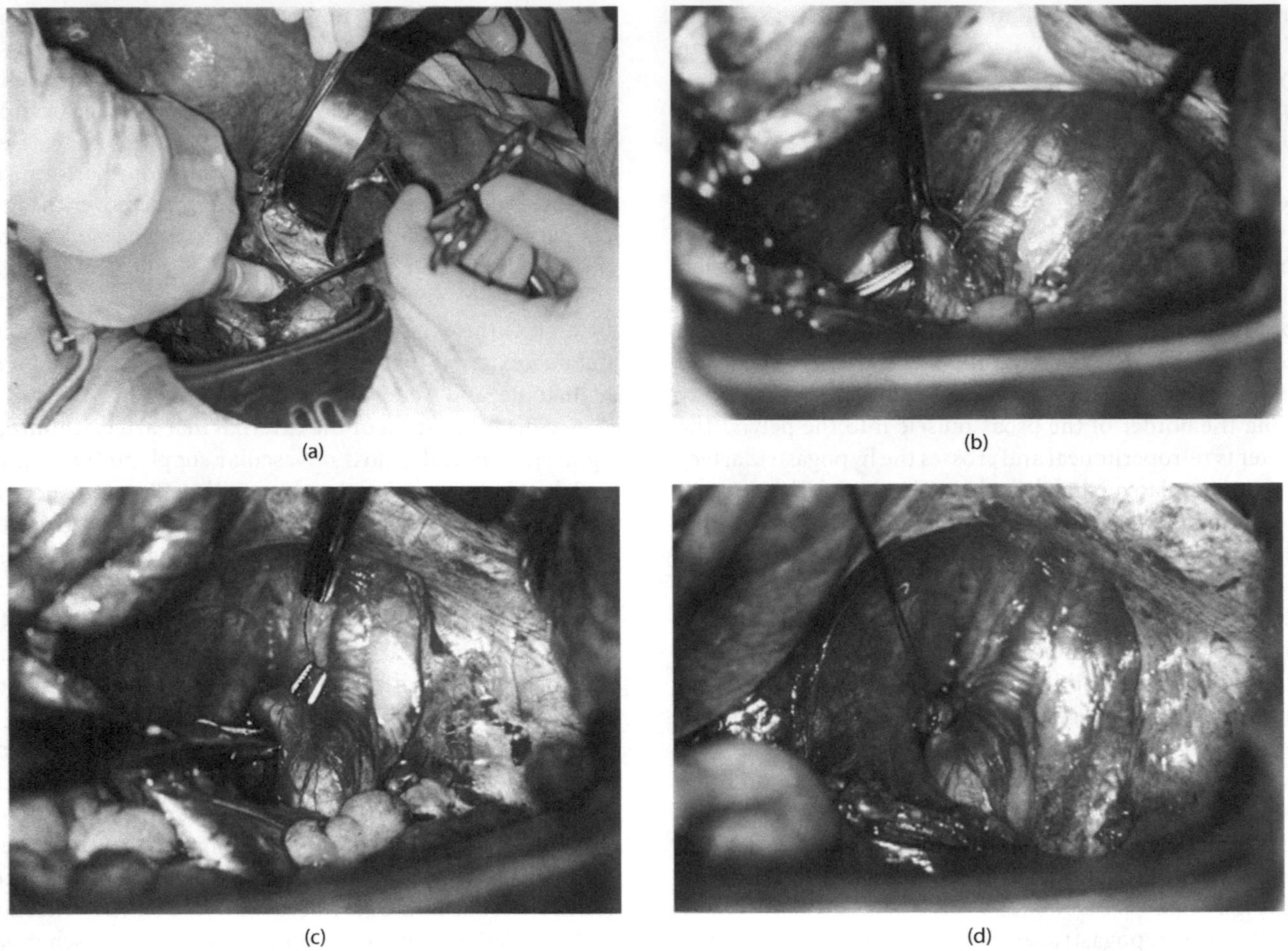

Figure 22.6 (a) Palpating for the pulsating external iliac artery through the opening of the peritoneum. (b) The Babcock clamp is picking up the right internal iliac artery at its origin from the common iliac artery. A right-angle clamp is to be passed under the vessel in a mediolateral direction. (c) The right-angle clamp having been passed under the internal iliac artery, a no. 0 silk thread is being fed into it. (d) The internal iliac artery has been ligated close to its origin from the common iliac artery.

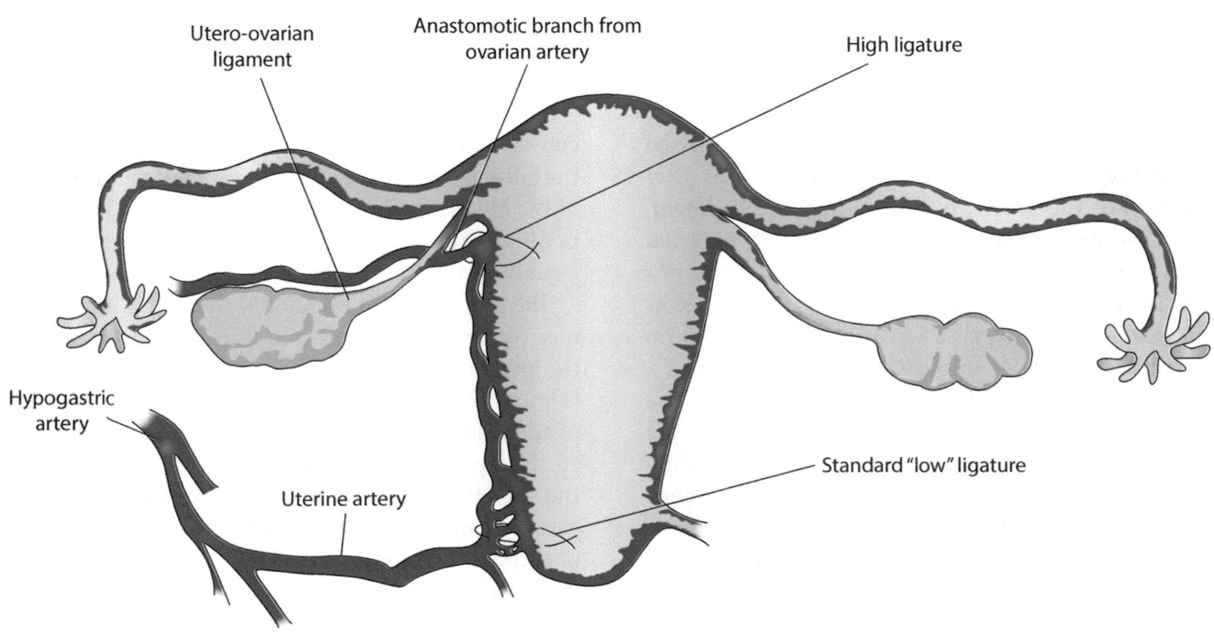

Figure 22.7 Ovarian arterial anatomy. Figure-of-8 represents area for ligation. (Courtesy CA Apuzzio.)

B-LYNCH SUTURE

If, after uterine exploration, the atony fails to resolve in response to medication and uterine massage, the B-Lynch suture may be effective.[90] In 1997, B-Lynch et al. reported the B-Lynch suturing technique as a new conservative treatment for PPH. This uterine compression procedure has been adopted throughout the world as an early intervention for the treatment of PPH due to uterine atony, with more than 1000 procedures reported in 2005.[91] The technique requires laparotomy and separation of the bladder peritoneum from the cervix. Despite a reported adverse experience, involving ischemic necrosis associated with it,[92] this procedure has gained considerable popularity in recent years. This technique should be used early in the course of hemorrhage management during cesarean delivery if the predominant cause is thought to be uterine atony. Typically, the procedure is performed after closure of the hysterotomy when refractory uterine atony is noted.

Utilizing a 70- to 80-mm, round-bodied needle with no. 2 polyglycolic suture or other delayed absorbable suture, Lynch recommends the placement of the suture 3 cm below the right end of the incision. Having penetrated the uterine cavity, the needle emerges 3 cm above the upper incision margin. At this point, the suture is carried over the body of the uterus at a distance of about 4 cm from its lateral border (Figure 22.8a). While an assistant compresses the uterus, the suture is carried to the posterior aspect of the organ and secured approximately at the level of the anterior incision by driving the needle through the posterior aspect of the lower uterine segment (Figure 22.8b). Then, once again, the suture is carried through the fundus of the uterus and passed through the uterine cavity at the left angle of the uterine incision in the same manner as previously described. The suture should then be securely tied in order to maintain uterine compression. When the operation is performed after vaginal delivery, Lynch recommends the opening of the lower segment of the uterus in the same manner as in case of a cesarean section in order to ensure that the anteriorly placed suture enters the uterine cavity.[90] This procedure has not been associated with an increase risk in future pregnancies.[93]

Other compression techniques such as the hemostatic multiple square suturing which uses a straight number 7 or number 8 needle and number 1 chromic catgut to approximate the anterior and posterior uterine walls in areas of heavy bleeding have also been described.[94]

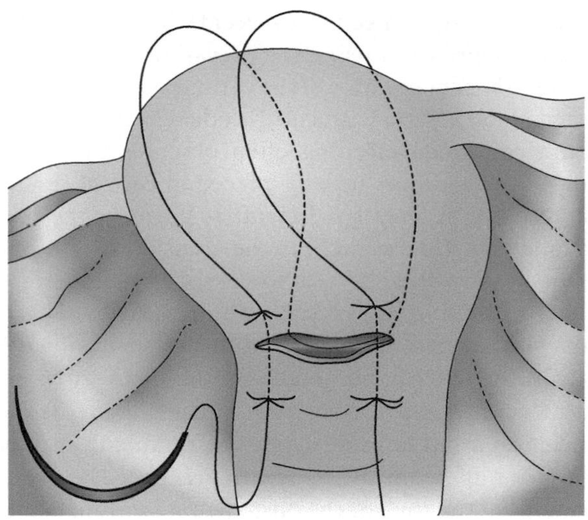

(a)

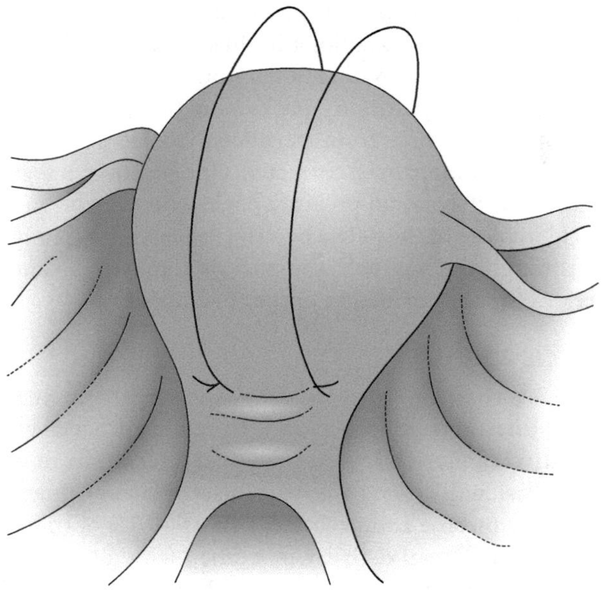

(b)

Figure 22.8 (a) Position and path of suture placement. (b) Position of suture prior to tightening.

PERIPARTUM HYSTERECTOMY

Emergency hysterectomy is the most common treatment when massive PPH fails to respond to sequential uterine devascularization and compression procedures. The incidence of emergency peripartum hysterectomy varies from 7 to 13 per 10,000 births.[95,96]

Removal of the uterus postpartum or in the course of a cesarean section requires essentially the same technical steps as a routine abdominal hysterectomy for gynecologic indications. However, since the former is usually performed under emergency conditions and on a patient who has already endured major blood loss, the surgeon is compelled to work under pressure and against narrow time limitations. The advantage of emergency hysterectomy in cases of massive hemorrhage, especially for the multiparous patient, is the ability to remove the source of bleeding. It must be remembered that the uterine arteries, which follow a spiral course in the nonpregnant state, are stretched out in advanced pregnancy. If severed, they tend to spring back to their original shape and, as a result, move away from the operative field. This fact makes ligation and cutting of the arteries a precarious and somewhat risky undertaking under certain emergency situations. The technical details described in connection with uterine artery ligation should generally be followed when the uterus is to be removed.

Under many, if not most, circumstances, a total hysterectomy may not be necessary for achieving hemostasis.

Good judgment is needed to decide between available operative approaches using the prevailing circumstances and the risk–benefit ratios of the various options as guides. Dilated blood vessels frequently hinder effective hemostasis and continued bleeding often obscures the surgical field. As the cervix is usually effaced in case of cesarean hysterectomy, it may be difficult to identify the cervicovaginal junction as well as the transition from lower uterine segment and corpus to cervix. Therefore, in the absence of significant cervical pathology, subtotal hysterectomy is the safest alternative for this lifesaving intervention. On the other hand, total removal may be attempted if clear delineation of structures is made, but care must be taken to avoid foreshortening the vagina. Even after a presumed total removal, the seemingly effaced cervix may re-emerge at the time of the postpartum examination as a cervical stump.

Hysterectomy does not guarantee control of bleeding especially if a coagulopathy has developed. In such instances following hysterectomy, intra-abdominal packing with large laparotomy packs may be appropriate to tamponade bleeding from peritoneal surfaces until the coagulation status can be corrected. One approach involves the use of transvaginal pressure pack, where Kerlix gauze in held in place in the pelvis by a sterile plastic bag brought out through the vaginal. The pack is removed 24 hours later or after the correction of the coagulopathy.[97]

UTERINE RUPTURE

While exceedingly rare in connection with an intact uterus, uterine rupture occurs with relative frequency in the setting of uterine hysterotomy scar after cesarean section, occasionally even before the onset of labor. Clinically significant uterine rupture occurs in 0.6–0.7% of trials of labor after cesarean delivery in women with a low transverse or unknown uterine scar.[98–100] The risk is particularly high after a classical incision and after surgical uterine reconstructive procedures such as myomectomy. Risk is further increased for women with multiple cesarean deliveries and shorter intervals between pregnancies of less than 18–24 months.[101]

The most common and usually unrecognized type of rupture is dehiscence of a lower segment scar. When it is recognized during a repeated cesarean delivery, the opening of the separated wound edges needs to be extended to allow the delivery of the fetus. In these cases the dehiscence may not be bleeding due to poor vascularization of the scar edges. Prior to repair, edges of the devascularized scar should be removed anteriorly and posteriorly to the point where vascularized tissues can then be approximated and repaired in the usual fashion. Compared with spontaneous labor, the use of labor induction or augmentation increases the risk for rupture in women undergoing a trial of labor with a prior cesarean scar and women should be counseled prior to trial of labor. In particular, the use of Misprostol for cervical ripening or induction for women attempting a trial of labor after cesarean should be avoided.[102,103]

After a previous cesarean section, rupture of the uterus usually involves the area of the incision. It creates a potentially catastrophic surgical emergency when the rupture extends to the parametrium and disrupts major blood vessels. Another serious potential injury is extension of the rupture to the cervix, not infrequently with coincidental damage to the bladder. The critical issues in this situation are the following:

1. Awareness of the retroperitoneal pelvic anatomy
2. Identification of the ureter
3. Hemostasis after visual identification of the bleeding vessel
4. Dissection of the bladder from the uterine isthmus and determination of the extent of the bladder injury
5. Decision about the optimum surgical management with due attention to the patient's realistic reproductive potential

If the uterus is considered salvageable after full control of the hemorrhage, repair is to be performed as circumstances permit, using a delayed-absorbing suture material. Frequently, the uterus is not salvageable and urgent hysterectomy must be performed in order to achieve hemostasis.

In the event of bladder injury requiring repair, the surgical correction must be established in such a manner that the organ remains watertight. This can be achieved by suturing the freshened edges of the musculature in two or more layers. To ensure adequate healing, the bladder must be kept empty using an indwelling transurethral or suprapubic catheter for at least 7 days.

After conservative surgery, the patient is to be instructed about the high risk of recurrent uterine rupture in case of a future pregnancy. The risk of recurrent rupture appears to be highest when the uterine fundus is involved.[104]

COAGULATION DISORDERS

Genetic and systemic diseases that interfere with the coagulation process may cause or contribute to PPH. These include von Willebrand's disease, blood dyscrasias, leukemia, and disseminated intravascular coagulopathy. The diagnosis is usually known prior to delivery on the basis of past personal or family history, or abnormal coagulation studies done upon admission to the labor and delivery suite. Usually, difficulty with bleeding is not encountered unless the coagulation abnormality is quite severe. Definitive management consists of replacement of the specific deficient coagulation factors. von Willebrand's disease is best treated with administration of factor VIII concentrate. If cryoprecipitate is not available, fresh frozen plasma (FFP) or fresh whole blood can be used. Platelet deficiency can be corrected by the administration of platelet concentrate. Consumptive coagulopathy may result from severe obstetric hemorrhage itself or from other underlying causes, such as placental abruption, amniotic fluid embolism, fetal death, and severe infection. Treatment of the underlying disease coupled with the usual measures to combat hemorrhage and shock, including replacement of blood and coagulation factors, make up the corrective therapy.

MEDICAL MANAGEMENT

Recombinant factor VIIa

Ongoing blood loss with severe hemorrhage can benefit from additional medical interventions. Human recombinant factor VIIa is effective in controlling severe, life-threatening hemorrhage. Recombinant factor VIIa is a 50-kD analog of the naturally occurring serine protease factor VII. Factor VII has a fundamental role in the initiation of coagulation following vascular injury. Recombinant factor VIIa acts on the extrinsic clotting pathway. It can be lifesaving and potentially prevent hysterectomy and the need for massive transfusion employed early in the course of management of severe hemorrhage.[105] A number of case reports and series describing the use of recombinant FVIIa for intractable PPH have been published.[106–108] The drug is given at a dosage of 50–100 µg/kg every 2 hours until hemostasis is achieved. Cessation of bleeding ranges from 10 to 40 minutes after administration. There is a potential for a paradoxical effect for subsequent thromboembolic events following factor VIIa use.[109]

Tranxemic acid

Tranexamic acid (TXA) is an antifibrinolytic agent that prevents clot breakdown by blocking lysine sites on the plasminogen molecule. It inhibits fibrinolysis and has no effect on clotting parameters. It appears that TXA does decrease postpartum blood loss. Thus far most trials assessing the use of TXA for PPH have been performed in low- or middle-income countries. While the use of TXA has shown promise in the prevention and treatment of PPH the body of evidence is inconclusive to recommend widespread use.[110] The WOMAN trial is a randomized, double-blind, placebo control among women with clinical diagnosis of PPH that will determine the reliability of the effects of early administration of TXA on death, hysterectomy, and other morbidities in women with PPH.[111,112]

Fibrinogen

A decreased fibrinogen level is associated with an increased risk for severe PPH. In a study by Charbit et al.,[113] a fibrinogen level <200 mg/dL had a 100% predicative value for severe PPH. Fibrinogen (Factor 1) is a soluble plasma glycoprotein that is converted by thrombin into fibrin during blood clot formation. Early replacement with fibrinogen can improve clot strength and survival, but randomized trials have not demonstrated the benefit of preemptive treatment of severe PPH in normofibrinogenemia.[114] However, use of fibrinogen concentrate 2 g IV may provide benefit based on literature from severe perioperative hemorrhage and traumatic hemorrhage.[115] The use of fibrinogen concentrate allows high-dose substitution without the need for blood type crossmatch. The belief in the benefits of early administration of fibrinogen substitution in cases of PPH has led to increased off-label use of fibrinogen. The FIB-PPH (Fibrinogen Concentrate as initial treatment for PPH) randomized controlled trial of fibrinogen concentrate as initial treatment for PPH is currently underway.[116]

BLOOD LOSS AND BLOOD REPLACEMENT

The consequences of acute blood loss may be immediate or delayed. Hypovolemic shock is an immediate threat. However, bleeding also reduces the patient's natural resistance and aggravates the risk of infection. Since the overall blood volume increases during gestation by an average of 60%, women's tolerance of blood loss is better in the pregnant than in the nonpregnant state.

Hypovolemia causes reduced cardiac output. This leads to a sympathetic reaction with increased vascular resistance and tachycardia. Major degrees of hypovolemia, sufficient to cause shock, also involve fluid deficit in the vascular space. Damage to the capillary endothelial layer increases permeability and permits the migration of fluid to the intercellular space and the cells. When hypovolemia prevails, the circulation of blood is diverted from nonvital organs (intestines, kidneys, and musculature) to vital ones (brain and heart). Oliguria is an early sign of hypovolemia. The severity of the latter is reflected in the degree of reduction of urine output. For this reason, insertion of a Foley catheter for continuous quantitative assessment of the same may be desirable. It is important to keep the output as at least 30 mL/hour. Administration of oxygen may help in maintaining adequate tissue oxygenation and, thus, preventing organ failure.

Acute hypovolemia may be overcome by the administration of lactated Ringer's or normal saline solution. One to two liters may be delivered intravenously in the course of 30–60 minutes until the blood pressure improves. However, newer approaches to hemostatic resuscitation involve three major principles:

1. Limiting early aggressive crystalloid use and considering permissive hypotension.
2. Early transfusion of pRBC, FFP, and platelets in a 1:1:1 ratio.
3. Early use of recombinant factor VIIa.

Additionally, point of care coagulation measures such as thromboelastography or thromboelastometry, in addition to traditional coagulation measurements, should be obtained early in order to begin targeted coagulation factor replacement.[117] There is current controversy regarding appropriate transfusion patterns in obstetric hemorrhage, as current guidelines are based on data from trauma-induced hemorrhage without adequate evidence in the obstetric hemorrhage population. The main disadvantage of these strategies is that donor blood products are obtained from nonpregnant donors who have lower circulating levels of fibrinogen and other clotting factors. Therefore, unmonitored transfusion may in fact lead to clotting factor dilution and lower level in the bleeding parturient.[118] Furthermore, the use of colloids, particularly hydroxyethyl starches may lead to further coagulopathy.[119] Despite these concerns, a dedicated massive transfusion protocol for early and aggressive blood product administration is recommended.[120]

The purpose of transfusing packed RBCs is to improve the oxygen-carrying capacity of the blood and to overcome orthostatic hypotension. FFP is to be given in case of liver disease, coagulation defect, disseminated intravascular coagulation, thrombotic and thrombocytopenic purpura, antithrombin deficiency, and association with massive transfusions. It contains all clotting factors, including factors V and VIII. It needs to be Rh compatible with the patient's blood. It is customary to give 2–4 U at a time. Each unit increases the amount of clotting factors by 2–3%.[121] Concentrated cryoprecipitate is prepared from fresh frozen plasma. It contains factor VIII, von Willebrand factor, and fibrinogen in high concentrations.

In case of inadequate number or function of the patient's own platelets, platelet transfusion is indicated. Transfusion is required if the platelet count falls below 20,000 or if major operation is contemplated and the count is less than 50,000. Critical thrombocytopenia predictably develops if the transfused blood exceeds the patient's own original blood volume by 50–100%. The usual amount of platelet transfusion is 1 U for every 10 kg body weight. If the blood group of the donor or donors is unknown, RhoGAM is to be given to Rh-negative women, since RBCs do occur among the platelets. The risk of infection is reduced only if platelets from one donor are used.

The appearance of thromboplastin and endotoxin in the circulation leads to DIC. These substances activate thrombin and aggregate platelets and fibrin in the capillaries. Fibrin degradation products consume platelets and activate coagulation factors (consumptive coagulopathy). Aggressive fluid replacement is conducive to coagulopathy but usually not before 80% of the original fluid volume has been replaced. As a result, even minor trauma results in microvascular hemorrhage. Apart from the blood loss, tissue hypoxia and ischemia contribute to the development of fibrin plugs in the capillary system. This leads to renal failure, pulmonary damage, and, occasionally, Sheehan's syndrome. The diagnosis of DIC should be considered if the laboratory parameters, including fibrin degradation products and D-dimers, remain abnormal after the administration of fresh frozen plasma.

Even after the patient has been stabilized after major blood loss, attention must be paid to the potential side effects deriving from the infusion of blood products. These include hemolytic febrile reactions, allergic manifestations, and pulmonary damage. Other untoward sequelas are renal insufficiency, cortical blindness, and adult respiratory distress syndrome. Naturally, these complications require the involvement in the management of a variety of specialists and subspecialists (Table 22.4).

In addition to donor blood transfusion, commercial systems for intraoperative cell salvage are available, although there is limited data for their use in obstetrics.[122] These systems are attached to the typical suction system during

Table 22.4 Duke hemorrhage protocols (by kind permission of Duke University Medical Center): (A) immediate OB blood pack, (B) laboratory evaluation, and (C) transfusion.

A. Immediate OB blood pack	
If type and screen are available	If type and screen are unavailable
4 U type-specific pRBCs	4 U O-negative pRBCs
4 U type-specific or AB thawed plasma	4 U thawed AB plasma
1 dose (10 U) cryoprecipitate	1 dose (10 U) cryoprecipitate
1 U apheresis platelets	1 U apheresis platelets
B. Laboratory evaluation	
Obstetric bleed hemostasis panel	
Type and screen	
Complete blood count[a]	
Prothrombin time[a]	
Activated partial thromboplastin time[a]	
Fibrinogen[a]	
Thromboelastography[a]	
C. Transfusion	
Platelets <50,000: transfuse one apheresis platelet dose	
Fibrinogen <125: transfuse 1 pool cryoprecipitate	
INR >1.5: transfuse 2–4 U FFP	
Massive hemorrhage (to be started after administration of initial OB blood pack)	
RBC to plasma (FFP) transfusion in 1:1 ratio	
After 6:6 U of RBC : plasma, give 1 U apheresis platelet dose	
After additional 6:6 RBC: plasma, give one 10 U pool of cryoprecipitate	
Continue alternating administration of 1 U platelets and one pool cryoprecipitate after every additional 6:6 RBC/plasma transfusion	

Abbreviations: FFP, frozen fresh plasma; INR, international normalized ratio; pRBC, packed red blood cell; RBC, red blood cell.

[a] To be repeated every 30 minutes.

surgery and pass through a filter system into a reservoir. This system is designed to remove cells and molecules such as tissue factor, alpha-fetoprotein, platelets, and procoagulant factors.[117] Initial concerns regarding the risk of amniotic fluid embolism are reduced, with more than 400 published case reports of transfusion of recovered allogeneic blood in obstetrics and the current opinion that amniotic fluid embolism is in fact not an embolic phenomenon and instead an anaphylactoid reaction to fetal antigens.[123] There is also concern for maternal alloimmunization to the Rh (D) antigen, but this can be prevented with adequate RhIG dosing.[123] Unfortunately, there is significant cost to equipment setup and blood collection. Currently, cell salvage is advocated as cost-effective for patients with a predictably high risk of transfusion, such as patients with placentation disorders.[124]

DELAYED POSTPARTUM HEMORRHAGE

Delayed or secondary PPH can manifest at any time in the puerperium. Secondary PPH is defined as excessive bleeding occurring between 24 hours and 12 weeks postpartum. In most instances, it occurs 7–14 days after delivery.[125] The incidence ranges from 0.2% to 2% in high-income countries.[126,127] Common causes are diffuse uterine atony or subinvolution of the placental site, retained fragments of placenta, and endometritis. A bleeding diathesis or coagulation disorder may also present as delayed PPH, particularly von Willebrand's disease.

Subinvolution results from failure or delay of the endometrium to return to its normal state after separation of the placenta. Histologic examination of noninvoluted vessels reveals thrombus formation, lack of an endothelial lining, and perivascular trophoblasts in the vessel walls.[128] Uterine atony and submucous myomas have also been implicated in the pathogenesis. The diagnosis is confirmed when curettage fails to recover placental fragments.

Subinvolution of the uterus or retained placental tissue causes bleeding when the necrotic tissue sloughs off the endometrium and opens previously thrombosed vascular channels. Patients with late PPH may present with a sudden gush of blood or intermittent spotting prior to an episode of profuse bleeding. On physical examination, the uterus usually appears large and boggy. If there is an associated infection, there is uterine tenderness, fever, and foul-smelling lochia. The diagnostic workup includes routine blood and coagulation studies for the assessment of the extent and nature of the blood loss, a thorough pelvic examination for old hematomas or lacerations, and sonographic study to detect retained placental parts.[129] The treatment depends upon the clinical presentation. In cases with profuse bleeding, hospital admission is mandatory and blood replacement is indicated. If endometritis is suspected, cervical-uterine and blood cultures can be obtained to help guide antibiotic therapy. If the bleeding continues or retained tissue is suspected, curettage should be performed. The procedure itself may cause severe blood loss and disseminated infection. Therefore, blood products should be available before it is performed and antibiotics should be administered preoperatively. The size, location, and consistency of the uterus must be assessed prior to the initiation of the procedure. The cervix is usually dilated to permit the insertion of instruments with relative ease; if not, it should be dilated to 12–13 mm in the usual manner. Ovum or sponge forceps may be used to remove placental tissue. A large, serrated curette can be utilized to empty the uterine cavity. Great care must be exercised so as to not perforate the uterine wall or curette too zealously. An uterotonic medication, usually oxytocin, is to be administered during the procedure.

Bleeding usually ceases within a short time after the completion of the curettage. Packing of the uterus, balloon insertion, or other surgical procedures are rarely required. Nonetheless, arrangements should be made for emergency hysterectomy if uncontrollable hemorrhage occurs. Consent for the same should be obtained from the patient before the operation, with due emphasis upon the fact that the need for such an intervention does arise on rare occasions. Curettage of the uterus, as described above, may exaggerate the bleeding and drive the patient into irreversible shock.

Fortunately, in most cases of secondary PPH the bleeding is not catastrophic. However, if bleeding is excessive on presentation, and/or a coagulopathy is suspected uterine artery embolization should be considered prior to proceeding with surgical management. Needless to say, the availability of large amounts of blood and close cooperation with the blood bank are critically important under these circumstances.

The postoperative follow-up should give due attention to some worrisome complications, such as Sheehan's syndrome and Asherman's syndrome. It deserves mention that the former is not necessarily associated with severe shock and can occur even if the blood pressure was successfully maintained above shock levels.

Pseudoaneurysm of the uterine artery[130] and arteriovenous malformations[128,131,132] are a rare cause of bleeding postpartum. However, this unusual alternative needs to be kept in mind when blood flow is demonstrated on sonographic examination. The anomaly can be congenital or acquired. In this setting, uterine curettage can cause catastrophic bleeding. Previous curettage, pregnancy termination, septic abortion, and gestational trophoplastic disease appear to predispose to such anomalies. High blood flow velocity (>96 cm/second) and low resistance to blood flow are suggestive of arteriovenous shunt or trophoplastic disease. High human chorionic gonadotropin concentrations are indicative of the latter alternative.[133]

For the identification of arteriovenous connection, the use of three-dimensional, color-Doppler ultrasound technology is helpful. This permits the recognition and localization of increased vascularity. It also generates waveforms that permit the measurement of systolic and diastolic blood-flow velocities.[134,135] Color-Doppler or gray-scale sonography facilitates the distinction between the vascular uterine wall and the retained product of conception. On gray-scale sonography, the placental tissue occupies the uterine cavity. In contrast, arteriovenous malformations often involve both the myometrium and the uterine cavity. The arteriovenous communications may regenerate; therefore, they can be managed expectantly.[136,137] When the bleeding is severe, uterine embolization usually permits the avoidance of hysterectomy.[135] Prior history of secondary or delayed history predisposes to a recurrence, and the clinician should be attentive to this possibility in subsequent pregnancy.[138]

ACKNOWLEDGMENT

This chapter contains material from the previous chapter authored by Akos Jakobovits and Jahir C. Sama.

REFERENCES

1. Hogan MC, Foreman KJ, Naghavi M et al. Maternal mortality for 181 countries, 1980–2008: A systematic analysis of progress towards Millennium Development Goal 5. *Lancet* 2010; 375: 1609–23.
2. AbouZahr C. Global burden of maternal death and disability. *Br Med Bull* 2003; 67: 1–11.
3. Creanga AA, Berg CJ, Syverson C et al. Pregnancy-related mortality in the United States, 2006–2010. *Obstet Gynecol* 2015; 125: 5–12.
4. Bateman BT, Berman MF, Riley LE, Leffert LR. The epidemiology of postpartum hemorrhage in a large, nationwide sample of deliveries. *Anesth Analg* 2010; 110: 1368–73.
5. World Health Organization. *Evaluating the Quality of Care for Severe Pregnancy Complications: The WHO Near-Miss Approach for Maternal Health.* Geneva, Switzerland: WHO, 2011.
6. Royal College of Obstetricians and Gynaecologists. *Green-Top Guideline No. 52:* Prevention and Management of Postpartum Haemorrhage. 2011. https://www.rcog.org.uk/en/guidelines-research-services/guidelines/gtg52/. Accessed August 31, 2015.
7. Abdul-Kadir R, McLintock C, Ducloy AS et al. Evaluation and management of postpartum hemorrhage: Consensus from an international expert panel. *Transfusion* 2014; 54: 1756–68.
8. Powers WF, Kiely JL. The risks confronting twins: A national perspective. *Am J Obstet Gynecol* 1994; 170: 456–61.
9. Bouvier-Colle MH, Ould El Joud D, Varnoux N et al. Evaluation of the quality of care for severe obstetrical haemorrhage in three French regions. *Int J Obstet Gynaecol* 2001; 108: 898–903.
10. Bouvier-Colle MH, Pequignot F, Jougla E. [Maternal mortality in France: Frequency, trends and causes]. *Journal De Gynecologie, Obstetrique et Biologie De la Reproduction* 2001; 30: 768–75.
11. Bouvier-Colle M, Varnoux N, Bréart G. *The Maternal Deaths in France.* Paris, France: Les Editions INSERM, 1994.
12. Lu MC, Fridman M, Korst LM et al. Variations in the incidence of postpartum hemorrhage across hospitals in California. *Matern Child Health J* 2005; 9: 297–306.
13. Callaghan WM, Kuklina EV, Berg CJ. Trends in postpartum hemorrhage: United States, 1994–2006. *Am J Obstet Gynecol* 2010; 202: 353 e1–6.
14. Pritchard J, Baldwin R, Dickey J, Wiggins K. Blood volume changes in pregnancy and the puerperium: 2. Red blood cell loss and changes in apparent blood volume during and following vaginal delivery cesarean section and cesarean section plus total hysterectomy. *Am J Obstet Gynecol* 1962; 84: 1271–82.
15. Brant HA. Precise estimation of postpartum haemorrhage: Difficulties and importance. *Br Med J* 1967; 1: 398–400.
16. Robson SC, Boys RJ, Hunter S, Dunlop W. Maternal hemodynamics after normal delivery and delivery complicated by postpartum hemorrhage. *Obstet Gynecol* 1989; 74: 234–9.
17. Joseph KS, Rouleau J, Kramer MS et al. Investigation of an increase in postpartum haemorrhage in Canada. *Int J Obstet Gynaecol* 2007; 114: 751–9.
18. Ford JB, Roberts CL, Simpson JM et al. Increased postpartum hemorrhage rates in Australia. *Int J Gynaecol Obstet* 2007; 98: 237–43.
19. MacDorman MF, Menacker F, Declercq E. Cesarean birth in the United States: Epidemiology, trends, and outcomes. *Clin Perinatol* 2008; 35: 293–307.
20. Smulian JC, Ananth CV, Kinzler WL et al. Twin deliveries in the United States over three decades: An age-period-cohort analysis. *Obstet Gynecol* 2004; 104: 278–85.
21. Belghiti J, Kayem G, Dupont C et al. Oxytocin during labour and risk of severe postpartum haemorrhage: A population-based, cohort-nested case–control study. *BMJ Open* 2011; 1: e000514.
22. Begley CM, Gyte GM, Devane D et al. Active versus expectant management for women in the third stage of labour. *Cochrane Database Syst Rev* 2015; (3): CD007412.
23. Myburgh JA, Mythen MG. Resuscitation fluids. *N Engl J Med* 2013; 369: 1243–51.
24. Haldar R, Samanta S. Post-partum sequential occurrence of two diverse transfusion reactions (transfusion associated circulatory overload and transfusion related acute lung injury). *J Emerg Trauma Shock* 2013; 6: 283–6.
25. Fiebig EW, Wu AH, Krombach J et al. Transfusion-related acute lung injury and transfusion-associated circulatory overload: Mutually exclusive or coexisting entities? *Transfusion* 2007; 47: 171–2.
26. Popovsky MA. Transfusion-related acute lung injury and transfusion-associated circulatory overload. *ISBT Sci Ser* 2006; 1: 107–11.
27. Sihler KC, Napolitano LM. Complications of massive transfusion. *Chest* 2010; 137: 209–20.
28. Fliegner JR. Third stage management: How important is it? *Med J Aust* 1978; 2: 190–3.
29. Hibbard BM. Obstetrics in general practice. The third stage of labour. *Br Med J* 1964; 1: 1485–8.

30. Golan A, Lidor AL, Wexler S, David MP. A new method for the management of the retained placenta. *Am J Obstet Gynecol* 1983; 146: 708–9.
31. Reddy VV, Carey JC. Effect of umbilical vein oxytocin on puerperal blood loss and length of the third stage of labor. *Am J Obstet Gynecol* 1989; 160: 206–8.
32. Fliegner JR, Hibbard BM. Active management of the third stage of labour. *Br Med J* 1966; 2: 622–3.
33. Westhoff G, Cotter AM, Tolosa JE. Prophylactic oxytocin for the third stage of labour to prevent postpartum haemorrhage. *Cochrane Database Syst Rev* 2013; (10): CD001808.
34. Dahlke JD, Mendez-Figueroa H, Maggio L et al. Prevention and management of postpartum hemorrhage: A comparison of 4 national guidelines. *Am J Obstet Gynecol* 2015; 213: 76 e1–10.
35. Maged AM, Hassan AM, Shehata NA. Carbetocin versus oxytocin for prevention of postpartum hemorrhage after vaginal delivery in high risk women. *J Matern Fetal Neonatal Med* 2016; 29: 532–6.
36. Moir DD, Amoa AB. Ergometrine or oxytocin? Blood loss and side-effects at spontaneous vertex delivery. *Br J Anaesth* 1979; 51: 113–7.
37. Prendiville W, Elbourne D, Chalmers I. The effects of routine oxytocic administration in the management of the third stage of labour: An overview of the evidence from controlled trials. *Br J Obstet Gynaecol* 1988; 95: 3–16.
38. Epperly TD, Fogarty JP, Hodges SG. Efficacy of routine postpartum uterine exploration and manual sponge curettage. *J Fam Pract* 1989; 28: 172–6.
39. Dildy GA, 3rd. Postpartum hemorrhage: New management options. *Clin Obstet Gynecol* 2002; 45: 330–44.
40. Combs CA, Murphy EL, Laros RK, Jr. Factors associated with postpartum hemorrhage with vaginal birth. *Obstet Gynecol* 1991; 77: 69–76.
41. Hendricks CH, Eskes TK, Saameli K. Uterine contractility at delivery and in the puerperium. *Am J Obstet Gynecol* 1962; 83: 890–906.
42. Weis FR, Jr., Markello R, Mo B, Bochiechio P. Cardiovascular effects of oxytocin. *Obstet Gynecol* 1975; 46: 211–4.
43. Hendricks CH, Brenner WE. Cardiovascular effects of oxytocic drugs used post partum. *Am J Obstet Gynecol* 1970; 108: 751–60.
44. Bigrigg A, Chissell S, Read MD. Use of intra myometrial 15-methyl prostaglandin F2 alpha to control atonic postpartum haemorrhage following vaginal delivery and failure of conventional therapy. *Br J Obstet Gynaecol* 1991; 98: 734–6.
45. Buttino L, Jr., Garite TJ. The use of 15 methyl F2 alpha prostaglandin (Prostin 15M) for the control of postpartum hemorrhage. *Am J Perinatol* 1986; 3: 241–3.
46. Hayashi RH, Castillo MS, Noah ML. Management of severe postpartum hemorrhage with a prostaglandin F2 alpha analogue. *Obstet Gynecol* 1984; 63: 806–8.
47. Douglas MJ, Farquharson DF, Ross PL, Renwick JE. Cardiovascular collapse following an overdose of prostaglandin F2 alpha: A case report. *Can J Anaesth* 1989; 36: 466–9.
48. Bakri YN, Amri A, Abdul Jabbar F. Tamponade-balloon for obstetrical bleeding. *Int J Gynaecol Obstet* 2001; 74: 139–42.
49. Georgiou C. Balloon tamponade in the management of postpartum haemorrhage: A review. *Int J Obstet Gynaecol* 2009; 116: 748–57.
50. Hutchon SP, Martin WL. Intrapartum and postpartum bleeding. *Curr Obstet Gynaecol* 2002; 12: 250–5.
51. Doolittle HH. Routine manual inspection of the postpartum uterus; study of the late effects. *Obstet Gynecol* 1957; 9: 422–5.
52. Endler M, Grunewald C, Saltvedt S. Epidemiology of retained placenta: Oxytocin as an independent risk factor. *Obstet Gynecol* 2012; 119: 801–9.
53. Smith GN, Brien JF. Use of nitroglycerin for uterine relaxation. *Obstet Gynecol Surv* 1998; 53: 559–65.
54. Altabef KM, Spencer JT, Zinberg S. Intravenous nitroglycerin for uterine relaxation of an inverted uterus. *Am J Obstet Gynecol* 1992; 166: 1237–8.
55. Axemo P, Fu X, Lindberg B, Ulmsten U, Wessen A. Intravenous nitroglycerin for rapid uterine relaxation. *Acta Obstet Gynecol Scand* 1998; 77: 50–3.
56. van Schalkwyk J, Van Eyk N, Society of Obstetricians and Gynaecologists of Canada Infectious Diseases C. Antibiotic prophylaxis in obstetric procedures. *J Obstet Gynaecol Can* 2010; 32: 878–92.
57. Mhyre JM, Shilkrut A, Kuklina EV et al. Massive blood transfusion during hospitalization for delivery in New York State, 1998–2007. *Obstet Gynecol* 2013; 122: 1288–94.
58. Breen JL, Neubecker R, Gregori CA, Franklin JE, Jr. Placenta accreta, increta, and percreta. A survey of 40 cases. *Obstet Gynecol* 1977; 49: 43–7.
59. Clark SL, Koonings PP, Phelan JP. Placenta previa/accreta and prior cesarean section. *Obstet Gynecol* 1985; 66: 89–92.
60. O'Brien JM, Barton JR, Donaldson ES. The management of placenta percreta: Conservative and operative strategies. *Am J Obstet Gynecol* 1996; 175: 1632–8.
61. Hull AD, Salerno CC, Saenz CC, Pretorius DH. Three-dimensional ultrasonography and diagnosis of placenta percreta with bladder involvement. *J Ultrasound Med* 1999; 18: 853–6.
62. Lam G, Kuller J, McMahon M. Use of magnetic resonance imaging and ultrasound in the antenatal diagnosis of placenta accreta. *J Soc Gynecol Invest* 2002; 9: 37–40.
63. Comstock CH. Antenatal diagnosis of placenta accreta: A review. *Ultrasound Obstet Gynecol* 2005; 26: 89–96.
64. Warshak CR, Eskander R, Hull AD et al. Accuracy of ultrasonography and magnetic resonance imaging in the diagnosis of placenta accreta. *Obstet Gynecol* 2006; 108: 573–81.

65. Baughman WC, Corteville JE, Shah RR. Placenta accreta: Spectrum of US and MR imaging findings. *Radiographics* 2008; 28: 1905–16.
66. Lee PS, Bakelaar R, Fitpatrick CB et al. Medical and surgical treatment of placenta percreta to optimize bladder preservation. *Obstet Gynecol* 2008; 112: 421–4.
67. Phelan JP. Uterine rupture. *Clin Obstet Gynecol* 1990; 33: 432–7.
68. Sebire NJ, Jolly M, Harris J et al. Risks of obstetric complications in multiple pregnancies: An analysis of more than 400 000 pregnancies in the UK. *Prenat Neonatal Med* 2001; 6: 89–94.
69. Brown BJ, Heaston DK, Poulson AM et al. Uncontrollable postpartum bleeding: A new approach to hemostasis through angiographic arterial embolization. *Obstet Gynecol* 1979; 54: 361–5.
70. Gilbert WM, Moore TR, Resnik R et al. Angiographic embolization in the management of hemorrhagic complications of pregnancy. *Am J Obstet Gynecol* 1992; 166: 493–7.
71. Ganguli S, Stecker MS, Pyne D et al. Uterine artery embolization in the treatment of postpartum uterine hemorrhage. *J Vasc Intervent Radiol* 2011; 22: 169–176.
72. Kirby JM, Kachura JR, Rajan DK et al. Arterial embolization for primary postpartum hemorrhage. *J Vasc Intervent Radiol* 2009; 20: 1036–45.
73. Heffner LJ, Mennuti MT, Rudoff JC, McLean GK. Primary management of postpartum vulvovaginal hematomas by angiographic embolization. *Am J Perinatol* 1985; 2: 204–7.
74. Hare WS, Holland CJ. Paresis following internal iliac artery embolization. *Radiology* 1983; 146: 47–51.
75. Ito M, Matsui K, Mabe K, Katabuchi H, Fujisaki S. Transcatheter embolization of pelvic arteries as the safest method for postpartum hemorrhage. *Int J Gynaecol Obstet* 1986; 24: 373–8.
76. Harris LJ. A new instrument for control of hemorrhage by aortic compression. A preliminary report. *Can Med Assoc J* 1964; 91: 128–30.
77. Cutler BS, Daggett WM. Application of the "G-suit" to the control of hemorrhage in massive trauma. *Ann Surg* 1971; 173: 511–4.
78. Pearse CS, Magrina JF, Finley BE. Use of MAST suit in obstetrics & gynecology. *Obstet Gynecol Surv* 1984; 39: 416–22.
79. Hall M, 3rd, Marshall JR. The gravity suit: A major advance in management of gynecologic blood loss. *Obstet Gynecol* 1979; 53: 247–50.
80. McBride G. One caution in pneumatic antishock garment use. *JAMA* 1982; 247: 1112.
81. O'Leary JL, O'Leary JA. Uterine artery ligation for control of postcesarean section hemorrhage. *Obstet Gynecol* 1974; 43: 849–53.
82. Waters EG. Surgical management of postpartum hemorrhage with particular reference to ligation of uterine arteries. *Am J Obstet Gynecol* 1952; 64: 1143–8.
83. Howard LR. Iatrogenic arteriovenous sinus of a uterine artery and vein. Report of a case. *Obstet Gynecol* 1968; 31: 255–7.
84. O'Leary JA. Pregnancy following uterine artery ligation. *Obstet Gynecol* 1980; 55: 112–3.
85. Clark SL, Phelan JP, Yeh SY, Bruce SR, Paul RH. Hypogastric artery ligation for obstetric hemorrhage. *Obstet Gynecol* 1985; 66: 353–6.
86. Mengert WF, Burchell RC, Blumstein RW, Daskal JL. Pregnancy after bilateral ligation of the internal iliac and ovarian arteries. *Obstet Gynecol* 1969; 34: 664–6.
87. Dubay ML, Holshauser CA, Burchell RC. Internal iliac artery ligation for postpartum hemorrhage: Recanalization of vessels. *Am J Obstet Gynecol* 1980; 136: 689–91.
88. Evans S, McShane P. The efficacy of internal iliac artery ligation in obstetric hemorrhage. *Surg Gynecol Obstet* 1985; 160: 250–3.
89. Cruikshank SH, Stoelk EM. Surgical control of pelvic hemorrhage: Method of bilateral ovarian artery ligation. *Am J Obstet Gynecol* 1983; 147: 724–5.
90. Chez R, B-Lynch C. The B-Lynch suture for control of massive postpartum hemorrhage. *Contemp Obstet Gynaecol* 1998; 43: 93–100.
91. Allam MS, B-Lynch C. The B-Lynch and other uterine compression suture techniques. *Int J Gynaecol Obstet* 2005; 89: 236–41.
92. Joshi VM, Shrivastava M. Partial ischemic necrosis of the uterus following a uterine brace compression suture. *Int J Obstet Gynaecol* 2004; 111: 279–80.
93. Cowan AD, Miller ES, Grobman WA. Subsequent pregnancy outcome after B-Lynch suture placement. *Obstet Gynecol* 2014; 124: 558–61.
94. Cho JH, Jun HS, Lee CN. Hemostatic suturing technique for uterine bleeding during cesarean delivery. *Obstet Gynecol* 2000; 96: 129–31.
95. Stanco LM, Schrimmer DB, Paul RH, Mishell DR, Jr. Emergency peripartum hysterectomy and associated risk factors. *Am J Obstet Gynecol* 1993; 168: 879–83.
96. Sturdee DW, Rushton DI. Caesarean and post-partum hysterectomy 1968–1983. *Br J Obstet Gynaecol* 1986; 93: 270–4.
97. Hallak M, Dildy GA, 3rd, Hurley TJ, Moise KJ, Jr. Transvaginal pressure pack for life-threatening pelvic hemorrhage secondary to placenta accreta. *Obstet Gynecol* 1991; 78: 938–40.
98. Chauhan SP, Martin JN, Jr., Henrichs CE et al. Maternal and perinatal complications with uterine rupture in 142,075 patients who attempted vaginal birth after cesarean delivery: A review of the literature. *Am J Obstet Gynecol* 2003; 189: 408–17.
99. Guise JM, McDonagh MS, Osterweil P et al. Systematic review of the incidence and consequences of uterine rupture in women with previous caesarean section. *Br Med J* 2004; 329: 19–25.
100. Landon MB, Hauth JC, Leveno KJ et al. Maternal and perinatal outcomes associated with a trial of labor after prior cesarean delivery. *N Engl J Med* 2004; 351: 2581–9.

101. Guise JM, Eden K, Emeis C et al. Vaginal birth after cesarean: New insights. *Evid Rep Technol Assess (Full Rep)* 2010: (191): 1–397.
102. Al-Zirqi I, Stray-Pedersen B, Forsen L, Vangen S. Uterine rupture after previous caesarean section. *Int J Obstet Gynaecol* 2010; 117: 809–20.
103. Committee on Obstetric Practice. Induction of labor for vaginal birth after cesarean delivery. *Int J Gynaecol Obstet* 2002; 99: 679–80.
104. Usta IM, Hamdi MA, Musa AA, Nassar AH. Pregnancy outcome in patients with previous uterine rupture. *Acta Obstet Gynecol Scand* 2007; 86: 172–6.
105. Magon N, Babu K. Recombinant factor VIIa in postpartum hemorrhage: A new weapon in obstetrician's armamentarium. *N Am J Med Sci* 2012; 4: 157–62.
106. Bouma LS, Bolte AC, van Geijn HP. Use of recombinant activated factor VII in massive postpartum haemorrhage. *Eur J Obstet Gynecol Reprod Biol* 2008; 137: 172–7.
107. Tanchev S, Platikanov V, Karadimov D. Administration of recombinant factor VIIa for the management of massive bleeding due to uterine atonia in the post-placental period. *Acta Obstet Gynecol Scand* 2005; 84: 402–3.
108. Ahonen J, Jokela R. Recombinant factor VIIa for life-threatening post-partum haemorrhage. *Br J Anaesth* 2005; 94: 592–5.
109. O'Connell KA, Wood JJ, Wise RP et al. Thromboembolic adverse events after use of recombinant human coagulation factor VIIa. *JAMA* 2006; 295: 293–8.
110. Sentilhes L, Lasocki S, Ducloy-Bouthors AS et al. Tranexamic acid for the prevention and treatment of postpartum haemorrhage. *Br J Anaesth* 2015; 114: 576–87.
111. Cook L, Roberts I, WOMAN Trial Collaborators. Post-partum haemorrhage and the WOMAN trial. *Int J Epidemiol* 2010; 39: 949–50.
112. Shakur H, Elbourne D, Gulmezoglu M et al. The WOMAN Trial (World Maternal Antifibrinolytic Trial): Tranexamic acid for the treatment of postpartum haemorrhage: An international randomised, double blind placebo controlled trial. *Trials* 2010; 11: 40.
113. Charbit B, Mandelbrot L, Samain E et al. The decrease of fibrinogen is an early predictor of the severity of postpartum hemorrhage. *J Thromb Haemost* 2007; 5: 266–73.
114. Wikkelso AJ, Edwards HM, Afshari A et al. Pre-emptive treatment with fibrinogen concentrate for postpartum haemorrhage: Randomized controlled trial. *Br J Anaesth* 2015; 114: 623–33.
115. Ducloy-Bouthors AS, Susen S, Wong CA et al. Medical advances in the treatment of postpartum hemorrhage. *Anesth Analg* 2014; 119: 1140–7.
116. Wikkelsoe AJ, Afshari A, Stensballe J et al. The FIB-PPH trial: Fibrinogen concentrate as initial treatment for postpartum haemorrhage: Study protocol for a randomised controlled trial. *Trials* 2012; 13: 110.
117. Pacheco LD, Saade GR, Gei AF, Hankins GD. Cutting-edge advances in the medical management of obstetrical hemorrhage. *Am J Obstet Gynecol* 2011; 205: 526–32.
118. Collis RE, Collins PW. Haemostatic management of obstetric haemorrhage. *Anaesthesia* 2015; 70(Suppl 1): 78–86, e27–8.
119. Perner A, Haase N, Guttormsen AB et al. Hydroxyethyl starch 130/0.42 versus Ringer's acetate in severe sepsis. *N Engl J Med* 2012; 367: 124–34.
120. Pacheco LD, Saade GR, Costantine MM et al. The role of massive transfusion protocols in obstetrics. *Am J Perinatol* 2013; 30: 1–4.
121. Shevell T, Malone FD. Management of obstetric hemorrhage. *Semin Perinatol* 2003; 27: 86–104.
122. Geoghegan J, Daniels JP, Moore PA et al. Cell salvage at caesarean section: The need for an evidence-based approach. *Int J Obstet Gynaecol* 2009; 116: 743–7.
123. Liumbruno GM, Liumbruno C, Rafanelli D. Intraoperative cell salvage in obstetrics: Is it a real therapeutic option? *Transfusion* 2011; 51: 2244–56.
124. Goucher H, Wong CA, Patel SK, Toledo P. Cell salvage in obstetrics. *Anesth Analg* 2015; 121: 465–8.
125. Dossou M, Debost-Legrand A, Dechelotte P, Lemery D, Vendittelli F. Severe secondary postpartum hemorrhage: A historical cohort. *Birth* (Berkeley, Calif.) 2015; 42: 149–55.
126. Alexander J, Thomas P, Sanghera J. Treatments for secondary postpartum haemorrhage. *Cochrane Database Syst Rev* 2002: (1): CD002867.
127. Hoveyda F, MacKenzie IZ. Secondary postpartum haemorrhage: Incidence, morbidity and current management. *Int J Obstet Gynaecol* 2001; 108: 927–30.
128. Aziz N, Lenzi TA, Jeffrey RB, Jr., Lyell DJ. Postpartum uterine arteriovenous fistula. *Obstet Gynecol* 2004; 103: 1076–8.
129. Khan A, Muradali D. Imaging acute obstetric and gynecologic abnormalities. *Semin Roentgenol* 2001; 36: 165–72.
130. Yun SY, Lee DH, Cho KH et al. Delayed postpartum hemorrhage resulting from uterine artery pseudoaneurysm rupture. *J Emerg Med* 2012; 42: e11–4.
131. Wiebe ER, Switzer P. Arteriovenous malformations of the uterus associated with medical abortion. *Int J Gynaecol Obstet* 2000; 71: 155–8.
132. Chang FW, Ding DC, Chen DC, Yu MH. Heavy uterine bleeding due to uterine arteriovenous malformations. *Acta Obstet Gynecol Scand* 2004; 83: 599–600.
133. Huang MW, Muradali D, Thurston WA et al. Uterine arteriovenous malformations: Gray-scale and Doppler US features with MR imaging correlation. *Radiology* 1998; 206: 115–23.
134. Jain KA, Jeffrey RB, Jr, Sommer FG. Gynecologic vascular abnormalities: Diagnosis with Doppler US. *Radiology* 1991; 178: 549–51.

135. Kwon JH, Kim GS. Obstetric iatrogenic arterial injuries of the uterus: Diagnosis with US and treatment with transcatheter arterial embolization. *Radiographics* 2002; 22: 35–46.
136. Nizard J, Pessel M, De Keersmaecker B et al. High-intensity focused ultrasound in the treatment of postpartum hemorrhage: An animal model. *Ultrasound Obstet Gynecol* 2004; 23: 262–6.
137. Timmerman D, Van den Bosch T, Peeraer K et al. Vascular malformations in the uterus: Ultrasonographic diagnosis and conservative management. *Eur J Obstet Gynecol Reprod Biol* 2000; 92: 171–8.
138. Thorsteinsson VT, Kempers RD. Delayed postpartum bleeding. *Am J Obstet Gynecol* 1970; 107: 565–71.

Forceps delivery

23

OWEN C. MONTGOMERY and JOSEPH J. APUZZIO

CONTENTS

There have been significant changes in the management of the labor process and delivery in the past 20 years with a marked increase in cesarean deliveries from 22% in 1992 to 32.9% in 2009[1] and a decrease in operative vaginal deliveries from 9% in 1992 to 3.3% in 2013.[2] Some of these changes were due to the perception of enhanced safety of cesarean delivery for both mother and fetus. In many hospitals, even those with obstetrical teaching services, there are few operative vaginal deliveries with forceps or vacuum extractors. Therefore, the opportunity to educate physicians in training in operative vaginal delivery is decreasing and seems to be becoming the lost art of operative obstetrics. Operative vaginal delivery now accounts for only about 3.3% of all deliveries in the United States.[2]

Operative vaginal delivery using forceps or one of the several vacuum extraction instruments is still one of the hallmarks of an obstetrician and, in the last 100 years, has probably saved more maternal and fetal lives than any other surgical instrument extant. Operative vaginal delivery does, however, have risks for both mother and infant just as there are also potential significant maternal risks with delivery by cesarean section. Operative vaginal delivery is no longer an elective procedure but requires an appropriate indication as well as consent. If a spontaneous vaginal delivery is imminent, no operative delivery is indicated. Therefore, the risk benefit ratio for patients who are candidates for operative vaginal delivery should be weighed against the alternative of a cesarean delivery and not a spontaneous vaginal delivery. In this era of "modern" obstetrics, with the potential maternal and fetal risks in mind, teaching residents the use of obstetric forceps has become increasingly difficult but can still be included in a complete curriculum.[3] Operative vaginal delivery with forceps or should only be performed by those who have the education and experience in the proper performance of their use.[4]

BRIEF HISTORY OF OBSTETRICAL FORCEPS

The fascinating history of the development of obstetric forceps has been reviewed in great detail elsewhere. (Those interested in a more detailed review are referred to the third edition of this book.) The following précis is based upon the third edition's references and upon three additional classic texts on forceps.[5–7]

The weight of the evidence points to the invention of the short, straight obstetric forceps which introduced the modern forceps era by some member of the Chamberlen family, probably Peter the Elder (1560–1631). Chamberlen's forceps, several models of which were discovered in 1813 and which now rest in a small glass case under the marble stairs in the museum of the Royal College of Medicine in London, was a simple but effective instrument. The forceps consisted of two branches, each about 12 inches long, having a fenestrated blade and a cephalic curve. The major innovation of these forceps was that the branches were separable and could be inserted singly; once applied to the fetal vertex, the branches were rejoined near the handles with a leather thong or a rivet. The forceps then functioned as a first-class lever, and extraction of the fetus without damage was possible.

The history and genealogy of the Chamberlen family, whose members practiced midwifery in England for three generations, constitute a fascinating example of professional life and ethics in the seventeenth century. The forceps were kept as a family secret for over 100 years. Hugh Chamberlen the elder did attempt to sell the family secret to Mauriceau in France in 1670; Mauriceau's interest waned when Chamberlen's forceps failed his critical test—the vaginal delivery of a rachitic dwarf after 3 hours of struggle; the poor woman died 24 hours later of a ruptured uterus. Nevertheless, the "secret" of Chamberlen's forceps was difficult to conceal over such a long interval, and similar instruments began to appear on the Continent. Around 1730, Hugh Chamberlen sold his family secret to Roonhuysen, a Dutch obstetrician; unfortunately, Roonhuysen purchased only a single branch of the forceps! The first publication of the "secret" in the medical literature was by Rathlaw of Holland in 1732. By the mid-eighteenth century, the form and use of the obstetric forceps had become public knowledge in England and on the Continent, and modifications of the original had begun to appear, the first of over 800 varieties of forceps that were described during the next 200 years.

In retrospect, the principles of forceps design seem simple. Most of the modifications in design or material introduced were elaborate but nonfunctional innovations. For example, in an effort to decrease the pressure of the forceps on the fetal head, Smellie (1754) recommended covering the forceps blades with leather; this suggestion was attacked almost immediately (fortunately) as "conveying humors which are infectious... from one patient to another." The concept reappeared in the twentieth century with the introduction of foam rubber and sterilizable "booties" that could be placed on the forceps blades.

A small number of significant design advances can be singled out. In 1734, Dusée described a movable, interlocking mechanism for joining the two branches of the forceps. Levret (1744) and Pugh (1954) independently designed forceps with a pelvic curve, which facilitated traction when the fetal head was arrested at a high station in the pelvis. This solved some of the mechanical problems of the "straight" forceps, but did not eliminate all of the difficulties associated with high and midforceps operations. It remained for Tarnier (1877) to develop a type of forceps traction in which the line of pull coincided with the pelvic axis. This "axis traction" was the first substantive modification in over 100 years, and its principles still are employed today not only in technique but also in axis traction handles[8,9] and in the addition of a pelvic curvature.[10] A return to a modified straight forceps,[11,12] specifically designed for application to an asynclytic head and permitting a new application technique to a vertex in transverse arrest, became possible with the development of improved anesthetic techniques (Figure 23.1).[13] An instrument designed specifically for application and traction in the anteroposterior diameter of the maternal pelvis was Barton's elegant solution to a problem over 300 years old.[14,15] Solid forceps blades were introduced in an attempt to reduce maternal vaginal trauma in forceps rotation, and the resultant problem of slippage on the fetal vertex was addressed by a semifenestrated modification.[15,16] There has been some interest in forceps designed solely for rotation of the fetal vertex. More recently, the use of parallel or divergent (rather than crossed) forceps was recommended by Luikhart and Lauffe to minimize fetal head compression, an inevitable concomitant of traction.[12,17,18]

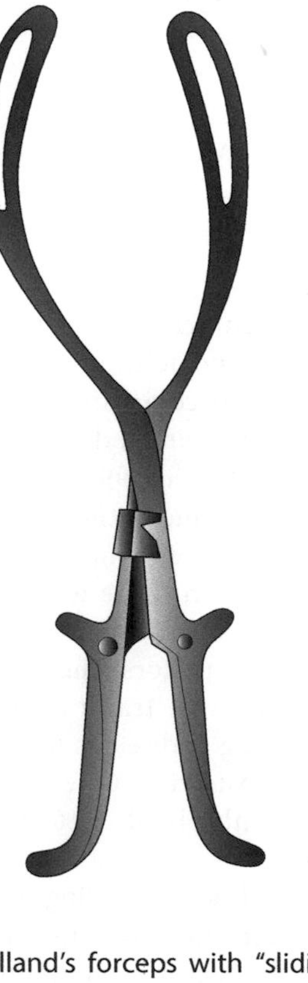

Figure 23.1 Kielland's forceps with "sliding lock." (From Burger K, *Operative Obstetrics*, Budapest, Hungary: Franklin Co, 1927.)

TYPES OF FORCEPS

Obstetric forceps consist of two blades that are labeled right or left, according to the side of the maternal pelvis in which they lie after application. The "rule" of forceps is as follows: left blade, left hand, to left side of pelvis; right blade, right hand, to right side of pelvis.

Forceps may be characterized by the relationship of their blades. Converging forceps are not in use today. The vast majority of obstetric forceps are of the crossed type. Forceps with overlapping shanks and slightly smaller blades are typified by Elliott's forceps (Figure 23.2). Forceps with separated parallel shanks and slightly longer blades are designed after Naegele's and Simpson's forceps (Figure 23.3). Regardless of their design, all forceps have the same parts: the blade, which fits around the fetal head and the maternal pelvis; the shank, which is the portion between blade and handle; and the handle, with which the instrument is manipulated. The blade has two curves: the cephalic curve permits the instrument to fit the fetal head accurately when applied to its lateral aspects; the pelvic curve adapts the instrument to the curved axis of the pelvis. Specialized forceps such as Kielland's have no pelvic curve. In all forceps except Barton's, the cephalic curve and pelvic curve are at right angles to each other; in Barton's forceps, the pelvic curve and cephalic curve are parallel. The blades themselves may be solid, fenestrated, or semifenestrated. The shanks may be short (as for outlet forceps) or long (for manipulation higher in the pelvis), parallel, or overlapping, and straight or with a perineal curve to facilitate axis traction.

After application, in the X-type of forceps, the two blades cross and articulate with each other, the articulation being known as the "lock." In the English lock, the articulation is composed of shoulders and flanges; in the French lock, of a notch in one branch into which fits a pin or screw of the other branch; and in the German lock, the most rigid of the three, a combination of both principles.

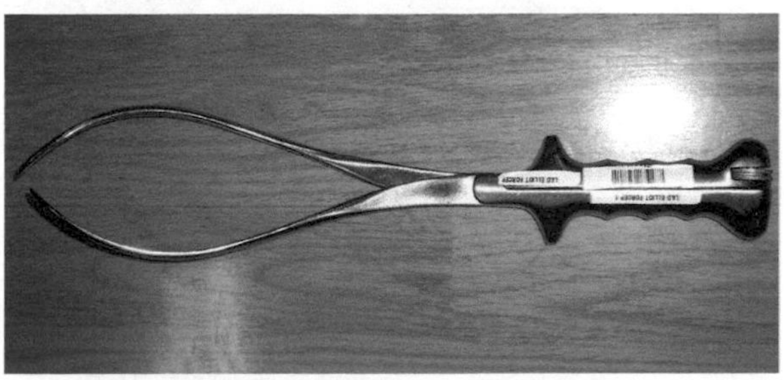

Figure 23.2 Elliott's forceps.

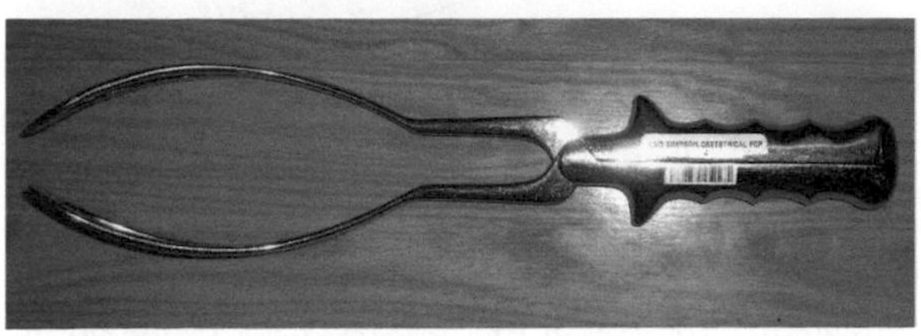

Figure 23.3 Simpson's forceps.

The sliding lock was introduced by Kielland (see Figure 23.1). It permits accurate application to an asynclytic head.

The handles of most forceps are similar. They are hollow (to reduce weight), have transverse projections at their junction with the shanks, and may or may not have lateral indentations to enhance the grip. Kielland's forceps handles are solid, narrow, and kept apart by a metal bar. Some forceps handles have a screw mechanism to prevent inadvertent compression during traction. The divergent forceps terminate in finger grips rather than handles.

The multiple forceps available, their minor differences, and the reasons therefore have been described in great detail.[19,20] There was always a reason for each modification that was introduced. Longer blades and separated shanks were deemed better for the grasp of a severely molded fetal head, but they distended and often tore the perineum prematurely. Overlapping shanks avoided this problem, but increased the probability of fetal head compression. Fenestrated blades permitted a good grip on the fetal head, but often left significant marks on the baby; in doing a forceps rotation, the fenestrated blades offered more opportunities for vaginal lacerations. Solid blades reduced these problems, but more frequently slipped on the vertex during difficult rotations; semifenestrated blades (indented toward the fetus, smooth toward the maternal side) were an attempt to alleviate this problem. Whether or not the forceps handles should be indented (Simpson's forceps) or smooth (DeLee's forceps) seems, in retrospect, insignificant and purely a matter of personal preference. Today, most of these variations are of little clinical importance.

TRADITIONAL CLASSIFICATION OF FORCEPS DELIVERIES

Based upon well-considered publications which analyzed both personal experience and reports in the obstetric literature, the following definitions for classification of forceps operations have been accepted.[21–25]

Outlet forceps

The application of forceps when the fetal scalp is visible at the introitus *without* separating the labia, the skull has reached the pelvic floor, and the sagittal suture is in the anteroposterior diameter of the maternal pelvis (Figure 23.4).

Midforceps

The biparietal diameter of the vertex has passed the plane of the pelvic inlet. This is the application of forceps when the head is engaged, but the conditions for outlet forceps have not been met. In the context of this term, any forceps delivery requiring forceps rotation regardless of the station is designated as a midforceps delivery. The term "low midforceps" is not an approved designation and should not be used (Figure 23.5).

High forceps

The application of forceps prior to the full engagement of the head is termed a "high-forceps" application. A high-forceps delivery is never justifiable (Figures 23.6 and 23.7).

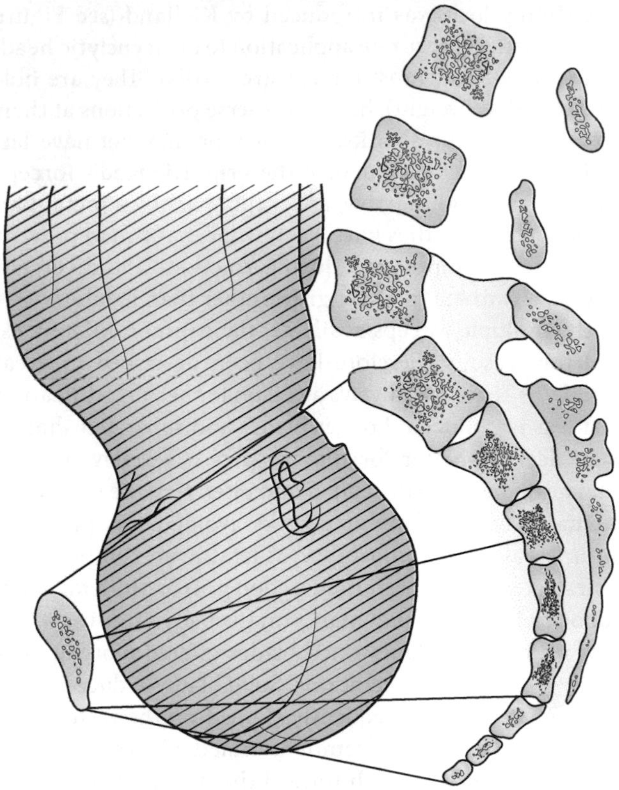

Figure 23.4 The head is deeply engaged. The sagittal suture has rotated into the anteroposterior diameter with the small fontanel directed toward the symphysis. Outlet forceps procedure can be performed at this point. (From Burger K, *Operative Obstetrics*, Budapest, Hungary: Franklin Co, 1927.)

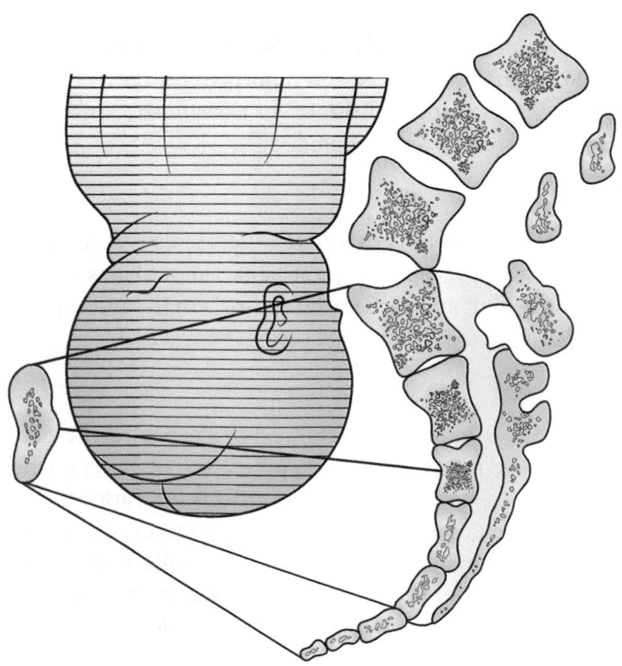

Figure 23.5 The greatest diameter of the fetal head has passed the plane of the pelvic inlet. By definition, a forceps procedure utilized at this point is "midcavity forceps." (From Burger K, *Operative Obstetrics*, Budapest, Hungary: Franklin Co, 1927.)

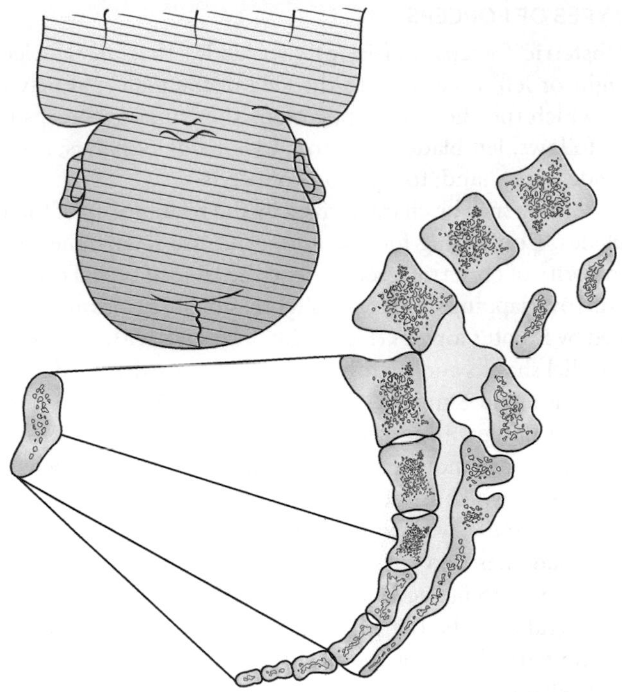

Figure 23.6 The head is high above the pelvic inlet (about – 5 station). Attempt at forceps delivery would require high-forceps procedure, which is absolutely contraindicated. (From Burger K, *Operative Obstetrics*, Budapest, Hungary: Franklin Co, 1927.)

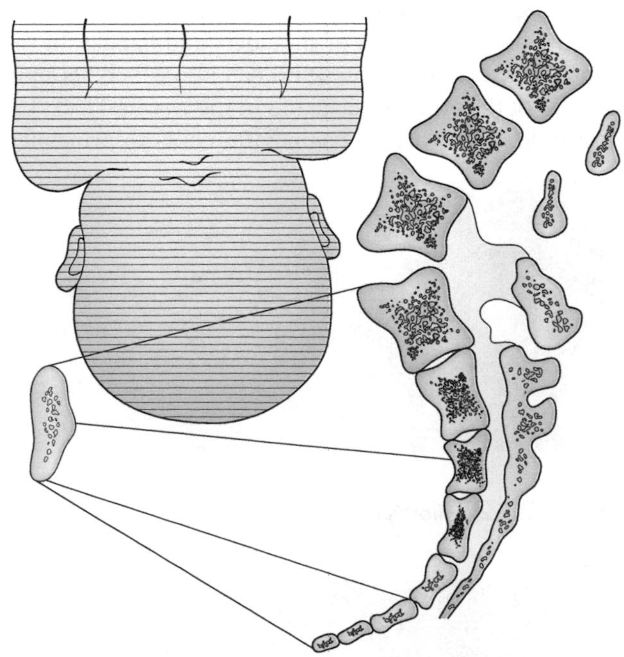

Figure 23.7 The greatest diameter of the fetal head is just entering the pelvis; according to British terminology, it is "engaging." The use of the forceps is still contraindicated at this point, and it would be, by definition, a "high-forceps" procedure.

MODERN CLASSIFICATION OF FORCEPS

Despite the fact that issues of both maternal and fetal safety had by no means been resolved definitively[24,26–37]; and that a marked difference in outcome for both patients is reported between forceps used only for traction to effect delivery or for rotation of more than 45° plus traction, in 1989, the Committee on Obstetrics: Maternal and Fetal Medicine of the American College of Obstetricians and Gynecologists[38] revised the definitions of forceps deliveries which continues to be used as the current definitions:

1. *Station:* the relationship of the estimated distance, in centimeters, between the leading bony portion of the fetal head and the level of the maternal ischial spines. In classifying midforceps procedures, the level of engagement of the fetal head must be stated as precisely as possible. Engagement of the vertex occurs when the biparietal diameter has passed through the pelvic inlet and is clinically diagnosed when the leading bony portion of the fetal head is at or below the level of the ischial spines (station 0 or more).
2. *Outlet forceps:* the application of forceps when (a) the scalp is visible at the introitus without separating the labia, (b) the fetal skull has reached the pelvic floor, (c) the sagittal suture is in the anteroposterior diameter or in the right or left occiput anterior or posterior position, and (d) the fetal head is at or on the perineum. According to this definition, rotation cannot exceed 45°. There is no documented difference in perinatal outcome when deliveries involving the use of outlet forceps are compared with similar spontaneous deliveries, and there are no data to support the concept that rotating the head on the pelvic floor 45° or less increases morbidity. Forceps delivery under these conditions may be desirable to shorten the second stage of labor.
3. *Low forceps:* The application of forceps when the leading point of the skull is at station +2 or more. Low forceps has two subdivisions: (1) rotation 45° or less (e.g., left occipitoanterior to occiput anterior, left occipitoposterior to occiput posterior), and (2) rotation of more than 45°.
4. *Midforceps:* The application of forceps when the head is engaged but the leading point of the skull is above station +2. Under very unusual circumstances, such as the sudden onset of severe fetal or maternal compromise, application of forceps above station +2 may be attempted while simultaneously initiating preparations for a cesarean delivery in the event that the forceps maneuver is unsuccessful. Under no circumstances, however, should forceps be applied to an unengaged presenting part or when the cervix is not completely dilated.

This change in nomenclature in no way modifies the risks inherent in these procedures. On the one hand, the relatively lower risk of forceps used for traction (with rotation limited to 45° from the vertical axis), now called "low forceps," is recognized and distinguished from "true" midforceps operations.

INDICATIONS OF FORCEPS DELIVERIES

Indications for the application of obstetric forceps may be fetal or maternal (ACOG guidelines Perinatal care 2012, pp. 190–192). Fetal indications primarily are related to fetal compromise such as Category 3 fetal heart tracings, Category 2 fetal heart tracings not responsive to conservative measures and remote from delivery, evidence of placenta abruption and others. Maternal indications for operative vaginal delivery are more numerous, most frequently based upon failure of descent in the second stage of labor, persistent occiput posterior, or maternal disease requiring shortening of the second stage of labor (e.g., cardiac disease). Prophylactic and other uses of forceps are of historical interest only.[39]

CONDITIONS FOR THE USE OF OBSTETRIC FORCEPS

It is the responsibility of the delivering provider who contemplates the use of forceps to ensure that the conditions for the safe use of these instruments have been fulfilled. These conditions are as follows:

1. The maternal bony pelvis must be clinically adequate, with no evidence of cephalopelvic disproportion.
2. The fetal vertex must be engaged.
3. The cervix must be completely dilated and retracted.
4. The fetal position and station must be known.
5. There must be no maternal bony or soft tissue obstruction (such as tumor or placenta previa).
6. The membranes must be ruptured.
7. The bladder and rectum must be empty.
8. Adequate and appropriate anesthesia must be available.

Of equal if not greater importance are the following *contraindications* for the application of forceps:

1. Hydrocephalic infant
2. Fetal position uncertain or unknown
3. Face presentation mentum *posterior*
4. Brow presentation
5. Fetal vertex not engaged.
6. Incomplete cervical dilation
7. Contracted maternal pelvis (or gross fetal macrosomia)
8. Lack of experience of the delivering provider!

FORCEPS PROCEDURES

Outlet forceps

To avoid the omission of essential steps, the obstetrician should carry out forceps operations in accordance with a specific and unvarying routine. In time, this routine becomes automatic. This routine will be detailed here and not repeated subsequently. Perhaps a checklist may be helpful at the time of the procedure and it can be added to the medical record at the conclusion of the delivery. Several checklists for operative deliveries have been published including the *ACOG Practice Bulletin 154*,[24] the Royal College of Obstetricians and Gynaecologists (RCOG) (Green-top guideline; no. 26) and individual teaching programs including Dartmouth and USCF (see further Video 23.1).

The indications and conditions should be reviewed to be certain that the forceps operation is appropriate and discussed with the patient. The patient should be placed on the delivery table in lithotomy position, with her buttocks a little past the lower end of the table. She should be anesthetized, cleansed, and draped in routine fashion for an aseptic delivery. The position and station of the fetal vertex should be rechecked by vaginal examination. In an outlet forceps procedure, the presentation will be cephalic; the sagittal suture will be in the anteroposterior diameter of the maternal pelvis, or no further than 45° in either direction. The occiput and posterior fontanel should be under the symphysis pubis. The head should be visible at the introitus without separating the vulva, and the presenting part should be at station +4 (e.g., 4 cm below the plane of the maternal ischial spines).

The locked forceps should be held outside the vagina, in front of the perineum, in the same position that they will occupy once applied to the fetal vertex (Figure 23.8); in the occipitoanterior position, both a perfect cephalic and an ideal pelvic application are possible. The forceps blades will be applied to the fetal vertex over the parietal bones bilaterally in an occipitomental application, with the concave edges of the blades toward the occiput. The left blade will be next to the left sidewall of the pelvis, and the right blade near the right side wall, with the concave edges pointing toward the pubis. The diameter of the forceps will be perpendicular to the sagittal suture, and in (or almost in) the transverse diameter of the pelvis (Figure 23.9).

The left forceps is inserted first. The handle is held in the left hand, near the mother's right groin. The fingers of the right hand are placed in the vagina between the fetal head and the left vaginal wall (Figure 23.10). The left blade is then inserted gently into the space between the fingers and the fetal head at about the 5 o'clock position. The handle is lowered slowly to the horizontal and toward the midline, while

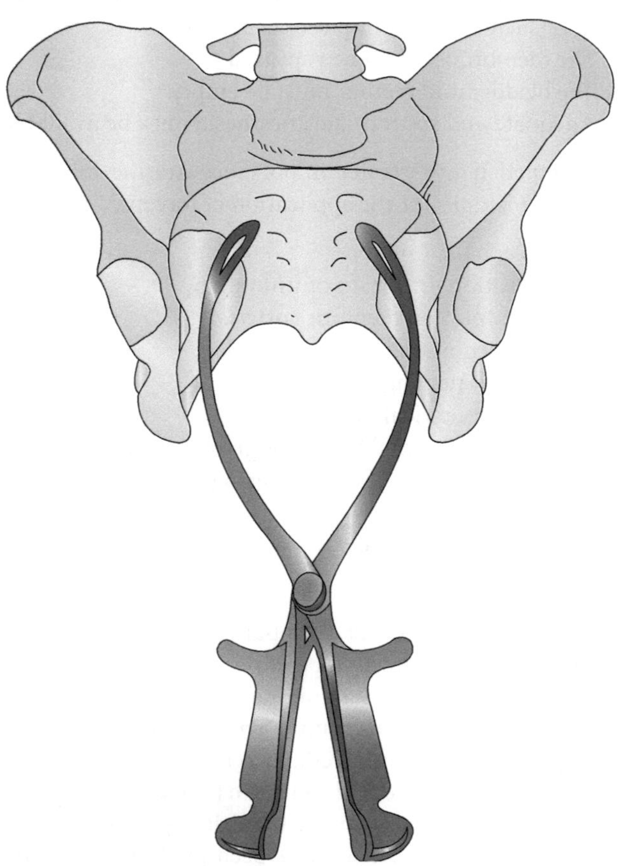

Figure 23.8 Contemplated application of the forceps in the transverse diameter of the pelvis. (Adapted from the original work of Ernst Bumm.)

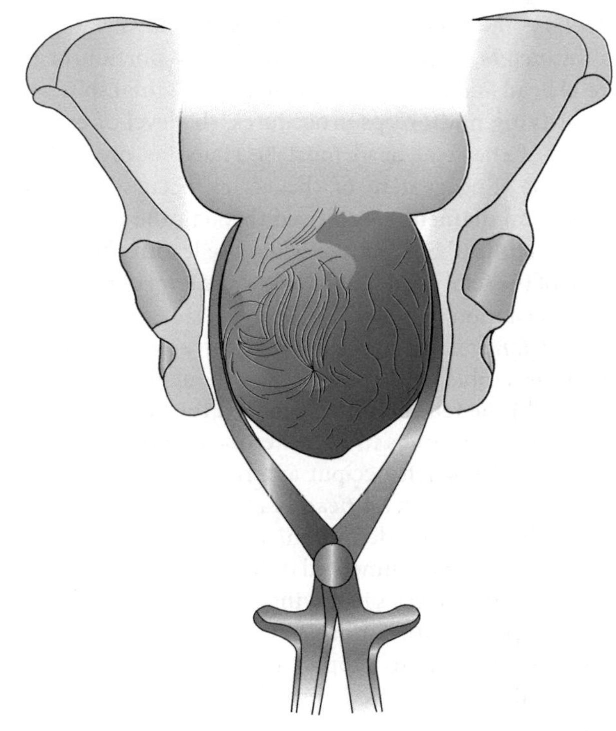

Figure 23.9 Actual application of the forceps in the transverse diameter of the pelvis. (Adapted from the original work of Ernst Bumm.)

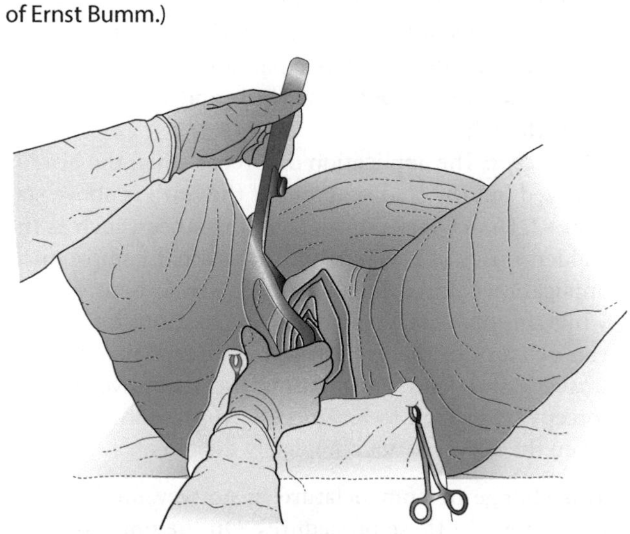

Figure 23.10 Introduction of the left blade in the course of application of the forceps. (From Burger K, *Operative Obstetrics*, Budapest, Hungary: Franklin Co, 1927.)

the blade is moved up by the fingers of the obstetrician's right hand over the left side of the fetal vertex toward an occipitomental application. When the obstetrician's fingers are removed, the forceps blade lies between the left parietal bone and the left pelvic wall. The forceps should be released by the operator and held in place by an assistant (Figure 23.11).

The right forceps blade is grasped in the right hand and held with the handle near the mother's left groin. The fingers of the left hand are inserted in the right side of the vagina between the fetal head and the vaginal wall. The right blade is inserted over the left blade, between the obstetrician's fingers and the fetal vertex, at about the 7 o'clock position (Figure 23.12). The handle is lowered to the horizontal and toward the midline, while the blade is moved up by the fingers of the obstetrician's left hand to an occipitomental position. When the obstetrician's fingers are removed, the forceps blade lies between the right parietal bone and the right pelvic wall (Figure 23.13). The forceps blades now are locked (Figure 23.14); if applied correctly, locking is easy; the handles must never be forced together (Figure 23.15).

As a routine, the fetal heart rate should be checked. The patient should be reexamined vaginally to be certain that nothing lies between the forceps and the fetal head, including umbilical cord, cervix, or fetal membranes. The application of the forceps must be rechecked. If the blades are a little off center, with one blade nearer the occiput and the other closer to the fetal face, the forceps must be unlocked and the blades repositioned. Now a gentle traction on the forceps should result in a slight advance of the vertex (Figure 23.16).

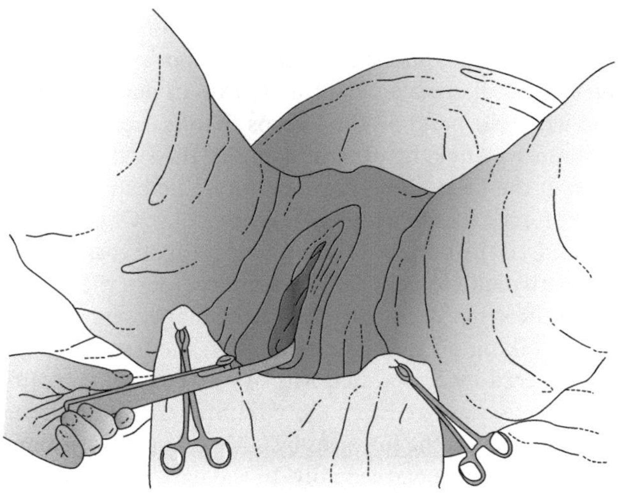

Figure 23.11 The left blade is in position and is held by an assistant. (From Burger K, *Operative Obstetrics*, Budapest, Hungary: Franklin Co, 1927.)

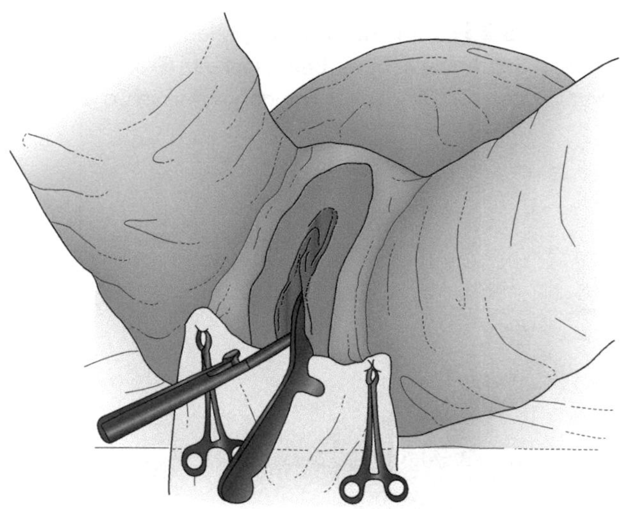

Figure 23.13 The position of the right blade following introduction and before the locking of the forceps. (From Burger K, *Operative Obstetrics*, Budapest, Hungary: Franklin Co, 1927.)

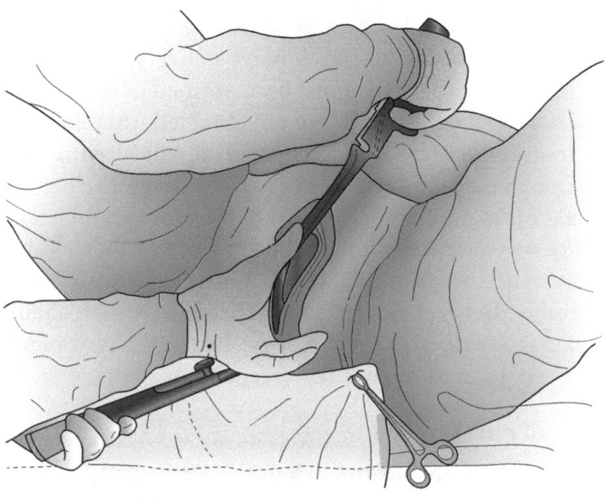

Figure 23.12 Introduction of the right blade. (From Burger K, *Operative Obstetrics*, Budapest, Hungary: Franklin Co, 1927.)

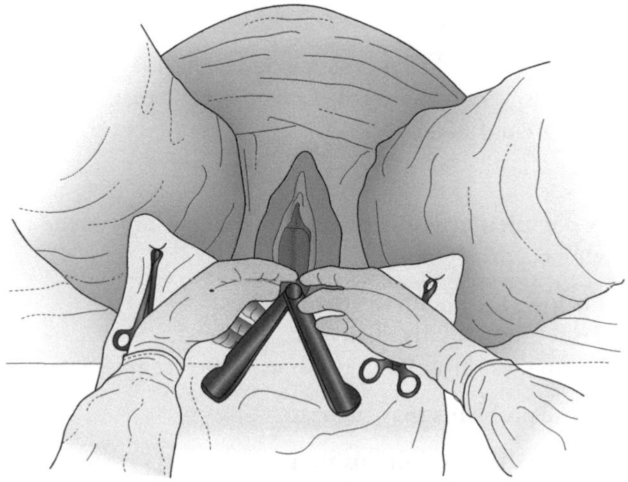

Figure 23.14 Locking the forceps after the two planes have been brought into the same plane. (From Burger K, *Operative Obstetrics*, Budapest, Hungary: Franklin Co, 1927.)

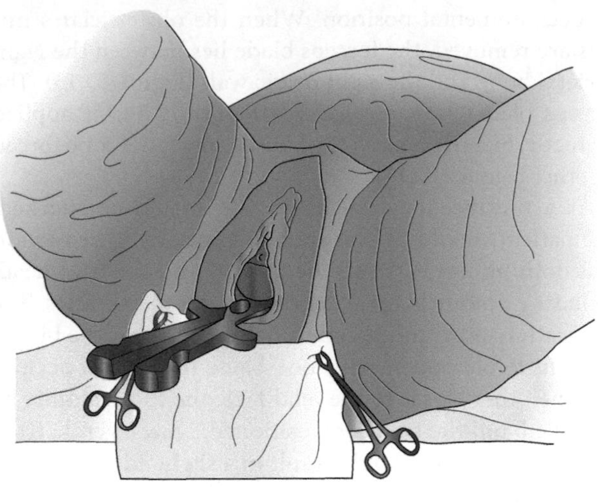

Figure 23.15 With the blades applied in the biparietal diameter, the forceps have been locked. (From Burger K, *Operative Obstetrics*, Budapest, Hungary: Franklin Co, 1927.)

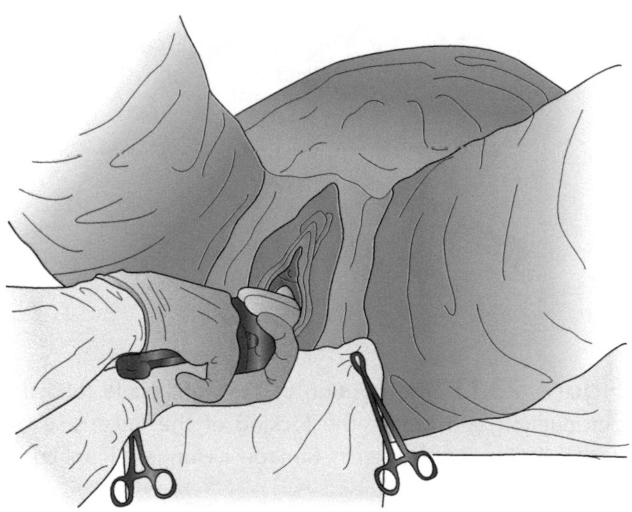

Figure 23.16 Traction is applied. Note the positions of the hands. (From Burger K, *Operative Obstetrics*, Budapest, Hungary: Franklin Co, 1927.)

A complete reassessment must ensue if any of the following occur:

1. Locking is difficult or impossible.
2. Trial traction fails to advance the head.
3. Vaginal examination reveals as incorrect application.

These problems may suggest

1. Wrong diagnosis of position
2. Incorrect application of forceps
3. Previously unrecognized cephalopelvic disproportion (including fetal macrosomia—the point to anticipate and prevent subsequent shoulder dystocia)
4. Cervical tissue between the blades and the fetal head (cervix incompletely dilated)
5. Uterine constriction ring

If the foregoing criteria are satisfied, the operator may proceed to extract the head. The operator may sit on a stool and grasp the forceps with both hands, one on the handles and the other on the shanks. The ends of the handles must never be compressed. Traction is applied intermittently at about 1- to 2-minute intervals for about 30 seconds. Between periods of traction, the forceps blades must be unlocked to relieve compression on the fetal head. The fetal heart should be auscultated after each traction. If possible, traction should be made during a uterine contraction and with the patient bearing down. The direction of traction must follow the birth canal (Figure 23.17). Initially, the pull should be outward and toward the rectum until the occiput comes under the symphysis and the nape of the neck pivots in the subpubic angle. In this maneuver (Saxtorph-Pajot's maneuver), the operator's hand on the forceps handles makes the traction in an outward direction while the hand on the forceps shanks exerts pressure posteriorly. After the occiput is under the symphysis, the birth of the head follows by extension and can be guided by the forceps before removal (Figure 23.18). Once the face has cleared the perineum, the forceps slip off easily. As an alternative, the forceps may be removed once the head is under the symphysis by reversing the maneuvers of application, taking off the right blade first; the head then can be delivered by a modified Ritgen's maneuver; removing the forceps early reduces the circumference of the part passing through the introitus by 0.50–0.75 cm, which may be of significance occasionally. In the past, almost all primigravidas and most multiparas had an episiotomy performed before forceps delivery. In the most recent *ACOG Practice Bulletin on Operative Vaginal Delivery*[24] and supported by a randomized trial published by Murphy et al.[40] routine episiotomy is now *not* recommended for all operative deliveries but a selected use at the judgment of the obstetrician. The decision to use a midline or mediolateral incision is discussed elsewhere in this text.

At the conclusion of any forceps delivery, the vagina, cervix, vulva, and uterus must be examined to rule out the presence of lacerations. If any are detected, they must be repaired unless they are too superficial, not bleeding and will not cause a cosmetic defect. To evaluate further the success of the forceps delivery, the operator should examine the newborn infant and record in the medical record any evidence of trauma as well as a detailed delivery note, preferably dictated as a surgical procedure, which should include the reason for the forceps delivery, the type of forceps used, lacerations and repair, episiotomy etc.

Low and mid-forceps

Delivery from any position when the fetal vertex is above the pelvic floor as indicated above, but particularly when rotation of the vertex is required, carries a degree of fetal and maternal risk which is a quantum jump removed from

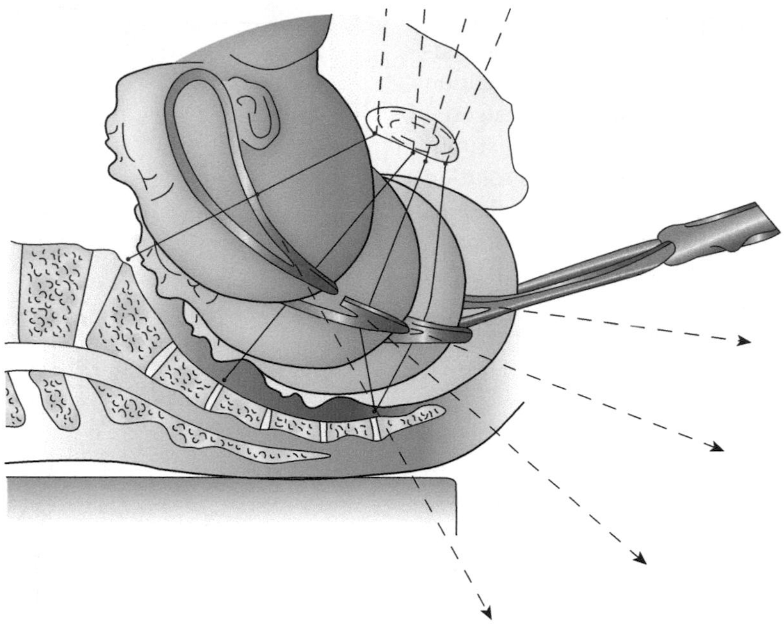

Figure 23.17 Direction of the traction in various forceps procedures. (From Hale R. (ed.), *Dennen's Forceps Deliveries*, Washington, DC: American College of Obstetricians & Gynecologists, 2001.)

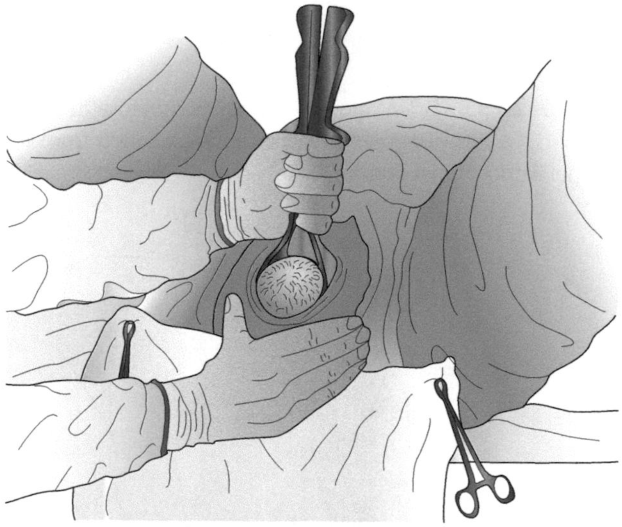

Figure 23.18 Delivery of the head with the use of forceps. In most clinical situations, this maneuver is preceded by episiotomy. (From Burger K, *Operative Obstetrics*, Budapest, Hungary: Franklin Co, 1927.)

delivery by outlet forceps. A more detailed analysis of the problem is required.

Assessment of pelvic dimensions and architecture

Pelvic capacity and configuration are critical determinants of obstetric management[41] even when clinical evidence suggests weak uterine contractility (e.g., secondary uterine inertia). In the presence of relative cephalopelvic disproportion, the arrest in labor usually will occur with the head at the +2 station or higher. If there has been considerable molding, the position of the presenting part may be obscured, and the level of the leading point not helpful. In such cases, even with the leading point of the vertex at station +2, the biparietal diameter still may be above the pelvic inlet and the fetal head not engaged. The pelvic architecture may determine the position of the vertex and dictate the options for delivery. In a platypelloid (flat) pelvis, the transverse position may be the normal mechanism of delivery until the vertex is crowning. In an android pelvis, the persistent straight sacrum and converging pelvic side walls may inhibit anterior rotation of the occiput. It would be folly to attempt to rotate the vertex into pelvic diameters that are even less suitable for passage. In the anthropoid pelvis, on the other hand, rotation to an occipitoanterior position brings the fetal vertex into an alignment with pelvic dimensions best suited for vaginal delivery.[41] In all types of pelvic architecture, it is important to remember that convergence of the pelvic side walls and/or the anteroposterior diameters may result in relative cephalopelvic disproportion in the midpelvis even though the pelvic inlet was adequate; in combination with the tendency for a parturient to deliver babies of increasing weight in successive pregnancies, this results in the infamous "multiparous trap" where the incorrect "assumption of success" delays the correct obstetrical intervention. These points must be clarified before the obstetrician takes instruments in hand for a forceps delivery.

Assessment of uterine and abdominal forces

Once the question of cephalopelvic disproportion has been eliminated, failure to progress in labor—to accomplish internal anterior rotation and to descend in the pelvis—results primarily from weak expulsive forces, stemming either from a secondary uterine inertia or inability of the abdominal musculature to contribute to the expulsive efforts. Failure of abdominal expulsive efforts may be the result of inborn or acquired conditions (e.g., poliomyelitis, spinal cord transection) or iatrogenic intervention (e.g., excessive maternal sedation, conduction analgesia) and maternal exhaustion. In such circumstances, stimulation of uterine contractions by an intravenous solution of oxytocin, with all of the precautions and stipulations ordinarily followed in such cases, is preferable to forceps delivery. In most cases, this will accomplish the desired results—anterior rotation of the occiput, and descent of the vertex in the pelvis—ending either with spontaneous vaginal delivery or delivery by outlet forceps with minimal rotation.

In some patients, the resistance of the pelvic floor (the levatorani muscle) is diminished because of inborn or acquired maternal neuromuscular defects, prior over distention as in the grand multipara, or injudicious iatrogenic intervention. In such patients, full flexion and internal anterior rotation of the occiput may be delayed until the vertex is at the pelvic floor and crowning. Pelvic floor inadequacy, in addition to pelvic architecture, may also result in rotation of the occiput into a direct posterior position. Delivery by forceps or spontaneously as a direct occiput posterior is preferable to any forceps rotation.

Delivery in occipitoanterior position

Delivery from an occipitoanterior position requires maneuvers similar to those described under outlet forceps (Figures 23.19 and 23.20). Because the vertex is higher in the pelvis, the risk to both infant and maternal tissues is increased—compression of the vertex resulting from traction and laceration of un-distended maternal structures. The actual delivery will take longer; thus, the fetal heart rate must be monitored after each tractive effort. With the head above the pelvic floor, it is more difficult manually to apply traction in the direction of the pelvis axis (e.g., the curve of Carus) consistently. Saxtorph-Pajot's maneuver, described above under outlet forceps, may not suffice, and the utilization of a mechanical method of providing axis traction is helpful. Such instruments include the Bill handle,[8] which can be attached to any standard forceps possessing transverse projections at the junction of the handles with the shanks; forceps such as the DeWees, in which the axis traction handle is a structural part of the forceps themselves; or forceps such as the Hawk-Dennen, in which the shape of the instrument's shanks places the handles in the axis of the maternal pelvis.

Delivery from an occipitotransverse position

Except when the maternal pelvis has an anthropoid or android configuration, the fetal vertex engages in and descends through the maternal pelvis most frequently in an occipitotransverse position. On abdominal examination, this position is suggested by the presence of a longitudinal fetal lie, with the vertex at or in the pelvis; the fetal back is directed laterally, toward the mother's flank; the fetal small parts are palpable on the opposite side of the maternal abdomen; the cephalic prominence (forehead)

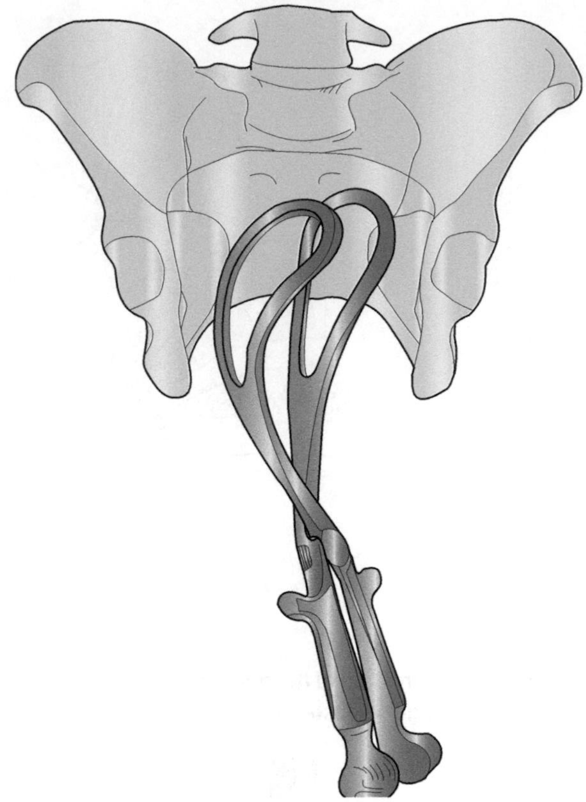

Figure 23.19 Orientation of the forceps before its application in the left oblique pelvic diameter. (Adapted from the original work of Ernst Bumm.)

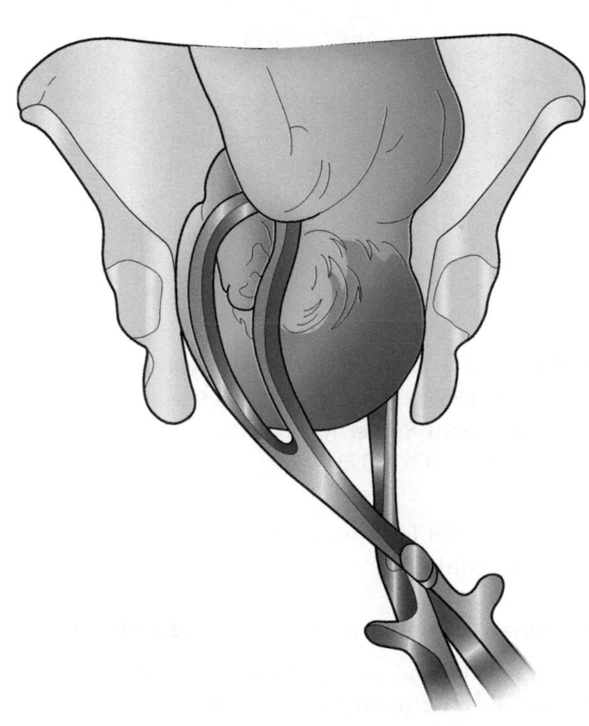

Figure 23.20 Actual application of the obstetric forceps in the left oblique diameter of the maternal pelvis. The position of the fetal head is left occipitoanterior (LOA). (Adapted from the original work of Ernst Bumm.)

is on the same side as the fetal small parts; and the fetal heartbeat is heard on the same side of the maternal abdomen as the fetal back. On vaginal examination, the sagittal suture is in the transverse diameter of the maternal pelvis (or within a few degrees thereof). The small posterior fontanel is on the same side as the fetal back—toward the mother's left in a left occiput transverse (LOT) position, and toward the mother's right in a right occiput transverse (ROT) position. The anterior fontanel and bregma lie on the opposite sides of the maternal pelvis. If the vertex is well flexed, the occiput is lower than the brow; if flexion is poor, the occiput and sinciput lie almost at the same level in the pelvis.

The normal evolution of an occiput transverse position is a result of the resistance of the pelvic floor to further downward descent of the vertex; there is an anterior rotation of the occiput of 90° (clockwise for ROT, counterclockwise for LOT), followed by delivery as an occiput anterior. Occasionally, no rotation occurs, and the vertex is arrested with the sagittal suture in the transverse diameter of the pelvis; infrequently, the occiput rotates posteriorly by 90° into an occiput posterior position. The diagnosis of transverse arrest can be made when there is a failure to rotate from the transverse position and to descend further in the pelvis for approximately one hour in the primigravida and for 30 minutes in the multipara. At this point, the patient and the labor must be reevaluated.

In patients in whom relative cephalopelvic disproportion has been ruled out, there are no problems of pelvic architecture, and stimulation of uterine contractions has not resulted in spontaneous evolution of the transverse position, manual maneuvers may facilitate anterior rotation of the occiput. Classically, persistent transverse arrest has been the major obstetric indication for forceps delivery.

Deep transverse arrest can be managed by any conventional type of forceps. Since rotation must be accomplished, instruments with long, overlapping shanks are preferable; forceps with separated and parallel shanks may unduly stretch or tear the maternal perineal and vaginal tissues. An instrument with a sliding lock is useful if any degree of asynclytism is present. The anterior forceps blade must be applied first to prevent elevation of the fetal vertex, which may result in encroachment of the more limited space in the anterior pelvic segment and possibly significant loss of station. A cephalic application is achieved by wandering the anterior blade over the face, and applying the posterior blade directly into the hollow of the sacrum. The handles of the forceps then are locked, and the application checked against the landmarks of the fetal skull. Rotation is performed by sweeping the handles in a wide arc of 90° to the symphysis (clockwise in the ROT position, counterclockwise in the LOT position). Rotation of the forceps handles through this wide arc is essential because of the pelvic curve of the conventional instrument. If the handles were merely twisted on their axis, the toes of the forceps blades would describe a wide and potentially injurious arc; moving the handles in a wide arc instead makes the toes of the blades the central axis of rotation. Once rotation is accomplished, the position of the fetal head must be rechecked to be certain that the sagittal suture has remained in the midline of the forceps; if necessary, the forceps application may be readjusted. Traction and extraction of the infant then are carried out as described previously.

Rotation of the fetal vertex must be achieved without the use of undue force. A well-molded vertex jammed forcefully into the deep pelvis may require slight elevation to facilitate easier rotation (Bill's maneuver), but care must be taken not to lose station significantly or to disengage the head. Resistance to rotation also may result from lack of full flexion of the vertex. Forceful rotation introduces shearing forces upon the fetal skull, whose deleterious effects are impossible to judge. It is the height of clinical acumen and experience to understand when excessive force is required for rotation and/or traction, to desist from further forced manipulation (trial forceps), and to move to delivery by cesarean section.

Special instruments have been designed to deal with special problems in transverse arrest.[14,42] The *Kielland's forceps* were designed specifically to facilitate biparietal application to the fetal vertex in any pelvic diameter and for rotation. Kielland's design eliminated the pelvic curve and provided a sliding lock for correction of asynclytism. They are the forceps of choice in cases of deep transverse arrest in the patient with a gynecoid or anthropoid pelvis. They should not be used in a patient with an android or platypelloid pelvis where further descent of the vertex in the transverse position is desirable. Kielland's forceps must never be used for traction before rotation in an occipito-transverse position! In such an instance, the anterior blade of the forceps rests directly against the base of the bladder, and vesicourethral injuries are easily produced.

The classic inversion technique of applying the anterior blade of the forceps was described originally by Kielland himself[14] and was designed to utilize the advantage in a tight pelvis of the triangular space in the lower uterine segment between the fetal shoulder and the vertex. The forceps must be oriented externally in the final position they will assume after application; markers on the forceps handles point toward the occiput. The anterior branch then is inverted and, with manual guidance, the blade is inserted along the anterior parietal bone inside the cervix and uterus, the cephalic side of the blade superior. (Since the blade is inverted, at this step the directional marker on the handle points toward the anterior fontanel.) The blade is inserted gently into the uterus until resistance is met and the forceps branch begins to turn spontaneously. Rotation of 180° toward the face, taking advantage of the curve of the blade, is performed by rotating the handle; the shank of the blade is in the axis of rotation. After rotation is completed, the blade drops against the anterior parietal bone in cephalic application. The posterior blade is inserted against the hollow of the sacrum, again with manual, intravaginal guidance to be certain there is no cervix between the blade and the vertex. Once a biparietal application is attained, the branches are locked; in the process, any asynclytism present is corrected. The application is checked with the landmarks of the fetal skull. Since Kielland's forceps have no significant pelvic curve, rotation can be performed in a limited arc, turning the vertex 90° to an occipitoanterior position. Once rotation is completed, Kielland's forceps have fulfilled their primary function, and the delivery may be completed by removal of the Kielland's forceps and application of a conventional instrument. Traction and extraction may be completed with Kielland's forceps if it is recognized that the forceps have no pelvic curve, and that extraction from midpelvis requires traction directed 45° or more below the horizontal plane of the pelvis.

Potential problems with this classic insertion technique include trauma to maternal tissues (especially the lower uterine segment), placental insertion site, and the umbilical cord. There must be no attempt to move the forceps during insertion against resistance. During the inverted insertion and rotation of the anterior blade, the arc traversed by the toe of the blade against the anterior lower uterine segment easily is palpable just above the symphysis of the mother. Problems such as this have resulted in the preference of some obstetricians for application of the anterior blade with the wandering technique (as with conventional forceps). Although this avoids the risks of intrauterine insertion and manipulation of the anterior blade, it sacrifices the very advantage that Kielland proposed in cases of deep transverse arrest which have occurred because of reduced transverse diameters of the pelvis.

The remaining problem in the occipitotransverse position is the case of transverse arrest in a platypelloid pelvis, in which the normal evolution of labor requires descent of the vertex in the transverse position to the introitus. *Barton's forceps* are the only obstetric instrument extant that can be used to apply traction to the vertex in a transverse position (Figure 23.21). The anterior blade, which is hinged to facilitate application to the anterior parietal bone under the symphysis pubis, is introduced into the hollow of the sacrum and wandered over the occiput to a position over the anterior parietal bone. If there is marked posterior asynclytism, the anterior blade may be inserted directly over the anterior parietal bone. The posterior blade then is inserted, with manual intravaginal guidance, along the hollow of the sacrum, and the branches are locked. Traction with Barton's forceps can be applied safely only with the use of Barton's traction handle, which

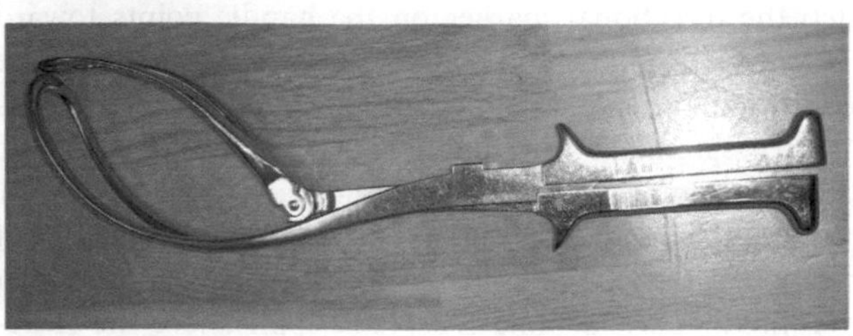

Figure 23.21 Barton's forceps with hinged anterior blade and traction handle.

is an integral part of the forceps, and which ensures that the resultant forces applied will be in the direction of the pelvic axis and not against the base of the bladder. In some patients, the vertex actually may deliver in the transverse position. Usually, when the vertex is under the pubic arch and beginning to crown, spontaneous rotation toward an occiput anterior position begins and can be assisted by a 90° rotation of the forceps handles in a wide arch. At this low level in the pelvis, spontaneous delivery usually ensues as soon as the forceps blades are removed.

Delivery from an occipitoposterior position

Occipitoposterior positions occur in about 15% of vaginal deliveries. Cephalopelvic disproportion is a frequent and serious complicating factor. Persistent occipitoposterior position may occur in any pelvis with a reduced transverse diameter and may be the normal mechanism of labor and delivery in an anthropoid and android pelvis. An occipitoposterior position also may result from the presence of prominent ischial spines, reduced capacity of the forepelvis, convergence of the lateral

Pelvic side walls, and a straight sacrum—all factors that inhibit anterior rotation. On abdominal examination, the presence of an occipitoposterior position is suggested by the presence of the fetal back in the maternal flank, often not clearly defined; fetal small parts filling the anterior maternal abdomen; a cephalic prominence which cannot be appreciated clearly; and a fetal heart that is auscultated most clearly on the side of the maternal abdomen opposite to the fetal back. On vaginal examination, the sagittal suture is in an oblique diameter of the maternal pelvis. The small fontanel is posterior, either to the right (ROP) or to the left (LOP); the anterior fontanel and bregma are in the opposite quadrants of the pelvis. Because failure of deep flexion is a concomitant of persistent occipitoposterior positions, the fontanels usually are at about the same level in the pelvis. In occipitoposterior positions, molding of the vertex results in some shortening of the occipitofrontal diameter and lengthening of the mentobregmatic diameter as the vertex becomes elongated. The diagnosis of position on vaginal examination may be obscured by molding and caput formation that mask the landmarks of the fetal skull; confirmation of position may require locating and identifying the pinna of the fetal ear and perhaps sonography.

The natural evolution of an occipitoposterior position in most cases is spontaneous internal anterior rotation of 135° to an occipitoanterior position, which occurs after the pelvic floor is reached and deep flexion established. In some cases, the occiput rotates in a small arc of 45° into the hollow of the sacrum, becoming a direct occipitoposterior position. Spontaneous delivery or extraction by forceps can occur from either position.

Indications for intervention in patients with persistent occipitoposterior position[42,43] of the fetus include absence of descent and prolonged second stage of labor. If there is evidence of cephalopelvic disproportion, cesarean section is indicated. For attempted operative vaginal delivery, the adequacy of the bony pelvis must be known, and a plan for extraction made out in advance. When the transverse diameters of the bony pelvis are reduced, as in an anthropoid or android pelvis, the vertex should not be rotated into or through less favorable pelvic dimensions but should be extracted as an occipitoposterior position. Techniques of manual rotation of the vertex are useful only when the head has reached the pelvic floor and the bony pelvis is clinically adequate.

A greater variety of instruments and procedures have been devised for the management of occipitoposterior positions than for any other malposition; only a few remain applicable in a modern context.[41–45] The simplest procedure is to deliver the vertex in a direct occipitoposterior position without any attempt at rotation. If the head is on the pelvic floor and beginning to distend the introitus, conventional outlet forceps may be used. A biparietal application of the forceps is accomplished, with the concave edges of the blades directed toward the face. Forceps with long, tapering blades and an ovoid cephalic curve can best accommodate the accentuated molding of the skull; Simpson's or Elliott's forceps are well suited for this purpose. Traction is made posteriorly to draw the sinciput beneath the pubic arch. As the handles of the forceps are raised, the occiput is borne over the perineum by increased flexion of the vertex. This is one of the clinical scenarios where an episiotomy may be necessary to permit passage of the larger diameters of the head which present in this position. The nose, face, and chin then are borne under the symphysis by extension of the head.

Kielland's forceps have a special utility as a rotator if needed. The directional markers on the handles must point toward the fetal occiput, so the forceps are applied in an inverted position with respect to the maternal pelvis. The blades are inserted with a wandering technique, the posterior blade always being applied first to prevent further posterior rotation of the occiput. The shanks of the blade form the axis of rotation, which is accomplished with pronation or supination of the forearm. Once an occipitoanterior position is attained, delivery may be carried out by substitution of a conventional forceps or by exerting traction with Kielland's forceps, bearing in mind that the forceps have no pelvic curve and that traction must be directed 45° or more below the horizontal plane of the pelvis.

Midforceps

Under the modern definitions of forceps deliveries, midforceps are forceps operations in which the leading point of the head is above station +2. By implication, since the leading point of the unmolded vertex is 3 cm ahead of the largest plane of the head, the biparietal diameter, that diameter has barely entered the bony pelvic inlet. With any significant degree of molding, there exists the probability that the fetal vertex is not truly engaged, and that this represents a "high-forceps" maneuver, which is proscribed. In these cases, the margin for error is very small. If any chance of a "high-forceps" situation exists, a more prudent course of action is to proceed directly to abdominal delivery by cesarean section.

Forceps delivery of an aftercoming head in breech presentation

The potential problems of vaginal delivery of a breech presentation in a current context have been reviewed in detail elsewhere.[46–48]

Though almost any obstetric forceps can be employed for the delivery of the aftercoming head, classic forceps, such as Simpson's or Elliott's, lack the advantage of a perineal curve and therefore tend to accentuate extension of the fetal body and neck, potentially increasing the risk of fetal injury. Forceps that have a perineal curve, such as the Hawks–Dennen instrument, or that have a compensated pelvic curve, such as Kielland's forceps, can be employed for this purpose. However, since its introduction, the standard instrument for delivery of the aftercoming head has been the forceps designed by Piper.[49,50] This instrument (Figure 23.22) is longer than the usual forceps, its handles are depressed below the arch of the shanks, the pelvic curve is reduced, and the shanks are long and curved. The tapered, shallow blades, with a spring-like quality, make for an easy application and a good fit to the vertex. More recently, the modified Piper's forceps were introduced; the newer instrument is somewhat shorter, and the conventional handles are replaced by a pivot lock and finger grips (Figure 23.23).

Forceps can be applied to the aftercoming head of the breech **only** after the shoulders and arms have been delivered and the head, with chin posterior, is well into the pelvis; the forceps must never be applied to a vertex above the pelvic brim. The principles of forceps delivery of an aftercoming head are three:

1. The forceps are inserted and applied from below upward;
2. The application is pelvic rather than purely biparietal; and
3. The mechanism of extraction is flexion of the fetal head, which is accomplished by elevating the handles of the forceps.

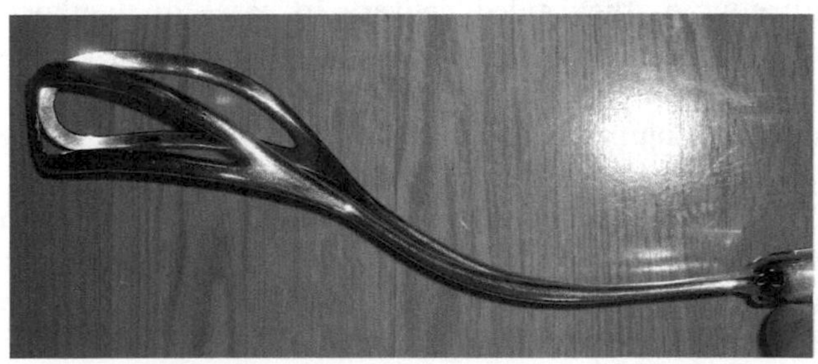

Figure 23.22 Piper's forceps.

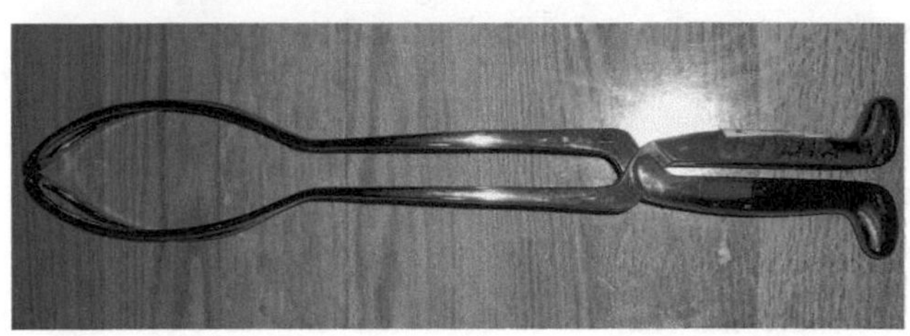

Figure 23.23 Piper's modified forceps.

Once the shoulders have been delivered, the baby's body is supported by an assistant and elevated slightly, but not to an extent that would hyperextend the neck. Vaginal examination should reveal the vertex deep in the pelvis, with the long axis of the head in the anteroposterior diameter of the pelvis; the occiput is anterior and the face (mentum) is posterior. The lower and upper limbs and the umbilical cord are kept out of the way. The left branch of Piper's forceps always is inserted first; this will permit locking of the branches without recrossing. The obstetrician assumes a position below the plane of the pelvic outlet, often kneeling on one knee. The handle of the left blade is grasped in the left hand, and the right hand is introduced between the hand and the left posterolateral wall of the vagina. The left blade is then inserted between the head and the fingers into a mento-occipital application, with the concave edge of the blade toward the occiput and the convex edge toward the face. The handle of the left blade is steadied by the assistant. The handle of the right blade is grasped in the right hand, and the left hand is introduced into the vagina between the head and the right posterolateral wall of the vagina. The right blade is inserted between the head and the fingers into a mento-occipital application. The forceps then are locked, and the application checked. Traction is outward and posterior until the nape of the neck is in the subpubic angle. The direction of force is then changed to outward and anterior, and the face and forehead are borne over the perineum by a process of flexion. Delivery usually is completed with the forceps still applied as the handles rise above the horizontal plane. Care must be exercised to prevent the head from dropping from between the blades as it is extracted.

CONTEMPORARY VIEW OF FORCEPS DELIVERY

Alternatives to forceps delivery

The utilization of obstetric forceps easily can be justified in an historic context. When obstetric forceps first were introduced, they aided delivery in cases of desultory, obstructed, or prolonged labor. They were employed primarily to salvage the mother, often with the recognition that fetal injury or demise would result. At that time there was no acceptable alternative to vaginal delivery.

Today, the risk of maternal mortality from a cesarean delivery is less than the mortality rate associated with appendectomy; cesarean delivery is safer the earlier in labor it is performed; and it is incontrovertible that the safest method of delivery for the infant is an elective cesarean section at term before the onset of labor or rupture of the membranes (eliminating iatrogenic errors of prematurity with modern diagnostic techniques).[51]

This fact is confirmed from the outcomes of the trial of labor after cesarean section study publications.[52,53]

Risk of forceps delivery

Maternal risks

The maternal risks of forceps delivery were recognized from their inception. Maternal injuries may include vaginal lacerations, episiotomy extensions, perineal and anal sphincter damage[54–56] bladder or urethral injuries, cervical tears, uterine rupture, and/or ureteral disruption. The primary cause of the most severe of these injuries was the high-forceps application and extraction, which has been proscribed for many years. The major problem area remains the low-forceps operation. Attempts have been made to distinguish in advance between "easy" and "difficult" procedures, not always successfully.

Fetal risks

The fetal risks of delivery by obstetric forceps are acceptable only in the context of greater maternal harm from any alternative. It is clear that these fetal risks, including facial bruising and lacerations, cephalohematomas, facial nerve paralysis, skull fractures, and intracranial tears and hemorrhages[57–70] occur primarily in low-forceps operations with rotations and in midforceps operations.

There is a consensus that outlet forceps delivery imposes no burden on the infant.[24,27] The assumed benefits of routine prophylactic forceps originally proposed in the past are not pertinent in this modern era. In contrast, forceps applied to the aftercoming head in breech delivery may be conducive to a reduction of perinatal mortality and morbidity,[59] probably because traction is applied to the skull rather than the shoulders or neck of the infant, and sudden decompression injury is prevented by a gradual and controlled delivery.

Current status of forceps delivery

Over fifty years ago, a trend toward the elimination of delivery by midforceps was already under way.[71] Although there have been dissenters to this transformation in obstetric practice,[71,72] the trend continued and has increasingly been accepted.[73–75] Midforceps operations carry significant risks for mother and infant. The risks for the mother of abdominal delivery by cesarean section probably are not greater and may be reducible by earlier intervention and improvements in clinical procedures. There is no comparison as to the safety of the infant at cesarean section. The process is becoming more inevitable with the declining opportunities for training in forceps techniques. Maximum safety for mother and infant rests in the hands of experienced providers of delivery services. The changing parameters of obstetric management in labor must be recognized, and should be accepted for the progress they denote. The rational application of obstetric forceps today should be reserved for the operations of outlet forceps, low forceps without rotation, and forceps delivery of the after coming head during a breech vaginal delivery.

High-forceps deliveries were proscribed decades ago. Midforceps delivery is disappearing from obstetric practice today. Low-forceps operations involving more than 45° rotation from the vertical axis may follow into oblivion shortly, its disappearance hastened by our litigious contemporary society.

In today's climate, the application of forceps purely as a training exercise is not indicated and cannot be countenanced. Even obstetricians already adequately trained in forceps delivery will lose their proficiency with the markedly reduced number of opportunities for operative vaginal deliveries unless educational opportunities are made available. The development of high fidelity operative delivery simulators and innovative educational curriculum such as developed by the ACOG Simulation Consortium may allow for a new generation of obstetricians proficient in operative deliveries as well as continued proficiency training for obstetricians already trained but needing repetition. In the future, operative delivery simulators may be used for primary education of obstetrical residents as well as recertification and credentialing.

ACKNOWLEDGMENT

This chapter contains material from the previous edition chapter coauthored by Joseph J. Rovinsky and Anthony Caggiano.

Video 23.1 Forceps-assisted vaginal delivery: reviving a lost obstetric art: https://goo.gl/OY05Kp.

REFERENCES

1. Menacker F, Hamilton, B. Recent trends in cesarean delivery in the United States. *NCHS Data Brief, No* 2010; (35): 1–8.
2. Martin JA, Hamilton BE, Osterman MJ, et al. Births: Final data for 2015. *Natl Vital Stat Rep* 2015; 64; 1–65.
3. Solt I, Jackson S, Moore T, et al. Teaching forceps: The impact of proactive faculty. *Am J Obstet Gynecol* 2011; 204(5): 448.e1–448.e4.
4. O'Mahoney F, Hofmeyer GJ, Menon V. Choice of instruments for assisted vaginal deliveries. *Cochrane Database Syst Rev* 2010; (11): CD005455.
5. Landis H. *How to Use the Forceps: With an Introductory Account of the Female Pelvis and the Mechanism of Delivery.* New York, NY: EB Treat, 1880.
6. Hale R (ed.). *Dennen's Forceps Deliveries.* Washington, DC: American College of Obstetricians & Gynecologists, 2001.
7. O'Grady JP. *Modern Instrumental Delivery.* Baltimore, MD: Williams & Wilkins, 1988.
8. Laufe LE. *Obstetric Forceps.* New York, NY: Hoeber Medical Division, Harper & Row, 1968.
9. Speert H. The obstetric forceps. *Clin Obstet Gynecol* 1960; 3: 761–6.
10. Bill AH. A new axis traction handle for solid blade forceps. *Am J Obstet Gynecol* 1925; 9: 606.
11. DeWees WB. New axis traction obstetric forceps. *JAMA* 1892; 19: 32.
12. Dennen EH. A new forceps with a traction curve. *Am J Obstet Gynecol* 1931; 22: 258.
13. Burger K. *Operative Obstetrics.* Budapest, Hungary: Franklin, 1927.
14. Kielland C. Über die Anlegung der Zange am nicht notierten Kopf mit Beschriebund eines neuen Zangermodelles und einer neuen Anlegungsmethode. *Monatsschr Geburtshilfe Gynak* 1916; 43: 48.
15. Laufe LE. Divergent and crossed obstetric forceps. Comparative study of compression and traction forces. *Obstet Gynecol* 1971; 38: 885–7.
16. Barton LG, Caldwell WE, Studdiford WE Sr. A new obstetric forceps. *Am J Obstet Gynecol* 1928; 15: 16.
17. Parry-Jones E. *Barton's Forceps.* Baltimore, MD: Williams & Wilkins, 1972.
18. Luikart R. A modification of the Kielland, Simpson, and Tucker–McLane forceps to simplify their use and improve traction and safety. *Am J Obstet Gynecol* 1937; 34: 686.
19. Laufe LE. A new divergent outlet forceps. *Am J Obstet Gynecol* 1968; 101: 509–12.
20. Seidenschnur G, Koepcke E. Fetal risk in delivery with the Shute parallel forceps. Analysis of 1503 forceps deliveries. *Am J Obstet Gynecol* 1979; 135: 312–17.
21. Davidson AC, Weaver JB, Davies P, et al. Relation between ease of forceps delivery and speed of cervical dilatation. *Br J Obstet Gynaecol* 1976; 83: 279–83.
22. Quilligan EJ, Zuspan F. *Douglas-Stromme's Operative Obstetrics* (4th edition). New York, NY: Appleton-Century-Crofts, 1982.
23. Dennen EH. A classification of forceps operations according to station of the head in the pelvis. *Am J Obstet Gynecol* 1969; 103: 470.
24. American College of Obstetricians and Gynecologists. Technical Bulletin. Operative vaginal delivery. No. 154, November 2015.
25. AAP Committee on Fetus and Newborn and ACOG Committee on Obstetric Practice. *Guidelines for Perinatal Care* (7th edition). Washington, DC: American Congress of Obstetricians and Gynecologists, 2012.
26. Nyirjesy L, Pierce WF. Perinatal mortality and maternal morbidity in spontaneous and forceps vaginal deliveries. *Am J Obstet Gynecol* 1964; 89: 568–78.
27. Broman SH, Nelson KB. Perinatal risk factors in children with serious motor and mental handicaps. *Ann Neural* 1977; 2: 371.
28. Cardozo LD, Gibb DMF, Studd JW, Cooper DJ. Should we abandon Kielland's forceps? *BMJ* 1983; 287: 315–17.
29. Dierker LJ, Rosen MG, Thompson K et al. The mid-forceps: Maternal and neonatal outcomes. *Am J Obstet Gynecol* 1985; 152: 176–83.
30. Healy DL, Quinn MA, Pepperell RJ. Rotational delivery of the fetus: Kielland's forceps and 2 other methods compared. *Br J Obstet Gynaecol* 1982; 89: 501.
31. O'Grady JP. *Modern Instrumental Delivery.* Baltimore, MD: Williams & Wilkins, 1988.
32. Miller E, Barber E, McDonald K, Gossett D. Association between obstetrician forceps volume and maternal and fetal outcomes. *Obstet Gynecol* 2014; 132(2): 248–54.

33. Richardson DA, Evans MI, Cibils LA. Mid forceps delivery: A critical review. *Am J Obstet Gynecol* 1983; 145: 621–32.
34. Traub Al, Morrow RJ, Ritchie JWH, Dornan KJ. A continuing use for Kielland's forceps? *Br J Obstet Gynaecol* 1984; 91: 894–8.
35. Nilsen ST. Boys born by forceps and vacuum extraction examined at 18 years of age. *Acta Obstet Gynecol Scand* 1984; 63: 549–54.
36. Chow SLS, Johnson CM, Anderson TD, et al. Rotational delivery with Kielland's forceps. *Med J Aust* 1987; 146: 616–19.
37. Burke N, Field K, Mujahid F, Morrison JJ. Use and safety of Kielland's forceps in current obstetric practice. *Obstet Gynecol* 2012; 120: 766–70.
38. Committee on Obstetrics. *Maternal and Fetal Medicine: Obstetric Forceps.* Washington, DC: ACOG, 1988, 1989.
39. DeLee JB. The prophylactic forceps operation. *Am J Obstet Gynecol* 1920; (1): 34.
40. Murphy DL, Macleod M, Goyder K, et al. A randomized control trial of routine versus restrictive use of episiotomy at operative vaginal delivery. A multicenter pilot study. *BJOG* 2008; 115: 1697–1702.
41. Feldman DM, Borgida AF, Somer F, et al. Rotational versus non-rotational forceps: Maternal and neonatal outcomes. *Am J Obstet Gynecol* 1999; 181: 1185–7.
42. Bill AH. The treatment of the vertex occiput posterior position. *Am J Obstet Gynecol* 1931; 26: 215.
43. DeLee JB. The treatment of the occiput posterior position after engagement of the head. *Surg Gynecol Obstet* 1928; 46: 696.
44. Krivak TC, Drewes P, Horowitz GM. Kielland vs. nonrotational forceps for the second stage of labor. *J Reprod Med* 2003; 44: 511–7.
45. King EL, Herring JS, Dyer I, King JA. The modification of the Scanzoni rotation in the management of persistent occipitoposterior positions. *Am J Obstet Gynecol* 1951; 61: 872–80.
46. Milner RDG. Neonatal mortality of breech delivery with and without forceps to the aftercoming head. *Br J Obstet Gynaecol* 1975; 82: 783–5.
47. Rovinsky JJ. Abnormalities of position, lie, presentation, and rotation. In: Iffy L, Kaminetzky HA (eds), *Principles and Practice of Obstetrics and Perinatology*, p. 907. New York, NY: Wiley, 1981.
48. Swartjes JM, Bleker OP, Schutte MF. The Zavanelli maneuver applied to locked twins. *Am J Obstet Gynecol* 1992; 154: 623.
49. Piper SB, Bachman C. The prevention of fetal injuries in breech delivery. *JAMA* 1929; 92: 217.
50. Laufe LE. An improved Piper forceps. *Obstet Gynecol* 1967; 29: 284–6.
51. O'Driscoll K, Foley M. Correlation of decrease in perinatal morbidity and increase in cesarean section rate. *Obstet Gynecol* 1983; 61: 1–5.
52. Landon MB, Hauth JC, Spong CY, et al. Maternal and perinatal outcomes associated with trial of labor after prior cesarean delivery. *NEJ* 2004; 16; 351(25): 2581–9.
53. ACOG Practice Bulletin No. 115, *Vaginal Birth after previous Cesarean Delivery.* Washington, DC: ACOG, 2015.
54. Bradley MS, Kaminski RJ, Streitman DC, et al. Effects of rotation on perineal lacerations in forceps assisted vaginal deliveries. *Obstet Gynecolo* 2013; 122(1): 32–7.
55. Ballard RC, Gardiner A, Duthie H, et al. Anal sphincter fecal and urinary incontinence: A 34-year follow-up after forceps delivery. *Dis Colon Rectum* 2003; 46: 1083–1088.
56. Chan SS, Cheung RY, Yiu LL, et al. Prevalence of levator ani muscle injury in Chinese priparous women after first delivery. *Ultrasound Obstet Gynecol* 2011.
57. Chiswick ML, James DK. Kielland's forceps: Association with neonatal mortality and morbidity *BMJ* 1979; 1: 7–9.
58. Cook WAR. Evaluation of the midforceps operation. *Am J Obstet Gynecol* 1967; 99: 327.
59. Stock SJ, Josephs K, Farquharson S, et al. Maternal and neonatal outcomes of successful Kieiland's rotational forceps delivery. *Obstet Gynecolo* 2013; 121: 1032–9.
60. Memon H, Blomquist J, Dietz H, et al. Comparison of levator ani muscle avulsion injury after forceps assisted and vacuum assisted vaginal birth. *Obstet Gynecol* 2015; 125(5): 1080–6.
61. Werner EF, Janevic TM, Illuzzi J, et al. Mode of delivery in nulliparous women and neonatal intracranial injury. *Obstet Gynecol* 2011; 118: 1239–46.
62. Evers EC, Blomquist JL, McDermott KC, Handa VL. Obstetrical and anal spinctor laceration and anal incontinence 5–10 years after childbirth. *Am J Obstet Gynecol* 2012; 207: 425.
63. Gei AF, Smith RA, Hankins GD. Brachial plexus paresis associated with fetal neck compression from forceps. *Am J Perinat* 1999; 20: 289–91.
64. Hellmann J, Vannucci RC. Intraventricular hemorrhage in premature infants. *Semin Perinatol* 1982; 6: 42–53.
65. Hepner WR. Some observations on facial paresis in the newborn infant: Etiology and incidence. *Pediatrics* 1951; 8: 494–7.
66. Mann LL, Carmichael A, Duchin S. The effect of head compression on fetal heart rate, brain metabolism, and function. *Obstet Gynecol* 1972; 39: 721–6.
67. O'Driscoll K, Meagher D, MacDonald D, Geoghegan F. Traumatic intracranial haemorrhage in firstborn infants and delivery with obstetric forceps. *Br J Obstet Gynaecol* 1981; 88: 577–81.
68. Painter MJ, Bergman I. Obstetrical trauma to the neonatal central nervous system and peripheral nervous system. *Semin Perinatol* 1982; 6: 89–104.
69. Rubin A. Birth injuries: Incidence, mechanisms, and results. *Obstet Gynecol* 1964; 23: 218–21.

70. Cohen WR. Influence of the duration of second stage of labor on perinatal outcome and puerperal morbidity. *Obstet Gynecol* 1977; 49: 266–9.
71. Danforth DD, Ellis AH. Midforceps delivery: A vanishing art? *Am J Obstet Gynecol* 1963; 86: 29–37.
72. de Vries B, Phipps H, Kuah S, et al. Transverse occiput position: Using manual rotation to aid normal birth and improve delivery outcomes. A study protocol for a randomized controlled trial. *Trials.* 2015; 16: 362.
73. Bowes WA Jr, Bowes C. Current role of the midforceps operation. *Clin Obstet Gynecol* 1980; 23: 549.
74. Nimmo RA, Murphy GA, Adhate A, et al. Factors affecting perinatal mortality in an urban center. *Natl Med Assoc J* 1991; 83: 147–52.
75. Park JS, Robinson JN, Norwitz ER. Rotational forceps: Should these procedures be abandoned? *Semin Perinat* 2003; 27: 112–20.

Vacuum-assisted vaginal delivery

24

ANNA LOCATELLI and ARMANDO PINTUCCI

CONTENTS

HISTORY

The use of a vacuum device to assist delivery was first attempted by James Yonge[1] in 1706, who attached a "cupping glass" to the fetal scalp by creating suction with an air pump. Simpson,[2] in Edinburgh, constructed a more practical suction instrument. His invention consisted of a pump that terminated in a metal cup over which a layer of leather was fitted. A double-valved piston pump working back and forth created the necessary vacuum.

Although this "suction tractor" was used by Simpson for both vertex and breech deliveries, it never gained much popularity, and it was later abandoned in favor of the forceps.

McCahey,[3] in Philadelphia, described an "atmospheric tractor" in which metal cups were attached to an air pump by tubing. Using a rubber suction cup reinforced with metal, Kuntzsch[4] delivered two infants; he was the first to introduce a pressure gauge into the system.

Torpin[5] developed a rubber plunger type of suction cup with a hollow rubber tube attached leading to a vacuum pump. The inner surface of this appliance was studded with rubber projections to prevent the fetal scalp from being sucked into the tubing and to aid the attachment of the rubber hemisphere to the fetal head. Castallo[6] produced a similar working model; however, both Castallo and Torpin used the instruments sparingly and never achieved great success with them.

Couzigou[7] described *la ventouse eutocique*, which used luminum cups ranging in diameter from 40 to 65 mm. His apparatus included a bottle between the vacuum cup and the pump to trap blood and amniotic fluid. Finderle's[8] horn-shaped instrument with traction handles was introduced in 1955. The cup was inserted into the vagina, and a terminal rubber cup was attached to the fetal head. Negative pressure of approximately 6 lbs (2.72kg) was produced by means of a 200- to 300-mL syringe. Between 1953 and 1957, Malmström developed a modification of the device. This device represents the current standard by which other vacuum extractors (VEs) are measured.[9,10] Shallow cups, varying in diameter, were constructed of stainless steel. The cups were flanged outward above the mouth so that the largest diameter was not at the opening proper, but, rather, higher in the interior of the cup.

In Malmström's department, the VE virtually took the place of the forceps. The experiences in other Continental

European, British, and Australian institutions were similar.[11–14]

Bird[15] modified the Malmström system by attaching the suction tube eccentrically, at the side of the cup dome, to allow for greater maneuver ability and more efficient traction by locating the traction chain at the center independently. An extensive review of the historical development of the VE may be found in Chalmers'[16] monograph and in Sjostedt's[13] review. Although the metal cup was quite successful in effecting vaginal delivery, concerns arose regarding the occurrence of serious lacerations to the scalp. This decreased the popularity of the VE. The development of soft cups was an attempt to decrease scalp injuries. Between 1969 and 1973, two plastic cups were introduced. The Kobayashi silastic cup is flexible and wide and almost completely covers the occiput.[17] This device does not require the formation of a chignon. The silastic cup has been proved to be less injurious to the fetal scalp[18]; however, it is associated with an increased failure rate,[19] especially in the setting of a synclitism or severe molding. By the end of the twentieth century, due to the high rate of failure rate, vacuum cup was manufactured using harder plastic. This was continued to be used widely.

COMPONENT INSTRUMENTATION

All current devices are based on Malmström's instrument. The Ventouse,[7] or VE, consists of several component parts. The cups are disk shaped. The convex surface of the disk is fitted with a hollow stem, which in turn communicates with the concave cavity (fetal surface) (Figure 24.1). The smooth shape of the cup diminishes the risk of trauma to the fetal scalp and facilitates sealing and the formation of an artificial caput succedaneum. This chignon, or button, is maximal inside the hemispheric walls above the cup edge (Figure 24.2). Rubber tubing attaches onto the stem located on the slightly convex surface of the cup (Figure 24.3). The second segment of rubber tubing extends to the inflow connection of the suction (trap) bottle. The third (final) section connects the outflows pigot of the suction bottle to the vacuum pump (Figure 24.4). A traction chain passes directly from the cup and is hooked onto a traction bar. The vacuum

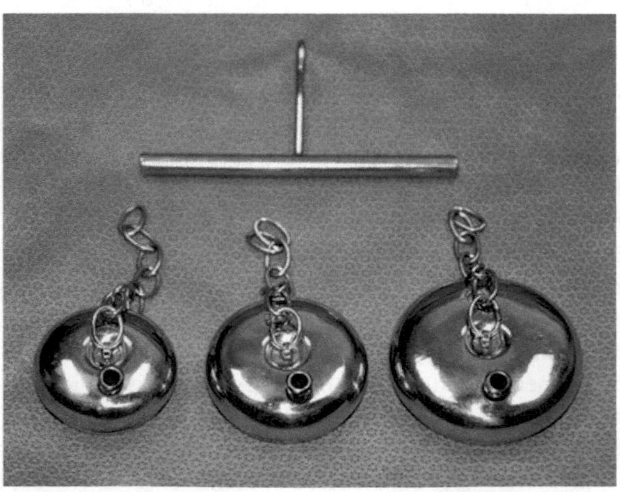

Figure 24.1 Malmström vacuum cups measure 4, 5, and 6 cm. The cups shown are made of stainless steel with the Bird modification, that is, eccentric fitting for suction tube attachment. The traction handle with hook couples directly to the cup chain.

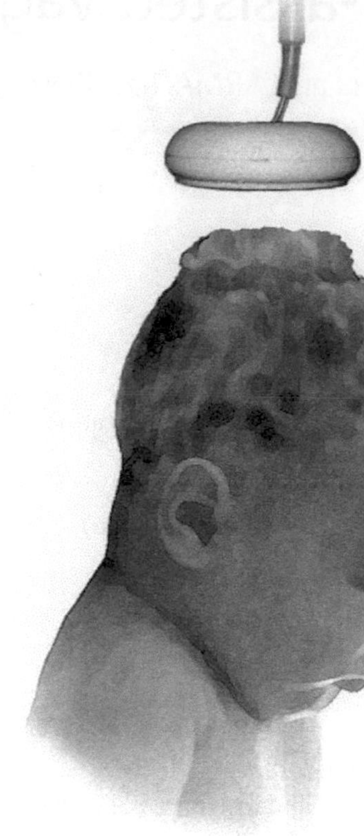

Figure 24.2 As suction is applied, a chignon, or button of scalp, is sucked.

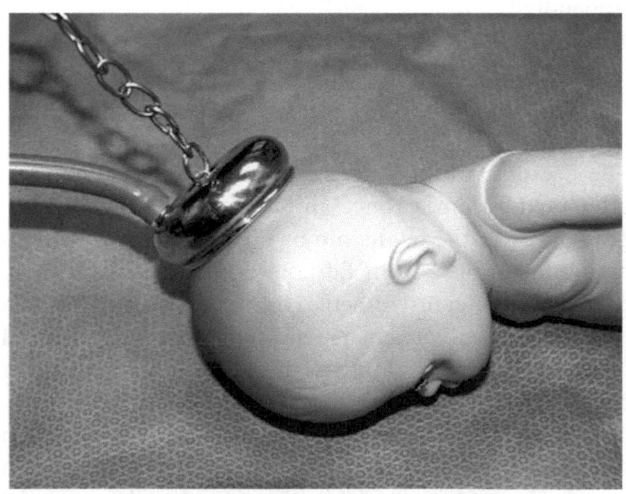

Figure 24.3 The 60-mm (6-cm) vacuum cup is attached to the head of a mannequin. The heavy-gauge tubing (left of image) is attached to a hollow stem on the convex surface of the cup. Traction is applied by the attached traction handle and transmitted to the chain and vacuum cup.

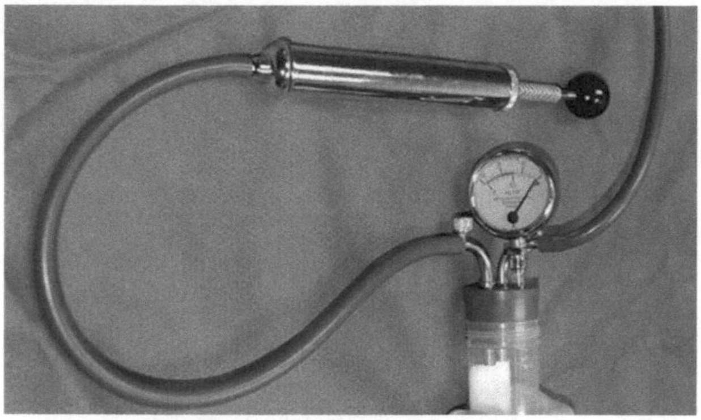

Figure 24.4 The tubing (see Figure 24.3) attaches to one of three fittings on a stopper, which in turn is plugged into a collecting jar. The three metal tubular fittings are as follows: (a) inlet that couples with tubing from the vacuum cup; (b) outlet with vacuum relief valve that couples with tubing leading to the hand vacuum pump; and (c) outlet to the vacuum-recording gauge.

tubing connects independently and eccentrically to a short-stem outlet built into the cup (Figure 24.3). A glass bottle is placed between the suction cup and the pump in order to collect blood, amniotic fluid, and other debris.

The bottle is sealed with a rubber stopper. The stopper is perforated by a gauge to record negative pressure (Figure 24.4). Current apparatuses use small hand pumps that connect disposable plastic cups and tubing with a filter that replaces the glass bottle. The Mityvac® device is an example of this (Figure 24.5). The cups could be semirigid or soft, mushroom shaped, or bell shaped. A disadvantage of this device is that the stem and cup are on a piece that is not very flexible, making proper application difficult in some cases. The Kiwi OmniCup® is a further modification; it is a disposable "all-in-one" instrument (Figure 24.6).

The plastic cup is rigid, mushroom shaped, and connected to a handle by tubing and a steel cable that runs through the tubing (Figure 24.7). This allows for flexibility and mobility of the cup similar to Bird's modification. The handle is integrated with a trigger that allows the operator to pump to a desired negative pressure. The pump on the handle contains the gauge and a pressure-release mechanism.

There is no ideal VE. In a randomized trial comparing Kiwi OmniCup and Malmström metal cup, Kiwi was associated with the same rate of success and a lower rate of subaponeurotic hemorrhage (1.0% vs. 1.2%).[20]

Some obstetricians use different type of VE according to the level of the presenting part, the fetal head position, and the level of difficulty of the procedure expected. A soft vacuum cup could be appropriate for low level deliveries because it is less traumatic for the scalp. Rigid cups may be preferable for occiput posterior (OP), occiput transverse (OT), and difficult occiput anterior deliveries because they are less likely to detach. As a rule of thumb, because the procedure is not frequent, a high level of confidence with the mean used is desirable, and sometimes our prediction of an easy procedure is not confirmed and so we suggest the use of the Kiwi OmniCup for all cases.

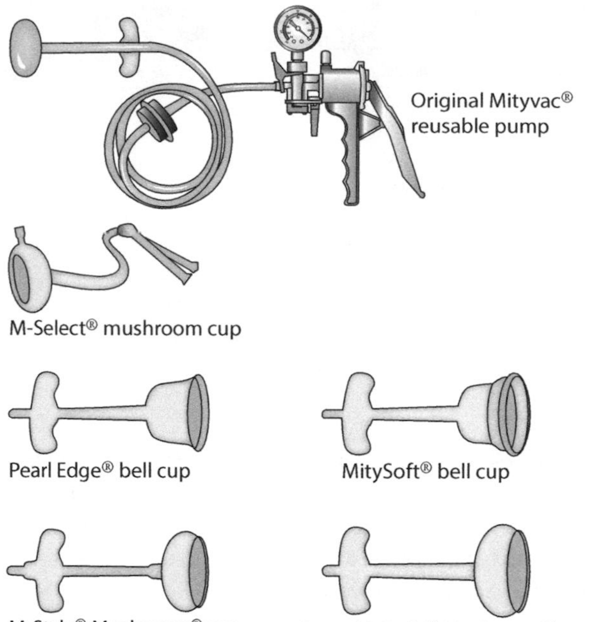

Figure 24.5 The Mityvac cup system is comprised of the reusable Mityvac pump and a variety of cup options. (Courtesy of Bacelar Equipamentos Medicos.).

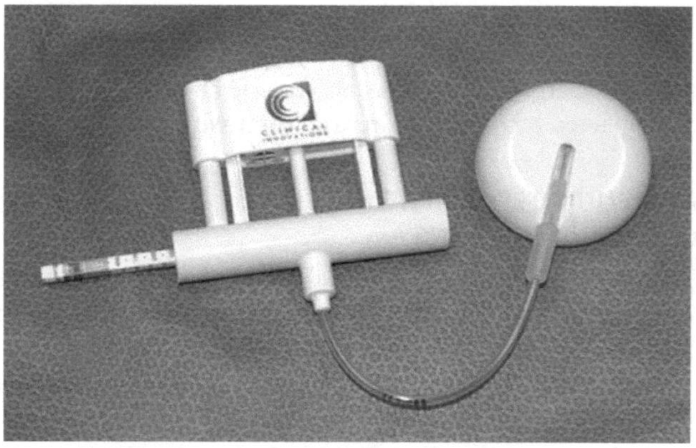

Figure 24.6 The Kiwi device has a Malmström-like cup attached to a combination handle and vacuum pump. The attachment is by flexible steel cable.

VACUUM USE

The objective of the operative vaginal delivery and of the vacuum use is to anticipate or allow a vaginal delivery with the minimum of morbidity. The decision to make an instrumental delivery should balance the maternal, fetal, and neonatal impact of the procedure against the alternative options of cesarean birth or expectant management.

The use of VE is largely variable across different countries and in the same country across hospitals, reflecting the assistance to the second stage of labor, including time allowed for pushing, use of fundal pressure, and the overall percentage of operative vaginal and abdominal delivery. In Italy, the rate of vaginal operative delivery is 3.4%, forceps use is uncommon, and the rate of cesarean delivery is as

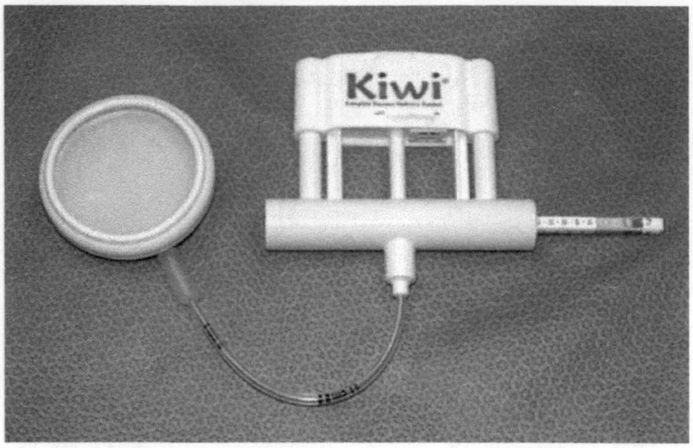

Figure 24.7 Same device as shown in Figure 24.6 with the cup reversed to show the interior. The cups, other than being constructed of plastic, are similar to Malmström cups. The vacuum pump handle of the Kiwi assembly is very convenient and includes a vacuum relief valve.

high as 38%. In other Europe countries, where the overall rate of vaginal delivery is higher, the use of VE is more frequent, e.g., in England the rate of VE is 7%, of forceps 3.3%, and of cesarean delivery 23%. In the United States, the overall rate of vaginal-assisted delivery is 3.3% (VE 2.7%, forceps 0.6%)[21] with a relevant decrease in the last years, corresponding to an increase of cesarean section (CS). Because a timely and reasonable rate of assisted vaginal delivery can avoid a CS in multiple clinical scenarios, its use should not be neglected by obstetricians and their patients.

PREREQUISITES, INDICATIONS, AND CONTRAINDICATIONS

The prerequisites for the use of the VE are listed in Table 24.1; the indications for the use of the VE are listed in Table 24.2.

Maternal indication is related to conditions that limit the desirability or ability to maternal effort or to maternal exhaustion that limits the effort and culminates in the need of assisted vaginal delivery. *Fetal indication:* Nonreassuring or abnormal fetal heart rate is a common indication, even if the indication is strictly dependent from the interpretation of the pattern and from the practice in the management of the second stage. Use of vacuum offers a shorter delivery with respect to CS, however, the obstetrician should consider that the combination between trauma and hypoxia is potentially dangerous. *Dystocia:* Time limits in the second stage at which point assisted delivery should be considered as not rigid, however, maternal and perinatal morbidity increase when the time is superior to 3 hours and the probability of spontaneous vaginal delivery is reduced.

American College of Obstetricians and Gynecologists' (ACOG) defined a prolonged second stage of labor as >2 hours without epidural analgesia or 3 hours with epidural analgesia in nulliparous women; and 1 hour without epidural analgesia or 2 hours with epidural analgesia for multiparous women.[22] In a document published in 2014

Table 24.1 Prerequisites for vacuum extraction.

Full cervical dilation
Ruptured membranes
Cephalic presentation
No cephalopelvic disproportion, estimation of fetal weight
Adequate pelvis
Station +2 or lower (engaged head)
Determination of fetal head position
Presence of experienced operator
Capability to perform a cesarean delivery
Willingness to abandon in case of failure
Empty bladder
Adequate anesthesia

Table 24.2 Indications for the use of the vacuum extractor.

Prolonged second stage of labor
Maternal conditions where voluntary expulsive efforts are contraindicated or impossible, such as cardiac, cerebrovascular, or neuromuscular disorders, overly dense epidural anesthesia
Fetal compromise

before diagnosing the arrest of labor in the second stage, if the maternal and fetal conditions permit, it is suggested to allow for the following: At least 2 hours of pushing in multiparous women and at least 3 hours of pushing in nulliparous women. Longer durations may be appropriate on an individualized basis (e.g., with the use of epidural analgesia or with fetal malposition) as long as progress is being documented.[22]

For a possible practical management of arrest/protraction of the second stage of labor in nullipara we propose the approach reported in a flow chart (Figure 24.8). For pluripara the overall time before a decision could be 2 hours, and oxytocin administered very cautiously if not previously used for induction or during the first stage of labor.

Contraindications to the use of the VE are listed in Table 24.3 and are the counterpart of the prerequisites for its application. There are no data in the literature that establish a safe lower limit of gestational age for use of the vacuum, since no trials have enrolled women for less than 34 weeks.

TECHNIQUES AND MANEUVERS

Forceps and vacuum are valid instruments for operative delivery and have similar indications.

In particular, forceps is the instrument of choice in face presentation (chin anterior) and for the delivery the after coming head after breech delivery; vacuum for the not-engaged second twin.

The choice of instrument is determined by the clinician's expertise. Vacuum delivery is generally less traumatic for the mother than forceps delivery, VE is easier to apply, places less force on the fetal head, requires less maternal anesthesia, is associated with less maternal soft tissue trauma, and

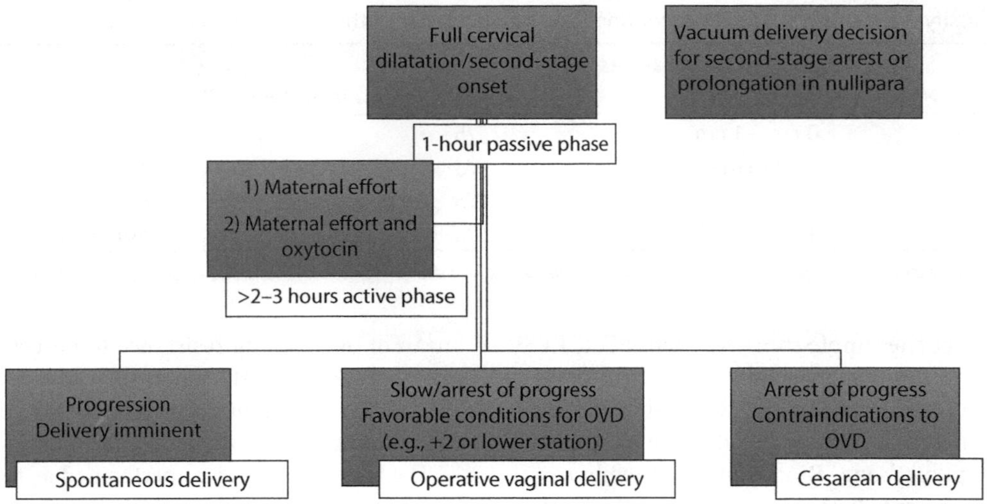

Figure 24.8 A practical management of arrest/protraction of the second stage of labor in nullipara.

does not compress the diameter of the fetal head. It does not take up additional space in the vagina.

It allows the fetal head to "seek its own space" rather than forcing its rotation. This "autorotation" can allow the fetal head to accommodate to the pelvis where the greatest space exists for exit.

The advantages of forceps are that they are unlikely to detach from the head during a difficult extraction, can be used on premature fetuses or to actively rotate the fetal head, result in fewer cases of cephalohematoma and retinal hemorrhage, and do not cause bleeding from scalp lacerations.

ACOG classification system for forceps deliveries is based on station and amount of rotation, which correlates with the degree of difficulty and risk of the procedure (e.g., lower fetal station and smaller degree of head rotation are associated with less risk of maternal and fetal injury).[23]

Vacuum deliveries do not have a separate classification system and the same classification can be adapted for its use (Table 24.4). A second classification is proposed by Vacca and based also on the abdominal evaluation of the level of the presenting part (Table 24.5).

Anesthesia

Because maternal cooperation is needed, the best results are obtained when uterine contractions and maternal bearing down efforts are combined with traction. Spinal or epidural anesthesia can be used but have the potential disadvantage of blocking maternal bearing-down reflexes. Local or pudendal blocks are usually adequate and in emergencies the vacuum can be used successfully in unanesthetized patients.

Standard procedure (with Kiwi OmniCup)

When a valid indication for vacuum delivery exists before the application a review of the history of the pregnancy and labor for factors that may influence the outcome of the vacuum should be made. For practical purposes it may

Table 24.3 Contraindications for the use of the vacuum extractor.

Operator inexperience
Inability to achieve proper application
Maternal refuse
Fetal prematurity (<34 weeks, although some recommend no <36 weeks)
Fetal scalp trauma or suspected fetal coagulation defects
Fetus with bone demineralization conditions
Incomplete cervical dilation
Cephalopelvic disproportion
Uncertain fetal head level and/or position
High station (i.e., higher than +2)
Prior failed forceps delivery

Table 24.4 Classification of operative delivery according to the level of the presenting part.

Outlet
The leading point of the fetal skull has reached the pelvic floor, and is at or on the perineum, the scalp is visible at the introitus without separating the labia.
The sagittal suture is in anteroposterior diameter or a right or left occiput anterior or posterior position.
Rotation does not exceed 45°.
Low
The leading point of the fetal skull is +2 cm beyond the ischial spines, but not on the pelvic floor (i.e., station is at least +2/5 cm)
Two subdivision
—Rotation ≤45°
—Rotation >45°
Midpelvis
The head is engaged (i.e., at least 0 station), but the leading point of the skull is not +2 cm beyond the ischial spines (i.e., station is 0/5 cm or +1/5 cm)

Source: Modified from Committee on Bulletins Practice—Obstetrics, *Obstet Gynecol*, 126, 1118–9, 2015.

Table 24.5 Classifying vacuum deliveries according to station and level of the head and visibility of the scalp.

Station of head	Level of the head respect to ischial spines	Fifths palpable abdominally	Visibility of the scalp
Mid-cavity vacuum	0 cm, +1 cm	1/5	Not visible
Low vacuum (a)	+2,+3 cm	0/5	Not visible
Low vacuum (b)	+3/+4 cm	0/5	Visible at introitus
Outlet	+5	0/5	Visible and distending introitus

Source: Modified from Vacca A, *Handbook of Vacuum Delivery in Obstetrics Practice* (3rd edition), Brisbane, Australia: Vacca Research, 2009.

be easy to remember the simple short acronym FORCEPS that includes all the variables to analyze.[24]: F as full cervical dilatation, O as only 1/5 or 0/5 head palpable abdominally and at vaginal visit engaged head using as referent ischial spines or pubic bone, R as ruptured membranes, C as contraction present, E as empty bladder, P as position known, and finally S as satisfactory analgesia. Before applying the cup, urinary catheters, fetal scalp electrodes, pulse oximeters, or any other device should be removed, especially if included in the cup. The level of the fetal head should be carefully assessed and the position of the fetal back and sinciput identified. Continuous fetal heart rate monitoring with external electrode is mandatory.

Before applying the vacuum, the position of the occiput and the exact localization of the flexion point should be achieved. The first step to identify the flexion point is to locate the posterior fontanel by moving the examining finger forward approximately 3 cm along the sagittal suture, so that the point can be marked. Figure 24.9 shows the correct application of the vacuum, while Figure 24.10 shows an incorrect application where the vacuum is located too anterior.

The cup insertion distance can be estimated by means of the first distance from the tip of the middle finger to the proximal interphalangeal joint and the second distance to the metacarpophalangeal joint. Prominent lines have been stamped on the suction tube of the Kiwi OmniCup at 6 and 11 cm, which corresponds, respectively, to the first and the second distance. The operator will find this information helpful to give an accurate indication of how far to insert the cup. At the time of insertion, the operator can lightly smear the outside of the cup with obstetric cream or oil, then should insert gently the cup through one single movement, retracting the perineum with two fingers to form a space into which the cup can be placed. Once the cup has passed through the introit it will automatically be pushed up against the fetal head by the maternal perineum. If the flexion point is displaced from the introitus region, as it could happen in OT or OP positions, a considerable additional maneuver should be required to achieve a correct application over the flexion point. The check if there is maternal tissue trapped between the cup and the scalp should be done later by moving the index finger around all the periphery of the cup.

When the operator has maneuvered the cup over the flexion point, the recommended vacuum pressure of 60–80 kPa (450–600 mmHg) may be attained in one step. The traction with the vacuum should be regarded as an adjunct to expulsive forces of labor and not as the primary mean of overcoming resistance to descent. Therefore, the traction should be started at the onset of a mother's contraction and be maintained smoothly for the duration, synchronously with the mother's expulsive efforts.

The traction should be performed as two-handed exercise with both hands working in unison, one providing the traction (the " pulling hand") and the other monitoring the progress (the "nonpulling hand") (Figure 24.11). Moreover, the "nonpulling hand" can be useful to prevent complete detachment of the cup by exerting counterpressure with the thumb on the cup and mainly to monitor the completion of autorotation of the fetal head during the maneuver as it happens in OP and/or OT positions.

At the beginning of the procedure, the direction of the traction should be parallel to the birth canal with the handle of the cup as straight as possible. Subsequently, when the head advances down the birth canal the direction should be more anterior as far as possible to keep the head moving along the axis of the pelvis. Finally, when the head begins to crown, the direction should be changed to an upward direction with an angle of 45° to the horizontal line to enable extension of perineum's muscles and the birth.

Restriction in the number of pulls has been the principal safety mechanism recommended for avoiding injury to the new born during the vacuum extraction. The limit of "three pulls plus three pulls": three pulls for the descent phase and three pulls for the perineal phase have been adopted as a general, acceptable, and safety rule. The signs of a successful progression are descent of the presenting part, flexion of the head, and correction of asynclitism, autorotation in OP and OT positions. After delivery of the head, the vacuum is released, the cup is eased off the scalp, and the birth is completed in the classic normal manner.

All infants will retain a characteristic chignon or caput (Figure 24.12). As soon as possible after the birth the operator should palpate the area over the chignon to exclude subgaleal by tapping the scalp with the finger tips. With a check to the position of the chignon the operator can evaluate if the application of the vacuum was correct and is mandatory to evaluate for cervical or vaginal or fourth-degree lacerations. The documentation of the details of the procedure should be done, and the form proposed by RCOG can be used as a guide (Appendix I).[25]

The day after the delivery the operator should reexamine the baby in the mother's presence to answer questions and discuss the procedure. About 5% of women who have an operative vaginal delivery will have a second operative vaginal delivery.[26,27]

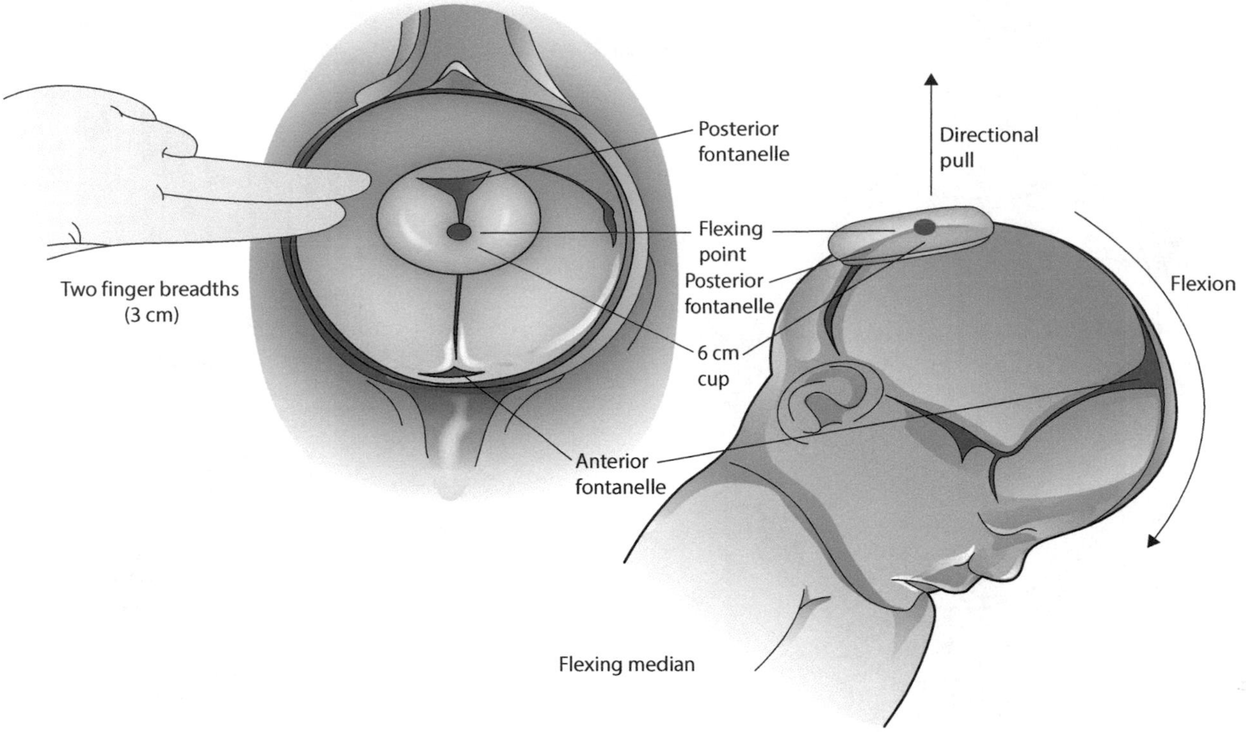

Figure 24.9 The cup is placed in the midportion of the sagittal suture and overlaps the posterior fontanelle. The center of the cup is two finger breadths forward of the posterior fontanelle. If the cup is properly positioned, traction will automatically produce flexion of the fetal head.

THE POSTERIOR CUP STANDARD PROCEDURE

Assisted vaginal delivery starting from an OT and/or OP fetal head position requires the finest clinical judgment.[24,28] The necessary rotation of OT and OP position increases the risks of maternal and fetal trauma. The technique for insertion of the vacuum is the same as for occipito-anterior position, but there are some differences on the techniques of applying the cup and exercising traction. Vaginal examination is similarly performed to confirm the flexion point and to estimate the cup insertion distance. In OP and OT positions, the fetal head is not visible. As a general rule, the operator should remember that the flexion point is at least 8 cm from the posterior furchette. Furthermore, in an obliquely OP position where the deflexion may be pronounced the insertion distance may be as much as 10 or 11 cm, therefore the operator should achieve during the insertion the maximum distance (Figure 24.13). When the cup has been applied a perpendicular direction of traction is frequently not possible to achieve with the initial pulls. For this reason, the operator should remember to apply an oblique angle to the cup in order to gain the axis traction. The oblique traction increases the risk of cup detachment; therefore, to prevent this complication the operator's thumb alone should be inserted into the vagina to press against the dome of the cup and obtain a counterpressure when the traction is applied.

The right application will result in the rotation of the head descending (autorotation) and at this time the traction should be directed in the line of the axis of the pelvis (Figure 24.14). No attempt should be made to complete the rotation of the cup manually or moving around because such maneuvers could dislodge the cup causing the detachment and increasing the risk of severe scalp lacerations. Another mistake could be to pull upward prematurely. In these fetal head positions the midpoint of the head is trailing approximately 6 cm behind the cup, so the fetal head will pivot around this point upward, and the traction should be delayed until the point emerged from beneath the pubic arch to maintain the correct axis of traction. The operator can observe the autorotation noting the shift in position of the groove on the surface of the OmniCup.

TRACTION FORCE AND DURATION OF THE PROCEDURE

When the fetal head passes through the birth canal, in a normal labor, the compression force acting depends on the friction between maternal tissues, the size of the baby, and the strength of the expulsive force. During the expulsive phase of a spontaneous labor, forces acting on the fetal head have been calculated to be between 8.4 and 15 kg. Many authors have tried to define what force constitutes a safe level of traction during an operative vaginal delivery and how long it should be applied but the difference between excessive, average, or minimum forces and limits in duration of traction actually depends on obstetrician's subjectivity. Petterson et al. suggested that obstetricians tend to underestimate the actual traction force applied and evaluated that no more than 2.5% of the operators,

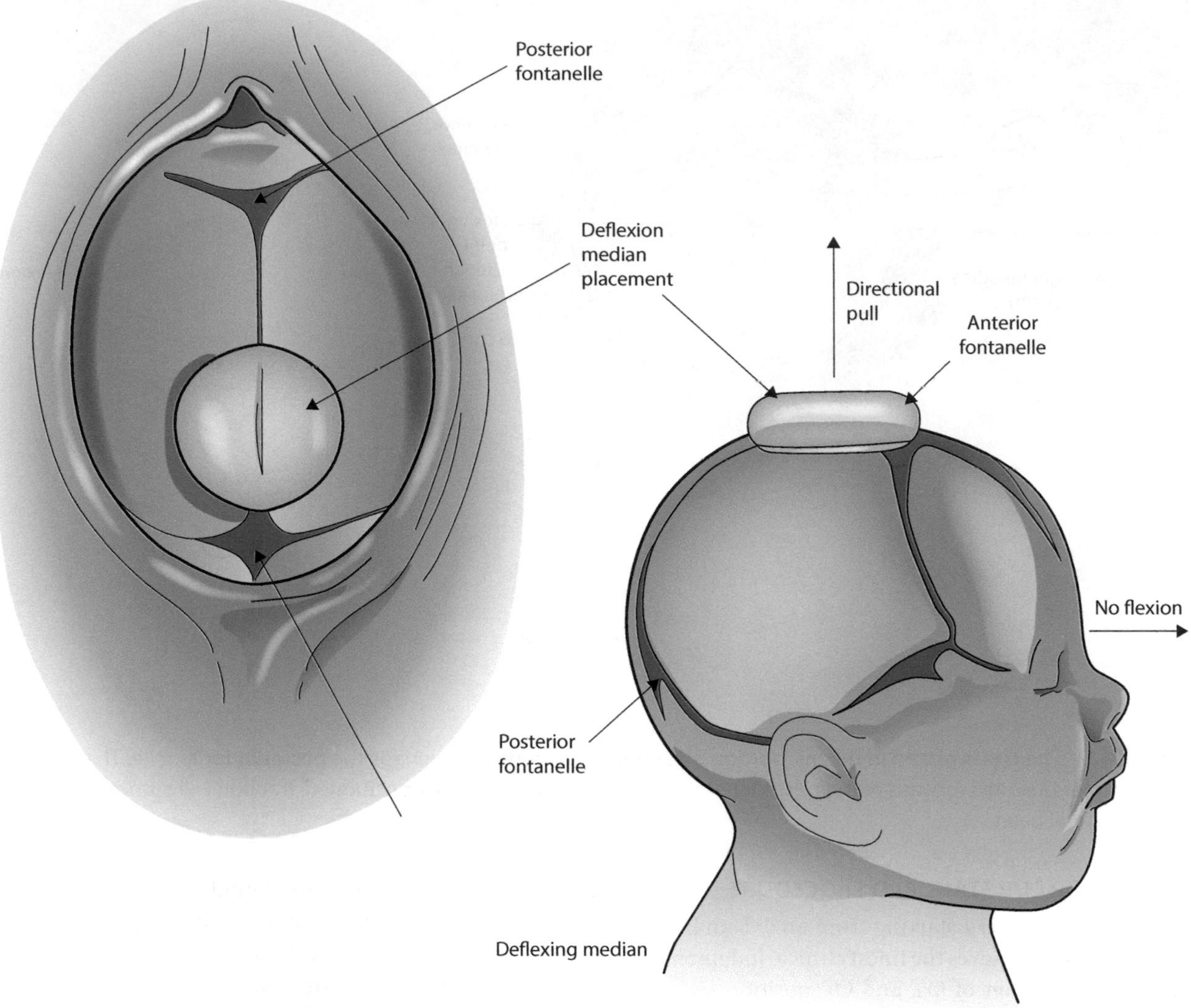

Figure 24.10 A cup placed too far anteriorly either in the midsagittal suture or farther toward the anterior fontanelle will with traction result in a deflexed or extended head.

regardless of experience, claimed to be aware of a maximum limit of the traction force to be used. A traction force of 225 N (corresponding to a mass equivalent of 23 kg) has been suggested as an upper safe limit for an operative vaginal delivery.[29]

Vacca et al. reported that a peak traction force <11.5 kg (equivalent to 113 N) would be sufficient in 80%–86% of vacuum extractions and instead reported a rate of 12% (3/24) of neonatal scalp abrasion and 16% (4/24) of cephalohematoma in infants delivered with traction that exceeded that limit, but there is no clear evidence of a relation between adverse neonatal outcome and high traction force employed. Vacca showed a high proportion of excessive traction force during the outlet phase.[30]

Petterson showed a decrease of force in the traction force employed with each successive pull.[29]

It is perhaps simplistic to talk about maximum traction force in isolation and not related to the duration of traction and the number of pulls. Many factors can be related to traction force and duration of the procedure: characteristics of the uterine contractions, epidural analgesia, operator's experience, parity, station, and position of fetal head. A significant increase in peak traction was noted in primiparous (209 N; confidence interval [CI] 63–452 N, $p < .05$) and in the case of OP position (335 N; CI 61–857 N, $p < .05$). Moreover, in the case of OP position there was an increased number of traction of pulls compared with those for occipital anterior (8 vs. 2). The average reduction of force is greater for minimum and average extraction compared with excessive vacuum extraction, and also the average time needed to reach the extraction is greater in the excessive compared with the average or minimum traction during the vacuum. If the duration of procedure is restricted to 15 minutes and the number of pulls is limited to three for descent phase and three for the perineal phase the vacuum-assisted vaginal delivery should be considered

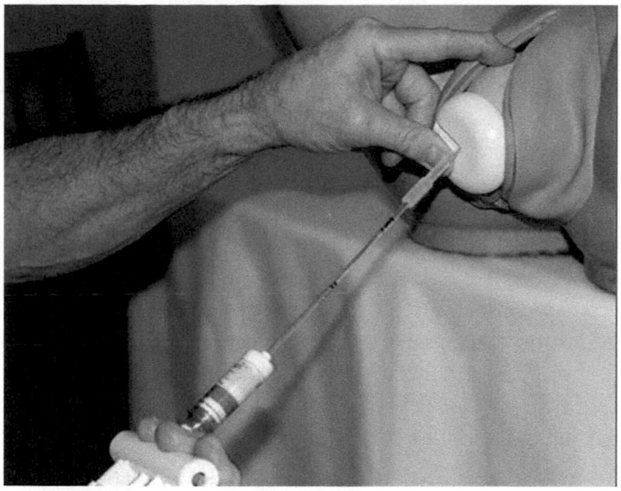

Figure 24.11 Prevention of cup detachment. (From Vacca A, *Handbook of Vacuum Delivery in Obstetrics Practice* (3rd edition), Brisbane, Australia: Vacca Research, 2009. With permission.)

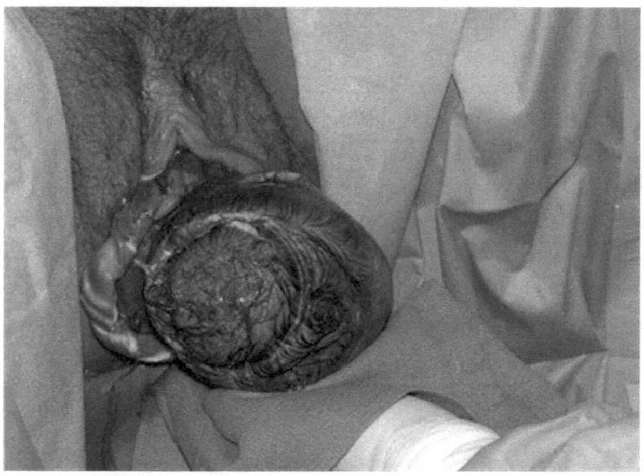

Figure 24.12 The cup has been removed. The cord has been released from around the baby's neck. Note the caput. The mother should be informed that the button is an expected result of the use of the vacuum device and will rapidly recede over 2–3 days.

relatively safe.[29,30] Unless the delivery is imminent, if the duration extends to or beyond 20 minutes the procedure should be discontinued and the baby delivered by CS.[24]

SPECIAL SITUATIONS

The vacuum instrument has special advantages, particularly for selected obstetric circumstances, including malpresentation, delivery of the second twin, and delivery at CS.

Malpresentation

Persistent OP position is the most common malposition of fetal head with an incidence ranging between 2% and 13%.[31] In a large series of OP and OT positions delivered by VE, the failure rate was 4% in each group.[32] OP positions rotated to the anterior in 96% of the cases and persisted in the remaining ones. For OT positions,

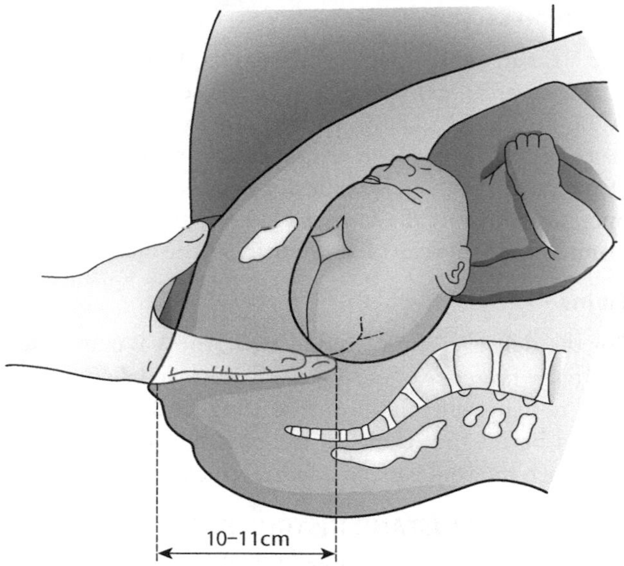

Figure 24.13 Insertion distance in posterior cup procedure. (From Vacca A, *Handbook of Vacuum Delivery in Obstetrics Practice* (3rd edition), Brisbane, Australia: Vacca Research, 2009. With permission.)

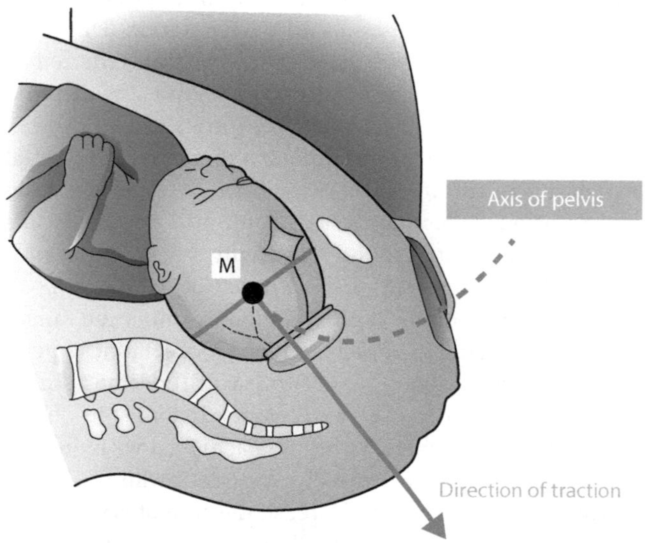

Figure 24.14 Rotation of the descending head in posterior procedure. (From Vacca A, *Handbook of Vacuum Delivery in Obstetrics Practice* (3rd edition), Brisbane, Australia: Vacca Research, 2009. With permission.)

96% also rotated anteriorly, 2% delivered faceup, and 2% persisted in the transverse. In a few cases, after VE rotation, forceps were used for delivery. The VE imposes no constraint to rotation, especially in the anthropoid pelvis. In the anthropoid pelvis, approximately one-third of the head rotates posteriorly when the traction is applied. While some authors do not view the vacuum favorably and prefer Barton's or Kielland's forceps formal positions of the fetal head,[33] others report that, if strict criteria are followed, the complication rate should approach zero when the VE is used.[34]

Cesarean section

The VE can be an effective adjunct to difficult extraction during cesarean delivery, e.g., in the presence of malpresentation or high presenting part or large myoma. The resistance of the uterine wound is less than that of the tissues of the birth canal, and the device takes less space than the operator's hand or the forceps blades. This approach could minimize in some cases the extension of the uterine incision.

Twins

For the delivery of the second twin, the VE may be useful in the presence of cord prolapse, delayed delivery with head not engaged, and nonreassuring fetal heart rate; VE should be the first choice if the obstetrician is not confident with internal version and breech extraction.

ULTRASOUND (US) AND INSTRUMENTAL DELIVERY

Correct diagnosis of fetal head position is a prerequisite for safe instrumental vaginal delivery. Suboptimal instrumental placement is associated with postpartum hemorrhage (odds ratio [OR] 1.94), increased risk of prolonged hospital stay (OR 2.28) and neonatal trauma (OR 4.25), and a greater use of sequential instruments (OR 3.99) and CSs after a failed attempt of instrumental delivery (OR 3.81).[35] Factors associated with suboptimal placement are fetal head malposition and mid-cavity station. Diagnosis of fetal malposition will determine the skill required of the operator, the place of delivery, the choice of delivery, and the success or failure of the procedure. However, even among experienced clinicians there is a substantial variability in the interpretation of the fetal head station and position, reflecting how difficult and unreliable this clinical evaluation can be, especially when caput and/or molding are present. The accuracy of fetal head position determination by vaginal digital examination ranges between 25% and 75%. Determination of fetal head position with US in labor is easier to learn. Indeed 82 digital vaginal examinations were necessary in order to obtain a low error rate, whereas this was achieved with only 32 examinations, all performed by a student who was in his learning curve.[62] US can decrease the rate of errors >45°, which has been reported in 53% of vaginal examinations during active labor.

In Table 24.6, a practical approach to US determination of the fetal head position is reported. A recent multicenter randomized trial shows that US assessment prior to instrumental delivery reduces the incidence of incorrect diagnosis of position without delaying the delivery.[36] On the contrary, US assessment of the OP of the fetal head or the level of the presenting part should neither be used to predict the mode of delivery nor should be used alone in the decision to perform vaginal operative delivery or not. Vaginal and abdominal evaluations are essential elements for a safe operative vaginal delivery. However, a US assessment prior to operative vaginal delivery can enhance the accuracy of diagnosis of fetal head position, then reducing the suboptimal instrumental placement which is an important factor related to maternal and/or neonatal morbidity.

EPIDURAL ANALGESIA (EA) AND INSTRUMENTAL DELIVERY

Labor EA is an increasingly used technique as the most effective for pain relief during labor. Since its introduction, the controversy about the relation between its effect and prolonged labor, instrumental delivery, and CS has continued.

During the second stage of labor, the fetal head descends, flexes, and rotates anteriorly. These cardinal movements are accomplished by effective uterine action and maternal expulsive efforts. After the first passive phase when uterine action causes the descent of the fetal head to the pelvic floor, the maternal effort is added to the active phase. Epidural analgesia blocks the Ferguson's reflex that is a normal endogenous source of oxytocin in the second stage of labor; moreover, the concomitant sensory blockade can diminish a women's urge to push.[28] The prevalence of prolonged second stage of labor occurs in 9.9% of nulliparous and 3.1% of multiparous with epidural analgesia in labor.[37] Compared with women who had spontaneous labor without epidural analgesia in the Consortium on Safe and Labor Study, nulliparous women who had epidural analgesia had a median duration of 66 minutes while those without had a median duration of 36 minutes.[38]

In addiction, some studies suggest that EA may be associated with fetal malposition such as OP or OT position as a result of fetal occiput malrotation during labor. A retrospective study which included 398 women found out that epidural analgesia applied when the fetal head is still "high" is associated with an increased rate of malposition during labor.[39]

Recently, a retrospective cohort of 1404 nulliparous women with spontaneous labor and EA did not show a clinically significant increase in the frequency of fetal head malposition at vaginal delivery compared with 1255 nulliparous with spontaneous labor without EA.[40]

A recent Dutch 10 years' population study found that EA was triplicated in 10 years but the rate of instrumental deliveries was relatively stable. Therefore, in the last years the relation between EA and operative vaginal delivery seems weaker than in the past.[41]

On the other side, in Netherlands, a randomized noninferiority trial on 488 women randomly allocated two groups: routine use of EA vs. use of EA on request showed a statistically significant difference in the rate of operative deliveries (difference 8.9%; 95% CI 0.4–17.4).[42]

Regarding the type of analgesia techniques there is no differences between the rate of operative vaginal delivery for combined spinal–epidural analgesia and standard techniques (OR 0.82; 95% CI 67–1.00) and the spontaneous delivery rate between patient controlled EA and continuous EA infusion.[25]

A retrospective case–control study on 3093 EA during labor using epidural bolus of 10–15 mL of bupivacaine with fentanyl followed by continuous infusion of bupivacaine with fentanyl at 7–10 mL/h found that women who requested for EA had need of oxytocin significantly more often: 80.3% vs. 58.3%, but there were no differences in the rate of instrumental delivery and in neonatal outcomes such as Apgar score and pH.[43]

The impact of EA on and in assisted vaginal delivery is still controversial probably because it influences maternal and fetal physiology, the course of labor, the duration of second stage, and affects the overall assistance and decision making during delivery.

Vacuum failure

There are two reasons to define the failure of vacuum procedure: continued detachment of the cups and/or lacking of fetal head descent. The rate of failed operative vaginal delivery has been reported to be 2.9%–6.5%.[23] The most common clinical factors associated with failed operative vaginal delivery are OP position (OR 12.7), macrosomia, nulliparity, higher station, excessive molding of the fetal head, protracted labor, and maternal obesity.[44]

In an analysis of 3798 cases, only birth weight and second-stage labor duration were significantly associated with failure, after controlling for operator experience.[54]

In case of a borderline cephalopelvic disproportion, excessive traction is likely, resulting in the detachment of the cup, and could be a protective mechanism of the VE.

The suboptimal placement of the primary instrument is associated with the greater use of sequential instruments (OR 3.20; 95% CI 1.71–5.95; $p < .001$), leading to longer delivery time and higher risk of an emergency CS. The incidence of suboptimal placement is in turn higher in case of fetal malposition (OR 2.44) and in case of midcavity station (OR 1.68) and twice as high if forceps were used as the primary instrument.[35]

Failure is more likely to occur with soft than with rigid vacuum cups (10% vs. 22%) even though the soft cups are associated with less fetal trauma.[44] The higher failure rate of soft cups is due to easy detachment usually in OP, asynclitic, and/or deflexed presentations.

Women who underwent cesarean delivery after an attempt of operative vaginal delivery are more likely to have wound complications and to undergo general anesthesia, and neonates had an increased incidence of an Apgar score less than 3 at 5 minutes and/or umbilical artery pH less than 7.[46] In a report of 1360 nulliparous women undergoing operative vaginal delivery, the use of sequential instruments was associated with increased anal sphincter tears and low umbilical artery pH.[47] Therefore, the sequential use of vacuum and forceps has been associated to increased neonatal complications and should be not routinely performed. A trial of a second attempt to operative vaginal delivery is an appropriate option only in the situation where the obstetricians feel the chance of success and where they must be ready to abandon faster the attempt and go to an emergency CS; i.e., proceeding to forceps after VE is feasible when there is a technical problem with the equipment, or where the fetal head is at the perineum and no macrosomia is suspected.

Episiotomy

Delivery may be controlled with the VE and be assisted over an intact perineum or may proceed after episiotomy. The use of episiotomy is controversial and should not be considered as routine as it does not appear to be always beneficial and may increase maternal morbidity.[48]

A large population-based study demonstrated that mediolateral episiotomy was protective against anal sphincter injury for both forceps and vacuum extraction and recommended that it should be used routinely to protect the anal sphincters.[49] Another study demonstrated that the incidence of sphincteric damage was 3.5% if mediolateral episiotomy was performed during VE and 15.6% if it was not.[50,51] A recent meta-analysis, however, suggests that only lateral episiotomy is protective.

If the decision to proceed to episiotomy has been done, a mediolateral or lateral incision should be preferred because a midline episiotomy is associated with higher probability of vaginal or anal sphincter injuries, and the direction of the incision is relevant.[52] A cooperation between obstetrician and midwife is essential.

Episiotomy could be protective in specific conditions:

- Nulliparity
- Delivery of a large baby (above all in a nullipara)
- Delivery of a baby in OP position
- Arrest of the descent at the outlet of the pelvis
- Detachment of the cup at the outlet
- High traction forces needed on the perineum
- Spontaneous tearing of the vagina or perineum for excessive stretching
- Incorrect cup application

If vacuum extraction is made without an episiotomy the operator should avoid excessive traction and perform one or two extra tractions for the perineum to distend over the head as it descends.

MATERNAL INJURIES AND MORBIDITY

Maternal complications associated with the use of the VE are rare,[23] nevertheless serious injuries have been reported, often occurring in mothers with predisposing factors. When we consider maternal complications we need to take into account that second-stage cesarean delivery is also associated with more complications than those performed in the first stage of labor.[53] Maternal complications include cervical and/or vaginal lacerations, vaginal hematomas, third or fourth degree lacerations, with consequent hemorrhage, pain, or infection. Established risk factors include nulliparity, high body mass index, high birth weight, difficult or obstructed labor, high station of fetal head, malposition of fetal head, incompleted dilated cervix, or failure of the procedure.[24,54,55] Cervical and/or vagina injury could be related to the procedure itself or caused by entrapment of the tissue under the suction cup.

Demisse et al.[56] reported severe perineal lacerations in 5.8% spontaneous delivery, 22% with forceps, 15% with vacuum, and 29% with forceps after failed vacuum. More recently Landy reports that VE is independently associated with a 2.7-fold and forceps with a 3.6-fold higher risk of third and fourth degree lacerations. Therefore an operative vaginal delivery has been recognized as a risk factor for perineal tears and anal sphincter injury, but it is difficult to separate its contribution to these injuries from other clinical factors associated to its use, such as prolonged second stage of labor, fetal size, fetal malposition, shoulder dystocia, and episiotomy.[48]

Fetal malposition has been shown to increase the risk of perineal trauma. A study of 1481 women found that any fetal position other than occipito-anterior was associated with a significant risk of perineal trauma (OR 1.30; 95% CI 1.14–1.48; $p < .005$).[45] Anal sphincter tears are more prevalent in case of fetal malposition, which is in turn an independent risk factor for failure of instrumental delivery.[44]

If anal sphincter lacerations happen with operative vaginal delivery, anal incontinence rates at 5–10 years after delivery are similar to those women who had a spontaneous delivery and the risk of recurrence rate of sphincter and/or anal sphincter tear is 3.2% but it could be increased if the second delivery requests another operative vaginal delivery.[49,53,61]

An inspection for lacerations after every instrumental delivery[57] is mandatory. Instrumental delivery does not seem to be associated per se with increased risk of persistent postpartum urinary incontinence compared with spontaneous vaginal delivery and does not appear to promote pelvic organ prolapse. Anyway, the presence of several perineal lacerations increases the risks of perineal diseases such as perineal pain, dyspareunia, and sexual diseases when compared with spontaneous vaginal delivery.[55] Unsuccessful attempt of instrumental delivery is associated with a higher risk of psychological maternal trauma. Women who have experienced a previous failed attempt are likely to opt for an elective CS rather than another attempt of vaginal birth.[54]

NEONATAL INJURIES AND MORBIDITY

Neonatal complications associated with the use of VE are more recurring, although in many cases these may be due to the complication of the labor that led to the necessity for the use of an instrumental vaginal delivery rather than to the procedure itself.

Alexander et al. reported data from a cohort of 3189 women disclosing that in the absence of a nonreassuring fetal heart rate tracing, an attempt at operative vaginal delivery before performing a caesarean delivery was not associated with adverse neonatal outcome. For this reason it could be better to classify neonatal complications according to clinical issue rather than a statistical issue. The neonatal complications should be classified[24]:

- Cosmetic scalp effects: Chignon (Figure 24.15), cup discoloration, and brushing.
- Clinically nonsignificant injuries: Retinal hemorrhage, blisters, superficial scalp abrasions, cephalohematoma, subcutaneous hematoma, and mild jaundice.
- Clinically significant injuries: Extensive or deep scalp lacerations, subgaleal hemorrhage, intracranial hemorrhage, and skull fracture.
- Indirect and coincidental effects: Brachial plexus injury and fracture of the clavicle associated with shoulder dystocia, neonatal respiratory depression.

The majority of neonatal effects are cosmetic, transient, and without any significance. These effects include the artificial caput succedaneum, named chignon, that develops inside the cup when the vacuum is induced. The chignon, which can be different in size, extension, and color due to the type of cup and the amount of traction decreases rapidly to become a diffuse swelling within 1 hour of birth and then behaves like a normal caput until 24–48 hours. According to Malmström,[58] ecchymoses are present on the fetal scalp 24 hours after delivery in 17% of the cases.

Scalp abrasion occurs in about 11% of vacuum, and the lesion always heals rapidly over a week without leaving any signs. Therefore, parents should be reassured the baby head does not show any residual markings on the scalp. The factors which could influence these lesions such as abrasion, ulceration, necrosis are prolonged traction, cup detachments, and failure of the procedure.

Retinal hemorrhage is a feasible manifestation that occurs in neonates after vaginal delivery, it is more common after instrumental delivery. The mechanism is still not well known but the low incidence in babies born after caesarean section suggests that forces associated with the passage of the fetal head through the birth canal predispose to the lesion. The lesions solve within 2–3 weeks in the easier cases or within 6 months in the more serious cases, leaving no residual effects. Evidence from randomized trials suggests that vacuum extraction is associated with more retinal hemorrhages than forceps delivery.[24]

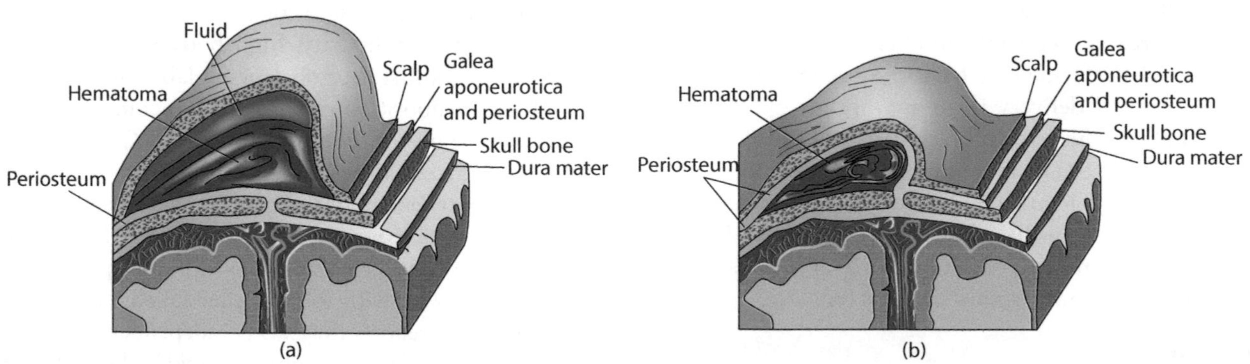

Figure 24.15 (a) Subgaleal hematoma is a serious injury. Blood collects between the galea and the table of the skull. Large volumes of blood can accumulate, leading to hypovolemia. (b) In contrast, cephalhematoma occurs under the tough, well-attached periosteum and is therefore self-limited.

Table 24.6 Ultrasound for determination of fetal position (transabdominal or suprapubic axial scansion).

Fetal head position	Image under symphysis	Occiput at "clock-face"
Occiput anterior	Cerebellum, cervical column	9:30/2:30
Occiput posterior	Nose, eyes	3:30/8:30
Occiput transverse	Midline	On the left 2:30/3:30 On the right 8:30/9:30

Cephalohematomas (Figure 24.15) are collections of blood under the periosteum of skull bone and are limited to the confines of a cranial bone, usually the parietal. It is more likely to occur as the duration of vacuum application increases. One study found out that cephalohematoma was diagnosed in 28% of neonates when the time from application to the delivery exceeded 5 minutes. Its incidence varies from 4% to 7% due to the type of cup, rising in the case of a rigid, metallic vacuum cup.

Resolution of subcutaneous hematoma occurs rapidly over a week. Clinical injuries such as subgaleal or intracranial hemorrhage are more severe complications. The subgaleal hemorrhage (Figure 24.15) is one of the most serious and potentially life-threatening complications of vaginal delivery, due to a bleeding which develops in the space between the periosteum and the galea aponeurotica. The hemorrhage can occur over several hours following delivery and unless careful observations are made, the bleeding may not become obvious until the hematoma is extensive. The subaponeurotic space has a capacity of about 250 mL; therefore, the symptoms of this condition are similar to a circulatory collapse characterized by pallor, hypotension, raised pulse, and fall of the hematocrit. The incidence of subgaleal hemorrhage is 1 in 2000–3000 spontaneous deliveries and 1 in 150–200 vacuum-assisted deliveries. The occurrence is the same for vacuum-assisted delivery with both rigid and soft cup and is likely to be increased with improper placement or with failed procedure.[28] The risk of rare intracranial hemorrhage rises after failed vacuum extraction mainly if it is followed by a forceps-assisted delivery. Clinical manifestations of serious intracranial bleeding are variable but neonates always show abnormal neurological signs such as increasing irritability, depression of breathing, apnoea, or convulsions. Estimates from large cohort studies have indicated that intracranial hemorrhage occurs in one of every 650–850 operative vaginal deliveries and neurologic complications occur in one of every 220–385 infants delivered using forceps or vacuum extraction.

Indirect and coincidental effects such as shoulder dystocia, brachial plexus injury, fractures of the clavicle, and/or humerus are more common after vacuum-assisted delivery, although in many cases these may be mainly due to fetal characteristics and related to a mild pelvic vacuum application. A recommendation is necessary for selective cases in which the fetal weight size was estimated to be above 4 kg and where there was an abnormal progress in labor.

Operative vaginal delivery was associated with a rate of neonatal encephalopathy of 4.2 per 1000 term neonates compared with 3.9 per 1000 delivered by cesarean delivery.[59] ACOG guidelines highlight that there are few data to assess the long-term consequences of operative vaginal delivery but the evidence indicates that they are equivalent to those of spontaneous vaginal delivery.

In another study no differences were seen in scholastic performance, speech, or neurologic abnormality between 295 children delivered by vacuum extraction and 302 children in the control group.[60]

TRAINING

VE has become the instrument of choice in vaginal-assisted delivery for many obstetricians. When utilized properly, it is an effective and important tool in the armamentarium and could contribute to reduce the rate of cesarean delivery. The danger of instrumental deliveries depends more on the operator's skill than on the instrument itself. As with any medical and obstetric devices, the following established guidelines minimize the risk of injury to mother and the infant. Training must ensure that obstetricians can identify indications and contraindications, knowledge of the instrument, of the technique, and correct use. Moreover, nontechnical skills are relevant like in other procedures, with more emphasis on situational awareness, relationship with the women, and cross-monitoring of performance. The usual training between teacher and trainees in the delivery room can be accompanied by simulations with mannequins that can reduce the problem that is experienced in a large number of procedures. The involvement of teachers and trainees obstetricians in these sessions may improve practice for both.

As sufficient experience is gained, more difficult procedures may be attempted, including use for malpositions, emergency deliveries, extraction at CS, and delivery of the second twin. In the case of forceps, it would be inappropriate to do rotational procedures before acquiring expertise in outlet techniques. The same logic should apply to the VE. Understandably, the complications occur early in training or, on the contrary, when a high confidence with the instrument can bring the operator to underestimate the relevance of the procedure.

We could summarize the vacuum operative delivery in 10 actions which include all the things to remember before, during, and after the procedure.

TEN ACTIONS TO DO IN VACUUM OPERATIVE DELIVERY

Before the procedure

1. Assessment of the indications and/or contraindications of the procedure.

2. Assessment of maternal–fetal conditions: Identification of any historical risk factors, preliminary analysis through semeiotic obstetric maneuvers, assessment of cervical dilatation.
3. Assessment of fetal head station and position.

During the procedure

4. Empty bladder, mother informed.
5. Application of the vacuum following the standard rules.
6. Check of gradual progression of fetal head during the procedure.
7. No more than three tractions: Possible fourth traction only if the head station is at perineum level.
8. No more than two applications if there is vacuum pop-off. In the second attempt involvement of a skilled operator.
9. No more than 15–20 minutes to conclude the procedure.

After the procedure.

10. Documentation of the procedure and assessment of the maternal and neonatal outcomes, remembering to reassure parents.

APPENDIX I*

Documenting operative vaginal delivery.

OPERATIVE VAGINAL DELIVERY							
Date		Patient historical details					
Operator							
Supervisor							
Midwife							
Indication(s) for OVD							
prolonged second stage of labor		fetal compromise		maternal exhaustion			
ACOG FHR category	Category I	Category II		Category III			
Rotation > 45°	Yes			No			
Classification of OVD	Outlet	Low		Midcavity			
Prerequisities for OVD							
F	Full cervical dilatation						
O	Only 1/5	Only 0/5		head palpable abdominally			
	engaged head			Yes	No		
R	ruptured membranes	Amniotic fluid		clear	meconium		
C	contractions present	Oxytocin infusion		Yes	No	___ml/h	
E	empty bladder	Catheterised	Yes	No	Mother's consent	Verbal	Written
P	Position known						
	Anterior	Bregma		Posterior			
	STATION	+2 / +3		0 / + 1			
	CAPUT	>	>>	>>>			
	MOULDING	>	>>	>>>			
S	Satisfactory analgesia	local	pudendal	regional	PLACE OF DELIVERY	room	theatre
OVD Procedure							
Vacuum extractor chosen	silastic	Kiwi		metal anterior	metal posterior		
Number of pulls:			Traction :	easy	moderate	strong	
Pop-off	Yes	No	Maternal effort	easy	moderate	strong	
HEAD POSITION AT DELIVERY	Anterior	Bregma		Posterior			
PLACENTA				Spontaneous	Manual		
EPISIOTOMY				Yes	No		
PERINEAL TEAR	1st degree	2th degree	3th degree	4th degree			
BLOOD LOSS:							
AFTER OVD Procedure							
BABY	M	F	Birth Weight		g		
			Apgar score	1min	5min	10min	
			Cord pH	Arterial		Venous	
			Base Excess				
Neonatal outcome(s)							
SIGNATURE				**DATE**			

Source: Modified from Royal College of Obstetricians and Gynaecologists, Green-top Guideline No. 26, Operative vaginal delivery, London, UK: RCOG, January 2011.

REFERENCES

1. Yonge J. An account of balls of hair taken from the uterus and ovaria of several women; by Mr. James Yonge, F.R.S. communicated to Dr. Hans Sloane, R.S. Secr. *Philos Trans R Soc* 1706; 25: 2387–2392.
2. Simpson JY. On a suction-tractor, or new mechanical power, as a substitute for the forceps in tedious labours. *Edinb Mon J Med Sci* 1849; 32: 556.
3. McCahey P. Atmospheric tractor: A new instrument and some new theories in obstetrics. *Med Surg Reporter* 1890; 43: 6319.
4. Kuntzsch D. Über geburtshilfische Extraktionen mit meinem Vakuumbelm. *Zentralbl Gynakol* 1912; 36: 893.
5. Torpin R. Preliminary report of obstetric device. *J Med Assoc Ga* 1938; 27: 96.
6. Castallo MA. Extractor instead of forceps. *Am J Obstet Gynecol* 1955; 70: 1375.
7. Couzigou Y. La Ventouse eutocique. *Bull Soc Med Paris* 1947; 152: 34.
8. Finderle V. Extractor instead of forceps. *Am J Obstet Gynecol* 1955; 69: 1148–53.
9. Malmström T. Vacuum extractor—An obstetrical instrument. *Acta Obstet Gynecol Scand Suppl* 1954; 33(4): 1–31.
10. Malmström T. Vacuum extractor: Indications and results. *Acta Obstet Gynecol Scand* 1964; 43 (Suppl 1): 5–52.
11. Bird GC. The use of the Malmström vacuum extractor inoperative obstetrics. *Aust N Z J Obstet Gynaecol* 1966; 6: 242.
12. Chalmers JA. The vacuum extractor. *Proc R Soc Med* 1960; 53: 753.
13. Sjostedt JE. The vacuum extractor and forceps in obstetrics, a clinical study. *Acta Obstet Gynecol Scand* 1967; 46 (Suppl 10): 1–208.
14. Snoeck J. The vacuum extractor (ventouse), an alternative to the obstetric forceps. *Proc R Soc Med* 1960; 53: 749.
15. Bird GC. Modification of Malmström's vacuum extractor. *BMJ* 1969; 3: 526.
16. Chalmers JA. *The Ventouse, the Obstetric Vacuum Extractor.* Chicago, IL: Year Book Medical Publishers, 1971.
17. Paul R, Saisch K, Pine S. The 'new' vacuum extractor. *Obstet Gynecol* 1973; 41: 800–2.
18. Kuit J, Eppinga H, Wallenburg H, Huikeshoven FJ. A randomized comparison of vacuum extraction delivery with a rigid and a pliable cup. *Obstet Gynecol* 1993; 82: 280–4.
19. Chenoy R, Johanson RB. A randomized prospective study comparing delivery with metal and silicone rubber vacuum extractor cups. *Br J Obstet Gynaecol* 1992; 99: 360–3.
20. Ismail NA, Saharan WS, Zaleha MA et al. Kiwi Omnicup versus Malmstrom metal cup in vacuum assisted delivery: A randomized comparative trial. *J Obstet Gynaecol Res* 2008; 34: 350.

21. Martin JA, Hamilton BE, Osterman MJ et al. Births: Final data for 2013. *Natl Vital Stat Rep* 2015; 64: 1–65.
22. American College of Obstetrics and Gynecology Committee on Practice Bulletins-Obstetrics. ACOG Practical Bulletin No. 49. Dystocia and augmentation of labor. *Obstet Gynecol* 2003; 102: 1445–54.
23. Committee on Bulletins Practice—Obstetrics. ACOG Practice Bulletin No. 154 Summary: Operative vaginal delivery. *Obstet Gynecol* 2015; 126: 1118–9.
24. Vacca A. *Handbook of Vacuum Delivery in Obstetrics Practice* (3rd edition). Brisbane, Australia: Vacca Research, 2009.
25. Royal College of Obstetricians and Gynaecologists. Green-top Guideline No. 26. Operative vaginal delivery. London, UK: RCOG, January 2011.
26. Bahl R, Strachan B, Murphy DJ. Outcome of subsequent pregnancy three years after previous operative delivery in the second stage of labour: Cohort study. *BMJ* 2004; 328: 311.
27. Melamed N, Ben-Haroush A, Chen R et al. Pregnancy outcome and mode of delivery after a previous operative vaginal delivery. *Obstet Gynecol* 2009; 114: 757.
28. Baskett TF, Calder AA, Arulkumaran S. *Munro Kerr's Operative Obstetrics* (12th edition). Philadelphia, PA: Saunders Elsevier, 2014.
29. Petterson K, Ajne J, Yousaf K et al. Traction force during vacuum extraction: A prospective observational study. *BJOG* 2015; 122: 1809–16.
30. Vacca A. Vacuum-assisted delivery: An analysis of traction force and maternal and neonatal outcomes. *Aust N Z J Obstet Gynaecol* 2006; 46: 124–7.
31. Caughey AB, Sharshiner R, Cheng YW. Fetal malposition: Impact and management. *Clin Obstet Gynecol* 2015; 58: 241–5.
32. Bird GC. The importance of flexion in vacuum extractor delivery. *Br J Obstet Gynaecol* 1965; 83: 893.
33. Nyirjesy I, Hawks BL, Falls HC et al. A comparative clinical study of the vacuum extractor and forceps. *Am J Obstet Gynecol* 1963; 85: 1071.
34. Simons EG, Philpott RH. The vacuum extractor. *Trop Doct* 1973; 3: 34–7.
35. Ramphul M, Kennelly MM, Burke G, Murphy DJ. Risk factors and morbidity associated with suboptimal instrument placement at instrumental delivery: Observational study nested within the Instrumental Delivery & Ultrasound randomized controlled trial ISRCTN 72230496. *BJOG* 2015; 122: 558–63.
36. Ramphul M, Ooi PV, Burke G et al. Instrumental delivery and ultrasound (IDUS): A multicenter randomized controlled trial of ultrasound assessment of the fetal head position versus standard care as an approach to prevent morbidity at instrumental delivery. *BJOG* 2014; 121: 1029–38.
37. Laughon SK, Branch DW, Beaver J et al. Changes in labor patterns over 50 years. *Am J ObstetGynecol* 2012; 206: 419; e1–9.
38. Zhang J, Landy HJ, Branch DW et al. Consortium on Safe Labor. Contemporary patterns of spontaneous labor with normal neonatal outcomes. *Obstet Gynecol* 2010; 116: 1281–7.
39. Le Ray C, Carayol M, Jaquemin S et al. Is epidural analgesia a risk factor for occiput posterior or transverse positions during labour? *Eur J Obstet Gynecol Reprod Biol* 2005; 123: 22–6.
40. Yancey MK, Zhang J, Schweitzer DL et al. Epidural analgesia and fetal head malposition at vaginal delivery. *Obstet Gynecol* 2001; 97: 608–12.
41. Wassen MM, Hukkelhoven CW, Scheepers HC et al. Epidural analgesia and operative delivery: A ten-year population-based cohort study in The Netherlands. *Eur J Obstet Gynecol Reprod Biol* 2014; 183: 125–31.
42. Wassen MM, Smits LJ, Scheepers HC et al. Routine labour epidural analgesia versus labour analgesia on request: A randomised non-inferiority trial. *BJOG* 2015; 122: 344–50.
43. Rimaitis K, Klimenko O, Rimaitis M et al. Labor epidural analgesia and the incidence of instrumental assisted delivery. *Medicina (Kaunas)* 2015; 5176: 8.
44. Wanyonyi SZ, Achila B, Gudu N. Factors contributing to failure of vacuum delivery and associated maternal/neonatal morbidity. *Int J Gynaecol Obstet* 2011; 115: 157–60.
45. Webb S, Sherburn S, Ismail KM. Managing perineal trauma after childbirth. *BMJ* 2014; 349: g6829.
46. Alexander JM, Leveno KJ, Hauth JC et al. Failed operative vaginal delivery. *Obstet Gynecol* 2009; 114: 1017–22.
47. Murphy DJ, Macleod M, Bahl R, Strachan B. A cohort study of maternal and neonatal morbidity in relation to use of sequential instruments at operative vaginal delivery. *Eur J Obstet Gynecol Reprod Biol* 2011; 156: 41–5.
48. Landy HJ, Laughon SK, Bailit JL et al. Consortium on Safe Labor Characteristics associated with severe perineal and cervical lacerations during vaginal delivery. *Obstet Gynecol* 2011; 117: 627.
49. Evers EC, Blomquist JL, McDermott KC, Handa VL. Obstetrical anal sphincter laceration and anal incontinence 5–10 years after childbirth. *Am J Obstet Gynecol.* 2012; 207: 425. e1–6.
50. De Leeuuw JW, de Vit C, Kulijken JPJA, Bruinse HW. Mediolateral episiotomy reduces the risk for anal sphincter injury during operative vaginal delivery. *BJOG* 2008; 115: 104–8.
51. De Vogel J, van der Leeuw-van Beek A, Gietelink D et al. The effect of a mediolateral episiotomy during operative vaginal delivery on the risk of developing obstetrical anal sphincter injuries. *Am J Obstet Gynecol* 2012; 206: 404.e1–5.
52. Sagi-Dain L, Sagi S. Morbidity associated with episiotomy in vacuum delivery: A systematic review and meta-analysis. *BJOG* 2015; 122(8): 1073–81.

53. Bailit JL, Grobman WA, Rice MM et al. Evaluation of delivery options for second-stage events. *Am J Obstet Gynecol* 2016; 214: 638.e1–10.
54. Aiken CE, Aiken AR, Brockelsby JC, Scott JG. Factors influencing the likelihood of instrumental delivery success. *Obstet Gynecol* 2014; 123: 796–803.
55. Vayssière C, Beucher G, Dupuis O et al. French College of Gynaecologists and Obstetricians. Instrumental delivery: Clinical practice guidelines from the French College of Gynaecologists and Obstetricians. *Eur J Obstet Gynecol Reprod Biol* 2011; 159: 43–8.
56. Demissie K, Rhoads G, Smulian J et al. Operative vaginal delivery and neonatal and infant adverse outcomes: Population based retrospective analysis. *BMJ* 2004; 329: 24–9.
57. Society of Obstetricians and Gynaecologists of Canada. SOGC clinical practice guidelines. Guidelines for vaginal birth after previous caesarean birth. Number 155 (Replaces guideline Number 147), February 2005. *Int J Gynaecol Obstet* 2005; 89: 319–31.
58. Malmström T, Jansson I. Use of the vacuum extractor. *Clin Obstet Gynecol* 1965; 8: 893.
59. Walsh CA, Robson M, McAuliffe FM. Mode of delivery at term and adverse neonatal outcomes. *Obstet Gynecol* 2013; 121: 122–8.
60. Ngan HY, Miu P, Ko L, Ma HK. Long-term neurological sequelae following vacuum extractor delivery. *Aust N Z J Obstet Gynaecol* 1990; 30: 111–4.
61. Basham E, Stock L, Lewicky-Gaupp C et al. Subsequent pregnancy outcomes after obstetric anal sphincter injuries (OASIS). *Female Pelvic Med Reconstr Surg* 2013; 19: 328–32.
62. Rozenberg P, Porcher R, Salomon LJ et al. Comparison of the learning curves of digital examination and trans abdominal sonography for the determination of fetal head position during labor. *Ultrasound Obstet Gynecol* 2008; 31: 332–7.

Fetal malpresentations

25

PIERRE F. LESPINASSE

CONTENTS

The labor process usually involves passage of the fetus through the birth canal in vertex presentation. In 2%–3% of pregnancies, the presenting part is the breech.[1] However, in about one in 300, the fetus is in transverse lie or presents by the shoulder. Malpresentations are pathologic, since they make vaginal delivery difficult or impossible. They are also associated with an increased incidence of birth injuries.

BREECH PRESENTATION

Breech presentation is common in early gestation, but its incidence decreases at term. The rate of breech presentation is still in the range of 7%–10% among fetuses weighing less than 2500 g. Therefore, factors that cause preterm labor increase the incidence of breech delivery.

Breech presentations may be subdivided into three categories: Frank breech, complete breech, and footling breech (Figure 25.1). The most common type is frank breech. Footling breech is seen relatively frequently in multiparas and in association with preterm labor.

The incidence of congenital malformations is about threefold higher among fetuses in breech presentation than those in cephalic presentation.[2] Malformations frequently associated with breech presentation include anencephaly, hip dislocation, hydrocephaly, spina bifida, trisomies 13, 18, and 21, and meningomyelocele.

Breech presentation can be diagnosed with abdominal palpation or pelvic examination during the third trimester.[3] In all suspected cases, an ultrasound examination should be performed to confirm the presenting part, the attitude of the fetal head, and the type of breech. It will also help determine the location of the placenta, the estimated fetal weight and gestational age, the amount of amniotic fluid, and the presence or absence of pelvic masses that, by obstructing the birth canal, may have caused the abnormal fetal presentation.

Previously virtually all breech presentations were managed by vaginal delivery,[4,5] the perinatal mortality rate for breech deliveries was three to five times higher than for vertex deliveries.[6,7] The main causes of fetal mortality and morbidity were prematurity, congenital malformations, intrapartum hypoxic insult, and birth trauma. Prolapse of the cord was and still remains a major problem with breech presentation. Whereas the incidence of cord prolapse is about 0.3% with cephalic presentation, it is in the range of 3%–5% with breech presentation. This risk is particularly high in footling breech. However, with a frank breech presentation, the incidence is close to that observed in cephalic presentation.

The gravest danger associated with breech delivery is arrest of the aftercoming head either by the pelvis or by the incompletely dilated cervix. The latter alternative is most threatening in premature deliveries, when the relatively small fetal body fails to dilate the cervix sufficiently for the passage of the head. It should be remembered that, whereas the progress of the head through the pelvis may take hours in cephalic presentation, the same must be accomplished within 2–3 minutes when the delivery of the head follows

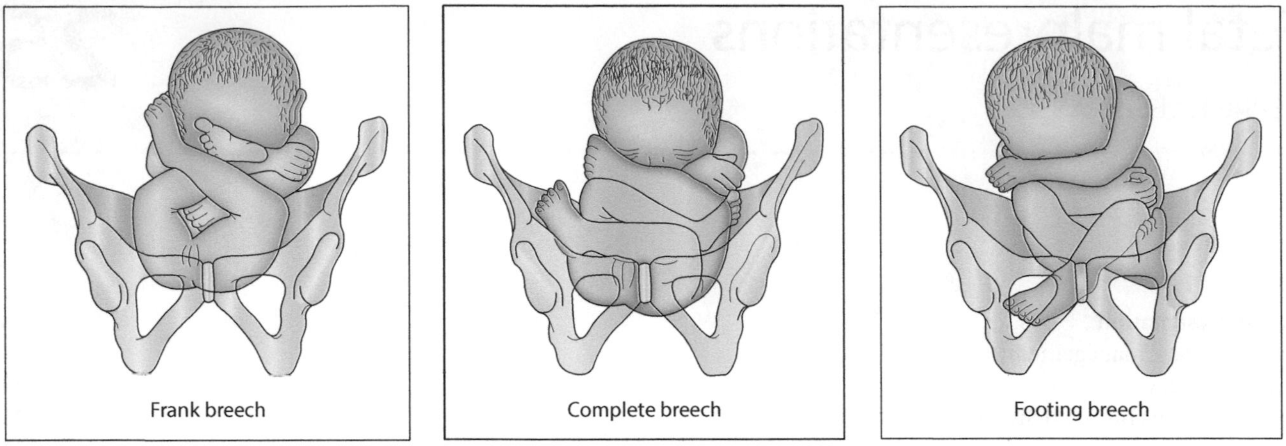

Figure 25.1 Various types of breech presentation. (Courtesy of Drs. Alvin Langer and Kay W. Kennedy, from Iffy L and Kaminetzky HA, eds., *Principles and Practice of Obstetrics & Perinatology*, p. 1521, New York, NY: Wiley, 1981. With permission from Leslie Iffy.)

that of the body. Passage of the head may be hindered further by deflexion of the head or by a nuchal arm or arms. This latter complication may occur as a result of either too rapid descent of the fetal body in the birth canal or traction applied upon the lower extremities by the accoucheur.

Traumatic fetal injuries associated with vaginal breech delivery include spinal cord laceration and even transection; intraventricular hemorrhage; tentorial tear; fracture of the skull, vertebrae, ribs, or long bones; rupture of the spleen or the liver; and bleeding in the adrenals.[8,9] Injuries may also involve the muscles, the scrotum, and the testes. The latter may lead to testicular atrophy.

The relatively high perinatal mortality and morbidity rates[10] attributed to vaginal delivery have resulted in the introduction of restrictions to elective breech vaginal delivery. The following factors have long been considered contraindications to attempted vaginal breech delivery:

1. Contracted pelvis[11]
2. Estimated fetal weight exceeding 3600 g
3. Poor obstetric history
4. First pregnancy in a >35-year-old woman
5. Placenta previa
6. Dysfunctional labor
7. Prolapse of the umbilical cord
8. Prolonged premature rupture of the membranes
9. Footling breech
10. Less than 32 weeks' gestation
11. Hydrocephaly
12. Scarred uterus
13. Deflexed fetal head

In recent decades, cesarean section has become the preferred method of delivery by most obstetricians. Some physicians and even medical organizations categorically reject the option of elective breech vaginal delivery currently and consider elective cesarean section the method of choice.[12,13] Others restrict elective breech deliveries to cases that fulfill certain specific criteria.[6,14–16]

CONTEMPORARY MANAGEMENT

Since opinions vary with regard to the place of vaginal breech delivery in contemporary obstetric practice,[17–21] elective cesarean section for breech presentation is always an acceptable management choice. It is advisable to inform the patient about the differing opinions about the mode of delivery and involve her in the decision making. In order to give informed consent, the patient should be told that intrapartum complications may necessitate abandonment of a planned vaginal delivery.

Irrespective of the contemplated management, patients with breech presentation need close follow-up during the antepartum period. They should be advised about the risks of premature rupture of the membranes and preterm labor. When the breech presentation persists, the patient should undergo ultrasound examination to exclude conditions conducive to persistent malpresentation, such as pelvic tumors or fetal malformations. In the absence of such abnormalities, external version around 35–36 weeks is the recommended contemporary management.[22,23]

Patients selected for a trial of labor need to be hospitalized early. The presentation of the fetus and the absence of deflexion of the head should be confirmed by ultrasound at the time of admission. It is important to remember that any degree of pelvic contraction is a contraindication to vaginal breech delivery. Computer tomography and magnetic resonance imaging can be used for pelvimetry, but their usefulness is disputed.[24] Before and after the procedure, the parturient must be monitored electronically. Rupture of the membranes must be avoided. Evidence of nonreassuring fetal heart rate or abnormal progress of labor is an indication for cesarean section.

Abdominal breech delivery can be performed under regional or general anesthesia. One should remember that extraction of the aftercoming head through a small incision can be as difficult as a complicated vaginal breech delivery. Fetal injuries, similar to those observed in connection with vaginal breech deliveries, can also occur with cesarean section. Complications such as extension of the uterine incision to the cervix or laterally to the uterine vessels may occur.

BREECH DELIVERY

Traditionally, the primary mode of delivering the breech fetus was through the vagina by a wide variety of techniques and maneuvers.[15] Maternal safety was the overwhelming concern, given the fact that modern antibiotics, blood banking, and safe anesthesia did not exist. In addition, techniques and facilities to sustain premature infants or those with congenital anomalies were not readily available.

To improve perinatal outcome, Hall and Kohl[25] suggested, in 1956, the routine use of cesarean section for breech presentation. Based on an analysis of 1456 breech-presenting fetuses, they concluded that cesarean section produced a lower perinatal mortality rate than vaginal delivery.[26] Since then, the rate of cesarean sections for breech presentation has risen from 5%–10% up to 80%–100%. On the ground of a large international study which involved a variety of obstetric centers with differing professional standards, Hannah et al.[27] in 2000 concluded that elective vaginal breech delivery involved unacceptable fetal risks.[21] Their view was endorsed virtually immediately by British authorities.[28] Although the protocol on which the findings of the investigators rested incorporated management patterns that had been considered unacceptable in the United States for decades, the American College of Obstetricians and Gynecologists soon followed.

The turnaround did not go unchallenged. Several authorities have presented the view that Hannah et al.'s data excluded reference to the effect of cesarean sections upon subsequent pregnancies and, thus provided inadequate evidence for the support of their far-reaching conclusions.[6,14,15,29] The perinatal mortality rate associated with breech presentation has decreased since the widespread application of cesarean section; however, there has been a concomitant concern about the maternal risks of cesarean section, including infectious morbidity and the danger of rupture of the uterus in subsequent pregnancies. Maternal death from elective cesarean delivery (CD) for breech has been reported. The latter complication along with a variety of others that occur with increased frequency after abdominal deliveries, such as placenta previa, placenta accreta, premature labor, and in utero fetal death, imposes substantial risks upon future siblings of babies delivered by the abdominal route.

In 2004, a follow-up study evaluating the outcome of children with the term Breech trial did not find that a planned CD was not associated with a reduction in fetal death or neurodevelopmental delay. Despite these findings the authors maintained their recommendation for a planned CD.

One alternative to abdominal delivery is external version.[23] Another alternative is selective trial of labor for breech fetuses. A randomized study which compared elective cesarean section with protocol-managed labor in frank breech fetuses at term found significant maternal morbidity when breech infants were delivered by cesarean section, with no dramatic improvement in the neonatal outcome.[30] Nonetheless, cesarean section is likely to remain the most frequent modality of delivery in breech presentation. When the opportunity arises for a selective trial of labor, the obstetrician must possess the skills necessary to conduct delivery vaginally. It is advisable to discuss the risks and benefits of the available options with the patient before any relevant decision making.

Although usually less conducive to birth trauma than a vaginal breech delivery, abdominal extraction of the fetus presenting by the breech can involve considerable technical difficulties. Since the lower uterine segment is often uneffaced, it may be difficult to cut a long enough transverse uterine incision for the delivery of the aftercoming head. Delay in completing the delivery process may cause fetal hypoxia, and undue force used during traction may result in traumatic injury.[31] In the same process, the incision may extend either laterally, involving the uterine blood vessels, or in the direction of the cervix, causing laceration that is difficult to repair. For this reason, careful inspection of the contemplated incision site is important. When necessary, there should be no hesitation to apply a lower segment vertical incision in order to minimize the risks of these complications and the incision can extend toward the fundus as necessary. If this opportunity has been forfeited, extension of the incision in an inverted "T" fashion may resolve the problem at the expense of leaving behind a weak and vulnerable scar in case of future pregnancy. Development of Bandl's ring secondary to protracted labor may make the extraction of the fetus virtually impossible. Extension of the incision into a long classical incision may be the only solution in such instances. In cases of premature cesarean breech delivery, when the lower uterine segment is not developed, a lower segment transverse incision may be insufficient to deliver the head. In such cases, a vertical lower segment incision may be preferable.

The manipulative procedures to be described evolved decades and even centuries ago as a result of extensive application in everyday practice. With regard to elective breech delivery, one must remember the importance of certain precautionary measures[6]: (1) labor should not be induced, (2) oxytocin should not be used for uterine stimulation, (3) the second stage should not extend beyond 60 minutes, (4) the estimated fetal weight should not exceed 3600 g.

Vaginal breech delivery may occur spontaneously or may require partial or complete breech extraction. Personnel critical to a safe vaginal delivery in breech presentation include: (1) an obstetrician skilled in the appropriate techniques; (2) an assistant to support the weight of the fetal body as the aftercoming head is delivered or, when needed, provide suprapubic pressure on the descending fetal head to maintain flexion; (3) a pediatrician to resuscitate the neonate if required; (4) an anesthesiologist to provide pain relief during the delivery; (5) appropriate nursing support; and (6) operating room personnel scrubbed and gowned for instant cesarean section. Based solely on the mode of vaginal delivery, the best perinatal outcome has been found in association with spontaneous birth. The more complicated the procedure and manipulation needed for vaginal breech delivery, the greater the perinatal morbidity and mortality risk.[4]

Spontaneous breech delivery

The only function of the obstetrician in spontaneous breech delivery is to support the body of the fetus as the uterine contractions and the bearing-down efforts of the mother effect vaginal birth. The expulsion of the legs precedes the emergence of the buttocks in partial or complete breech presentations. As the fetal buttocks distend the perineum, episiotomy usually is required to prevent undue delay and maternal perineal lacerations. As the fetal body descends to the umbilicus, the physician supports, but does not place traction on, the fetal torso. With a few additional contractions, the fetal arms and shoulders are delivered. It is important to allow sufficient time for spontaneous delivery, bearing in mind, however, that once the body is expelled to the scapula, the umbilical cord becomes compressed between the head and the bony pelvis.

Assisted breech delivery

In the process of birth, the delivery of the fetal body occurs relatively quickly once the breech has emerged through the pelvic outlet and the trunk has begun its rotation. In the presence of adequate uterine contractions, reflected by the fact that the process of labor has followed Friedman's curve,[32] not more than one or two contractions are required for the delivery of the trunk up to the level of the scapula. The accomplishment of this process requires unimpeded uterine action and is facilitated by the parturient's abdominal and pelvic muscles. This important factor is bound to be lost or reduced if conduction or general anesthesia is used.[33]

When, prior to the delivery of the breech, cervical dilation and descent of the presenting part have been progressing at the normal rate, spontaneous delivery of the body up to the level of the shoulders occurs rather predictably without need for intervention on the part of those attending. Such a development provides the most favorable outcome. Interference prior to the delivery of the trunk, whether elective or indicated, increases the risks involved with the delivery of the head.[6,34] It is at the time of the birth of the fetus up to the shoulders that the greatest diameter of the head reaches the level of the pelvic inlet. In most instances, the need exists for providing assistance with the delivery of the aftercoming head. The various maneuvers that facilitate this process will be discussed in some detail in the following sections.

Despite favorable cephalopelvic proportions, the premature fetus is liable to be stressed excessively or suffer birth injuries due to its fragile physical structure. Additional risks are introduced by the fact that the relative diameters of the breech, as compared with the head, are small, and the presenting part can pass through the cervix at a lesser degree of dilation than that required for the passage of the head. Thus, chances are high that the powerful musculature of the cervix will prevent delivery of the caput for a prolonged period of time. The delay is conductive to fetal hypoxia, and the physician's effort to overcome the resistance of the cervix and may cause birth injuries.

On rare occasions, the normal rotation of the fetus is reversed and the chin instead of the occiput rotates toward the symphysis after the delivery of the body. In this situation, the chin interlocks with the symphysis; a collision which is bound to deflex the head. The end result is an almost insurmountable impasse. Ideally, the malrotation should be prevented by facilitating the anterior rotation of the back before the full delivery of the trunk. Alternatively, an attempt should be made to correct the malrotation. This can be begun by an external maneuver; a fist over the symphysis displaces the chin toward one side. The effort is to be completed internally; a hand inserted into the vagina tries to rotate the occiput toward the desired direction. If this maneuver fails, as it often does, the "reverse Prague maneuver" is the last resort. One hand grasps the fetal extremities and brings them, with gentle force, toward the abdomen of the mother. The other hand grasps the neck much in the same manner as in Mauriceau's maneuver, and traction is applied in an upward direction. If the effort succeeds, the fetus is born as if it turned a somersault. Since the use of some force is likely to be required under these exceedingly unfavorable circumstances, the maneuver involves considerable fetal risks. Therefore, it is more of historical than clinical interest. In contemporary practice, "abdominal rescue"[35] seems to be the preferable approach.

Partial breech extraction

Partial breech extraction involves the spontaneous delivery of the fetus to the umbilicus and the employment of obstetric maneuvers thereafter for delivery of the upper torso, shoulders, arms, and aftercoming head.[9,36] When spontaneous delivery of the fetus to the umbilicus is accomplished by the uterine contractions and maternal bearing-down efforts, the obstetrician places both hands around the fetal thighs with both thumbs over the sacrum and parallel to the fetal lumbar spine (Figure 25.2). The key to success is steady, gentle, sharp downward traction at the time of contraction

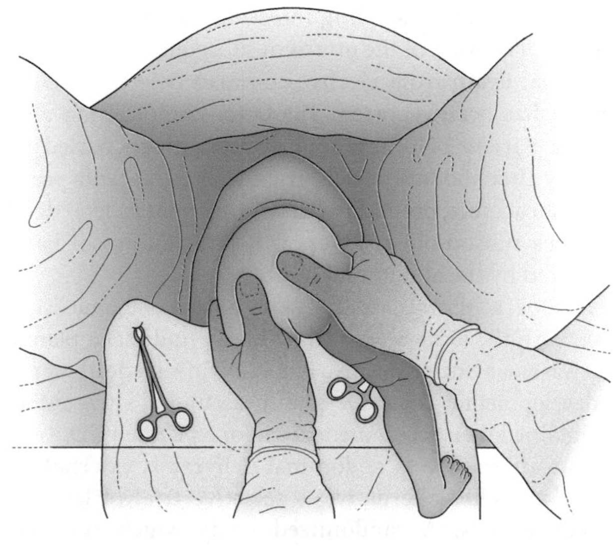

Figure 25.2 The initial step for partial breech extraction. (From Burger K, *Obstetric Surgery*, Budapest, Hungary: Franklin Társulat, 1927.)

at about a 60° angle with the back in the transverse diameter until the scapulae are outside the vulva. Care must be taken to avoid the birth injuries ascribed to this procedure. Although partial breech extraction may be necessary in some instances, the advisability of waiting until spontaneous delivery of the body up to the shoulder blades has been accomplished cannot be overemphasized.

Delivery of the shoulders and arms

Continuous traction upon the fetus is likely to entail unimpeded delivery of the shoulder girdle and arms, a mechanism traditionally attributed to Müller. An alternative, highly effective, and time-proven maneuver is somewhat more involved and requires careful observance of a series of steps.[9,34]

The classical method emphasizes the fact that there is more room in the space provided by the sacrum than under the symphysis. This approach stipulates that: (1) extraction of the retained arm should be carried out in the space provided by the sacrum; (2) the right arm should be extracted with the right hand and the left arm with the left hand; (3) the arm should be brought out in front of the fetus and never behind the body; and (4) any traction or pressure exerted upon the arm must be directed against a joint, usually at the elbow.

The procedure itself is carried out as follows. When the tendency of the rotation is such that the left shoulder is anterior and the right one is posterior, the legs of the fetus are grasped with the left hand, and, with a semicircular swing, they are lifted up to rest against the right inguinal area of the mother. The index and middle fingers of the right hand are inserted into the vagina over the perineum in such a manner that they follow the shoulder and upper arm and reach out for the elbow joint of the right arm. With pressure and traction upon the joint, the arm is swept out under the body in the space provided by the curve of the sacrum. The arm having been delivered, the limbs are grasped now with the right hand and brought with a broad 270° downward swing to the opposite inguinal area of the mother (Figure 25.3). Now the left hand is introduced into the vagina and the index and middle fingers sweep out the left arm in the same manner as described before. The delivery of the arms having been completed, that of the head follows. This procedure is highly useful for the prevention, as well as for the correction, of extension of the arm above the head. By the same token, rotation of the body in the wrong direction is likely to result in extension of the arm and difficulties with delivery of the head.[38]

Delivery of the head

Delivery of the head is a routine procedure required in most cases of breech delivery. It should be attempted without awaiting spontaneous birth. Thus, by definition, this is "assisted breech delivery", part of the expected process when breech delivery is an elective procedure. Several excellent methods are available, probably equally satisfactory in experienced hands.

Mauriceau's maneuver. Interestingly, the maneuver was described, but not practiced, by Mauriceau. It was through the contributions of Levret, Smellie, and Veit that it achieved great popularity during the last three centuries. In the absence of spontaneous delivery up to and including the shoulders and the arms, the Mauriceau maneuver (as well as the other comparable techniques) follows the extraction of the arms immediately. The body of the fetus rests upon one arm as if the fetus was riding upon the forearm of the surgeon (Figure 25.4). The other arm holds the

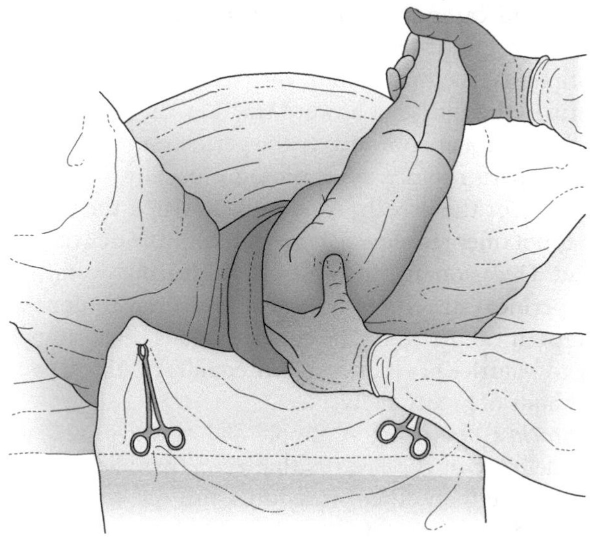

Figure 25.3 The classical method of extracting the arm during assisted breech delivery. (From Burger K, *Obstetric Surgery*, Budapest, Hungary: Franklin Társulat, 1927; Hourihane MJ. *Obstet Gynecol* 1968; 32: 512–9.)

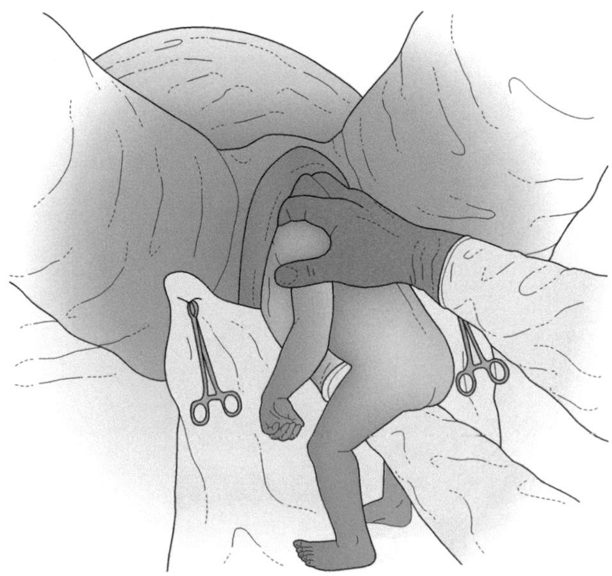

Figure 25.4 Extraction of the fetal head by the Mauriceau–Smellie–Veit maneuver. Note that the left hand simply supports the body of the fetus while the right one is used for traction. (From Burger K, *Obstetric Surgery*, Budapest, Hungary: Franklin Társulat, 1927; Hourihane MJ, *Obstet Gynecol* 1968; 32: 512–9.)

shoulders with the index and middle fingers surrounding the neck of the fetus. One finger (usually the index) of the supporting hand is inserted into the mouth of the fetus (Figure 25.5). The purpose of this hold is not traction (in fact, traction should be avoided very carefully), but flexion of the fetal head in order to permit the passage of the most favorable diameter of the vertex through the pelvis. Traction is exercised only by the upper hand and invariably in a downward direction, in the axis of the fetal spinal column, as depicted in Figure 25.4. With flexion of the fetal head carefully maintained throughout the traction, as the occiput is felt to clear the resistance offered by the symphysis, the direction of the pull is changed gradually until, in the course of upward traction, the nose, forehead, and cranium are borne over the perineum.

The performance of episiotomy usually precedes the delivery of the breech. Alternatively, when the perineum does not offer resistance, it may precede the delivery of the head. Occasionally, in cases of multiparous women with lax perineal structures, breech delivery may be done without perineal incision. The considerations that are applicable to Mauriceau's maneuver are equally pertinent to other methods of breech delivery.

Bracht's maneuver. A simple and effective method for the delivery of the head is that recommended by Bracht. Even more than other procedures, this one mandates that the bladder be emptied immediately before the delivery. The technique requires the cooperation of two persons, one who handles the fetus and another who exercises pressure over the lower abdomen of the mother upon the fetal head. In Germany, where the technique enjoys particular popularity, the role of the person exercising pressure above the symphysis is perceived as the crucial one. Therefore, it is generally the attending physician who applies the pressure and the assistant, or assisting midwife, who holds and delivers the fetus. In general, the procedure is considered suitable for the completion of spontaneous birth, but not for one that requires partial or complete extraction. Accordingly, those attending should refrain from any action until the fetus is delivered up to the neck. If necessary, the arms are brought down with one of the earlier discussed methods. The assistant simply supports the body of the fetus in such a manner that with the birth of the upper body, the trunk is lifted up first to the level of and then above the symphysis. When the full delivery of the body is accomplished, with two fists placed over the symphysis, the physician applies firm, continuous pressure against the head of the fetus. The latter is felt distinctly at this point immediately above the pubic bone. Under constant pressure and elevation of the body by the attending physician or the assistant, the fetus is delivered finally in a head-down position.[2] Undue pressure should be avoided, since it may result in "cannonball"-type extrusion of the head from the pelvis, a high-risk situation for the sudden changes in intracranial pressure and their sequelae. In the practice of many European obstetricians, the Bracht maneuver is the first-line procedure. They resort to the Mauriceau maneuver on those rare occasions when the procedure fails.

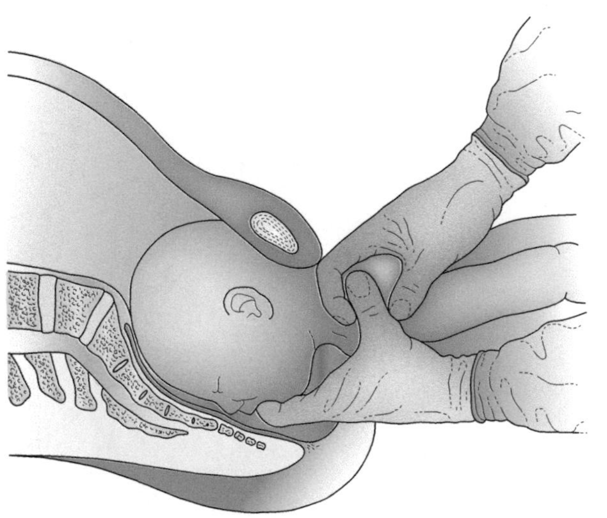

Figure 25.5 Lateral view of the extraction of the fetal head by the technique of Mauriceau. The index finger of the inside hand ensures flexion of the head and is not used for traction. (From Burger K, *Obstetric Surgery*, Budapest, Hungary: Franklin Társulat, 1927.)

Delivery by Piper's forceps. Instead of manual extraction, forceps may be applied to the aftercoming head. Piper's forceps[40] are used because of their wide shanks, fenestrations, cephalic curve, and reverse handle angle. Before the application of forceps to the aftercoming head, the fetus must be held by an assistant with some degree of extension at the neck. The feet are elevated upward above the plane of the abdomen and the arms are held by the assistant's other hand behind the back of the fetus. Some operators prefer to assume a kneeling position before introducing the left blade upward and diagonally across the introitus along the mento-occipital line of the fetal head. A large episiotomy is essential so that during the introduction of the forceps blade, extension of the head is avoided. Before locking the forceps, it is important to be certain that the blades have been inserted with sufficient depth to have a good purchase on the fetal head. Traction is then made in a downward curve and in a continuous fashion until delivery is completed, with the forceps shanks not rising above the horizontal plane, as in the case of a reverse-curved Kielland's forceps delivery.

Piper's forceps were developed in 1924 for delivery of the aftercoming head. These forceps are designed to prevent injury to the fetal neck, to decrease compression of the fetal head, and to give the needed axis traction. Because of the absence of pelvic curve, one may encounter injury to the perineum.

HEAD ENTRAPMENT

In premature fetus the head maybe entrapped by an insufficient dilated cervix. In order to expedite delivery it maybe necessary to perform cervical incisions at 2, 10, and 6 o'clock as described by Duhrsen.

Nuchal arms

Nuchal arms are a significant complication during breech delivery that may be prevented to a large degree. Rapid extraction of the fetal body should be avoided. It has been shown that umbilicus-to-mouth delivery times of up to 240 seconds (4 minutes) are usually associated with 5-minute Apgar scores of 7 or greater. If nuchal arms are present, the infant should be raised or lowered in the direction opposite to the nuchal arm and flexed over the opposite groin or buttocks of the mother. The operator's fingers should then be inserted along the humerus to the elbow, avoiding hooking the fetal arm, and, with the fingers as a splint, sweep the arm downward through the vulva. The trunk is then rotated so that the opposite nuchal arm is swept along the chest wall and the splinting maneuver repeated. The rule of delivering left arm with left hand and right arm with right hand must be remembered.

TOTAL BREECH EXTRACTION

Total breech extraction is associated with a significant incidence of hypoxic and traumatic fetal injury. It should be performed only when the child is in jeopardy and CD is not immediately available. During this procedure, no part of the fetal body other than the leg is delivered spontaneously. The operator places a hand in the birth canal, locates by palpation both or at least one of the fetal feet, and delivers the lower extremities by gentle traction. The fetal thighs are next grasped as in partial breech extraction and the fetal torso is delivered to the scapulae. The shoulder, arms, and aftercoming head are delivered as in partial breech extraction (Figure 25.2).

The anesthesiologist in the delivery room may be called upon to administer general anesthesia during total breech extraction in the absence of sufficient maternal pain relief. Hardly ever used in connection with elective delivery of singleton fetuses presenting by the breech, the technique is favored by some obstetricians for the delivery of the second twin, sometimes after the performance of an internal version.

INTERNAL VERSION

In contemporary obstetrics, the procedure of internal version is no longer an acceptable maneuver except for the delivery of the second twin. Although, even relatively recently, internal version and extraction have been used widely for the delivery of the second twin presenting as a vertex, such a stressful fetal manipulation is rarely justifiable. Spontaneous vertex delivery usually follows artificial rupture of the membranes; if not, delivery can be accomplished with the vacuum extractor. Thus, transverse lie of the second twin is probably the only good reason for internal version and extraction in modern obstetrics.[41]

The procedure requires general or conduction anesthesia. It consists of three steps: (1) introduction of the hands, (2) grasping the lower extremity or extremities, and (3) version of the body.

Ideally, the membranes are intact until the hand is introduced to effect internal version of the body; then, they must be ruptured. The hand to be introduced is the one that corresponds with the side of the fetal legs—the left hand if the lower limbs are on the mother's right side, and the right hand if they are on the mother's left. If there is a choice, the upper foot is to be grasped when the fetal abdomen or chest is presenting, whereas the extraction of the lower limb is preferable when the presenting area is the fetal back. This promotes anterior rotation of the back and prevents anterior rotation of the chin and its earlier mentioned sequelae. In the absence of a choice, the leg that can be reached easiest is to be used for traction. Occasionally, it is possible to grasp both lower limbs, a circumstance that facilitates the procedure. While one hand is being introduced, the assisting hand holds the uterine fundus in order to prevent colporrhexis (Figure 25.6a).

The limb having been reached, traction is exerted upon it. The direction of the pull is toward the midline. Meanwhile, the external hand may divert the head from its lateral position toward the middle part of the fundus (Figure 25.6b).

The conclusion of internal version is identical with that of breech extraction as described earlier in this chapter. Internal uterine manipulations carry the risks of uterine rupture and cervical damage as well as that of colporrhexis. Therefore, exploration of the uterine cavity after the delivery of placenta and thorough inspection of the cervix and the vaginal vault are integral parts of the total operative procedure.

EXTERNAL VERSION

External version can result in up to 70% reduction in the incidence of breech presentation at term.[42–45] Since many physicians favor the use of tocolysis, in order to facilitate the performance of this procedure, it should be remembered that major cardiac disorders and arrhythmia represent contraindications to the use of tocolytic agents.[21] Hibbard and Schulmann[46] effectively practiced prophylactic external version at week 34.[47–48] Van Dorsten et al.[49] conducted a randomized, controlled trial in which the external version was performed under terbutaline tocolysis at 37–39 weeks' gestation. It was successful in 68% of the cases, and all of these presented in labor subsequently with vertex presentations. Nulliparity, maternal obesity, engagement of the breech, and uterine anomaly tended to reduce the success rate of external version. In the control group, only 18% of the presenting breeches converted to vertex beyond week 37 of the pregnancy. Transient fetal heart rate decelerations were noted during version in 36% of the attempts (24% of successes and 63% of failures). These decelerations responded to cessation of manipulation. External cephalic version is less successful in cases of frank breech, where the splinting action of the extended fetal legs makes version difficult to perform. Studies have shown that regional anesthesia increase the success rate of version.

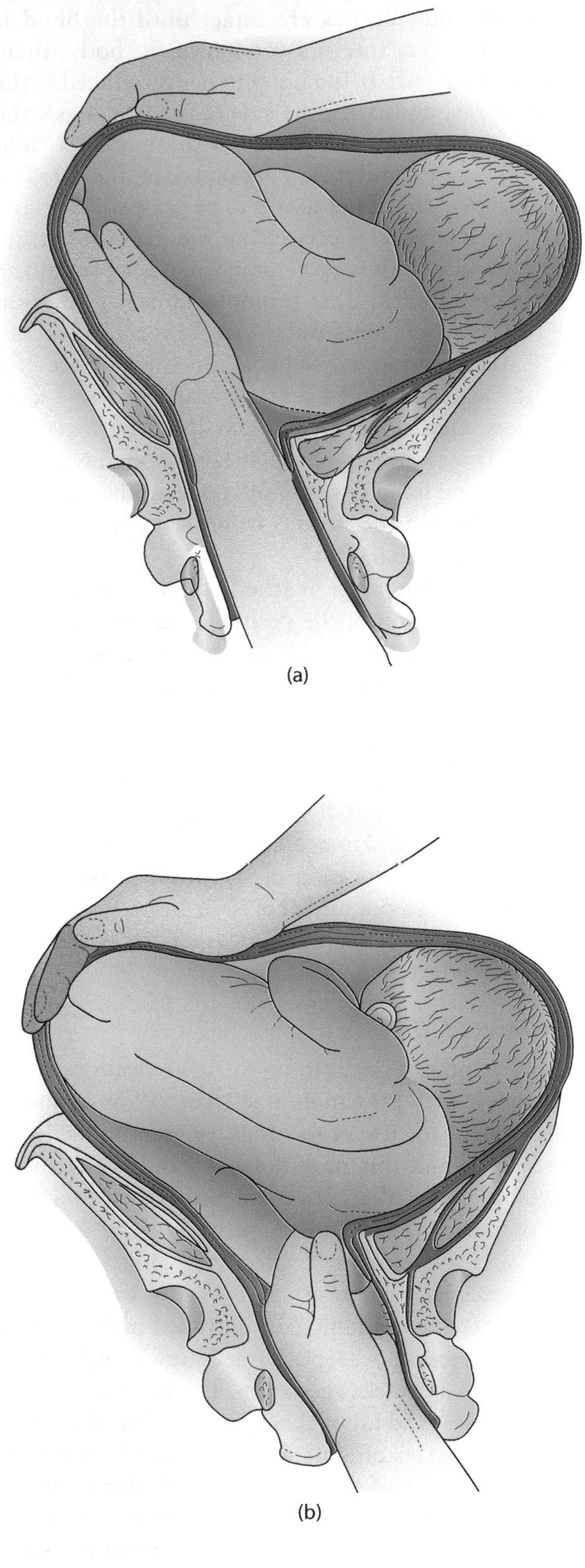

(a)

(b)

Figure 25.6 Internal version for the correction of transverse lie. (a) Introduction into the uterus of one hand while counterpressure is exerted by the assisting (outside) hand of the operator. (b) Traction applied toward the midline. (A classical nineteenth-century illustration by Halban-Seitz, reproduced from Iffy L and Kaminetzky HA, (eds.) *Principles and Practice of Obstetrics & Perinatology*, New York, NY: Wiley, 1981. With permission from Leslie Iffy.)

Successful version is associated with an increased need for cesarean section on account of dystocia.[46] There is a relative contraindication in Rh-negative women because of the risk of accidents leading to fetomaternal transfusion. Other complications of external version include fetal distress; twisting, knotting, or laceration of the cord; placental separation; uterine rupture; premature labor; premature rupture of the membranes; and spinal cord transection in utero. For reasons mentioned above, Rh-negative mothers should be have a Kleihauer–Betke test ordered after the procedure and should receive RhoGAM if evidence of fetomaternal transfusion is documented. Parity, sufficient amniotic fluid, and unengaged presenting part are conducive to a successful version. Previous cesarean or other penetrating uterine scar is a contraindication.

It is recommended that the external version procedure be carried out according to a prearranged protocol.[47,48] Although it can be attempted at any time before the occurrence of labor,[49] it is best to wait until the fetal lung has achieved maturity, yet the amount of the amniotic fluid has not decreased to such an extent as to hinder the manipulation of the fetus. This optimum time is probably the weeks 35–36 of gestation. It is necessary to have facilities for electronic monitoring, ultrasound, and easy access to the operating room for CD if circumstances require. The availability of at least one assistant for the performance of the procedure is considered essential.

For the performance of external version, the patient should take nothing by mouth for at least 6 hours before the procedure. The blood indices should be tested in anticipation of the procedure. The bladder must be empty. The placement of the patient into a head-down Trendelenburg position (about 15°) is conducive to the disengagement of the presenting breech from the pelvis. It is considered advantageous by some to spread fine talc powder over the abdomen in order to facilitate the maneuver. As mentioned earlier, the performance of a nonstress test at the end of the procedure is indicated in order to avoid overlooking fetal distress resulting from the version.

After the exact position of the fetus has been established by ultrasound, the physician performing the procedure positions himself/herself in such a manner that he/she faces the fetus. The procedure itself begins with the operator lifting out the presenting breech from the pelvis and elevating it as high as possible without the use of undue force. Thereafter, the breech is displaced toward the direction of the fetal back, away from the pelvic inlet. At the same time, the other hand of the operator attempts to drive the head forward and downward as if encouraging the fetus to do a somersault. A useful alternative approach is to entrust the assistant with the elevation and displacement of the breech in order to permit the operator to use both hands for driving the head through 180° into the pelvic inlet while the breech is moved gently upward in the opposite direction. It is to be remembered that the direction of version is counterclockwise in case of first breech presentation (fetal back turned to the mother's left side) and clockwise when the presentation is second breech (fetal back turned to the right side of the mother). It is axiomatic in good obstetric practice not to force the version in the absence of success with one or two attempts or when, after what appears to have been an accomplished external version, the fetus repeatedly returns to its original position. It is to be remembered, furthermore, that a breech presentation carries less risk than a transverse lie. Accordingly, care must be taken not to leave the fetus, initially presenting by the breech, lying in transverse or oblique position.

Contrary to what one might expect, external version in the case of transverse lie is more difficult than when the presentation is breech. Particularly, when permitted to prevail until the late third trimester, the shape of the uterus adjusts to the transverse lie of the fetus. Thus, when the axis of the body changes from transverse to longitudinal, it hinders the maintenance of the desired presentation. Whereas after a successful external version from breech presentation the fetus usually remains in vertex presentation, it tends to return to transverse hours or days after the procedure when version is attempted from a transverse lie.

If external version is employed, a number of rigid criteria must be met. The fetus must be judged normal, with no oligohydramnios or placenta previa demonstrated by standard sonography. External fetal monitoring should be utilized before and after the procedure. The breech should preferably be unengaged. It is performed at a gestation of 35–36 weeks so that, in the event of an accident requiring delivery, the fetal outcome will not be compromised by prematurity. The uterus must be nontender and not irritable. This is best ensured by a tocolytic agent,[50] such as 0.25 mg terbutaline administered 15–30 minutes before the attempt.

That difficulties arising during the labor process can be resolved by cesarean section is an old concept. On the other hand, it was accepted up to the last decades of the twentieth century that difficulties leading to the demise of the child may arise during the process of delivery in a variety of clinical situations. The latter include shoulder dystocia in the process of delivering a fetus presenting by the vertex, interlocking of the heads of twins (thus preventing the delivery of the first one), arrest of delivery of conjoined twins, and inability to deliver the aftercoming head in breech presentation. Fetal death or catastrophic injury deriving from these complications has generally been considered inevitable by obstetricians until recently.

The double-setup for delivery of breech presentations and twin deliveries along with the development of some contemporary techniques discussed elsewhere in this volume provides an opportunity for overcoming some difficulties during the vaginal delivery process that had previously led to fetal death or gross injury in the past. Relevant to breech presentation, "abdominal rescue" represents a desperate, last-ditch effort to save fetal life in a situation when extraction of the aftercoming head or upper body appears impossible without potentially catastrophic fetal injury.[35,51] This maneuver requires the elevation of the body of the fetus by an assistant in order to improve circulation in the brain, and quick performance of a hysterotomy, typically by a vertical uterine incision, followed by extraction of the head, and the rest of the body abdominally. Under double setup, the same technique may be a practical solution whenever delivery of the aftercoming head becomes impossible for some unforeseen reason, such as deflexion of the fetal head during the process of delivery, resistance offered by an incompletely dilated cervix,[52] or interlocking of the heads of twins.

GENERAL CONSIDERATIONS

Some experts believe that cesarean section offers improved outcome for the premature breech fetus weighing less than 1500–2000 g. It is thought that the vaginal delivery of the premature breech fetus creates an increased risk of brain damage due to intracranial hemorrhage and birth trauma.[53] The studies result are contradictory. A randomized control trial done in Great Britain was closed because it failed to recruit enough participants. For fetuses above 2000 g, the benefit of cesarean section is less apparent.[30,54,55]

However, for a term fetus, a specific protocol must be implemented for selection of patients for vaginal breech delivery. This should include (1) frank breech position; (2) immediate availability of cesarean section (including anesthesiologist and nursing staff); (3) estimated fetal weight 2000–3600 g; (4) adequate clinical pelvimetry, (5) absence of hyperextension of the fetal head; (6) absence of fetal distress; (7) absence of postmaturity; (8) normal progress of labor; (9), in case of second twin presenting by the breech, absence of a difference exceeding 3–4 mm between the biparietal diameters in favor of twin B.

It is an important principle that the membranes in breech labor must be left intact as long as possible. Since the small presenting parts permit the escape of much of the amniotic fluid after their rupture, breaking the membranes artificially is an invitation for cord-related complications.

The establishment of a plan with regard to the method of delivery by term (i.e., week 38) is of utmost importance. Labor frequently is preceded by rupture of the membranes, an event that carries the risk of prolapse of the cord and its dire sequelae. Since no tangible improvement in prenatal mortality and morbidity rates derives from continued fetal maturation beyond completed week 38, the risk/benefit ratio of procrastination beyond this time, in cases where vaginal delivery in contraindicated, is bound to be unfavorable. Accordingly, the recommended time for elective abdominal delivery is completed week 38 of gestation.

TRANSVERSE LIE

When the long axis of the fetus is perpendicular to the axis of the mother, the technical term of transverse lie applies. The head or the breech occupies the iliac fossa. The shoulder presents and it is the point of designation. With regard to the definition of the position of the fetus, it needs to be determined whether the fetus is in a dorsoanterior or dorsoposterior position.

The incidence of transverse lie is about one in 300 pregnancies. Those risk factors known to be conducive to breech presentation are also conducive to this entity.[56–62] Transverse lie can be easily detected by the Leopold maneuvers alone. On palpation, the maternal corpus is wide and the fundal height is shortened. The fetal head is palpated in one of the maternal flanks or iliac fossae. On pelvic examination, no presenting part is felt. A suspicion of transverse lie requires careful evaluation. The risks of early labor or rupture of membranes need to be brought to the attention of the patient. The exact presentation should be confirmed by ultrasound with the same considerations in mind that have been described for breech presentation.

It is advisable to attempt the external version maneuver earlier with a transverse lie than in breech presentation since it becomes extremely difficult, if not impossible, by the last few weeks of gestation. By that time, the shape of the uterus has adjusted to the position of the fetus, and with the amount of amniotic fluid reduced, it can no longer accommodate the child in the longitudinal lie. For the same reason, versions that appear to be successful initially may often prove to be a failure a few days later.

Presumably on account of the loss of most of the amniotic fluid, fetuses in transverse lie fare poorly after the membranes have ruptured. For this reason, prolonged observation in connection with premature rupture of the membranes is not a viable option in transverse lie.

Because of the high risk of prolapse of the cord (10%), elective delivery at week 37 by cesarean section is recommended. If the fetal back is turned downward, a lower vertical or classical incision is needed. If the back is turned upward, the technique of abdominal delivery is essentially the same as in breech presentations.

ACKNOWLEDGMENT

This chapter contains material from the previous chapter coauthored by Leslie Iffy.

REFERENCES

1. Cruiskshank DP, White CA. Obstetric malpresentation: Twenty years' experience. *Am J Obstet Gynecol* 1973; 116: 1097.
2. Braun FHT, Jones KL, Smith DW. Breech presentation as an indicator of fetal abnormality. *J Pediatr* 1975; 86: 419–21.
3. Thorp J, Jenkins T, Watson W. Utility of Leopold maneuvers in screening for malpresentation. *Obstet Gynecol* 1991; 78: 394–6.
4. Morgan ES, Kane SH. An analysis of 16,327 breech births. *JAMA* 1964; 187: 262–4.
5. Moore WT, Steptoe PP. The experience of the Johns Hopkins Hospital with breech presentation. An analysis of 1,444 cases. *South Med J* 1943; 36: 295.
6. Alarab M, Regan C, O'Connell MP et al. Singleton vaginal breech delivery at term: Still a safe option. *Obstet Gynecol* 2004; 103: 407–12.
7. Eide MA, Oyen N, Skjaerven R et al. Breech delivery and intelligence: A population-based study of 8,738 breech infants. *Obstet Gynecol* 2005; 105: 4–11.
8. Brenner WE, Bruce RD, Hendricks CH. The characteristics and perils of breech presentation. *Am J Obstet Gynecol* 1974; 118: 700–12.
9. Weingold AB. The management of breech presentations. In: Iffy L, Charles D (eds), *Operative Perinatology*, p. 537. New York, NY: Macmillan, 1984.
10. Ventura SJ, Martin JA, Curtin SC. Birth: Final data for 1997. *Natl Vital Stat Rep* 1999; 47: 1–96.
11. Bhagwanani SG, Price HV, Laurence KM, Ginz B. Risks and prevention of cervical cord injury in the management of breech presentation with hyperextension of the fetal head. *Am J Obstet Gynecol* 1973; 115: 1159–61.
12. American Academy of Pediatrics and American College of Obstetricians and Gynecologists. *Guideline for Perinatal Care* (5th edition), p. 109. Washington, DC: American Academy of Pediatrics and American College of Obstetricians and Gynecologists, 2002.
13. Kotaska A. Inappropriate use of randomised trials to evaluate complex phenomena: Case study of vaginal breech delivery. *BMJ* 2004; 329: 1039–42.
14. Apuzzio J, Iffy L, Weiss G. Mode of delivery in breech presentation. *Acta Obstet Gynecol Scand* 2002; 81: 1091.
15. Apuzzio J, Iffy L, Weiss G. Mode of term singleton breech delivery. *Obstet Gynecol* 2002; 99: 1131–3.
16. Van Roosmalen J, Rosendaal F. There is still room for disagreement about vaginal delivery of breech infants at term. *Br J Obstet Gynaecol* 2002; 109: 967–9.
17. Green PM, Walkinshaw S. Management of breech deliveries. *Obstet Gynaecol* 2002; 4: 87.
18. Gimovsky ML, Wallace RL, Schifrin BS, Paul RH. Randomized management of the non-frank breech presentations at term: A preliminary report. *Am J Obstet Gynecol* 1983; 146: 34–40.
19. Giuliani A, Scholl WM, Basver A Tamussino. Mode of delivery and outcome of 699 term singleton breech deliveries at a single center. *Am J Obstet Gynecol* 2002; 187: 1694–8.
20. Sibony O, Luton D, Oury JF, Blot P. Six hundred and ten breech versus 12,405 cephalic deliveries at term: Is there any difference in the neonatal outcome? *Eur J Obstet Gynecol Reprod Biol* 2003; 107: 140–4.
21. Wong WM, Lao TT, Liu KL. Predicting the success of external cephalic version with a scoring system. A prospective, two-phase study. *J Reprod Med* 2000; 45: 201–6.
22. American College of Obstetricians and Gynecologists. ACOG Practice Bulletin No. 13. External cephalic version. *Obstet Gynecol* 2000; 95: 1–7. Reaffirmed 2014.
23. Hansen GF. Version of the fetus. In: Iffy L, Charles D (eds), *Operative Perinatology*, p. 471. New York, NY: Macmillan, 1984.

24. Van Loon AJ, Mantingh A, Serlier EK et al. Randomized controlled trial of magnetic resonance pelvimetry in breech presentation at term. *Lancet* 1997; 350: 1799–804.
25. Hall JE, Kohl S. Breech presentation: A study of 1,456 cases. *Am J Obstet Gynecol* 1956; 72: 977–90.
26. Hall JE, Kohl SG, O'Brien F et al. Breech presentation and perinatal mortality. *Am J Obstet Gynecol* 1965; 91: 655.
27. Hannah ME, Hannah WJ, Hewson SA et al. Planned caesarean section versus planned vaginal birth for breech presentation at term: A randomized multicenter trial. *Lancet* 2000; 356: 1375–83.
28. Lumley J. Any room left for disagreement about assisting breech birth at term? *Lancet* 2000; 356: 1369–70.
29. Hauth LT, Cuningham FG. Vaginal breech delivery is still justified. *Obstet Gynecol* 2002; 99: 1115–6.
30. Collea JV, Chein C, Quilligan EJ. The randomized management of frank breech presentation: A study of 208 cases. *Am J Obstet Gynecol* 1980; 137: 235–44.
31. Schutte JM, Steegers EA. Maternal deaths after elective cesarean section for breech presentation in the Netherland. 2007; 86: 240–3.
32. Whyte H, Hannah M. Outcomes of children at 2 years after planned cesarean birth versus planned vaginal delivery. *Am J Obstet Gynecol* 2004; 191: 864e71.
33. Alexander J, Gregg JEM, Quinn MW. Femoral fractures at cesarean section. Case reports. *Br J Obstet Gynaecol* 1987; 94: 273.
34. Friedman EA. *Labor: Clinical Evaluation and Management* (2nd edition). New York, NY: Appleton-Century-Crofts, 1978.
35. Whyte H, Hannah ME, Saigal S et al. Term Breech Trial Collaborative Group; outcomes of children at 2 years after planned cesarean birth versus planned vaginal birth for breech presentation at term: The International Randomized Term Breech Trial. *Am J Obstet Gynecol* 2004; 191: 864–71.
36. Iffy L, Toliver CW. Manual extraction procedures. In: Iffy L, Kaminetzky HA (eds), *Principles and Practice of Obstetrics & Perinatology*, p. 1521. New York, NY: John Wiley, 1981.
37. Burger K. *Szülészeti Mütéttan*, p. 117. Budapest, Hungary: Franklin Társulat, 1927.
38. Iffy L, Apuzzio JJ, Cohen-Addad N et al. Abdominal rescue after entrapment of the aftercoming head. *Am J Obstet Gynecol* 1986; 154: 623.
39. Hourihane MJ. Etiology and management of oblique lie. *Obstet Gynecol* 1968; 32: 512–9.
40. Martius G. *Lehrbuch der Geburtshilfe* (9th edition), p. 299. Stuttgart, Germany: Georg Thieme, 1977.
41. Beischer NA. Pelvic contraction in breech presentations. *J Obstet Gynaecol Br Commonw* 1966; 73: 421–7.
42. Piper EB, Bachman C. The prevention of fetal injuries in breech delivery. *JAMA* 1929; 92: 217.
43. Winn HN, Cimino J, Powers J et al. Intrapartum management of nonvertex second-born twins: A critical analysis. *Am J Obstet Gynecol* 2001; 185: 1204–8.
44. Siddiqui D, Stiller RJ, Collins J, Laifer SA. Pregnancy outcome after successful external cephalic version. *Am J Obstet Gynecol* 1999; 181: 1092–5.
45. Zhang J, Bowes WA, Fortney JA. Efficacy of external cephalic version including safety cost benefits analysis and impact on the cesarean section rate. *Obstet Gynecol* 1993; 82: 306–12.
46. Hibbard LT, Schumann WR. Prophylactic external version in an obstetric practice. *Am J Obstet Gynecol* 1973; 116: 511–8.
47. Goetzinger K. Harper L. Effect of regional anesthesia on the success rate of external cephalic version: A systematic review and meta-analysis. *Obstet Gynecol* 2011; 118(5): 1137–44.
48. Khaw KS, Lee SW, Ngan Kee et al. Randomized trial of anaesthetic interventions in external cephalic version for breech presentation. *Br J Anaesth* 2015; 114: 944–50.
49. Van Dorsten JP, Schifrin BS, Wallace RL. Randomized control trial of external cephalic version with tocolysis in late pregnancy. *Am J Obstet Gynecol* 1981; 141: 417–24.
50. Vezina Y, Bujold E, Varin J et al. Cesarean delivery after successful external cephalic version of breech presentation at term: A comparative study. *Am J Obstet Gynecol* 2004; 190: 763–8.
51. Hellstrom AC, Nilsson B, Stange L, Nylund L. When does external cephalic version succeed? *Acta Obstet Gynecol Scand* 1990; 69: 281–5.
52. Mancuso KM, Yancey MK, Murphy JA et al. Epidural analgesia for cephalic version: A randomized trial. *Obstet Gynecol* 2000; 95: 648–51.
53. Impey L, Lissoni D. Outcome of external cephalic version after 36 weeks' gestation without tocolysis. *J Matern Fetal Med* 1999; 8: 203–7.
54. Yanny H, Johanson R, Balwin KJ et al. Double-blind randomized controlled trial of glyceryl trinitrate spray for external cephalic version. *Br J Obstet Gynaecol* 2000; 107: 562–4.
55. Swartjes JM, Bleker OP, Schutte MF. The Zavanelli maneuver applied to locked twins. *Am J Obstet Gynecol* 1992; 166: 532.
56. Tchabo J, Tomai T. Selected external version of the second twin. *Obstet Gynecol* 1992; 79: 421–3.
57. Gravenhorst JB, Schreuder AM, Veen S et al. Breech delivery in very preterm and very-low-birth infants in the Netherlands. *Br J Obstet Gynaecol* 1993; 100: 411–5.
58. Penn ZJ, Steer PJ, Grant A. A multicentre ramdomised controlled trial comparing elective and selective caesarean section in preterm Breech infant. *BJOG* 2014; 121 (Suppl 7): 48–53.

59. Thomas PE, Petersen SG. The influence of mode of birth on neonatal survival and maternal outcomes at extreme prematurity. A retrospective cohort study. *Aust N Z J Obstet Gynaecol* 2016; 56: 60–8.
60. Alfirevic Z, Milan SJ. Caesarean section versus vaginal delivery for preterm birth in singleton. *Cochrane Database Syst Rev* 2013; (4): CD008991.
61. Bergenhenenegoowen L, Vlemmix F. Preterm breech presentation: A comparison of intended vaginal delivery and intended vaginal delivery. *Obstet Gynecol* 2015; 126(6): 1223.
62. Collea JV. Malpresentations and cord accidents. In: Pernoll ML, Benson RC (eds), *Current Obstetric and Gynecologic Diagnosis and Treatment*, p. 23. Norwalk, CT: Appleton & Lange, 1987.

Delivery of twins and higher-order multiples

26

ISAAC BLICKSTEIN

CONTENTS

Changes in the epidemiology of multiple gestation influence the decision of how and when to deliver twins. The dramatic increase in the frequency of multiple birth has affected preterm deliveries.[1] The 2002 U.S. vital statistics show that the twin birth rate reached a remarkable 3.1% of all live births; a 65% increase over the past two decades and a 38% increase since 1990.[2] In 2002, the incidence of triplets and higher-order multiples was 1.84 per 1000 live births compared with about 1:10,000 births after spontaneous conceptions.[2]

This trend continues over the years. In 2013, the U.S. national Vital Statistics Reports indicated that the birth rate increased to 3.37%, a U.S. record, for a 76% increase from 1980 to 2009, a steady state between 2009 and 2012.[3]

Data from the 2010 European Perinatal Health Report[4] clearly show that in all but three European countries participating in the Euro-Peristat project, the incidence of multiple birth rate increased from 2004 to 2010.

The increased rates of multiple birth inevitably increase those of preterm deliveries because 12% of twins, 36% of triplets, and 60% of quadruplets are born before 32 weeks' gestation.[2] According to the U.S. Centers for Disease Control, the main reason for the increase in preterm births is multiple gestation secondary to assisted reproductive technologies (ART), with 16% of all preterm deliveries in the United States (79,684 in 2002) being due to multiple births.[2] Tul et al.[5] found a twofold increased incidence of twins from 1987 to 2010, and a threefold increased incidence of twins born after ART. Twins after ART born at <32 weeks comprised 0.05% of all births (range 0.004%–0.11%) and increased 27-fold from 1987 to 2010.

Another important change is the increasing age of the mothers of multiples.[6] U.S. data indicate that fewer mothers in the age group 15–29 years delivered their firstborn in 2002 than in 1990, whereas the first birth rate increased 25%–30% in the age group 30–44 years.[2] In the past, pregnancies at older age were primarily unintended, and women usually delivered their last baby at an earlier age. At present, however, many women intentionally postpone childbirth until they achieve personal milestones. Because of the reduced fecundity associated with older age, there is a significant need for ART to achieve the desired pregnancy. Thus, social trends and available therapy act in concert to increase the risk of multiple births. Loos et al.,[7] using data from the East Flanders Prospective Twin Survey, noted that in 1976 there was one induced twin maternity for every 32 spontaneous twins. In contrast, by 1996, this ratio was 1:1.02. With increasing frequencies of *iatrogenic* pregnancies, the proportion of previously infertile women delivering twins is increasing, leading to higher rates of "premium pregnancies," for which any mode of delivery except a cesarean (justified or not) may be declined.[8]

The decision of how to deliver multiples may be further modified by recent publications demonstrating the reduced risk of elective cesarean, mainly in terms of maternal mortality, and describing the potential benefits of elective cesarean for both mothers and children in terms of reduced morbidity.[9] It could be inferred that if a cesarean section upon a woman's request is medically[9] and ethically[10] permissible (although not necessarily advisable), it would be logical to opt for a cesarean delivery of multiples, although the indication may seem subtle or unfounded by evidence.

The second consideration comes from a study documenting the advantage of a planned cesarean section for the term fetus in breech presentation without increasing the maternal complication rate compared with vaginal breech delivery.[11] As a result of this study based on singletons, many centers extrapolated its conclusions to twin births with any presentation other than vertex–vertex, and no longer undertake breech deliveries by the vaginal route irrespective of plurality. Consequently, many young residents presently lack the training, experience, and manual dexterity required for breech delivery. Indeed, a secondary analysis of the Term Breech Trial cited the presence of an experienced clinician at delivery among the significant factors that reduced the risk of adverse perinatal outcome among vaginal breech deliveries.[12] Because twin pairs include at least one breech or transverse lying twin in 50%–60% of cases, assisted or operative deliveries are the rule rather than the exception. Indeed, a direct relationship exists between the cesarean section rate in twins and the combined delivery rate, suggesting that those who perform more abdominal deliveries in twins and are, thus, less experienced in vaginal deliveries of twins, are more likely to decide on a cesarean for the second twin.[13] In summary, because twin gestations frequently involve maternal and fetal complications, and are quite often considered "premium" pregnancies, many clinicians prefer to deliver twins by the abdominal route for subtle reasons rather than clear-cut indications.[8]

CESAREAN SECTION FOR ALL TWINS

The U.S. cesarean delivery rate increased by 13% between 1989 and 1991 and 1997 and 1999 among twins delivered at >22 weeks and weighing >500 g.[14] This value represents average increases of 52%, 28%, and 9%, among twin pregnancies delivered at 22–27, 28–33, and >34 weeks' gestation, respectively. Although the rates increased to a greater extent at earlier than at later gestational ages, the absolute number of cesareans was much higher at later gestational ages.[14] These rates are quite similar to the commonly cited rates of 50%–60% abdominal births among twins and nearly 100% among triplets.[8] In the United Kingdom, the 2001 cesarean rate for twin deliveries was 59%.[15] Barber et al.[16] found that the indication for cesarean section in the United States for multiple gestation increased at a much faster rate than the incidence of multiples in the population, with an estimate of 200% higher than would be expected based on population figures. However, the clinician's problem is not reduction of the overall cesarean rate but avoiding unnecessary operations. In this respect, one addresses two important questions. First, are there specific maternal risks associated with abdominal delivery of twins?[17] Second, is there any solid evidence that cesarean section is safer for twins than vaginal delivery?

Regrettably, the first question has not been addressed in the literature adequately. On the other hand, the potential beneficial effect of cesarean section for twins has been studied extensively by case–control methodology. Hogle et al.[18] recently reported their systematic review and meta-analysis aimed to determine whether a policy of planned cesarean section or vaginal delivery is favorable for twins. Their literature research ranging from 1980 through 2001 included studies that compared planned cesarean section to planned vaginal birth for babies weighing >1500 g or reaching at least 32 weeks' gestation. Only four studies with a total of 1932 infants were included in the analysis. A low, 5-minute Apgar score occurred less frequently in twins delivered by planned cesarean section (odds ratio [OR] 0.5; 95% confidence interval [CI] 0.3, 0.9) principally because of a reduction among pairs with twin A in breech presentation. Twins delivered by planned cesarean section spent longer time in the hospital, but, there were no significant differences in perinatal or neonatal mortality, neonatal morbidity, or maternal morbidity.

It follows that the decision for a cesarean in twins, intentionally or not, is based on qualitative variables. The quantitative variables suggest no advantage for abdominal delivery in the majority of cases.[8]

VAGINAL DELIVERY OF TWINS

Malpresentation

Each twin may present as vertex or breech, or assume a transverse lie. To simplify the discussion, twins are vertex/vertex roughly 40% of the time; vertex/nonvertex 30% of the time; nonvertex/vertex 20% of the time; and nonvertex/nonvertex 10% of the time.[19] In many ways, decision making related to fetal presentation seems to be the easy way to deal with the optimal manner to deliver twins.

Vertex–vertex

Vertex–vertex pairs are generally considered *suitable* candidates for vaginal delivery albeit with a *few* exceptions related to size and/or gestational age. During the labor and delivery process of the first twin, the only sure thing to say is that twin B is likely to remain in the vertex presentation. This reservation emerges from the observation that what appears to be vertex twin B is, in fact, more similar to an oblique presentation, because the position of twin A in the pelvis does not allow a true vertex presentation of twin B. Moreover, when twin B is surrounded by polyhydramnios, it might easily revert to a transverse lie after the delivery of its firstborn co-twin.

In the optimal setting, labor is allowed to progress under dual external monitoring of the twins. Most modern cardiotocographic machines can distinguish simultaneous signals from the two fetuses and record an adequate dual fetal heart rate tracing. However, this frequently necessitates the use of three belts on the maternal abdomen. Therefore, once the membranes of the presenting twin are ruptured, an internal (scalp) electrode is often used to replace one external Doppler electrode. The dual fetal heart rate tracing enables individual attention to the well-being of each fetus.

The preferred method of pain relief is regional anesthesia by epidural block.[20,21] Lumbar epidural anesthesia is recommended when vaginal delivery is anticipated. It also provides adequate anesthesia for interventions such as instrumental or cesarean delivery.

Once the first twin is delivered, the clamped umbilical cord should be marked in order to recognize it as belonging to twin A when the placenta is examined postpartum. Arguments favoring cord clamping in singletons suggest that this procedure enhances the separation of the placenta, an undesirable event before the delivery of twin B. To our knowledge, the practice of cord clamping for twin A has not been studied vis-à-vis the documented higher frequency of intrapartum placental abruption in twins.[22] A supporting argument of cord clamping of twin A refers to the possibility of blood loss from twin B via open vascular connections that are invariably found in monochorionic placentas. Cord clamping in this circumstance may avoid acute intrapartum twin-to-twin transfusion. For the same reason, umbilical cord-blood gases should be sampled from a segment of the cord distal to the clamp.

Immediately after the birth of twin A, the uterus often undergoes a strong, but brief, contraction. This is usually followed by a period of uterine quiescence, lasting a minute or two, before contractions resume for the delivery of twin B. This short period provides a window of opportunity for external manipulation of twin B, if necessary. In the case of vertex–vertex presentation, this may be used to perform external semiversion from oblique lie into longitudinal lie. To be able to do this, however, one needs three hands: one to perform a vaginal examination to establish the station of the presenting part, another to palpate the uterine fundus to determine the period of uterine relaxation, and a third one to hold a bedside ultrasound transducer to establish the correct presentation. Obviously, assistance is needed. When twin B is in the vertex position, a diluted solution of oxytocin should be administered via an infusion pump to ensure the resumption of uterine contractions. Amniotomy is expected to reduce the time interval between the deliveries of the twins. However, with a high station of the head, prolapse of the umbilical cord may occur if the membranes are ruptured intentionally or inadvertently. In one study, 26% of emergent cesareans for twin B, when both twins were in vertex presentation, resulted from cord prolapse of twin B.[23] It is, therefore, recommended that amniotomy be deferred until the head of twin B becomes engaged or a presenting umbilical cord is excluded.

At times, the head of twin B remains high above the pelvic inlet. This circumstance makes it clear that after the delivery of twin A, one is not dealing with an otherwise usual vertex delivery of a (remaining) singleton, but with the delivery of twin B. It is debatable whether the interdelivery interval should be more than the traditionally recommended 20 minutes. Leung et al.[24] found that umbilical cord blood values of pH, pCO_2, and base excess deteriorate with increasing twin-to-twin delivery interval. In their series, none of the second twins delivered within 15 minutes of the birth of twin A had a pH value under 7. However, 5.9% had such a value when delivered within 16–30 minutes, and 27% had this low pH value when delivered after an interval of over 30 minutes. Importantly, 73% of the twins with an interval of over 30 minutes had signs of fetal distress that required operative delivery. Erdemoglu et al.[25] found a linear relationship between the delivery interval and the 5-minute Apgar score. Pons et al.[26] compared expectant to active management in the delivery of the second twin and found similar neonatal results. These data support the concept that prevailed before the 1980s, namely, that the time interval between the deliveries of the twins should not exceed 20 minutes. Therefore, extension of this time limit to a maximum of 30 minutes should be subject to documentation of reassuring heart rate pattern of twin B by close electronic or ultrasonic surveillance.

Because twins are smaller than singletons, absolute cephalopelvic disproportion is rarely present. More commonly, relative disproportion is seen as a result of compound presentation. This is managed, as in the case of singleton birth, by gentle sweeping of the forelying extremity backward.

Delayed birth due to inadequate uterine contraction should be rare with the judicious use of oxytocin. After decompression caused by the expulsion of the presenting twin, abruption of the placenta of the second twin may occur.[22,23] This needs emergency intervention by either the vaginal or the abdominal route.

Throughout the interval between births, the heart rate of twin B should be carefully monitored, and any sign of fetal distress should be effectively assessed. In the common scenario, the most relevant question is how soon the delivery of twin B is anticipated. When the cervix is fully dilated and the head is engaged, a vacuum extraction is a good option. Delivery of the second twin is the only circumstance where high-station vacuum extraction is permissible. However, this procedure should be reserved for special circumstances because the unengaged head of twin B has not undergone the necessary molding, and it may be difficult to place the vacuum cup on an unengaged head. Alternatively, internal podalic version (see below) and breech extraction can sometimes be performed. Thus, if prompt delivery of twin B is necessary, skillful instrumental delivery or internal version may be the first option, rather than abdominal delivery. If worst comes to worst, however, a combined twin delivery should be performed (see below).

Vertex–nonvertex

Vertex–nonvertex pairs were always considered *possible* candidates for vaginal delivery, with *many* exceptions related to size and/or gestational age.[27] The ultimate goal is the safe delivery of twin B in breech presentation.[12] When twin B is in a transverse lie, it must first undergo version into the longitudinal lie (usually breech). Historically, this combination of presentations was subject to innumerable studies. Delivery of vertex–nonvertex twins is one of the highest challenges in manual dexterity (Figure 26.1).

When twin B presents by the breech, birth can be accomplished either by assisted breech delivery or by total breech extraction. In the former, amniotomy is delayed as much as possible to use the pressure effect of the amniotic sac on the cervix. Quite often, episiotomy is performed, and the breech presentation of twin B should be reconfirmed. It has been found that 52% of cesarean sections performed for twin B in the "safest" configuration (vertex A–vertex B) were done for change in presentation of twin B, with inability to perform version and extraction.[23]

Quite often, cervical dilation decreases after the delivery of twin A. This "clamping down" of the cervix is attributed to the sudden decompression of the uterine cavity. However, the cervix in this case is different from a cervix with the same dilation in the active phase. Here, when "clamping down" occurs, the time required to achieve again full dilation is relatively short. With adequate uterine contractions, the cervix will usually regain its previous dilation within 5–15 minutes.

Alternatively, the feet of twin B are grasped with intact membranes, and then the membranes are ruptured, and the fetus is delivered by total extraction. Another alternative approach applies external version (EV) to the vertex. The pros and cons for each method are related to the size of twin B. Some authors recommend that the nonvertex second twin over 24 weeks' gestation and under 1700 g estimated fetal weight should undergo external cephalic version (ECV). If unsuccessful, a cesarean section should be performed. In contrast, in the nonvertex twin B over 1700 g, either EV or assisted breech extraction might be appropriate.[28] Others use a weight cutoff of 1500 g to select cases for vaginal birth.[29] It follows that breech delivery should not be performed on premature or growth-restricted twins with estimated weight under 1500 g.

When the nonvertex second twin is much larger than the firstborn twin, delivery in breech presentation may prove difficult. According to various sources, the uppermost tolerable difference ranges between 2 mm, as stated in the second edition of this volume, and 4 mm[30] in terms of biparietal diameter.

Numerous case series have developed methods of delivery of the nonvertex twin B. While failing to reach a solid conclusion, the majority of authorities favor total breech extraction of the nonvertex second twin over external cephalic version.[31–34] It is crucial to know the exact presentation of twin B immediately after the vaginal delivery of twin A. Bedside sonography can establish the relationship of the fetal back to the maternal pelvis. In addition, the position of the fetal head (right or left) should be known.

When twin B is in transverse lie, the fetus should be turned into a longitudinal lie. This may be performed either by EV or by internal podalic version. Both maneuvers are easiest accomplished under adequate anesthesia. This may mean that an anesthetist should be present in the delivery room for any emergency.

A transverse lie is either dorsoinferior or dorsosuperior when the back is directed downward toward the pelvis or upward, respectively. A dorsosuperior transverse lie requires a 90° version; a dorsoinferior lie may necessitate either a 270° somersault or a 90° version (backward somersault). Without ultrasound, neither maneuver is easy. Ideally, this procedure should be performed within the short period of uterine quiescence following the delivery of twin A. One may facilitate external or internal versions of the second twin by using intravenous nitroglycerin for uterine relaxation.[35] In one study, high-dose (0.1–0.2 mg/10 kg pregnant weight) intravenous nitroglycerin was used for internal podalic version of the second twin in transverse lie with intact membranes. Twenty of the 22 attempts were successful.[35]

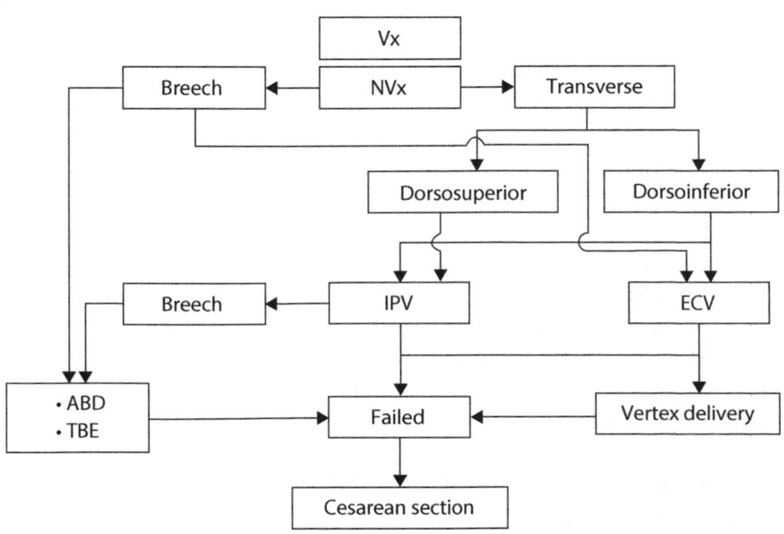

Figure 26.1 Options for vaginal birth of vertex–nonvertex (Vx–NVx) twins. ECV, external cephalic version; IPV, internal podalic version; ABD, assisted breech delivery; TBE, total breech extraction.

Internal podalic version refers to the introduction of the operator's hand into the birth canal in order to grasp the fetal legs after amniotomy and adequate episiotomy. In the past, this procedure was dependent on transabdominal palpation of the fetus. Currently, it is best performed under sonographic guidance. Once the legs are grasped, the fetus is gently turned into the breech presentation and delivered by total breech extraction. Like EV, internal podalic version is easier and might prove less traumatic in the dorsosuperior lie. Uterine manipulation of the second twin does not increase the risk of postpartum metritis or neonatal sepsis, nor does the time interval between the deliveries of the twins. The rate of endometritis has been reported to be higher with twins delivered by cesarean section than in the general population of cesarean deliveries.[36,37]

Following numerous studies, none of which randomized, the question of how to deliver a vertex-first twin gestation seems to be settled.[38] This study showed that between 32 + 0 and 38 + 6 weeks' gestation, the rate of cesarean delivery was 90.7% in the planned-cesarean delivery group (i.e., some 10% delivered before the planned cesarean) and was 43.8% in the planned-vaginal delivery group (i.e., 56% of planned vaginal births ended vaginally). Planned cesarean delivery did not significantly decrease or increase the risk of fetal or neonatal death or serious neonatal morbidity, as compared with planned vaginal delivery. On the other hand, planned cesarean delivery did not significantly increase the risk of maternal morbidity, as compared with planned vaginal delivery. Thus, this prospective randomized multicenter trial pleases those who advocate vaginal birth as well as those who advocate planned abdominal delivery.

Nonvertex first twin

Cesarean section is almost universally performed when the first twin presents as nonvertex.[39] A multicenter study of a large sample of breech-first twin pairs delivered in 13 European centers indicated that when the twins weighed under 1500 g, there was a 2.4-fold increased risk of depressed (<7) 5-minute Apgar scores and a 9.5-fold increased risk of neonatal mortality among pairs delivered vaginally compared with those delivered by cesarean section. However, when the breech-first twin weighed >1500 g, there was no difference in outcome.[40] As a rule of thumb, the criteria for singleton breech delivery could and should be applied to twin breech delivery also.

The potential complication of "locked twins" (also known as "entangled twins" or "interlocking twins") is often cited as an argument against vaginal births of breech–vertex pairs. In this rare presentation, the chin of the breech-first twin is above the chin of the vertex-second twin. When the breech-first twin starts its descent, the chins become "locked" and, with further descent, the heads become entrapped above or within the pelvis. Some ambiguity exists about which pairs are indeed "locked." For instance, twins that appear to be interlocking on imaging are not, in fact, locked but have the *potential to become* locked (Figure 26.2). The term "locked twins" should be reserved for those cases where the breech of the first twin has been delivered halfway, and locking

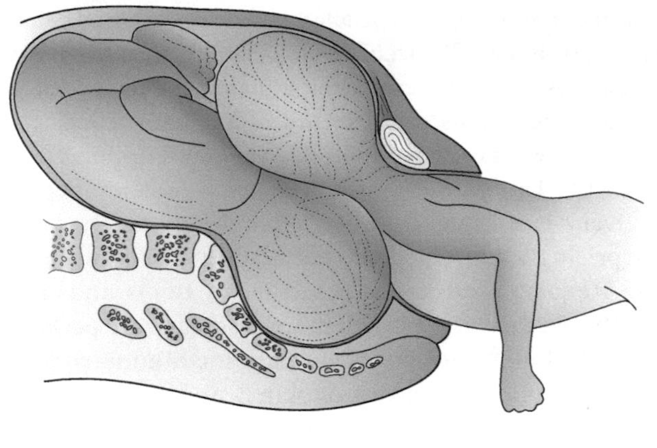

Figure 26.2 The mechanism of interlocking of fetal heads in breech–vertex combination in the course of attempted twin delivery.

obstructs further descent of both twins. This devastating situation is rare, with an estimated prevalence of about 0.1%. It is not entirely clear whether the cited frequencies for cesarean births for "locked twins" refer to twins that were actually "locked," or whether imaging (probably radiography) led to an assumed "dangerous" proximity between the chins. Because size matters in such an event, entrapment of the fetal heads is more likely in premature (and small) twins. Interestingly, no case of "locked twins" was encountered in the large cohort compiled by Blickstein et al.[40] In Sweden, Rydhstrom and Cullberg[41] identified 29 cases in 26,428 (0.15%) twin pregnancies. Interlocking was attributed to growth restriction, birth weight under 2000 g, and antenatal fetal death. The intrapartum mortality was high: 38.9%. In order to facilitate unlocking, uterine relaxation may be achieved by beta-mimetic drugs[42] or nitroglycerin.[43] There is no generally accepted procedure to alleviate this obstetric emergency or that deriving from the accoucheur's inability to extract the aftercoming head arrested by entrapment by the cervix, deflexion of head, or absolute cephalopelvic disproportion. A modification of the Zavanelli maneuver employed in shoulder dystocia has been described to overcome this potentially catastrophic situation.[44] This involves pushing the partially delivered fetus back into the birth canal and then prompt classical cesarean section to effect emergent "abdominal rescue" of the arrested first twin. Thereafter, the second twin is extracted in the usual manner. This new technique has gained some acceptance since its introduction almost two decades ago.[45]

Combined twin delivery

This term refers to cesarean section performed for twin B after the vaginal delivery of twin A. In its purest sense, combined twin delivery should thus be discussed under the subheading of cesarean delivery.[13] Jill Walton described this situation as "the worst of both worlds—a tiring and often risky pregnancy, a tiring labour, a major abdominal operation, two lots of stitches and two new babies to care for" (*British Medical Journal*, November 5, 2002). It is safe to assume that no one intentionally plans a combined delivery. In a typical case, it occurs unexpectedly after the delivery of twin A, when an emergent situation is recognized, and the operator, in his/her best clinical judgment, considers an emergency cesarean for twin B as the safest option.

In the United States, the frequency of combined twin delivery is estimated to be 9.5%.[46] Interestingly, but not surprisingly, a direct, linear correlation was found between the frequency of cesarean section in twins and that of combined delivery.[13] When more cesareans are performed for both twins, less experience is gained in managing the often complicated delivery of twin B, and, thus, more combined twin deliveries are performed. Other investigators[47] demonstrated a statistically significant increase in combined vaginal cesarean and elective cesarean deliveries, with a decrease in the rate of vaginal deliveries.

Combined twin deliveries may occur in all combinations of presentation in which vaginal delivery is appropritate.[13] Using data from the large U.S. multiple birth file, Wen et al.[46] found that the cesarean rate for twin B increased when the mothers had medical or labor and delivery complications. Breech and other malpresentations were the most important predictors of emergent combined deliveries (population-attributable risk 33.2%). The need for emergent cesarean delivery of the second twin after vaginal delivery of the first twin was increased four-fold in such combinations. Operative vaginal delivery of the first twin was associated with a decreased rate of cesarean delivery for the second twin. In one study, the frequency of cesarean section for the second twin increased 7.6-fold if twin A was in vertex rather than breech presentation.[23]

It is important to remember that a prolonged interval between the vaginal delivery of twin A and the abdominal delivery of twin B may cause the uterus to contract around the malpresenting fetus, leading to difficult extraction during cesarean section. In this situation, nitroglycerin is the agent of choice in managing the "entrapped" second twin.

In summary, it is not possible to avoid combined deliveries entirely unless cesarean section is performed in all twins. The operator must acknowledge the limits of his/her manual dexterity in what deserves to be included among the most formidable obstetric situations. If—for whatever reason—safe vaginal delivery of twin B cannot be expected, there is no need to test one's ability to handle cataclysmic situations. To avoid addition stress and distress, the operator may choose to perform a twin delivery under double setup, in an operating room fully prepared for an abdominal operation on 1- to 2-minute notice. All personnel required for the operation must be scrubbed and gowned before the attempted vaginal twin delivery.

Vaginal birth after cesarean section

As a result of the currently high cesarean rates, there is a 1:3–1:6 chance that a given multipara carrying twins had a previous cesarean. The combination of a uterine scar with a multiple pregnancy and its associated uterine overdistention and fetal malpresentation constitutes a contraindication for a vaginal birth after cesarean (VBAC) in the opinion of most clinicians, even if the evidence does not entirely support this policy.[48–50] Therefore, when the patient is well motivated and is willing to accept the recognized risks of an attempted vaginal delivery,[29] and after the patient gives informed consent, VBAC can be accomplished in carefully selected cases. Both vertex–vertex and some vertex–nonvertex pairs may be candidates for vaginal delivery. However, when manipulations to deliver the second twin are anticipated, cesarean section is probably a better choice. The frequency of combined deliveries is likely to be higher than in the general population. This fact should be included in the counseling process.

SPECIAL CIRCUMSTANCES RELATED TO MULTIPLE BIRTHS

Delivery of small twins

Currently, no prophylactic measure can reduce prematurity in multiple gestations, except fetal reduction. Generally, twins are delivered earlier and are smaller than singletons. Two-thirds of all twins are delivered before week 36 of gestation (14% under 33 weeks), and half of them weigh less than 2500 g (10% weighing under 1500 g).[2] Any planned mode of delivery should take these facts into consideration. One population-based study found that the overall chances of one or both twins weighing less than 1500 g were 10.8% and 5.9%, respectively. There was a significantly higher incidence of low-birth-weight (LBW) twins among nulliparous than among multiparas (16.1% vs. 7.5%).[51]

The presence of small twins, especially when they weigh under 1500 g and are before week 32, is a frequent argument against vaginal delivery. While ample data support the safety of vaginal deliveries of small singletons in the vertex presentation, few studies describe outcomes for small, vertex-presenting twins. Thus, decisions are frequently based on extrapolation from singleton series.

Recent population-based studies of very LBW infants compared the outcomes of singletons, twins, and triplets[52] and those of twins A and B.[53] In this large Israeli database, the mode of delivery (vaginal vs. abdominal) did not significantly influence the neonatal outcome. Importantly, the mode of delivery had no effect on the neurologic findings in the neonates.[52] In contrast, a French hospital-based study found a significantly higher incidence of periventricular leukomalacia among vaginally delivered LBW twins than among twins delivered by cesarean section.[54]

It should be realized that the data on outcomes of preterm or LBW twins come from retrospective studies, some of which with unexcluded confounders, and the results are at best conflicting. Yet, many neonatologists prefer to get premature twins "intact" by the forces of labor, even without solid evidence.

Delayed interval delivery

At times, one of the members of a multiple pregnancy is completely aborted or delivered remote from term. The uterus occasionally spontaneously ceases to contract after the birth of one or more grossly premature infant or infants. At this stage, one must decide whether to terminate the entire pregnancy or to perform the initial steps for a delayed interval delivery (also termed "asynchronous delivery"). Such a procedure involves ligation of the umbilical cord as high as possible, preferably at the level of the external cervical os, and leaving the placenta of the aborted/delivered fetus in situ. The cervix then usually contracts while the pregnancy continues under close supervision.[55]

This heroic intervention is primarily used to salvage the remaining fetus(es) from the dismal outcome associated with extreme prematurity. The most serious concern is the fear of infection that may have caused the expulsion of the first fetus. Nevertheless, the literature is replete with cases and small series describing prolongation of the pregnancy after expulsion of the first fetus.

The following three points have been raised since the first reports on delayed interval delivery.

First, in selected cases, the attempt to prolong the rest of the pregnancy may be justified,[56] since even modest prolongation at critical gestational ages can improve neonatal survival.[57] Yet, the selection criteria remain unclear and obviously, this daring intervention is better reserved for "premium" pregnancies or for women with a history of infertility.[56]

Second, the prognosis is not bright. Although some studies show favorable outcome, this may reflect "reporting bias," whereby failures remain unpublished.[58] Even if pregnancy is prolonged by several weeks, the outcome, in terms of risk of neurologic disability, is not favorable if the first twin was delivered at around 20 weeks. In other words, the time gained may save the retained fetus from mortality, but not from prematurity-related morbidity.[59,60] In a retrospective analysis of 80 multiple pregnancies with the birth of one child at a gestational age of 16–31 weeks, van Doorn et al.[59] were able to postpone the delivery of the second (and third) infant in 10 out of 15 attempts, with a mean delay of 12 days, and a mean gestational age at the delivery of the remaining fetuses of 27 5/7 weeks. There was no difference in outcome between the first-born and the retained infant when the procedure was performed after 28 weeks. A recent U.S. study found that asynchronous delivery occurred at a rate of 0.14 per 1000 births, mainly (86%) as a result of second-trimester rupture of membranes. The mean gestational age of the first delivered fetus was 21 ± 2.0 weeks and the median latency was 2 days (range <1–70 days). Of the 19 retained fetuses, 2 died in utero, 10 died between birth and day 57 of life, and 7 (37%) survived until hospital discharge. Six of the survivors had major prematurity-related sequelae, and only one (5%) was discharged without major consequences. More than half of the mothers suffered infectious morbidity, including one case of septic shock.[60]

Thirdly, the exact protocol for delayed deliveries has not been established. After the birth of the first infant, most practitioners keep the patient on bed rest until the pregnancy is completed, under close observation for signs of impending infection. Prophylactic antibiotics and tocolysis are the mainstay of therapy. There is dispute about the role of cervical cerclage. A survey of seven case series that previously identified all delayed interval deliveries found that despite routine prophylactic use of broad-spectrum antibiotics, intrauterine infection occurred after the first delivery in 36% of the cases. The incidence of maternal sepsis was 4.9%. The survey further indicated that cerclage was associated with a longer latency period than in cases without cerclage (median, 26 vs. 9 days). The cerclage did not significantly increase the risk of intrauterine infection.[61] Interestingly, patients who already had a cerclage had shorter latency intervals.

In summary, the data indicate that delayed interval delivery is a feasible procedure and may prolong pregnancy beyond the limit of viability. Naturally, it should not be attempted without full disclosure to the patient of the serious maternal and fetal risks. These should be included in the patient's written informed consent in considerable detail.

Delivery of discordant twins

Significant intertwin size differences, per se, do not indicate cesarean section.[62] Nonetheless, as discussed elsewhere, discordance is an argument against vaginal delivery of vertex–nonvertex twins in whom twin B is significantly larger than twin A.

Delivery of monochorionic twins

Monochorionic (MC) twins deserve special consideration for three reasons. The first concerns the MC-diamniotic variety with or without the twin–twin transfusion syndrome (TTTS). To date, despite extensive research on antepartum management of TTTS, the preferential mode of delivery has not been determined. In the case of treated or untreated TTTS, it would seem that the burden of labor and delivery should not be imposed on these twins, who may be either seriously anemic (as part of the twin anemia–polycythemia sequence) or have decompensated cardiac function.

Another concern is the association of MC twinning with bizarre anomalies. One example is the delivery of the acardiac, acephalic twin (the so-called twin reversed arterial perfusion sequence [TRAP]) (Figure 26.3). The umbilical cord of the acardiac, acephalic twin is usually very short, and the diameters of this ovoid-shaped mass often are larger than the pelvic outlet or the 10- to 12-cm uterine incision performed at cesarean section. Accordingly, because extraction might prove traumatic and cause rupture of cord and exsanguination of the normal (pump) twin, it seems reasonable to seek the welfare of the normal twin first. This may be accomplished only through cesarean section. Thus, after the uterine incision and the delivery of the normal twin, there is no rush to deliver the acardiac, acephalic mass. Sometimes, despite the elastic nature of the mass, extraction through a narrow incision may be difficult. It is advisable to have a good grip on the mass in order to perform a controlled, slow delivery. Care must be taken to avoid lateral extension of the

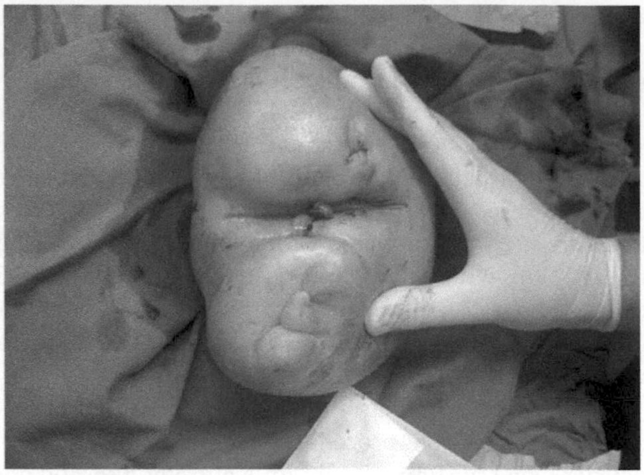

Figure 26.3 Acardiac, acephalic twin. The shortest diameter may be larger than the uterine incision, causing difficult extraction during cesarean section.

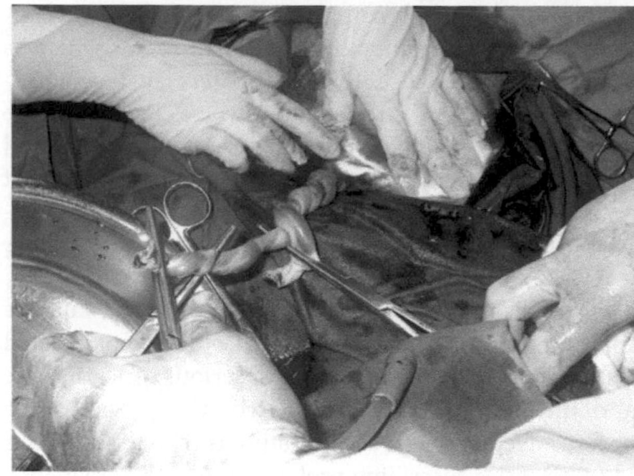

Figure 26.4 Cord entanglement in case of monoamniotic twins seen at cesarean section.

uterine incision toward the uterine arteries. One may use a "corkscrew" device attached into the mass in order have a firm grasp and a safe extraction. The cutting of a "smile" incision into the lower uterine segment is often warranted.

Another problem is the delivery of conjoined twins. In such rare circumstances, and particularly if the twins are to be spared a traumatic and destructive birth, cesarean section is preferred. Often, a classical incision is required for a safe dual delivery.

A matter of concern is the delivery of MC-monoamniotic (MA) twins. Before the era of sonography, very few MA twins survived, because the diagnosis was not made in a timely manner. Cord entanglement is almost invariably present and may occur as early as week 12 of pregnancy. When such entanglement becomes sufficiently tight, one or both twins die (Figure 26.4). For many authorities, this "ticking bomb" situation warrants delivery at 32 weeks, even without proving lung maturity. The wisdom of this protocol was questioned[57] by a series of 17 sets of MA twins delivered after 30 weeks with at least one twin still alive. The risks of early delivery in these pregnancies appear to outweigh the risk of fetal death. The argument used in defending this latter view is that twins of over 30 weeks' gestational age are too large to move around in the uterine cavity and are therefore unlikely to tighten the entangled cords. Most authors hold that the balance of the risks is in favor of delivery when pregnancy reaches 32 weeks.[63,64]

Labor induction and augmentation

About 20% of twin gestations may require induction of labor for fetal and/or maternal reasons. However, the overdistended uterus is a relative contraindication for labor induction by means that may cause uterine hyperstimulation. Although pregnancy is often terminated by cesarean section, it seems that unfavorable cervical condition is no impediment for trial of labor in appropriate candidates. There is a report describing the effective use of an intrauterine balloon catheter for the induction of labor in carefully selected cases.[65] Likewise, Simões et al.[66] evaluated the use of oral misoprostol in near term (≥35 weeks) twin pregnancies in nulliparous. Compared with nulliparous delivered by planned cesarean section, the two groups were comparable in most aspects, except for fetal malpresentation, which was the major reason for avoiding induction. A total of 76.8% had a vaginal birth, 4.3% had a combined twin delivery, and 18.8% had a cesarean during labor.

The conflicting results in the older literature related to oxytocin induction or augmentation[67,68] were questioned in a recent study of 62 twin gestations matched with singleton controls.[69] Women with twin pregnancies and those with singletons responded similarly regarding maximum needed oxytocin dosage, time from oxytocin administration to delivery, and successful vaginal deliveries (90% in both groups). It is clear from these studies that labor induction in twins is not contraindicated and might be used in carefully selected cases.

Defining "term" for twins

The discussion about the definition of "term" in twins has been revitalized in the last few years. Since "term" occurs earlier in twins than in singletons, one may argue that twins delivered later are exposed to risks associated with post-term pregnancy. This concept explains the increased risk of cerebral palsy observed in twins weighing more than 2500 g or delivered after 37 weeks.[70] The following lines of evidence suggest that "term" occurs in twin pregnancies at 37–38 weeks[70]: (1) statistical deductions shows that the proportion of twins born after 38 weeks is similar to that of singletons born after 40 weeks; (2) growth curves of twins do not demonstrate a significant increase in size after 37 weeks (Figure 26.5); (3) fetal pulmonary and neurologic maturity appears to be achieved by completed week 37; and (4) perinatal mortality and morbidity rates decrease until 36 weeks but increase again thereafter.

In the last decade, a series of studies attempted to quantify the excess risk of intrauterine fetal demise (IUFD) in monochorionic–diamniotic (MCDA) twins despite being

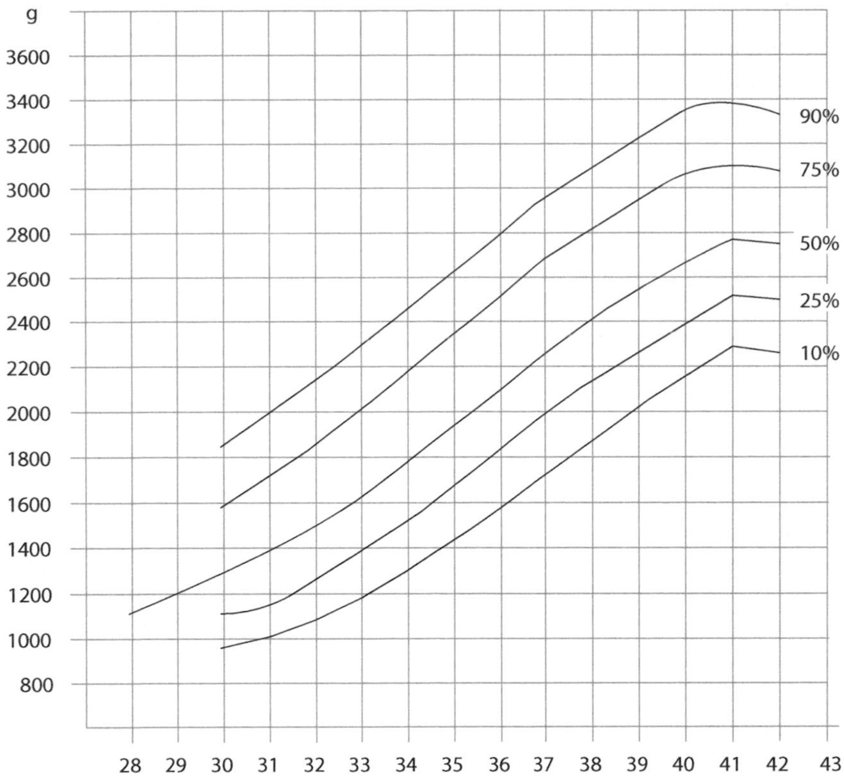

Figure 26.5 The average rate of growth of twins during the third trimester of gestation. Horizontal line: gestational age in weeks; vertical line: birth weight in grams. (Adapted from Bazsó J et al., *Magy Noorv Lapja*, 32, 248, 1969; Bazsó J et al., *Zentralbl Gynakol* 1970; 92: 628–33.)

apparently "uncomplicated." In general, the numerous studies showed a risk of 1.5%–2% per pregnancy after 33 weeks' gestation. This alarming incidence, however, seems to be higher in population-based datasets[72] compared with data coming from dedicated centers with specific interest in monichorionicity.[73–75] Simply put, a significant excess risk of unexpected deaths in monochorionic biamniotic (MCBA) twins exists and might indeed outweigh the risks of prematurity, and hence be an indication for elective preterm delivery. The ample circumstantial evidence supports the contention that bichorionic twins should be delivered during week 38 of gestation[76] and monochorionic twins at 36–37 weeks.

Delivery of triplets

Triplet delivery is more complex than that of twins. Therefore, the abdominal route is generally preferred.[50] However, it should be realized that in some centers the option of vaginal delivery of triplets has never been discarded.[77]

As the number of triplets increased worldwide due to the epidemic of multiple births,[1] and with the advent of sonography, fewer cases of triplets were misdiagnosed, and more centers gained experience with more triplets in a shorter time span[77–85] (Figure 26.6).

Delivery of triplets, by either route, is a logistic endeavor. As each of the infants deserves its own immediate postpartum care, there must be three neonatology teams. The obstetric team must include at least two operators, supported by an anesthesiologist. Including the midwives and nurses, a triplet delivery may require as many as 15–20 persons. The logistics involved in recruiting the necessary staff may be difficult. As the time of spontaneous birth cannot be predicted, a planned, daytime, elective cesarean section offers the simplest solution to the logistic problem.

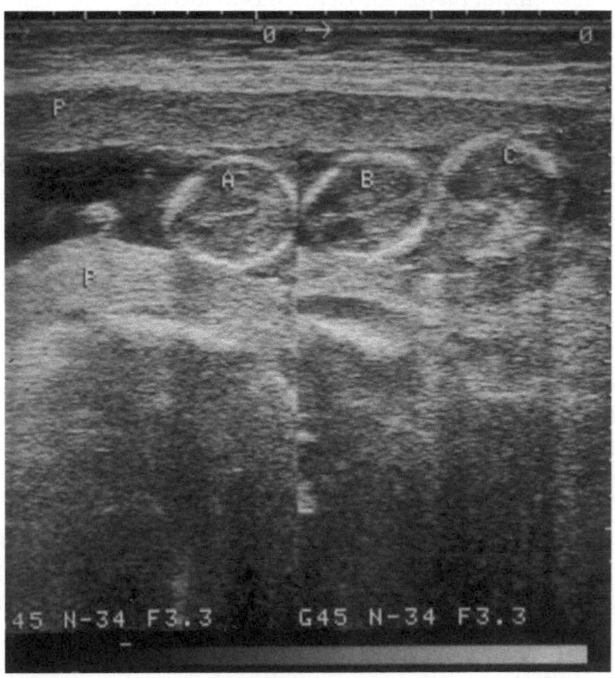

Figure 26.6 Demonstration of triplets by sonographic examination at 17 weeks' gestation.

EPILOGUE

"And it came to pass in the time of her travail, that, behold, twins were in her womb. And it came to pass, when she travailed, that the one put out his hand: and the midwife took and bound upon his hand a scarlet thread, saying, This came out first. And it came to pass, as he drew back his hand, that, behold, his brother came out: and she said, How has thou broken forth? This breach be upon thee . . . And afterward came out his brother, that had the scarlet thread upon his hand" (Genesis 38:27–30).

The description of the delivery of Pharez and Zarah is a vivid documentation of the complexity of twin birth.[86] The midwife must have been experienced since she made the diagnosis of twins intrapartum; otherwise she could not have been ready to apply the scarlet thread to the firstborn. This biblical narrative summarizes the concept of the delivery of multiples: good clinical judgment and skills.

Generally speaking, cesarean section is the simplest and most efficient way to deliver multiples. This statement is especially true for a "premium" pregnancy. A recent study from Germany[87] indicated that cesarean rates changed from 63.6% (<28 weeks), 88.9% (28–31 weeks), 59.6% (32–36 weeks), and 40% (>36 weeks) in 1990 to 74.2%, 95.5%, 76.9%, and 68.7% in 2012, respectively. The lowest increase (16.8%) was found in university hospitals with perinatal units and the highest (22.1%) was noted in smaller hospitals without perinatal units. As already predicted in 1991 by Blickstein et al.,[13] this dramatic increase of nearly 25% in abdominal births for twins was associated with almost doubling of combined twin deliveries, from 3.9% in 1990 to 7.0% in 2012.

These data reiterate the idea that in any particular case, the fact that vaginal delivery is *permissible* makes little sense if the operator is inexperienced in breech delivery. With training opportunities diminishing, the admission of lack of expertise should cause no embarrassment even for fully qualified obstetricians.

Indeed, the results of the Twin Birth Study[38] suggests that even in centers skilled enough in the art of vaginal twin birth, the chance to complete a vaginal twin birth was roughly 50%. Even so, some women might enjoy the freedom of choice between vaginal and cesarean births that is provided by the results of these studies.[88]

REFERENCES

1. Blickstein I, Keith LG. The spectrum of iatrogenic multiple pregnancy. In: Blickstein I, Keith LG (eds), *Iatrogenic Multiple Pregnancy: Clinical Implications*, p. 1. New York, NY: Parthenon, 2001.
2. Martin JA, Hamilton BE, Sutton PD et al. Births: Final data for 2002. *Natl Vital Stat Rep* 2003; 52: 1.
3. Martin JA, Hamilton BE, Osterman MJ et al. Births: Final data for 2013. *Natl Vital Stat Rep* 2015; 64(1): 1–65.
4. Euro-Peristat. The European Perinatal Health Report 2010, 2010. http://www.europeristat.com/reports/european-perinatal-health-report-2010.html. Accessed September 1, 2016
5. Tul N, Lucovnik M, Verdenik I et al. The contribution of twins conceived by assisted reproduction technology to the very preterm birth rate: A population-based stud. *Eur J Obstet Gynecol Reprod Biol* 2013; 171: 311–3.
6. Blickstein I. Motherhood at or beyond the edge of reproductive age. *Int J Fertil Wom Med* 2003; 48: 17.
7. Loos R, Derom C, Vlietinck R et al. The East Flanders Prospective Twin Survey (Belgium): A population-based register. *Twin Res* 1998; 1: 167.
8. Blickstein I. Cesarean section for all twins? *J Perinat Med* 2000; 28: 169.
9. Minkoff H, Chervenak F. Elective primary cesarean delivery. *N Engl J Med* 2003; 348: 946.
10. Minkoff H, Powderly KR, Chervenak F et al. Ethical dimensions of elective primary cesarean delivery. *Obstet Gynecol* 2004; 103: 387.
11. Hannah ME, Hannah WJ, Hewson SA et al. Planned caesarean section versus planned vaginal birth for breech presentation at term: A randomised multicentre trial. Term Breech Trial Collaborative Group. *Lancet* 2000; 356: 1375.
12. Su M, McLeod L, Ross S et al.; Term Breech Trial Collaborative Group. factors associated with adverse perinatal outcome in the Term Breech Trial. *Am J Obstet Gynecol* 2003; 189: 740.
13. Blickstein I, Zalel Y, Weissman A. Cesarean delivery of the second twin after the vaginal birth of the first twin—Misfortune or mismanagement? *Acta Genet Med Gemellol* 1991; 40: 389.
14. Ananth CV, Joseph KS. Impact of obstetric intervention on trends in perinatal mortality. In: Blickstein I, Keith LG (eds), *Multiple Pregnancy: Epidemiology, Gestation, and Perinatal Outcome* (2nd edition), pp. 651–9. London, UK: Parthenon, 2004.
15. The National Sentinel Caesarean Section Audit Report. October 2001. RCOG Clinical Effectiveness Support Unit.
16. Barber EL, Lundsberg L, Belanger K et al. Contributing indications to the rising cesarean delivery rate. *Obstet Gynecol* 2011; 118: 29–38.
17. Blickstein I. Maternal mortality in twin gestations. *J Reprod Med* 1997; 42: 680.
18. Hogle KL, Hutton EK, McBrien KA et al. Cesarean delivery for twins: A systematic review and meta-analysis. *Am J Obstet Gynecol* 2003; 188: 220.
19. Blickstein I, Smith-Levitin M. Twinning and twins. In: Chervenak FA, Kurjak A (eds), *Current Perspectives on the Fetus as a Patient*, p. 507. London, UK: Parthenon, 1996.
20. Redick LF. Anesthesia for twin delivery. *Clin Perinatol* 1988; 15: 107.
21. Williams KP, Galerneau F. Intrapartum influences on cesarean delivery in multiple gestation. *Acta Obstet Gynecol Scand* 2003; 82: 241.
22. Ananth CV, Smulian JC, Demissie K et al. Placental abruption among singleton and twin births in the United States: Risk factor profiles. *Am J Epidemiol* 2001; 153: 771.

23. Kurzel RB, Claridad L, Lampley EC. Cesarean section for the second twin. *J Reprod Med* 1997; 42: 767.
24. Leung TY, Tam WH, Leung TN et al. Effect of twin-to-twin delivery interval on umbilical cord blood gas in the second twin. *Br J Obstetrics Gynaecol* 2002; 109: 63.
25. Erdemoglu E, Mungan T, Tapisiz OL et al. Effect of inter-twin delivery time on Apgar scores of the second twin. *Aust N Z J Obstet Gynaecol* 2003; 43: 203.
26. Pons JC, Dommergues M, Ayoubi JM et al. Delivery of the second twin: Comparison of two approaches. *Eur J Obstet Gynecol Reprod Biol* 2002; 104: 32.
27. Blickstein I, Schwartz Z, Lancet M et al. Vaginal delivery of the second twin in breech presentation. *Obstet Gynecol* 1987; 69: 774.
28. Houlihan C, Knuppel RA. Intrapartum management of multiple gestations. *Clin Perinatol* 1996; 23: 91.
29. Chervenak FA, Johnson RE, Berkowitz RL et al. Is routine cesarean section necessary for vertex-breech and vertex-transverse twin gestations? *Am J Obstet Gynecol* 1984; 148: 1.
30. Colon J, Apuzzio JJ, Evans H et al. Obstetric considerations of premium iatrogenic multiple pregnancy. In: Blickstein I, Keith LG (eds), *Iatrogenic Multiple Pregnancy*, p. 117. Cranford, NJ: Parthenon, 2000.
31. Fishman A, Grubb DK, Kovacs BW. Vaginal delivery of the nonvertex second twin. *Am J Obstet Gynecol* 1993; 168: 861.
32. Gocke SE, Nageotte MP, Garite T et al. Management of the nonvertex second twin: primary cesarean section, external version, or primary breech extraction. *Am J Obstet Gynecol* 1989; 161: 111.
33. Hutton EK, Hannah ME, Barrett J. Use of external cephalic version for breech pregnancy and mode of delivery for breech and twin pregnancy: A survey of Canadian practitioners. *J Obstet Gynaecol Can* 2002; 24: 804.
34. Barrett J. Randomised controlled trial for twin delivery. *BMJ* 2003; 326: 448.
35. Dufour P, Vinatier D, Vanderstichele S et al. Intravenous nitroglycerin for internal podalic version of the second twin in transverse lie. *Obstet Gynecol* 1998; 92: 416.
36. Suonio S, Huttunen M. Puerperal endometritis after abdominal twin delivery. *Acta Obstet Gynecol Scand* 1994; 73: 313.
37. Alexander JM, Gilstrap LC 3rd, Cox SM et al. The relationship of infection to method of delivery in twin pregnancy. *Am J Obstet Gynecol* 1997; 177: 1063.
38. Barrett JFR, Hannah ME, Hutton EK et al. A randomized trial of planned cesarean or vaginal delivery for twin pregnancy. *N Engl J Med* 2013; 369: 1295–305.
39. Blickstein I, Weissman A, Ben-Hur H et al. Vaginal delivery for breech-vertex twins. *J Reprod Med* 1993; 38: 879.
40. Blickstein I, Goldman RD, Kupermine M. Delivery of breech-first twins: A multicenter retrospective study. *Obstet Gynecol* 2000; 95: 37.
41. Rydhstrom H, Cullberg G. Pregnancies with growth-retarded twins in breech-vertex presentation at increased risk for entanglement during delivery. *J Perinat Med* 1990; 18: 45.
42. Sevitz H, Merrell DA. The use of a beta-sympathomimetic drug in locked twins. Case report. *Br J Obstet Gynaecol* 1981; 88: 76.
43. Johansson BG, Helgadottir EA. A case of locked twins successfully treated with nitroglycerin sublingually before manual reposition and vaginal delivery. *Acta Obstet Gynecol Scand* 2001; 80: 275.
44. Iffy L, Apuzzio JJ, Cohen-Addad N, et al. Abdominal rescue after entrapment of the aftercoming head. *Am J Obstet Gynecol* 1986: 154: 623.
45. Swartjes JM, Bleker OP, Schutte MF. The Zavanelli maneuver applied to locked twins. *Am J Obstet Gynecol* 1992; 166: 532.
46. Wen SW, Fung KF, Oppenheimer L et al. Occurrence and predictors of cesarean delivery for the second twin after vaginal delivery of the first twin. *Obstet Gynecol* 2004; 103: 413.
47. Persad VL, Baskett TF, O'Connell CM et al. Combined vaginal-cesarean delivery of twin pregnancies. *Obstet Gynecol* 2001; 98: 1032.
48. Sansergret A, Bujold E, Gaauthier RJ. Twin delivery after a caesarean: A twelve-year experience. *J Obstet Gynecol Can* 2003; 25: 294.
49. Delaney T, Young DC. Trial of labour compared to elective caesarean in twin gestations with a previous caesarean delivery. *J Obstet Gynecol Can* 2003; 25: 289.
50. ACOG. ACOG Practice Bulletin No. 54. Vaginal birth after previous cesarean delivery. *Obstet Gynecol* 2004; 104: 2003.
51. Blickstein I, Goldman RD, Mazkereth R. Risk for one or two very low birth weight twins: A population study. *Obstet Gynecol* 2000; 96: 400.
52. Shinwell ES, Blickstein I, Lusky A et al. Excess risk of mortality in very low birth weight triplets: A national, population based study. *Arch Dis Child Fetal Neonatal Ed* 2003; 88: F36.
53. Shinwell ES, Blickstein I, Lusky A et al. Effect of birth order on neonatal morbidity and mortality among very low birth weight twins: A population based study. *Arch Dis Child Fetal Neonatal Ed* 2004; 89: F145.
54. Salomon LJ, Duyme M, Rousseau A et al. Periventricular leukomalacia and mode of delivery in twins under 1500 g. *J Matern Fetal Neonatal Med* 2003; 13: 224.
55. Platt JS, Rosa C. Delayed interval delivery in multiple gestations. *Obstet Gynecol Surv* 1999; 54: 343.
56. Tzafettas JM, Farmakides G, Delkos D et al. Asynchronous delivery of twins and triplets with an interval period ranging from 48 hours to 19 weeks. *Clin Exp Obstet Gynecol* 2004; 31: 53.

57. Farkouh LJ, Sabin ED, Heyborne KD et al. Delayed-interval delivery: Extended series from a single maternal-fetal medicine practice. *Am J Obstet Gynecol* 2000; 183: 1499.
58. Fayad S, Bongain A, Holhfeld P et al. Delayed delivery of second twin: A multicentre study of 35 cases. *Eur J Obstet Gynecol Reprod Biol* 2003; 109: 16.
59. van Doorn HC, van Wezel-Meijler G, van Geijn HP et al. Delayed interval delivery in multiple pregnancies. Is optimism justified? *Acta Obstet Gynecol Scand* 1999; 78: 710.
60. Livingston JC, Livingston LW, Ramsey R et al. Second-trimester asynchronous multifetal delivery results in poor perinatal outcome. *Obstet Gynecol* 2004; 103: 77.
61. Zhang J, Johnson CD, Hoffman M. Cervical cerclage in delayed interval delivery in a multifetal pregnancy: A review of seven case series. *Eur J Obstet Gynecol Reprod Biol* 2003; 108: 126.
62. Blickstein I. The definition, diagnosis, and management of growth-discordant twins: An international census survey. *Acta Genet Med Gemellol* 1991; 40: 345.
63. Carr SR, Aronson MP, Coustan DR. Survival rates of monoamniotic twins do not decrease after 30 weeks' gestation. *Am J Obstet Gynecol* 1990; 163: 719.
64. Sau AK, Langford K, Elliott C et al. Monoamniotic twins: What should be the optimal antenatal management? *Twin Res* 2003; 6: 270.
65. Manor M, Blickstein I, Ben-Arie A et al. Case series of labor induction in twin gestations with an intrauterine balloon catheter. *Gynecol Obstet Invest* 1999; 47: 244.
66. Simões T, Condeço P, Dias E et al. Induction of labor with oral misoprostol in nulliparous mothers of twins. *J Perinat Med* 2006; 34: 111–4.
67. Leroy F. Oxytocin treatment in twin pregnancy labour. *Acta Genet Med Gemellol* 1979; 28: 303.
68. Price JH, Marivate M. Induction of labour in twin pregnancy. *S Afr Med J* 1986; 70: 163.
69. Fausett MB, Barth WH Jr, Yoder BA et al. Oxytocin labor stimulation of twin gestations: Effective and efficient. *Obstet Gynecol* 1997; 90: 202.
70. Blickstein I. Is it possible to reduce the incidence of neurological complications in multiple pregnancies? In: Carrera JM, Chervenak FA, Kurjak A (eds), *Controversies in Perinatal Medicine. Studies on the Fetus as a Patient*, p. 161. New York, NY: Parthenon, 2003.
71. Bazsó J Dolhany B, Pohánka O. Weight increase in twins during the 28th to 42nd week of pregnancy. *Zentralbl Gynakol* 1970; 92: 628–33.
72. Tul N, Verdenik I, Novak Z et al. Prospective risk of stillbirth in monochorionic–diamniotic twin gestations: A population based study. *J Perinat Med* 2011; 39: 51–4.
73. Hack K, Derks J, Elias S et al. Perinatal mortality and mode of delivery in monochorionic biamniotic twin pregnancies ≥32 weeks of gestation: A multicentre retrospective cohort study. *BJOG* 2011; 118: 1090–97.
74. Van Klink JMM, Van Steenis A, Steggerda SJ et al. Single fetal demise in monochorionic pregnancies: Incidence and patterns of cerebral injury. *Ultrasound Obstet Gynecol* 2015; 45: 294–300.
75. Simões T, Queirós A, Marujo AT et al. Prospective risk of intrauterine death of monochorionic twins: Update. *J Perinat Med* 2015. pii: /j/jpme.ahead-of-print/jpm-2015-0319/jpm-2015-0319.xml.
76. Dodd JM, Crowther CA. Elective delivery of women with a twin pregnancy from 37 weeks' gestation. *Cochrane Database Syst Rev* 2003; (2): CD003582.
77. Pheiffer EL, Golan A. Triplet pregnancy. A 10-year review of cases at Baragwanath Hospital. *S Afr Med J* 1979; 55: 843.
78. Ron-El R, Caspi E, Schreyer P et al. Triplet and quadruplet pregnancies and management. *Obstet Gynecol* 1981; 57: 458.
79. Thiery M, Kermans G, Derom R. Triplet and higher-order births: What is the optimal delivery route? *Acta Genet Med Gemellol* 1988; 37: 89.
80. Feingold M, Cetrulo C, Peters M et al. Mode of delivery in multiple birth of higher order. *Acta Genet Med Gemellol* 1988; 37: 105.
81. Clarke JP, Roman JD. A review of 19 sets of triplets: The positive results of vaginal delivery. *Aust N Z J Obstet Gynaecol* 1994; 34: 50.
82. Wildschut HI, van Roosmalen J, van Leeuwen E et al. Planned abdominal compared with planned vaginal birth in triplet pregnancies. *Br J Obstet Gynaecol* 1995; 102: 292.
83. Bakos O. Birth in triplet pregnancies. Vaginal delivery—How often is it possible? *Acta Obstet Gynecol Scand* 1998; 77: 845.
84. Alamia V Jr, Royek AB, Jaekle RK et al. Preliminary experience with a prospective protocol for planned vaginal delivery of triplet gestations. *Am J Obstet Gynecol* 1998; 179: 1133.
85. Ziadeh SM. Perinatal outcome in 41 sets of triplets. *Gynecol Obstet Invest* 2000; 50: 162–5.
86. Blickstein I, Gurewitsch ED. Biblical twins. *Obstet Gynecol* 1998; 91: 632.
87. Kyvernitakis A, Kyvernitakis I, Karageorgiadis AS et al. Rising cesarean rates of twin deliveries in Germany from 1990 to 2012. *Z Geburtshilfe Neonatol* 2013; 217: 177–82.
88. Blickstein I. Delivery of vertex/nonvertex twins: Did the horses already leave the barn? *Am J Obstet Gynecol* 2016; 214: 308–10.

Maternal birth injuries

27

SHIMON GINATH and ABRAHAM GOLAN

CONTENTS

A substantial risk to the mother always existed at parturition. In the not-too-distant past, parturition was a very dangerous event in a woman's life, and many babies lost their mothers at birth. With the improvement of obstetric services, availability of blood transfusions, antibiotics, modern anesthetic methods, and the increasing popularity of hospital deliveries, maternal death has almost disappeared. There is a tendency today to abandon potentially traumatic vaginal deliveries and use cesarean sections whenever difficulties are expected, for the sake of both mother and fetus. However, maternal morbidity and injury during labor unfortunately still exist, especially in underdeveloped parts of the world where medical surveillance of deliveries is less effective than in the more developed countries. Iatrogenic or elective injury, such as episiotomy, may be still needed, sometimes in order to avoid more extensive birth trauma.

PROCEDURES

Episiotomy

Although its popularity has been declining, episiotomy is described at length in another chapter, and it is not discussed here any further.

Symphysiotomy

Symphysiotomy is also very rarely performed in modern obstetrics, and mainly in low- and middle income countries. First used by Sigault in Paris in 1777, this operation consists of division of the symphysis pubis in order to increase the pelvic diameters and allow vaginal delivery in minor degrees of cephalopelvic disproportion.[1] The operation is performed with the patient in the lithotomy position, with both legs supported by an assistant on each side, limiting abduction and external rotation to avoid further accidental trauma to the pelvis. The bladder is emptied, and the catheter is left in place during the operation.

After infiltration with 1% lidocaine solution, a short midline longitudinal incision of the skin over the symphysis is made, and the symphysis pubis is divided with a long, solid scalpel from behind forward and from above downward, introducing the knife behind the symphysis pubis at its upper border and keeping strictly to the midline. The surgeon uses a finger in the vagina to displace the urethra and the bladder neck laterally well to one side of the symphysis before cutting. The assistants continue to support the legs during the assisted delivery. A large episiotomy is performed. Traction is always directed away from the symphysis. A firm strapping or binding of the legs is applied for the support of the pelvis for 1 week.

In the majority of cases, proper healing takes place and the pelvis regains its former stability. However, complications such as injury to the urethra, stress incontinence, infection, hemorrhage, and pelvic instability have been reported.

Data on long-term problems after 40 years, in patients undergoing symphysiotomy were reported in 37 Irish women. The most common problems were back problems (94/6%), bladder problems (78.4%), hip (77.8%), and psychological problems (75.7%). Bowel and kidney problems were also reported, however to a lesser degree.[2] An attempt to issue a Cochrane review on symphysiotomy yielded no randomized controlled trials (RCTs).[3]

This operation probably has no place in developed countries nowadays when operating room facilities and personnel are readily available whenever necessary. However, it is still performed in rural areas in Africa and other underdeveloped regions. It has, in these cases, the advantages of avoiding a cesarean section for a moderately contracted pelvis and not weakening the uterus for future pregnancy. It also permanently increases the pelvic dimensions at all levels, allowing easier subsequent vaginal delivery.[4,5]

INJURY TO THE PERINEUM AND VULVA

Some degree of injury to the soft tissues of the external part of the birth canal is almost inevitable in primiparas and sometimes even in multiparas. The reasons for the injury of the perineum and vulva are, in general, quite similar:

1. Large fetal measurements, such as a large head or broad shoulders, occipitoposterior rotation, and face presentation
2. Precipitated labor and delivery, which do not allow gradual dilation of the tissues
3. Narrow bony passage due either to narrow subpubic angle or to a straight sacrum
4. Narrow soft tissue passage, as in very young parturients, or extremely high perineum, whether primary or due to previous repair
5. Hasty or otherwise improper use of instrumentation or manual techniques
6. Insufficient control of the delivery due to an uncooperative patient or technical difficulties

Injury to the vulva

The most frequent lacerations of the vulva are longitudinal on either side of the labium minor. They are usually shallow and bleed only slightly. Poor wound approximation has been demonstrated in women who had not been sutured.[6] Therefore, it is preferable to close even a small superficial wound with a few stitches of rapidly absorbed polyglactin (Vicryl Rapide) 2-0, threaded on an atraumatic needle.

Periurethral lacerations are another variety of vulvar injury. These should always be sutured after inspection of the urethral orifice. In deeper lacerations, care has to be taken not to damage the urethra during repair. This can be done by the insertion of a catheter. Longitudinal laceration of the upper part of the vulva may include the clitoris or its preputium. Such a tear is often accompanied by bleeding. The ligation of all actively bleeding vessels is essential before the repair of the tear itself; otherwise, a hematoma will arise or continuous bleeding will require a secondary repair. Proper analgesia and use of very fine suture materials of Vicryl Rapide are important in this particular area due to its extensive vascularization and innervation.

Another site of vulvar lacerations is along the edge of the perineum in a transverse direction. These are not very common by themselves and sometimes represent a continuation of labial lacerations. More frequent is damage to this part of the vulva in combination with either a vaginal or a perineal tear. In most cases, its direction is longitudinal into the vagina, down to the perineum, or both.

Injury to the perineum

Tears of the perineum are longitudinal, extend from the vulva, and can reach the rectal canal.[7] It is of major importance to recognize the full extent of the damage, since the repair must be meticulous in order to avoid unnecessary complications. They are classified into four grades according to their extent[8]:

1. *First-degree tear.* This is a short tear involving only the upper portion of the perineal body and the superficial tissues.
2. *Second-degree tear.* This involves the whole length of the perineum and includes the perineal body. It reaches the sphincter ani, but does not involve it.
3. *Third-degree tear.* This includes the anal sphincter, but does not extend into the anorectal canal.
4. *Fourth-degree tear.* Sometimes called a complete perineal tear, this tear extends into the anorectal canal.

As this classification does not include the depth of external anal sphincter rupture or the involvement of the internal sphincter, it has been modified[9] as follows to allow differentiation between injuries to the external anal sphincter, the internal anal sphincter, and the anal epithelium:

1. *First*: Injury to the skin only
2. *Second*: Injury to the perineum involving perineal muscles but not the anal sphincter

3. *Third*: Injury to perineum involving the anal sphincter complex
    a. Less than 50% of external anal sphincter thickness torn
    b. More than 50% of external anal sphincter thickness torn
    c. Internal anal sphincter torn
4. *Fourth*: Injury to perineum involving the anal sphincter complex and anal epithelium

This classification has been adopted by the International Consultation on Incontinence and the Royal College of Obstetricians and Gynaecologists (RCOG).[10] The term Obstetric Anal Sphincter Injuries (OASIS) encompasses both third- and fourth-degree perineal tears.

Following vaginal delivery, anal sphincter and anorectal mucosal injury cannot be excluded without performing a rectal examination. Visual assessment of the extent of perineal trauma to include the structures involved, the apex of the injury and assessment of bleeding should be followed by a rectal examination to assess whether there has been any damage to the external or internal anal sphincter or if there is any suspicion that the perineal muscles has been damaged.[10]

The following are principles of repair[10]:

- Suture as soon as possible after delivery to reduce bleeding and risk of infection.
- Check equipment and count swabs prior to commencing the procedure and count again after completion of the repair.
- Good lighting is essential to visualize and identify the structures involved.
- Ask for consultation if in doubt regarding the extent of trauma or structures involved.
- Repair of third- and fourth-degree tears should be conducted by an appropriately trained clinician or by a trainee under supervision.
- Repair should take place in an operating theatre under regional or general anesthesia.
- Insert an indwelling catheter for 24 hours to prevent urinary retention.
- Ensure good anatomic alignment of the wound and give consideration to cosmetic results.
- Rectal examination after completing the repair will ensure that suture material has not been accidentally inserted through the rectal mucosa.
- After completion of the repair, inform the woman regarding the extent of trauma and discuss pain relief, diet, hygiene, and the importance of pelvic floor exercises.

The repair of a first-degree tear is simple since the damage is superficial. After the wound is cleansed, hemostasis is ensured, and the edges of the wound are approximated with rapidly absorbed polyglactin (Vicryl Rapide) 2-0.

In second-degree tears, after hemostasis is secured, the torn perineal body exposes the edges of the two pillars of the pubococcygeal portion of the levator ani, and often the outer wall of the rectum becomes visible. The repair includes three or four interrupted sutures of rapidly absorbed polyglactin (Vicryl Rapide) 2-0, approximating the two separate portions of the levators. If the rectum is exposed, these sutures have to include its outer layer. Special care has to be taken not to enter the rectal cavity. After the tying of these sutures, the perineal body is approximated with interrupted sutures. Finally, the skin is closed with another layer of absorbable sutures (Vicryl Rapide 2-0). In patients with a thin subcutaneous layer, the two external layers, namely, the perineal body and fascia, and the skin may be sutured in one layer. The proper closure of the separated levators is important, since inadequate repair may be followed by rectocele at a later stage of the patient's life.

The first step in the repair of a fourth-degree tear is the suturing of the rectal mucosa. This is performed by approximating the torn edges of the rectal mucosa by sutures using either the continuous or interrupted technique. With interrupted sutures the knot can be tied either within or outside the anal canal. Polyglactin (Vicryl) 3-0 is usually used. Whichever technique is used for the repair, figure of eight sutures should be avoided during repair of the anal mucosa as they may cause ischemia.[10]

The repair of a third-degree tear preceded by the repair of the anal mucosa and followed by the stages of a second-degree repair. In order to reunite the external anal sphincter, its two edges have to be exposed. This is not always an easy task, since the torn edges usually retract. Nevertheless, they have to be pulled out from their retracted position on the sides of the anus in the direction of the retracted end, which is then elevated into view. It is essential to recognize the tissue and hold its whole thickness to achieve a good result.

The repair of a third-degree perineal tear, according to the RCOG classification,[10] requires the following steps. The internal anal sphincter, which appears as a glistening, white, fibrous structure between the rectal mucosa and the external anal sphincter, should be closed separately with interrupted or mattress sutures without any attempt to overlap.[11] Monofilament sutures such as 3-0 PDS or 2-0 polyglactin (Vicryl) can be used with equivalent outcomes. The external anal sphincter, which appears as a band of skeletal muscle with a fibrous capsule, can be sutured in an end-to-end manner. Alternatively, it can be repaired by overlapping the edges of the torn sphincter, using larger surface area of tissue contact between the two torn ends.[12] The overlap technique can only be used for full thickness external sphincter tears to allow the torn ends to be overlapped without tension. As two free ends of the muscle are needed for a proper overlap repair, overlapping of partial thickness external anal sphincter tears would exert undue tension on the repair. Therefore, an end-to-end repair should be performed in a partial thickness external anal sphincter tear; tear grades 3a (less than 50% of external anal sphincter thickness), and some of 3b (more than 50% of external anal sphincter thickness).[13] Although colorectal surgeons prefer to use the overlapping method to repair the sphincter remote from delivery, a recent Cochrane review demonstrated no difference in outcomes between an end-to-end and an overlap repair.[14] This Cochrane review on the method of repair for third- and fourth-degree tears examined six trials involving 588 women. It was recommended to use monofilament sutures such as 3-0 PDS or 2-0 polyglactin (Vicryl) with equivalent outcomes[10] The repair of the sphincter is followed by that of the perineum, as described in the second-degree tear repair.

Many deliveries are performed under epidural anesthesia, and this is also efficient for perineal repair. Alternatively, local anesthesia can be used in first and second-degree tears, while general anesthesia is preferred in the more extensive variations. Postoperative care includes analgesics, prophylactic antibiotic therapy, sitz bath, and stool softeners, which are continued for about two weeks after the repair. Diet is normal, and no special local care is given except for the sitz bath. The patient is discharged when full anal control is ensured. Some stool softeners may be needed for a few weeks.

All women who have had a third- and fourth-degree tear repaired should be offered a follow-up examination at 6–12 months by a gynecologist or a colorectal surgeon. Endoanal sonography and anorectal manometry may prove useful as additional means for diagnosis and follow-up.[10]

Prevention of perineal tears

Many authors believe that the repair of an episiotomy, like that of any other surgical incision, is simpler than that of an uncontrolled tear. This classical belief has been challenged recently.[15] The preventive measures include allowance of gradual dilation of the tissues, controlled use of instruments, and, last but not least, assurance of good cooperation of the patient during delivery. Two meta-analyses of RCTs of perineal protection techniques[16,17] found no difference in the incidence of OASIS between "hands-on" and "hands-off" approaches. The Cochrane review found no significant difference when the Ritgen maneuver was also used.[16] However, warm perineal compresses were beneficial in reducing the incidence of OASIS. Although the mechanism of action remains uncertain, this approach may well reduce perineal edema.[16]

Several studies in Norway compared the impact incorporation of manual perineal protection/"hands-on" technique versus hands-off approaches in time series analyses.[18–21] The perineum protection program consisted of four components when the baby's head is crowning: (a) slowing the delivery of the baby's head with one hand, (b) supporting perineum with the other hand and squeezing with fingers (first and second) from the perineum lateral parts towards the middle in order to lower the pressure in middle posterior perineum, (c) asking the delivering woman not to push, and (d) performing correct episiotomy only when indicated. A significant reduction in the incidence of OASIS was observed in all women after implementing the training program for perineal protection.[20,21] Nonetheless, the "hands-on" technique was associated with no benefits in the meta-analysis of studies on this issue.[17]

A variety of other preventive measures have been suggested by midwives in an attempt to protect against perineal trauma.[22] Kegel exercises, taking vitamins C and E to improve skin elasticity, avoiding the use of soap on the perineum during the last few weeks to avoid dryness of the skin's natural emollients, and prenatal perineal massage are all of questionable value. The Cochrane review of four trials (2497 women) showed that perineal massage undertaken by the woman or her partner was associated with an overall reduction in the incidence of trauma requiring suturing, but there was no differences in the incidence of third-/fourth-degree perineal trauma.[23] Warm packs placed on perineum during the second stage have also been associated with decreased incidence of OASIS.[16]

Subsequent vaginal delivery may worsen anal incontinence. All women who had a third- and fourth-degree tear in their previous pregnancy should be counseled regarding the risk of developing anal incontinence or worsening symptoms with subsequent vaginal delivery.[24]

VAGINAL LACERATIONS

During labor and delivery, the vaginal tissues are under strain, as they are stretched and compressed at the same time or alternately. This is a natural occurrence, and if labor progress is normal, acute or permanent damage to the tissues is minimal. However, the following obstetric situations or interventions predispose to damage of the vagina:

1. Overt lacerations at different locations often combined with tears of other adjacent structures (cervix, perineum, and vulva)
2. Hematoma formation due to submucous tear of blood vessels

Lacerations of the vagina occur more often with precipitated labor when gradual dilation of the tissue cannot occur, in cases of difficult vaginal delivery combined with a large fetus or pathologic presentations, in cases of instrumental delivery, and in prolonged labor when prolonged pressure on the tissues makes them edematous and brittle.

One of the rarest forms of vaginal laceration, namely, colporrhexis, or vault rupture, is a tear of the posterior cul-de-sac, with protrusion of intestines into the vagina. Colporrhexis necessitates careful repair under general anesthesia and excellent visualization. The intestine has to be carefully cleansed before replacing it into the peritoneal cavity, and the vaginal opening is then sutured with rapidly absorbed polyglactin (Vicryl Rapide) 2-0.

Longitudinal tears of the vagina are common. They follow the axis of the vagina, more frequently at the posterior wall. They can occur at normal spontaneous deliveries, but are more frequent in instrumental deliveries and prolonged and difficult labors. All detectable tears should be carefully visualized and sutured, care being taken for good hemostasis. The initial stitch must be taken well above the upper edge of the tear in order to include any retracted vessel that may bleed later if not closed. Vaginal tears combined with laceration of other structures may occur at both ends of the vagina.

Cervical tears may extend laterally and include the lateral fornix. This form may cause severe bleeding, since a branch of the uterine artery may be included. Repair of tears in this variety needs full operative conditions—anesthesia and perfect exposure by assistants and lights. Possible occult bleeding into the parametria has to be kept in mind. The vaginal tear is sutured from the side toward the cervix, followed by full repair of the cervical tear. Care must be taken not to damage the ureter, which can be in close proximity to an extensive tear.

Spontaneous vulvovaginal and combined perineo-vulvo-vaginal tears, and vaginal tear as an extension of episiotomy are another variety of vaginal lacerations. The same principles of treatment already described are applied.

Rarely, multiple vaginal abrasions and lacerations occur. Some of these can be sutured, but the mucosa can be so extensively damaged that suturing is impossible. In such cases, the best way to overcome the problem is tight tamponade of the vagina after inspection of the cervix and the fornices. The packing remains in place for up to 24 hours. Usually, good healing follows. A Foley catheter can be left in the uterine cavity to facilitate drainage.

Most vaginal lacerations heal quickly to full anatomic and functional integrity. One less noticed complication which can disturb the patient during the puerperium or later is granulation tissue formation. This tends to form at the edges of mucosal surfaces that have not been united. Its symptoms are spotting, contact bleeding, discharge, and, when sexual activity is resumed, dyspareunia. This minor complication can cause much discomfort. At the postnatal examination, small foci of granulation may be overlooked. Symptomatic patients are treated for vaginitis, bleedings are attributed to cervical erosion or uterine dysfunction, and the dyspareunia is often accepted as a "normal" result of childbirth.

Careful search for granulation tissues must be a part of any postpuerperal examination. The vaginal parts of an episiotomy, sutured vaginal tears, and the complete surface of the vagina, even where no suturing was performed, must be examined. The treatment is simple; electrocautery as an office procedure, without the need of anesthesia, gives excellent results.

Hematoma formation

Hematomas may occur in the vulva, vagina, and, much less frequently, subperitoneally above the pelvic floor. Most hematomas become evident after delivery; however, rarely, the vaginal type may start during labor and disturb the progress of childbirth. If this is the case and correct diagnosis is made, incision and drainage of the hematoma may enable birth, but the lacerated vessels must be sutured immediately afterward.[25]

As stated, hematomas usually become evident after delivery, but since their symptoms and signs develop slowly, most of them are discovered only hours later. The exception to this is the very rare instance of hematoma caused by laceration of a large vessel, often above the pelvic floor, which leads to blood volume decrease of significant degree, causing anemia and shock before giving any local signs or symptoms. The diagnosis of this situation is based mainly on the blood loss evident in progressive anemia and development of hypotension and shock, without any external loss through the birth canal. Sometimes some bulging of the fornix or parametria on the affected side may be detectable on vaginal palpation, accompanied by tenderness. Hematoma of this kind should be promptly treated, since the blood vessels must be tied. This can be best achieved by laparotomy by the retroperitoneal approach. In cases when the development of the hematoma is slow, it is sometimes self-limited and resolves spontaneously. This is often accompanied by fever due to resorption or infection; therefore, antibiotic treatment is indicated. Persistent fever during the puerperium in the presence of a parametrial mass is an indication for incision and drainage, which is preferentially performed abdominally. A parametrial hematoma may also evolve after cesarean section due to insufficient hemostasis and extravasation of the blood into the parametria.

Vulvar hematomas of smaller extent appear a short time after the completion of delivery. They usually result from incomplete hemostasis at suturing vulvar damage or from pricking of a vein during the procedure of repair. They are usually mild, cause little discomfort, and resolve spontaneously. Less frequently, vulvar hematoma results from a vaginal hematoma which dissects through the loose tissue into the vulvar region. These hematomas are usually unilateral and may reach considerable size if left untreated. They require surgical incision and drainage, and, most important, the torn vessels in the vagina have to be ligated.

The vaginal tissues, including the blood vessels, are under considerable strain during delivery. The tissues are stretched and compressed by the forces of labor and by the passage of the fetus. The congested blood vessels burst easily by pressure or tear in spontaneous delivery, but more often, at instrumental delivery. The hematoma formation usually starts during the second stage of labor, since, at this stage, the vessels are under maximal strain. However, even if ruptured, they are compressed, and blood effusion is slow or nil. After delivery, the intravaginal pressure decreases, and the open vessels, more often veins, start bleeding and cause hematoma formation. The extent of the hematoma and the rate of its growth depend on the location of the torn vessel and its size. Most hematomas remain undetected for a few hours after delivery, until the patient complains about intense pain and a tearing sensation in the vagina, about the rectum, and the perineal region. The pain increases, tenesmus can be felt, and, if the hematoma dissects its way under the bladder, difficulty in urination can be a symptom.

One must be attentive to the patient's complaints and be aware of the possibility of a hematoma formation at any stage of the puerperium. The diagnosis can then be made easily by vaginal and rectal palpation, and immediate treatment implemented. Surgical incision, under anesthesia with good exposure and illumination, facilitates clearing of the clots, after which the wound must be carefully searched for the bleeding vessels. All detectable bleeders must be ligated; however, this is sometimes a difficult task since the damage done by the hematoma itself causes secondary injury to capillaries, leading to diffuse oozing. Electrocoagulation can sometimes be used to overcome some of the difficulty. In some cases, tight vaginal packing for 24 hours may prove the only effective way to overcome the difficulties. Drainage of the wound is usually helpful.

Two additional types of vaginal hematomas must be kept in mind. First, a hematoma may develop in a repaired vaginal tear or episiotomy when hemostasis was inadequate. The open bleeding vessel can be anywhere in the wound, but the most probable site is a retracted vessel at its upper edge. Hence, it is most important to start any vaginal repair (tear or surgical incision) above the upper end of the wound. The usual pitfall causing delay in the diagnosis is that the pain arising from it is attributed to the sutured wound, and patients are given pain relievers and not examined sufficiently.

Second, a rather late form of hematoma formation is due to the delayed burst of a vessel, damaged by pressure necrosis during labor or delivery but bleeding only at a later stage. The symptoms are the same as in the other forms, but their onset is delayed. Thus, hematoma has to be thought of, even if previous vaginal and rectal examinations were normal.

The obstetrician is aware of the dangers of overt bleeding, searches for its cause, and applies treatment. Although occult bleeding is less frequent, the same awareness is necessary, since, if not discovered and treated, it may complicate an otherwise normal childbirth.

Attention is called to any complaint of pain in the vagina, rectum, or perineum, or pressure on the bladder—in cases of both a repaired wound and a woundless delivery—at any stage of the puerperium. Such pain must not be attributed to any cause before a thorough examination of the patient is performed.

CERVICAL TEARS

In normal labor, the cervix is gradually dilated, and the passage of the newborn causes only minimal damage that changes the appearance of the cervical os after involution. More severe tears occur when dilation is rapid or forceful, often accompanied by premature pushing of the newborn through an incompletely dilated cervix, as is sometimes the case in breech presentation or with an uncooperative patient. Manual displacement of the cervical edge during labor also causes cervical damage, as does an attempt at instrumental delivery before the cervix is completely dilated.[26]

Scarring due to previous operations or cervical rigidity may also predispose to cervical tears. Special attention must be paid to parturients who had a cervical cerclage during pregnancy. It is customary to remove the McDonald-type cerclage at 37 weeks in order to enable healing of the cervix until labor starts. However, sometimes labor starts before the suture is removed, and the damage may become serious if the suture is not removed instantly. Many cervices are cicatrized or torn after cerclage, and the more worn off they are, the more they tend to tear. In such cases, abdominal delivery may be considered in order to prevent extension of a tear into the uterus or parametria.

Prolonged labor can weaken the cervical structure, and pressure necrosis occurs if a part of the cervix is compressed between the fetal head and the pelvic wall. In modern obstetrics, care is taken to prevent vaginal delivery in unfavorable conditions; thus, this type of injury is rare. Nonetheless, one must be acquainted with its symptoms and treatment.

In most cases, the injury is limited to the vaginal portion of the cervix; however, in some instances, the laceration may extend higher into the isthmic part of the uterus and thus form one of the variants of uterine rupture. Another possible extension is into the vaginal fornix.

The usual direction of a cervical laceration is longitudinal; however, a few cases of circular damage with complete ablation of the cervical ring have also been described. In such a case, if bleeding occurs, an attempt must be made to reconstruct the cervical lip along its entire circumference by approximating the endo- and exocervical mucosal lining, preferably with a continuous buttonhole stitch. However, although the damage is considerable since it usually results from prolonged compression, the lesion may not bleed at all and can be left to heal spontaneously.

Another unusual type of cervical damage can result from careless use of forceps, or of the vacuum cup when it is applied on an elongated part of the cervix and that portion is torn out at the delivery. The repair of such a lesion is a variation or a combination of the repairs of a circular ablation and a longitudinal tear; the tendency to one direction or the other depends on the extent of the absent tissue.

The most common cervical laceration is longitudinal, or radial; it can be single, or even multiple. The frequency of these lesions is higher than those diagnosed after delivery; since some do not bleed, their edges heal spontaneously and are discovered only later at a postnatal examination. The usual location of the radial cervical tear is lateral, although anterior or posterior locations are possible. These are usually connected with instrumental deliveries.

Cervical tear (and/or another lesion of the lower birth canal) should be suspected in any case of persistent bleeding in the presence of a well-contracted uterus. The vaginal canal and the whole circumference of the cervix must be visually explored. At least one but preferably two assistants should be available. In all delivery units, prepared sets containing the necessary instruments should be ready: four broad-bladed retractors at least 10 cm long, six ring forceps or sponge holders, two long needle holders, and two long, surgical tissue forceps.

The retractors are carefully inserted in the vagina and pushed up toward the fornices under visual control. The edge of the cervix is gripped by a ring forceps, and then another is applied about 60° in one direction and one more in the opposite one. The rest are applied successively in the same way; thus, the whole circumference of the cervix is held by the instruments. Any tear thus must become visualized between two forceps, and repaired immediately. The remaining forceps are taken off. The tear is well exposed by pulling the cervix to the opposite direction and toward the vaginal outlet. The suturing must start above the apex of the tear in order to include all retracted blood vessels and muscular tissue. We prefer one layer of interrupted, rapidly absorbed polyglactin (Vicryl Rapide) 2-0 sutures for this kind of repair. Interrupted suturing takes more time but enables good adaptation of tissues and prevents tension (Figure 27.1). Continuous and especially buttonhole sutures are usually too tight and often cause necrosis, which interferes with unification of the wound edges, resulting in a residual defect that has to be repaired later.

UTERINE RUPTURE

Etiology, classification, and prophylaxis

Rupture of the uterus is one of the major catastrophes seen in obstetric practice (Figure 27.2). It carries a high rate of fetal and maternal mortality, of which it still is a major cause in developing countries. In a large series, the rate of uterine rupture was reported as 1:2900–1:4300 deliveries.[11,27,28] Rupture of an unscarred uterus is a rare event involving 1:17,000 deliveries.[29] In contrast, the reported rate of symptomatic uterine rupture of the scarred uterus in prospective cohort studies was 3.8 per 1000 trials of labor.[30] In a large series of ruptured uteri reported in 1980, there was a distinct difference in both fetal and maternal outcomes between the group with a previously scarred uterus, usually a previous cesarean section scar (approximately one-third of all uterine ruptures), and the group with no previous scarring[31] (Table 27.1).

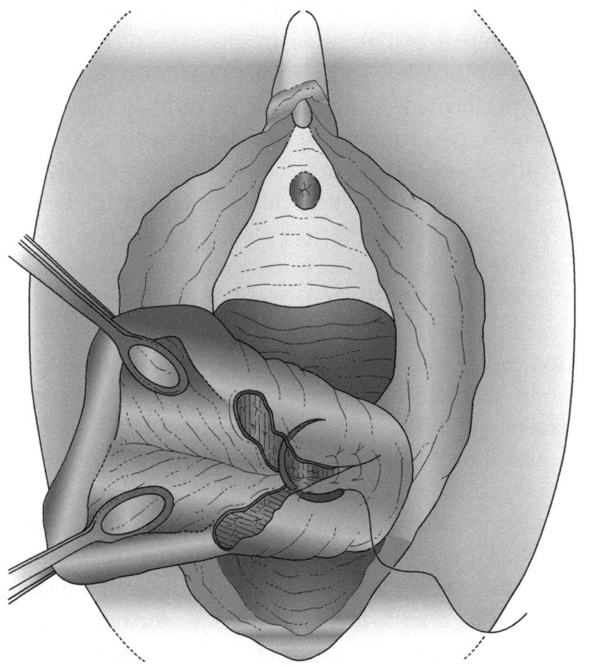

Figure 27.1 Repair of a cervical tear.

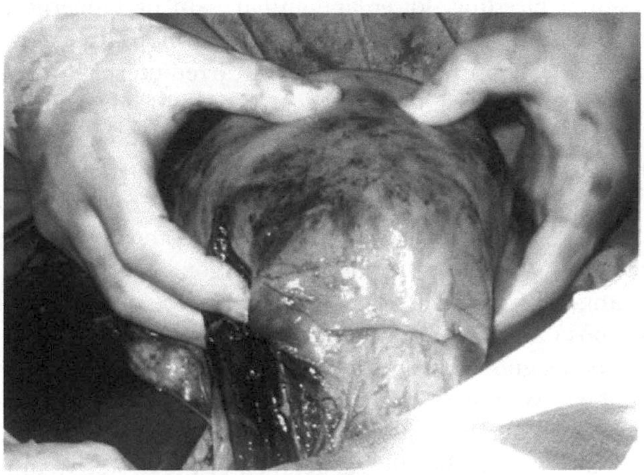

Figure 27.2 Ruptured uterus: unscarred, longitudinal tear.

The majority of reports of unscarred uterine ruptures come from rural areas in developing countries where poor antenatal care and obstetric facilities contribute to the occurrence of this grave complication. Common incriminating factors in previously unscarred uteri are cephalopelvic disproportion and grand multiparity (Table 27.2), but uncontrolled use of oxytocin is probably the leading etiologic factor these days. Special care should be exercised when oxytocin is used in the presence of any predisposing factor, such as grand multiparity, malpresentation, or a previous cesarean section scar, conditions that are relative contraindications to the use of oxytocin. Cephalopelvic disproportion is a major contraindication.

Abruptio placentae and, in particular, Couvelaire uterus, with its extravasation of blood in the stretched and disrupted uterine wall, may predispose to uterine rupture. In our series, as many as 18% of the unscarred uterine ruptures were associated with abruptio placentae. The use of oxytocin in these patients may be particularly hazardous. One must realize that a patient with shock and tender abdomen, and without audible fetal heart sounds, diagnosed as having abruptio placentae, may have a ruptured uterus.

In Golan's et al.[31] series, about one-third of uterine ruptures occurred after previous cesarean section. A small number of these involved classical cesarean section scars. The incidence of rupture in these longitudinal, upper-segment scars was reported as 2.2%–13% as compared to 0–0.5% in lower-segment scars.[32,33] The rupture of the latter usually takes place in labor, whereas a classic scar may rupture during pregnancy.

Uterine rupture after previous scarring due to hysterotomy or uterine perforation at operative hysteroscopy and dilation and curettage has been reported but is uncommon. The same is true of uterine rupture during difficult operative deliveries, malpresentations, and destructive operations, which are hardly seen these days.

Prophylaxis is the main way to fight this catastrophic obstetric complication. Improving medical facilities and antenatal care in rural areas and in developing countries, and implementation of family planning programs will probably lower the incidence of rupture of the uterus. Great effort must be made in any obstetric unit in diagnosing even minor degrees of cephalopelvic disproportion or malpresentation, and in treating the grand multipara and all

Table 27.1 Clinical features of uterine rupture.

Clinical features	Previously scarred uterus (*n* = 32)	Unscarred uterus (*n* = 60)	Total
Tachycardia only	1	4	5
Shock	3 (9%)	24 (40%)	27
Scar (or abdominal) tenderness or pain	9 (28%)	14 (23%)	23
Uterine bleeding	13 (40%)	40 (66%)	53
Hematuria	1	1	2
Cessation of contractions		4	4
Change in fetal position	2	6 (10%)	8
Disappearance of fetal heart sounds	3	17 (28%)	20
Routine examination of scar	9	47 (28%)	15

Source: Reproduced from Golan A et al., *Obstet Gynecol*, 56, 549–54, 1980. With permission from Lippincott Williams & Wilkins.

Table 27.2 Etiologic factors involved in uterine rupture.

Unscarred uterus	Cephalopelvic disproportion
	Oxytocin misuse
	Grand multiparity
	Abruptio placentae
	Malpresentations (face, brow, shoulder)
	Operative deliveries (forceps, internal version)
	Destructive operations
Previously scarred uterus	Cesarean section scar
	Hysterotomy scar
	Uterine perforation scar
	Myomectomy or metroplasty scar
	Previous repair of a ruptured uterus

patients with suspected abruptio placentae as very high-risk patients. They should be attended and treated in a special high-risk intensive care zone in the labor ward by specially trained personnel. Difficult operative deliveries should be abandoned and replaced by cesarean sections. Vaginal birth after cesarean delivery (VBAC) should be attempted only on a patient who has had a previous transverse, lower-uterine-segment cesarean section, and after a careful assessment was favorable for delivery by the vaginal route. Previous postcesarean section sepsis can be an indicator of poor scar healing. Routine hysterosalpingograms in women who had cesarean sections demonstrate relatively often deficiencies of the uterine scars.[34] High correlation has been found between measurements of the lower uterine segment thickness by ultrasound preoperatively and by inspection intraoperatively.[35,36] However, such radiography or sonographies provides no absolute reassurance for the future resistance of the scar under the stress of labor; thus, each case should be assessed carefully and the management individualized. When vaginal delivery is decided upon, careful monitoring of labor is required along with adequate analgesia for an assisted second stage, if required.

A previous classical cesarean section should always be followed by a repeat section, and the same should be the case after repair of a uterine rupture.

Induction of labor is a common obstetric practice and is often performed in women with an unfavorable cervix. Although vaginal birth after cesarean section is associated with a low risk of uterine rupture, its management is controversial. A recent review of eight studies, examined pregnancy outcome in induced versus spontaneous labor in women with previous cesarean section. Uterine rupture/dehiscence has occurred in 136 out of 17,412 women attempting vaginal birth after previous cesarean section, with a 0.7% incidence. Women with induction of labor were more likely to experience uterine rupture/dehiscence compared with spontaneous labor (46/4,038, 1.1% and 90/13,374, 0.6%, respectively [odds ratio {OR}: 1.62; 95% confidence interval {CI}: 1.13–2.31]).[37]

In a review comparing single versus double layers for uterine closure of low transverse cesarean incision, two RCTs studies reported no significant difference between single- versus double-layer closure for uterine dehiscence (relative risk: 1.86; 95% CI: 0.44–7.90; p = .40) or uterine rupture (no case).[38]

Clinical presentation, diagnosis, and pathology

Vaginal bleeding, lower abdominal pain or tenderness, fetal distress, and shock are the most common clinical features. The rupture of a previously scarred uterus is a less dramatic event. Shock appears to be rare, vaginal bleeding and abdominal tenderness and pain being the main features. Obviously, less bleeding occurs from a separated uterine scar than from the fresh, torn edges of a primary uterine rupture. Other reported signs and symptoms include tachycardia, hematuria, cessation of contractions, change in fetal position, and disappearance of fetal heart sounds (Table 27.1).

The diagnosis of rupture of the uterus is usually a clinical one. Awareness of the risk of this condition is important in all high-risk patients. VBAC deserves special care and awareness. The clinical acumen of the obstetrician is of prime importance. Suspected rupture of the uterus is an indication for surgery.

The uterine tear may be complete, penetrating through the serosal layer of the uterus and communicating with the peritoneal cavity, or incomplete (dehiscence), leaving the serosa intact. It can be longitudinal, transverse, or compound. The most common type of tear in the unscarred uterus is the longitudinal one, which is usually complete. Rupture of the previously scarred uterus is usually transverse and incomplete, as most ruptures are in fact dehiscent scars.[31] In 12%–22% of the cases, bladder lacerations accompany ruptures. These are almost always related to a previous cesarean section scar. The main symptoms are hematuria or meconium-stained urine.[39–41]

Treatment and outcome

The basic treatment of a patient with a ruptured uterus is immediate resuscitation and surgery.[25]

Especially in young women, there may be good reasons for preserving the uterus. In general, the surgical procedure employed must be individualized, and it is dependent upon the type, location, and extent of the laceration. The decision to perform a total or a subtotal hysterectomy should depend on whether the cervix or vagina is involved and on the patient's condition. When the dehiscence of a previous cesarean section scar is repaired, the edges should be excised prior to the repair. The repair is performed with polyglactin (Vicryl) 2-0 sutures, two continuous layers for a lower-segment rupture repair and three continuous layers for an upper-segment rupture repair. Special care must be taken to secure hemostasis at the apexes of the tear. Repair of a ruptured uterus is mainly considered when future fertility is desired. When there is only slight dehiscence of a uterine scar, or when a tear is linear and easily reparable in a young patient of low parity, further pregnancies may be allowed after adequate repair.

Careful postoperative attention and support are needed, as, even after surgery is completed, the patient is still at risk of complications of hemorrhage, sepsis, and thromboembolic phenomena. In case of damage to the bladder, drainage with an indwelling catheter is needed for 5–7 days. It is an important means of preventing fistula formation.

Rupture of the uterus is still an important cause of maternal death in obstetric practice. In a publication describing the trends in pregnancy-related mortality and risk factors for pregnancy-related deaths in the United States for the years 1991–7, uterine rupture accounted for 1.7% of all maternal deaths.[42] In the United Kingdom, it accounted for 1.9% of all maternal deaths for the years 1994–6.[43] It is worth noting that there are considerably fewer maternal deaths among ruptured scarred uteri than among ruptured unscarred uteri. No maternal deaths were reported in the former group. In the unscarred group, the maternal mortality was 6.5%–10% in various large series.[31,44] The fetal mortality rate was high as a result of separation of the placenta; in the unscarred group, it was 46%–74%, but only 22%–28% in the scarred group.[31]

EARLY MISCELLANEOUS INJURY

Symphysiolysis

Peripartum pubic symphysis separation is a recognized complication of pregnancy, estimates of its incidence ranging from 1:300 to 1:30,000.[45] Some degree of relaxation of the pelvic joints is present in all pregnant women. It is regarded as a preparatory process for delivery. The peptide hormone relaxin, structurally related to insulin and insulin-like growth factor, and primarily secreted by the corpus luteum and the placenta during pregnancy, is involved in a variety of functions.[46] It was isolated and studied as a substance that dissolved the anterior pelvis in guinea pigs late in pregnancy.[47] Although there is no proof for this role of relaxin in human subjects, the genetic machinery for production of relaxin does exist in humans, and may explain this phenomenon.[48]

The amount of relaxation of the pelvic joints during pregnancy may be quite considerable. The two pubic bones may become separated by a few centimeters without any symptom, complaint, or other difficulty for the pregnant woman. However, in other cases, a much smaller separation may be very painful and severely debilitating. This sometimes occurs during the later part of pregnancy and probably is combined with relaxation of the two sacroiliac joints.

Symphysiolysis is an infrequent affliction of the pelvic joint. It is characterized by loosening of the ligamentous support of the joint, and hence, a free sliding movement of the bones, mainly in the direction of the body axis. This comes into effect most prominently during gait and is accompanied by severe pain, which often interferes with mobilization. During walking, the body weight is alternately shifted from one leg to the other, this shift being transferred through the pelvic girdle. In the case of a loose symphysis pubis, at each step the pelvic bone is elevated in relation to the opposite side. This can be demonstrated by radiography if exposures are taken as the patient stands on each of her legs (Figure 27.3). The source of the pain can be of dual origin, due to friction of the bones or to excessive stretching of the joint ligaments.

The most prominent symptom of symphysiolysis is pain in the joint at any movement involving the pelvis. Gait is most severely inhibited, and even movements in bed often cause severe discomfort. Pressure on the joint usually elicits pain. Another diagnostic measure is to adduct and abduct the thighs against external counterpressure exerted by the examiner. In normal condition, this is painless; if the joint is affected, the procedure is painful. As already stated, radiologic proof can be documented by special techniques.

Symphysiolysis often occurs after difficult delivery, either spontaneous or instrumental. It is possible that in some cases the ligaments supporting the joint are ruptured during a traumatic or forceful delivery. Recovery from symphysiolysis usually occurs within 6–8 weeks.

The treatment of pelvic relaxation is mainly symptomatic, both during pregnancy and after delivery. Tight

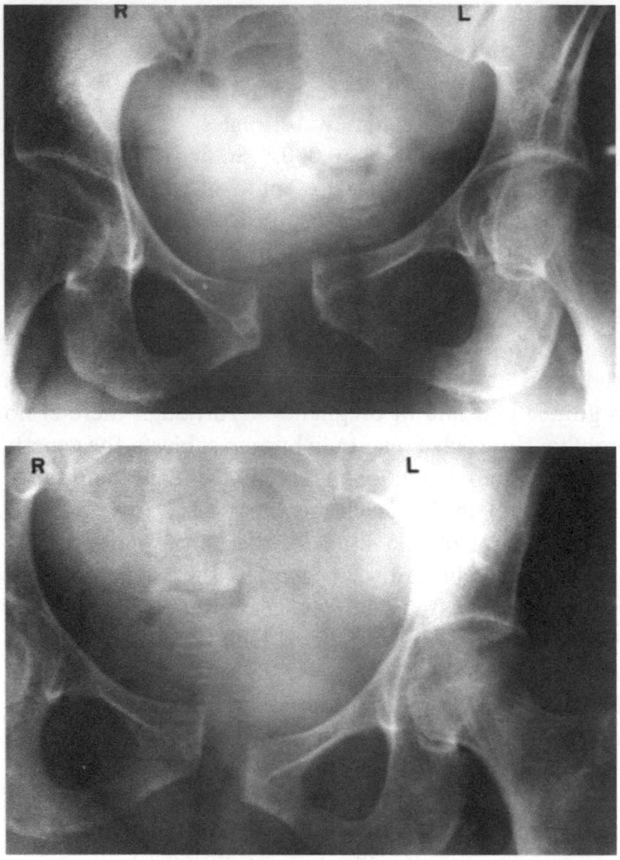

Figure 27.3 Radiographs of patient with symphysiolysis, standing alternately on each leg. Note change of joint as body weight shifts (anteroposterior plane).

binding of the pelvis usually permits free movement, although sometimes it is accompanied by discomfort. The puerpera should be encouraged to move in order to prevent other complications. Nonsteroidal anti-inflammatory drugs (NSAIDs) are in common use. Injection of corticosteroids into the joint has been tried, but the results are controversial. Local injection of anesthetics is of help in difficult cases and may promote mobilization. Orthopedic repair of the joint is very rarely needed in patients whom conservative management is unsuccessful or the sacroiliac joints remain unstable. Those patients may benefit from open reduction and internal or external skeletal fixation. Women who have had peripartum symphyseal separations may be at risk for subsequent separations.[49]

Damage of the coccyx

During delivery, the coccyx is pushed backward in order to enlarge the pelvic outlet. This physiologic movement, if exaggerated, can cause tearing of the sacrococcygeal joint or, in some cases, fracture of the coccyx. This is most likely to occur in cases of difficult deliveries of large infants, occipitoposterior positions, and instrumentation, or if the coccyx points sharply forward. Damage to the joint or the bone itself is usually painful. It disturbs the patient mainly in the sitting position, but also when she lies in bed or defecates.

Diagnosis is by combined rectal and external examination. This procedure discloses tenderness and sometimes swelling of the surrounding tissues. A lateral radiograph of the sacroiliac joint can be helpful. Spontaneous healing is the rule in most cases; however, sometimes healing is by ankylosis, often with a coccyx directed anteriorly, a result which can obstruct the next labor. In some cases, pain continues for prolonged periods. It can be treated by injection of local anesthetics, but surgery may be indicated in severe cases.

Peroneal palsy

Peroneal palsy is a rare complication attributable to improper and prolonged strapping of the legs during delivery. If the legs are strapped too tightly and externally to the supportive poles, pressure on the peroneal nerve may cause palsy, with foot drop resulting. Today, when strapping is no longer popular and supportive poles are used infrequently, this complication is hardly seen. Usually, no permanent damage is left; however, this preventable complication unnecessarily prolongs puerperal convalescence. Treatment is by physiotherapy combined with foot support to facilitate free movement. Even if wide abduction is needed for delivery, the legs can be freed for the third stage and, if necessary, strapped again for any further procedure.

Miscellaneous cervical damage

In most instances, obstetric trauma of the cervix is diagnosed soon after delivery or in the early puerperium. In these detected cases, the lesion should be repaired upon diagnosis. Unfortunately, in some cases, cervical damage is unsuspected and spontaneous healing takes place, resulting, albeit infrequently, in permanent damage to the structural and functional integrity of the cervix.

The factors contributing to such cervical damage include mainly those also causing cervical incompetence. Previous cervical surgery predisposes to damage during labor and delivery. Cervical cerclage is a quite frequent cause of inconspicuous cervical tears, fenestration, and fibrosis.

Most of the injuries, mainly lateral tears, partial muscular retractions, and eversion of endocervical mucosa, are detected at postpartum examination. They should be corrected at the earliest occasion, since further involvement may be expected at a future delivery. Infrequently, cervical damage is undetectable at first examination, and its existence becomes obvious only at some later stage. Cervical scarring and fibrosis may result in cervical dystocia due to rigidity and failure to dilate. If neglected, new tears, often severe, or even annular detachment of the cervix may occur. Cervical damage may cause problems of infertility due to chronic cervicitis or extensive damage to the endocervical glands.

Urinary fistula

Urinary incontinence after childbirth may herald the formation of a urinary fistula. In his monograph on vesicovaginal fistula, Chassar-Moir[50] reported that almost one-third of the fistulas he operated on were of obstetric origin. Mahfouz,[51] reporting on 758 cases in Egypt, found that obstetric trauma was the most common cause of urinary fistulas. These were also the findings in two large series reported from South Africa.[52,53] The main causes of urinary fistulas were protracted labors, difficult forceps deliveries, cesarean sections, ruptured uterus, and symphysiotomy. However, it seems that with the improvement of obstetric services, obstetric trauma as the predisposing factor for urinary fistulas is becoming rare.

Two types of fistulas occur. The most common type is caused by pressure necrosis. In prolonged labor with cephalopelvic disproportion, the bladder neck and urethra are compressed between the fetal head and the symphysis pubis. When this compression is prolonged, these tissues become ischemic and undergo necrosis. This leads to urinary incontinence, usually appearing 7–10 days later when the necrotic tissue sloughs out, forming a hole in the bladder base communicating with the vagina. It is usually located between the cervix and the external urethral meatus, involving the bladder neck and the anterior vaginal wall. Such fistulas vary in size, from some that hardly admit a probe to large ones easily recognized on vaginal inspection.

The second type is the traumatic fistula caused by direct injury to the bladder at difficult forceps delivery, craniotomy, or whenever a uterine or large anterior cervical tear involving the bladder is overlooked. Such circumstances are rare today. At cesarean section, especially at a repeat operation, damage can be done to the bladder during its downward displacement and, also on opening the uterus or its subsequent suturing. Blood stained urine is a warning sign.

Immediate effective continuous drainage of the bladder is mandatory. Small obstetric vesicovaginal fistulas may heal spontaneously if the bladder is effectively drained by an indwelling catheter. If no healing occurs within 3 months, surgical repair is necessary. It was always considered unwise to attempt surgical repair too soon after the causative trauma. Apart from achieving reduction in size by spontaneous healing, in time the local blood supply improves, the slough separates, and the inflammation subsides, providing better conditions for surgery.

Sometimes ureterovaginal fistula may occur. Injury to a ureter during cesarean section or a repair of a ruptured uterus may result in ureterovaginal or ureterocervical fistula. Corrective surgery is usually the treatment. The urologist should be involved in the management of such fistulas.

Rectovaginal fistula

Although less common than the vesicovaginal fistula, the rectovaginal fistula is a very distressing consequence of birth trauma. Fortunately, this complication has become extremely rare. Three main situations are considered to cause rectovaginal fistula. The first is prolonged and firm compression of the posterior vaginal wall by the presenting part toward the bony birth canal. This continuous compression causes impairment of the circulation, edema, and necrosis of the tissues, leading finally to a fistula formation. Such a fistula may appear any time during the puerperium. The second causative factor is faulty repair or healing process of a fourth-degree perineal tear. The third is unnoticed damage of the rectum during repair of a third-degree tear, an episiotomy, or a deep vaginal tear. Gynecologic or colorectal surgeons should be involved in the management of such fistulas.

Genital prolapse

Pelvic organ prolapse is a major health issue for women. Women with normal life expectancy have an 20% chance of undergoing at least one operation for pelvic organ prolapse or urinary incontinence during their lifetime.[54] The causal basis of genital prolapse is multifactorial. Birth trauma to the pelvic floor and other surrounding tissues supporting the uterus and adjoining structures is of basic and major importance.[55,56]

In a longitudinal cohort study, women with spontaneous vaginal birth were associated with a significantly greater odds of prolapse to or beyond the hymen compared women with cesarean without labor, 5–10 years after first delivery (OR: 5.6, 95% CI: 2.2–14.7). Operative vaginal birth significantly increased the odds for prolapse (OR: 7.5, 95% CI: 2.7–20.9).[57] In the Swedish Pregnancy, Obesity and Pelvic floor (SWEPOP) study, pelvic floor function was evaluated 20 years after one single pregnancy terminating either in by VD or by CS. The prevalence of pelvic organ prolapse, two decades later, was doubled after one vaginal delivery compared with one caesarean section.[58]

Genital prolapse also occurs in other mammals, but is much less frequent in quadrupeds. The erect posture of the human female exerts a dual influence on the pathogenesis of genital prolapse. First, the evolutionary process of the erect posture of the human species caused an adaptational strengthening of the pelvic girdle. This structure has to carry the weight of the body, transferred to the legs; therefore, the bones became stronger and thicker, resulting in the narrowing of the internal measures of the bony birth canal. The relatively large human fetus, as compared to other species, further increases the problem of passage through the tightly fitting birth canal. The birth process in most species is much easier and less traumatic due to larger space and smaller fetal size, thus resulting in less damage to the pelvic musculature and fascia.

Second, the fascial and muscular support of the human pelvic floor is under continuous strain from intra-abdominal pressure, which in the erect posture is also influenced by the forces of gravity. In order to resist this continuous strain, the pelvic floor has to be strong and undamaged; otherwise, its supportive function of the pelvic organs fails. Some amount of damage to the floor is almost inevitable in childbirth, and the additional pressure due to the erect posture exacerbates the condition.

Genital prolapse may occur shortly after childbirth if the damage is extensive, but it is far more frequent with advancing age when additional contributing factors come into effect. These include general weakening of connective and estrogen-dependent tissues in the pelvis, often aggravated by recurrent or chronic abdominal pressure due to constipation, chronic cough, or obesity.

DeLee[59] explained the principles of pelvic floor damage as follows:

1. The head advancing through the hiatus genitalis stretches the vagina radially and longitudinally—sometimes it also wipes the vagina off its fascial anchorings, sliding it downward and outward.
2. The head stretches the pelvic fascia over the levator ani and, between the rectum and the vagina and the layer behind the rectum, also radially and longitudinally, and this also permits the rectum to be wiped downward and slide off its fascial attachments to the levator ani.
3. The head often tears or overstretches the fascia over the levator ani, especially those bundles which hold the pillars of the muscle in position at the sides of the rectum, spanning the hiatus genitalis, and this permits the pillars to separate, diastasis of the levator pillars resulting—the disorder is similar to that of diastasis recti abdominalis. This diastasis of the levator pillars and the wiping or sliding of the rectum and vagina downward and outward are the essential features of most pelvic floor injuries, and have been, we think, the least noticed by current writers.
4. The tears in the levator ani muscle are usually due to improper treatment, and they occur, least commonly, near the insertion of the muscle on the pubic ramus (usually due to cutting by the forceps) and more commonly at the sides of the rectum, behind, near the raphe.
5. Labor always ruptures the urogenital septum, tearing it in all directions, and also from its ramifications with the endopelvic fascia, both above and below the levator ani.
6. The fascia between the rectum and the bladder is also stretched or torn, also radially and in a downward direction, tearing the vagina and bladder off its anchoring to the upper surface of the endopelvic fascia over the levator ani and the posterior surface of the pubis.

It is thus evident that most of the damage resulting from labor is due to injury, rupture, distraction, and displacement of the fascia, and less to tearing of the muscles. The more difficult childbirth is, the more damage is to be expected. Macrosomia, constitutional or as seen with postmaturity or diabetes, is an important factor. Too conservative obstetric practice and prolonged trials of labor could be involved. Occipitoposterior and difficult breech deliveries, shoulder dystocia, and hastily managed instrumentation due to emergency situations all contribute to pelvic floor damage.

The site of the late disorder depends on the site of the initial injury. The most common lesion is the diastasis of the levator ani pillars, which destroys the posterior and lateral support of the vagina, resulting in a relaxed and atonic vaginal inlet with a tendency to rectocele formation. The atonic vagina itself may cause, at any stage, sexual insufficiency and, in combination with a sagging perineum, recurrent vaginal infections.

This form of injury to the pelvic floor is usually due to large fetal parts, but its extent depends on the preventive measures taken. The performance of episiotomy and good repair may be of importance, and so may judicious management of the second stage of labor, allowing gradual relaxation of the pelvic and perineal structures.

An even deeper tear affects the muscular bundles of the pubococcygeus, which, in combination with detachment of the rectum from its superior anchorage to the pelvic fascia, leads to the formation of a high rectocele as the vaginal wall slides along with the loosened rectum.

Damage to the posterior part of the pelvic support arises more commonly in cases of continuous pressure and tension at this region. Undetected and prolonged anterior asynclitism may be of importance.

Affliction of the fascia supporting the bladder and the urethra causes, at a later stage, anterior vaginal wall prolapse, combined with cystocele, urethrocele, or both. In some instances, this leads to functional disturbances of the bladder and its control, resulting in stress incontinence.

Untimely pushing or pulling of the fetus through an insufficiently prepared birth canal often damages the uterine anchorage and the ligamentous support of the uterus. This predisposes to uterine prolapse at a later stage. Solitary damage to the ligaments is less common and leads to cervical elongation or uterine prolapse. More commonly, it is combined with additional damage to the pelvic floor, resulting later in prolapse, combined with other forms of vaginal relaxation.

Although many of these injuries can be prevented by proper obstetric management, some will occur due to the large size of the fetus. As only a small part of this damage can be detected immediately after delivery, the rest will remain obscure until a later stage, when additional strain is exerted on the pelvic support.

Urinary incontinence

Urinary incontinence can occur at any age; however, it is much more common in parous women late in their reproductive years. Obstetric injury to the urethrovesical support is the most common factor predisposing to the development of stress incontinence, although many years may intervene between childbirth and the onset of symptoms. Vaginal birth may increase the risk of stress and mixed urinary incontinence, but not of urge urinary incontinence and overactive bladder.[60,61] In the Norwegian EPINCONT (Epidemiology of Incontinence in the County of Nord-Trøndelag) study,[62] the risk of any urinary incontinence was higher after vaginal delivery than cesarean section and nulliparous women (21%, 15.9%, 10.1%, respectively).

Stress incontinence and mixed-type incontinence were associated with mode of delivery in the same manner as any incontinence. However, urge incontinence was not associated with mode of delivery. In a recent SWEPOP (Swedish Pregnancy, Obesity and Pelvic Floor) study, the prevalence of stress urinary incontinence, urge urinary incontinence and mixed urinary incontinence was 15.3%, 6.1%, 14.4%, respectively, and was higher for all subtypes after VD versus CS.[63] In a difficult labor, the bladder is compressed between the advancing fetal head and the symphysis pubis, and its fascial supports may be weakened. Some degree of stress incontinence may also appear during pregnancy, but this is only temporary and usually disappears after delivery.[64]

Dyspareunia

Dyspareunia resulting from childbirth can occur either shortly after resuming sexual activity or at any later stage of the woman's life. At the later stage, additional components usually play an important role, such as hormonal deficiency and aging of the tissues. In its milder forms, dyspareunia is probably quite common; however, women tend to accept it as a result of childbirth. They do not complain, and many times its pathologic meaning is brought to their attention only by the physician.

Damage to the birth canal and its repair accounts for these cases of dyspareunia. Too tight a repair of a vaginal tear or of an episiotomy can make coitus difficult and uncomfortable, a too tightly repaired perineum can make sexual relations almost impossible, and, if insisted on, very painful. One must be careful in repair of multiple lacerations, since here lies the danger of a too perfect repair and multifocal fibrosis.

A frequent, but often overlooked, cause of coital discomfort soon after the puerperium is formation of granulation tissue in the vagina. Causes of deep dyspareunia resulting from childbirth include organized hematomas and scars in the parametria or the vaginal vault.

In many instances, no interference with sexual activity appears during the fertile age; however, when additional factors resulting from aging appear, mainly atrophy and tightening due to hormonal deprivation, dyspareunia becomes evident.

Allen–Masters syndrome

In 1955, Allen and Masters[65] described the syndrome, named after them, of a tear in the posterior leaf of the broad ligament, extreme retroversion of the uterus, and a freely movable cervix termed a "universal joint cervix." They established an anatomic basis for the pelvic congestion syndrome described earlier by Taylor,[66] showing that the anatomic defect is a tear at the base of the broad ligament, on one or both sides, which can also include the sacrouterine ligaments. They assumed that the loss of support of the blood vessels leads to kinking and subsequently venous congestion. In the majority of cases, a conglomerate of congested veins is visible through the defect in the broad ligament, and almost invariably some amount of serous fluid is found in the pouch of Douglas. The venous congestion produces softness of the lower part of the uterus, which further weakens the uterine support, resulting in the "universal joint cervix," with hypermobility of the cervix in relation to the uterus.

The clinical features of the syndrome include dysmenorrhea, menorrhagia, dyspareunia, continuous pelvic pain and discomfort, pain on defecation, general weakness, emotional instability, and headaches. The syndrome is not difficult to diagnose on a clinical basis; however, laparoscopy can be a helpful diagnostic aid. Endometriosis might be an alternative in the differential diagnosis.

A traumatic obstetric event has been suggested as the etiologic factor involved in the majority of these cases. Compromise of the uterine support usually follows some traumatic obstetric incident such as a difficult instrumental delivery, breech extraction, prolonged labor, manual removal of placenta, and puerperal curettage. As most of the complaints of this syndrome are nonspecific, the gynecologist must be aware of its existence.

Birth trauma may have an impact on a woman's health far beyond its immediate influence. It is imperative that such trauma be promptly and properly diagnosed and treated in order to avoid further complications and modifications of the woman's health, sexual life, and social well-being.

REFERENCES

1. Dumont M. [The long and difficult birth of symphysiotomy or from Severin Pineau to Jean-Rene Sigault]. *J Gynecol Obstet Biol Reprod (Paris)* 1989; 18(1): 11–21.
2. Shaarani SR, van Eeden W, O'Byrne JM. The Irish experience of symphysiotomy: 40 years onwards. *J Obstet Gynaecol* 2016; 36(1): 48–52.
3. Hofmeyr GJ, Shweni PM. Symphysiotomy for fetopelvic disproportion. *Cochrane Database Syst Rev* 2012; (10): CD005299.
4. Bjorklund K. Minimally invasive surgery for obstructed labour: A review of symphysiotomy during the twentieth century (including 5000 cases). *BJOG* 2002; 109(3): 236–48.
5. Armon P. Symphysiotomy. *Trop Doct* 2015; 45(2): 60–7.
6. Fleming VEM, Hagen S, Niven C. Does perineal suturing make a difference? The SUNS trial. *BJOG* 2003; 110(7): 684–9.
7. Signorello LB, Harlow BL, Chekos AK, Repke JT. Midline episiotomy and anal incontinence: Retrospective cohort study. *BMJ* 2000; 320(7227): 86–90.
8. Cunningham FG, Hauth CJ, Leveno JK et al. *Williams Obstetrics* (22nd edition). New York, NY: McGraw-Hill Professional, 2001.
9. Sultan AH. Obstetrical perineal injury and anal incontinence. *Clinical Risk* 1999; 5: 193–6.
10. Royal College of Obstetricians and Gynaecologists. *Management of Third and Fourth-Degree Perineal Tears Following Vaginal Delivery.* RCOG Guideline No. 29. London, UK: RCOG Press, 2015.

11. Ofir K, Sheiner E, Levy A, Katz M, Mazor M. Uterine rupture: Risk factors and pregnancy outcome. *Am J Obstet Gynecol* 2003; 189(4): 1042–6.
12. Leeman L, Spearman M, Rogers R. Repair of obstetric perineal lacerations. *Am Fam Physician* 2003; 68(8): 1585–90.
13. Sultan AH, Monga AK, Kumar D, Stanton SL. Primary repair of obstetric anal sphincter rupture using the overlap technique. *Br J Obstet Gynaecol* 1999; 106(4): 318–23.
14. Fernando RJ, Sultan AH, Kettle C, Thakar R. Methods of repair for obstetric anal sphincter injury. *Cochrane Database Syst Rev* 2013; (12): CD002866.
15. Carroli G, Mignini L. Episiotomy for vaginal birth. *Cochrane Database Syst Rev* 2009; (1): CD000081.
16. Aasheim V, Nilsen AB, Lukasse M, Reinar LM. Perineal techniques during the second stage of labour for reducing perineal trauma. *Cochrane Database Syst Rev* 2011; (12): CD006672.
17. Bulchandani S, Watts E, Sucharitha A, Yates D, Ismail KM. Manual perineal support at the time of childbirth: A systematic review and meta-analysis. *BJOG* 2015; 122; (9): 1157–65.
18. Laine K, Pirhonen T, Rolland R, Pirhonen J. Decreasing the incidence of anal sphincter tears during delivery. *Obstet Gynecol* 2008; 111(5): 1053–7.
19. Hals E, Oian P, Pirhonen T et al. A multicenter interventional program to reduce the incidence of anal sphincter tears. *Obstet Gynecol* 2010; 116(4): 901–8.
20. Laine K, Skjeldestad FE, Sandvik L, Staff AC. Incidence of obstetric anal sphincter injuries after training to protect the perineum: Cohort study. *BMJ Open* 2012; 2(5): pii: e001649.
21. Fretheim A, Odgaard-Jensen J, Rottingen JA et al. The impact of an intervention programme employing a hands-on technique to reduce the incidence of anal sphincter tears: Interrupted time-series reanalysis. *BMJ Open* 2013; 3(10): e003355.
22. Bruce E. Everything you need to know to prevent perineal tearing. *Midwifery Today Int Midwife* 2003; (65): 10–13.
23. Beckmann MM, Stock OM. Antenatal perineal massage for reducing perineal trauma. *Cochrane Database Syst Rev* 2013; (4): CD005123.
24. Harvey MA, Pierce M, Alter JE et al. Obstetrical Anal Sphincter Injuries (OASIS): Prevention, recognition, and repair. *J Obstet Gynaecol Can* 2015; 37(12): 1131–48.
25. Mirza FG, Gaddipati S. Obstetric emergencies. *Semin Perinatol* 2009; 33(2): 97–103.
26. Devine PC. Obstetric hemorrhage. *Semin Perinatol* 2009; 33(2): 76–81.
27. Gardeil F, Daly S, Turner MJ. Uterine rupture in pregnancy reviewed. *Eur J Obstet Gynecol Reprod Biol* 1994; 56(2): 107–10.
28. Waterstone M, Bewley S, Wolfe C. Incidence and predictors of severe obstetric morbidity: Case-control study. *BMJ* 2001; 322(7294): 1089–93; discussion 93–4.
29. Miller DA, Goodwin TM, Gherman RB, Paul RH. Intrapartum rupture of the unscarred uterus. *Obstet Gynecol* 1997; 89(5 Pt 1): 671–3.
30. Guise JM, McDonagh MS, Osterweil P et al. Systematic review of the incidence and consequences of uterine rupture in women with previous caesarean section. *BMJ* 2004; 329(7456): 19–25.
31. Golan A, Sandbank O, Rubin A. Rupture of the pregnant uterus. *Obstet Gynecol* 1980; 56(5): 549–54.
32. Dewhurst CJ. The ruptured caesarean section scar. *J Obstet Gynaecol Br Emp* 1957; 64(1): 113–8.
33. Halperin ME, Moore DC, Hannah WJ. Classical versus low-segment transverse incision for preterm caesarean section: Maternal complications and outcome of subsequent pregnancies. *Br J Obstet Gynaecol* 1988; 95(10): 990–6.
34. Poidevin LO, Bockner VY. A hysterographic study of uteri after caesarean section. *J Obstet Gynaecol Br Emp* 1958; 65(2): 278–83.
35. Rozenberg P, Goffinet F, Phillippe HJ, Nisand I. Ultrasonographic measurement of lower uterine segment to assess risk of defects of scarred uterus. *Lancet* 1996; 347(8997): 281–4.
36. Tanik A, Ustun C, Cil E, Arslan A. Sonographic evaluation of the wall thickness of the lower uterine segment in patients with previous cesarean section. *J Clin Ultrasound* 1996; 24(7): 355–7.
37. Rossi AC, Prefumo F. Pregnancy outcomes of induced labor in women with previous cesarean section: A systematic review and meta-analysis. *Arch Gynecol Obstet* 2015; 291(2): 273–80.
38. Roberge S, Demers S, Berghella V et al. Impact of single- vs. double-layer closure on adverse outcomes and uterine scar defect: A systematic review and meta-analysis. *Am J Obstet Gynecol* 2014; 211(5): 453–60.
39. Raghavaiah NV, Devi AI. Bladder injury associated with rupture of the uterus. *Obstet Gynecol* 1975; 46(5): 573–6.
40. Ewen SP, Notley RG, Coats PM. Bladder laceration associated with uterine scar rupture during vaginal delivery. *Br J Urol* 1994; 73(6): 712–3.
41. Ho SY, Chang SD, Liang CC. Simultaneous uterine and urinary bladder rupture in an otherwise successful vaginal birth after cesarean delivery. *J Chin Med Assoc* 2010; 73(12): 655–9.
42. Berg CJ, Chang J, Callaghan WM, Whitehead SJ. Pregnancy-related mortality in the United States, 1991–1997. *Obstet Gynecol* 2003; 101(2): 289–96.
43. Crowhurst JA, Plaat F. Why mothers die. Report on confidential enquiries into maternal deaths in the United Kingdom 1994–1996. *Anaesthesia* 1999; 54(3): 207–9.
44. Schrinsky DC, Benson RC. Rupture of the pregnant uterus: A review. *Obstet Gynecol Surv* 1978; 33(4): 217–32.
45. Snow RE, Neubert AG. Peripartum pubic symphysis separation: A case series and review of the literature. *Obstet Gynecol Surv* 1997; 52(7): 438–43.

46. Baccari MC, Calamai F. Relaxin: New functions for an old peptide. *Curr Protein Pept Sci* 2004; 5(1): 9–18.
47. Hisaw FL. Experimental relaxation of the pubic ligament of the guinea pig. *Proc Soc Exp Biol Med* 1926; 23: 661–3.
48. Ziel HK. A guest editorial: Dialog between basic and clinical science: Relaxin as a possible cause of symphyseal separation. *Obstet Gynecol Surv* 2001; 56(8): 447–8.
49. Jain N, Sternberg LB. Symphyseal separation. *Obstet Gynecol* 2005; 105(5 Pt 2): 1229–32.
50. Chassar-Moir J. *The Vesico-Vaginal Fistula* (2nd edition). London, UK: Bailliere Tindall and Cassell, Ltd., 1967.
51. Mahfouz N. Urinary fistuale in women. *J Obstet Gynaecol Br Emp* 1957; 64(1): 23–34.
52. Coetzee T, Lithgow DM. Obstetric fistulae of the urinary tract. *J Obstet Gynaecol Br Commonw* 1966; 73(5): 837–44.
53. Lavery DW. Vesico-vaginal fistulae: A report on the vaginal repair of 160 cases. *J Obstet Gynaecol Br Emp* 1955; 62(4): 530–9.
54. Wu JM, Matthews CA, Conover MM et al. Lifetime risk of stress urinary incontinence or pelvic organ prolapse surgery. *Obstet Gynecol* 2014; 123(6): 1201–6.
55. Dannecker C, Anthuber C. The effects of childbirth on the pelvic-floor. *J Perinat Med* 2000; 28(3): 175–84.
56. Sze EH, Sherard GB 3rd, Dolezal JM. Pregnancy, labor, delivery, and pelvic organ prolapse. *Obstet Gynecol* 2002; 100(5 Pt 1): 981–6.
57. Handa VL, Blomquist JL, Knoepp LR et al. Pelvic floor disorders 5–10 years after vaginal or cesarean childbirth. *Obstet Gynecol* 2011; 118(4): 777–84.
58. Gyhagen M, Bullarbo M, Nielsen TF, Milsom I. Prevalence and risk factors for pelvic organ prolapse 20 years after childbirth: A national cohort study in singleton primiparae after vaginal or caesarean delivery. *BJOG* 2013; 120(2): 152–60.
59. DeLee JB. The prophylactic forceps operation. *Am J Obstet Gynecol* 1920; 1(1): 34–44.
60. Burgio KL, Zyczynski H, Locher JL et al. Urinary incontinence in the 12-month postpartum period. *Obstet Gynecol* 2003; 102(6): 1291–8.
61. Parazzini F, Chiaffarino F, Lavezzari M, Giambanco V. Risk factors for stress, urge or mixed urinary incontinence in Italy. *BJOG* 2003; 110(10): 927–33.
62. Rortveit G, Daltveit AK, Hannestad YS, Hunskaar S. Urinary incontinence after vaginal delivery or cesarean section. *N Engl J Med* 2003; 348(10): 900–7.
63. Gyhagen M, Bullarbo M, Nielsen TF, Milsom I. A comparison of the long-term consequences of vaginal delivery versus caesarean section on the prevalence, severity and bothersomeness of urinary incontinence subtypes: A national cohort study in primiparous women. *BJOG* 2013; 120(12): 1548–55.
64. Viktrup L, Lose G, Rolff M, Barfoed K. The symptom of stress incontinence caused by pregnancy or delivery in primiparas. *Obstet Gynecol* 1992; 79(6): 945–9.
65. Allen WM, Masters WH. Traumatic laceration of uterine support: The clinical syndrome and the operative treatment. *Am J Obstet Gynecol* 1955; 70(3): 500–13.
66. Taylor HC, Jr. Life situations, emotions and gynecologic pain associated with congestion. *Res Publ Assoc Res Nerv Ment Dis* 1949; 29: 1051–6.

Puerperal inversion of the uterus

28

JOHANNA QUIST-NELSON and REBECCA JACKSON

CONTENTS

References to uterine inversion can be found in Hindu Ayurvedic literature (2500–600 BC), but Hippocrates is said to be the first to give an accurate description of the problem and offer a treatment regimen.[1] In the first half of the twentieth century, puerperal inversion of the uterus was associated with high mortality (12%–40%) because of delay in diagnosis, lack of anesthesia, and inadequate management of hemorrhage, shock, and infection.[2–6] Since 1960, the outcome for puerperal uterine inversion has improved remarkably as a result of early diagnosis, adequate treatment of shock, and prompt manual reinversion of the uterus.[6–16]

CLASSIFICATION

The following classification is based on the time of diagnosis[15] and the relationship of the inverted uterine fundus to the cervix and the perineum:

1. *Acute puerperal inversion.* The inversion is noted shortly after delivery and before there is significant contraction of the cervix (usually within a few hours of delivery).
2. *Subacute puerperal inversion.* The inversion is noted within 4 weeks after delivery and after contraction of the cervix has occurred.
3. *Chronic inversion.* More than 4 weeks have elapsed since the inversion and cervical contraction occurred.
4. *Incomplete inversion.* No part of the corpus of the uterus extends past the cervix.
5. *Complete inversion.* The inverted corpus extends beyond the cervix.
6. *Prolapsed inversion.* The inverted uterus extends beyond the introitus.

This chapter is devoted to the diagnosis and management of acute or subacute puerperal uterine inversion.

INCIDENCE

In 11 studies performed in North America, and recently abroad in the Netherlands, and India complicated by puerperal inversion of the uterus that has occurred since 1960 (Table 28.1), the incidence varied from 1 in 1,739 to 2 in 20,312 deliveries (average 1/4,195).[6–16] The problem, therefore, remains sufficiently uncommon that any single practitioner may encounter only one or two such complications in a professional lifetime and no obstetric service or individual gains enough experience to test management protocols in any reasonable prospective study. Consequently, the assessment of this problem depends upon the retrospective review of case reports and series with small numbers of patients.

EPIDEMIOLOGY

There is no consistent epidemiologic characteristic of puerperal inversion of the uterus, with the possible exception of parity. In several studies, the proportion of nulliparous patients has been higher in cases of uterine inversion than in the total birthing population. Other series have not confirmed the association of acute puerperal inversion with primiparity.[6–8]

ETIOLOGY

The etiology of acute puerperal uterine inversion is not known with certainty. The following conditions have been suggested as predisposing or causal factors: manual removal of the placenta, improper fundal pressure, excessive cord traction, injudicious use of oxytocics, short umbilical cord, abnormally adherent placenta, and fundal implantation of the placenta. In almost all cases of uterine inversion in which the site of implantation of the placenta was recorded, it was noted to be in the fundus of the uterus.[3,4,7,11] Fundal implantation of the placenta occurs

Table 28.1 Acute inversion of the uterus.

Author and site	Years of study	Number of patients and incidence	Method of reinversion	Placental management (removal or leave intact)	Tocolytics
Kitchen et al., University of Virginia[6]	1960–74	11 1/2,284	All replaced vaginally	No data. Discussion advises removal if replacement difficult without doing so	Tocolytics not used
Watson et al., University of Colorado[7]	1969–78	18 1/1,739	All replaced vaginally	All replacements occurred after placenta had been separated from uterine wall	Tocolytics not used
Cumming and Taylor, University of Calgary[8]	1966–77	9 1/2,176	7 replaced vaginally 1 laparotomy 1 hysterectomy	8 removed before replacement 1 no information given	Tocolytics not used
Platt and Druzin University of Southern California[9]	1972–7	28 1/2,148	27 replaced vaginally 1 laparotomy	No data or discussion of management of the placenta	$MgSO_4$ recommended but no data given
Brar et al., University of Southern California[10]	1977–86	54 1/2,495	52 acute inversions replaced vaginally 2 subacute inversions replaced with laparotomy	No data. Statement that less blood loss noted if placenta left intact	18 treated with tocolytics (terbutaline or $MgSO_4$)
Shah-Hosseini and Evrard, Women and Infants Hospital of Rhode Island[11]	1978–88	11 1/6,407	9 replaced vaginally 1 Huntington procedure, 1 hysterectomy	No data. Discussion mentioned the oft-repeated notion that blood-loss is less if uterus replaced before the placenta is removed	No data or discussion about use of tocolytics
Catazarite et al., University of New Mexico[12]	1983–4	6 1/1,200	All replaced vaginally	No data or discussion of management of placenta	2 treated with terbutaline 2 treated with MgSO4
Abouleish et al., University of Texas, Houston[13]	1987–93	18 1/3,643	All replaced vaginally	No data or discussion of management of placenta	5 received terbutaline
Baskett, Dalhousie University of Halifax, NS[14]	1977–2000	40 1/3,737	27 cases of acute inversion after vaginal delivery, all replaced vaginally 13 cases of acute inversion with cesarean delivery	No data or discussion of management of placenta	No data
Witteveen et al., VU University Amsterdam, Netherlands[15]	2004–6	16 1/20,312	14 cases replaced vaginally 1 case Rusch balloon to prevent recurrence	No data or discussion of management of placenta	No data
Gupta et al. New Delhi, India[16]	2007–13	6 No data	6 cases of acute inversion All replaced manually; reinversion prevented with a hydrostatic method of warm saline infusion	No data or discussion of management of placenta	No data

in only approximately 10% of pregnancies. The uterine wall (myometrium) beneath the placental implantation site is thin in comparison to the remainder of the uterus. It is presumed that when this thin area of endometrium is in the fundus of the uterus, a slight inward dimpling of the uterus may occur as the placenta begins to separate. Thereafter, a progressive inversion ensues, with each contraction extending the inversion as the uterus virtually delivers itself inside out. Such maneuvers as fundal pressure or traction on the umbilical cord may enhance the inversion tendency, but they are probably not independent causal factors. A substantial proportion of uterine inversions occur spontaneously where there has been no uterine or cord manipulation.[2,3]

There are several reports of uterine inversion occurring at the time of cesarean delivery.[14,19–21] Among the 40 cases of uterine inversion reported by Baskett,[14] 13 occurred at the time of cesarean delivery. The author noted that inversion of the uterus at the time cesarean occurred in each case immediately after manual removal of the placenta. Although this may be evidence that manual removal of the placenta is a cause of puerperal uterine inversion, there was no control group of cesarean deliveries performed with spontaneous delivery of the placenta.

PATHOPHYSIOLOGY

Acute puerperal inversion of the uterus is almost always associated with uterine hemorrhage and shock. Some authorities have suggested that the degree of cardiovascular collapse is out of proportion to the hypovolemia resulting from blood loss[2,5]; however, it is probable that blood loss does account for the hypotension and tachycardia experienced by many of these patients.[7] The placenta is frequently attached to the inverted fundus, suggesting that the inversion process begins before separation of the placenta has occurred by cleavage along the decidua basalis.

If a complete inversion occurs, the cervix forms a ring or collar around the inverted fundus. This results in edema and vascular congestion, promoting additional blood loss and further edema, which, in turn, aggravates the cervical constriction. Prolonged inversion may result in tissue necrosis and infection, but, with prompt recognition and treatment, these complications are seen only rarely in modern obstetric services.

MORTALITY

Reviews of the literature that included predominantly cases reported prior to 1940 record maternal mortality rates of 13%–70%.[1,3,4] Kitchin et al.[6] quoted one report from the Committee on Maternal Health of the Ohio Medical Association in 1963 listing six maternal deaths from uterine inversion. The obstetric population in which these six deaths occurred is not known; therefore, the maternal mortality rate represented by these cases cannot be determined.

Selected series of cases suggest there was no improvement in the mortality rate of puerperal uterine inversion until 1960. McCullagh[4] summarized 233 cases from 1911 to 1924 and found a mortality rate of 16%. Bell et al.[2] reported 76 cases from the literature from 1940 to 1952 and found 13 (17%) deaths. Burke and Hofmeister[22] reviewed 22 cases published in the literature from 1957 to 1962 and added 19 cases from nine Milwaukee hospitals with an accumulated death rate of 23%.[18] However, in 11 series reviewed in Table 28.1, there were 217 cases of puerperal inversion of the uterus with no deaths being reported (Table 28.1).[6–16]

PREVENTION

Measures to prevent uterine inversion include recognizing those patients who are at a high risk of the complication and avoiding any of the precipitating factors in their management. Fundal implantation of the placenta is the single most common prerequisite of uterine inversion. With the use of ultrasound, which is now common in the third trimester of pregnancy, those patients with fundal implantation, in many cases, will be identified prior to labor. In such patients, there should be no more than minimal traction on the umbilical cord and only very gentle pressure on the uterine fundus during the third stage of labor. These patients must also be observed carefully for signs of spontaneous inversion during and after the third stage of labor.

There is debate among experts on the role of oxytocin in either precipitating[5,6,23] or preventing uterine inversion.[14] Active management of the third stage of labor, which involves giving intravenous (IV) oxytocin after delivery of the infant's shoulder, has been shown to reduce blood loss, postpartum hemorrhage, and the need for blood transfusion.[24] Baskett[14] studied a series of 40 pregnancies complicated by acute post-delivery inversion of the uterus at a regional tertiary-level maternity hospital in Nova Scotia (1977–2000). When the period 1989–2000 was compared to the period 1977–1989, there was a fourfold decrease in the incidence of acute inversion of the uterus after vaginal delivery. This decrease followed the introduction of active management of the third stage of labor. In one large series of 10,082 patients in which oxytocin was given prior to delivery of the placenta, there were no uterine inversions.[25] These studies suggest that giving oxytocin after delivery of the infant's shoulders is a useful measure to reduce the risk of uterine inversion.

DIAGNOSIS

Successful management of puerperal inversion of the uterus depends upon early recognition and diagnosis, prompt and efficient treatment of hemorrhage and shock, and reinversion of the uterus at the earliest opportunity.

Diagnosis is straightforward if an acute, total inversion occurs in the third stage of labor. The dramatic appearance of the placenta adherent to the inverted uterine corpus protruding through the introitus is an unforgettable sight (Figure 28.1). Even in cases where the placenta separates immediately before the inversion occurs, the beefy red tumor, the size of an infant's head, protruding through the introitus is recognized as an inverted uterus. Routine visual examination of the cervix after delivery of the placenta will result in the early detection of some cases of

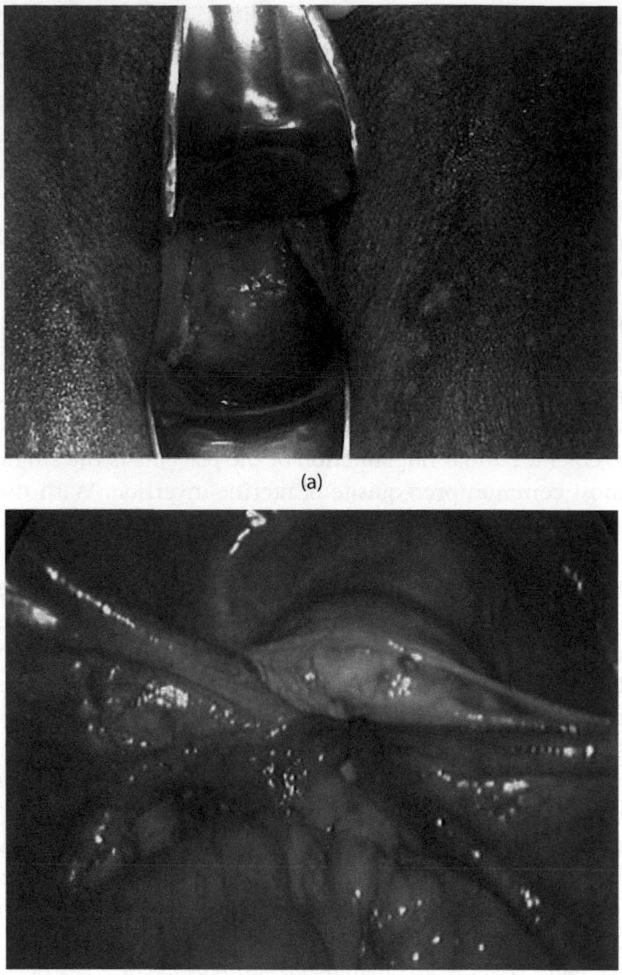

(a)

(b)

Figure 28.1 (a) Inverted uterus at introitus. (b) Inverted uterus viewed on laparoscopy. (Reprinted from *Journal of Minimally Invasive Gynecology*, 16, Sardeshpande NS, Sawant RM, Sardeshpande SN, Sabnis SD, Laparoscopic correction of chronic uterine inversion, 646–646, 2009, with permission from Elsevier.)

incomplete inversion. More difficult is the diagnosis of a nonprolapsed or incomplete inversion which occurs after the third stage of labor.[26] At times transvaginal ultrasound may aid in diagnosis (Figure 28.2). Lewin and Bryan[22] reported a case of puerperal inversion of the uterus in which magnetic resonance imaging was used to confirm the diagnosis when physical examination and sonograms were equivocal. Some authors have also advocated manual exploration of the uterus immediately after delivery of the placenta as a means of making the earliest possible diagnosis of uterine inversion.[6]

The only symptoms may be hemorrhage and shock. In all cases of puerperal hemorrhage, uterine inversion must be kept in mind if subtle cases are not to be misdiagnosed. Palpation of the abdomen may reveal a suspicious absence of the uterine fundus, a sign that should always raise suspicions for uterine inversion. Thereafter, a careful inspection of the vagina, both visually and manually, will discover the cause of the hemorrhage in cases of inversion of the uterus. Occasionally, physicians have been misled by assuming that the prolapsed fundus is a large leiomyomata or cervical polyp.[4] Whenever a mass is visualized or palpated in the cervix or vagina in the immediate postpartum period, especially when there is unexplained blood loss or hypotension, the diagnosis of uterine inversion should be suspected. Delay in recognizing this complication increases the difficulty of reinverting the corpus because of cervical contraction and edema, which may enhance blood loss and shock and increase the chance of infection and tissue necrosis.

TREATMENT

All physicians, nurse midwives, and nurses entrusted with the care of women in labor should be familiar with the diagnosis and management of acute inversion of the uterus because its infrequent occurrence precludes the supervised training of each individual in the technique of manual replacement. Since prompt therapy is the key to successful replacement and low morbidity, treatment will often have to be initiated by the practitioner at hand, who may have never personally managed such a case.

A major reason for the high mortality reported in earlier series of uterine inversion was inadequate therapy for blood loss and shock. Modern use of prompt replacement of blood volume, using crystalloid or colloid solutions and blood products, can usually be accomplished before the serious side effects of prolonged hypotension occur. Immediately upon making the diagnosis of inverted uterus, or in cases of acute postpartum hemorrhage, more than one large-bore, IV infusion lines should be established. An infusion of a crystalloid solution, such as 5% dextrose/lactated Ringer's, is begun, while whole blood and packed red cells are obtained. Vital signs, including pulse and blood pressure, should be monitored frequently, as well as urine output. As soon as blood volume is restored, efforts should be made to replace the uterus in its normal anatomic position. Restoration of the uterus to its normal position will frequently require general anesthesia, and an anesthesiologist should be summoned at the time of diagnosis.

Before administering inhalation anesthesia, tocolytic drug can be administered; this will often allow manual reinversion of the uterus.[9,10,12,13,28] As noted in the series listed in the Table 28.1, tocolytic drugs, such as magnesium sulfate (4 g, IV) or terbutaline (0.25 mg, intramuscular [IM]), have been used for treatment of acute puerperal uterine inversion. There is also enthusiasm for the use of nitroglycerine, which has been used in a variety of clinical situations requiring acute emergency uterine relaxation.[29] Although there are a number of case reports demonstrating that nitroglycerin (100 μg, IV) is effective in providing transient uterine relaxation during manual replacement of the inverted uterus,[30–33] there are insufficient data to establish one or another tocolytic drug as being superior in either effectiveness or safety for treatment of the inverted uterus. Moreover, tocolytic therapy is not successful in all cases, and inhalation anesthesia

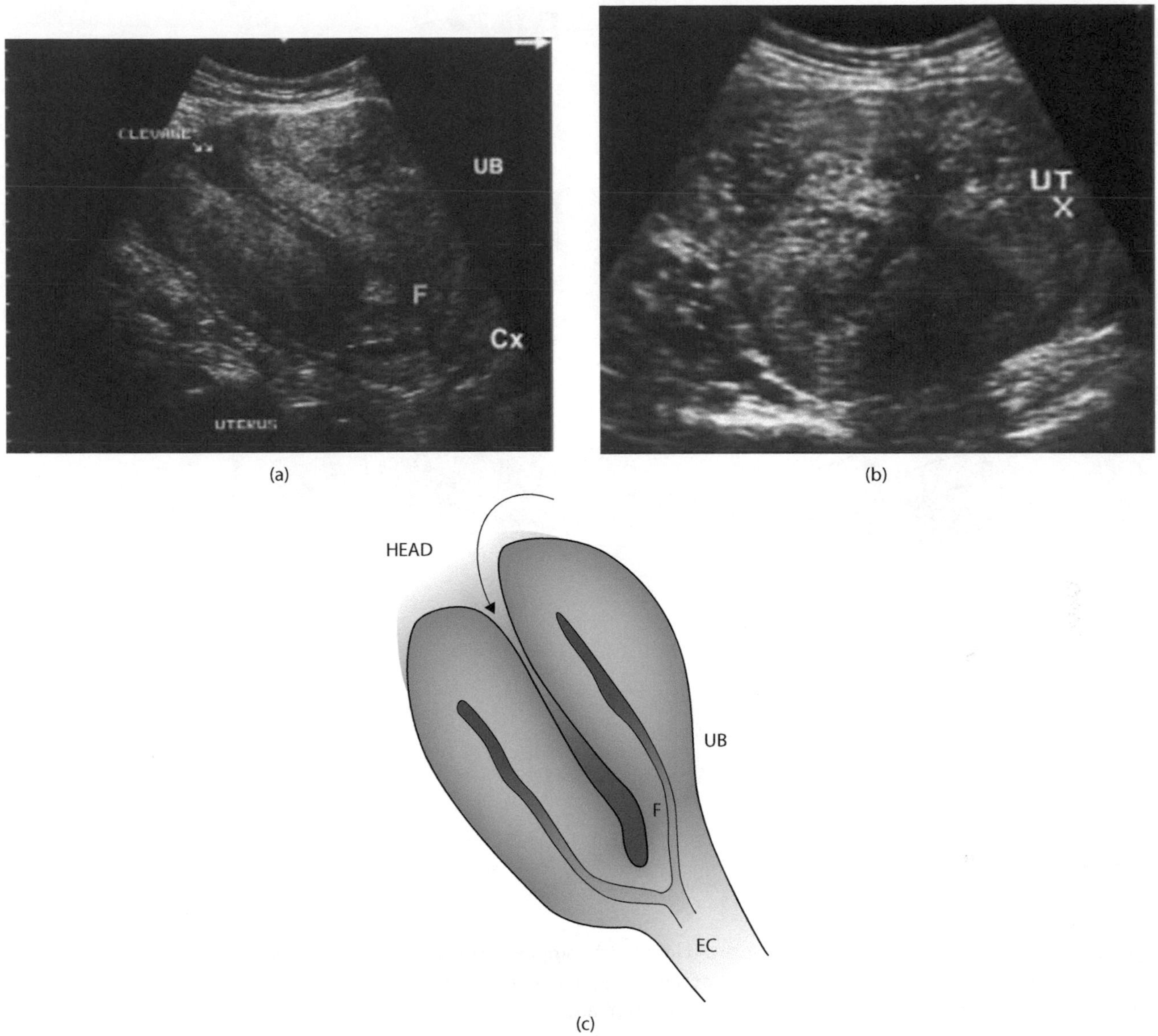

Figure 28.2 Sonographic evidence of uterine inversion. (a) Longitudinal transabdominal sonogram shows bulky uterus with fundal inversion. Central cleavage (small arrows) represents path of inversion. Cx, cervical region; F, inverted fundus; UB, location of urinary bladder. (b) Transverse transabdominal sonogram at the level of lower segment shows X-shaped hypoechoic center corresponding to folded endometrial cavity. UT, uterus. (c) Sketch demonstrating incomplete inversion. UB, urinary bladder; F, fundus; EC, endometrial canal. (Photograph by Momin AA et al., Sonography of Postpartum Uterine Inversion from Acute to Chronic Stage. *Journal of Clinical Ultrasound*, 2009, 37[1], 53–56. Copyright Wiley-VCH Verlag GmbH & Co. KGaA. Reproduced with permission.)

may be necessary in refractory situations. It is our recommendation to commence with the method first described by Johnson[34] in 1949 (Figure 28.3). This method is most widely used and most likely to be successful for manually replacing the uterus.

To replace the inverted uterus using Johnson's method, the entire hand is placed in the vagina with the tips of the fingers at the uterocervical junction and the fundus uteri in the palm of the hand. The entire uterus is then lifted out of the pelvis and forcefully held in the abdominal cavity above the level of the umbilicus. It is necessary to hold the uterus in this position for a period of 3–5 minutes, at which time the fundus recedes from the palm of the hand. It is emphasized that in order to accomplish this procedure the entire hand and two-thirds of the length of the forearm must be placed in the vagina; otherwise the pull and tension of the ligaments are not sufficient to correct the condition.

Johnson explained that the mechanism of fundal replacement by this method depends upon traction, which occurs on the uterine ligaments when the uterus is elevated into the abdomen. Among the nine patients treated by Johnson, there were two chronic inversions, one subacute inversion, and six acute inversions. All patients survived. Table 28.1 as well as a recent prospective cohort study from the Netherlands[15] confirms the effectiveness of this method. In the Netherlands, over a 2-year period there were 16 acute puerperal inversions, all of which were

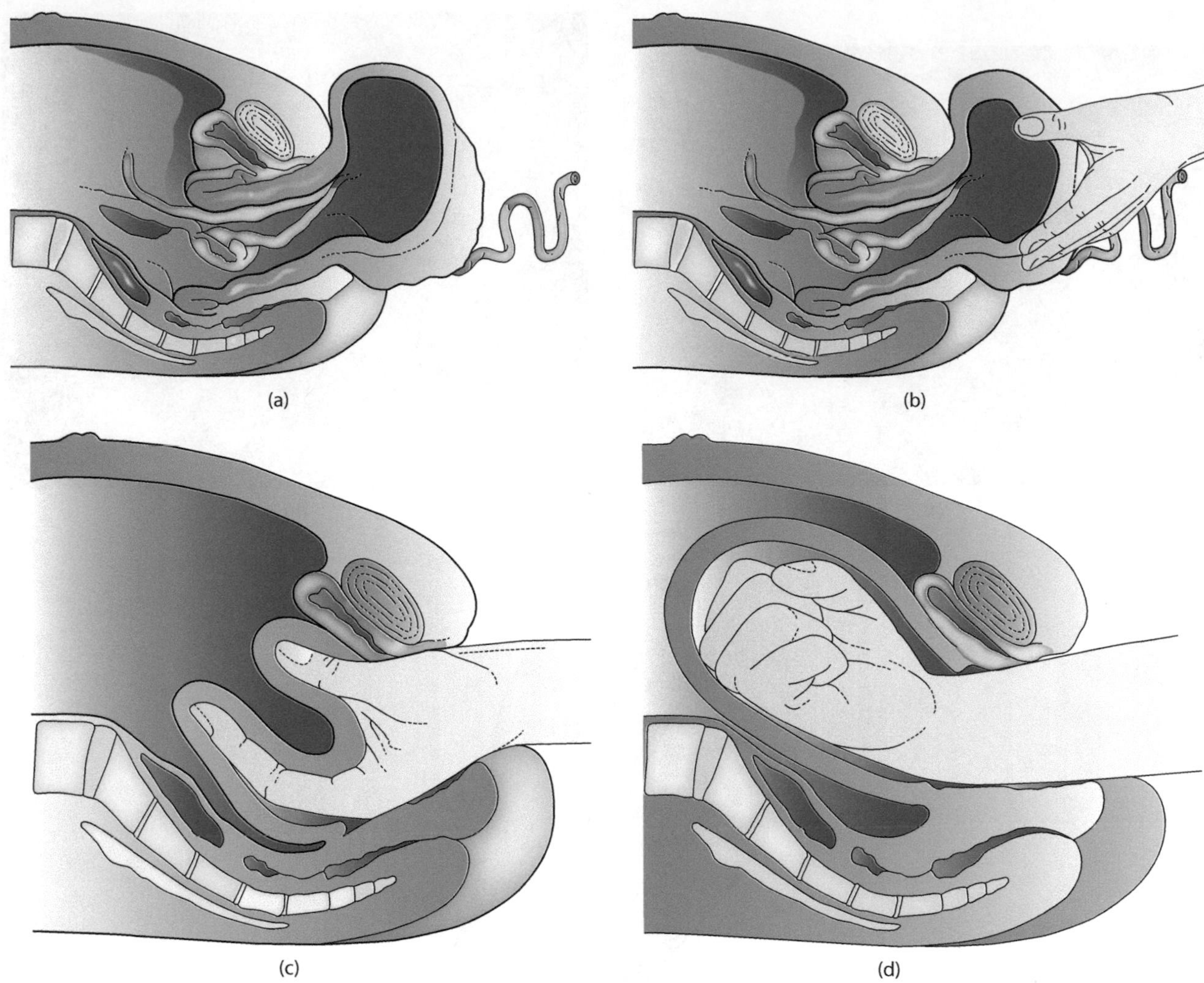

Figure 28.3 Manual replacement of the inverted uterus. (a) Complete acute inversion of the uterus with the placenta attached to the uterine fundus. (b) The inverted fundus is grasped in the palm of the hand with the fingers directed toward the posterior fornix. (c) The uterus is lifted out of the pelvis and directed with steady pressure toward the umbilicus. (d) The fundus is held in position for 3 minutes. (Reproduced from Watson P, Besch N, Bowes WA Jr: Management of acute and subacute puerperal inversion of the uterus, *Obstet Gynecol*, 55, 12–167, 1980 with permission from Lippincott Williams & Wilkins.)

able to be replaced manually without need for further surgery in the postpartum period.

A hydrostatic method of inducing replacement of the inverted uterus was first described by O'Sullivan[35] in 1945. This method involves infusion of 1000–2000 mL warm saline into the vagina with the patient in the lithotomy position. Fluid is prevented from escaping from the vagina by blocking the introitus with the operator's hand. Momani and Hassan[36] reported five consecutive cases of acute puerperal uterine inversion that were successfully reduced within 5–10 minutes by this method. Although reported as being used with success in the United Kingdom, Australia, and the Middle East, the hydrostatic method has not been reported in recent series from North America.

Once the uterus is manually replaced, there are several measures that may be taken to avoid reinversion and need for surgery. In all cases, prompt administration of a uterotonic medication is necessary after successful restoration of anatomy.[12,36] Recent case reports[37,38] suggest that tamponading balloons used in cases of uterine atony (e.g., Bakhri balloon) may also serve a role in the conservative management of uterine inversion as well as to reduce the risk of reinversion. One case report[38] also utilized a McDonald cerclage to hold the tamponading balloon in position. These methods have not been widely established but are to be considered depending on the clinical context.

There is no consensus in the medical literature whether to remove an adherent placenta from the uterine fundus before attempting manual replacement. Several authors strongly advise against removing the placenta prior to manual replacement,[17,39] while others suggest that its removal is not dangerous,[8] and still others claim that removal of the placenta will actually facilitate replacement of the inverted fundus.[6] As noted in the series summarized in Table 28.1, there are remarkably little data about management of the placenta upon which to establish an evidence-based opinion. In the absence of such data, perhaps the most practical advice is to remove the placenta if that can be accomplished easily and with minimal trauma and blood loss. But if the placenta seems unusually adherent, or if its removal will cause an appreciable delay, manual elevation of the uterus should be accomplished with the placenta intact. The placenta can then be removed manually when the fundus is repositioned.

On rare occasions, manual replacement fails. In these situations, surgery is necessary. Huntington[40] and Huntington et al.[41] reported the successful treatment of five cases of acute puerperal inversion with this procedure. The operation is accomplished by performing a laparotomy incision in the lower abdomen. The inverted fundus will be apparent (Figure 28.4), with the round ligaments disappearing into the inverted crater. The uterus is

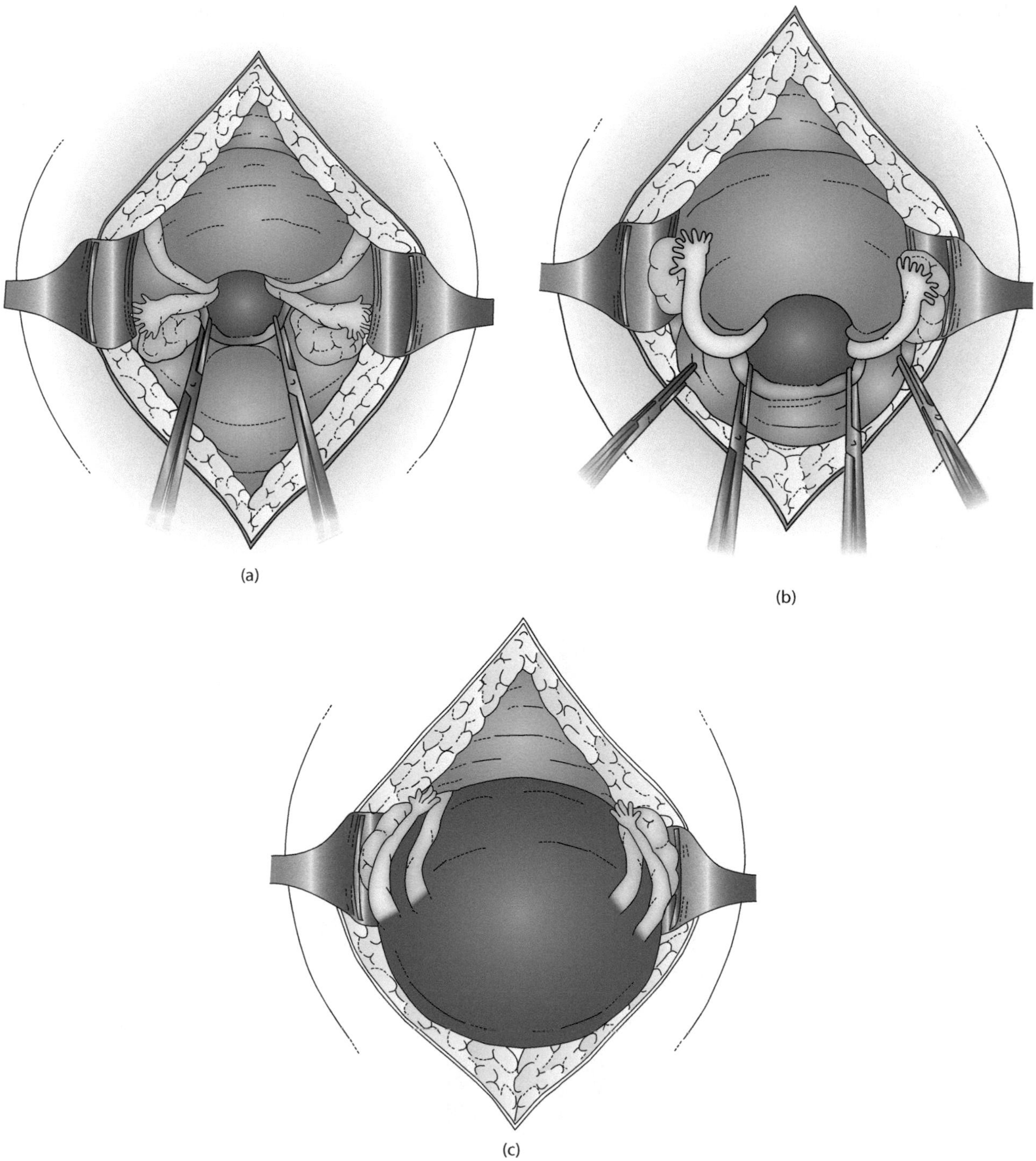

Figure 28.4 Huntington procedure for correction of uterine inversion. (a) The surface of the uterus is grasped with two Allis or Ochsner clamps approximately 1 inch (2.54 cm) within the crater, and gentle traction is applied. Pressure on the inverted fundus through the vagina by an assistant may facilitate the procedure. (b) As the uterine corpus is drawn out of the crater, an additional set of clamps is used to grasp the round ligaments 1 inch beyond the first set of clamps. (c) The uterine corpus after resolution of the inversion. (Adapted from Douglas RG and Stromme WB, *Operative Obstetrics* (3rd edition), New York, NY: Appleton-Century-Crofts, 1976.)

grasped in two places with clamps 1 inch (2.54 cm) within the crater, and gentle traction is exerted. A second set of clamps is then placed an inch beyond the first clamps, and so on, until the fundus is repositioned. Occasionally, pressure on the inverted fundus from an assistant's hand in the vagina will aid in the repositioning procedure. Tews et al.[42] described a modification of the transabdominal approach in which the bladder is dissected away from the cervix and a longitudinal incision is made into the vagina below the contraction ring. Two fingers inserted through this incision assist in applying upward pressure on the invaginated uterus.

If the traction method described by Huntington[40] does not succeed in repositioning the fundus because the cervix is too tightly contracted, as may occur with subacute uterine inversion, a vertical incision is made through the posterior wall of the uterus where the inversion disappears from the abdomen. The inversion is then corrected by upward pressure from within the vagina by an assistant, a procedure described by Haultain[43] (Figure 28.5). Modifications

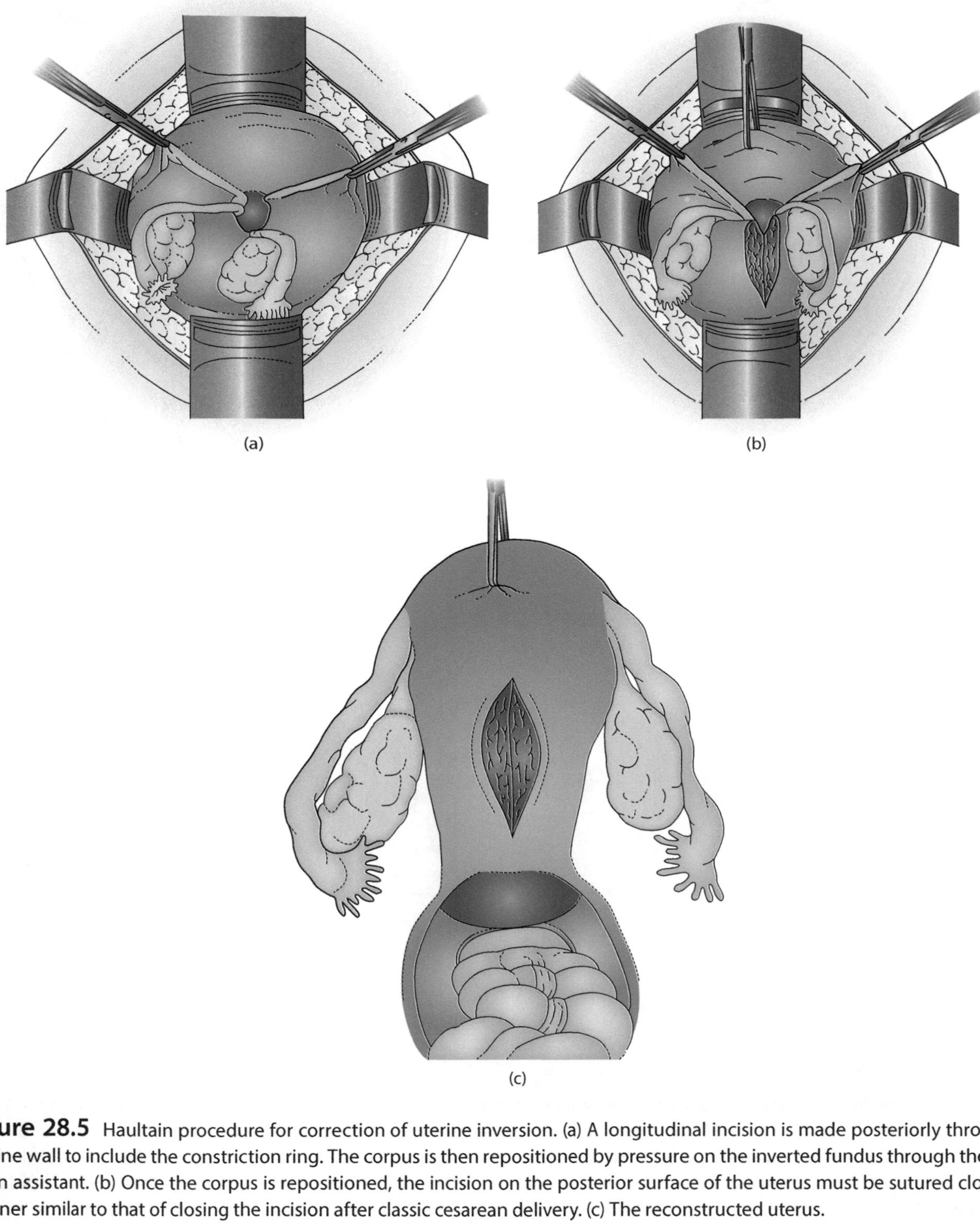

Figure 28.5 Haultain procedure for correction of uterine inversion. (a) A longitudinal incision is made posteriorly through the uterine wall to include the constriction ring. The corpus is then repositioned by pressure on the inverted fundus through the vagina by an assistant. (b) Once the corpus is repositioned, the incision on the posterior surface of the uterus must be sutured closed in a manner similar to that of closing the incision after classic cesarean delivery. (c) The reconstructed uterus.

of this procedure have been described in which an anterior incision is made in the uterus.[24] In addition, the Spinelli procedure (transvaginal incision in the anterior wall of the inverted and prolapsed uterus) has been reported for replacement of the uterine fundus in some cases of refractory inversion.[2] There have also been reports of successful laparoscopic approaches to the Huntington and Haultain procedures for cases of uterine inversion refractory to attempted manual replacement.[44]

Bell et al.[2] collected 76 cases of puerperal inversion of the uterus reported in the U.S. and U.K. literature from 1940 to 1952. Fifteen (20%) of these cases were treated surgically, five with the Huntington procedure, one with the Haultain method, three with the Spinelli procedure, and six with hysterectomy. Among 182 cases of puerperal inversion of the uterus after vaginal delivery reported in Table 28.1, surgical therapy was required in only seven (4%).[6–14] It is difficult to estimate a more recent incidence of surgical management in patients with puerperal uterine inversion given the lack of recent evidence on the topic. It is likely that earlier recognition, tocolytic drugs, improved anesthesia, and prompt use of the manual procedure to reposition the uterus have reduced the need for surgical intervention, as evidenced by the prospective cohort study from 2012 in which none of the 16 cases of uterine inversion required surgical management.[15] It is reasonable to administer a course of broad spectrum antibiotics, such as cefazolin, after either manual or surgical treatment of uterine inversion. Blood loss, contamination of the endometrium, and tissue trauma all predispose the patient to puerperal infection.

RECURRENCE

The precise risk of recurrence of puerperal uterine inversion is not known. There are isolated reports of recurrent uterine inversion after manual repositioning. Some of these occurred in the postpartum period of the same pregnancy,[2,45] and others occurred in subsequent pregnancies.[16,19] Miller[46] reported the incidence of recurrence of inversion in subsequent pregnancies to be 26% and found the recurrence risk was higher when the inversion had been corrected manually (40%) than when it had been treated surgically (0%). However, recurrence of uterine inversion after surgical repair has been reported.[47] Even if future studies demonstrate a lower risk of recurrence than that given by Miller,[46] a patient with a history of uterine inversion must be considered to be at a greater risk of recurrence in subsequent pregnancies. Such a history would justify an ultrasound examination to determine the location of placental implantation. If fundal implantation is identified, intrapartum management of this patient should include use of oxytocin after delivery of the shoulders of the infant and minimal cord traction or fundal pressure in delivery of the placenta. There is no evidence that a history of uterine inversion necessitates cesarean delivery in subsequent pregnancies.

ACKNOWLEDGMENTS

Inasmuch there are no randomized controlled trials and no well-designed cohort or case–control analytic studies on puerperal inversion of the uterus, statements regarding etiology, pathophysiology, diagnosis, and management in this chapter are based upon level II-3 and level III evidence, that is, evidence obtained from multiple time series and opinions of respected authorities based on clinical experience and descriptive studies. Recommendation for management should be regarded as level B, that is, based on limited or inconsistent scientific evidence.[48]

This chapter contains material from the previous edition chapter coauthored by Watson A. Bowes, Jr. and Peter T. Watson.

REFERENCES

1. Fenton AN, Singh BP. Acute puerperal inversion of the uterus. *Obstet Gynecol Surv* 1950; 5: 781–95.
2. Bell JE Jr, Wilson F, Wilson L. Puerperal inversion of the uterus. *Am J Obstet Gynecol* 1953; 66: 767–80.
3. Das P. Inversion of the uterine. *Br J Obstet Gynaecol* 1940; 47: 525–48.
4. McCullagh WMH. Inversion of the uterus. A report on three cases and an analysis of 223 recently recorded cases. *J Obstet Gynaecol Br Emp* 1925; 32: 280–5.
5. Schaeffer G, Veprovsky EC. Inversion of the uterus. *Surg Clin North Am* 1949; 29: 599–610.
6. Kitchin JD III, Thiagarajah S, May HV, Thornton WN. Puerperal inversion of the uterus. *Am J Obstet Gynecol* 1975; 123: 51–8.
7. Watson P, Besch N, Bowes WA Jr. Management of acute and sub-acute puerperal inversion of the uterus. *Obstet Gynecol* 1980; 55: 12–16.
8. Cumming DC, Taylor JT. Puerperal uterine inversion: Report of nine cases. *Can Med Assoc J* 1978; 118: 1268–70.
9. Platt LD, Druzin MKL. Acute puerperal inversion of the uterus. *Am J Obstet Gynecol* 1981; 141: 187–90.
10. Brar HS, Greenspoon JS, Platt LD et al. Acute puerperal uterine inversion: New approaches to management. *J Reprod Med* 1989; 34: 173–7.
11. Shah-Hosseini R, Evrard JR. Puerperal uterine inversion. *Obstet Gynecol* 1989; 73: 567–70.
12. Catanzarite VA, Moffit KD, Baker ML et al. New approaches to the management of acute puerperal uterine inversion. *Obstet Gynecol* 1989; 68: 7S–10S.
13. Abouleish E, Ali V, Joumaa B et al. Anaesthetic management of acute puerperal uterine inversion. *Br J Anaesth* 1995; 75: 486–7.
14. Baskett TF. Acute uterine inversion: A review of 40 cases. *J Obstet Gynaecol Canada* 2002; 24: 953–6.
15. Witteveen T, van Stralen G, Zwart J, vam Roosmalen J. Puerperal uterine inversion in the Netherlands: A nationwide cohort study. *Acta Obstet Gynecol Scand.* 2013; 92: 334–7.

16. Gupta P, Sahu RL, Huria A. Acute uterine inversion: A simplified modification of hydrostatic method of treatment. *Ann Med Health Sci Res.* 2014; 4: 264–7.
17. Kellogg FS. Puerperal inversion of the uterus. Classification for treatment. *Am J Obstet Gynecol* 1929; 18: 815–17.
18. Henderson H, Alles RW. Puerperal inversion of the uterus. *Am J Obstet Gynecol* 1948; 56: 133–42.
19. Kriplani A, Relan S, Kumar RK et al. Complete inversion of the uterus during caesarean section: A case report. *Aust N Z J Obstet Gynaecol* 1996; 36: 17–9.
20. Rudloff U, Joels LA, Marshall N. Inversion of the uterus at ceasarean section. *Arch Gynecol Obstet* 2003; 3: 224–6.
21. Banerjee N, Deka D, Roy KK et al. Inversion of uterus during cesarean section. *Eur J Obstet Gynecol Reprod Biol* 2000; 91: 75–7.
22. Burke JW, Hofmeister FJ. Uterine inversion obstetrical entity or oddity. *Am J Obstet Gynecol* 1965; 91: 934–40.
23. Heyl PS, Stubblefield PG, Phillippe M. Recurrent inversion of the puerperal uterus managed with 15(s)-15-methyl prostaglandin F2a and uterine packing. *Obstet Gynecol* 1984; 63: 263–4.
24. Penderville W, Elbourne D, Chalmers I. The effects of routine oxytocic administration in the management of the third stage of labour: An overview from controlled trials. *Br J Obstet Gynaecol* 1988; 95: 3–16.
25. Fleigner JR, Hibbart BM. Active management of the third stage of labour. *BMJ* 1966; 2: 622–3.
26. Romo MS, Grimes DA, Strassle PO. Infarction of the uterus from subacute incomplete inversion. *Am J Obstet Gynecol* 1992; 166: 878–9.
27. Lewin JS, Bryan PJ. MR imaging of uterine inversion. *J Comput Assist Tomogr* 1989; 13: 357–9.
28. De Villiers VP. Intravenous hexoprenaline in the reduction of acute puerperal inversion of the uterus. *S Afr Med J* 1977; 51: 664–5.
29. Smith GN, Brien JF. Use of nitroglycerin for uterine relaxation. *Obstet Gynecol Surv* 1998; 53: 559–65.
30. Altabef KM, Spencer JT, Zinberg S. Intravenous nitroglycerin for uterine relaxation of an inverted uterus. *Am J Obstet Gynecol* 1992; 16: 1237–8.
31. Dayan SS, Schwalbe SS. The use of small-dose intravenous nitroglycerin in a case of uterine inversion. *Anesth Analg* 1996; 82: 1091–3.
32. Bayhi DA, Sherwood CDA, Campbell CE. Intravenous nitroglycerin for uterine inversion. *J Clin Anesth* 1992; 4: 487–8.
33. Thiery M, Delbeke L. Acute puerperal uterine inversion: Two-step management with a B-mimetic and a prostaglandin. *Am J Obstet Gynecol* 1985; 153: 891–2.
34. Johnson AB. A new concept in the replacement of the inverted uterus and a report of nine cases. *Am J Obstet Gynecol* 1949; 57: 557–62.
35. O'Sullivan JV. Acute inversion of the uterus. *BMJ* 1945; 2: 282–3.
36. Momani A, Hassan A. Treatment of puerperal uterine inversion by the hydrostatic method: Reports of five cases. *Eur J Obstet Gynecol Reprod Biol* 1989; 32: 281–5.
37. Ida A, Ito K, Kubota Y, Nosaka M et al. Successful reduction of acute puerperal uterine inversion with the use of a Bakri postpartum balloon. *Case Rep Obstet Gynecol* 2015, 2015: 424891.
38. Marasighe J, Epitawela D, Cole S, Senanayake H. Uterine balloon tamponade device and cervical cerclage to correct partial uterine inversion during puerperium: Case report. *Gynecol Obstet Invest* 2015; 80: 67–70.
39. Campbell J, Pash J, Walters WAW. Acute inversion of the uterus and its management. *Med J Aust* 1972; 2: 475–6.
40. Huntington JL. Acute inversion of the uterus. *Boston Med Surg J* 1921; 15: 376.
41. Huntington JL, Irving FC, Kellogg FS. Abdominal reposition in acute inversion of the puerperal uterus. *Am J Obstet Gynecol* 1928; 15: 34.
42. Tews G, Ebner T, Yaman C et al. Acute puerperal inversion of the uterus—Treatment by a new abdominal uterus preserving approach. *Acta Obstet Gynecol Scand* 2001; 80: 1039–40.
43. Haultain FWN. The treatment of chronic uterine inversion by abdominal hysterectomy with a successful care. *BMJ* 1901; 2: 974.
44. Sardeshpande NS, Sawant RM, Sardeshpande SN, Sabnis SD. Laparoscopic correction of chronic uterine inversion. *J Minim Invasive Gynecol* 2009; 16: 646–8.
45. Silver DF, Heyl PS, Linfert JB. Delayed uterine reinversion: A unique symptom complex. *Am J Obstet Gynecol* 2004; 191: 378–9.
46. Miller NF. Pregnancy following inversion of the uterus. *Am J Obstet Gynecol* 1927; 13: 307–22.
47. Steffen E. Puerperal inversion of the uterus occurring in consecutive pregnancies in the same patient. *Am J Obstet Gynecol* 1957; 74: 655–7.
48. American College of Obstetricians and Gynecologists. *Reading the Medical Literature: Applying Evidence to Practice.* Compendium of Selected Publications, pp. 259–70. Washington, DC: ACOG, 2004.

Wound healing, sutures, knots, needles, drains, and instruments

29

ROBYN T. BILINSKI and JESÚS R. ALVAREZ-PEREZ

CONTENTS

It is imperative for a surgeon to have a basic understanding of the mechanisms that control wound healing. Understanding the normal process and molecular basis allows surgeons to manipulate the wound for healing to occur in a timely and aesthetic fashion.

NORMAL WOUND HEALING

Wound healing is a homeostatic response to injury in an effort to restore function and integrity. Different tissues will heal in a different manner. Tissue loss or damage causes either regeneration or repair by scar tissue, or a combination of both. Human tissue heals by scarring with the exception of the epidermis, bone, liver, and the mucosa of the intestinal tract, which heal by regeneration.

Wound healing occurs through several concurrent events. The biologic events involved in wound healing are conceptually defined as *inflammation*, *proliferation*, and *remodeling*. These steps occur simultaneously and should not be seen as separate processes. These are nonspecific mechanisms activated by the tissue injury.

Inflammation

The first step in normal wound healing involves inflammation and hemostasis. This phase starts immediately after injury and its role is to limit the amount of blood loss and remove necrotic tissue and bacteria. When tissue injury occurs, vasoconstriction traps platelets at the wound site. The coagulation cascade is stimulated, forming a stable clot at the site of injury. The vasoconstriction lasts approximately 10 minutes and is followed by vasodilation, which causes edema. Blood loss is controlled by vasoconstriction and clot formation. Clearing bacteria and tissue debris is achieved by polymorphonuclear cells (PMN) and leukocytes, which, in response to the presence of potent chemotactic factors, arrive immediately after injury and achieve their maximum number 24 hours after the initial injury. Monocytes then differentiate into macrophages, which are crucial to wound healing. Their function is to remove debris and bacteria by active phagocytosis and complement-induced lysis. Macrophages continue to consume tissue and bacterial debris but, more importantly, also secrete a plethora of growth factors and cytokines.[1] Lymphocytes also appear in the wound at this time, but their exact role is not completely understood.

Proliferation

As platelets degranulate, biologically active products are generated, stimulating the converting fibroblasts and endothelial cells into reparative entities. These further stimulate fibroblasts and epithelial cells to initiate granulation tissue formation. The main role of this phase is to create a scaffold for healing.

During this phase, fibroblast proliferation (fibroplasia), endothelial cell division, and angiogenesis occur. This process produces a new, loose, extracellular matrix composed of collagen (mostly types I and III), fibronectin, hyaluronic acid, and adhesion glycoproteins that maintain the matrix together.

Epithelialization occurs by migration of marginal basal cells. These cells are derived from the fixed basal layer zone adjacent to the tissue injury site. The daughter cells migrate over the new wound matrix in an immature form. They release type IV collagen and mature epithelial cells that move under the scab. Glycoproteins in the matrix and hemidesmosomes maintain the integrity of these cells, and a watertight seal is produced 24 hours after tissue injury. The process of fibroplasia and angiogenesis leads to the formation of new blood vessels, which gives the wound its characteristic beefy-red color.

Remodeling

Fibroplasia is the step in wound healing that ultimately forms a fibrous scar secondary to collagen deposition. Once collagen synthesis reaches a plateau, the remodeling phase starts. Fibroblasts migrate to the site of tissue injury secondary to the chemo-attractants released by macrophages. These fibroblasts deposit collagen on the fibrin and fibronectin sheets after the clot forms. New collagen fibers can be appreciated 3 days after injury. Fibroblasts also release mucopolysaccharides and glycoproteins. They are the major contributors to the new extracellular matrix formed.

NONHEALING WOUNDS

Occasionally, the wound healing process may become arrested in one of its stages and not progress as expected. This arrest may occur secondary to multiple causative entities, but the most common causes are local factors such as necrotic tissue, infection, and edema, and systemic factors such as malnutrition, previous radiation treatment, and diabetes mellitus.

Presence of necrotic tissue

While the presence of a large amount of devitalized tissue is a cause for wound closure delays secondary to an increased risk of infection, it is important to recognize that small amounts of necrotic tissue along the edges can also contribute to delayed wound closure. Necrotic tissue causes the continuous release of proinflammatory mediators. Functional aberrancy in chemokines and chemokine receptor systems is recognized as one of the important mechanisms underlying the pathology of impaired wound healing.[2]

Infection

A wound will not heal if the bacterial colony is over $10^{(5)}$. Bacteria and endotoxins can lead to a prolonged elevation of proinflammatory cytokines leading to an increased level of metalloproteases (MMPs), increasing the degradation of the extracellular matrix. This shift in protease activity leads to a chronic degradation of growth factors characteristic in chronic nonhealing wounds.[3]

Edema

Edema impairs local oxygen delivery leading to ischemia. This occurs through the collapsing of capillaries secondary to an increased interstitial and venous pressure, thereby causing postcapillary obstruction. An early hypoxic state stimulates the release of angiogenic and growth factors for wound healing, but the presence of oxygen is then required to maintain the healing process. Furthermore, hypoxia may amplify the inflammatory response, thereby prolonging injury by increased levels of oxygen radicals.

Malnutrition

Protein is one of the most important nutrient supplementats required for normal wound healing. A patient with an albumin level of less than 2.0 g/dL may experience wound dehiscence.[4] A deficiency in protein will lead to impaired angiogenesis and fibroblast proliferation, collagen synthesis, and wound remodeling. Several vitamins such as A and C are essential in the hydroxylation of lysine/proline and collagen cross-linking. Vitamin A in particular reverses the glucocorticoid effects on collagen.

Diabetes mellitus

Diabetics have decreased blood inflow, and thus decreased oxygen delivery to the wound. Diabetic wounds also have a chronic antiangiogenic state. In hyperglycemic conditions, the levels of matrix metalloproteinases (MMPs) are increased leading to a breakdown of the extracellular matrix and an increased susceptibility to infection. These conditions are detrimental for wound healing.

Medications

Chemotherapy agents impair wound healing secondary to a delay in cell migration to the wound, decreased protein synthesis, decreased fibroplasia and angiogenesis, and decreased collagen and extracellular matrix formation. Many of these medications induce anemia, thrombocytopenia, neutropenia, and decreased oxygen delivery to the wound.[5]

The use of systemic glucocorticoids may lead to an incomplete granulation tissue and decreased wound contraction.[5] The anti-inflammatory state of systemic steroids may increase the risk of wound infection.

TYPES OF WOUND HEALING

Wound healing is classified as healing by primary, secondary, or tertiary (delayed primary) intention (Figure 29.1).

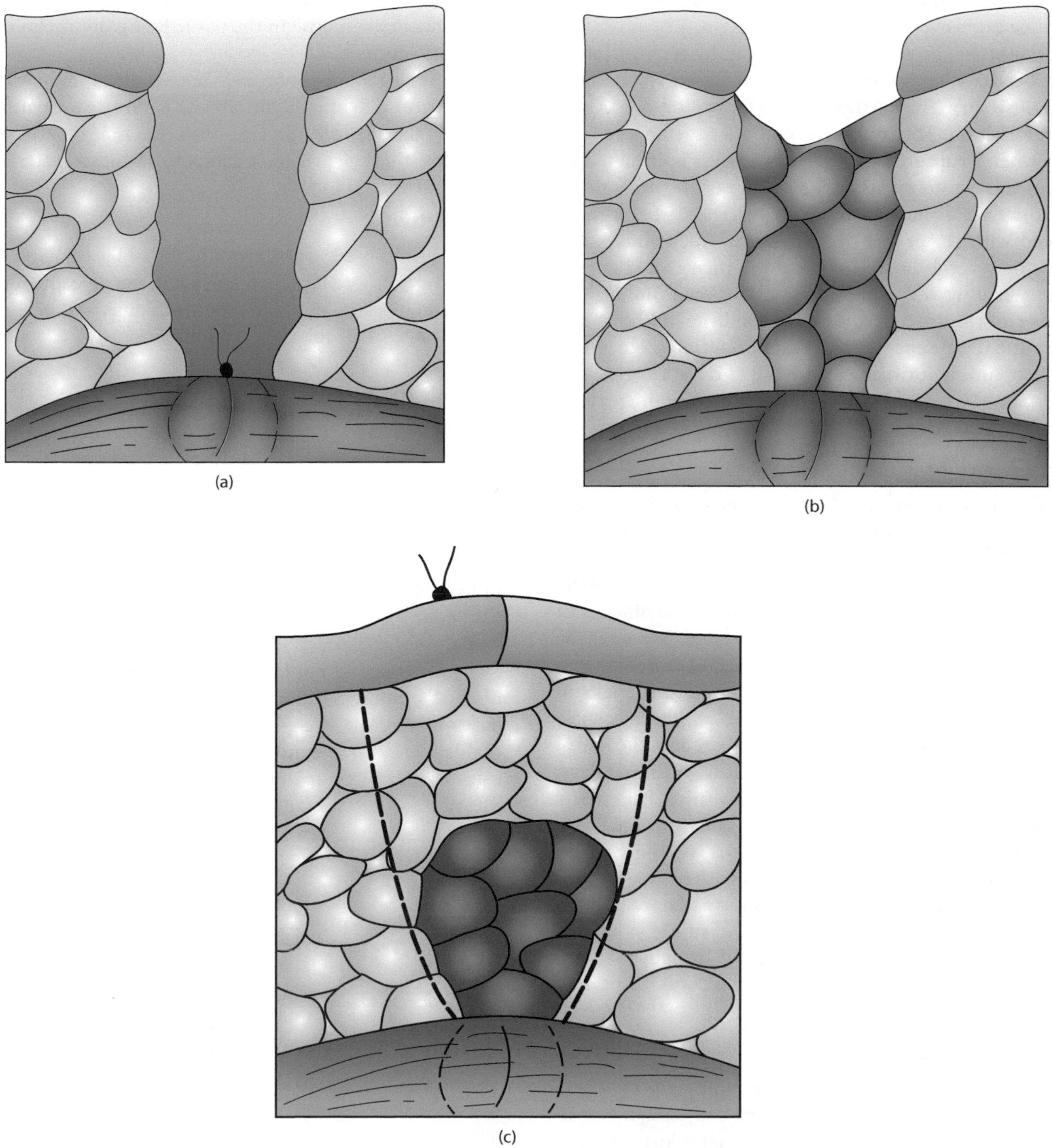

Figure 29.1 Wound healing by (a) primary, (b) secondary, and (c), and tertiary intention.

Primary or first intention healing occurs when the edges of a wound are approximated, such as a surgical skin incision closed with sutures. The apposition of the tissue layers permits a rapid re-epithelialization sealing of the incisional defect with minimal scarring.

Secondary intention type of healing occurs when the wound edges are not approximated and are left open to granulate and heal. This is seen in burns, in punch biopsies, or in cases of infected wounds or incisions left open to allow closure spontaneously. With a combination of contraction and granulation, the wound eventually epithelializes. However the healing process can be slow and may produce extensive scarring.

Delayed primary closure, or healing by tertiary intention, occurs when an open wound is closed several days after the injury. This method is used for wounds with gross contamination. This type of wound management may be used when a ruptured tuboovarian abscess is encountered during a laparotomy. After the closure of the peritoneum and the fascia, the subcutaneous layer and the skin are packed with sterile wet dressings, and the wound is left open for several days. The wound is then closed several days later after the contamination has been diminished. Successful closure depends on the condition of the wound edges and the absence of significant bacterial colonization. The best timing for such closure is 3–4 days. Delayed closures after 1 week do not heal well due to an increase of collagen deposition.[6]

SUTURE MATERIAL

The Edwin Smith papyrus from 3000 BC describes the use of linen strips and animal sinews for simple wound closure. Celsus, the Roman physician, advocated ligation of blood vessels. Although sutures have been used for many centuries, it was only in the second half of the nineteenth century that suturing became practical and safe, after the introduction of asepsis by Semmelweis and Pasteur.[7]

The suture is characterized by the type of material and the gauge of the suture, according to the U.S. Pharmacopeia (USP) system. This characterization is based on the rate of absorption. If the tensile strength is lost within 60 days, the suture is categorized as *absorbable*. This term implies that eventually the suture will disappear from the tissue implantation site. *Nonabsorbable sutures* are those which maintain their tensile strength for more than 60 days.

A surgeon has a wide choice of suture materials available today. The decision of which type of suture to be used should be based on the knowledge of the physical and biologic properties of the suture material, and the healing ability of the sutured tissue.

Absorbable sutures

Absorbable material may be either organic (catgut) or synthetic. The organic sutures are lysed by body enzymes.[8,9] In the first stage, the strength of the material is lost, and later the suture is totally absorbed.

The *organic absorbable sutures* used in operative obstetrics are chromic catgut or plain sutures. Catgut may be chromicized.

(Chromic catgut) or plain. The difference is in the strength of the suture material and the time needed for absorption. The manufacturers used to mark catgut with the number of days it was supposed to take until it was completely absorbed. The strength of the knot of both types of catgut is lessened by 50% after 1 week. Plain material is absorbed within 12 days, while the chromic suture lasts for about 28 days. Catgut suture absorption is caused by a proteolytic enzymatic reaction. This causes a marked inflammatory response in the tissue that is approximated with this suture.

Although a number of papers have claimed to show the superiority of synthetic absorbable sutures over natural ones,[10,11] the majority of U.S. obstetric and gynecologic surgeons still prefer chromic catgut to any other material.[7]

Plain catgut

This suture is used in obstetrics for tubal ligation and for approximation of the subcutaneous tissue. It is the ideal material (2.0 plain gut) for a modified Pomeroy tubal ligation because of its quick absorption.[12]

Chromic suture

This suture may be used when performing bilateral uterine artery ligation, closure of the uterine incision, approximation of the peritoneal surfaces, tubal ligation, and closure of episiotomies and lacerations after vaginal delivery. It is customary to use no. 1.0 chromic suture for a nonpermanent hypogastric artery ligation, because it is unlikely to lacerate the tissue, and is quickly absorbed in the body.[13]

The *synthetic absorbable suture* material is absorbed by hydrolysis, and not by enzymatic reaction.[7,8] Because of this, synthetic sutures provoke less tissue reaction, have great tensile strength, and are absorbed less rapidly (Table 29.1). These synthetic absorbable sutures can be categorized further into braided and monofilament sutures.

Table 29.1 Comparison of the biomechanical properties of absorbable suture materials.

Absorbable suture	50% Tensile strength	Complete absorption
Plain	3 days	10 days
Chromic	7 days	21 days
Monocryl	7 days	21 days
Vicryl	14 days	60–90 days
PDS	>42 days	>6 months

Abbreviation: PDS, polydioxanone.

Since the 1970s, two types of braided absorbable sutures have been used. Braided sutures have great tensile strength but may induce bacterial infection.

Polyglactin 910 (Vicryl)

This is a braided, absorbable, synthetic suture material similar to Dexon, composed of 90% polyglycolic acid and 10% lactic acid. Breakdown is by hydrolysis, causing minimal inflammatory reaction. After 14 days, Vicryl has a tensile strength of 50%. It is usually absorbed after 60–90 days. Since braided sutures induce bacterial infection, an antibiotic-coated Vicryl suture was developed, but it failed to decrease infection rates. This suture may be used for cystotomy and bowel repair, occasionally used for closure of the uterine incision, and for fascial closure of a transverse or Pfannenstiel incision.

Polyglactin 910 (Vicryl Rapide)

This braided suture was first used in Europe and is available now in the United States. It is chemically similar to Vicryl, but has lower molecular weight. Its absorption is by hydrolysis. It has a tensile strength of 1 week, similar to that of catgut. Vicryl Rapide is mostly used in episiotomies for skin closure.

Poliglecaprone 25 (Monocryl)

This is a monofilament suture similar in absorption time to chromic catgut. The tensile strength of this suture is 50%–60% in 7 days. It is absorbed by hydrolysis, causing minimal inflammatory response. After 21 days, it has lost all its tensile strength, so it is not recommended for fascial closure. This suture is mostly used for closure of the uterine incision, B-Lynch suture, peritoneal and muscle approximation, and subdermal or subcuticular skin closure.

Polyglyconate (Maxon) and polydioxanone (PDS)

These sutures have similar characteristics and biologic properties. They are monofilament polymers with a slow absorption rate. Both have a tensile strength of 80% by 2 weeks and of 50% by 4 weeks. Since they are monofilament and not braided, bacterial infection secondary to the suture material is not common.

It is rare for an inflammatory response to this suture material to occur even though its complete absorption may take months. PDS is a synthetic polymer monofilament suture material. It has high tensile strength and long duration, making it ideal for fascial closure. PDS maintains its integrity even in the presence of a bacterial infection. Its disadvantages are that it is stiff, is difficult to handle, and has poor knot security.

Synthetic absorbable sutures are frequently used in modern operative obstetrics. Vicryl suture is the one most frequently used for uterine incision closure, hysterectomy, ligament and vessel suture ligation, skin closure, and episiotomy repair. Because it causes minimal inflammatory reaction, episiotomy repair with Vicryl is less likely to cause short-term perineal pain than chromic catgut. Nevertheless, the length of time taken for the synthetic material to be absorbed is of concern.

Polyglycolic acid (Dexon)

Dexon is braided, absorbable, synthetic suture material with greater tensile strength than catgut. This suture causes minimal tissue reaction, retains 50%–60% of its tensile strength for 14 days, and is reabsorbed by hydrolysis after 60–90 days. Dexon is useful for the closure of fascia, tendons, muscle, and capsules. Vicryl Rapide and Monocryl are probably the best sutures for episiotomy closure, since they have minimal inflammatory response and have the same properties as chromic catgut.

Monocryl suture is widely used for closure of uterine incisions, myomectomies, reapproximation of peritoneal surfaces and the subcutaneous layer, episiotomies, and skin closure. Because of its short tensile strength, it should never be used in fascial closure. It creates minimal inflammatory tissue response, making it ideal for myomectomy (decreasing the risk of adhesions) and episiotomy repair.

Nonabsorbable sutures

Nonabsorbable sutures maintain their tensile strength for over 60 days and are absorbed only after a long period of time.

Polypropylene (Prolene)

This is a monofilament linear polymer suture. Prolene causes the least immune reaction of any suture materials. It is frequently used for cervical cerclage. This suture has been retrieved after 2–6 years and still maintained its tensile strength.[14]

Nylon

Nylon suture is available as a monofilament (Ethilon, Dermalon) or a multifilament (Neurolon, Surgilon). Neither form causes tissue reaction and may be used in the presence of bacteria since nylon is inert. Nylon is usually absorbed after 2 years. Its disadvantage is knot slippage, so careful attention should be used when tying it.

Polyester

These types of sutures have great strength and durability, but since they are braided, they are not recommended in the presence of bacteria. Mersilene is an uncoated type of suture. It is frequently used for cervical cerclage. The advantage of this suture is that it possesses great knot security.

Silk

This is a protein filament obtained from silkworm larvae. It is braided, has great tensile strength, and is easy to handle. The major advantage of this suture is its knot security.

However, silk may act as a nidus of infection, and therefore its popularity has diminished.

Staples

Skin staples are frequently used in obstetrics for closure, especially in a vertical skin incision. The only benefit of staples over subcuticular stitches is speed. However, skin staples may cause more pain and a less favorable cosmetic result.[14–18] Internal stapling devices are rarely used in obstetrics.

For fascial closure, the suture must be chosen by its tensile strength, the type of laparotomy incision made, and the quality of the fascial layer to be approximated. When performing a fascial closure, one should not lock the suture, since this causes necrosis and weakens the fascia. If a vertical incision is performed, the fascia should always be reapproximated either with PDS, or with a nonabsorbable suture, such as nylon. Neither Vicryl nor Dexon should be used for a vertical fascial closure. The best fascial closure for a vertical incision is a continuous, running mass closure because it has a significantly greater wound strength, and decreases closure time when compared to the interrupted technique.[15,19] If a transverse incision is performed and the patient has no medical problems, the fascial closure can be performed with Vicryl or Dexon. If the patient has diabetes, is morbidly obese, or had previous surgery, closure of the fascia should be done with PDS.

KNOTS

Surgery is both a science and an art. Dexterity and speed in tying knots constitute an art which only practice can make perfect.[15]

The surgical knots used in operative obstetrics can be divided into two categories: sliding knots (identical or nonidentical) and flat knots (square and surgeon's). A sliding knot is formed when two half-hitches are tied, applying greater tension on one segment of the suture. A flat knot is formed when two half-hitches are tied applying the same tension to both segments of the suture.

Sliding knots have a tendency to slip and are less secure. However, they are easy to make and are frequently used in operative obstetrics.[20] It is better to use a sliding knot in certain situations, as when tying deep in the pelvis. The addition of several throws to a sliding knot improves the knot's security.[21]

Flat knots are the most secure of the surgical knots if the number of throws is adequate.[22] When unnecessary throws are used, the risk of infection increases. Studies have shown that a minimum of four throws should be used to achieve optimum knot-holding capacity when using a flat knot on a non-monofilament absorbable suture.[23]

Investigations to determine the security of knots tied with one looped end and one free end versus knots with two free ends have been done. It has been demonstrated that knots with one looped and one free end are weaker than those tied with two free ends.[23] Therefore, a continuous suture line is best tied with a knot having two free ends (Figure 29.2).

NEEDLES

Currently, the needle is attached to the suture material by the manufacturer and is atraumatic; therefore, the type of eye of the needle meticulously described in former textbooks is no longer relevant.

Curved needles are usually used for sutures. The diameter of the curve depends on the bulk of the material to be sutured. The profile of the needle (transverse section) is of two main types: round and cutting. Cutting needles may be of different shapes, such as reverse cutting with the point away from the curve, tapering in the form of a spatula, and so forth. Needles may be of various lengths, usually in the range of 13–50 mm. Several sutures have needles attached to each end. Soft and friable tissue should be sutured with round needles, and thick or hard tissue with a cutting needle. Therefore, the uterus and the peritoneum are transfixed with round needles, while the cutting needles are recommended for the fascia and the skin. The use of different types of cutting needles and straight needles will depend on the preference of the surgeon. Hand needles, which require no needle holder, shorten operation time and are therefore popular in the United Kingdom. They have gained little acceptance, however, in the United States.

DRAINS

The earliest documented use of a drainage system was by Celsus in the first century AD. He placed lead and bronze tubes into the abdominal cavity as gravity drains. In contemporary surgery, the use of prophylactic drains for peritoneal contamination has been abandoned because they are quickly surrounded by bowel and omentum.[24]

Currently, there are four type of drains used: (1) the Penrose drain, (2) the closed-suction drain, (3) the sump drain, and (4) the closed-suction Penrose drain. In obstetrics, the Penrose drain and the closed-suction drain are most frequently used. These drains are brought through a separate stab wound, not through the surgical incision, to prevent infection in the suture line, weakness of the fascia, and subsequent hernia.

Penrose drain

This is a very efficient drain; however, it increases the risk of secondary infection.[25] It is a latex drain which varies in size and diameter. It is used for drainage of blood, pus, or serosanguineous fluid from a cavity.

Closed-suction drain (Jackson Pratt or Blake Drain)

Closed-suction drains of silicone are minimally irritating to tissues. These drains have a low incidence of secondary infection, but tend to clog and cease functioning earlier than the Penrose drain.[26,27]

To drain or not to drain is still an area of controversy. Some studies in surgery have shown no benefit from intra-abdominal drains. Besides, intra-abdominal drains can

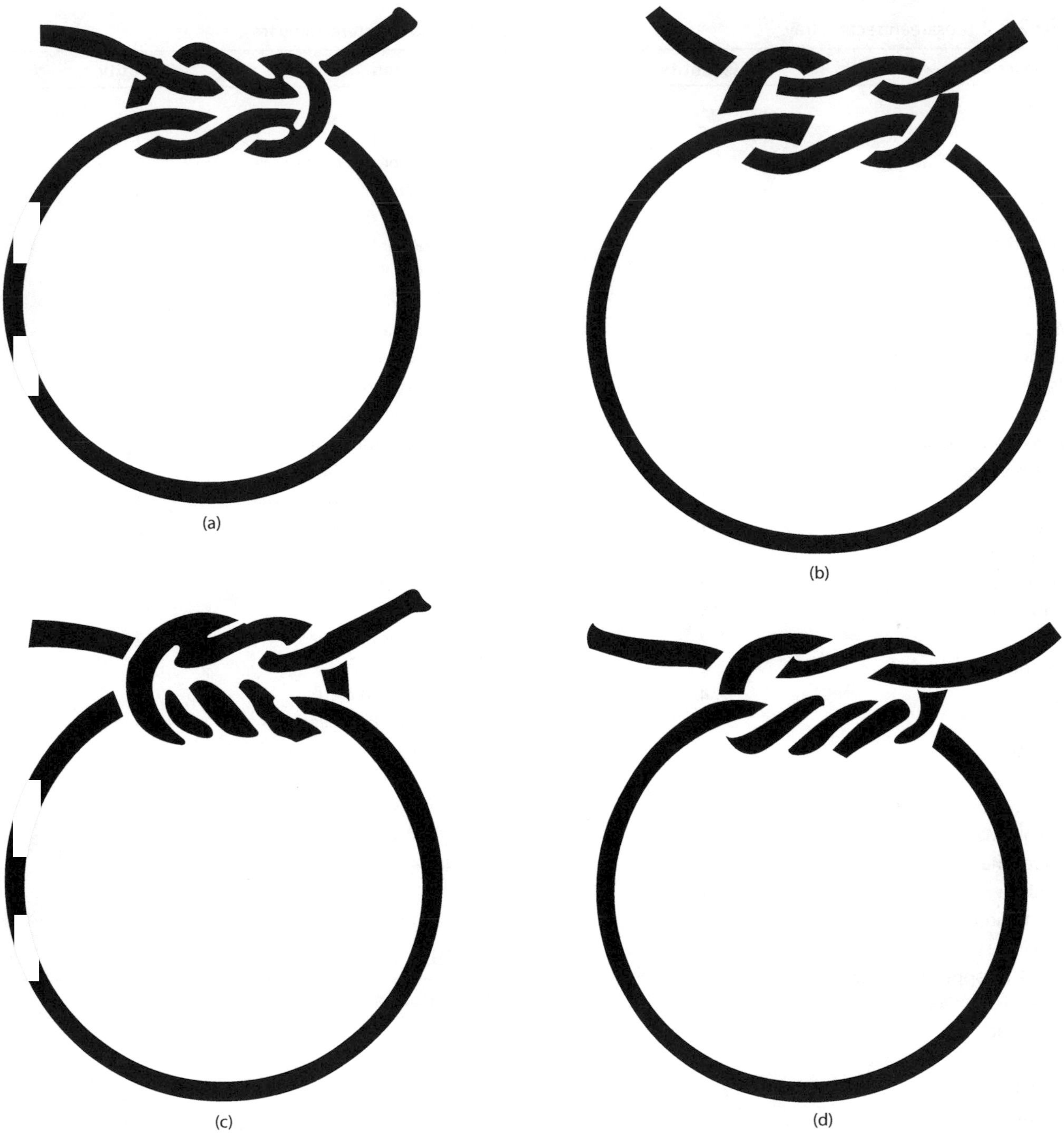

Figure 29.2 (a) Square knot, (b) granny knot, (c) surgeon's square knot, and (d) surgeon's granny knot. (Drawing by Julian Gaspar.)

cause adhesions and possibly bowel obstruction. However, it is advisable to place an intra-abdominal drain whenever hemostatic control is not optimal during a cesarean section. This may occur in cases of ruptured uterus, uterine rupture severe preeclampsia, and superimposed HELLP syndrome (Hemolysis, Elevated Liver enzymes, Low Platelets), and in patients on anticoagulation therapy. It can also be helpful in the testing for creatinine for cases like invasive placentation in which bladder injury may occur and a cystotomy closure was made.

Some studies have suggested that the use of drains in the subcutaneous space may reduce the incidence of postoperative complications in obese women who have at least 2 cm of subcutaneous tissue.[28] Nevertheless, suture closure of the subcutaneous fat during a cesarean section is probably better than placement of a subcutaneous drain.[29]

INSTRUMENTS FOR OPERATIVE OBSTETRICS

The instrument table should include the proper armamentarium and drapes for operative obstetrics. The following lists of instruments (Tables 29.2–29.5) include the equipment necessary to perform a cervical cerclage, dilation and curettage, cesarean section, and hysterectomy. Other

Table 29.2 Cesarean section tray.

Item description	Quantity
Knife handle	2
Sponge sticks	5
Retractors	
Balfour blade	1
Richardson (large)	2
Richardson (small)	2
Roux	2
Forceps	
Mouse tooth	2
Adson forceps with teeth	2
Tissue with teeth (large)	1
Russian (large)	1
De Bakey vascular	1
Needle holders	
Large	1
Small	1
Clamps	
Towel	6
Hemostat	14
Kelly	7
Babcock	4
Kocher	4
Allis	4
T-clamp	10
Scissors	
Metzenbaum	2
Straight Mayo	2
Curved Mayo	2
Bandage	1
Kidney basin	1
Light handles	2
Stat pack (wrapped separately in a surgical towel)	
Hemostat	6
Kelly	4
Kocher	2
T-clamps	5
Knife handles	2
Suture scissors	1
Curved Mayo	1
Bandage scissors	1
Metzenbaum scissors	1
Allis clamp	2
Needle holder	2
Forceps (plain and toothed)	2

Table 29.3 Hysterectomy tray.

Item description	Quantity
Knife handle	2
Knife handle long	1
Balfour retractor and blade	1
Ribbon retractor small	1
Ribbon retractor medium	1
Ribbon retractor large	1
Roux retractor	2
Bookwalter retractor	1
Richardson retractor small	2
Richardson retractor medium	2
Richardson retractor large	2
Deaver retractor small	2
Deaver retractor medium	2
Deaver retractor large	2
Carmalt forceps curved	4
Needle holder, 8 inches	2
Needle holder, 6 inches	2
Tissue forceps with teeth, 8 inches	2
Dressing forceps plain, 8 inches	2
Adson forceps with teeth	2
Babcock clamps, 8 inches	4
Kocher clamps	6
Allis clamps	8
Heaney clamps	4
Right angle clamps	4
Tonsil clamps	6

Table 29.4 Cerclage set.

Item description	Quantity
Ring forceps	4
Long Heaney needle holder	1
Kelly	2
Scissors (long straight Mayo)	1
Retractors—lateral (Sims)	2
Heavy weighted speculum	1
Forceps plain	1
Forceps with teeth	1
Russian forceps	1
Sound	1
Sims retractor	1
Briesky or lateral retractors	2
Disposable scalpel, Size 10	1
Disposable scalpel, Size 12	1
Disposable scalpel, Size 15	1

Table 29.5 D & C tray.

Item description	Quantity
Lateral retractor, L-shaped blades	1
Heavy-weighted speculum	1
Leaves speculum (medium or large)	1
Hank dilators	
Set no. 1	
9/10	1
11/12	1
13/14	1
15/16	1
17/18	1
19/20	1
Set no. 2	
17/18	1
19/20	1
21/22	1
23/24	1
25/26	1
27/28	1
Uterine curette sharp no. 1	1
Uterine curette sharp no. 2	1
Uterine curette sharp no. 3	1
Uterine curette sharp no. 4	1
Uterine curette sharp no. 5	1
Curette, Heaney endometrial (serrated cup)	1
Curette, endocervical (tip end is square)	1
Uterine sound (tip end has a ball tip)	1
Thumb tissue forceps	1
Thumb dressing forceps	1
Baum's tenaculums	2
Allis tissue clamps	2
Polyp forceps	1
Mayo Hegar needle holder	1
Mayo dissecting scissors	1
Forrester sponge forceps straight	4
Curved Allis	1

Abbreviation: D&C, dilation and curettage.

surgeons may use different instruments, according to their own preferences and experience.

REFERENCES

1. Rappolee DA, Mark D, Banda MJ et al. Wound macrophages express TGF-alpha and other growth factors in vivo: Analysis by mRNA phenotyping. *Science* 1989; 241: 708–12.
2. Su Y, Richmond A. Chemokine regulation of neutrophil infiltration of skin wounds. *Adv Wound Care (New Rochelle)* 2015; 4(11): 631–40.
3. Guo S, DiPietro LA. Factors affecting wound healing. *J Dent Res* 2010; 89(3): 219–29.
4. Kolb BA, Buller RE, Connor JP et al. Effects of early postoperative chemotherapy on wound healing. *Obstet Gynecol* 1992; 79: 988–92.
5. Franz MG, Steed DL, Robson MC. Optimizing healing of the acute wound by minimizing complications. *Curr Probl Surg* 2007; 44: 691–763.
6. Edlich RF, Rogers W, Kasper G et al. Studies on the management of the contaminated wound. I. Optimal time for closure of contaminated open wounds. *Am J Surg* 1969; 117: 323–9.
7. Stroumtsos A. *Perspectives on Sutures*. Pearl River, NY: David and Geek, American Cyanamid Company, 1978.
8. Hartko WJ, Ghanekar G, Kemmann E. Suture materials currently used in obstetric-gynecologic surgery in the United States. *Obstet Gynecol* 1982; 9: 241.
9. Holmlund D, Tera H, Wiberg Y et al. *Sutures and Techniques for Wound Closure. Medical and Surgical Publications*. New York, NY: Naimark and Barba, 1978.
10. Gallitano AL, Kondi ES. The superiority of polyglycolic acid sutures for closure of abdominal incision. *Surg Gynecol Obstet* 1973; 37: 794–6.
11. Kronborg O. Polyglycolic acid (Dexon) versus silk for fascial closure of abdominal incision. *Acta Chir Scand* 1976; 142: 9–12.
12. Bishop E, Nelms WF. A simple method of tubal sterilization. *N Y State J Med* 1930; 30: 214.
13. Kettle C, Johanson RB. Absorbable synthetic versus catgut suture material for perineal repair. *Cochrane Database Syst Rev* 2000; (2): CD000006.
14. Parell GJ, Becker GD. Comparison of absorbable with nonabsorbable sutures in closure of facial skin wounds. *Arch Facial Plast Surg* 2003; 5: 488–90.
15. Edgerton MT. *The Art of Surgical Technique*. Baltimore, MD: Williams & Wilkins, 1988.
16. Eldrup J, Wied U, Andersen B. Randomised trial comparing Proximate stapler with conventional skin closure. *Acta Chir Scand* 1981; 147: 501–2.
17. Ranaboldo CJ, Rowe-Jones DC. Closure of laparotomy wounds: Skin staples versus sutures. *Br J Surg* 1992; 79: 1172–3.
18. Frishman GN, Schwartz T, Hogan JW. Closure of Pfannenstiel skin incisions. Staples vs. subcuticular suture. *J Reprod Med* 1997; 42: 627–30.
19. Seid MH, McDaniel-Owens LM, Poole GV Jr, Meeks GR. A randomized trial of abdominal incision suture technique and wound strength in rats. *Arch Surg* 1995; 130: 394–7.
20. Bashir Z. *Ethicon Knot Tying Manual*. Someville, NJ: Ethicon, 1996.

21. Trimbos JB. Security of various knots commonly used in surgical practice. *Obstet Gynecol* 1984; 64: 274–80.
22. Ivy JJ, Unger JB, Mukherjee D. Knot integrity with nonidentical and parallel sliding knots. *Am J Obstet Gynecol* 2004; 190: 83–6.
23. Brouwers JE, Oosting H, Haas D, Kloppers PJ. Dynamic loading of surgical knots. *Surg Gynecol Obstet* 1991; 173: 443–8.
24. Brown RP. Knotting technique and suture materials. *Br J Surg* 1992; 79: 399–400.
25. Annunziata CC, Drake DB, Woods JA et al. Technical considerations in knot construction. I. Continuous percutaneous and dermal suture closure. *J Emerg Med* 1997; 15: 351–6.
26. Stylianos S, Martin, EC, Starker PM et al. Percutaneous drainage of intra-abdominal abcesses following abdominal trauma. *J Trauma* 1989; 29: 584–8.
27. Berlin RB, Javna SL. Closed suction wide area drainage. *Surg Gynecol Obstet* 1992; 174: 421.
28. Allaire AD, Fisch J, McMahon MJ. Subcutaneous drain vs. suture in obese women undergoing cesarean delivery. A prospective, randomized trial. *J Reprod Med* 2000; 45: 327–31.
29. Chelmow D, Rodriguez EJ, Sabatini MM. Suture closure of subcutaneous fat and wound disruption after cesarean delivery: A meta-analysis. *Obstet Gynecol* 2004; 103: 974–80.

Cesarean delivery

30

GEORGE F. GUIRGUIS and JOSEPH J. APUZZIO

CONTENTS

Cesarean delivery has had a tumultuous and controversial history. The procedure was seldom used before the end of the nineteenth century because of its prohibitive maternal mortality. However, a dramatic rise in abdominal deliveries has occurred over the past five decades. The cesarean delivery rate in the United States in 1970 was 5.5% compared with 32.7% in 2013.[1–3] This is the latest available statistic at the time of this writing and this rate resulted in 1,284,339 cesarean deliveries in 2013. Several factors have contributed to this change[4–6]:

1. Women are delaying childbearing, leading to more births among women of older age. This group has a high rate of cesarean deliveries and medical complications.
2. A higher proportion of births are occurring in nulliparous women who are at a higher risk for cesarean delivery.
3. Continuous fetal monitoring during labor has increased the cesarean delivery rate for category II and III tracings.
4. There are concerns about medical legal action in the event of an adverse fetal outcome if a cesarean is *not* performed.
5. A diagnosis of dystocia is made more frequently and managed by cesarean delivery.
6. Term vaginal breech delivery has been discouraged by the medical literature.
7. Routine scheduled repeat cesarean birth is more commonplace.
8. There is cesarean delivery secondary to "Maternal Request."
9. However, the final goal of any surgery is that the necessity of performing the surgery would appear as valid in retrospect as it does in prospect. Although this goal may never be achieved in all cases, it should be sought.

INDICATIONS FOR CESAREAN DELIVERY

Cesarean delivery may be performed for maternal, fetal, or combined indications. Maternal indications include those done in the mother's best interest when vaginal birth is dangerous or impossible. Cesarean delivery would be done for fetal indication when the fetal risk is less with abdominal delivery than with vaginal birth. When it is in the interest of both mother and fetus to have a cesarean, there is a combined indication.

The four most common indications for cesarean delivery that account for approximately 70% of these deliveries are as follows:

1. Failure to progress in labor
2. Concerning fetal status (antepartum fetal testing by nonstress test, biophysical profile, Doppler assessment, contraction stress test, fetal heart rate monitoring, etc.)
3. Previous cesarean delivery or uterine surgery such as myomectomy
4. Fetal malpresentation for breech, transverse lie, etc.

Sometimes the best interest of the mother and fetus do not always coincide. The decision to perform surgery requires experience, clinical judgment, logic, and considering the wishes of the parents. The correct decision results from understanding all factors, rather than relying on just a tabulated list of indications. Decisions should take into account any conflict between the interests of the mother and the fetus.

Maternal indications

From the maternal perspective, the crucial questions are as follows:

- How soon must the pregnancy be terminated by delivery for the health and well-being of the mother, i.e., severe preeclampsia?
- How soon can vaginal birth be accomplished?
- What are the chances of severe complications arising as a result of any delay in delivery?
- To what extent will a major operation (cesarean delivery) be dangerous for the mother?

Indications

1. Patients with a complete placenta previa should always be delivered by cesarean delivery even with a fetal demise. Low-lying placenta previa is considered by many as an indication for cesarean, although, as a maternal indication, the imperativeness of the indication varies somewhat with the degree of the previa.
2. Placental abruption is an indication for cesarean delivery if the hemorrhage is severe and the fetus is not immediately deliverable. In this situation, cesarean delivery may be indicated even in the presence of fetal death. However, if the fetus is immediately deliverable, vaginal birth may be preferable for the mother's benefit.
3. Marginal abruption ("marginal sinus rupture"), on the other hand, is not a maternal indication for cesarean delivery because complications such as severe hemorrhage, clotting disorders, and renal failure, sometimes associated with placenta abruption, do not usually arise.
4. Most neurologists feel that cesarean delivery should be performed if the patient has had cerebral hemorrhage or has an untreated aneurysm because any form of second-stage bearing-down effort is usually contraindicated.
5. Mechanical obstruction to vaginal birth (such as large leiomyoma or large condyloma acuminata, severely displaced pelvic fracture, large cervical myoma, or pedunculated ovarian tumor). All myomas do not require cesarean delivery, however, some will be drawn upward as the lower uterine segment develops. Clinical correlation is necessary on a case-by-case basis.
6. Virtually everyone agrees that the cervix should not be dilated with invasive carcinoma of the cervix. Pregnant women with carcinoma in situ or microinvasive disease (up to 3 mm in depth, having undergone full evaluation during pregnancy with a conization showing negative margins) may be followed to term and delivered vaginally, with reevaluation and treatment at 6 weeks postpartum.[7] Recurrences have been reported at the episiotomy site in women who delivered

vaginally; this area should be inspected and palpated during post-treatment surveillance.[8,9] Delivery in women with larger-volume, invasive cervical cancer should undergo a classical cesarean delivery to avoid potential cervical hemorrhage and possible dissemination of tumor cells during labor and vaginal birth, although the latter risk is controversial.[8,9] A classical cesarean and radical hysterectomy with therapeutic lymphadenectomy may be the treatment of choice for early lesions, after fetal pulmonary maturity is established.

7. Repaired and healed vesico-vaginal fistulas may be considered potential indications, since the stretching of the vagina during birth may reopen the fistula. The exceptions are repairs close to the introitus, which may be protected by episiotomy.
8. Some abnormal fetal presentations and positions constitute strong maternal indications for cesarean delivery. A transverse lie is one example because of the danger of uterine rupture. A face presentation with a persistent mentum posterior position is also an indication because the fetus is undeliverable in that position. Other face presentations such as mentum anterior do not necessarily imply that a section should be performed. During early labor, a brow presentation does not indicate immediate operative birth because there is often spontaneous conversion to an occiput or face presentation but it is an indication if the brow presentation persists.
9. Cephalopelvic disproportion is so pronounced that vaginal birth would be almost impossible. This indication for cesarean delivery is more fetal than maternal. The key question is whether or not the mother would be injured by waiting longer, stimulating the labor with oxytocin, or attempting vaginal birth.

Relative indications

1. Gestational hypertensive diseases such as preeclampsia, eclampsia, and HELLP (hemolysis, elevated liver enzymes, low platelet count) syndrome are relative maternal indications for delivery and possibly cesarean delivery, depending upon severity of the disease and how soon delivery must occur. Most clinicians would choose induction of labor if time permitted; however, if the condition is rapidly progressing, cesarean delivery is a means of immediate delivery.
2. Maternal cardiac disease is not an absolute indication for cesarean section. The stress of major surgery should not be superimposed upon a failing or potentially failing heart. The goal for these patients is a short second stage, with minimal bearing down. The mother should give birth with the least possible stress. Obviously, if there is indication for cesarean delivery, such as disproportion, the surgery need not be avoided.
3. It is estimated that 2.5% of all births in the United States are cesarean deliveries on maternal request. However, delivery should not be performed for this reason until 39 weeks and is not recommended for patients desiring several children given the risks of abnormal placentation following each cesarean delivery.[10,11]

Fetal indications

When the fetus is jeopardized by an attempt at vaginal birth, there is a *fetal* indication for cesarean delivery. An example of a fetal indication without a maternal component is a prolapsed umbilical cord. The fetus is seriously threatened, but the mother's life or health is not. A cesarean delivery is indicated unless the fetus is immediately deliverable vaginally or the fetus is not alive.

Fetal indications can be grouped into several categories. Some indications are obligatory, such as a category II or III tracing that does not respond to resuscitative fetal interventions in labor. Sometimes there is a fetal indication when the pregnancy is complicated by diabetes mellitus, preeclampsia, or renal disease and tests for fetal well-being become ominous. In this situation, a "hostile" intrauterine environment may warrant delivery without delay.

Other signs of "hostile" intrauterine environment include oligohydramnios; thick, pea-soup amniotic fluid (not merely stained fluid); and evidence of fetal bleeding during labor. The use of the deepest vertical pocket measurement as opposed to amniotic fluid index (AFI) to diagnose oligohydramnios is associated with a reduction in unnecessary interventions without an increase in adverse perinatal outcomes.[12] Most clinicians would consider these conditions as fetal indications for cesarean delivery.

Other recognized indications include the threat of birth trauma. Cephalopelvic disproportion and failure to progress often are used as a wastebasket diagnosis. This group may include patients who have labored in the second stage with ruptured membranes for several hours without descent of the head. At the other extreme are patients with dysfunctional contractions in the latent stage who in retrospect were not even in labor.

Most fetuses in the breech presentation are delivered by cesarean delivery. Providers should counsel and recommend external cephalic version at the completion of 37 weeks' gestation.[13] The American Congress of Obstetricians and Gynecologists' (ACOG) committee on obstetric practice recommended that planned vaginal delivery of a term singleton breech was no longer appropriate. Currently, the recommendation regarding a planned vaginal delivery of a term singleton breech fetus being managed by an experienced provider may be a reasonable option. Informed consent should be obtained including discussion of increased perinatal and neonatal mortality with vaginal breech delivery.[14]

Currently, cesarean delivery often is utilized for twins mainly to provide the second twin with maximum safety at birth. Mortality and morbidity rates usually are higher for the second twin than for the first twin. This is not because all second-twin vaginal births are traumatic but because there are few good solutions when trouble arises. The optimal route of delivery in women with twin gestaions depends on the type of twins, fetal presentation, gestational age, and experience of the clinician.[15–17] When a concerning category II or III tracing is encountered, the clinician must choose between vaginal birth and emergency cesarean delivery for the second twin. Vaginal birth is the desirable choice only when there is a good chance of success without trauma, and emergency delivery is impossible. This is a difficult choice and depends upon specific circumstances at the time. If a cesarean delivery for the second twin is necessary after vaginal delivery of the first twin, one should not forget to repair the episiotomy if it was performed.

Cesarean delivery is almost always utilized for triplet and quadruplet births in the interest of fetal survival if pregnancy has progressed to the point of fetal viability.

In certain clinical circumstances, an abruptio placentae is a fetal indication. When part of the placenta is separated, immediate fetal death results if the remaining functioning placenta is insufficient to support life. In some cases, a portion of placenta remains functional and will sustain life only for a short time. For these, delivery can be lifesaving for the fetus. In other cases, the abruption is so small that the feto-maternal exchange is not really compromised. Since there is no accurate way to determine placental reserve, delivery is often the best method to ensure the birth of a live fetus.

In cases of placenta previa, fetal survival is unlikely with vaginal birth. In addition, the methods used for vaginal birth with placenta previa were often directly traumatic to the fetus.

Certain fetal presentations can expose the fetus to birth trauma. Even in early labor, transverse presentations are extremely dangerous to the fetus because of the risk of prolapsed cord. The potential trauma of version and extraction thus provide an absolute fetal indication.

Maternal infection

Maternal infection such as active genital herpes vulvovaginitis is a fetal indication for cesarean delivery. Also, elective cesarean delivery should be discussed and recommended for all human immunodeficiency virus (HIV)-infected pregnant women with viral loads above 1000 copies/mL.[18] If the decision is made to perform an elective cesarean delivery, it is recommended to be done at 38 weeks' gestation, due to the potential risk of labor and membrane rupture before the woman reaches 39 weeks' gestation, which is the standard recommended time for operative deliveries in women without HIV infection. Zidovidine (ZDV) prophylaxis should be provided regardless of the mode of delivery, as the available data indicate that ZDV provides an additional protective effect in women undergoing elective operative delivery. Intravenous ZDV should begin 3 hours prior to surgery. Because of the potential for increased postoperative maternal morbidity in HIV-infected women undergoing operative delivery, clinicians may opt to administer perioperative antibiotic prophylaxis.

In women at very low risk of transmission, such as those with low or undetectable viral load, the additional benefit provided by elective cesarean delivery may be marginal. The potential benefit of elective cesarean delivery should be discussed with all HIV-infected pregnant women and the decisions regarding operative delivery will need to be individualized according to the woman's clinical, immunologic, and virologic status.

The influence of the mode of delivery on perinatal transmission of hepatitis C virus (HCV) is incompletely understood. However, cesarean delivery is associated with a reduced risk of HCV transmission in women who are HCV/HIV coinfected.[19,20]

A difficult clinical situation arises when there is an indication for delivery and several days of induction have been unsuccessful. Whether or not a cesarean delivery is indicated depends upon the strength of the indication for delivery, not upon the fact that there is failed induction. However, one should not induce patients without an appropriate indication for delivery, expecting that an easy induction will ensue.

Some data indicate that grossly premature fetuses do not withstand the stress of labor well. Accordingly, obstetricians tend to use relatively liberal criteria for cesarean delivery when the gestation is very preterm, but the fetus is considered viable, particularly when tracings of the fetal heart rate monitoring indicate significant and recurrent cord compression, a circumstance predisposing to intracerebral hemorrhage.

If the fetus is not alive, the mother should be delivered vaginally unless there is a maternal indication for cesarean delivery. Similiary, if the fetus estimated fetal weight is less than 23 weeks' gestation, a cesarean delivery should not be performed for a fetal indication. When there is no reasonable chance for fetal survival, the mother should not be exposed to the risk of an operation.

Combined indications for cesarean delivery

There are combined indications for cesarean section with maternal and fetal components that can be additive. Abruptio placentae and placenta previa are such examples.

Years ago, there were few cesarean deliveries for fetal indications because the operation was dangerous for the mother. Her interests always superseded those of the fetus. Now, the procedure is safe enough; nonetheless, it endangers the mother in the interests of the fetus. This being the case, what should be done when the fetus has little chance of survival no matter how delivered? In the very preterm pregnancy, there may be strong fetal indication for cesarean delivery with relatively little chance of survival, and in some cases, increased maternal danger. There is no easy answer, but the clinician's dilemma brings up the third consideration: Legal liability for results. Legal liability has increased in all areas of medicine, but obstetrics is considered one of the most serious areas for several reasons. There is a certain irreducible fetal morbidity, yet society expects perfect results. Performing a cesarean delivery has been safer from a legal point of view than persisting with a vaginal birth. The impression has developed that if a section was performed, everything possible was done and that any untoward results with vaginal birth could not be defended. Whether or not true from a legal point of view, this impression has had a great impact clinically.

The increase in the number of cesarean deliveries for dystocia, fetal distress, and breech presentation probably reflects an increased concern for the fetus and an effort to reduce perinatal mortality and morbidity. Since cesarean delivery increases the danger to the mother, there is crucial need to ensure that every procedure performed is necessary for one or both of the patients. Critical understanding of the indications and a logical decision-making process should help clinicians to attain this goal.

Repeat cesarean delivery

The dictum "once a cesarean always a cesarean" was stated in 1916 because the risk of uterine rupture after a previous section was considered unduly high.[21] It took more than half a century before the concept was almost totally accepted.[19] In the ensuing decade, clinicians have decided that the dictum is not true and that most patients with previous sections can be delivered vaginally safely.

The US national enthusiasm for vaginal birth after cesarean delivery (VBAC) led to a decrease in the cesarean delivery rate, which reached 20.7% in 1996. During the same period (1989–1996), the VBAC rate increased from less than 18.9%–28.3%. Some third-party payers and managed-care organizations even mandated that all women who had a previous cesarean undergo a trial of labor. Many physicians were pressured into offering VBAC to unsuitable candidates or to women who wanted to have a repeat cesarean delivery. As the VBAC rate increased, so did the number of well-publicized reports of uterine rupture and other complications during trials of labor after previous cesarean deliveries. As a result, many physicians and hospitals have discontinued the practice altogether. The cesarean delivery rate in the United States is increasing again, reaching 32.7% in 2013, while most published series of women attempting a trial of labor after a previous cesarean delivery demonstrate a 60%–80% success rate.[22–24]

CANDIDATES FOR TRIAL OF LABOR AFTER CESAREAN DELIVERY

The ACOG guidelines for identifying women who are potential candidates for trial of labor after a cesarean delivery (TOLAC) include the following criteria[24]:

- No traditional contraindication to labor or vaginal birth.
- One or two previous low transverse uterine incisions. However, an ACOG Task Force on Evaluation of Cesarean Delivery recommended restricting VBAC attempts to women with only one previous low transverse incision[22].
- No other uterine surgical scars.
- No history of previous uterine rupture.
- A clinically adequate pelvis.
- TOLAC is not contraindicated for women with previous cesarean delivery with an unknown scar unless clinical suspicion of a previous classical incision.
- Induction of labor for maternal or fetal indication remains an option for TOLAC.[25]
- A physician immediately available throughout active labor who is capable of making the decision for and performing an emergency cesarean delivery.
- Availability of anesthesia and nursing personnel for emergency cesarean delivery with delivery within 30 minutes of the decision to operate.
- Pregnancy of 37–40 weeks' gestation.

More data are required before recommendations can be made for women with two or more previous cesarean deliveries, unknown uterine scar, multiple gestation, postterm or preterm pregnancy, low vertical incision, induction, or suspected macrosomia.[21–24]

Contraindications to trial of labor

TOLAC should not be attempted in women at high risk for uterine rupture or with contraindications to labor or vaginal birth. Contraindications for TOLAC include the following:

- Prior classical or inverted T-shaped uterine incision or other transfundal uterine surgery (such as myomectomy)
- Previous uterine rupture
- Medical or obstetric complication that precludes vaginal birth (such as placenta previa)
- Inability to perform emergency cesarean delivery due to factors related to the facility, surgeon, anesthesia, or nursing staff

Most unknown uterine incisions at term are the result of low transverse incisions. Women with an unknown incision in the setting of risk factors for a previous classical or T incision (preterm birth before 28 weeks of gestation and transverse lie) should be considered at higher risk of uterine rupture with a trial of labor.

If TOLAC is appropriately offered, experience shows that about 50%–70% of the attempts will be successful.[22]

TYPES OF CESAREAN DELIVERY INCISIONS

Each type of cesarean has advantages and disadvantages. Obstetricians should be experienced with the different types of operations as well as cesarean hysterectomy. Both of the lower-segment techniques to be discussed are useful depending on gestational age and the clinical situation.

Abdominal skin incisions

Both transverse and vertical skin incisions are used for cesarean deliveries. Vertical incisions have the advantage of providing rapid entry into the peritoneal cavity and good exposure. The midline incision is commonly used, as it is easy to effect and to close. This results in minimal dissection of cleavage planes between muscle and fascia helps prevent wound infections.

All vertical skin incisions place stress on the suture line, making postoperative hernia formation more common than with the transverse incision. However, this does not appear to be an important practical factor, since patients with cesarean deliveries are usually young and have a good musculature.

Transverse skin incisions are popular for entry into the abdominal cavity. For cosmetic purposes, the Pfannenstiel incision is often used. This incision, which can often be made within the pubic hairline, is barely visible postoperatively. One problem with this incision may be exposure. Because anterior rectus fascia must be dissected from the muscle, there is opportunity for wound infection. If exposure is inadequate with a classic Pfannenstiel, the Cherney modification (rectus tendons divided at pubis) will provide generous exposure. Excellent exposure is also obtained with the Maylard incision, a transverse incision through all layers, but this necessitates cutting through the rectus muscles and ligating the inferior epigastric vessels.

Sometimes, with a Pfannenstiel incision, the intact rectus muscles hinders the delivery of the head. In this case, the medial two-thirds of each rectus can be cut without worrying about the inferior epigastric vessels. If this is done, one should resuture the rectus muscles so that they heal in an intact manner.

The choice of abdominal incision seems to depend primarily upon how the clinician was trained and what the custom is in the area of practice. Individuals trained to utilize Pfannenstiel incisions often use this incision almost exclusively. Irrespective of the original incision, the peritoneum usually is opened vertically.

Lower-segment transverse cesarean delivery

Lower-segment transverse uterine incisions is the standard routine procedure, which is easy to perform, as the incised area is less vascular and the uterus at this area is easy to suture. However, there are potential problems. The length of the incision is limited by the width of the anterior lower uterine segment between the round ligaments. Any lateral extension of the incision could result in tearing of the uterine arteries and veins, resulting in hemorrhage and/or hematoma. Therefore, the incision may be difficult to use for premature birth where the lower uterine segment is underdeveloped and narrow. In these cases, a lower-segment vertical incision may be preferable. If, at operation, there is insufficient space for a transverse incision, a vertical incision can be made in the middle of the superior flap to form an inverted "T." The junction joint of both incisions is difficult to close and probably is always weak, so a T incision should be used only as a last resort to deliver the fetus.

If either or both of the ascending uterine arteries at the lateral angles of the incision are torn, they can easily be repaired. The vessels (both artery and veins may be injured) should be temporarily clamped to prevent bleeding, and ligated superior and inferior to the incision with an encircling mattress suture. Removal of the clamps should result in no bleeding. Then the urine incision can be closed in the usual manner. This technique provides far better hemostasis for major vessels than merely trying to stop bleeding by the usual closure of the incision. With upward traction on the uterus, the ureters are far away from the torn vessels so need not be a concern.

In summary, the lower-segment transverse incision is usually ideal for most patients (Table 30.1).

Operative technique

After the abdomen is opened, the peritoneal reflection between the bladder and uterus is identified. A bladder flap is developed to mobilize the loose visceral peritoneum between the bladder and uterus; the peritoneum is picked up about 1 cm below its firm attachment to the uterus and incised laterally toward the round ligaments (Figure 30.1). This step should be carried out under direct vision with a bladder retractor inferiorly and Richardson retractors laterally so that the round ligaments can be seen. Note should be made of any uterine rotation to assist in later extension of the uterine incision.

With the bladder peritoneum grasped with thumb forceps and stretched away from the uterus, blunt finger dissection with the fingertip against the uterine surface is used to separate the posterior surface of the bladder from the anterior surface of the lower uterine segment (Figure 30.2). Sharp dissection may be necessary if the patient has had a previous cesarean delivery; otherwise, blunt finger dissection will usually cause less bleeding.

At this point, any rotation of the uterus is noted and a transverse incision is made in the midline of the uterus. Extension of the incision may be made with bandage scissors or by placing one and then two fingers into the incision and extending it laterally by "tearing" the muscles, since the muscle bundles separate easily (Figure 30.3).

Each method of uterine incision has pros and cons. Cutting the lower uterine segment with bandage scissors allows a precise termination of the lateral margin of the incision, so that there is no injury to major vessels. A

Table 30.1 Advantages, problems, and dangers of lower-segment transverse incision.

- Advantages
    - Incision lies entirely in lower segment
    - Incisional area less vascular than upper segment
    - Lower segment easier to suture than upper
    - Easy to cover incision with bladder peritoneum
    - Technical problems
    - Incision length limited by lateral margins of uterus
        - Problem with premature birth
        - Problem with abnormal presentation
    - Angles may be difficult to suture
- Specific dangers
    - Injury to vessels at lateral margins of uterus
    - Hemorrhage and hematoma at angles

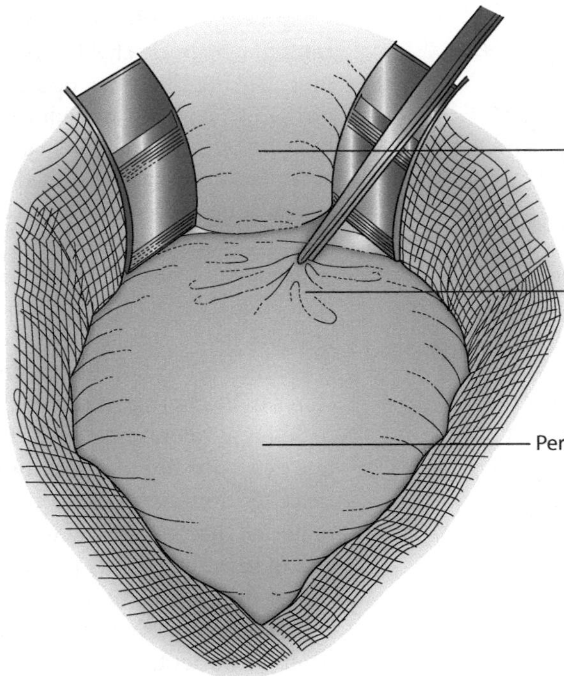

Figure 30.1 Mobilization of bladder flap; peritoneum on the anterior surface of the uterus is picked up just below (caudad) its firm attachment and incised laterally from the midline to each round ligament.

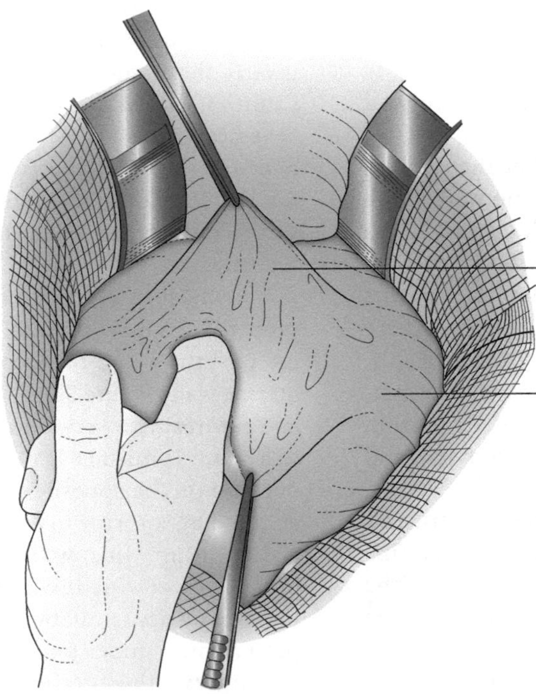

Figure 30.2 Mobilization of bladder flap; the inferior edge of peritoneum is elevated with forceps and put on stretch. Blunt finger dissection separates the peritoneum and bladder from the lower uterine segment.

problem is that several arcuate arteries may run transversely across the uterus, resulting in increased blood loss. Enlarging the initial incision by tearing usually avoids injury to the arcuate arteries. Experience is necessary to enlarge the initial incision symmetrically and yet not tear into the ascending uterine artery and vein. When tearing, it is important to pull toward the fundus of the uterus (cephalad), as well as laterally. This will ensure that the lateral ends of the resulting incision curve upward where the lower uterine segment between the round ligaments is

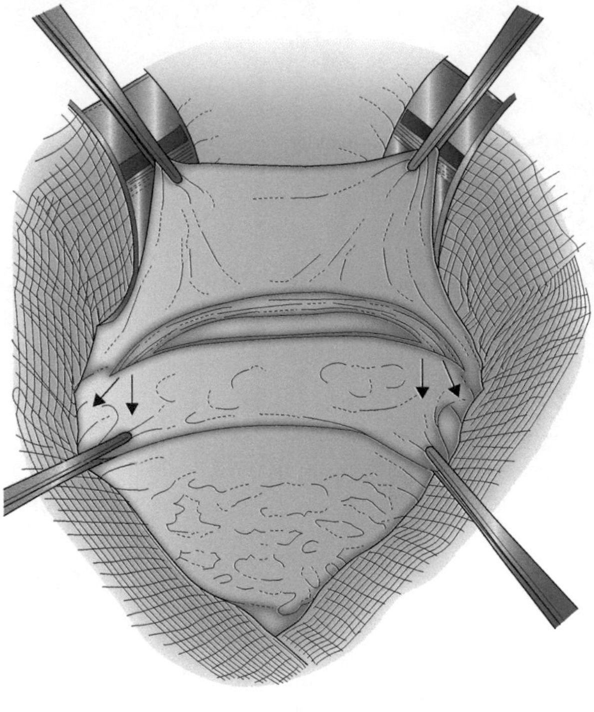

Figure 30.3 Transverse incision into the uterus; after the uterus is opened in the midline by means of a small incision, the opening is enlarged laterally by "tearing" with fingers in a lateral and cephalad direction (arrows).

wider. How well the incision has been made is determined by observation after delivery.

With either method, it is important that the original incision be made through the entire uterine wall. There is a plexus of arteries and veins about one-third of the way through the uterine wall. If the incision is inadvertently enlarged by either blunt or sharp dissection in this plane, it can cause severe hemorrhage. Sometimes, there is concern about injuring the fetus by cutting too deeply. In this case, the lateral margins of the transverse incision can be picked up with Allis clamps after the incision has started to hold the uterine tissue away from the fetal head.

Another method is routinely used by some obstetricians to avoid fetal injury. The central, small, transverse uterine incision is made through almost the entire thickness of the uterine wall. Then a hemostat is used to tease through the remaining few millimeters of uterine wall. When amniotic fluid appears, the incision can be enlarged by either of the previously mentioned techniques.

It is crucial with any cesarean delivery that the uterine incision be large enough for atraumatic delivery. When the delivery is performed to prevent the stress of labor with a fragile premature fetus, it would be absurd to have a traumatic birth because the incisions were too small. The incision must not be extended so far laterally as to injure arteries and veins, but if it seems too small for atraumatic birth, the incision can be enlarged by incising vertically in the center of the superior flap to create an inverted T.

Immediately after delivery but before the placenta separates, the operative field is usually bloodless for a few minutes. During this time, operative bleeding from the edges of the incision can be reduced by mobilizing the uterine incision with T and Allis clamps and beginning the closure. T clamps can be placed at the angles of the incision and at other areas where bleeding is active. Traditionally, the placenta is removed first and then suturing begins. Alternatively several sutures could be placed beginning immediately from the angle before the placenta separates and the field becomes covered with blood (Figure 30.4). After the removal of the placenta, the suturing of the incision can be continued rapidly.

Some surgeons exteriorize the uterus, which may facilitate exposure and may result in a quicker repair. However, there is some evidence that exteriorization increases maternal discomfort and nausea, but does not increase the risk of infection.[26] This point is controversial.

The uterus can be closed in a single layer, a method which decreases operating time.[27] However, it is not clear whether patients who have a single-layer closure are at increased risk of complications during the next pregnancy compared with those who undergo a two-layer closure.

To close the uterus in two layers, a continuous running suture is used. Care must be taken to avoid the endometrium and to invert the two flaps so that both edges of the myometrium are juxtaposed (Figure 30.5). After one again inverts the tissue, a second line of continuous running sutures is placed to cover the first one. When suture lines have been placed properly, the first is covered by the second, and the only sutures visible are the ties at each angle for the second layer. Some operators utilize a Lembert suture rather than a continuous running suture for the second layer.

Care must be given to suturing the angles of the uterus properly. The most common mistake is to neglect the uterine curvature and thus not suture perpendicular to the uterine wall (Figure 30.6). This may result in vessel injury and sutures with very little myometrium tissue. It is easy to avoid this mistake if each angle suture is placed by the operator on the opposite side of the table, and the incision is closed by suturing to the midline.

The suture line will become loose in a few days because of uterine involution. The aspect of healing in the face of tissue catabolism and involution is normally present only under one circumstance in the entire field of surgery—the uterine incision of cesarean section! This raises the point of continuous compared with interrupted sutures for uterine closure. Poidevin's work in the 1960s[36] seemed to show that there is less chance of a uterine scar defect if interrupted sutures are used. This would seem logical, yet, few operators ever use interrupted sutures. With the emphasis on vaginal birth after a previous section, this entire area of investigation should possibly be renewed.

Factors that may affect the strength of the closure also need to be studied. These include choice of suture material,

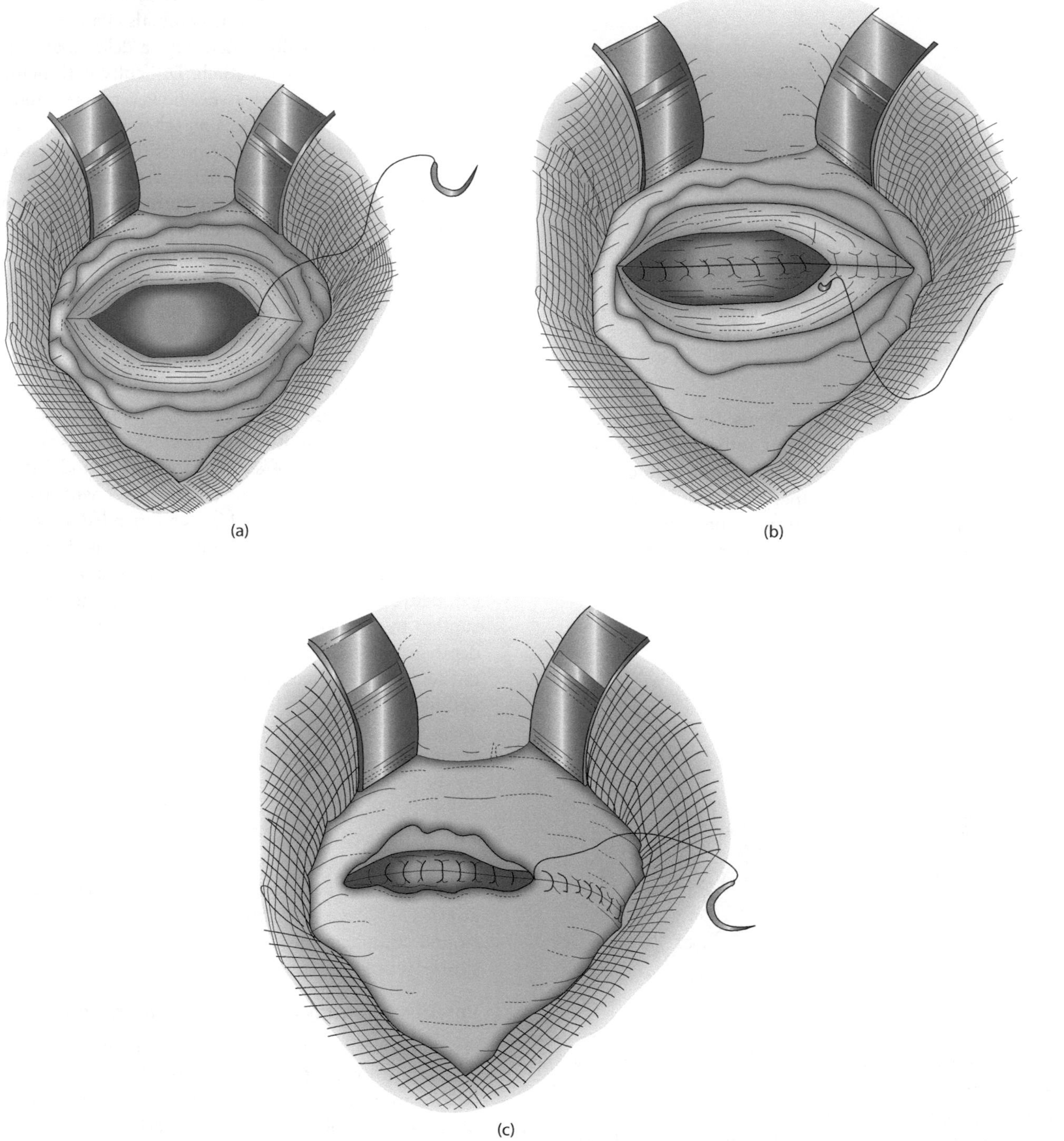

(a) (b) (c)

Figure 30.4 Closing the uterus; a low-segment transverse incision is usually closed in two layers. Care is taken to place angle sutures lateral to the apex of the incision and approximate myometrium (a). The second layer should cover the first suture line (b). The peritoneum is closed so that the lower flap covers the incision (c).

closure technique, and presence of postoperative infection. In women contemplating subsequent pregnancies, the surgeon should consider using a polyglactin suture and/or a double layer closure.

Since vascular muscle tissue is easily torn, suturing the uterus may be difficult. A fairly heavy suture with a large diameter is best (no. 1–0 or 0) because it will not cut through the muscle even though it is tied snugly. The diameter of the heavy suture, rather than its strength, is the critical factor. To avoid tearing apart or cutting through the myometrial fibers, each bite should be large enough so that the suture gets a good purchase on the tissue. When bleeding points remain after the second row of sutures, they can best be controlled by figure-of-8 stitches over the site tied snugly but not tightly. The sutures should be placed away from,

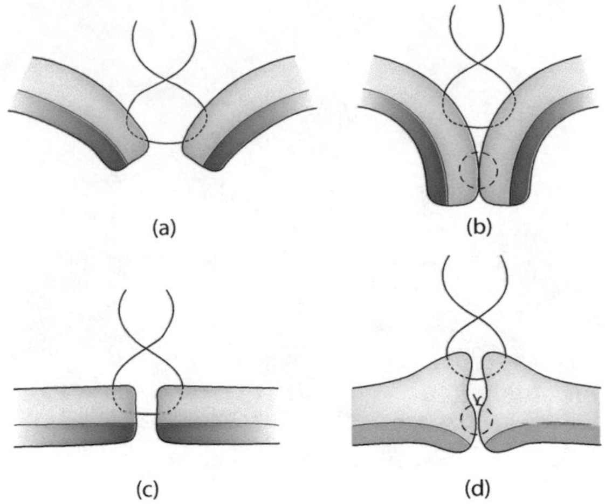

Figure 30.5 Suturing the uterus; the uterus should be sutured so that the myometrium, rather than the endometrium, is approximated and that the second suture line covers the first. The uterine tissue, therefore, should be inverted—panels (a) and (b) show how this can be accomplished even when the uterine wall is thin; (c) and (d) show the technique when the two edges are thicker.

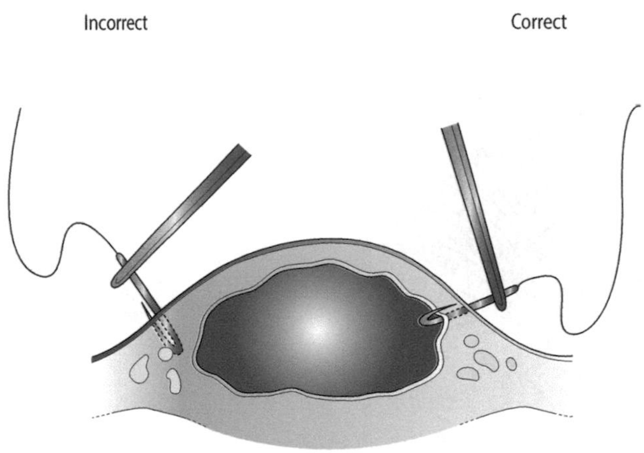

Figure 30.6 Suturing the angles; the lower uterine segment is convex after birth, although the peritoneum on the anterior surface of the broad ligament makes it appear flat. Care must be taken, therefore, to place angle sutures into the uterine muscle rather than into the peritoneum and vessels at the lateral margins.

but still around, the bleeding site and tied to compress the tissue.

Closure of the peritoneal bladder flap or the parietal peritoneum is not generally performed, as there is no conclusive evidence that such closure has benefits such as reduction in infectious morbidity, analgesia requirements, or bowel function. The effect on adhesion formation is unclear. Discordant results have been reported[28–31]; thus, if the peritoneum is closed to prevent adhesions, it should be done by a fine 3:0 suture. Intra-abdominal irrigation does not reduce maternal morbidity beyond the reduction achieved with preoperative prophylactic antimicrobials alone.[32]

The fascia is typically closed with a delayed-absorbable suture using a continuous stitch. Difficulty with hemostasis is usually not a major issue; however, care should be taken to avoid too much tension when closing the fascia: Approximation, not strangulation, is the appropriate goal. A delayed-absorbable monofilament (such as polydiaxanone [PDS] or polyglyconate) or permanent monofilament suture (such as polypropylene or polybutester) is recommended for patients at high risk of fascial dehiscence, especially with a vertical incision. These patients include those who are obese, diabetic, immunosuppressed, or undernourished, as well as women with a history of prior fascial herniation. A running Smead-Jones closure can be considered in such cases to enhance the tensile strength of the incision.[33]

Appropriate antimicrobial use, careful handling of tissue,[34] and judicious use of electrical cautery appear to decrease the risk of seroma formation and infection. Closure of the subcutaneous adipose layer with plain catgut suture is also helpful and is recommended if the layer is deep. This was illustrated by a meta-analysis showing that suture closure of the subcutaneous adipose layer at cesarean delivery decreased the risk of subsequent wound disruption by one-third in women with subcutaneous tissue depth greater than 2 cm but not less than 2 cm.[35,36] Closure of the dead space seems to inhibit accumulation of serum and blood, which can lead to a wound seroma and subsequent wound breakdown. This occurrence is a major cause of morbidity, can be costly, and lengthens the recovery time for the patient.

Finally, reapproximation of the skin may be performed with staples or suture.[44] If the skin incision was transverse, the staples may be removed in about 3–5 days. If a vertical incision was performed, the staples are left in place for at least 5–7 days, and longer in a patient at high risk of wound complications, since there is more tension on the skin edges of a vertical incision.

Vascular anatomy and uterine hemorrhage control

A major contributing factor in uterine hemorrhage control is lack of knowledge about the vascular anatomy. Several factors are important to keep in mind. The uterus is supplied by four major arteries—two uterine and two ovarian. To shut off all blood flow, one would need to ligate all four arteries, as well as the two ascending vaginal branches of the pudendal arteries. In addition, arterial anastomoses are such that the uterus should be considered as one system in equilibrium. Blood freely flows from one area or one vessel to any other vessel. Arcuate arteries originate from the uterine arteries at the lateral margins and course around the uterus (back and front) with multiple anastomoses in the midline.

From an operative point of view, this means that a bleeding point is best controlled by placing fairly deep mattress sutures around the site of hemorrhage, since ligation of a specific vessel is often impossible. These sutures should be placed about 1 cm away from the bleeding site.

If there is injury to the uterine arteries or veins along the lateral margin of the uterus, all the vessels in the area can be safely ligated.

To control bleeding, a horizontal mattress suture may be placed that passes through the uterine muscle and around the vessels. A large suture (no. 1–0) should be used so that it can be tied snugly and still not cut through the muscle. A suture is placed above and below the injury, and these two sutures should control all bleeding in the ascending vessels. Any attempt to dissect and ligate vessels individually will produce more tissue injury and hemorrhage.

The risk of extensive uterine injury or extension of the incision into the uterine vessels is usually low; only 1%–2% of all patients having cesarean deliveries require blood transfusion.[41] Hemorrhage may be due to uterine atony, placenta accreta, or lacerated vessels. Lacerations extending into the lateral vagina and broad ligament should be evaluated carefully and repaired with meticulous attention to the position of the ureter.

Lower segment vertical cesarean delivery

A vertical uterine incision is still sometimes utilized for cesarean deliveries and in some instances has clear advantages over the transverse incision (Table 30.2). The vertical incision can be enlarged easily, since its length is not limited by vital structures such as the major vessels on the lateral margin of the uterus. It is useful for the delivery of premature infants because it is not limited by the size of the lower uterine segment. With abnormal presentations, such as breech or transverse, these advantages are significant.

There are also some disadvantages. The lower-uterine segment is short, unless the patient has been in labor, and, without due care, the bladder may be injured in making the uterine incision or from extension during birth. Moreover, with a short lower segment, it may be necessary to continue the incision into the upper segment. Because muscle in this area must be incised rather than separated, the vertical incision may be more vascular than the transverse one and potentially bleed more.

Operative technique

The procedure is started the same way as the lower-segment transverse procedure. The peritoneum between uterus and bladder is picked up just below its firm attachment to the uterus and incised transversely toward the round ligaments. Blunt dissection is used to separate the bladder from the uterus. A small incision is made through the uterine wall in the midline after noting any rotation of the uterus. Large bandage scissors are used to extend this incision. First, the incision is extended downward to a point 1 or 2 cm above the bladder reflection (Figure 30.7). This is a critical distance because, if the incision is carried to the reflection, the bladder may be injured when the baby is born. Then, with bandage scissors, the incision is extended upward to a length sufficient for delivery.

If only the lower segment is involved, closure is done with two layers of running sutures.

Table 30.2 Advantages, problems, and dangers of the lower-segment vertical incision.

Advantages	
	Lower-segment incision
	Incision easy to outline
	Incision length not limited
Technical problems	
	Extensive bladder dissection
	Upper-segment extension
	Upper segment difficult to suture specific dangers
	Bladder injury from extension
	Poor scar in upper-segment extension

Classical cesarean delivery

There are few indications for the classical operation in contemporary obstetrics. In this operation, the entire uterine incision is placed in the upper segment, so structures over the bladder should not be disturbed (Table 30.3).

Pregnant women with invasive carcinoma of the cervix should have a classical delivery in order to avoid areas potentially involved with tumor. Other indications may be a major degree of placenta previa or placenta accreta, when the operator wishes to avoid cutting through the placenta attached to the lower segment or neglected transverse lie, or possibly a transverse lie with the back turned downward. A classical delivery might be desirable after previous vesico-vaginal fistula repair when there are extensive bladder adhesions to the uterus, and in some cases of

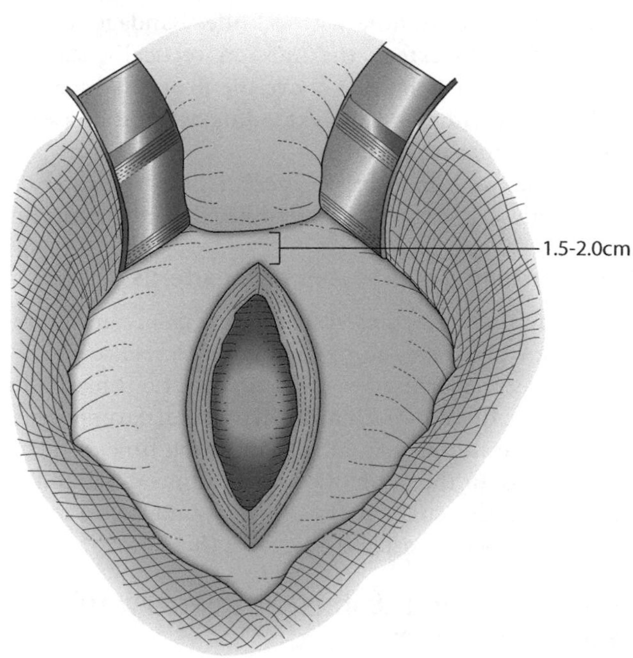

Figure 30.7 Uterine incision with lower-segment vertical section; the uterus is opened by making a small incision in the midline. This incision is extended downward to a point 1–2 cm above the bladder reflection. This will help ensure that the bladder is not injured as the fetus is delivered.

Table 30.3 Advantages, problems, and dangers of classical cesarean incision.

Advantages	
	Cervix and bladder not dissected (carcinoma of the cervix, fistulas)
	No limitation in uterine incision length
Technical problems	
	Closing incision difficult
	Vascular incision hemorrhage
Specific dangers	
	Poor uterine closure
	Subsequent uterine rupture
	Adhesion of bowel to incision wound, postoperative ileus

uterine sacculation. The advantage to the procedure is that the operative field avoids the bladder and the lower segment. Since the lower segment vertical incision can always be extended superiorly for exposure, there is little indication for a classical cesarean delivery today unless there is a cogent need to exclude the entire lower segment from the operative site. The classical cesarean operation has several disadvantages. An incision in the upper part of the uterus is more likely to rupture in a subsequent pregnancy than one in the lower segment, and such ruptures tend to occur prior to the onset of labor.

Operative technique

Technically, opening the uterus is less difficult than a low vertical section. The uterus is incised through its full thickness in the midline with a knife. Bandage scissors may be used to extend the incision vertically, starting from an inferior point just above the firm attachment of the bladder peritoneum and extending as far as necessary to provide exposure for birth.

After delivery, the uterine incision must be carefully closed with several layers of interrupted or running sutures.

Extraperitoneal approaches to the uterus

Physick first described extra-peritoneal cesarean delivery more than 150 years ago in an attempt to reduce mortality.[37] It was mainly used to decrease infectious morbidity at that time; this approach has fallen into disfavor because of its technical difficulty, longer operating time, and lack of advantage in the antibiotic era, and thus it will not be discussed in this chapter. Those who are interested in this topic should see the second edition of this book.

TECHNICAL COMPLICATIONS ASSOCIATED WITH CESAREAN DELIVERY

Adherent bladder

Unless the patient has had a previous cesarean delivery, there is usually an excellent cleavage plane between the uterus and bladder, and bladder mobilization is easy. However, bladder dissection may be a problem if there is scarring from a previous cesarean section or if there are varicosities on the surface of the uterus or bladder. If blunt dissection is used to mobilize the bladder, these veins, which are friable, often rupture. An avascular cleavage plane usually exists between the two structures, but sharp dissection must often be employed for this mobilization (Figure 30.8). This is not difficult technically, if the bladder is picked up with a tissue forceps and placed on a stretch away from the uterus to expose the vesicouterine plane. Since sharp dissection is not difficult for one with experience, the surgeon should be competent in the technique so that it can be utilized when blunt dissection would be impossible.

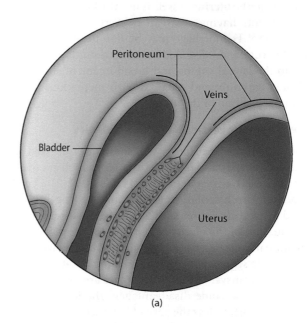

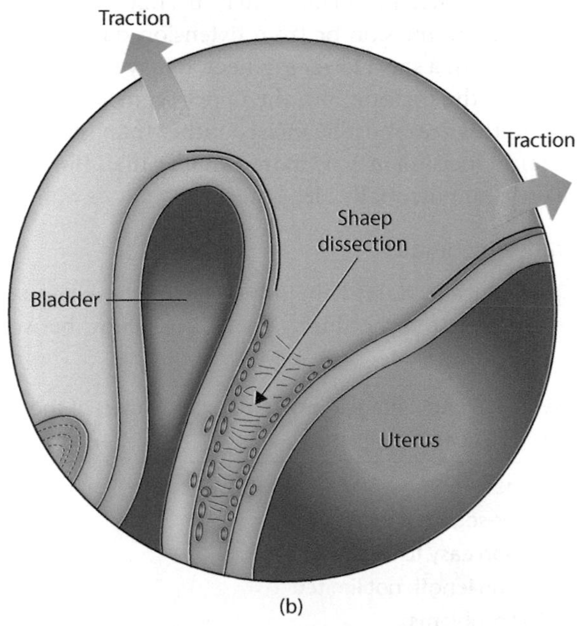

Figure 30.8 Sharp dissection of adherent bladder; there is an avascular, fascial cleavage plane between bladder and uterus that can be identified if the bladder and uterus are separated by traction on both at a 60° angle. The plane for sharp dissection lies halfway between the two organs.

One last resort would be an intentional bladder dome cystotomy to help delineate the bladder from the uterus and therefore perform a clean, sharp dissection. This approach would prevent multiple, small serosal or muscularis, or full-thickness injuries during a difficult dissection and thus decrease the risk of vesicouterine fistula formation.

Placental obstruction at cesarean delivery

Sometimes the placenta is encountered upon opening the uterus when performing a cesarean delivery. This occurs in the following two situations: (1) with a classical section, when the placenta is on the anterior wall of the uterus; (2) with a low cervical delivery done for placenta previa.

The management of this problem is controversial. Many operators cut through the placenta, but this opens the fetal circulation, and even a small amount of fetal bleeding may be dangerous. The umbilical cord should be clamped immediately if the placenta is incised. Perhaps a safer procedure is to push the placenta to the side or actually remove it first. There is more maternal bleeding, but it is less dangerous to the infant than fetal hemorrhage.

Difficulties in delivering the fetus

There may be difficulty in delivering the fetal head if it has become tightly wedged into the mid-pelvis after prolonged labor. In this situation, someone in the operating theater can provide upward pressure on the head by inserting two fingers from a sterile gloved hand in the vagina. If this difficulty is expected, preparation for this maneuver should be made in advance. In addition, the operator can push his or her hand down into the pelvis between the fetal head and the symphysis, elevate the head and deliver it from the uterus. Some obstetricians use forceps or a vacuum extractor to help deliver the head. Difficulties with fetal delivery can arise with breech or transverse presentations. It is helpful to remember that the inferior pole of the fetus must be delivered first through any lower uterine segment incision, but the superior pole may come first through a classical incision.

Incision into the vagina

One important question for the surgeon at cesarean delivery is where to make the transverse incision into the uterus. If it is too high, it may be near the thicker upper muscular uterine segment. An incision that is low is not usually a problem. However, incisions have actually been made into the vagina rather than the uterus.[45] In such cases, the patients had been in the second stage of labor for several hours, and the cesarean delivery was done for disproportion. The lower uterine segment was thin and the bladder was easily mobilized. However, once the anatomy is recognized after delivery, the repair is usually easy and patients have uneventful recovery.

A somewhat similar situation may arise in the event of sacculation of the uterus. In this event, both the vagina and the bladder may be drawn up as high as the level of the navel. The uterine incision under such circumstances is likely to involve both the bladder and the vagina. This complication is to be suspected when the cervix is high in the vaginal canal and cannot be reached by the examining finger during pelvic examination. When diagnosed in advance, inadvertent placement of the incision and thus injury of the bladder and vagina can be avoided by utilizing a higher midline skin incision in anticipation of a uterine entry at or above the level of the umbilicus.

Fetal monitoring at cesarean delivery

Electronic fetal monitoring is commonplace in labor and delivery units and is particularly necessary in high-risk pregnancies or at times when there is a category II or III tracing. The most effective way to monitor prior to cesarean is a subject of much concern and discussion. Often there is a hiatus in fetal monitoring from the time when the electrode is removed until the time when the baby is born. This time interval should be minimized, but time may be lost in preparing and draping the patient. Sometimes, after draping, a regional anesthetic will not be satisfactory and the anesthesiologist will recommend waiting for a few more minutes. The result is that the fetus is not monitored at a potentially crucial time.

Certain procedures may prevent this problem:

- If an internal scalp electrode if applied, may be left on until the head is delivered at section; then the wire is cut and pulled out vaginally.
- Regional anesthesia is checked while the external monitor is applied prior to draping.
- A clock is started when the external or internal electrode is removed, and the obstetrician is notified about time.

Obstetric conditions affecting cesarean delivery

Certain obstetric conditions affect cesarean delivery from a technical point of view; the clinician should understand the pathophysiology and be prepared. In addition to being an indicator for section, placenta previa may complicate the procedure. There is less myometrium in the thinned-out lower segment, and since muscular contraction is the basis of uterine hemostasis postpartum, there may be severe uncontrolled hemorrhage with placenta previa. Sometimes one can visualize large vessels that may be covered only with peritoneum and endometrium. If seen, these vessels can be ligated with sutures running through the entire thickness of the uterine wall if necessary. There is such an abundance of the uterine blood supply that a small area of the wall can be isolated to control hemorrhage without fear. If the placental site is denuded of myometrium and mattress sutures may not stop bleeding, internal iliac ligation or even hysterectomy may be necessary.

There is controversy about the management of abruptio placentae at cesarean delivery. Traditionally, it was said that hysterectomy was necessary when there was bleeding into the myometrium (Couvelaire uterus). It is now known that most of the time the Couvelaire uterus contracts well and that removal is rarely necessary. This is common sense because Couvelaire uterus is diagnosed only at cesarean delivery, although it must occur and remain undiagnosed in patients who give birth vaginally with a placenta abruption. The critical point with abruption is whether or not the uterus contracts sufficiently to provide hemostasis after delivery.

This raises another point of uterine physiology: A uterus may contract well after it is sutured and yet remain flaccid as long as the incision is open. With uterine atony, a further operation would be valid only after oxytocics medication had been utilized and the uterus had been closed. This physiologic fact is the counterpart of the observation that when cesarean delivery is performed for tetanic contraction, the uterus often relaxes as soon as the incision is made.

Finally, abnormal placental adherence such as placenta accreta may complicate a cesarean section. In this situation, there is no cleavage plane between placenta and uterus. As a result, the placenta cannot be removed without injury to the myometrium with resulting hemorrhage. When the condition involves more than a minor area of attachment, hysterectomy is indicated. A multidisciplinary approach in the management of placenta accreta involving obstetricians, anesthesiologists, radiologists is recommended. In selected patients who feel that another pregnancy is important, one might consider leaving the placenta in place, suturing bleeding sites with mattress sutures, and using drugs such as methotrexate to promote placental death. However, the risks of this approach are considerable and unacceptable to most patients.[38]

Cesarean delivery in the obese patient

Obese women are at an increased risk of needing a cesarean delivery. This may be related to a higher incidence of pregnancy complications necessitating induction of labor or soft tissue dystocia in the maternal pelvis.[39,40] In one large, prospective study, the cesarean delivery rates in primigravid women with first-trimester body mass index of <30 (controls), 30–34.9 (obese group), and >35 (morbidly obese group) were 21%, 34%, and 47%, respectively.[40]

The optimal surgical approach for the morbidity obese patient is not clear. A high (supraumbilical) transverse incision is one option, as it has the strength of the transverse repair, avoids burying the incision under a large panniculus, and affords excellent exposure. However, may not be safer than a low transverse incision.[41] The supraumbilical incision is often anatomically directly over the lower uterine segment because the large pannus draws the umbilicus caudally.

Although the Pfannenstiel incision is sometimes unsatisfactory because it provides limited exposure even in the thin patient, Cherney's modification provides excellent exposure. If any of the transverse incisions are chosen, the upper flap can be turned back upon itself and suspended with skin clips so that it is held entirely out of the operative field.

Another contributing factor to wound infections in the obese patient is subcutaneous bleeding or serous oozing. Closure of the subcutaneous fat tissue with 3:0 plain catgut has been shown to decrease seroma formation by one-third.

For the prevention of thromboembolic complications in obese patients, the prophylactic use of heparin perioperatively is usually indicated. Weight-based dosing of enoxaparin for venous thromboembolism prophylaxis following cesarean delivery may be more effective in achieving adequate anti-Xa concentrations; its use may be considered in the obese population.[42,43]

Remote effects of cesarean delivery

There are some short- and long-term sequelae to cesarean delivery. An enormous physical effort is required to care for a newborn during the first few months of life. When a woman is also recovering from major surgery, the difficulty is compounded. A protracted convalescence is expected. Woman delivered by cesarean also must take care of a baby. In the presence of a chronic illness, she is under tremendous stress during the postpartum period. Some patients with chronic cardiac disease remain compensated with protected care during pregnancy but promptly go into circulatory failure after returning home with the baby.

The average blood loss at delivery is about twice as great with cesarean delivery as with a vaginal birth and there is a higher incidence of transfusion and hence of transfusion-related complications.

One long-term consequence of cesarean delivery is a high likelihood of future repeat operations and the fact that these operations may be increasingly difficult. Once delivered abdominally, many women will have repeat operations for subsequent pregnancies. After cesarean, there is an increased chance of uterine rupture, which may result in fetal death and frequently requires hysterectomy. Cesarean delivery, therefore, can compromise long-term childbearing ability.

Certain complications of cesarean delivery can lead to other operations. Adhesions and pelvic pain may necessitate exploratory celiotomy. An incisional hernia can require a second operation years after the first one. Cesarean delivery can make a subsequent operation more problematic. There may be difficulty in dissection of the bladder from the cervix, and there is an increased possibility of bladder injury. In the presence of a weak scar, the risk of uterine perforation during dilation and curettage, or other methods of induced abortion, increases. The risk of placenta implantation abnormalities, such as accreta, increta, and percreta, is also increased with each cesarean delivery. Because cesarean delivery can have deleterious long-term consequences, it should be performed only when there is a valid indication.

Postoperative infection

The most common infections after cesarean are endometritis (endomyometritis), urinary tract infection, respiratory tract infection, wound infection, septic pelvic thrombophlebitis, and rarely pelvic abscess.

The most frequent postoperative infection after cesarean delivery is endometritis. The risk of postoperative endometritis after cesarean delivery is 35%–40% in the absence of prophylactic antibiotics.[44] This rate is as low as 4%–5% after scheduled cesarean delivery with intact membranes and as high as 85% after an extended labor with ruptured membranes without prophylactic antimicrobials.[43] Prophylactic antibiotics reduce the overall rate of infection by approximately 60%.[45]

The classical definition of febrile morbidity is an elevated oral temperature of 100.4°F (38°C) or more on two occasions at least 6 hours apart from day 2 to day 10 postpartum. However, it is recognized that postpartum day 1 should not be excluded from this definition, since some organisms, such as group B b-hemolytic streptococcus, tend to cause temperature elevation within the first 12–24 hours of cesarean delivery. The patient who satisfies the definition of febrile morbidity after cesarean delivery must be examined completely for any other focus of infection or atelectasis. Typical findings of endometritis include uterine and abdominal tenderness; but these are "soft" signs of infection, since a recent, normal postcesarean patient would also be expected to have a tender uterus and abdomen. Therefore, the most important aspect of the diagnosis of endometritis is that it is a diagnosis by exclusion of other causes of febrile morbidity.

Risk factors for endometritis are listed in Table 30.4. However, the most important risk factor is the mode of delivery. Patients delivered by cesarean are 10–20 times more likely to develop infection than those with similar risk factors delivered vaginally.

The standard laboratory workup for endometritis includes a complete blood count with differential, blood, urine, and endocervical specimens for culture; and blood urea nitrogen and serum creatinine. The causative organisms of endometritis are multiple and the infection is considered polymicrobial. The more common pathogens include peptococcus and peptostreptococci, group B b-hemolytic streptococcus, *Escherichia coli*, and the *Bacteroides* group of organisms. Approximately 10%–14% of patients with endometritis after cesarean delivery also have an associated bacteremia. If the group B b-hemolytic streptococcus is determined to be the causative organism, the pediatrician should be notified, since this organism may cause devastating, fulminant neonatal sepsis.

Antimicrobial therapy for endometritis after cesarean delivery should include a broad-spectrum antibiotic appropriate for a polymicrobial infection. Standard therapy is clindamycin and gentamicin, but other antibiotics are also effective as a single-agent therapy. A suggested scheme is seen in Table 30.5. Patients treated for endometritis with appropriate antibiotics should show improvement within 48 hours. A worsening of the clinical condition as determined by clinical examination, increasing white blood cell count, and so on requires a reevaluation of the patient. If available, the bacteriology reports from previously obtained culture specimens should guide further antibiotic therapy. If the initial antibiotic regimen included clindamycin and gentamicin, the addition of ampicillin for enterococcal coverage is prescribed. If the initial antibiotic coverage was an extended-spectrum penicillin, such as Timentin, Unasyn, Zosyn, or a cephalosporin, the addition of an aminoglycoside is appropriate. It is advisable to obtain peak and trough serum values to guide aminoglycoside dosage if gentamicin is prescribed every 8 hours. Alternatively, gentamicin may be prescribed once a day at a dose of 5 mg/kg body weight per day with no need to obtain peak and trough serum levels.

A small percentage of patients with endometritis will fail to respond to the adjusted antibiotic therapy. This group of patients should be evaluated for septic pelvic thrombophlebitis and/or a pelvic abscess. A heparin challenge test may be prescribed in these cases along with the triple antibiotic regimen of clindamycin, gentamicin, and ampicillin. If septic pelvic thrombophlebitis is present, the patient usually responds rather rapidly to heparin. The dose of heparin should be adjusted so that the partial thromboplastin time (PTT) is approximately 1.5–2 times normal. If the patient fails to respond to triple antibiotics and heparin, one should search for other causes such as pelvic abscess or wound infection. Reexamination of the patient and appropriate diagnostic tests, including pelvic sonography and computed tomography (CT) should be ordered if appropriate. Should an abscess or wound infection be present, drainage is usually required.

Table 30.4 Risk factors for endometritis.

Cesarean delivery
Prolonged duration of labor
Prolonged duration of rupture of membranes
Frequent pelvic examination intrapartum
Obesity
Internal uterine monitoring

Cesarean hysterectomy

Indications for cesarean hysterectomy are relatively rare except as an emergency lifesaving procedure. The most common indication is intractable uterine bleeding that cannot be controlled by other, more conventional means.

Table 30.5 Antimicrobial therapy for post-cesarean endometritis.

- Clindamycin 900 mg every 8 hours and gentamicin 3–5 mg/kg body weight per day IV or IM divided every 8 hours *or* gentamicin 5–7 mg/kg body weight IV every 24 hours
- Cefoxitin 1–2 g IV or IM every 6 hours (or equivalent cephalosporin)
- Ticarcillin and clavulanate (Timentin®) 3.1 g IV every 4–6 hours
- Ampicillin plus sulbactam (Unasyn®) 1.5–3 g IV or IM every 6 hours
- Piperacillin plus tazobactam (Zosyn®) 3.375–4.5 g IV every 6 hours
- Ertapenem (Invanz®) 1 g IV or IM every 24 hours

Severe forms of placenta previa sometimes necessitate hysterectomy. When the placenta is implanted upon the thin lower segment, there may be too little muscle to provide uterine hemostasis after birth. In these cases, the operation is particularly difficult because the tissues around the cervix are even more vascular than they are with a normal pregnancy. Placenta accreta (increta, percreta) may also coexist with placenta previa, necessitating hysterectomy. This complication should always be kept in mind when the placenta fails to separate easily or in patients who are having repeat cesarean delivery with an anterior low placenta.

Another indication for cesarean hysterectomy is rupture of the uterus. However, the uterus sometimes may be saved if the patient is anxious to have more children, and conservative surgery is possible technically, since the uterus can function even after major operations. Some other conditions provide valid indications for hysterectomy but do not occur commonly. Large uterine myomas are one example. There may be an indication for cesarean hysterectomy in cases of severe uterine infection not responsive to antimicrobials.

For the purpose of sterilization, cesarean hysterectomy is a more extensive and potentially morbid procedure than section and tubal ligation. Thus, only in association with other indications for removal of the uterus can cesarean hysterectomy be considered as the procedure of choice.

Technically, the cesarean hysterectomy proceeds as any other cesarean section until after the baby is born. Thereafter, the same principles of abdominal hysterectomy apply with certain particularities that emerge from the gravid uterus and the emergent situation. Usually, the uterus is closed quickly in one layer to attempt to decrease blood loss so one could move on with the hysterectomy. The pelvic tissues are usually edematous and "rough" application of clamps may cause tearing. The uterus is usually exteriorized and placed under tension. Then the round ligaments are divided first, followed by the cornual region of the fallopian tubes and the utero-ovarian ligaments. Next, the uterine vessels are skeletonized and the bladder is dissected off the lower uterine segment and the cervix, utilizing sharp or blunt dissection as appropriate. As the uterus enlarges during pregnancy, it stretches the broad ligaments, so that there is considerable slack immediately postpartum. This change in anatomic configuration makes it easy to clamp the broad ligament more laterally than usual during cesarean hysterectomy and thus to potentially endanger the ureter (Figures 30.4 and 30.9).

Supracervical hysterectomy is preferred whenever possible in this setting due to its decreased morbidity in a patient

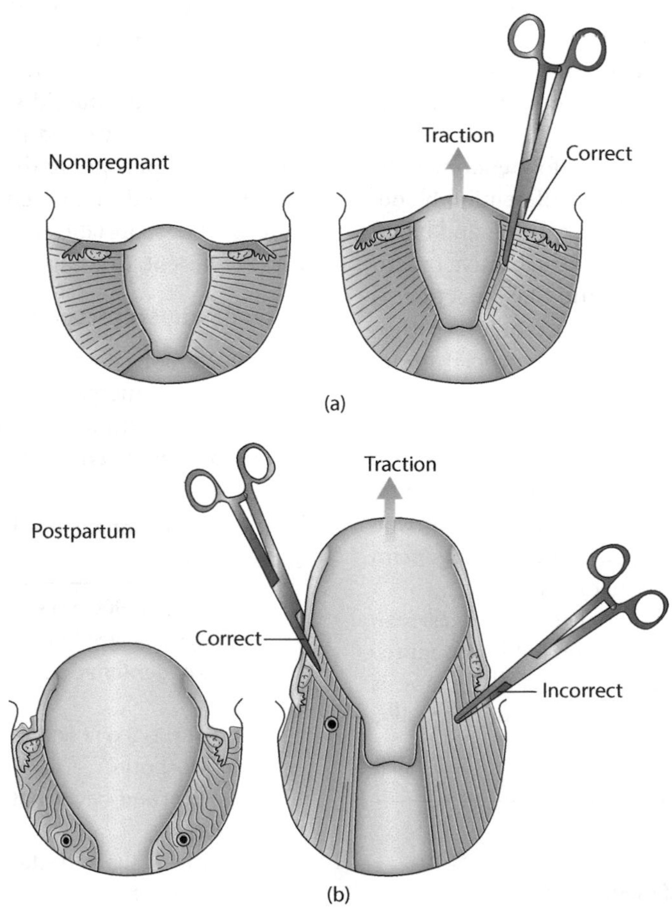

Figure 30.9 Instead of being taut (a), the broad ligaments are slack (b), allowing inadvertent placement of clamps to endanger vital structures.

who is already hemodynamically compromised and unstable. In this case, the uterosacral ligaments are identified and the uterus amputated above their level. If total hysterectomy is needed because of placenta previa, placenta accreta, cervical lesions, bleeding from the cervix, and so on, the next problem is identifying the boundary between cervix and vagina and attaining vaginal hemostasis (Figure 30.10). Cervical boundaries are difficult to determine after advanced labor when the cervix is very thin. However, they can be identified by pinching the upper vagina between thumb and forefinger, moving the hand superiorly, and determining where the cervix extends into the vagina. Another method involves palpating the inside of the vagina to identify the cervical lip. The vagina is entered after the cervix is identified and incised with scissors. A last resort would be empirically to transect the tissue 0.5–1 cm below the lower edge of the uterosacral ligaments insertion.

The postpartum vagina is always vascular and heavy bleeding may ensue. Usually, this can be controlled by temporary application of ring forceps. If not, figure-of-8 sutures can be placed in the vaginal cuff as it is incised. Care must be taken to identify both ureters if total hysterectomy is undertaken.

OPERATIVE COMPLICATIONS

Injury to the urinary tract

Urinary tract injuries are uncommon with cesarean delivery, occurring in approximately 1% of cesarean deliveries. When recognized during the operation, most are easily repaired and the "cure rate" is excellent.

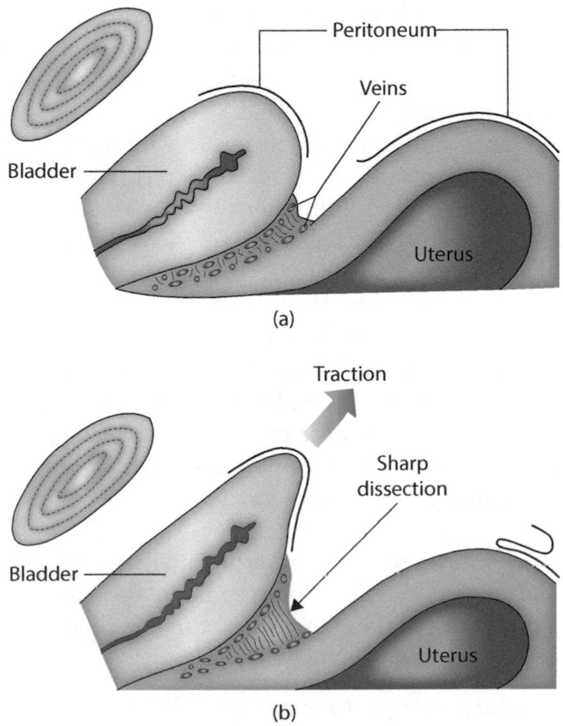

Figure 30.10 With bladder and uterine varicosities (a), sharp dissection (b) is mandatory to separate the structures without bleeding.

Bladder injuries

Bladder injuries are at times almost inevitable. Risk factors include previous pelvic surgery such as previous cesarean delivery and cesarean hysterectomy. Another problem is that there may be marked engorgement of the veins on both the bladder and the uterus. These veins rupture easily, requiring the operator to dissect in a bloody field. When these anatomic variations are combined with the necessity for haste in delivering a potentially compromised fetus, it is apparent that an unavoidable laceration of the bladder is more probable.

It is important to make a firm diagnosis and to outline the extent of the injury. A finger inserted through the laceration can do this. It is a mistake to begin suturing the rent before its extent has been assessed. When there is any doubt about bladder injury, methylene blue dye in normal saline or sterile milk can be instilled into the bladder through the indwelling Foley catheter. Either of the two will quickly identify the point of leakage, but milk has the added advantage that it can be used repeatedly, so the bladder can be tested again after the repair.

Sometimes only the muscularis layer of the bladder is injured and the mucosa is intact. These injuries may not be identified unless the bladder is filled with fluid (100–200 ml). Identification is important as fistulas may ensue if the muscularis is not oversewn and if the bladder is not immobilized postoperatively. This type of injury is easily repaired with a fine suture such as 2:0 or 3:0 Vicryl, or 2:0 or 3:0 chromic suture.

Basically, repair of bladder injuries involves inverting the tissue with two layers of sutures and immobilizing the bladder postoperatively. The suture lines should be free from tension. When fistulas develop after primary injuries that have been diagnosed and repaired it is almost always because the sutures have been placed under tension (Figure 30.11). Before suturing, the bladder should be mobilized for 1.5–2.0 cm all around the injury so that there is sufficient tissue to invert (Figure 30.11). Two layers of continuous running suture, such as 2:0 Vicryl or 2:0 chromic suture, are used to close the defect. The bladder should be immobilized for 7–10 days with catheter drainage. If the laceration is well sutured without tension and the bladder is immobilized, there is little risk of fistula formation.

Usually, abdominal drains are not needed, but if they are present, there is no problem if some urine leaks through the repair. The problem occurs when there is leakage and no drain. If the operator is not absolutely sure that there is no leakage, it is safer to use drains.

Ureteral injuries

See the section on "Ureteral injury" in Chapter 37.

Intestinal injuries

Injuries to the large and small bowel are uncommon with cesarean delivery. Most patients are young and have had few previous operations, and the adhesions from previous sections are anterior to the uterus. Bowel is uncommonly

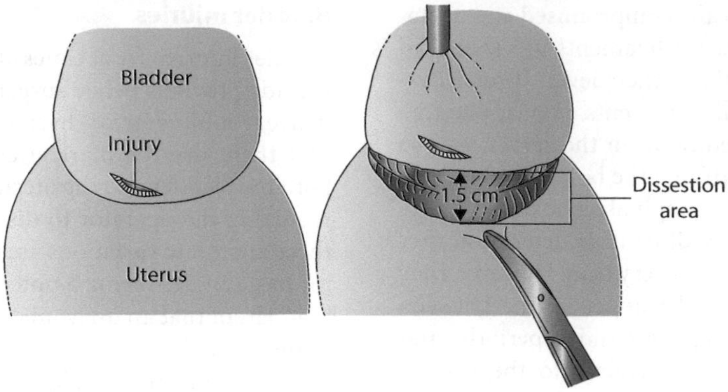

Figure 30.11 Before repair of the bladder, tissue around an injury is dissected in such a manner that the rent can be closed without tension on the sutures.

involved in these adhesions. Even with cesarean hysterectomy, when the cul-de-sac is included in the operative field, adhesions are rare. The chance that bowel will be injured is much less with section than with hysterectomy for the usual gynecologic indications.

However, with operative bowel injury, the diagnosis is crucial. An undiagnosed injury will result in serious postoperative complication and peritonitis. The diagnosis is made by inspection of the area of possible trauma. Unless there is a cogent reason to proceed with the operation, it is usually wise to stop and examine the bowel at the time of the suspected injury. If this cannot be done (as when the section must proceed to deliver a fetus in distress), the injured loop of bowel should be marked in some way. It is easy to "lose" a traumatized area and have difficulty finding it subsequently.

Another method that can be used to survey the bowel (both large and small) in the true pelvis for even the smallest perforation is as follows: The pelvis is filled with physiologic saline (approximately 100 mL may be required) and the bowel submerged. After a few moments, air from the rent will rise to the surface, and if the bowel is "milked," gas coming from any injury through the bowel wall will be evident. This method will help to pinpoint the site of the perforation more precisely than simple inspection.

The principles of the repair of surgical injuries to the bowel are quite different from those employed in gynecologic surgery. First, the closure must be done precisely and meticulously so that it is absolutely watertight. Repair of the bowel is usually based on the inversion of the tissue, so that serosa is approximated with serosa. This is important, since there is little margin for error in suturing. A mistake cannot be "oversewn." The sutures must be placed precisely as to depth. A suture in the external layer should not penetrate through the bowel wall, since that would make a potential tract for microbial contamination with bowel flora.

It is important to preserve an adequate bowel lumen. This is a greater problem with small than with large bowel. One technique for this is to close all injuries transversely if at all possible. Thus, consideration should be given to closing a longitudinal injury transversely if it is not too long. Suture bites must be small so that an unnecessarily large amount of bowel wall is not to be used in the repair.

During the course of the repair of both large and small bowel, the contaminated operative field should be packed off with laparotomy pads and atraumatic rubber-shod clamps should be placed on each side of the injury to prevent continuous contamination during the procedure. Stay sutures used as guides and also for traction are placed beyond the ends of the rent. These sutures of no. 3:0 Vicryl will subsequently be the angle sutures of the inside layer (Figure 30.12). Fine atraumatic bowel suture, such as 4:0 Vicryl, is used for the inner layer of continuous running sutures. Stitches are taken in such a manner that the edges are inverted, with no suture material between the two serosal edges. A running Lembert suture is useful for this. Care is to be taken to ensure that the edges are not everted when the suture is tied at the end.

The inner suture line is reinforced with a second row of Lembert sutures (3:0 silk or 3:0 Vicryl) (Figure 30.12), which should not pass through the entire wall but only into the muscularis layer. After this part of the operation is complete, a thumb and forefinger are used to feel that the lumen is open. They should touch freely without any surrounding constriction. As soon as the injury is repaired, the potentially contaminated packs around the field should be removed, and the operator and assistants should change gloves, since they may have been contaminated with bowel flora. The upper abdomen should not be explored after bowel surgery unless there is a compelling reason.

Bowel injuries requiring resection and anastomosis are beyond the scope of this discussion. The operator who is not experienced in these surgical techniques should have a general surgical consultant when necessary.

Incidental pelvic pathology

It is unusual to find significant pathology at cesarean delivery since most patients are young and healthy. In general, a decision and plan of management are based upon the pathology encountered, the indication for section,

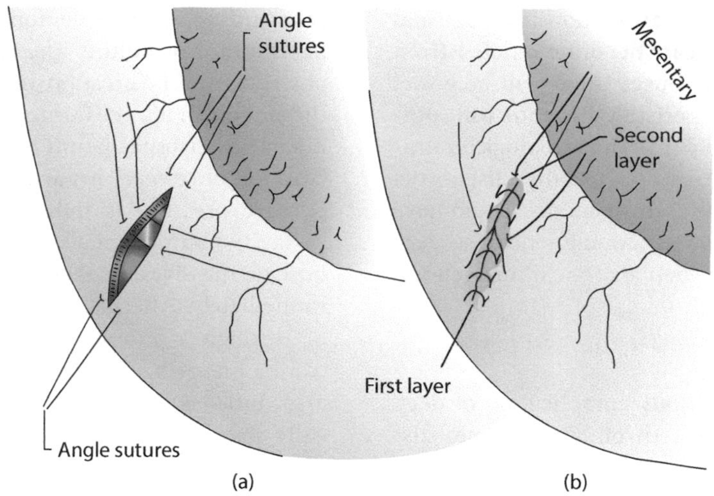

Figure 30.12 Bowel injuries are closed in two layers (a and b) by carefully inverting the bowel wall.

and the condition of the patient. The last is usually no deterrent to treatment unless it is an emergency section for maternal reasons with a hemodynamically unstable patient. The serious potential for infection is an important consideration.

Ovarian tumors are the most common pathologic lesions encountered at the time of cesarean section. For the most part, they should be treated as they would be at any other abdominal operation. Cystectomy or oophorectomy is not contraindicated, but many feel that myomectomy is because of its predilection for morbidity. Small pedunculated myomas or those actually involved in the incision should be removed.

There has been controversy about elective appendectomy during cesarean section. Theoretically, it would seem to be contraindicated because of potential contamination by bowel contents. On the other hand, there are large reported series indicating that appendectomy can be done safely at the time of a routine section.

POSTOPERATIVE COURSE AND MANAGEMENT

Patients who deliver by cesarean delivery are not generally ill before the operation, and they recover quickly afterward. They should be ambulated on the day of the operation if possible to decrease the risk of postoperative morbidity such as deep vein thrombosis. The next day, they can have a diet as tolerated.

The Foley catheter can be removed immediately after the operation when the patient is able to void or the next day. Physiologically, a urinary catheter is probably unnecessary during the postoperative period. An important aspect of postoperative care is deep breathing and coughing, particularly after general anesthesia. Thus, prophylactic incentive spirometry is important to prevent pulmonary complications particularly for those receiving general anesthesia.

Vaginal bleeding should be observed, and if it is excessive, evaluation and treatment can be given.

POSTOPERATIVE COMPLICATIONS

With the exception of infection, severe postoperative complications after cesarean delivery are uncommon. Atelectasis especially after general anesthesia is one of the most common problems and should be suspected when there is a fever spike within the first 24 hours after delivery. Diagnosis is made by auscultation of the chest and radiologic examination if needed. Treatment consists of incentive spirometry and deep breathing every couple of hours, coughing, and sometimes intermittent positive-pressure breathing four times a day for 15 minutes.

Urinary tract infections are also common postpartum. Bacteriuria and urinary tract infection are common during pregnancy, and they can be treated effectively postpartum if they were not treated prior to delivery.

Ileus and obstruction

Ileus does not usually develop after cesarean delivery unless the bowel has been handled extensively or there is infection. In order to prevent the occurrence of the latter, the abdomen should probably not be explored at the time of cesarean delivery unless there is a specific indication. The upper abdomen should not be explored in an infected patient without a compelling reason. The upper abdomen is difficult to explore before the fetus is removed from the uterus, and the potential danger of spreading infection after the section is completed contraindicates routine exploration.

Postoperative ileus can be diagnosed when the abdomen is quiet on auscultation and becomes distended. Any oral intake should be stopped when ileus is suspected and nasogastric suction initiated if the patient is vomiting. If the condition is secondary to peritonitis, the primary infection needs to be treated with appropriate antibiotics. When bowel sounds return and the patient is passing gas, the tube can be clamped and then removed, and the patient can take sips of clear fluid.

Bowel obstruction after cesarean section is an unusual but serious complication. It can be differentiated from paralytic ileus because at the onset there will be bowel sounds present and often the peristaltic sounds will coincide with crampy abdominal pain. The radiologic examination (CT scan with contrast) is usually diagnostic. Patients with a suspected bowel obstruction should have bowel rest and nasogastric tube suction. General surgery consultation may be needed when a surgical intervention is contemplated.

Pulmonary embolism

Pulmonary embolism is a serious complication of deep venous thrombosis in which a thrombus becomes dislodged and passes through the vena cava and the right heart into the pulmonary arterial tree. The clinical picture will depend upon the size of the clot. A small clot will pass to the periphery of the lung and produce a small wedge-shaped infarct. There may be a few symptoms or mild chest pain. Often there is tachycardia, chest pain, cyanosis, and dyspnea. Subsequently, there will be a transient pleural friction rub, bloodstained sputum, and, finally, pleural effusion. A radiologic examination 12 hours after the initial symptoms will usually demonstrate the lesion. Even small infarcts are likely to be followed by others; thus, they are serious.

Diagnosis of a pulmonary embolism is made by spiral CT, pulmonary arteriography, ventilation perfusion scan, and occasionally pulmonary angiography. Venous Doppler studies of the lower extremities are noninvasive and may be helpful. Arterial blood gases are also mandatory to quantify the degree of hypoxia and direct the resuscitation effort.

If a large clot blocks the pulmonary arterial tree, the signs and symptoms are more dramatic. Chest pain, acute cyanosis, dyspnea, and shock may be apparent. The patient may not be stable enough for CT scan or ventilation perfusion scans. An electrocardiogram (ECG) and a bedside echocardiogram will demonstrate the acute, right-sided heart strain or failure. The clot could be so large that it obstructs the bifurcation of the pulmonary artery, and the embolism may be immediately fatal. The clot produces intense arteriospasm and vagal stimulation. The administration of oxygen, heparin, morphine, and intermittent positive pressure is indicated as emergency measures. Today, in many hospitals, embolectomy is a feasible procedure for massive embolism if the patient does not succumb immediately. Alternatively, thrombolysis, either systemic or through a pulmonary arterial angiography catheter, can be lifesaving. Heparin or low-molecular-weight heparin anticoagulation is the treatment for hemodynamically stable patients with postoperative thromboembolic complications as soon as the diagnosis is entertained. Diagnostic studies can then be performed.

Wound disruption

Wound disruption is another rare but significant complication of abdominal surgery. It may occur without any warning. Slight abdominal pain and a serous or serosanguineous discharge from the wound are ominous signs. The skin may open up so that the bowel can be palpated upon exploration or the abdomen may break open during a cough. Whenever wound disruption is suspected, the incision should be explored in the operating room under anesthesia.

Closure is a debatable question. In general, surgeons use a permanent suture, and most prefer monofilament material such as Prolene or PDS. Some close with through-and-through sutures either including or excluding the peritoneum. Others employ a layer closure with meticulous suturing of peritoneum, fascia, subcutaneous tissue, and skin. A few imbricate the fascia so that there is a larger area for adhesion. For imbrication, the fascial flaps are freed of subcutaneous fat for 1–2 cm. The flaps are overlapped by about 1 cm for suturing (Figure 30.13a). The fascia is closed with two rows of mattress sutures, making a double layer of fascia at the suture line (Figure 30.13b).

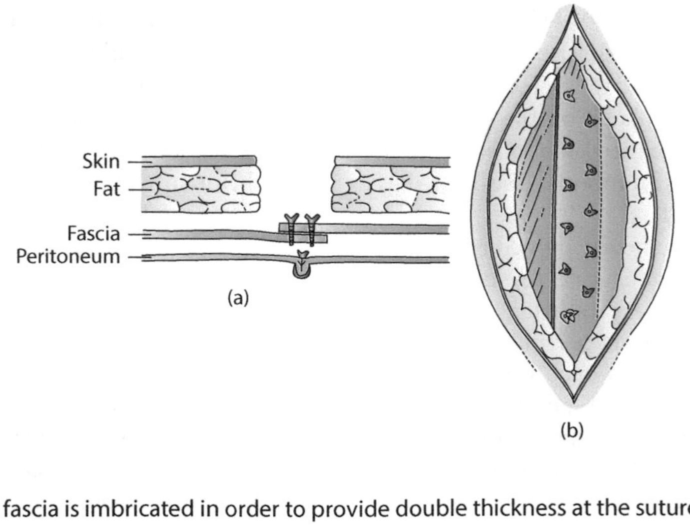

Figure 30.13 (a and b) The fascia is imbricated in order to provide double thickness at the suture line.

POSTMORTEM CESAREAN DELIVERY

Occasionally providers of obstetrical services may be called upon in an emergency situation to evaluate a pregnant woman who has been pronounced dead but is still receiving life support. When this occurs time is of the essence if there is to be an attempt at salvaging a potentially viable fetus. However, there is little guidance in the literature about postmortem cesarean delivery (PMCD).[46-48] It has been poorly studied because of its rarity and the cases that have been reported are of variable circumstances and the information and recommendations seem to be conflicting as to how soon after the pronouncement of death should the delivery be considered. PMCD when performed has the potential to save the life of both mother and fetus. Occasionally patients who were pronounced dead suddenly respond to resuscitative measures after delivery of the fetus.

There are several factors that should be considered prior to making the decision regarding the performance of a PMCD. The estimated gestational age of the fetus is important to rapidly determine since candidates should have a potentially viable fetus. This might be obtained by history or from the patient's medical record if available. Alternatively a clinical assessment of the uterine fundal height measuring from the patient's pubic symphysis may help. An ultrasound examination to determine gestational age may or may not be feasible in an emergency setting unless the event takes place in the ED of a hospital and the ultrasound machine is readily available. Most would consider a fetal gestational age of 23 or more weeks to be a potentially viable fetus. However, most often an ultrasound machine is not readily available so time should not be wasted trying to find an ultrasound machine. An attempt should be made to auscultate the fetal heart rate with the bell portion of the stethoscope in order to determine if the fetus is still alive. Ideally, if the estimated gestational age is 23 weeks or more then the procedure may be considered. Adequate surgical instruments should be available although usually only a surgical scalpel is all that is needed to perform the cesarean delivery since bleeding should be minimal.

It is imperative for cardiopulmonary resuscitation (CPR) to continue as maternal resuscitative measures and advanced cardiac life support (ACLS) without interruption while preparing for surgery as well as during the PMCD. The best neonatal outcomes based on limited information appear to occur when the infant is delivered within 5 minutes of maternal cardiac arrest. The decision to perform a PMCD should then must be made about 4 minutes into the arrest regardless of the cause, although case report have indicated that even after this time period fetus delivered may survive neurologically intact. Pregnant patients who are not candidates are those less than 23 weeks' gestation, or if there is documented intrauterine fetal demise. Occasionally patients who were pronounced dead and are delivered as above may suddenly respond to resuscitative measures. This may subsequently be termed a perimortum cesarean delivery, for which there is little guidance in the medical literature.

ACKNOWLEDGMENT

We particularly thank Charbel Solomon, MD, for his assistance with the previous edition of this chapter.

REFERENCES

1. Bottoms SF, Rosen MG, Sokol RJ. The increase of cesarean birth rate. *N Engl J Med* 1980; 302: 559–63.
2. Petitti D, Olson RO, Williams RL. Cesarean section in California: 1960 through 1975. *Am J Obstet Gynecol* 1979; 133: 391–7.
3. Centers for Disease Control. *National Vital Statistics Reports*. November 5, 2014; 63(6).
4. Cunningham FG, McDonald PC, Gant NF, et al. *Williams' Obstetrics* (21st edition). New York, NY: McGraw-Hill, 2001.
5. NIH Consensus Development Conference Statement. Vaginal birth after cesarean: New insights. *Obstet Gynecol* 2010; 115: 1279–1295.
6. O'Driscoll KO, Foley M. Correlation of decrease in perinatal mortality and increase in cesarean section rates. *Obstet Gynecol* 1983; 61: 1–5.
7. ACOG Practice Bulletin No. 140. Management of Abnormal Cervical Cancer Screening Test Results and Cervical Cancer Precursors. *ACOG*, December 2013. Washington, DC, pp. 1338–67.
8. Van der Vange N, Weverling GJ, Ketting, BW, et al. The prognosis of cervical cancer associated with pregnancy: A matched cohort study. *Obstet Gynecol* 1995; 85: 1022–6.
9. Sood AK, Sorosky JI, Mayr N et al. Cervical cancer diagnosed shortly after pregnancy: Prognostic variables and delivery routes. *Obstet Gynecol* 2000; 95: 832–8.
10. ACOG Committee opinion no. 559. Cesarean delivery on maternal request. *Obstet Gynecol* 2006; 107: 1226–32.
11. NIH State-of-the-science conference statement on cesarean delivery on maternal request. *NIH Consensus Statement* 2006; 23: 1–29.
12. ACOG Practice Bulletin No 145. Antepartum fetal surveillance. Washington, DC. 2014.
13. Guirguis GF, Andrew Haddad, Williams S. External cephlic version. *Topics in Obstetrics & Gynecology* July, 2016; 36: 10, 1–4.
14. ACOG Committee Opinion No. 340. Mode of term singleton breech delivery, 2015.
15. ACOG Practice Bulletin No. 144. Multifetal gestation: twin, triplet and higher order mulifetal gestation. Washington, DC. 2014.
16. Miller DA, Diaz FG, Paul, RH. Vaginal birth after cesarean: A 10-year experience. *Obstet Gynecol* 1994; 84: 255–8.
17. Miller DA, Mullin P, Hou D, Paul RH. Vaginal birth after cesarean section in twin gestation. *Am J Obstet Gynecol* 1996; 175: 194–8.

17. ACOG Committee opinion No. 234. Scheduled cesarean delivery and the prevention of vertical transmission of HIV infection. Washington, DC. 2000.
18. Thomas SL, Newell ML, Peckham CS, et al. A review of hepatitis C virus (HCV) vertical transmission: Risks of transmission to infants born to mothers with an without HCV viremia or HIV infection. *Int J Epidemiol* 1998; 27: 108–17.
19. ACOG Committee Opinion No. 220. Breastfeeding and the risk of hepatitis C virus transmission. Committee on Obstetric Practice. *American College of Obstetricians and Gynecologists* 1999.
20. Yeh S, Huang X, Phelan JP. Postterm pregnancy after previous cesarean section. *J Reprod Med* 1984; 29: 41–4.
21. ACOG Practice Bulletin No 110. Vaginal birth after previous cesarean delivery. Washington, DC. 2014.
22. Phelan JP, Clark SL, Diaz F et al. Vaginal birth after cesarean. *Am J Obstet Gynecol* 1987; 157: 1510–5.
23. Elkousy MA, Sammel M, Stevens E, Peipert JF. The effect of birth weight on vaginal birth after cesarean delivery success rates. *Am J Obstet Gynecol* 2003; 188: 824–30.
24. Sondgeroth KE, Stout MJ, Graseck AS, et al. Progress of induced labor in trial of labor after cesarean delivery. *Am J Obstet Gynecol* 2015; 213: 420.e1–5.
25. Wilkinson C, Enkin MW. Uterine exteriorization versus intraperitoneal repair at caesarean section. *Cochrane Database Syst Rev* 2000; CD000085.
26. Bujold E, Bujold C, Hamilton EF, et al. The impact of a single-layer or double-layer closure on uterine rupture. *Am J Obstet Gynecol* 2002; 186: 1326–30.
27. Poidevin LOS. The value of hysterography in the prediction of cesarean section wound defects. *Am J Obstet Gynecol* 1961; 81: 67–71.
28. Wilkinson CS, Enkin MW. Peritoneal non-closure at caesarean section. *Cochrane Database Syst Rev* 2000; CD000163.
29. Cheong YC, Bajekal N, Li TC. Peritoneal closure to close or not to close. *Human Reprod* 2001; 16: 1548–52.
30. Lyell D, Caughey A, Hu E, Daniels K. Peritoneal closure at primary cesarean section decreases adhesion formation. *Am J Obstet Gynecol* 2004; 189: S61.
31. Harrigill KM, Miller HS, Haynes DE. The effect of intraabdominal irrigation at cesarean delivery on maternal morbidity: A randomized trial. *Obstet Gynecol* 2003; 101: 80–5.
32. Wallace D, Hernandez W, Schlaerth JB, et al. Prevention of abdominal wound disruption utilizing the Smead–Jones closure technique. *Obstet Gynecol* 1980; 56: 226–30.
33. Lyon JB, Richardson AC. Careful surgical technique can reduce infectious morbidity after cesarean section. *Am J Obstet Gynecol* 1987; 157: 557–62.
34. Chelmow D, Rodriguez EJ, Sabatini MM. Suture closure of subcutaneous fat and wound disruption after cesarean delivery: A meta-analysis. *Obstet Gynecol* 2004; 103: 974–80.
35. Alderdice F, McKenna D, Dornan J. Techniques and materials for skin closure in caesarean section. *Cochrane Database Syst Rev* 2003; CD003577.
36. Physick P. In Dewees WP (ed.), *A Compendious System of Midwifery*, p. 580. HC Carey & I Lea: Philadelphia, 1824.
37. ACOG Committee Opinion No. 529. *Placenta accreta*. Washington, DC. 2010.
38. Weiss JL, Malone FD, Emig D, et al. Obesity, obstetric complications and cesarean delivery rate—A Population-based screening study. *Am J Obstet Gynecol* 2004; 190: 1091–7.
39. Kaiser PS, Kirby RS. Obesity as a risk factor for cesarean in a low-risk population. *Obstet Gynecol* 2001: 97; 39–43.
40. Postoperative morbidity in the morbidly obese parturient woman; supraumbilical and low transverse abdominal approaches. *Am J Obstet Gynecol* 2000; 182: 1033–5.
41. Overcash, R; Somers, A. Enoxaparin dosin after cesarean delivery in morbidly obese women. *Obstet Gynecol* 2015; 125:1371–6.
42. Ghaffari N, Sindhu S, Durnwald, C. The multidisciplinary approach to the care of the obese parturient. *Am J Obstet Gynecol* 2015; 213: 318–25.
43. Duff P. Pathophysiology and management of postcesarean endomyometritis. *Obstet Gynecol* 1986; 67: 269–76.
44. Hopkins L, Smaill F. Antibiotic prophylaxis regimens and drugs for cesarean section. *Cochrane Database Syst Rev* 2000; CD001136.
45. Dekruif H, Rockwood H, Norman H, David J, Sanderson MD. Postmortem cesarean section with survival of infant. *J Am Med Assoc* 1957; 162: 938–9.
46. Arthur, R. Postmortem cesarean section. *Am J Obstet Gynecol* 1978; 132:175–9.
47. Ritter, J. Postmortem cesarean section. *J Am Med Assoc* 1961; 175:715–6.

Prevention of surgical site infections

31

DIANA EL-NEEMANY and MARK MARTENS

CONTENTS

Postoperative surgical site infections (SSIs) are a major cause of prolonged hospitalization, morbidity, and mortality. In 2009, the U.S. Department of Health and Human Services initiated a steering committee solely dedicated to the elimination of hospital-acquired infections (HAIs)[1] and created standardized definitions to assist in surveillance (Table 31.1). The national survey included 183 hospitals of small, medium, and large sizes to calculate the incidence of HAI. The data from this survey showed that SSIs ranked as the number one cause of HAIs along with pneumonia with an estimated cases of 157,500 SSIs in 2011.[2]

In this chapter, the various methods and practices used to prevent SSIs will be discussed in addition to specific details pertaining to cesarean sections' recommendations for SSI in obese patients and other obstetrical procedures.

SURGICAL ATTIRE

Personal protective equipment (PPE) used to decrease exposure of the patient and operating room personnel to chemical and infectious agents during surgery include surgical mask, eye protection (goggles, face shields, etc.), surgical cap, shoe covers, scrubs, sterile gown, and gloves.

Scrub suits

Protective clothing (scrub suits) should be worn to prevent contamination from street clothing and to protect the skin of healthcare personnel from exposure to blood and body secretions. Guidelines and regulations for laundry practices and restrictions regarding wearing scrub uniform outside the surgical area vary extensively from institution to institution. While some studies show that home laundering is more economical, significantly higher bacteria counts were isolated from home-laundered and unwashed scrubs than from new, hospital-laundered, disposable scrubs.[4] All protective clothing should be changed when it becomes visibly soiled and as soon as feasible if contaminated by blood or other potentially infectious fluids. Scrub suits should also be removed before leaving the hospital.

Table 31.1 National healthcare network criteria for defining an SSI.

Superficial incisional	Occurs within 30 days postoperatively and involves skin or subcutaneous tissue of the incision and at least *one* of the following: 1. Purulent drainage from the superficial incision 2. Organisms isolated from an aseptically obtained culture of fluid or tissue from the superficial incision 3. At least one of the following signs or symptoms of infection: pain or tenderness, localized swelling, redness, or heat, **and** superficial incision is deliberately opened by surgeon and is culture positive 4. Diagnosis of superficial incisional SSI by the surgeon or attending physician
Deep incisional	Occurs within 30 days postoperatively if no implant is left in place or within 1 year if implant is in place and the infection appears to be related to the operative procedure, involves deep soft tissues (i.e., fascial and muscle layers) of the incision, and at least *one* of the following: 1. Purulent drainage from the deep incision, but not from the organ/space component of the surgical site 2. A deep incision spontaneously dehisces or is deliberately opened by a surgeon and patient has one of the following signs or symptoms: fever (>38°), localized pain or tenderness, or culture positive 3. An abscess or other evidence of infection involving the deep incision is found on direct examination, during reoperation, or by histopathologic or radiologic examination 4. Diagnosis of a deep incisional SSI by a surgeon or attending
Organ/space	Occurs within 30 days postoperatively if no implant is left in place or within 1 year if implant is in place and the infection appears to be related to the operative procedure, involves any part of the body, excluding the skin incision, fascia, or muscle layers, that is opened or manipulated during the operative procedure and at least *one* of the following: 1. Purulent drainage from a drain that is placed through a stab wound into the organ/space 2. Organisms isolated from an aseptically obtained culture of the fluid or tissue in the organ/space 3. An abscess or other evidence of infection involving the organ/space that is found on direct examination, during reoperation, or by histopathologic or radiologic examination 4. Diagnosis of an organ/space SSI by the surgeon or attending physician

Source: Horan T et al., *Am J Infect Control*, 36, 309–32, 2008.
Abbreviation: SSI, surgical site infection.

Eye protection, surgical mask, shoe covers, and surgical caps

Surgical masks and eye protection provide barriers to blood-borne pathogen exposure to the mucous membranes of the eyes, nose, and mouth. While a recent Cochrane study showed that there is limited data regarding contamination of surgical incisions by masked versus unmasked wearers, it continues to be a standard practice in the operating room to protect from splashes, sprays, or splatters of blood.[5,6] Masks should be changed between surgical cases if the outer surface becomes contaminated with either secretions or from touching the mask with contaminated fingers. When airborne infection isolation precautions are necessary (e.g., tuberculosis [TB] patients), a National Institute for Occupational Safety and Health (NIOSH)-certified particulate filter respirator (such as N95, N99, or N100) should be used.[7]

There are various forms of eye protection including goggles and face shields. They should be comfortable, allow for sufficient peripheral vision and adjustable to ensure a secure fit. Goggles have the benefit of having various options for fit and size and some have the ability to fit over prescriptions glasses with minimal gaps. However, for optimal infection control, face shields provide better protection of other facial areas as they extend around the face and reduce the likelihood of a splash reaching the eyes. Removal of eye protection should be from the part of the equipment that secures the device to the head (side ties, elastic band, etc.) rather than the front or side of the device as this is the "clean" portion of the equipment.[8]

Shoe covers and surgical caps are also routinely used during surgery though neither has proven to decrease rates of SSIs. Nonetheless, disposable shoe covers prevent contamination by preventing displacement of microorganisms when moving from one area to another and surgical caps prevent contamination of the incision with hair from the surgeons' scalp.[9,10]

Sterile gowns and drapes

Sterile gown and drapes are used to separate and protect the surgical field from contaminants. There is great heterogeneity regarding the characteristics of available products. Nonetheless, a level of liquid barrier protection must be approved by the Association for the Advancement of Medical Instrumentation guidelines. Gowns and drapes can be disposable or made of reusable fabric. Surgical gowns are worn by and should adequately fit every member of the surgical team participating in the procedure so that the back of the gown is completely closed and the sleeve length long enough to prevent cuff exposure outside the glove. The front of the gown is sterile from the chest to the level of the sterile field and gown sleeves are sterile from 2 inches above the elbow to the cuff, circumferentially (Figure 31.1). The gown cuff should be at the level of or slightly below the wrist to maintain sterility and to prevent its exposure outside the glove. Sterile drapes are used to cover the patient, furniture, and equipment that is included in the surgical field.[11]

Gloves

Gloves serve a dual purpose: (1) they protect healthcare workers (HCWs) from becoming contaminated by microorganisms transmissible through mucous membranes, blood, and secretions and (2) they prevent transmission of microorganisms from the HCWs' hands to the patient during physical examination and performance of procedures. The quality of medical gloves, both patient examination and surgeon's gloves, is regulated by the Food and Drug Administration (FDA) and required to meet general control, or Class I, requirements—the most basic regulations applied to medical devices to ensure their safety and effectiveness.[12] Additionally, sterile gloves, both patient examination gloves and surgical gloves, must meet standards for sterility assurance established by the FDA.[13]

Medical gloves, are manufactured as single-use, disposable items that should be used for only one patient and discarded. Sterile surgical gloves are put on after donning sterile gowns and replaced and discarded when contaminated, torn, or punctured. Using two layers of gloves, glove liners, or thicker orthopedic gloves is a common practice by surgeons. A Cochrane review of double gloving showed that this practice does not reduce SSIs, though there was insufficient power for this outcome. However, double/triple gloving, knitted outer gloves, and glove liners significantly reduced perforation of the inner gloves. Additionally, perforation indicator systems significantly increased detection of innermost glove perforations.[15,16] While some believe that double gloving decreases tactile sensation during surgery, studies show wearing double gloves has minimal impact in manual dexterity and tactile sensitivity.[16,17] The type of suture needle also impacts the risk for glove punctures. A meta-analysis showed that the use of blunt needles appreciably reduced the risk of exposure to blood and bodily fluids for surgeons and their assistants.[18] There was no difference between sharp and blunt needle glove perforations in cesarean sections, while studies regarding episiotomy and repair of obstetrical lacerations are controversial. Regardless, surgeons found more satisfaction with sharp surgical needles and found increased difficulty with blunt needles.[19–21]

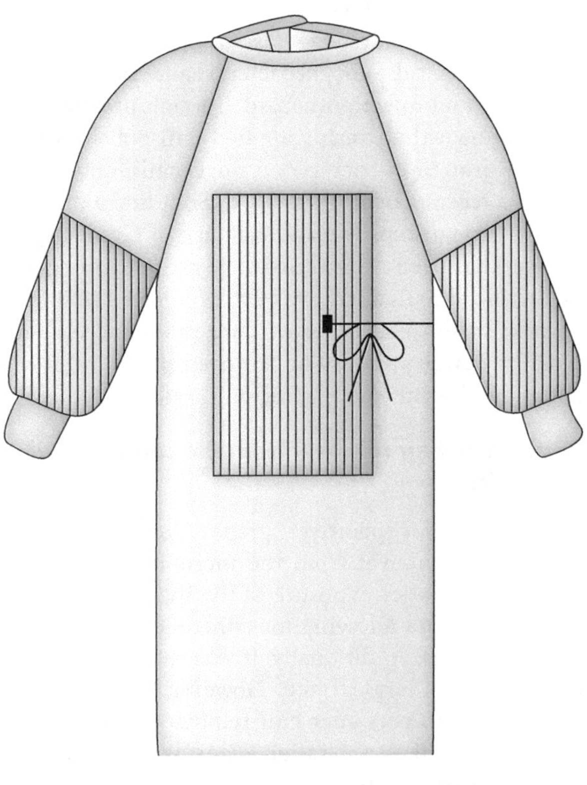

Figure 31.1 Sterile portions of surgical gown. (From www.medsupplier.com. With permission.)

PERIOPERATIVE INTERVENTIONS

Hand wash

Since the last century and Ignatz Semmelweis discovery, hand hygiene has been accepted as a primary mechanism of infection control. In the last few decades, new technologies have been developed to improved hand hygiene efficacy and compliance. Current World Health Organization (WHO) guidelines recommend alcohol-based handrub as the preferred means of hand antisepsis. Plain hand soap, with water, assists with cleaning through its detergent properties, however, it has minimal antimicrobial activity.[22] There are different forms of antiseptic agents with different action spectra as outlined in Table 31.2. Alcohol-based handrubs have several benefits, including elimination of a majority of bacteria and viruses, short time required for application, portability of the product and its presence at the point of care, better skin tolerability, and no need for a particular infrastructure (sink, water supply, etc.). Without a doubt, plain soap and water should be used when hands are visibly dirty or soiled with blood or other bodily fluids or when there is exposure to potential spore-forming pathogens, such as *Clostridium difficile*.[23]

However, frequent use of the various forms of antiseptic agents may lead to development of skin irritation in the form of irritant contact dermatitis or allergic contact dermatitis. Signs and symptoms of irritant contact dermatitis include dryness, itching, cracking, and sometimes bleeding, as opposed to allergic contact dermatitis, which can be mild or severe ranging from a rash to respiratory distress, respectively. Of the various forms of antiseptics, alcohol-based handrubs are better tolerated while iodophors are more commonly associated with irritant contact dermatitis. Additionally, frequent use of plain soap and water has

Table 31.2 Antimicrobial activity and summary of properties of antiseptics used in hand hygiene.

Antiseptics	Gram-positive bacteria	Gram-negative bacteria	Viruses (enveloped)	Viruses (nonenveloped)	Mycobacteria	Fungi	Spores
Alcohols	+++	+++	+++	++	+++	+++	–
Chloroxylenol	+++	+	=	±	+	+	–
Chlorhexidine	+++	++	++	+	+	+	–
Hexachlorophene[a]	+++	+	?	?	+	+	–
Iodophors	+++	+++	++	++	++	++	±[b]
Triclosan[c]	+++	++	?	?	±	±[d]	–
Quaternary ammonium compounds[e]	++	+	+	?	±	±	–

Source: WHO, *WHO Guidelines on Hand Hygiene in Health Care: A Summary*, Geneva, Switzerland: WHO, 2009. With permission.

Notes: good, +++, moderate, ++, poor, +, variable, ±, none, –.

[a] Bacteriostatic.

[b] In concentrations used in antiseptics, iodophors are not sporicidal.

[c] Mostly bacteriostatic.

[d] Activity against *Candida* spp., but little activity against filamentous fungi.

[e] Bacteriostatic, fungistatic, and microbicidal at high concentrations.

a greater risk of causing skin irritation. Other common causes of contact dermatitis include washing before and after use of alcohol-based handrubs, using hot water when hand washing, and rubbing rather than patting when using towel for drying hands. In order to minimize skin irritation, the least irritating product should be chosen, hand moisturizers should be used, and unnecessary hand washing should be discouraged.[23]

Surgical scrub

Participating members of the surgical team who will have contact with the sterile field should perform a surgical hand scrub immediately before gowns and gloves are fitted. Rings, wrist watches, and bracelets must be removed before beginning surgical preparation. Hands should be washed with antiseptic soap and water for at least 1 minute if they are visibly soiled prior to using surgical hand scrub. The form of surgical hand scrub is chosen according to the operating team member's preference. A Cochrane review of surgical hand antisepsis for reduction of SSI concluded that alcohol rubs with additional active ingredients were as effective as aqueous scrubs in reducing SSIs.[24] However, alcohol rubs containing chlorhexidine was more effective in reducing the amount of bacteria on hand than povidone-iodidne.[24] If using an antimicrobial soap, the length of time recommended by the manufacturer should be referenced and it is usually between 2 and 5 minutes. When using alcohol-based surgical handrub product with sustained activity, refer to manufacturer's instruction for applications times. The technique for surgical hand preparation using alcohol-based handrubs is illustrated in Figure 31.2. Additionally, several studies in this review showed that chlorhexidine gluconate (CHG)-based aqueous scrubs are more effective than povidone-iodine-based aqueous scrubs in terms of the numbers for colony-forming units on hands.[23,24]

Fingernails and rings

Currently, there is insufficient evidence regarding length of fingernails and whether removal of nail polish, finger rings, or artificial nails prevents wound infection.[22,25] However, a study by McGinley et al.[26] showed that subungual areas of the hand harbor high concentrations of bacteria, most commonly coagulase-negative staphylococci, Gram-negative rods, corynebacteria, and yeast and thus pose a potential infection hazard. Though previous studies have shown that freshly applied nail polish does not affect the growth of bacteria on fingernails, and chipped nails do, a recent Cochrane study did not find a difference between these groups.[25] Hand carriage of Gram-negative organisms has been determined to be greater among wearers of artificial nails and have been implicated in multiple outbreaks in hospital intensive care units and operating rooms.[27–30] Jewelry should be removed prior to initiating surgical hand scrub and putting on surgical gloves.[23]

Preoperative hair removal from the surgical incision site

Traditionally, preoperative preparation for surgery included hair removal from the incision site, providing surgeons with better exposure of the incision and subsequent wound, and allowing for adherence of drapes and wound dressings. Additionally, it was thought to prevent infection at the surgical site. However, evidence shows microscopic skin cuts after hair removal can become the foci for bacterial proliferation, causing an increase in operative site infections.[31]

There are three forms of hair removal prior to surgery: shaving, clipping, and chemical depilation. Shaving

The handrubbing technique for surgical hand preparation must be performed on perfectly clean, dry hands. On arrival in the operating theater and after having donned theater clothing (cap/hat/bonnet and mask), hands must be washed with soap and water.
After the operation when removing gloves, hands must be rubbed with an alcohol-based formulation or washed with soap and water if any residual talc or biological fluids are present (e.g., the glove is punctured).

Surgical procedures may be carried out one after the other without the need for hand-washing, provided that the hand-rubbing technique for surgical hand preparation is followed (Images 1 to 17).

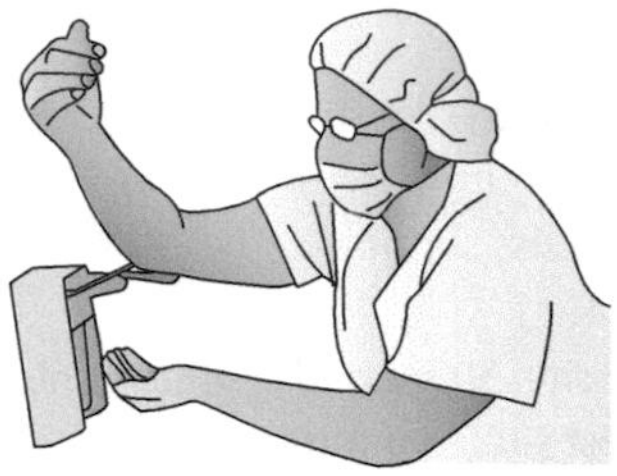

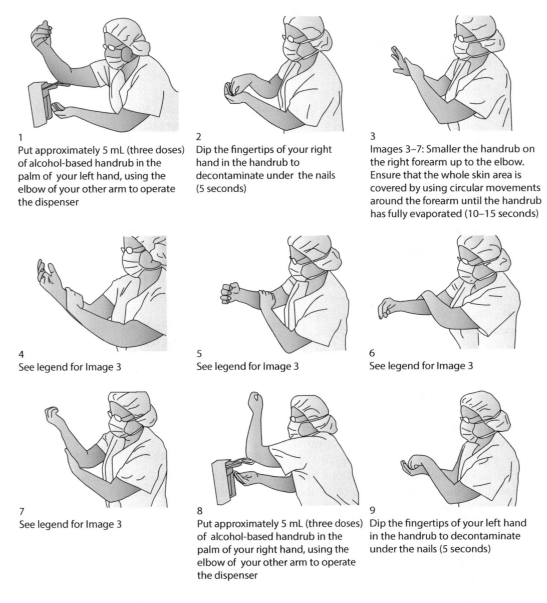

1
Put approximately 5 mL (three doses) of alcohol-based handrub in the palm of your left hand, using the elbow of your other arm to operate the dispenser

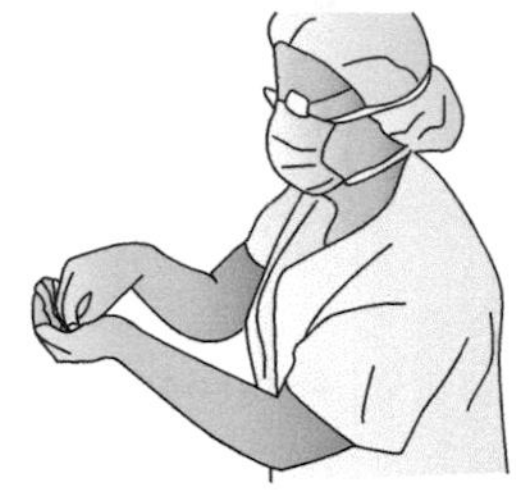

2
Dip the fingertips of your right hand in the handrub to decontaminate under the nails (5 seconds)

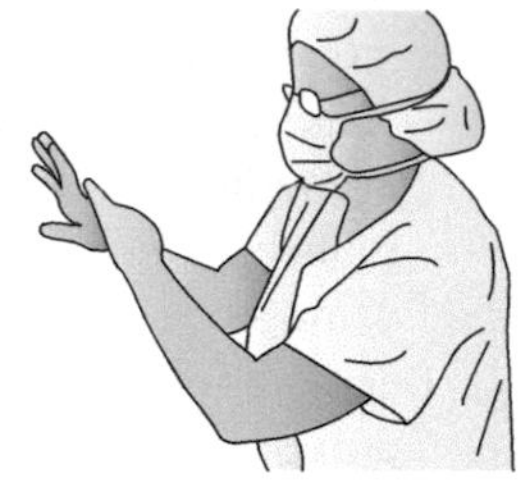

3
Images 3–7: Smaller the handrub on the right forearm up to the elbow. Ensure that the whole skin area is covered by using circular movements around the forearm until the handrub has fully evaporated (10–15 seconds)

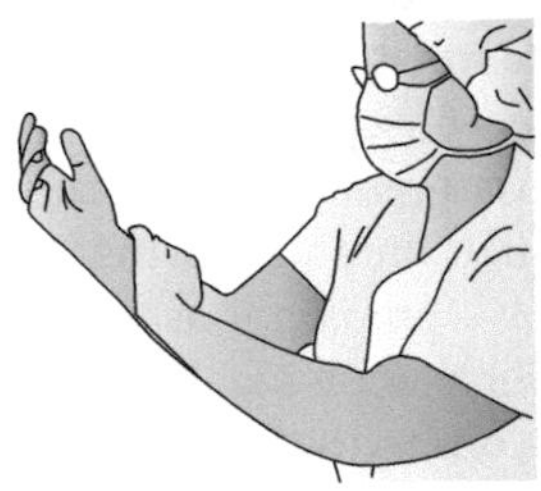

4
See legend for Image 3

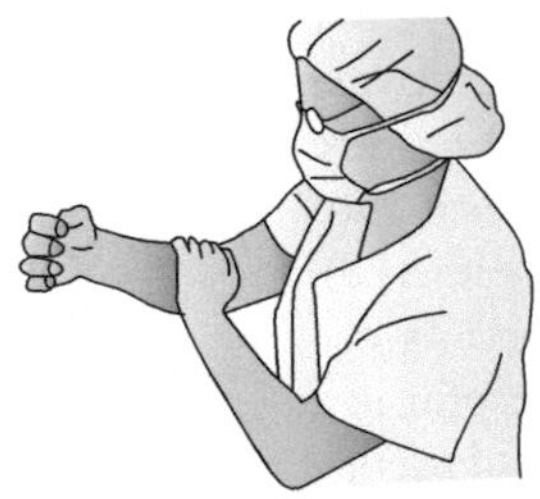

5
See legend for Image 3

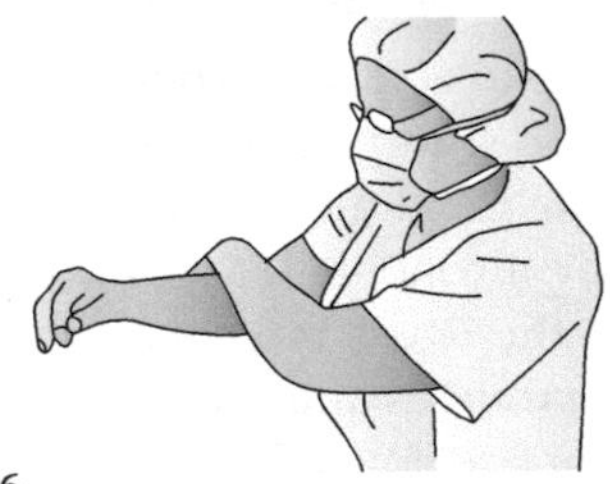

6
See legend for Image 3

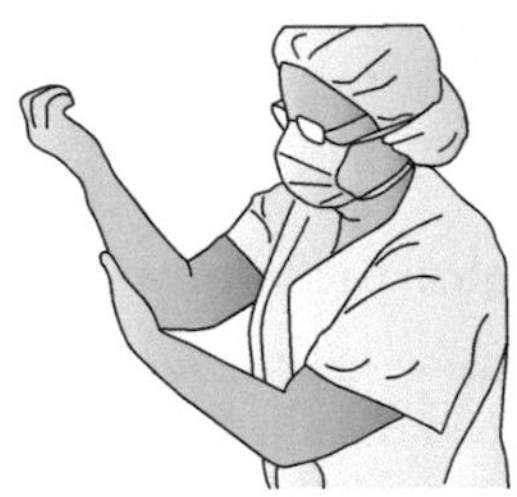

7
See legend for Image 3

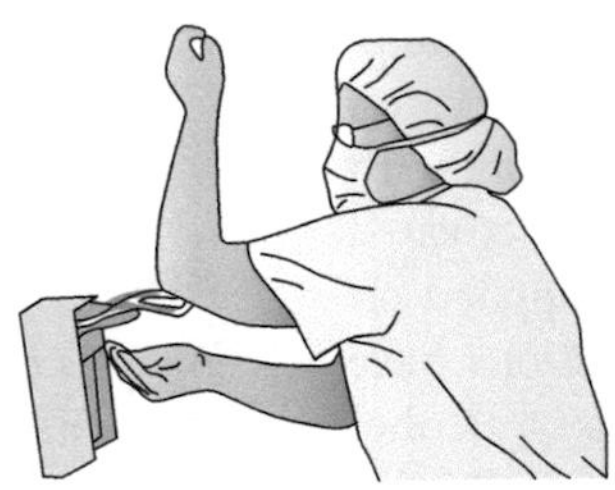

8
Put approximately 5 mL (three doses) of alcohol-based handrub in the palm of your right hand, using the elbow of your other arm to operate the dispenser

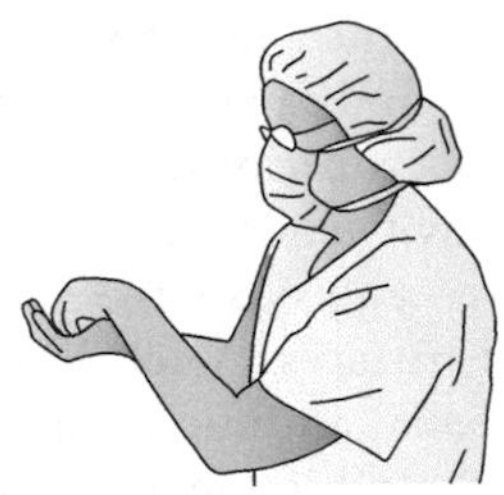

9
Dip the fingertips of your left hand in the handrub to decontaminate under the nails (5 seconds)

Figure 31.2 Surgical hand preparation technique with an alcohol-based handrub formulation. (From WHO, *WHO Guidelines on Hand Hygiene in Health Care: A Summary*, Geneva, Switzerland: WHO, 2009. With permission.)

involves using a razor to cut the hair close to the skin, while clipping uses an electric razor to cut, usually leaving approximately 1 mm of hair. Chemical depilatories require application of a cream to dissolve hair.[32]

A meta-analysis of literature regarding different methods of hair removal showed that there were significantly fewer SSIs with clipping, chemical depilation, or no depilation in comparison to shaving. The meta-analysis of literature also confirmed no benefit from depilation to prevent SSI and the higher risk of SSI with shaving.[33] The optimal timing for hair removal is yet to be determined; however, review of literature suggests that there is a greater risk of SSI when hair removal was performed on the day before the surgery than when it is performed on the day of and immediately prior to the surgery; however, these statistics are not significant.[33] For these reasons, it is recommended that hair removal not be performed unless surgical incision cannot be adequately visualized.

Table 31.3 Characteristics of antiseptic solutions.

Antiseptics	Mechanism of Action	Onset	Duration	Application	Examples
Aqueous iodophor	Free iodine—protein, DNA damage	Intermediate	2 hours	Two-step scrub and paint	Betadine, scrub care
Aqueous CHG	Disrupts membranes	Intermediate	6 hours	Two-step scrub and dry, repeat	Hibiclens
Alcohol iodophor	Denatures protein, free iodine—protein, DNA damage	Rapid	48 hours (DuraPrep), 96 hours (Prevail-FX)	One-step paint dry time, minimum of 3 minutes on hairless surface	DuraPrep solution, Prevail-FX
Alcohol CHG	Denatures protein, disrupts membranes	Rapid	48 hours	Dry site; 30-second scrub Moist site: 2-minute scrub Dry time, minimum of 3 minutes on hairless surface	ChloraPrep

Source: Hemani M and Lepor H, *Rev Urol*, 11(4), 190–5, 2009.
Abbreviation: CHG, chlorhexidine gluconate.

Skin preparation in the operating room

Several agents are available for preoperative skin preparation. Most common skin preparation agents utilized are povidone-iodine or CHG and are further classified into either aqueous or alcohol-based solutions (Table 31.3). Chlorhexidine is the agent of choice when patients are allergic to iodine products and additionally is becoming a common form of antiseptic for hand scrubbing and preoperative showering prior to surgery.

The benefits of using aqueous iodophors such as povidone-iodine include their broad-spectrum antimicrobial properties, efficacy, and safety in nearly all skin surfaces. Aqueous CHG has a superior reduction in skin flora with more sustained activity and furthermore is not inactivated by blood. However, aqueous CHG cannot be applied on vaginal epithelial surfaces. Alcohol-based solutions have the advantage of dual antimicrobial activities of alcohol with chlorhexidine and iodophors. Alcohols usually dry a few minutes after application and thus can be applied in one step. Despite its immediate evaporation, antimicrobial activity of chlorhexidine or iodophor is sustained. However, an important disadvantage of alcohol-based solutions is its contraindication in cleansing of mucosal surfaces and its flammability.[34]

In comparing the most commonly used forms of antiseptics, several studies show alcohol-based chlorhexidine is superior to aqueous povidone-iodine.[35–37] A study by Darouiche et al.[35] comparing preoperative skin preparation with aqueous povidone-iodine versus alcohol-based chlorhexidine showed preparation with chlorhexidine-alcohol is superior for preventing superficial and deep SSIs after clean-contaminated surgery. Riley et al.[37] replaced iodine-povidone with alcohol-based CHG for skin preparation prior to low transverse cesarean section and provided patients with no-rinse CHG cloths for preoperative skin preparation the night before surgery and found they reduced their SSI rate by two-thirds.

Preparation of the surgical skin site begins after removing all gross contamination that could interfere with the application of the antiseptic solution. Traditionally, the skin is prepared in concentric circles, beginning at the area of the proposed incision and moving outward. However, alcohol-based CHG preparations require a "back-and-forth" motion when applying to optimize its activity. Certain modifications to the traditional preoperative skin preparation have been described, including removal or wiping of the antiseptic solution applied and utilization of antiseptic impregnated adhesive drapes among others. However, none of these variations have been demonstrated to represent an advantage.[38]

Asepsis and surgical technique

Asepsis is an extension of the concept of hygiene based on the awareness of the various routes by which infection can spread. This notion includes many different methods to prevent transmission of pathogenic organisms. Rigorous adherence to the principles of asepsis by all scrubbed personnel is the foundation of SSI prevention.[38] Traffic patterns and personnel moving in and around the operating room should be at a minimum, since an association between the number of people moving and levels of microbial counts in the air exists.[39,40] Checklists to help improve intraoperative behaviors for prevention of SSIs have also showed to increase compliance and decrease SSIs.[41,42] Optimal surgical environment and reduction in distractions are also essential as lapses have been shown to increase the rate of SSIs.[43,44] Minimizing blood loss and tissue trauma during surgery, removing necrotic tissue, and avoiding injury to neighboring structures and hypothermia represent basic principles of surgical technique directly associated with SSI prevention.[38] Foreign bodies, including suture material, may promote an inflammatory reaction and a subsequent infection. Recent evidence suggests suture material has the potential of harboring microbial biofilms. A study by Edmiston et al. recovered sutures (nonabsorbable and absorbable) from infected and noninfected sites and found that approximately 50% of all sutures harbored bacteria. While sutures from noninfected patients were found to have commensal skin flora, sutures from infected patients grew *Staphylcoccus epidermis*, *Staphylococcus aureus*, coagulase-negative staphylococci, *Poststreptococcus* spp., *Bacteroides fragilis*, *Escherichia coli*, *Enterococcus* spp., *Pseudomonas aeruginosa*, and *Serratia* spp. Additionally, there is no difference in quantitative microbial recovery between monofilament and multifilament sutures from infected patients.[45]

Postoperative care

Most incisions after obstetric surgery are closed primarily with staples or sutures. The incision usually is covered with a sterile dressing for several days. Immobilization provided by the sterile dressing contributes to the healing process. However, data are lacking to assess the value of covering the incision after that period of time. Several studies have shown that there is no detrimental outcome from removing the dressing prior to 48 hours.[46] Currently, there are insufficient data regarding showering or bathing after surgery; however, a study by Heal et al.[47] reports no significant difference of rate of SSI between those who shower within or after 48 hours of surgery.[48] The incision should be assessed on a daily basis and surgical staples are removed usually on the fourth day after surgery. Recent studies have shown increased rates of wound separation when staples are removed before 4 days. There remains no difference between rates of wound infection, pain, or cosmesis when staples are compared with sutures.[49,50] Ambulation is encouraged by the first 24 hours postoperatively; the patient should get out of bed briefly with assistance, and by the second day, walking is expected. Bladder catheters are usually removed the next morning after surgery with verification of adequate urinary output. Early discharge is advised; however, adequate discharge planning requires individualization of care. Many patients return home before surgical incisions are fully healed; therefore, instruction on signs and symptoms of infection or other complications must be stressed.

OPERATIVE ROOM ENVIRONMENT

Ventilation systems

Operating room air may contain microbial-laden dust, respiratory droplets, skin particles, and other microscopic contaminants. Levels of microorganisms in the air are associated with the number of healthcare personnel and movement in the operating room.[51] Operating rooms should be maintained at positive pressure with respect to adjacent areas. All ventilation or air-conditioning systems should have two filter screens in series, with the efficiency of the first filter screen being over 30% and that of the second being over 90%. Air should be introduced from the ceiling and exhausted near the floor. A minimum of 15 air changes of filtered air per hour should be produced, of which 20% should be fresh air. Recommended relative humidity ranges are 30%–60%, with room temperatures between 68°F and 73°F (depending on normal ambient temperatures). A more comprehensive review on ventilation parameters in the operating room is available from the American Institute of Architects in collaboration with the U.S. Department of Health and Human Services.[52] Laminar airflow is designed to mobilize ultraclean air at a constant velocity, producing a sweeping action over microscopic particles. Recirculated air is passed through a high efficiency particulate air filter, which can remove particles larger than 3 μm in diameter (e.g., *Aspergillus* spores) with efficiency superior to 99%. Currently, several studies have questioned the benefit of having laminar airflow ventilation systems as cost is becoming an important factor in health care.[53] This measure has been demonstrated to marginally reduce infections in orthopedic surgery.[54] A recent study by Brandt et al.[55] is one of few studies that include abdominal surgery and report a higher SSI rate in departments with laminar airflow operating room ventilation (as compared with turbulent operating room ventilation) for all studied procedures including, hip and knee prosthesis, appendectomy, cholecystectomy, and herniorrhaphy, but not for colon surgery. Other interventions for room decontamination include ultraviolet and hydrogen peroxide systems. Ultraviolet light decontamination technologies can break molecular bonds in DNA in certain wavelengths. For example, an automated, mobile ultraviolet unit has been shown to eliminate vegetative bacteria and *C. difficile*. Hydrogen peroxide systems have been shown to eliminate methicillin-resistant *Staphylococcus aureus* (MRSA), vancomycin-resistant enterococci (VRE), *M. tuberculosis*, spores, viruses, and multidrug-resistant Gram-negative bacilli. Both these decontamination systems cost a substantial amount, require removal of personnel and patients from the room, adequate staff to transport the system to rooms that require decontamination and monitor its use, and require the removal of dust and debris in the room. Hydrogen peroxide systems require more time for decontamination but have been shown to be better at removing spore-forming organisms.[56]

Environmental disinfection

An important component of infection control includes thorough cleaning and disinfection of hospital surfaces and surgical instruments. While visualization of a clean environment was thought to be an adequate method of infection control, studies in recent years have shown that HAIs can be transmitted by organisms that are invisible to the naked eye.[57] These infectious pathogens notorious for causing outbreaks in different hospital facilities have the capability of remaining on surfaces for prolonged periods of time without adequate decontamination. These culprits include MRSA, *C. difficile*, VRE, *Acinetobacter* spp., and norovirus.[58,59]

There are different levels of decontamination. Cleaning is the removal of visible soil, both organic and inorganic, from objects and surfaces, and is an essential step prior to high-level disinfection or sterilization. This process usually requires manual or mechanical use of water with detergents or enzymatic products. Disinfection is performed to allow for handling of instruments and surfaces so that microorganisms are not transmitted from one patient to another. An U.S. Environmental Protection Agency (EPA)-registered hospital disinfectant, such as alcohols, iodophors, hydrogen peroxide, etc., is used during this process and many pathogenic microorganisms are eliminated, except for spore-forming bacteria. Sterilization is a process that destroys all forms of microbial life and utilizes specialized physical or chemical methods. This process is essential for medical devices penetrating sterile body sites, as well as all parenteral fluids and medications. When visible soiling or large blood spills occur during surgery, an EPA-approved hospital disinfectant effective against hepatitis B virus (HBV) and human immunodeficiency virus (HIV) or an EPA-registered hospital tuberculocidal disinfectant should be used before the next operation as part of the Occupational Safety and Health Administration (OSHA) requirements. In settings where resources are limited, a 1:100 dilution of sodium hypochlorite (approximately 1/4 cup of 5.25% household chlorine bleach to 1 gallon of water) is an inexpensive and effective alternative.[60]

STANDARD PRECAUTIONS

HCWs are in constant contact with bodily and bloody fluids that place them at an increased risk of acquiring a blood-borne infection, such as HIV, HBV, and other blood-borne pathogens. "Universal Precautions," a concept created by the Center for Disease Control and Prevention (CDC) in the 1987 document "Recommendations for Prevention of HIV Transmission in Health-Care Setting," made recommendations to apply blood and body fluid precautions to all patients regardless of blood-borne infection status. Under this protocol, all patients were considered potential carriers of human immunodeficiency virus (HIV), hepatitis B virus (HBV), and other blood-borne pathogens[61] and thus were required to wear PPE for prevention. This was further modified with guidelines for "Body Substance Isolation," which stated that healthcare workers should protect themselves not only from bodily fluids but also from other modes of transmission of diseases, such as respiratory secretions and urine.

The combination of both of the above concepts of universal precautions and body substance isolation evolved into "standard precautions" and operate under the principle that all blood, body fluids, secretions, excretions (except sweat), nonintact skin, and mucous membranes may contain transmissible infectious agents (Table 31.4). There are several elements within standard precautions that make them unique from universal precautions including, respiratory hygiene/cough etiquette, safe injection practices, and the use of masks during insertion of catheters or injection of material into spinal or epidural spaces via lumbar puncture procedures. Through these new changes, the current standard precautions not only seek to protect healthcare workers from infection, but also protect patients.[62]

Standard precautions apply to vaginal secretions as well. Since the obstetric practice is often faced, during emergencies or at the time of delivery, with a potential risk of exposure to hazardous secretions, strict adherence to standard precaution practices must be followed in all cases.

Consistent utilization of protective barriers such as gloves, masks, and protective eye wear or face shields should be used to reduce the risk of exposure of the HCWs' skin or mucous membranes to potentially infective materials.

PERIOPERATIVE PROPHYLACTIC ANTIBIOTICS

The trend in the rates of performing cesarean section has increased every year from approximately 20% in 1996 to 32% in 2013,[63] and the operation is one of the most common abdominal procedures performed in the United States.

Postpartum infections are one of the top causes of pregnancy-related deaths in the United States ranging between 10% and 14% of all deaths.[64,65] Postoperative infectious complications after cesarean delivery include postoperative fever, chorioamnionitis, endometritis, wound infection, urinary tract infection, pneumonia, and other serious infectious complications. In a population-based retrospective cohort study by Liu et al.,[66] postpartum morbidity was significantly increased in patients undergoing primary cesarean delivery compared with vaginal delivery, with major puerperal infection contributing to this increased risk. The greatest risk for developing uterine infection in the postpartum period is cesarean section, with most infections occurring in emergent or nonelective situations.[67] An increased risk of chorioamnionitis is more likely in women undergoing a cesarean during the second stage of labor, especially in women with a body mass index (BMI) >40 kg/m^2 undergoing trial of labor after cesarean (TOLAC).[67] Additionally, this risk is compounded in patients with prolonged rupture of membranes, prolonged labor with multiple vaginal examinations, postpartum fever, anemia and poor nutrition, and low socioeconomic status possibly due to inadequate prenatal care.[68]

Increasing rates of cesarean section necessitate proper preventative methods for SSI. A meta-analysis by McKibben et al. found several studies with good quality data and strong evidence that showed three interventions that significantly reduced SSIs: (1) perioperative antibiotic prophylaxis, (2) preoperative vaginal cleansing, and (3) several surgical techniques. These include a Joel-Cohen incision as superior to Pfannenstiel incisions, suture closure of skin more superior than staple closure, suture closure of subcutaneous tissue with thickness >2 cm, and cord traction of placenta superior to manual removal.[69]

Vaginal preparation prior to cesarean section has been shown to decrease the risk of endometritis. A Cochrane study including 2816 women was evaluated for effect of vaginal cleansing with povidone-iodine and showed that postcesarean endometritis was reduced from 8.3% in

Table 31.4 Recommendations for applications of standard precautions for the care of all patients in all healthcare settings.

Component	Recommendations
Hand hygiene	After touching blood, body fluids, secretions, excretions, contaminated items; immediately after removing gloves; between patient contacts.
Personal protective equipment	For touching blood, body fluids, secretions, excretions, contaminated items; for touching mucous membranes and nonintact skin.
Gloves	During procedures and patient care activities when contact of clothing/ exposed skin with blood/body fluids, secretions, and excretions is anticipated.
Gown, mask, eye protection (goggles), face shield	During procedures and patient care activities likely to generate splashes or sprays of blood, body fluids, secretions, especially suctioning, endotracheal intubation
Soiled patient care equipment	Handle in a manner that prevents transfer of microorganisms to others and to the environment; wear gloves if visibly contaminated; perform hand hygiene.
Environmental control	Develop procedures for routine care, cleaning, and disinfection of environmental surfaces, especially frequently touched surfaces in patient care areas.
Textiles and laundry	Handle in a manner that prevents transfer of microorganisms to others and to the environment.
Needles and other sharps	Do not recap, bend, break, or hand-manipulate used needles; if recapping is required, use a one-handed scoop technique only; use safety features when available; place used sharps in puncture-resistant container.
Patient resuscitation	Use mouthpiece, resuscitation bag, other ventilation devices to prevent contact with mouth and oral secretions.

Source: Siegel J et al., Guideline for Isolation Precautions: Preventing Transmission of Infections Agents in Healthcare Settings, http://www.cdc.gov/hicpac/pdf/isolation/Isolation2007.pdf, 2007.

control groups to 4.3% in vaginal cleansing groups, especially in women who were already in labor at the time of cesarean or had a rupture of membranes.[70] No recommendations are currently in place to support this as a standard method of surgical preparation prior to a cesarean section; however, it is easy to perform in preparation for surgery and should be performed if the opportunity is available.

Surgical techniques vary by surgeon, institution, and urgency of cesarean. There is currently no consensus regarding the different methods used for performing cesarean sections, however, studies have attempted to study differences in technique and the disadvantages and advantages of the method in question. Transverse and midline vertical incision are the two options for skin incision during a cesarean section, though transverse incisions are commonly performed. Advantages of transverse incision include better cosmetic results from following Langer's lines, decreased rates of postoperative pain, fascial wound dehiscence, and incisional hernia. In cases where greater exposure is needed, vertical incisions are usually performed.[71] As transverse incisions are more common, recent studies have compared Joel-Cohen-based incisions versus Pfannenstiel incision and have found the former was associated with less postoperative fevers, less blood loss, shorter operating times, and shorter hospital stay.[72,73]

Antimicrobial prophylaxis has played a large role in reducing SSIs after cesarean. A Cochrane review of placebo versus antibiotic prophylaxis prior to cesarean, which included 95 studies with a total of 15,000 women, showed that the latter reduced endometritis, wound infection, and other serious infectious complications by 60%–70% and recommend prophylaxis in all cesareans, emergent or nonemergent[74] as cesarean section is considered a clean-contaminated surgical procedure with exposure to microbes from the skin, abdomen, and vagina (Table 31.5). The drug of choice should be one that covers Gram-positive and Gram-negative bacteria. Several drug regimens have been studied, including penicillins and first-, second-, and third-generation cephalosporins, and several studies support that there is no difference between pencillins and cephalosporins in affecting rates of SSIs.[75] Due to the narrow-spectrum activity, low cost, and efficacy of first-generation cephalosporins, such as cefazolin, it is the drug of choice advocated by the American College of Obstetrics and Gynecology (ACOG) and the American Academy of Pediatrics.[68,76] A single 1 g cefazolin dose is sufficient and lasts approximately 3–4 hours. This dose may need to be increased in obese patients; this is discussed further below. Several new studies have attempted extending the spectrum of antibiotics to include coverage for *Ureaplasma* and *Mycoplasma* with the addition of azithromycin, doxycycline, or metronidazole and have found reductions in infection rates and duration of hospital stay; however, more studies are needed to identify if this difference is significant.[77,78] It is important to note that the evidence of the effect of these antibiotics on neonatal outcome, such as infant sepsis or oral thrush, is insufficient and require further research.[74,75] Prophylactic antibiotics should ideally be administered 60 minutes prior to incision in order to achieve adequate tissue penetration at the site of the incision. However, this is a controversial topic due to the unknown effects of antibiotics on neonatal outcome and has led institutions to administer the antibiotics

Table 31.5 Microorganisms associated with cesarean section.

Skin flora	*Staphylococcus aureus*
	Staphylococcus epidermidis
Abdominal	*Escherichia coli*
	Enterococci
Vaginal	*Staphylococci*
	Streptococci
	Enterococci
	Lactobacilli
	Diphtheroids
	E. coli
	Anaerobic streptococci
	Bacteroides
	Fusobacterium
	Ureaplasma

Source: Bratzler D et al., *Am J Health Syst Pharm*, 70(3), 195–283, 2013.

after cord clamping. A meta-analysis including 10 studies and 5041 women showed administration of prophylactic antibiotics prior to incision halved the risk of endometritis and wound infection as opposed to women who received antibiotics after cord clamping.[79] Although no difference in neonatal outcomes were noted in this meta-analysis, more research is needed, especially in light of the potential effect of these antibiotics to the neonatal microbiome.

In cases of severe penicillin allergies, such as anaphylaxis, angioedema, respiratory distress, or urticaria, clindamycin with an aminoglycoside, such as gentamicin, is an appropriate alternative.[76]

There is no consensus regarding additional antibiotic prophylaxis in women who are in labor and already receiving antimicrobial prophylaxis for Group B *Streptococcus* or are being treated for chorioamnionitis and require a cesarean section. More randomized controlled trials are required for the development of an algorithm or guidelines.

ANTIBIOTIC PROPHYLAXIS FOR OTHER OBSTETRIC PROCEDURES

Repair of third or fourth degree laceration and operative vaginal delivery

Currently, the use of prophylactic antibiotics in the repair of third and fourth degree lacerations is not standard due to the limited amount of studies available. Some physicians prescribe them because of the proximity of the incision to the rectum and the potential of transmitting bacteria from the rectum to the laceration. A prospective randomized controlled study performed by Duggal et al. included 147 women with 83 patients receiving placebo and 64 patients receiving antibiotic prophylaxis with a second-generation cephalosporin. Of those who received antibiotics and returned for a 2-week postpartum check as required for the study ($n = 49$), 8.2% or 4 out of 49 people developed an infection, compared with the placebo population, where 24.1% or 14 of 58 patients developed an infection. Due to the high dropout rate, these results are difficult to generalize to the population.[76,80,81]

There are also limited amount of research regarding antibiotic prophylaxis in patients undergoing operative vaginal delivery. Currently, there are no evidence-based recommendations for antibiotic prophylaxis.[82]

Cervical cerclage

Cervical cerclage placement is indicated for three reasons: (1) examination or emergency indicated, where the patient is noted to have advanced cervical dilation without signs or symptoms of labor or abrupted placenta in the second trimester, (2) history indicated, where a patient has a history of second trimester delivery with painless cervical dilation, and (3) ultrasound indicated with history of preterm delivery before 34 weeks with finding of shortened cervix (<25 mm) prior to 24 weeks in the current pregnancy. However there are several risks associated with cervical cerclage placement, including chorioamnionitis, preterm premature rupture of membranes, preterm delivery, displacement of sutures, and cervical lacerations. Transabdominal cerclage placement also has additional risks that normally exist for abdominal surgery. Cerclage placement is contraindicated in patients who exhibit signs of labor or chorioamnionitis. The risk of developing intra-amniotic infection is increased in patients with emergency, indicating cerclage placement; however, no recommendations currently exist for the use of antibiotic prophylaxis. In patients with cerclage placement due to history or ultrasound finding, the risk of developing intra-amniotic infection is rare and no antibiotic prophylaxis is indicated.[83]

Manual removal of the placenta

Manual extraction of the placenta at the time of cesarean section is associated with an increase in postcesarean section endometritis, even in the presence of antibiotic prophylaxis. It is also associated with increased blood loss and longer hospital stay. Therefore, it is recommended that cord traction be used as the method of delivering the placenta during a cesarean.[84] There are no published studies to support antibiotic prophylaxis for the manual removal of retained placenta after a vaginal birth.[85]

Cesarean hysterectomy

Rates of cesarean hysterectomy average about 0.5 in 1000 deliveries, but this operation is increasing as a result of the rising cesarean section rate. Cesarean hysterectomy is performed for several indications including, uncontrolled postpartum hemorrhage, abnormal placentation, uterine rupture, leiomyoma, cervical laceration, invasive cervical cancer, or ovarian neoplasia. In recent years, the predominant reason for cesarean hysterectomy has been abnormal placentation, followed by uterine atony and uterine rupture. The morbidities associated with this procedure include blood transfusion, fever, perinatal death, bladder injuries, wound infection, disseminated intravascular coagulation, and postoperative ileus. Maternal mortality ranged between 1% and 2%. In patients, where placental accreta disorders are detected in the intrapartum period, preparations are made in anticipation of these risks and lead to decreased blood loss, less requirement for transfusion, and less disruption of the urinary tract system. In cases where the procedure is performed as an emergency, blood loss prior to the procedure compounds the blood loss associated with the procedure itself.[86,87]

As long as the procedure remains a clean-contaminated procedure, routine prophylactic antibiotics may be administered. However, additional doses may be administered when there is a blood loss greater than 1500 mL or if the procedure is longer than 4 hours.[68] Additionally, necrotic tissues, soaked lap pads, and other materials that can contaminate the sterile field should be immediately be removed to prevent risk of SSIs.

OBESITY IN PREGNANCY

Obesity has become a pandemic in the United States. Between 2011 and 2012, 68.5% of adults above the age of 20 were considered to be overweight or obese, with 34.9% of those adults being obese.[88] In 2006, the CDC published recommendations for improving women's health before and between pregnancies. As part of that initiative, data were collected to study the different maternal behaviors, health conditions, and experiences for women in the United States who had a live birth. The mean prevalence of being overweight and obese was 13.2% and 21.9%, respectively. Prevalence was noted to be higher among women aged 20 years old or greater, and among black and Hispanic women.[89]

Obesity in pregnancy increases the risk for developing hypertensive disorders, GDM, and thromboembolic disorders.[90–92] Additionally, there is an association between obese women having macrosomic fetuses leading to greater risk of intrapartum interventions including labor inductions and cesarean sections.[90–92] As a surgical candidate, the obese patient is at an increased risk from intra-/postoperative complications including anesthesia risk, blood loss, prolonged surgical time, and wound infections[93–95] and these risks are further compounded if the patient had multiple cesareans with prior pregnancies.[96] In a study by Stamilio and Scifres,[95] extremely obese patients, defined as having a BMI of 45 or higher, had nearly a threefold increase in the rate of composite postoperative infectious morbidity outcome, i.e., endometritis and wound infection, compared with nonobese patients. A retrospective cohort study by Conner et al.[93] also found that there is a dose–response relationship between increasing BMI and risk for wound infection.

With evidence showing increased rates of wound-related complications in obese pregnant women, recommendations for wound infection prevention include antibiotic prophylaxis with consideration for a higher dosage.[91] In nonpregnant obese patients, recommendations are for 1 g cefazolin in patients weighing 80 kg or more and 2 g in patients weighing 120 kg or more.[68] The American College of Obstetrics and Gynecology (ACOG) recommends the increase of prophylactic antibiotic dosage in women with a BMI > 30 or an absolute weight of 10 kg or more,[76] however, no recommendations for the standard higher dosage currently exist. Most hospital institutions have 2 g cefazolin dosing as the standard recommended higher dose. Adequate antibiotic levels at the incision site in pregnant obese patients are affected by a greater volume of distribution and increased glomerular filtration rate. A study performed by Pevzner et al.[97] showed that the 2 g cefazolin dosing provides insufficient antimicrobial coverage in pregnant obese patients undergoing cesarean section. Maggio et al.[98] showed that 3 g cefazolin dosing did not significantly increase the concentration in adipose tissue at the incision site required to provide adequate antibiotic prophylaxis in comparison to the 2 g dosing. Another small study showed 4 g cefazolin dosing provided increased antibiotic concentrations in adipose but it did not study whether it decreased infection rates.[99] More studies with larger samples sizes are required to determine the appropriate dose of antibiotic prophylaxis in obese patients.

Other methods appropriate for infection prevention include closure of the subcutaneous layers with plain suture when it is greater than 2 cm for prevention of wound separation and its associated complications.[91,100,101] A recent study by Corbacioqlu et al.[102] showed that the rate of wound complications was not significantly different between subcutaneous and nonsubcutaneous closure in patients with a Pfannenstiel skin incision, unless the subcutaneous layer was greater than 4 cm and if the mother had diabetes. Several studies have also examined drainage systems in conjunction with subcutaneous closure in reducing wound infection and found no difference.[103,104,105]

ACKNOWLEDGMENTS

This chapter contains material from the previous edition chapter authored by Javier Garcia and Joseph J. Apuzzio.

REFERENCES

1. Health and Humans Services. health.gov. National Action Plant to Prevent Health Care-Associated Infections: Road Map to Eelimination. http://health.gov/hcq/prevent-hai.asp. Accessed September 2015.

2. Magill S, Edwards J, Bamberg W et al. Multistate point-prevalence survey of health care–associated infections. *N Engl J Med* 2014; 370: 1198–208.
3. Horan T, Andrus M, Dudeck M. CDC/NHSN surveillance definition of health care associated infection and criteria for specific types of infections in the acute care setting. *Am J Infect Control* 2008; 36: 309–32.
4. Nordstrom J, Reynolds K, Gerba C. Comparison of bacteria on new, disposable, laundered, and unlaundered hospital scrubs. *Am J Infect Control* 2012; 40(6): 539–43.
5. Lipp A, Edwards P. Disposable surgical face masks for preventing surgical wound infection in clean surgery. *Cochrane Database Syst Rev* 2014; (2): CD002929.
6. Administration OS&H. Surgical Suite. www.OHSA.gov. https://www.osha.gov/SLTC/etools/hospital/surgical/surgical.html#BloodbornePathogens. Accessed September 18, 2016.
7. Jensen P, Lambert L, Iademarco M, Ridzon R. Guidelines for preventing the transmission of Mycobacterium tuberculosis in health-care settings. *MMWR Recomm Rep* 2005; 54(RR-17): 1–141.
8. CDC. Workplace Safety and Health Topic: Eye Protection for Infection Control. CDC.gov, 2004. http://www.cdc.gov/niosh/topics/eye/eye-infectious.html. Accessed September 18, 2016.
9. Santos A, Lacerda R, Graziano K. [Evidence of control and prevention of surgical infection by shoe covers and private shoes: A sytematic literature review]. *Rev Lat Am Enfermagem* 2005; 13(1): 86–92.
10. Reichman D, Greenberg J. Reducing surgical site infections: A review. *Rev Obstet Gynecol* 2009; 2(4): 212–21.
11. AORN Recommended Practices Committee. Recommended practices for maintaining a sterile field. *AORN J* 2006; 83(2): 402–16.
12. FDA. U.S. Department of Health and Human Services. 2014. http://www.fda.gov/MedicalDevices/DeviceRegulationandGuidance/Overview/GeneralandSpecialControls/ucm055910.htm. Accessed September 18, 2016.
13. Center for Devices and Radiological Health. *Medical Glove Guidance Manual*. Rockville, MD: FDA, 2008.
14. www.medsupplier.com. Medical equipment and supplies.
15. Tanner J, Parkinson H. Double gloving to reduce surgical cross-infection. *Cochrane Database Syst Rev* 2006; (3): CD003087.
16. Mischke C, Verbeek J, Saarto A et al. Gloves, extra gloves or special types of gloves for preventing percutaneous exposure injuries in healthcare personnel. *Cochrane Database Syst Rev* 2014; 3: CD009573.
17. Fry D, Harris W, Kohne E, Twomey C. Influence of double-gloving on manual dexterity and tactile sensation of surgeons. *J Am Coll Surg* 2010; 210(3): 325–30.
18. Parantaine A, Verbeek J, Lavoie M, Pahwa M. Blunt versus sharp suture needles for preventing percutaneous exposure incidents in surgical staff. *Cochrane Database Syst Rev* 2011; (11): CD009170.
19. Stitely M, Close J, Ferda A, et al. Glove perforations with blunt versus sharp surgical needles in Caesarean delivery: A randomized control trial. *W V Med J* 2013; 109(5): 32–6.
20. Wilson L, Sullivan S, Goodnight W, et al. The use of blunt needles does not reduce glove perforations during obstetrical laceration repair. *Am J Obstet Gynecol* 2008; 199(6): 641.e1–3.
21. El-Rafaie T, Sayed K, El-Shourbagy MAE. Role of blunt suture needle in episiotomy repair at uncomplicated vaginal deliveries in reducing glove perforation rate: A randomized controlled trial. *J Obstet Gynecol Res* 2012; 38(5): 787–92.
22. Boyce J, Pittet D. Guideline for hand hygiene in health-care settings: Recommendations of the Healthcare Infection Control Practices Advisory Committee and the HICPAC/SHEA/APIC/IDSA Hand Hygiene Task Force. *MMWR Recomm Rep*; 51(RR-16): 1–45.
23. WHO. *WHO Guidelines on Hand Hygiene in Health Care: A Summary*. Geneva, Switzerland: WHO, 2009.
24. Tanner J, Swarbrook S, Stuart J. Surgical hand antisepsis to reduce surgical site infection. *Cochrane Database Syst Rev* 2008; (1): CD004288.
25. Arrowsmith V, Taylor R. Removal of nail polish and finger rings to prevent surgical site infection. *Cochrane Database Syst Rev* 2014; (8): CD003325.
26. McGinley K, Larson E, Leyden J. Composition and denisty of microflora in the subungual space of the hand. *J Clin Microbiol* 1988; 26: 950–3.
27. McNiel S, Foster C, Hedderwick S, Kauffman C. Effect of hand cleansing with antimicrobial soap or alcohol-based gel on microbial colonization of artifical fingernails worn by health care workers. *Clin Infect Dis* 2001; 32: 367–72.
28. Hedderwick S, McNiel SLM, Kauffman C. Pathogenic organisms associated with artificial fingernails worn by healthcare workers. *Infect Control Hosp Epidemiol* 2000; 21: 505–9.
29. Parry M, Gran B, Yukna M et al. Candida osteomyelitis and diskitis after spinal surgery: An outbreak that implicates artificial nail use. *Clin Infect Dis*. 2001; 32: 352.
30. Moolenaar R, Crutcher J, San Joaquin V et al. A prolonged outbreak of Pseudomonas aeruginosa in a neonatal intensive care unit: Did staff fingernails play a role in disease transmission? *Infect Control Hosp Epidemiol* 2000; 21(2): 80–5.
31. Kjonniksen I, Anderson B, Sondenaa V, Segadal L. Preoperative hair removal: A systematic literature review. *AORN J* 2002; 75(5): 928–40.
32. Tanner J, Norrie P, Melene K. Preoperative hair removal to reduce surgical site infection. *Cochrane Database Syst Rev*. 2011; (11): CD004122.

33. Lefebvre A, Saliou P, Lucet J et al. Preoperative hair removal and surgical site infections: Network meta-analysis of randomized controlled trials. *J Hosp Infect* 2015; 91(2): 100–8.
34. Hemani M, Lepor H. Skin preparation for the prevention of surgical site infection: Which agent is best? *Rev Urol* 2009; 11(4): 190–5.
35. Darouiche R, Wall MJ, Itani K et al. Chlorhexidine-alcohol versus povidone-iodine for surgical-site antisepsis. *N Eng J Med* 2010; 362(1): 18–26.
36. Maiwald M, Chan E. The forgotten role of alcohol: A systematic review and meta-analysis of the clinical efficacy and perceived role of chlorhexidine in skin antisepsis. *PLoS ONE* 2012; 7(9): e44277.
37. Riley M, Suda D, Tabsh K et al. Reduction of surgical site infections in low transverse cesarean section at a university hospital. *Am J Infect Control* 2012; 40: 820–5.
38. Mangram A, Horan T, Pearson M et al. Guideline for prevention of surgical site infections, 1999. Centers for Disease Control and Prevention (CDC) Hospital Infection Control Practices Advisory Committee. *Am J Infect Control* 1999; 27: 97–132.
39. Andersson A, Bergh I, Karlsson J et al. Traffic flow in the operating room: An explorative and desriptive study on air quality during orthopedic trauma implant surgery. *Am J Infect Control* 2012; 40(8): 750–5.
40. Scaltriti S, Cencetti S, Rovesti S et al. Risk factors for particulate and microbial contamination of air in operating theatres. *J Hosp Infect* 2007; 66(4): 320–6.
41. Tartari E, Mamo J. Pre-educational intervention survey of healthcare practitioners' compliance with infection prevention measures in cardiothoracic surgery: Low compliance but internationally comparable surgical site infection rate. *J Hosp Infect* 2011; 77: 348–51.
42. Van der Slegt J, Van der Laan L, Veen E et al. Implementation of a bundle of care to reduce surgical site infections in patients undergoing vascular surgery. *PLoS ONE* 2013; 8: e71566.
43. Healy A, Sevdalis N, Vincent C. Measuring intra-operative interference from distraction and interruption observed in the operating theatre. *Ergonomics* 2006; 49: 589–604.
44. Beldi G, Bisch-Knaden S, Banz V et al. Impact of intraoperative behavior on surgical site infections. *Am J Surg* 2009; 198: 157–62.
45. Edmiston C, Krepel C, Marks R et al. Microbiology of explanted suture segments from infected and non-infected surgical patients. *J Clin Microbiol* 2013; 51: 417–21.
46. Toon C, Lusuku C, Ramamoorthy R, Davidson BGK. Early versus delayed dressing removal after primary closure of clean and clean-contaminated surgical wounds. *Cochrane Database Syst Rev* 2015; (9): CD010259.
47. Heal C, Buettner P, Raasch B et al. Can sutures get wet? Prospective randomised controlled trial of wound management in general practice. *BMJ* 2006; 332: 1053–6.
48. Toon C, Sinha S, Davidson B, Gurusamy K. Early versus delayed post-operative bathing or showering to prevent wound complications. *Cochrane Database Syst Rev* 2015; (7): CD010075.
49. Mackeen A, Berghella V, Larsen M. Techniques and materials for skin closure in caesarean section. *Cochrane Database Syst Rev* 2012; (9): CD003577.
50. Figueroa D, Jauk V, Szychowski I et al. Surgical staples compared with subcuticular suture for skin closure after cesarean delivery: A randomized controlled trial. *Obstet Gynecol* 2013; 121(1): 33–8.
51. Birgand G, Saliou P, Lucet J. Influence of staff behavior on infectious risk in operating rooms: What is the evidence? *Infect Control Hosp Epidemiol* 2015; 36(1): 93–106.
52. Sehulster L, Chinn R, CDC, HICPAC. Guidelines for environmental infection control in health-care facilities. Recommendations of CDC and the Healthcare Infection Control Practices Advisory Committee (HICPAC). *MMWR* 2003; 52(No. RR-10): 1–48.
53. Lipsett P. Do we really need laminal air flow ventilation in the operating room to prevent surgical site infections? *Ann Surg* 2008; 248(5): 701–3.
54. Diab-Elschahawi M, Berger J, Blacky A et al. Impact of different-sized laminar air flow versus no laminar air flow on bacterial counts in the operating room during orthopedic surgery. *Am J Infect Control* 2011; 39(7): e25–9.
55. Brandt C, Hott U, Sohr D et al. Operating room ventilation with laminar airflow shows no protective effect on the surgical site infection rate in orthopedic and abdominal surgery. *Ann Surg* 2008; 248(5): 695–700.
56. Rutala W, Weber D. Disinfectants used for environmental disinfection and new room decontamination technology. *Am J Infect Control* 2013; 41: S36–S41.
57. Dancer S. The role of envronmental cleaning in the control of hospital-acquired infection. *J Hosp Infect* 2009; 73: 378–85.
58. Dancer S. Importance of the environment in methicillin-resistant Staphylococcus aureus acquisition: The case for hospital house cleaning. *Lancet Infect Dis* 2008; 8: 101–13.
59. Weber D, Rutala W, Miller M et al. Role of hospital surfaces in the transmission of emerging health care-associated pathogens: Norovirus, Clostridium difficile, and Acinetobacter species. *Am J Infect Control* 2010; 38(5): S25–33.
60. Rutala W, Weber D, HICPAC. *Guideline for Disinfection and Sterilization in Healthcare Facilities*, 2008.
61. CDC. Perspectives in disease prevention and health promotion update: Universal precautions for prevention of transmission of human immunodeficiency virus, hepatitis B virus, and other bloodborne pathogens in health-care settings. *MMWR* 1988; 37(4): 377–88.

62. Siegel J, Rhinehart E, Jackson M et al. 2007 Guideline for Isolation Precautions: Preventing Transmission of Infections Agents in Healthcare Settings, 2007. http://www.cdc.gov/hicpac/pdf/isolation/Isolation 2007.pdf. Accessed September 18, 2016.
63. Osterman MJ, Martin JA. Trends in low-risk cesarean delivery in the United States, 1990–2013. *Natl Vital Stat Rep* 2014; 63(6): 1–16.
64. CDC. Pregnancy Mortality and Surveillance System: Pregnancy-Related Deaths, 2015. http://www.cdc.gov/reproductivehealth/maternalinfanthealth/pmss.html. Accessed September 18, 2016.
65. Berg C, Callaghan W, Syverson C, Henderson Z. Pregnancy-related mortality in the United States, 1998–2005. *Obstet Gynecol* 2010; 116(6): 1302–9.
66. Liu S, Liston R, Joseph K et al. Maternal mortality and severe morbidity associated with low-risk planned cesarean delivery versus planned vaginal delivery at term. *CMAJ* 2007; 176(4): 455–60.
67. Hammad I, Suneet P, Magann E, Abuhamad A. Peripartum complications with cesarean delivery: A review of Maternal-Fetal Medicine Units Network publications. *J Matern Fetal Neonatal Med* 2014; 27(5): 463–74.
68. Bratzler D, Dellinger E, Olsen K et al. Clinical practice guidelines for antimicrobial prophylaxis in surgery. *Am J Health Syst Pharm* 2013; 70(3): 195–283.
69. McKibben R, Pitts S, Suarez-Cuervo C et al. Practices to reduce surgical site infections among women undergoing cesarean section: A review. *Infect Control Hosp Epidemiol* 2015; 36(8): 915–21.
70. Hass D, Morgan S, Contreras K. Vaginal preparation with antiseptic solution before cesarean section for preventing postoperative infections. *Cochrane Database Syst Rev* 2014; 12: CD007892.
71. Cunningham F, Leveno K, Bloom S et al. Cesarean delivery and peripartum hysterectomy. In: Cunningham F, Leveno K, Bloom S (eds), *Williams Obstetrics* (24th edition). New York, NY: McGraw-Hill, 2013.
72. Mathai M, Hofmeyr G, Mathai N. Abdominal surgical incisions for cesarean section. *Cochrane Database Syst Rev* 2013; 5: CD004453.
73. Hofmeyr G, Mathai M, Shah A, Novikova N. Techniques for cesarean sections. *Cochrane Database Syst Rev* 2008; 201: 431–44.
74. Smaill F, Grivell R. Antibiotic prophylaxis versus no prophylaxis for preventing infection after cesarean section. *Cochrane Database of Syst Rev* 2014; 10: CD007482.
75. Gyte G, Dou L, Vazquez J. Different classes of antibiotics given to women routinely for prevention infection at cesarean section. *Cochrane Database Syst Rev* 2014; (11): CD008726.
76. American College of Obstetricians and Gynecologists. ACOG Practice Bulletin Number 120: Use of prophylactic antibiotics in labor and delivery. *Obstet Gynecol* 2011; 117: 1472–83.
77. Tita A, Hauth J, Grimes A et al. Decreasing incidence of postcesarean endometritis with extended-spectrum antibiotic prophylaxis. *Obstet Gynecol* 2008; 111: 51–6.
78. Tita A, Owen J, Stamm A et al. Impact of extended-spectrum antibiotic prophylaxis on incidence of postcesarean surgical wound infection. *Am J Obstet Gynecol* 2008; 199(3): 303.e1–3.
79. Mackeen A, Packard R, Ota E et al. Timing of intravenous prophylactic antibiotics for preventing pospartum infectious morbidity in women undergoing cesarean delivery. *Cochrance Database Syst Rev* 2014; (12): CD009516.
80. Buppasiri P, Lumbiganon P, Thinkhamrop J, Thinkhamrop B. Antibiotic prophylaxis for third- and fourth-degree perineal tear during vaginal birth. *Cochrane Database of Syst Rev* 2014; (10): CD005125.
81. Duggla N, Mercado C, Daniels K et al. Antibiotic prophylaxis for prevention of postpartum perineal wound complications: A randomized controlled trial. *Obstet Gynecol* 2008; 111(6): 1268–73.
82. Liabsuetrakul T, Choobun T, Peeyananjarassri K, Islam Q. Antibiotic prophylaxis for operative vaginal delivery. *Cochrane Database Syst Rev* 2014; (10): CD004455.
83. American College of Obstetricians and Gynecologists. ACOG Practice Bulletin Number 142: Cerclage for the management of cervical insufficiency. *Obstet Gynecol* 2014; 123: 372–9.
84. Anorlu R, Maholwana B, Hofmeyr G. Methods of placenta delivery at cesarean section. *Cochrane Database Syst Rev* 2008; (3): CD004737.
85. Chongsomchai C, Lumbiganon P, Laopaiboon M. Prophylactic antibiotics for manual removal of retained placenta in vaginal birth. *Cochrane Database Syst Rev* 2014; (10): CD004904.
86. Shellhaas C, Gilber S, Landon M et al. The frequency and complication rates of hysterectomy accopanying cesarean delivery. *Obstet Gynecol* 2009; 114(2, Part 1): 224–9.
87. Machado L. Emergency peripartum hysterectomy: Incidence, indications, risk factors and outcome. *N Am J Med Sci* 2011; 3(8): 358–61.
88. Ogden C, Carroll M, Kit B, Flegal K. Prevalence of childhood and adult obesity in the United States, 2011–2012. *JAMA* 2014; 311(8): 806–14.
89. D'Angelo D, Williams L, Morrow B et al. Preconception and interconception health status of women who recently gave brith to a live-born infant—Pregnancy risk assessment monitoring system (PRAMS), United States, 26 Reporting Areas, 2004. *MMWR* 2007; 56(SS10): 1–35.
90. Marshall N, Spong C. Obesity, pregnancy complications and birth outcomes. *Semin Reprod Med* 2012; 30: 465–71.
91. American College of Obstetricians and Gynecologists. ACOG Committee opinion no. 549: Obesity in pregnancy. *Obstet Gynecol* 2013; 121: 213–7.

92. Yu C, Teoh T, Robinson S. Review article: Obesity in pregnancy. *Br J Obstet Gynecol* 2006; 113(10): 1117–25.
93. Conner S, Verticchio J, Tuuli M et al. Maternal obesity and risk of post-cesarean wound complications. *Am J Perinatol* 2014; 31(4): 299–304.
94. Girsen A, Osmundson S, Nagvi M et al. Body mass index and operative times at cesarean delivery. *Obstet Gynecol* 2014; 124(4): 684–9.
95. Stamilio D, Scifres C. Extreme obesity and postcesarean maternal complications. *Obstet Gynecol* 2014; 124(2-Part 1): 227–32.
96. Mourad M, Silverstein M, Bender S et al. The effect of maternal obesity on outcomes in patient undergoing tertiary or higher cesarean delivery. *J Matern Fetal Neontal Med* 2015; 28(9): 989–93.
97. Pevzner L, Swank M, Krepel C et al. Effects of maternal obesity on tissue concentrations of prophylactic cefazolin during cesarean delivery. *Obstet Gynecol* 2011; 117: 877–82.
98. Maggio L, Nicolau D, DaCosta M et al. Cefazolin prophylaxis in obese women udergoing cesarean delivery. *Obstet Gynecol* 2015; 125: 1205–10.
99. Stitely M, Sweet M, Slain D et al. Plasma and tissue cefazolin concentrations in obese patients undergoing cesarean delivery and receiving differing pre-operative doses of drug. *Surg Infect* 2013; 14: 455–9.
100. Anderson E, Gates S. Techniques and materials for closureof the abdominal wall in cesarean section. *Cochrane Database Syst Rev* 2004; (4): CD004663.
101. Chelmow D, Rodriguez E, Sabatini M. Suture closure of subcutaneous fatand wound disruptionafter cesarean delivery: A meta-analysis. *Obstet Gynecol* 2004; 103(5 Pt 1): 974.
102. Corbacioqlu E, Goksedef P, Akca A et al. Role of subcutaneous closure in preventing wound complications after cesarean delivery with Pfannestiel incision: A randomized clinical trial. *J Obstet Gynecol Res* 2014; 40(3): 728–35.
103. Ramsey P, White A, Guinn D et al. Subcutaneous tissue, reapproximation, alone or in combination with drain, in obese women undergoing cesarean delivery. *Obstet Gynecol* 2005; 105(5 Pt 1): 967–73.
104. Hellums E, Lin M, Ramsey P. Prophylactic subcutaneous drainage for prevention of wound complications after cesarean delivery—A meta-analysis. *Am J Obstet Gynecol* 2007; 197(3): 229–35.
105. Mackeen A, Schuster M, Berghella V. Suture versus staples for skin closure after cesarean: A meta-analysis. *Am J Obstet Gynecol* 2015; 212(5): 621.e1–10.

Cesarean scar pregnancy

32

ANA MONTEAGUDO, JOANNE RAMOS, and ILAN E. TIMOR-TRITSCH

CONTENTS

INTRODUCTION: THE SCOPE OF THE PROBLEM

Cesarean scar pregnancy (CSP) is a "new, manmade medical condition" of the twentieth century. It can occur only after a prior cesarean delivery or deliveries or after a prior CSP[1,2]; it is essentially an iatrogenic and late consequence of an earlier cesarean delivery (CD). Over the latter part of the twentieth century, and indeed in the past several decades, CDs have dramatically increased. In 1965, the total CD rate was 4.5%; by 1985, the rate rose to 22.7%, reaching a peak of 32.9% in 2009; however, during the last several years this rate has slowly decreased and the preliminary data for 2014 revealed that the overall CD is 32.2%.[3,4] Complications of CD include both maternal complications at the time of the first or repeat surgical procedures. In a subsequent pregnancy, complications can occur during the antenatal period such as bleeding from a placenta previa and/or abnormally adherent placenta or even uterine rupture. Regardless of the gestational age many of these complications can be catastrophic for both mother and neonate.[5] In the continuum, or spectrum, of placental attachment disorders CSP is a common starting point and eventually progresses to early second-trimester placenta accreta, ultimately resulting in the well-known clinical picture of morbidly adherent placenta (MAP) classically seen in the late second and third trimesters.[6–8] Placental adherence disorders are discussed in a separate chapter.

BACKGROUND AND THE ROLE OF THE CESAREAN DELIVERY SCAR

The accepted estimated rate of CSP ranges from 1:1800 to 1:2500 in all patients with a history of a previous CD, although its true rate is unknown.[1] In 2004, Seow et al. estimated that the rate of CSP to be 0.15% of all pregnancies with a history of a previous CD.[9] More recently, Maymon et al.[10] reported that the rates of CSP for the general obstetric population in their institution to be 1:3000, and 1:531 among patients with at least one CD. Nevertheless, the actual rates may be different, because of factors such as CSPs are diagnosed as cervical pregnancies or just by simply not being recognized. Furthermore, it is estimated that CSP represent 6% of ectopic pregnancies.[9,11] The question is, is whether CSP is an ectopic pregnancy? Many would argue that CSP is not a true ectopic pregnancy since it is located within the uterine cavity, although the placenta may be implanted within the prior CD scar or niche, which is still part of the uterine cavity. It can also be located in the upper cervical canal. Furthermore, if the CSP is allowed to continue, eventually the gestational sac and the fetus will "move up" and develop within the uterine cavity as in any intrauterine gestation and for the most part may result in a live neonate.[7] Last, many of the treatments that are designed for "classic" ectopic pregnancies may not necessarily work in CSP and could result in catastrophic complications. Notwithstanding this argument in the literature one can find terms such as "cesarean ectopic," "cesarean section ectopic pregnancy," and others.

After one or more CDs all uteri have a distinct scar which is demonstrable by ultrasound (US). At times in the area of the scar a niche of variable size and shape or a dehiscence may be seen (Figure 32.1). A niche is defined as an anechoic defect in the anterior low myometrium in the area of the prior incision. It is usually referred to as a dehiscence mainly when there is a large and total defect without covering myometrium. This niche can be easily seen at the time of a saline infusion sonohysterography[12] (Figure 32.2). The typical sonographic appearance of the niche is that of a triangle with the apex pointing toward the myometrial/bladder interphase. The myometrial roof

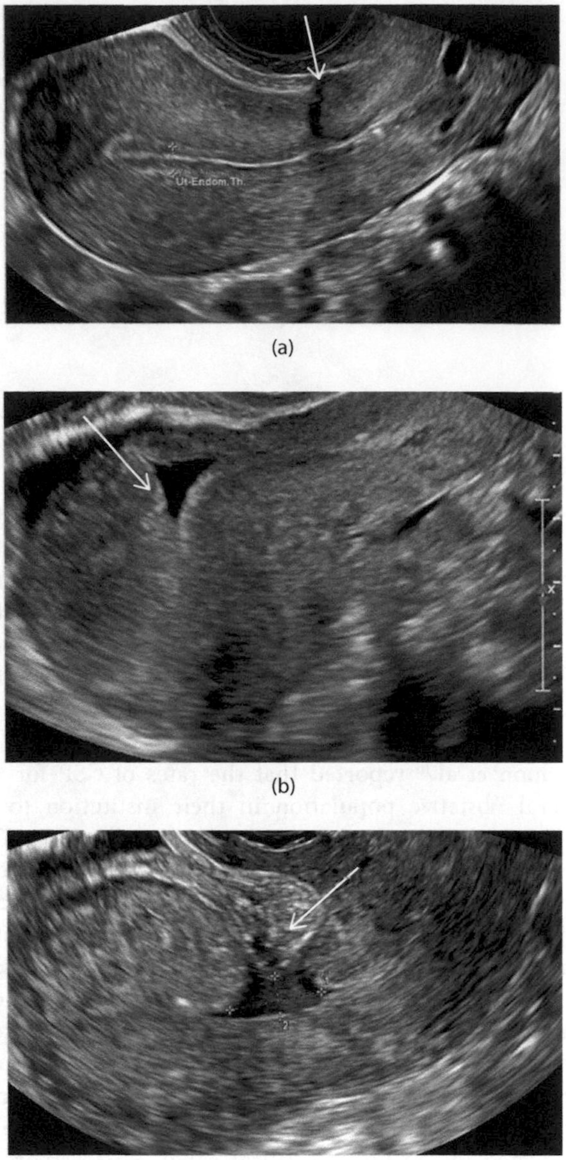

Figure 32.1 Long-axis view of three different uteri after cesarean delivery. (a) The CD scar is evident as an anechoic linear structure (arrow). (b) A niche is evident as a triangular anechoic structure (arrow). (c) The dehiscence is seen at the site of the CD scar. There is no myometrial tissue covering the defect (arrow).

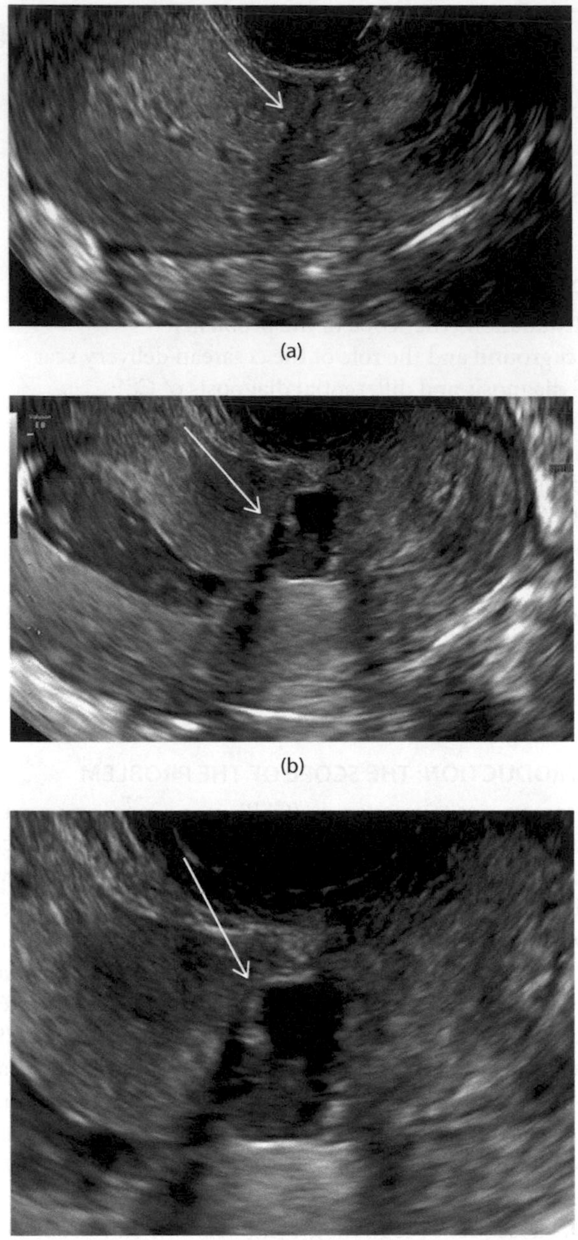

Figure 32.2 Long-axis view of the uterus after two prior cesarean deliveries before and after saline infusion. (a) The area of the CD scar is not clearly seen (arrow) prior to the saline infusion. (b) After the saline infusion the scar and the thin covering myometrium is clearly seen (arrow). (c) Zooming reveals the relatively thin myometrial roof of this "large" niche is evident (arrow).

is thinner than the myometrium just above or below the CD scar (Figure 32.2). In many cases, the niche can be so prominent that it may be seen even without instilling saline (Figure 32.1). This niche is typically depicted in a longitudinal sagittal view of the uterus. When the probe is rotated to a transverse plane or when a 3D volume of the uterus is obtained; the niche's width can be seen and usually will appear to be wider than expected (Figures 32.3, 32.4). This finding is consistent with the fact that in most CDs the incision is made in the transverse fashion (Kerr incision). Osser et al. (2009)[13] found that in a series of 287 patients undergoing transvaginal US 6–9 months after a delivery, of which 162 had undergone one or more CD, the scar could be identified by transvaginal US. After one CD, a defect (niche) was seen in 61% of the cases, a large defect (large niche) was seen in 14% of the cases, and a total defect (dehiscence) in 6% of the cases; in patients who had undergone two prior CDs the numbers were 81%, 23%, and 7%, respectively, and in those patients with at least three prior CDs the numbers were 100%, 45%, and 18%, respectively. When the patient's history shows more previous CDs, there is higher probability that the defects (niches) will be detected. Large defects (large niches)

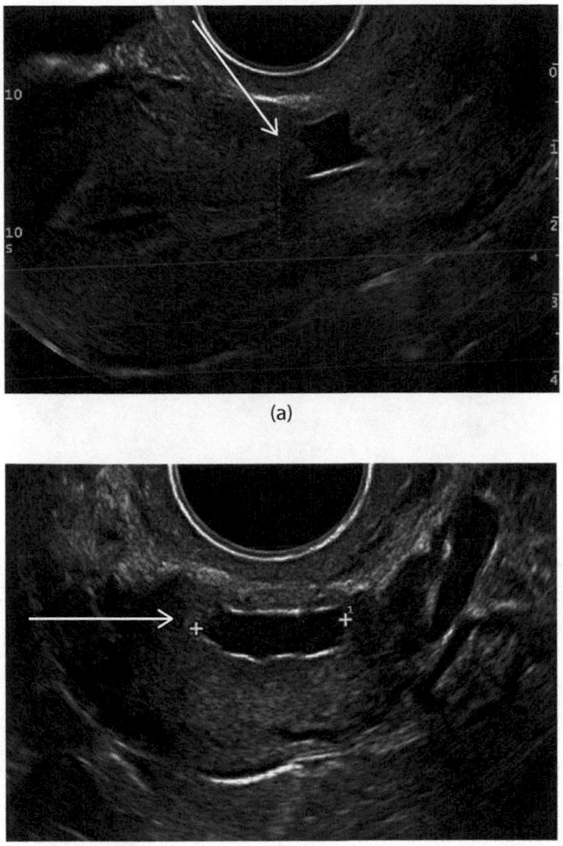

(a)

(b)

Figure 32.3 Uterus after cesarean delivery demonstrating the niche. (a) The long-axis, sagittal view of the uterus demonstrates a box like anechoic niche in the area of the prior CD (arrow). (b) After rotating the probe 90° around its axis the transverse view of the uterus is seen. The anechoic niche is wider than seen on the sagittal plane (arrow). It now measures 1.75 cm.

or total dehiscences also become more common with multiple CDs (Figure 32.2). In addition, large niches or total scar defects (dehiscences) are more frequently seen in retroflexed uteri than those in anteflexion (Figure 32.1b). Although niches can occur in any place along the prior CD scar in a study of 124 scar defects, 110 (89%) were noted to be centrally located by US while the balance was divided equally to the right or left of the midline.[13] Bij De Vaate et al.[14] performed a systematic review of the prevalence, potential risk factors for the development, and symptoms related to the presence of the niches. They found that the prevalence varied between 56% and 84% of the studied prior CDs. The shape of the niches or dehiscence can vary from triangular, round, or oval, at times it may be extensive and reaching the anterior uterine wall or the area below the bladder in the shape of a fistulous connection between the uterine cavity and the uterine surface. In other instances, the niche may be deep and extremely wide. Since the prevalence of niches is relatively high one can speculate that the possibility of the blastocyst implanting in or on the niche is all too realistic. The above systematic review also revealed that there is no definition of what is considered a large niche. Several descriptions for large niches have been used such as "the niche penetrating to a depth of at least 50% or 80% of the anterior myometrium," or "the remaining myometrial thickness is ≤2.2 mm when evaluated by transvaginal sonography (TVS)" and "≤2.5 mm when evaluated at the time of a saline infusion." A total defect was defined as no remaining myometrium covering the defect; in our practice we typically refer to this as a "dehiscence." If the dehiscence is large and no myometrium is detected the term "window" can also be used. The Bij De Vaate study also identified several risk factors for development of niches such as the technique of repair, location of the incision, wound healing, and probably the number of layers included in the closure as well as multiple CDs and uterine retroflexion. The practical importance of the above is that in order to correctly evaluate a niche it is imperative that the US image is obtained not only in the sagittal but also in the transverse plane.

US DIAGNOSIS AND DIFFERENTIAL DIAGNOSIS OF CSP

At presentation, the correct diagnosis of a CSP can be challenging to the OB/GYN practitioner. Commonly, CSP is undiagnosed, misdiagnosed as a cervical pregnancy or a pregnancy that is in the process of passing through the cervix as part of a spontaneous abortion. In a review of 751 cases of CSP from the literature,[8] it was estimated that at least 13.6% of the cases of CSP were undiagnosed. Timor-Tritsch et al. suggested an easy method for the obstetrical practitioners to differentiate between an intrauterine pregnancy and a CSP. In a patient with a prior CD and a positive pregnancy test, a long-axis, sagittal view, of the uterus is obtained in which the uterine fundus, the gestational sac, and the cervix are seen. A line is drawn from an opening in the center of the ectocervix (external cervical os) to the external surface of the uterine fundus. A second line is drawn at a 90° angle at the half point of the previous line to divide the uterus into two (Figure 32.5). If the center of the gestational sac in question is seen above the line (closer to the fundus) it is most likely a normal implantation; however, if the center of the sac is below the above mid-line (closer to the cervix), it is almost surely a CSP. The sensitivity, specificity, and positive and negative predictive values for the cervix-to-sac-center in the study were 93%, 98.9%, 96.4%, and 97.9%. respectively.[15] However, it is important to note that this method also "works" for a cervical pregnancy since in this case the sac will also be below the line; however, in a cervical pregnancy usually there is no prior history of CD. In a cervical pregnancy, the placenta and the entire gestational sac containing an embryo/fetus are present centrally within the endocervical canal below the level of the internal os. The internal os can be identified by the level of the approach and insertion of the uterine arteries into the cervix, which is observed on a coronal section by US using color/power Doppler. The cervical canal and the cervix are dilated and barrel-shaped while the uterine cavity is empty.[16] A pregnancy that is "passing" through the cervical canal as part of a spontaneous abortion can be differentiated from a normal pregnancy, a CSP, or a

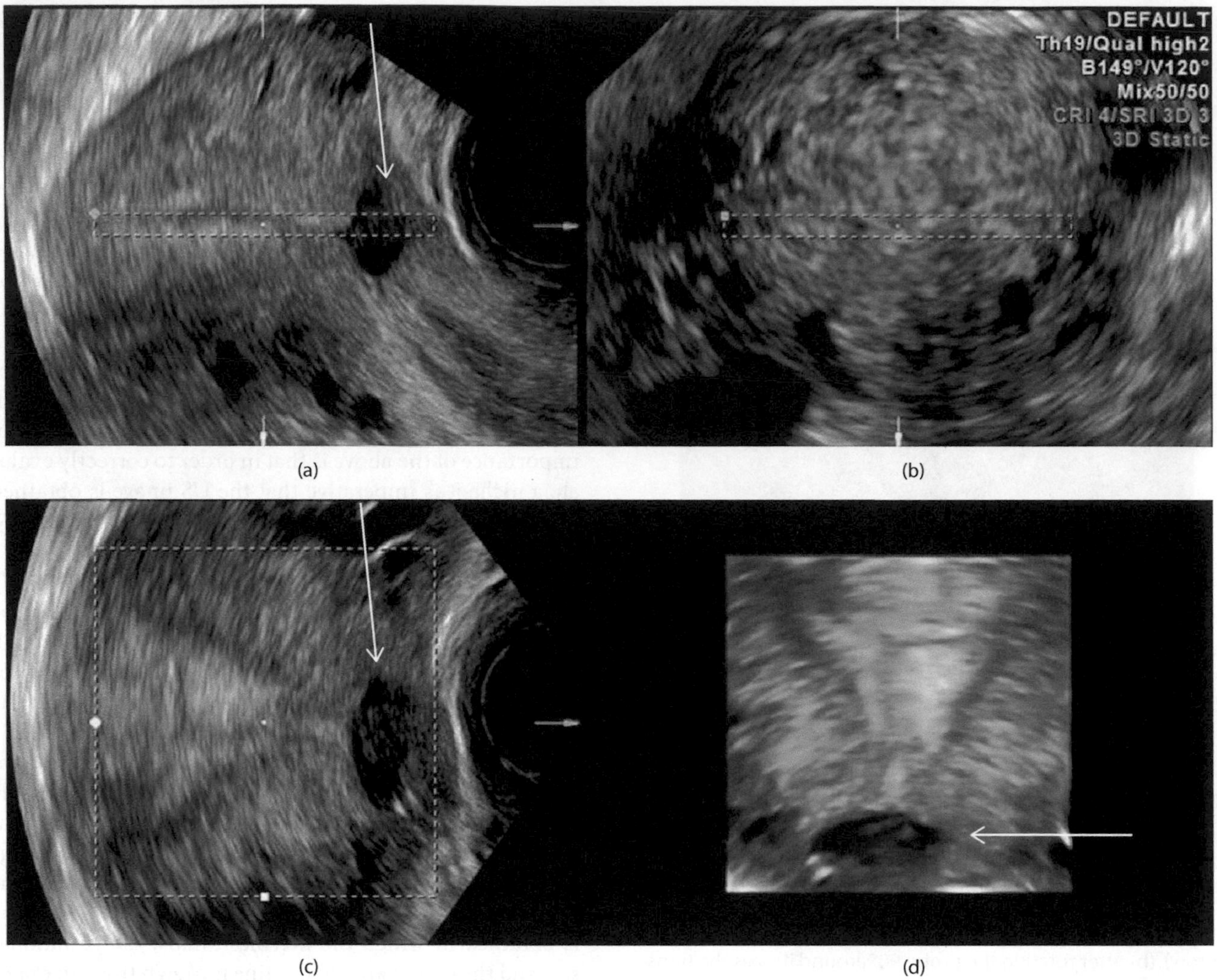

Figure 32.4 Three-dimensional multiplanar image of a uterus after cesarean delivery demonstrating a large niche (arrows). (a) Sagittal plane, (b) axial plane, and (c) coronal plane. The 3D reconstruction (d) shows the large defect in the area of the scar.

cervical pregnancy by the absence of cardiac activity and blood flow surrounding the gestational sac when using color/power Doppler. Under real-time US, the sac may be seen moving within the cavity spontaneously or when pressure is exerted on the anterior uterus (Table 32.1).[17]

Various and at times slightly different criteria have been proposed to diagnose CSP.[18–20] However, they all include an empty uterus and cervical canal and a low anteriorly located gestational sac positioned in or on the prior scar or niche. Our group has taken into consideration additional clinical and sonographic criteria when diagnosing a CSP.[1,8] The clinical criteria include a history of at least one prior CD with a positive human chorionic gonadotropin (hCG) test. The sonographic criteria include the following observations: an endometrial and endocervical canal without a gestational sac; a gestational sac and/or placenta with a viable or nonviable embryo implanted in the prior CD scar or niche; detection of a CSP below the line dividing the uterus in half (close to the cervix) by using cervix-to-sac-center method; and a triangularly shaped gestational sac filling the niche of the scar in pregnancies of <8 postmenstrual weeks (Figures 32.6, 32.7, and 32.8). At ≥8 postmenstrual weeks the sac shape may become rounded or even oval and may be seen "moving up" into the lower uterine segment (Figure 32.8). Depending on the appearance and size of the prior CD niche a 1- to 5-mm myometrial layer between the gestational sac and the bladder may be apparent; if there was a dehiscence present no myometrium will be seen between the sac and the bladder. Using color/power Doppler we strongly rely on the presence of a prominent, and at times rich, vascular blood flow pattern that can be detected at the implantation site of the tiny placenta (Figures 32.6c, 32.7c and d) (Table 32.1).

The role of 3D ultrasound in the diagnostic process and management of CSP is controversial. Nonetheless, it can provide information regarding the precise location of the gestational sac, its vascularity, and the volume of the gestational sac. Vascularization of the placenta implantation site can be expressed in a quantitative fashion (Figures 32.9, 32.10). These quantitative blood flow measurements can be used to serially monitor the healing process of treated cases. In addition, they can serve as baseline measurement

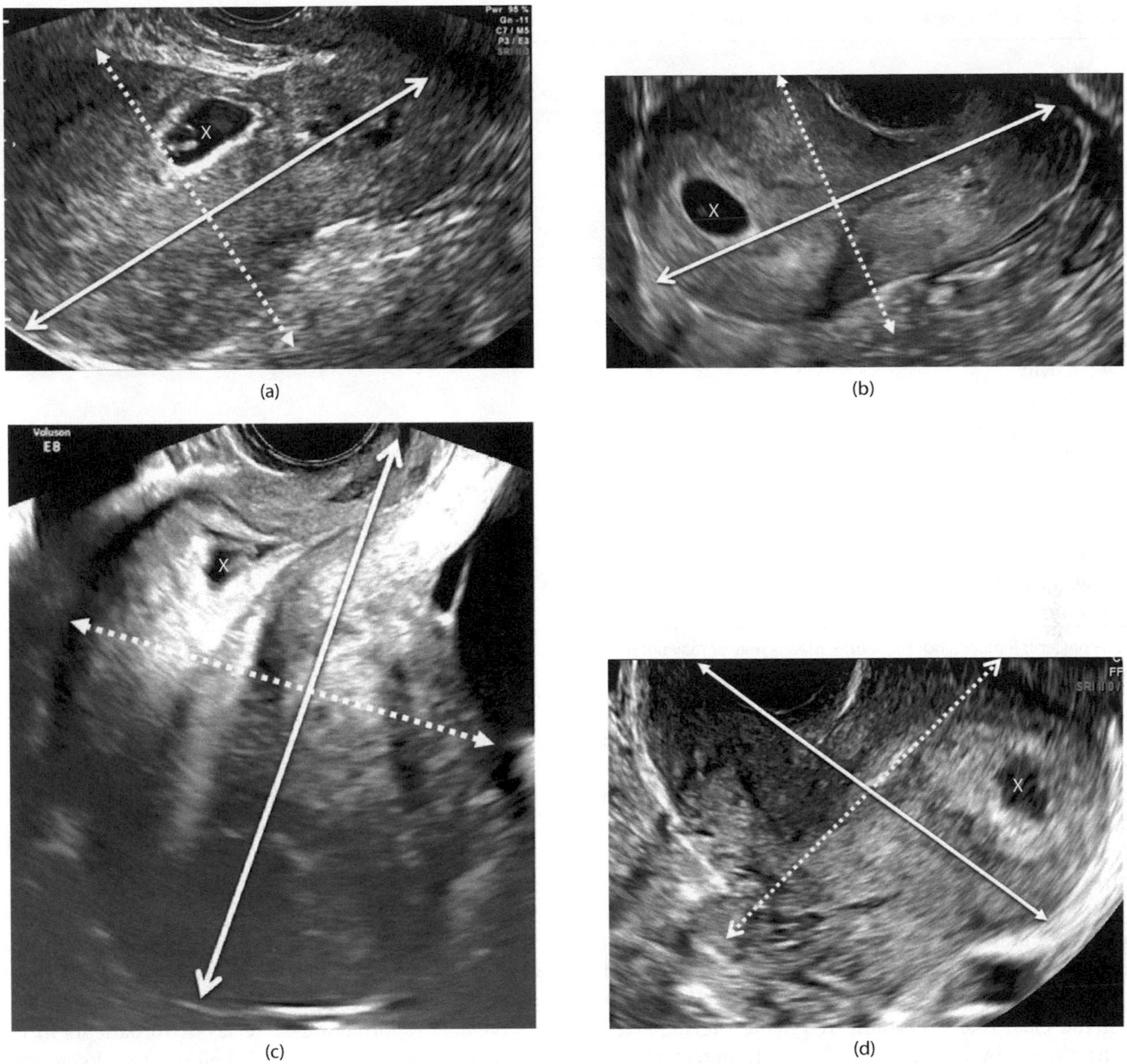

Figure 32.5 CSP versus IUP—The location of the sac center marked by "X" in relation to the midpoint of the uterus (dotted lines) determined along the external cervical os to the uterine fundus on the sagittal images of the uterus (solid lines). (a) CSP in an anteverted uterus. (b) IUP in an anteverted uterus. (c) CSP in a retroflexed uterus. (d) IUP in a retroflexed uterus.

of flow velocities in cases of looming formation of arteriovenous malformation (AVM) at the site of the treated CSP (Figure 32.11).

OUTCOMES AND NATURAL HISTORY OF CSP

Before 2012, there were only a handful of articles reporting on successful deliveries of third-trimester neonates when a CSP was diagnosed in the first trimester. There were numerous articles discussing severe bleeding, shock, uterine rupture, and hysterectomies in patient reaching only the second trimester. Based upon the above severe complications and dismal outcomes patients were counseled almost exclusively for termination of the pregnancy to avoid life-threatening complications resulting from the abnormal implantation into the scar.

Complications of CSP include but are not limited to profuse hemorrhage, uterine dehiscence/rupture, throughout all three trimesters, and permanent loss of fertility due to hysterectomy. There is typically an urgency to terminate the pregnancy as soon as the decision to terminate is reached. The reason is that as the pregnancy is allowed to grow larger and further in gestation, it may cause more complications at the time of the treatment (Table 32.2). In addition, with deeper placental invasion, there is progressive and faulty invasion of the placenta into the scar, resulting in an abnormal and at times deeply invading placentation, typically referred to as placenta accreta. Nonetheless, as more information about the natural history of the CSP is slowly emerging, our evidence-based counseling is changing or becoming more individualized

Table 32.1 Differential diagnosis of a viable CSP.

	IUP 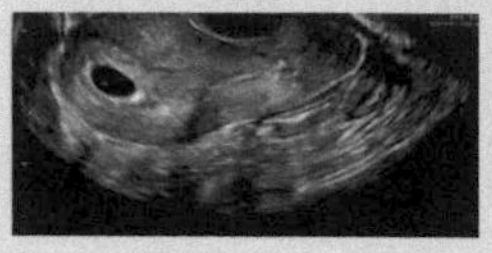	CSP 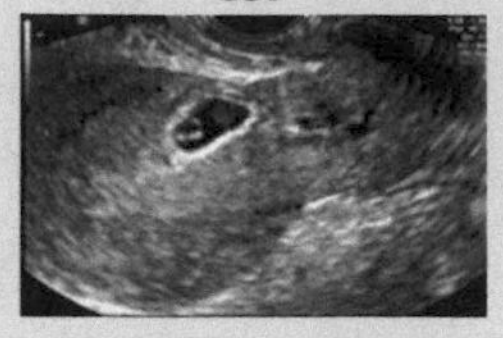	Cervical pregnancy 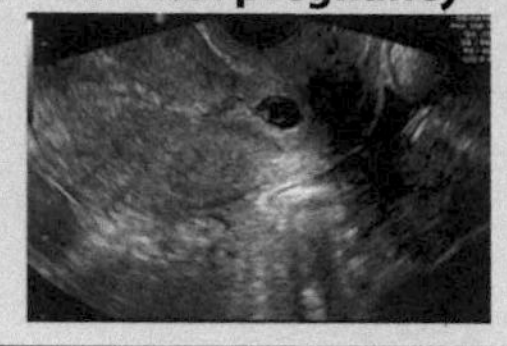	Ab "in transit" 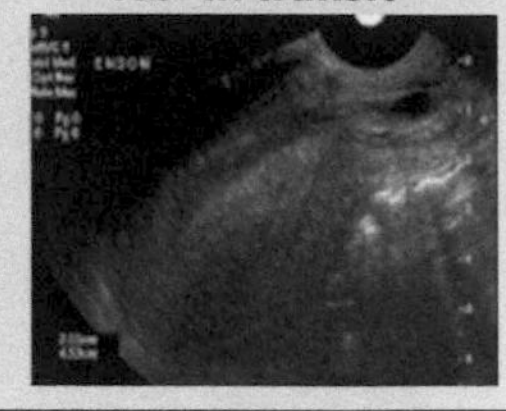
Positive BHCG	+	+	+	+
H/o prior CD	±	+	±	±
Empty uterus	–	+	+	+
Cardiac activity	+	+	+	–
GS in the cervix	–	–	+	+
Blood flow around GS	+	+	+	–
GS anterior/close to the bladder	–	+	–	–
GS central/below the uterine arteries	–	–	+	+
GS below the half point of the uterus	–	+	+	+

+ means present; – means not present; ± means may or may not be present.
Abbreviations: Ab, abortion; BHCG, Beta hCG; GS, gestational sac.

enabling a select group of patients who understand the involved risk to continue their pregnancy.

We published on the outcome of 60 cases of CSP managed in our department. Forty-eight of the patients at presentation had a viable CSP and 12 nonviable CSP[7] (Figure 32.12). Ten of the twelve nonviable pregnancies were treated with conservative management and all resolved without any severe and long-lasting complications. The other two who presented with intractable bleeding were eventually diagnosed with an AVM at the site of the CSP, one eventually requiring uterine artery embolization (UAE) and the other a hysterectomy. In the group of 48 patients presenting with viable CSP, 33 patients elected termination of the CSP by local injection, of which 31 resolved without complications and 2 developed an AVM requiring UAE with eventual resolution. Ten patients elected to continue the pregnancy, of which five had significant second-trimester complications, three had uterine rupture, one had uterine dehiscence and bulging membranes, and all five eventually needing a hysterectomy. However, 3 of the 10 patients who continued the pregnancy delivered a viable baby by elective cesarean section, but all three had a hysterectomy. In summary, of the original 60 cases with CSP, 47 (78.3%) resolved, 11 (18.3%) had hysterectomy, 5 (8%) developed an AVM, and 4 (7%) needed UAE. All 33 (100%) cases managed with transvaginally guided local intragestational sac injection resolved without the need for hysterectomy. Among the 10 patients that opted to continue the pregnancy 4 (40%) delivered a viable neonate and 5 (50%) had second-trimester complications resulting in hysterectomy. In conclusion, 78.3% of the 60 patients had a favorable outcome while 18.3% had hysterectomy (3.4% were lost to follow-up).

Michaels et al.[21] studied 34 cases of CSP at Brigham and Women's Hospital, Harvard Medical School; their results were comparable with our results described earlier. In 14 of the 24 CSP with positive cardiac activity, which was treated minimally invasively, all resolved without hysterectomies. Amid these cases, eight patients continued the pregnancy of which five (62.5%) delivered live neonates in the third trimester with three (37.5%) requiring hysterectomy; the other three had a pregnancy loss of which two required UAE, but none had a hysterectomy.

We also reported a case series of 10 patients in which the diagnosis of CSP was made before 10 weeks' gestation.[6] After extensive counseling, all patients elected to continue the pregnancy. By the second trimester all the patients demonstrated the typical sonographic features of the morbidly adherent placenta (MAP); 9 of the 10 (90%) patients delivered live-born neonates between 32 and 37 weeks. One of the patients had a gravid hysterectomy due to second-trimester complications (cervical shortening and severe bleeding); pathology confirmed placenta percreta in this case. All nine patients underwent hysterectomy for an abnormally adherent placenta and the pathology confirmed placenta percreta in all nine cases.

In summary, the literature has mounting evidence that patients with viable CSP who opt for early treatment using puncture injection of the CSP with immediate termination of the cardiac activity typically have resolution of the CSP without the need for hysterectomy. However, after extensive counseling patients decide to continue the pregnancy and there is growing evidence that under certain circumstances and precautions taken this is possible. In a significant number of cases by the second trimester and sometimes earlier, the typical sonographic features

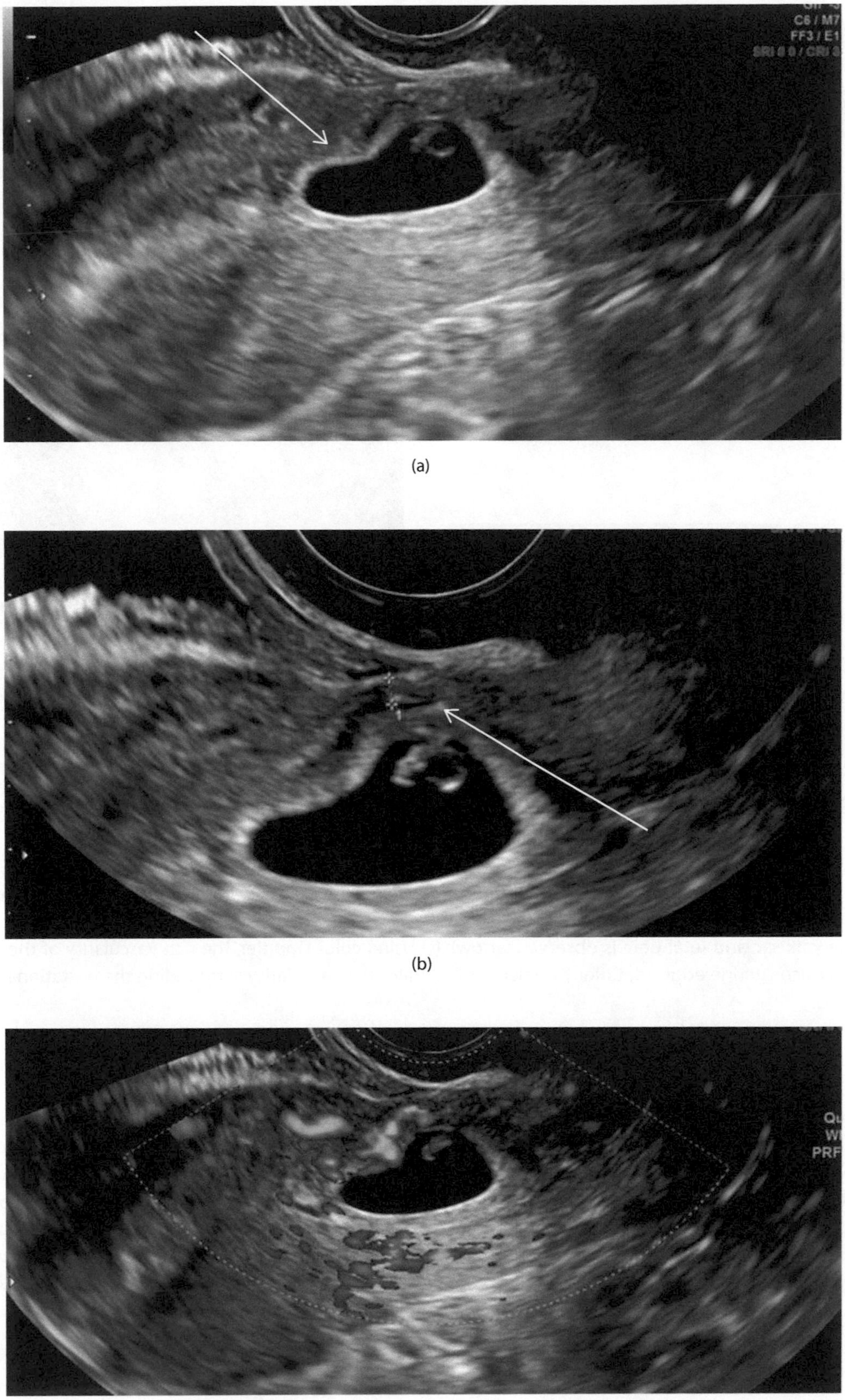

(a)

(b)

(c)

Figure 32.6 Diagnostic US criteria for the sonographic diagnosis of CSP. (a) Endometrial and endocervical canal without a pregnancy. The gestational sac with a live embryo and yolk sac at 6 5/7 weeks is seen anterior in close proximity to the bladder (arrow). (b) The gestational sac is triangularly shaped with a thin myometrial roof measuring 2.1 mm (arrow). (c) Using Power Doppler, the blood vessels of the placenta are seen invading the myometrial roof of the defect (arrow).

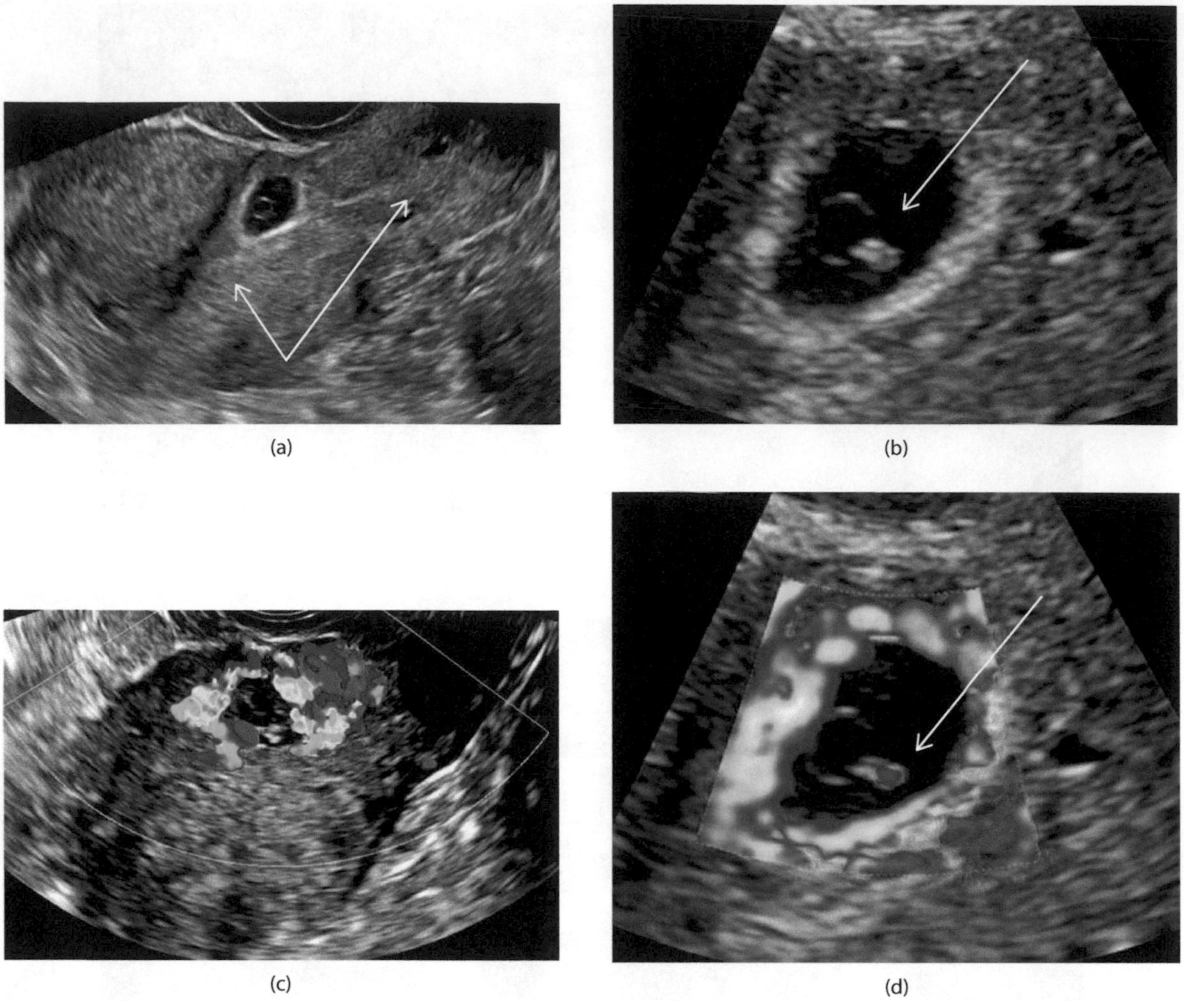

Figure 32.7 CSP at 5 5/7 weeks of gestation. (a) The long-axis view of the uterus demonstrates empty fundus and endocervical canal (arrow). The gestational and yolk sac are seen "tucked" in the niche and in very close proximity to the bladder (b). (b) Zooming in on the CSP, the yolk sac and fetal pole is observed (arrow). (c) Using color Doppler, the rich vascularity of the placenta is seen extending to the vesico-uterine edge. (d) Color Doppler demonstrates the vascularity surrounding the gestational sac and the cardiac activity (arrow).

suggestive of a MAP are already present.[6,17,22] Though, in most of these cases the pregnancy can progress resulting in a live-born neonate at the expense of a hysterectomy. Histology of the uteri in nearly all of the above cases confirmed the presence of the adherent placenta. Furthermore, there is growing evidence that some patients with CSP who continue the pregnancy are at risk of severe obstetrical complications during the second trimester, at times resulting in hysterectomy and a fetal demise.

TREATMENT OPTIONS

Management of the patients with CSP depends upon the clinical scenario at presentation as well as the wishes for the couple of preserving fertility. In the literature there are numerous treatment options, some of which are associated with significant rates of complications (Table 32.3).

Based upon the literature a total of 31 primary treatment modalities for CSP were identified.[8] The overall complication rate in this cohort was 331/751 (44.1%). Complications were defined first and foremost as the immediate or delayed need for a secondary treatment. Other most common indications for the secondary treatments were failure to stop the heart rate by a primary treatment, blood loss requiring transfusion of greater than 200 mL, shock, and hemoperitoneum. Secondary treatments included surgical interventions such as laparoscopy, hysteroscopy, laparotomy, hysterectomy, or procedures that required general or regional anesthesia or embolization of the uterine arteries.

Among all of the treatment modalities, three were identified to have the largest complications rates: dilation and curettage (D&C) alone or in combination with any other treatment had a complication rate of 61.9% and single injection of systemic intramuscular (IM) methotrexate (MTX) alone, usually of 1 mg/kg body weight or even 100 mg, had a 62.1% complication rate mostly due to the fact that it did not stop the beating fetal heart. UAE alone or in combination with other treatments carried a complication rate of 46.9%.

It is interesting to note that these three treatments that are commonly used to treat obstetrical complications of

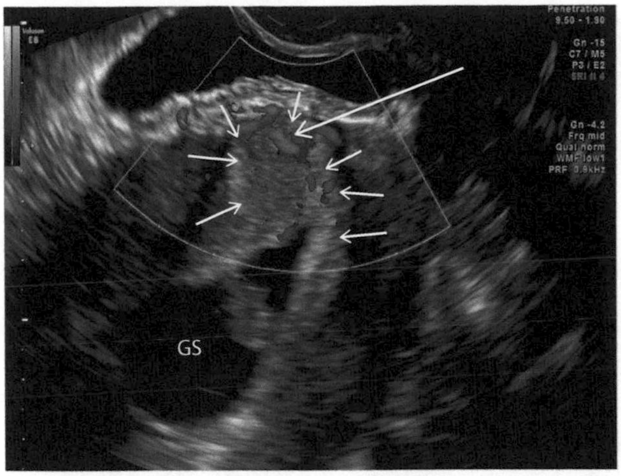

Figure 32.8 CSP at 8 2/7 weeks of gestation. The gestational sac (GS) is seen elongated extending into the uterine cavity. The placenta is clearly seen marked by small arrows. Using color flow Doppler the vascularity of the placenta is seen in the area of the prior scar in very close proximity to the bladder (long arrow). Note the blood vessels traversing the myometrial/bladder interphase—this scan is almost pathognomonic for an abnormally adherent placenta (accreta).

pregnancies have a high complication rate when applied to the CSP. The reasons for the high complication/failure rates may be multiple and complex, depending on a number of variables such as gestational age, expertise of the operator, the specific treatment applied, and other factors. Dilatation and curettage have high complication rates because the scar tissue where the CSP has implanted, unlike the uterine body, does not contain a grid of three myometrial layers, which quell bleeding by contracting after curettage; therefore, profuse bleeding occurs in the implantation site in the scar. IM MTX is usually the first drug that is administered by the practitioners. Its high complication rate may stem from the fact that it takes several days for the drug to take effect; therefore, while waiting for the drug to take effect the CSP is continuing to grow and its placenta further invading the scar and the uterus. If it does not stop the heart activity (and in many cases it does not do so) the patient has to be treated by another or secondary treatment, which carries higher complication rates. Multidose MTX regimens have also been used. While they were somewhat more effective than single-dose treatment, they may also fail. Of note, in the treatment of unruptured tubal ectopic pregnancy it is a well-accepted fact that the presence of cardiac activity is a relative contraindication for MTX usage due to its relatively high failure rate.[23] Barnhart et al.[24] in a meta-analysis comparing single-dose versus multidose regime of MTX for the treatment of tubal ectopic pregnancies found that the presence of embryonic cardiac activity documented by US was significantly associated with treatment failure with an odds ratio (OR) of 9.09 (95% confidence interval [CI] 3.76, 21.95). However, UAE is not an effective single first-line treatment; it is effective when used as an adjunct prior to other treatments to minimize bleeding or as a rescue procedure when there is profuse bleeding after other procedures.

Several treatment modalities have acceptable complication rates; among these is the hysteroscopic removal of CSP with a complication rate of 18.4%. However, treatment modalities with the lowest complication rates were those in which KCl or MTX is directly injected into the gestational sac or intrafetally under real-time US guidance using either transabdominal or TVS. Only 8 of 81 (9.6%) published cases treated in this fashion had complications. In a subsequent review of the literature encompassing the years 2012 and 2015,[25–32] an additional 63 cases of CSP treated by local intragestational injection under real-time US guidance were identified; in addition to KCl and MTX some cases were injected with intragestational/intrafetal ethanol and the pooled complication rates from these cases ranged from 0% to 5.8%. The most likely reason for the effectiveness of this treatment modality is that there is complete and immediate cessation of the cardiac activity and growth of the pregnancy. Systemic injection of MTX given in conjunction with intragestational sac/intracardiac injection of MTX or KCl has probably the highest success rate; however, the numbers are still too low to advocate its use. Insertion and inflation of a single balloon Foley catheter after local intra-gestational sac injection of MTX was successful to prevent and/or stop post-treatment bleeding.[33] The least invasive treatment of CSP appears to be that of insertion of a cervical double ripening balloon catheter to compress the chorionic sac and the embryo stopping the heart activity and at the same time prevent bleeding.[34]

The scope and the format of this chapter does not allow for a detailed analysis of the more than 30–35 different treatment modalities published as a single case series. The complete review of them is available in the literature.[8]

MANAGEMENT PROTOCOL AND PATIENT SELECTION

In Figure 32.13, a practical management approach is presented for patients with CSP. Based on the initial US findings, the patient can be triaged to the most appropriate treatment protocol.

In a case where there is CSP with yolk sac and no embryo or cardiac activity, before any treatment is instituted, the patient should be rescanned every 2–3 days. If after 7–10 days there is no visible embryo with heart-beats or if the embryo's crown-rump length is measuring >7 mm with no heart-beats, the pregnancy is consistent with a failed CSP. At this point, weekly US and hCG should be planned until the serum hCG test is negative. It is debated if these cases need systemic MTX treatment; some management protocols call for the systemic administration of MTX even if the pregnancy has been deemed nonviable. The amount of systemic MTX given in the absence of any contraindications should be calculated using the standard single-dose regime for ectopic pregnancies of 50 mg/m^2 intramuscularly.[23] Patients should be followed serially, initially weekly after which the interval may be increased to every other week depending on the

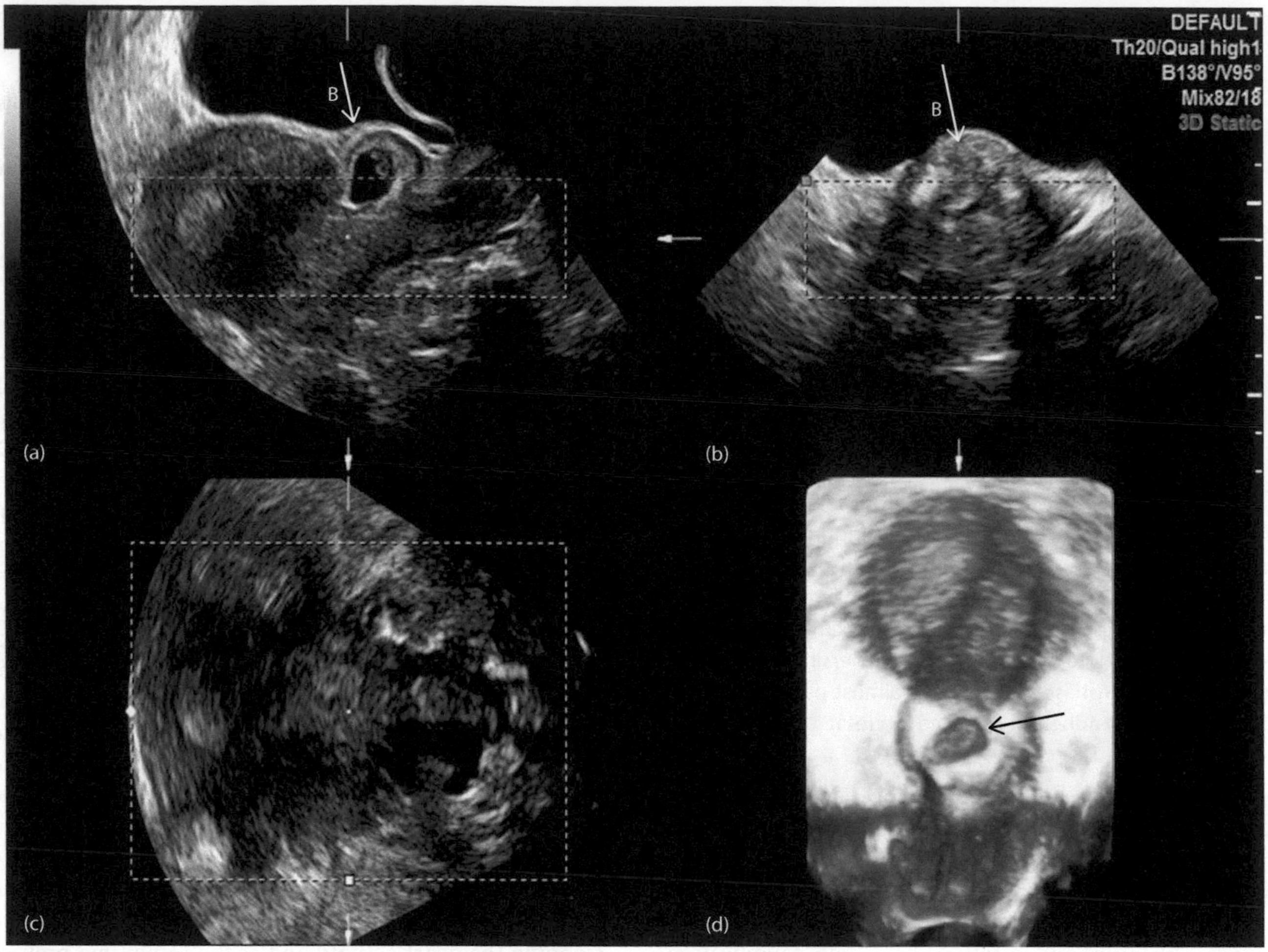

Figure 32.9 Three-dimensional US and 3D reconstruction of a CSP. (a,b) The bladder B contains a small amount of urine. The CSP is seen bulging into the bladder (arrows). 3D reconstruction (d) of the uterus demonstrates the empty uterine cavity with the CSP (black arrow).

hCG level and the sonographic appearance of the CSP. The hCG should decrease by at least 15% after 7 days. If during the post-op period the hCG level plateaus or increases a second dose of systemic MTX should be considered. Typically, we follow these patients until the hCG is negative and the CSP appears to be resolving as judged by US. Dilatation and curettage are not indicated since it can result in severe bleeding needing blood transfusion, UAE, and at times even hysterectomy. As noted in our series of 60 CSPs, the majority of these cases will spontaneously resolve.[7] If increased vascularity is detected at the site of the CSP by color/power Doppler, a peak systolic velocity (PSV) measurement of the vascular region is indicated to exclude an acquired AVM. In an AVM, the PSV of the vessels are typically higher than 30–40 cm/s and the vessels linger for weeks.

CSP containing yolk sac and an embryo with cardiac activity

In a situation where CSP with yolk sac and embryo with cardiac activity is seen, a detailed counseling session is needed since there are two possible options with very different outcomes. The first option is for the patient to continue the pregnancy and the second is to terminate the CSP immediately before the pregnancy progresses any further. Patients who typically select to continue the pregnancy are typically those who want more children and/or those who clearly understand that due to the ensuing placental pathology they might have to undergo a cesarean hysterectomy.[6,7] Given the fact that CSP is a risk factor for abnormal placentation it is important to follow these patients closely and to make the diagnosis of the degree of abnormally adherent placenta as early as possible. Detailed bleeding precautions should be given to these patients and their management should be similar to those with an abnormally adherent placenta (see Chapter 18). A multidisciplinary team with experience in managing and delivering patient with abnormally adherent placenta should be involved in the care and delivery. Blood products should be available since US may not predict the blood loss at surgery. Some advocate preventive inflatable balloons to be inserted into the hypogastric arteries to inflate them if needed by the interventional radiologist.

The second option for a patient with a viable CSP is to terminate the pregnancy. This should be done soon

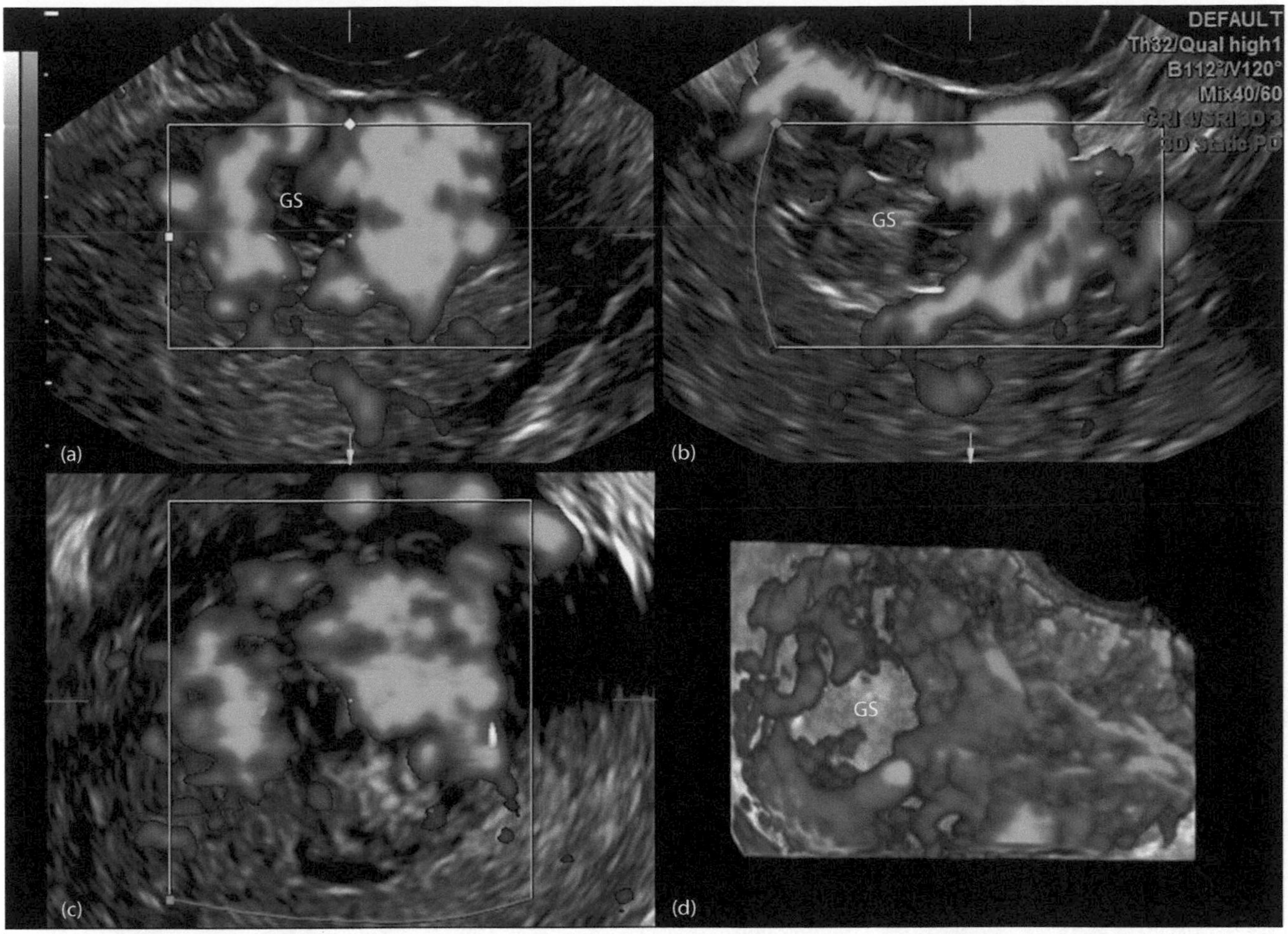

Figure 32.10 Three-dimensional power Doppler US of a CSP. The rendering box (d) generated from the multiplanar images (a), (b), and (c) demonstrate the rich vascularity surrounding the sac (GS). This image explains why the structure is bleeding heavily when disturbed by curettage.

without any delay, almost immediately after the decision to do so is agreed upon. As mentioned before the most reliable method to stop the heart activity is imperative. Intragestational and/or intrafetal MTX injection is our preferred method to treat CSPs. There are many reasons for our choice: there is no need for anesthesia since the injection is relatively painless and most patients reporting only cramping, there is no need for patient hospitalization and most patients can be followed up as outpatients, and last, based on our experience and the growing experience from the literature, it is associated with a high success rate with the lowest reported complication rates. The literature is replete with various treatment regimens and or combinations thereof.[8] Several of the treatment methods use the combination of both major and minor surgical as well as minimal invasive methods. Intragestational injection of CSP as well as systemic MTX have been previously described and reviewed above (Table 32.3).

In this chapter, we describe our treatment protocol implemented for the last several years. Once the patient has made the decision to proceed with the minimally invasive treatment this procedure is performed on the same day. A written informed consent is obtained from the patient. Before the procedure is performed a baseline hCG, metabolic profile, type and screen, hemoglobin, and hematocrit are drawn. A Foley balloon catheter (5–30 mL) is always available in the event of bleeding during or immediately after the procedure. At times the catheter is placed as an elective prophylactic measure at the completion of the local injection.[35] A TVS is performed to plan the best approach to terminate the CSP. During the US examination, placenta location, and vascularity surrounding the CSP and along the planned needle path are determined. If significant vascularity is seen along the planned needle path an alternate path is chosen. Under direct TVS US guidance, the needle is inserted into the gestational sac as close as possible to the embryo and 1–2 mL of MTX is injected directly in the sac or intrafetally. We usually turn the needle several times around its axis to take advantage of the mechanical destructive effect of the beveled needle tip. After the cessation of cardiac activity, the needle is slowly withdrawn and an additional 1–2 mL is injected along the needle path. Without removing the US probe we confirm the presence of a fetal demise as well as assess if there is any active bleeding into the sac or around it. Some practitioners use 1–2 mL of 2 mEq/L KCl solution instead

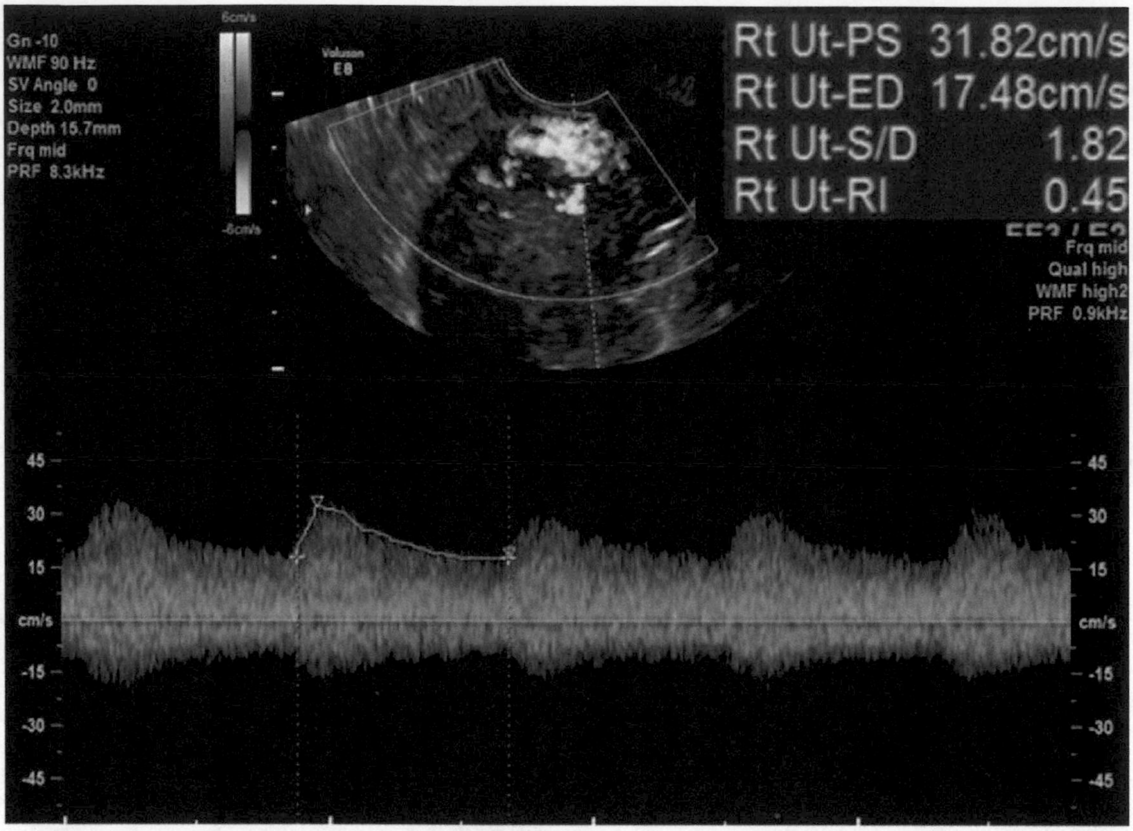

(a)

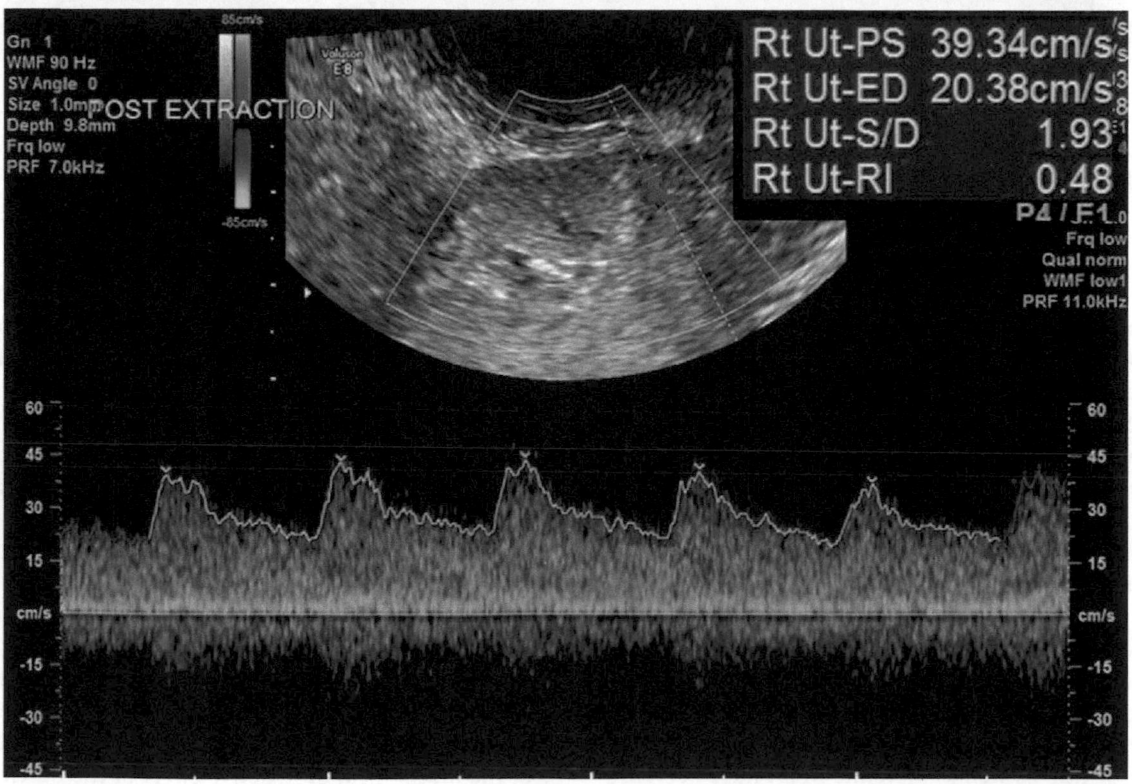

(b)

Figure 32.11 Color Doppler evaluation of two different patients immediately after treatment showing baseline Doppler flow velocity and resistance index values. (a) Long-axis view of the uterus demonstrates the abundant vascularity at the site of the placenta implantation. Note the baseline PSV of 31.82 cm/s. RI is low at 0.45. (b) Zoomed view of the scar after treatment and extraction of the Foley balloon. Note the PSV of 39.34 cm/s. Resistance index is low at 0.48.

Table 32.2 Clinical outcome of patients with CSP as a function of gestational age at first treatment.

	Gestational age, weeks				
Outcome[a]	**5–6**	**7**	**8**	**9**	**10–15**
No complications	51	35	14	4	4
Complications	12	16	26	6	16

[a] Number of cases.
Source: Timor-Tritsch IE et al., *Am J Obstet Gynecol* 207: 1–13, 2012. With permission.

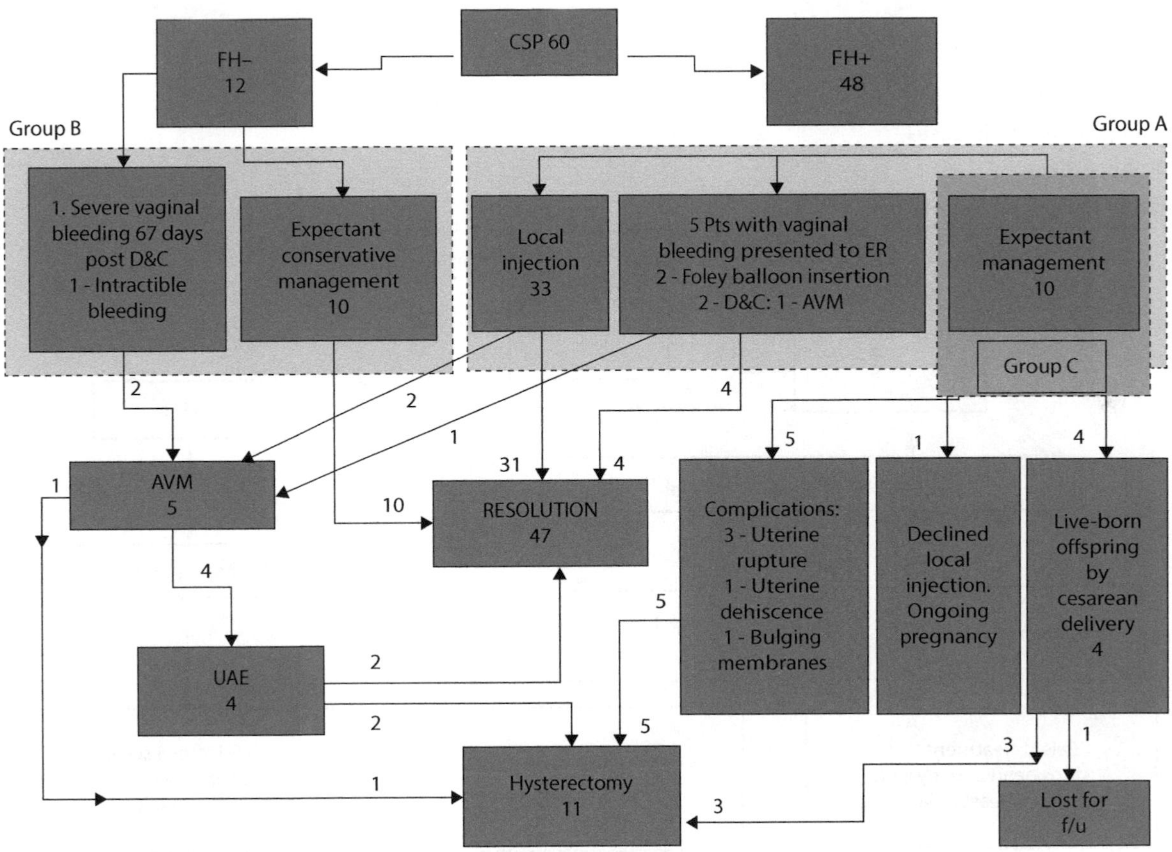

Figure 32.12 Flowchart of the major groups (A and B), including our 60 cases of cesarean scar pregnancies and subgroup C with their treatments and outcomes. ER, emergency room; FH, fetal heartbeat, f/u, follow-up; UAE, uterine artery embolization. (From Timor-Tritsch IE et al., *Journal of Ultrasound in Medicine: Official Journal of the American Institute of Ultrasound in Medicine* 34: 601–610, 2015. With permission.)

of the MTX.[21] If systemic MTX is given, the usual accepted dose is 50 mg/m^2 of body surface. After the procedure, the patient is observed for 2 hours, vital signs and bleeding are monitored, and the US is repeated to reassess the area of injection (Figure 32.14). The patient is given prophylactic oral antibiotics and is discharged home with bleeding precautions. The patient is rescanned 48 hours later as well as 7–10 days later. A repeat serum hCG is also drawn. An increase in the hCG level may be seen within 2–3 days after the procedure before the hCG starts trending down. This initial increase in the hCG does not necessarily means a failed treatment or that a second dose of systemic MTX is needed; the reason for this maybe an increased release of hCG from the affected placenta.

Subsequently, the hCG should start decreasing rapidly by at least 15% after 7 days; however, it may take several weeks for the hCG to reach nonpregnant levels. In tubal ectopic pregnancies managed conservatively the average number of days until the hCG drops below 2 IU/L is 20–31 days and in cases treated with medical management the average number is 30 days (range 27–33 days).[36] In 1994, Timor-Tritsch et al.[16] published an article on a series of five cervical pregnancies between 5 and 8 weeks' gestation treated by intrafetal MTX injection. In these five cases, the mean number of days for the hCG to normalize was 47.2 days (range 17–112 days).[16] Recently, we published 16 cases of CSP and 2 cervical pregnancies treated with Foley balloon catheters and IM MTX. In 16 cases, there

Table 32.3 Treatment options in the management of viable CSP.

Major surgical procedures (requiring general or regional anesthesia)
• Laparotomy (hysterectomy or local excision)
• Laparoscopy, hysteroscopy, or by vaginal surgery
• Dilatation of the cervix and sharp or blunt curetting
• Suction aspiration without dilatation of the cervix
Minimally invasive surgical procedures (not requiring general or regional anesthesia)
• Local injection of MTX or KCl.
• Vasopressin (has also been used)
• UAE
• Foley balloon placement
Systemic medication
• MTX single or multiple doses
• Etoposide (not in the USA)
Combination of the above treatments

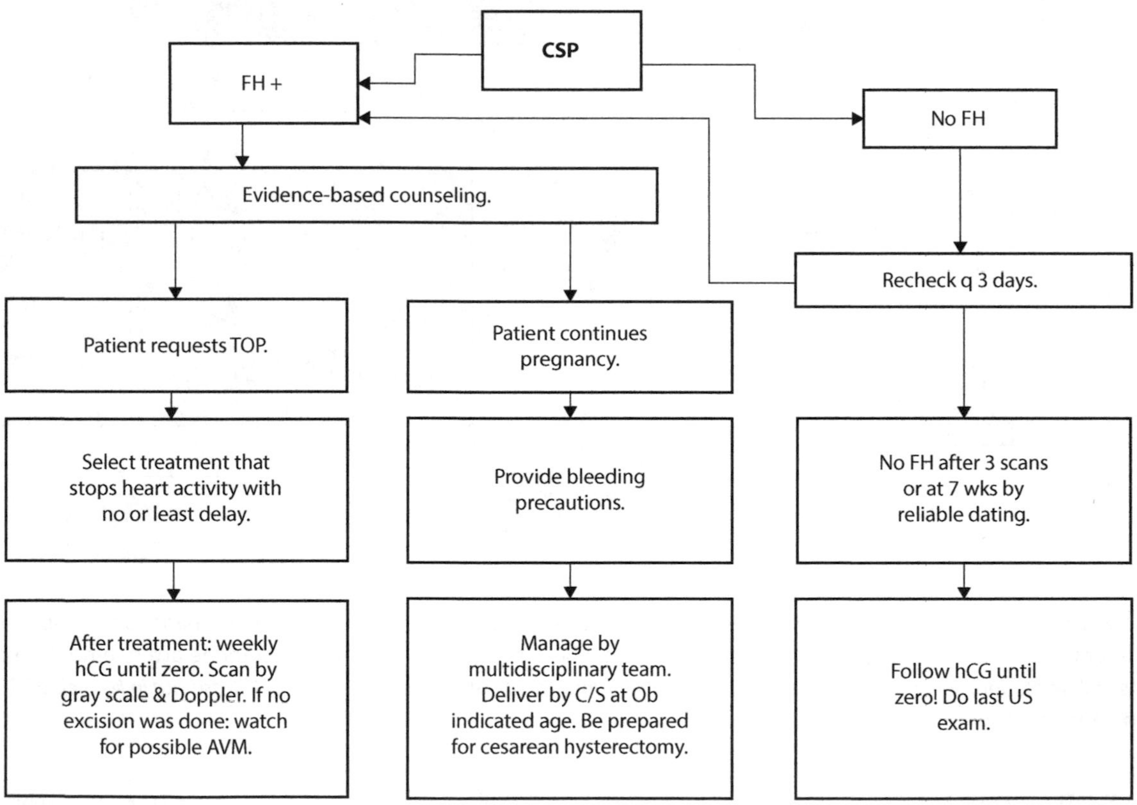

Figure 32.13 Triage and management of patients with CSP by the presence or absence of fetal heartbeat (FH). (From Timor-Tritsch IE, In: Abramowicz JS, ed., *First-Trimester Ultrasound*. Switzerland: Springer, 2015. With permission.)

was information available regarding the length of time for the hCG to become negative. The mean number of days was 39.1 (range 15–82 days).[35] In 2014, Yamaguchi et al.[32] reported on eight cases where CSP was treated using the intragestational injection of MTX. The mean number of days to normalization of the hCG was 78.5 days (range 42–166 days). Nguyen-Xuan et al.[29] published on six cases of CSP in which the mean number of days for the resolution of the hCG was 96 days (range 69–148 days).

Current data show that the recovery period for CSP, or the time to a nonpregnant level of hCG, appears to be longer for CSP than was reported for tubal ectopic pregnancies: ranging from 15 to 148 days. During the post-op period if the hCG level plateaus or increases, a second dose of MTX is considered. In the absence of significant bleeding, the patient is followed biweekly until the hCG reaches nonpregnant levels and the vascularity of the CSP is resolved.

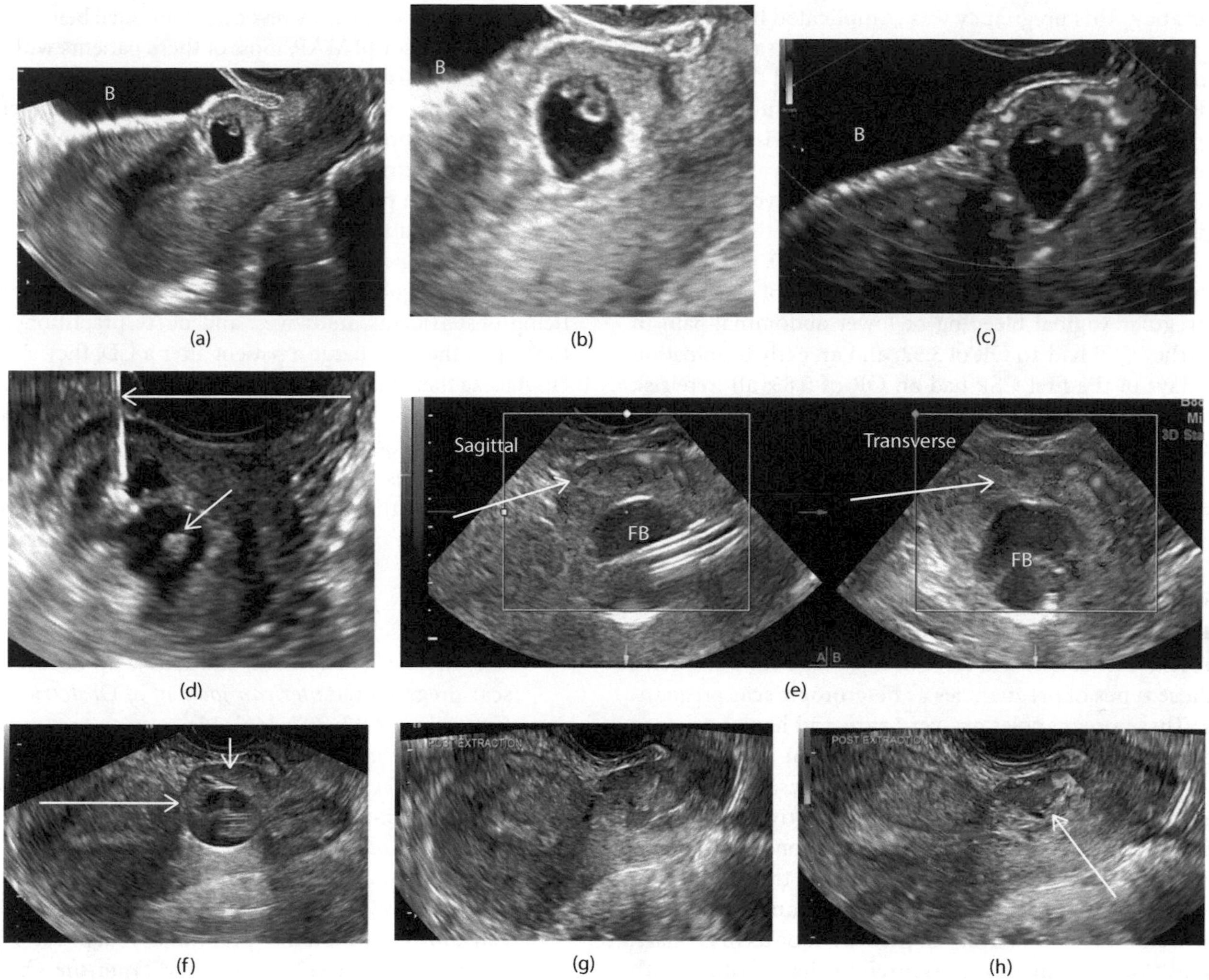

Figure 32.14 CSP before and after minimally invasive treatment using intragestational MTX injection and Foley balloon catheter to prevent bleeding (B: bladder). (a) The placenta of the CSP is seen in the area of the scar. (b) The CSP is bulging into the bladder. (c) Using color Doppler, the vessels of the placenta are seen almost penetrating into the bladder. (d) The needle (long arrow) and the prophylactically inflated balloon (arrow). (e) Enlarged sagittal and transverse images of the compressed gestational sac (long arrows) by the Foley balloon (FB) seen at the end of the treatment. (f) One-and-a-half hours after the procedure the FB (long arrow) is seen filling the niche. The remnants of the gestational sac appear as a bright echogenic line (small arrow). (g) After the Foley was removed the gestational sac is no longer visible on this gray-scale image. (h) Color Doppler after removal of the Foley demonstrates the vascularity of the injected area.

SECONDARY TREATMENTS

As mentioned before, in cases of postprocedure bleeding or at times even prophylactically an 8- to 10-French silicon Foley catheter with an inflatable balloon volume capacity of 5–30 mL can be inserted.[35] The catheter is inserted by exposing the cervix by a speculum and using a sponge forceps once in the cervix, the speculum is removed and the catheter is advanced under transvaginal US guidance.

The balloon is inflated under real-time observation until the pressure compresses the sac. This usually stops the bleeding or if it was electively inserted it prevents bleeding. Patients can be discharged home with the Foley left in place for 1–6 days. They may shower and do not need bed rest. Single balloon Foley catheters may slip out necessitating reinsertion if bleeding is still occurring. Patients during the resolution of the CSP may experience some spotting; however, this does not necessary require any secondary treatment. However, should severe bleeding occur and cause a drop in the hematocrit or if the patient becomes symptomatic, a secondary treatment may be necessary. UAE may be the best treatment in these cases.

SUBSEQUENT PREGNANCY

The risk of a recurrent CSP has been estimated to be 1% of all CSP. In a recent study among eight patients with a prior history of a CSP, two (25%) had a recurrent CSP.[10] Gupta et al.[2] reported on a patient with four recurrent live CSP all treated with intragestational sac injection of MTX. Subsequently, this patient returned with a fifth CSP; however, this time the patient decided to continue the pregnancy. This pregnancy was complicated by a placenta previa and MAP. The patient delivered a near-term live-born neonate by cesarean hysterectomy and the histology confirmed the presence of placenta percreta (unpublished).

Qian et al.[37] reported on how to identify risk factors for recurrent CSP. In their study, which was carried out in China, they found that having a history of delivering in rural community hospitals had an OR of 4.75, a thinner lower uterine segment of ≤5 mm had an OR of 7.10, a gestational sac bulging into the uterovesical fold an OR of 6.25, history of irregular vaginal bleeding or lower abdominal pain in an earlier CSP had an OR of 3.52, and an early termination ≤56 days of the first CSP had an OR of 5.85; all were risk factors for recurrent CSP. Although all of these risk factors that they identified may not be true in other countries, thinner lower uterine segment, a gestational sac bulging into the uterovesical fold, and a prior CSP should all raise flags and result in close monitoring of the index pregnancy.

THE DILEMMA OF TWINS WITH A CSP

Twins in which one twin is in the uterus and the other is in the cesarean section scar have been described. Many refer to these types of pregnancies as heterotopic scar pregnancies. These pregnancies are very rare and have been seen after assisted reproduction techniques. In the literature, there are only case reports describing these pregnancies. They have been managed mostly by selective injection of the CSP by local intragestational injection of KCl or by laparoscopic or hysteroscopic excision of the CSP.[38–41] In most cases, the intrauterine pregnancy can be preserved after treatment and delivery of near term or term neonate. In addition, similar to the counseling that a patient with single CSP is given conservative management of the twin pregnancy with a CSP can be offered to the patient after extensive risk/benefit counseling. Kim et al.[42] reported on the successful delivery of a twin pregnancy after the diagnosis of a CSP and intrauterine pregnancy had been made at 5 weeks. The pregnancy progressed to 37 weeks' gestation with a low-lying placenta previa; the patient delivered by elective cesarean section at term and at the time of the delivery the bladder was noted to be severely adherent to the lower uterine segment and the placenta was bulging toward the vesicoperitoneal reflection. After delivery of the twins, bleeding ensued which was managed by the complete excision of the anterior lower uterine segment along with bilateral uterine arteries ligation; pathology revealed a placenta accreta.[42]

CONCLUSION

The goal of this chapter was to bring CSP to the forefront and offer the obstetrician useful information about this condition. CSPs are increasing in number. This increase parallels the increasing number of CDs. The most important issue regarding CSP is to establish the diagnosis early in order for the patient to be adequately counseled and undertake appropriate management of the CSP. There is growing evidence that patients with CSP who desire to continue the pregnancy can and in many cases succeed to deliver a living neonate; however, as mentioned before since CSP is a precursor of MAP, most of these patients will face the complications related to MAP and may undergo hysterectomy. At this point, evaluation of the prior CD scar before the subsequent pregnancy is not routinely performed; however, given the growing information about the CD scar and the relative high prevalence of small as well as large niches or dehiscences it may become imperative to assess the CD scars before the next planned pregnancy and definitely very early in a subsequent pregnancy. A practical advice to practicing obstetricians, midwives, and nurse practitioners is that when they discharge a patient after a CD, they should emphasize that at the very beginning of a subsequent pregnancy (5–6–7 weeks) they should present for a TVS scan to evaluate the location of the pregnancy. Surely most of these pregnancies will be intrauterine; however, if a CSP is diagnosed early, they can make an informed and evidence-based decision to continue or terminate the pregnancy.

REFERENCES

1. Timor-Tritsch IE, Monteagudo A, Santos R, et al. The diagnosis, treatment, and follow-up of cesarean scar pregnancy. *American Journal of Obstetrics and Gynecology* 2012; 207: 44e1–13.
2. Gupta S, Pineda G, Rubin S, Timor-Tritsch IE. Four consecutive recurrent cesarean scar pregnancies in a single patient. *Journal of Ultrasound in Medicine: Official Journal of the American Institute of Ultrasound in Medicine* 2013; 32: 1878–1880.
3. Hamilton BE PhD, Martin JA, Osterman M MHS, Curtain S MA. Births: Preliminary data for 2014. *National Vital Statistics Reports: From the Centers for Disease Control and Prevention, National Center for Health Statistics, National Vital Statistics System* 2015; 64: 1–19.
4. Taffel SM, Placek PJ, Liss T. Trends in the United States cesarean section rate and reasons for the 1980–1985 rise. *American Journal of Public Health* 1987; 77: 955–959.
5. Spong CY, Berghella V, Wenstrom KD, et al. Preventing the first cesarean delivery: Summary of a joint Eunice Kennedy Shriver National Institute of Child Health and Human Development, Society for Maternal-Fetal Medicine, and American College of Obstetricians and Gynecologists Workshop. *Obstetrics and Gynecology* 2012; 120: 1181–1193.
6. Timor-Tritsch IE, Monteagudo A, Cali G, et al. Cesarean scar pregnancy is a precursor of morbidly adherent placenta. *Ultrasound in Obstetrics and Gynecology: The Official Journal of the International Society of Ultrasound in Obstetrics and Gynecology* 2014; 44: 346–353.
7. Timor-Tritsch IE, Khatib N, Monteagudo A, et al. Cesarean scar pregnancies: Experience of 60 cases. *Journal of Ultrasound in Medicine: Official Journal of the American Institute of Ultrasound in Medicine* 2015; 34: 601–610.

8. Timor-Tritsch IE, Monteagudo A. Unforeseen consequences of the increasing rate of cesarean deliveries: Early placenta accreta and cesarean scar pregnancy. A review. *American Journal of Obstetrics and Gynecology* 2012; 207: 14–29.
9. Seow KM, Huang LW, Lin YH, et al. Cesarean scar pregnancy: Issues in management. *Ultrasound in Obstetrics and Gynecology: The Official Journal of the International Society of Ultrasound in Obstetrics and Gynecology* 2004; 23: 247–253.
10. Maymon R, Svirsky R, Smorgick N, et al. Fertility performance and obstetric outcomes among women with previous cesarean scar pregnancy. *Journal of Ultrasound in Medicine: Official Journal of the American Institute of Ultrasound in Medicine* 2011; 30: 1179–1184.
11. Rheinboldt M, Osborn D, Delproposto Z. Cesarean section scar ectopic pregnancy: A clinical case series. *Journal of Ultrasound* 2015; 18: 191–195.
12. Monteagudo A, Carreno C, Timor-Tritsch IE. Saline infusion sonohysterography in nonpregnant women with previous cesarean delivery: The "niche" in the scar. *Journal of Ultrasound in Medicine: Official Journal of the American Institute of Ultrasound in Medicine* 2001; 20: 1105–1115.
13. Osser OV, Jokubkiene L, Valentin L. High prevalence of defects in Cesarean section scars at transvaginal ultrasound examination. *Ultrasound in Obstetrics and Gynecology: The Official Journal of the International Society of Ultrasound in Obstetrics and Gynecology* 2009; 34: 90–97.
14. Bij de Vaate AJ, van der Voet LF, Naji O, et al. Prevalence, potential risk factors for development and symptoms related to the presence of uterine niches following cesarean section: Systematic review. *Ultrasound in Obstetrics and Gynecology: The Official Journal of the International Society of Ultrasound in Obstetrics and Gynecology* 2014; 43: 372–382.
15. Timor-Tritsch I, Arslan A, Monteagudo A, Cali G, Refaey HE. How to avoid misdiagnosis of cesarean scar pregnancy: An easy method for sonographic differentiation of the 5–10 completed weeks intrauterine and cesarean scar pregnancies. Unpublished.
16. Timor-Tritsch IE, Monteagudo A, Mandeville EO, et al. Successful management of viable cervical pregnancy by local injection of methotrexate guided by transvaginal ultrasonography. *American Journal of Obstetrics and Gynecology* 1994; 170: 737–739.
17. Comstock CH, Bronsteen RA. The antenatal diagnosis of placenta accreta. *BJOG: An International Journal of Obstetrics and Gynaecology* 2014; 121: 171–181; discussion 81–82.
18. Godin PA, Bassil S, Donnez J. An ectopic pregnancy developing in a previous caesarian section scar. *Fertility and Sterility* 1997; 67: 398–400.
19. Vial Y, Petignat P, Hohlfeld P. Pregnancy in a cesarean scar. *Ultrasound in Obstetrics and Gynecology: The Official Journal of the International Society of Ultrasound in Obstetrics and Gynecology* 2000; 16: 592–593.
20. Seow KM, Hwang JL, Tsai YL. Ultrasound diagnosis of a pregnancy in a Cesarean section scar. *Ultrasound in Obstetrics and Gynecology: The Official Journal of the International Society of Ultrasound in Obstetrics and Gynecology* 2001; 18: 547–549.
21. Michaels AY, Washburn EE, Pocius KD, et al. Outcome of cesarean scar pregnancies diagnosed sonographically in the first trimester. *Journal of Ultrasound in Medicine: Official Journal of the American Institute of Ultrasound in Medicine* 2015; 34: 595–599.
22. Ballas J, Pretorius D, Hull AD, et al. Identifying sonographic markers for placenta accreta in the first trimester. *Journal of Ultrasound in Medicine: Official Journal of the American Institute of Ultrasound in Medicine* 2012; 31: 1835–1841.
23. American College of O, Gynecologists. ACOG Practice Bulletin No. 94: Medical management of ectopic pregnancy. *Obstetrics and Gynecology* 2008; 111: 1479–1485.
24. Barnhart KT, Gosman G, Ashby R, Sammel M. The medical management of ectopic pregnancy: A meta-analysis comparing "single dose" and "multidose" regimens. *Obstetrics and Gynecology.* 2003 ; 101: 778–784.
25. Yin XH, Yang SZ, Wang ZQ, et al. Injection of MTX for the treatment of cesarean scar pregnancy: Comparison between different methods. *International Journal of Clinical and Experimental Medicine.* 2014; 7: 1867–1872.
26. Uysal F, Uysal A, Adam G. Cesarean scar pregnancy: Diagnosis, management, and follow-up. *Journal of Ultrasound in Medicine: Official Journal of the American Institute of Ultrasound in Medicine* 2013; 32: 1295–1300.
27. Berhie SH, Molina RL, Davis MR, et al. Beware the scar: Laparoscopic hysterectomy for 7-week cesarean delivery scar implantation pregnancy. *American Journal of Obstetrics and Gynecology* 2015; 212: 247 e1–2.
28. Shao MJ, Hu M, Hu MX. Conservative management of cesarean scar pregnancy by local injection of ethanol under hysteroscopic guidance. *International Journal of Gynaecology and Obstetrics: The Official Organ of the International Federation of Gynaecology and Obstetrics* 2013; 121: 281–282.
29. Nguyen-Xuan HT, Lousquy R, Barranger E. [Diagnosis, treatment, and follow-up of cesarean scar pregnancy]. *Gynecologie, Obstetrique and Fertilite* 2014; 42: 483–489.
30. Pang YP, Tan WC, Yong TT, et al. Caesarean section scar pregnancy: A case series at a single tertiary centre. *Singapore Medical Journal* 2012; 53: 638–642.

31. Seow KM, Wang PH, Huang LW, Hwang JL. Transvaginal sono-guided aspiration of gestational sac concurrent with a local methotrexate injection for the treatment of unruptured cesarean scar pregnancy. *Archives of Gynecology and Obstetrics* 2013; 288: 361–366.
32. Yamaguchi M, Honda R, Uchino K, et al. Transvaginal methotrexate injection for the treatment of cesarean scar pregnancy: Efficacy and subsequent fecundity. *Journal of Minimally Invasive Gynecology* 2014; 21: 877–883.
33. Timor-Tritsch IE, Cali G, Monteagudo A, et al. Foley balloon catheter to prevent or manage bleeding during treatment for cervical and cesarean scar pregnancy. *Ultrasound Obstet Gynecol* 2015; 46: 118–123.
34. Timor-Tritsch IE, Monteagudo A, Bennett TA, et al. A new minimally invasive treatment for cesarean scar pregnancy and cervical pregnancy. *Am J Obstet Gynecol* 2016; 215: 351.
35. Timor-Tritsch IE, Cali G, Monteagudo A, et al. Foley balloon catheter to prevent or manage bleeding during treatment for cervical and Cesarean scar pregnancy. *Ultrasound in Obstetrics and Gynecology: The Official Journal of the International Society of Ultrasound in Obstetrics and Gynecology* 2015; 46: 118–123.
36. Capmas P, Bouyer J, Fernandez H. Treatment of ectopic pregnancies in 2014: New answers to some old questions. *Fertility and Sterility* 2014; 101: 615–20.
37. Qian ZD, Guo QY, Huang LL. Identifying risk factors for recurrent cesarean scar pregnancy: A case-control study. *Fertility and Sterility* 2014; 102: 129–134 e1.
38. Ugurlucan FG, Bastu E, Dogan M, et al. Management of cesarean heterotopic pregnancy with transvaginal ultrasound-guided potassium chloride injection and gestational sac aspiration, and review of the literature. *Journal of Minimally Invasive Gynecology* 2012; 19: 671–673.
39. Demirel LC, Bodur H, Selam B, et al. Laparoscopic management of heterotopic cesarean scar pregnancy with preservation of intrauterine gestation and delivery at term: Case report. *Fertility and Sterility* 2009; 91: 1293 e5–7.
40. Wang CJ, Tsai F, Chen C, Chao A. Hysteroscopic management of heterotopic cesarean scar pregnancy. *Fertility and Sterility* 2010; 94: 1529 e15–18.
41. OuYang Z, Yin Q, Xu Y, et al. Heterotopic cesarean scar pregnancy: Diagnosis, treatment, and prognosis. *Journal of Ultrasound in Medicine: Official Journal of the American Institute of Ultrasound in Medicine* 2014; 33: 1533–1537.
42. Kim ML, Jun HS, Kim JY, et al. Successful full-term twin deliveries in heterotopic cesarean scar pregnancy in a spontaneous cycle with expectant management. *The Journal of Obstetrics and Gynaecology Research* 2014; 40: 1415–1419.

Anesthetic procedures in obstetrics

33

JOEL MANN YARMUSH, JONATHAN DAVID WEINBERG, and SOHEILA JAFARI

CONTENTS

Obstetric anesthesia is a subspecialty with many unique features not found in other areas of anesthetic practice. The altered physiology of pregnancy increases the risk of anesthetic morbidity in otherwise healthy patients. In addition, the obstetric population increasingly includes older and sicker patients, further complicating their anesthetic management. Often, labor management decisions directly affect anesthesia requirements and vice versa. Each patient's labor course may suddenly require emergency surgical intervention with accompanying anesthetic considerations. Obstetricians and anesthesiologists must coordinate plans for management in order to facilitate delivery, while minimizing the risk to the mother. It behooves every obstetrician to become aware of the benefits, alternatives, and risks of obstetric anesthesia procedures.

Procedures covered in this chapter include spinal anesthesia for cerclage insertion, general anesthesia for general surgery, epidural analgesia for labor and delivery, and epidural and general anesthesia for cesarean sections. Postoperative pain management techniques, as well as aspects of obstetric critical care, will be covered. Fetal surgery procedures will not be covered.

CERCLAGE

A cerclage is usually inserted in the late first or early second trimester. Anesthesia for a cerclage may be problematic because of the fragile state of the embryo or fetus. A spinal anesthetic is generally considered the anesthesia of choice, for several reasons.[1] Of the possible anesthetic techniques, a spinal anesthetic uses the least amount of medication, thus reducing the possibility of systemic and teratogenic effects from the local anesthetic. Unlike a general anesthetic, a spinal anesthetic does not irritate the airways and precipitate cough reflexes in the postoperative patient. It also seems that the sacral nerve roots, which innervate the cervix and vagina, are more easily blocked with a spinal than with an epidural anesthetic.

There are different "flavors" of spinal anesthesia. Some spinal anesthetics (usually just referred to as a "spinal") can cause major hemodynamic changes in the mother, which can affect the uteroplacental blood flow, in turn affecting the fetus.[2] A spinal anesthetic can block sensation from the chest to the toes with major hemodynamic consequence or can block the sensation in the inner thighs and perineum (the so-called saddle block) with minimal hemodynamic consequence, or can block anywhere in between those two.[3] The local anesthetic injected in a spinal canal is often mixed with glucose to increase its specific gravity so that it is greater than that of cerebrospinal fluid (CSF; the term "hyperbaric" is used to indicate a greater specific gravity than CSF). This enables you to use gravity to control the spread of the anesthetic within the spinal canal, much as a bartender uses gravity to control where the grenadine syrup goes in a tequila sunrise. If you perform the spinal procedure in the sitting position and lay the patient down, the local anesthetic spreads cephalad, generally settling at the central portion of the thoracic kyphosis. If you keep the person sitting upright for about 15 minutes after injection, the spinal injectate will become confined to the portion of the spinal canal inferior to the lumbar lordosis, resulting in a saddle block that leaves the rest of the body unanesthetized. The dermatomal innervation of the cervix is such that regardless of the type of spinal (i.e., saddle block or regular spinal anesthetic) procedure, the cervix is certain to be anesthetized, although a saddle block will potentially fail to block the pudendal nerve, which arises from L1 and L2. A cerclage may be facilitated by letting the patient sit for a somewhat shorter period of time to allow some blockade of the lumbar dermatomes.

In Yoon, Hong, and Kim's randomized controlled study,[4] the investigators found no change in pre- and post-cerclage serum oxytocin level that could be attributed to either a regional or general anesthetic technique; similarly, anesthetic technique did not seem to be significantly related to increased uterine activity in the immediate postoperative period.

Procedure

The spinal anesthetic is usually performed in the sitting position. It can be performed in the lateral position but it is technically more difficult, particularly if a saddle block is contemplated (Figure 33.1).

Let's start with sterility. We stick needles everywhere with just a quick swipe of the skin with an alcohol swab. This degree of antisepsis may be adequate for placement of an intravenous (IV) catheter, but the veins contain swarms of leukocytes which will destroy any stray microbes that may be accidentally injected. In the case of a spinal procedure, the injection is going into the CSF, beyond the blood–brain barrier. There is no swarm of leukocytes—just a warm liquid with a little bit of sugar and some electrolytes. In other words, the CSF makes a terrific bacterial growth medium. Consequently, strict asepsis is of paramount importance.[5]

The patient should be seated on a flat surface, with the knees elevated a bit by placing her feet on a stool or tilting the table backward. Her gown or other clothes should be secured out of the way. The patient's back must be first cleaned of any obvious surface dirt and then scrubbed with a sterilizing solution. Povidone iodine works just fine but becomes effective only after it has dried. Apply it widely to the lower back and let it dry by evaporation. Blotting or wiping it dry defeats the purpose. A sterile gown is probably not necessary but sterile gloves, a mask, and a hat for both practitioner and patient are.

While the povidone iodine is drying (applying the prep solution first is most efficient), draw up your medications from a kit. The medication selected for the spinal is dependent on the time needed for the procedure. A cerclage is usually a relatively short procedure, and the drug most often used in the past was lidocaine. Over the last several years, lidocaine spinals have fallen out of favor because of reports of transient neurologic syndrome (TNS).[6,7]

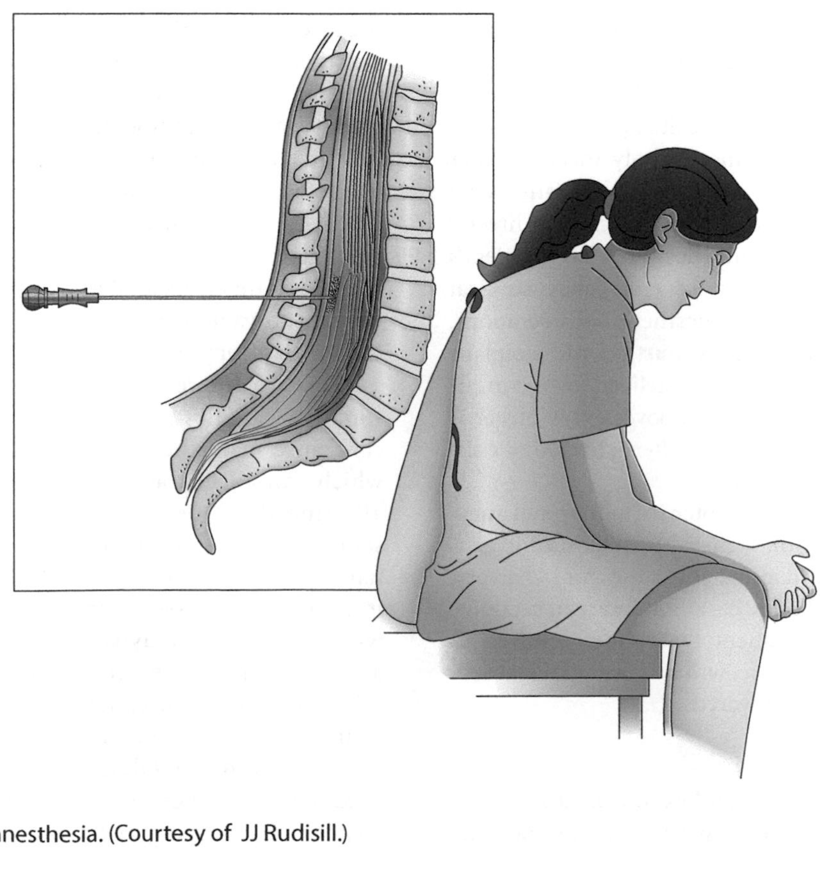

Figure 33.1 Spinal anesthesia. (Courtesy of JJ Rudisill.)

The most common alternative medication to lidocaine is bupivacaine. The effects of a bupivacaine spinal will last longer than a lidocaine spinal, which may be disturbing to the patient and result in an inefficient use of Recovery Room resources. Another alternative is tetracaine whose effects last even longer than bupivacaine.

In our practice a third alternative is the charm, namely meperidine. Meperidine is an opioid with local anesthetic properties (one of the authors disagrees, insisting on calling it a local anesthetic with opioid properties).[8] Its local anesthetic properties are short-lived but should be sufficient for a cerclage (~45 minutes). It can be added to glucose to make it hyperbaric and can be prolonged with the addition of a small amount of epinephrine (we use 100 μg of epinephrine for this purpose). In our experience, meperidine often gives a block that, relative to a lidocaine spinal, features a motor block and hypotension that are often reduced and delayed. In other words, although the sensory block is present after 5 minutes or so, the patient may not lose strength in her legs for 15 or 20 minutes, or not at all. There is also more pruritus and nausea with a meperidine spinal than there is with a lidocaine spinal but, on the upside, there is enhanced postoperative analgesia.

Another alternative is to abandon the hyperbaric spinal altogether and use an isobaric solution instead. This involves injecting a local anesthetic—usually lidocaine—that has a similar specific gravity to CSF, and therefore largely stays where it is placed. This places a greater importance on the specifics of the injection (the direction that the aperture of the needle is facing and the speed of injection) in determining how high a dermatomal level is achieved. TNS seems to be seen more often after a hyperbaric spinal than an isobaric one.[9]

Next is the placement of the needle. With the patient sitting on the operating room (OR) bed as before with the legs dangling, the patient's upper body stoops forward to flatten out the lumbar lordosis, increasing the space between the spinous processes. This can be achieved by giving the patient a pillow to hug, or asking her to push out her back like a cat, or to bend forward like she is tying her shoes, or any of a number of other ways.

The posterior superior ischial spines are palpated which is approximately the level of the L3–L4 interspace. That level may be as high as the L2–L3 interspace and should set the practical maximum cephalad position of the spinal needle, as the inferiormost extent of the spinal cord is essentially never lower than L2. The lumbar intervertebral spaces get slightly larger as you move caudad as well.

The skin and subcutaneous tissue is then anesthetized with a small amount of lidocaine using a fine needle (e.g., 25 gauge). This needle may be as long as 1½ inches and can also be used to confirm that you are indeed in the interspace and to feel for the spinous processes. The layers that must be traversed are the skin, subcutaneous fat, supraspinous ligament, intraspinous ligament, ligamentum flavum, and the dura.

The spinal needle used should be a 25- to 27-gauge "pencil point" needle with an obturator. It was originally postulated that the pencil point needle splits the fibers rather than cutting them. Electron microscopy seems to indicate that trauma from the pencil point needle causes swelling, which prevents leakage, which minimizes post-dural puncture headaches (discussed later).[10] Because the needles are 3½ inches (and longer if needed) in length, a larger gauge 1½ inch introducer needle is usually warranted. Going through the different layers, especially the *ligamentum flavum* and the dura mater can generate a classic "pop" sensation. However, this is often not appreciated and is an unreliable marker. The authors recommend methodical, incremental advancement of the needle with frequent removal of the obturator to visualize the CSF flow. Pencil point needles often need to be advanced a bit (~1 mm) after the CSF is seen in order to get the entire aperture past the dura and into the CSF. The patient sits for ~5 minutes after administration of the spinal and is then positioned supine with a wedge under the right hip to prevent compression of the vena cava by the abdominal contents. Compression of the vena cava is a greater issue in patients with greater abdominal mass, e.g., third-trimester pregnancy or morbid obesity.[11,12]

GENERAL SURGERY

A woman may need a surgical operation requiring general anesthesia during her pregnancy. The safest time for the fetus would be during the second trimester. General anesthesia may be necessary at other times as well.

A number of pregnancy-related changes of the airway and the upper gastrointestinal tract render general anesthesia more challenging for the anesthesia provider and more dangerous for the patient.[13,14] The patient is presumptively considered to have a "full stomach" for most of her pregnancy. That means that she is expected to have a greater chance of regurgitation—both active and passive—and aspiration and that the severity of aspiration would be worse. This is due to increased intragastric pressure, to a delay in gastric emptying, and to the decrease in tone of the lower esophageal sphincter, all of which are associated with pregnancy. There is also a greater likelihood of having difficulty securing a patient's airway, as edema and increased friability of the tissues of the pharynx and larynx may make exposure of the vocal cords by laryngoscopy more difficult. Later in pregnancy, the gravid uterus displaces the diaphragms cephalad, reducing the functional residual capacity of the lungs, and decreasing the length of time that the patient can be apneic before hypoxia sets in. A rapid sequence induction of a pregnant patient is thus fraught with peril and should be attempted by the most experienced practitioners with immediate availability of all of the necessary special airway management equipment (e.g., fiberoptic bronchoscope, jet ventilator, laryngeal mask airway.).[15]

A question often arises whether the fetus should be monitored.[16] If circumstances are such that a cesarean section (C-section) is a potential option in the event of fetal distress, then the fetus should be monitored. A plan must be developed ahead of time for the possible C-section and a separate (anesthetic, obstetric, and pediatric/neonatal) team must be present. Additionally, if surgical technique and equipment might reversibly compromise perfusion of the uterus and placenta, then intraoperative fetal monitoring can guide the surgeon to minimize adverse effects on the fetus. Finally, the fetal heart monitor can also serve as an early warning system for the mother's well-being.

Procedure

The patient is positioned supine with a wedge underneath the right hip to minimize compression of the vena cava. The patient's head should be at the head of the OR table to facilitate airway management. She is given high flow 100% oxygen by a mask with an occlusive seal to replace the nitrogen in her lungs with oxygen. If possible, this preoxygenation should last for around 4 minutes. Alternatively, an end-tidal oxygen of 90% or greater can be used to indicate that nearly all the nitrogen in her lungs has been replaced by oxygen. The anesthesia provider gives an induction agent and a rapid-acting neuromuscular blocker (e.g., propofol and succinylcholine) in rapid sequence while a second person applies pressure to the cricoid cartilage to indirectly occlude the esophagus and prevent passive regurgitation. Ideally, laryngoscopy should last no longer than 15 seconds and a cuffed endotracheal tube should be seated in the larynx with the cuff inflated below the vocal cords, protecting the trachea from any liquids that may pool in the pharynx. A gastric tube should be inserted via either the nose or the mouth to decompress the stomach and remove any liquid that may have accumulated. The actual anesthetic is similar to any general anesthetic. Nitrous oxide has been demonstrated to be teratogenic and is associated with a greater incidence of fetal loss, and should probably be avoided in most circumstances.[17] Other inhalational anesthetics have not been shown to cause problems. Opioids are considered fairly harmless, as the worst side effect, namely transient respiratory depression, is not relevant to an embryo or fetus that is oxygenated via the placenta.

Because of the danger associated with airway management, the authors feel that is best to use regional anesthesia whenever possible.[18] If general anesthesia must be used, there are many new and old aids to help with laryngoscopy. The gold standard is a fiberoptic bronchoscope. The new and relatively inexpensive videolaryngoscope is widely available and user friendly and seems to work nearly as well.[19,20] Other aids include a jet ventilator to use with a needle cricothyroidotomy; laryngeal mask airways, of which there are many types; and an esophageal obturator airway (commonly known as a "Combi-tube").

ANALGESIA FOR LABOR AND DELIVERY

Pain of the pelvic viscera is carried via autonomic nervous system pathways to the dorsal horn of the spinal cord (Figure 33.2). These fibers are thin and unmyelinated, and transmission is easily blocked with dilute local anesthetic solutions at the appropriate level.

In the first stage of labor, pain is caused by uterine contractions, cervical dilation, and distention of the lower uterine segment. Action potentials conveying the information about these painful stimuli travel via sympathetic fibers at the T10–Ll dermatomes. A bilateral selective sympathetic block of these dermatomes would provide analgesia for this stage but is generally impractical. A paracervical block could also provide analgesia for this stage, but it has its own drawbacks, namely rapid absorption of anesthetics and the risk of injection into the fetus.[21] A lumbar epidural block, hereafter known simply as an epidural block, typically is administered at the L3–L4 level and can easily be used to deliver analgesic medications to the T10–L1 dermatomal level.[22]

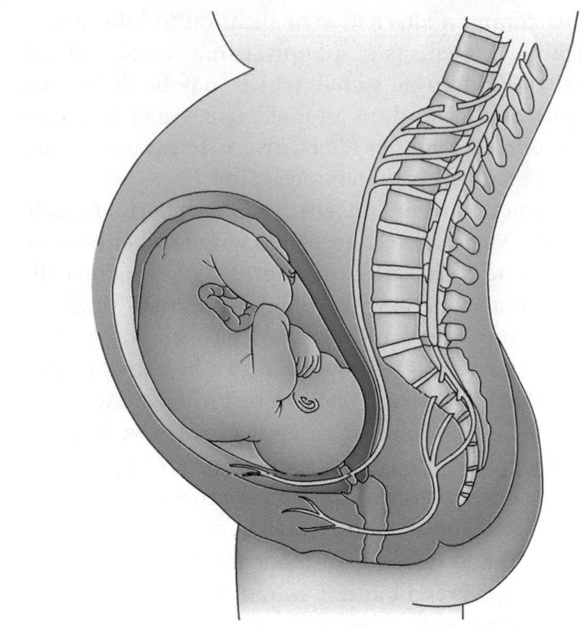

Figure 33.2 Autonomous nerve pathways for noxious stimuli.

In the second stage of labor, pain is caused by the above factors, but additionally by distention of the vagina and perineum as the fetus descends. These additional pain impulses travel via S2–S4 parasympathetic fibers. A pudendal block could provide analgesia for most, but not all, of the pain during this stage.[23] The epidural block may require additional volume or additional concentration to affect analgesia at these lower levels, but it can usually provide complete analgesia for this stage.[24] A caudal block, which is an epidural block inserted at the space between the sacrum and the coccyx, can also be used for the second stage of labor, although it has fallen out of favor in the Western world.

Procedure

Insertion of an epidural is similar to a spinal anesthetic in many ways. It is usually performed in the sitting position and the landmarks and sterile technique are the same. It can be performed in the lateral position but it is technically easier to do with the patient sitting (Figure 33.3).

The epidural needle is usually a blunt large bore needle with an obturator that is inserted into the space just

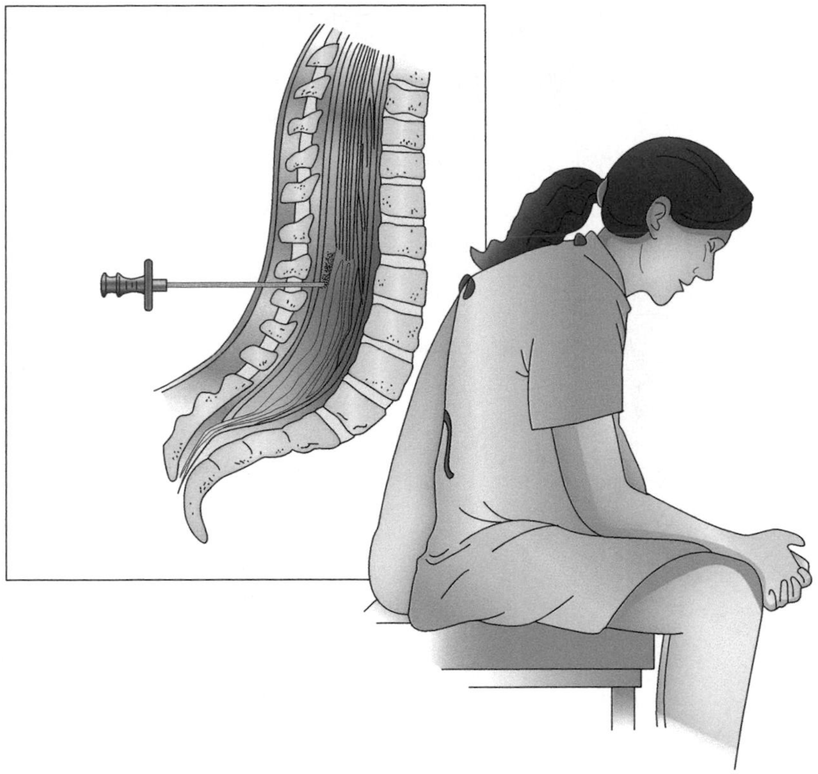

Figure 33.3 Epidural anesthesia. (Courtesy of JJ Rudisill.)

outside the dura. A catheter can be introduced to facilitate multiple dosing. The placement of the needle is usually aided by the loss of resistance technique. The epidural needle with obturator is first placed through the sterilized skin and subcutaneous tissue into the supraspinous ligament. At this point, the obturator is removed and a syringe with normal saline or air is connected to the needle.[25] The plunger of the syringe is lightly tapped and the resistance to injection of the fluid in the syringe is noted. The needle and syringe are incrementally advanced together, and the plunger is tested again to assess resistance. Intermittent advancement and resistance testing continue through the intraspinous ligament and the *ligamentum flavum*—where the resistance to both advancing the needle and injecting the fluid increases. When the needle tip passes beyond the *ligamentum flavum*, the injection of normal saline or air no longer encounters significant resistance. This loss of resistance signifies that the needle is in the epidural space. The syringe is carefully removed and a flexible epidural catheter is advanced through the needle. Once the needle has been removed, the catheter can be secured in place and capped. The catheter can be used for multiple dosing of the neuraxial block.

Alternatively, after inserting the needle into the epidural space but before inserting the epidural catheter, a fine pencil point spinal needle can be inserted down the barrel of the epidural needle and placed through the dura and into the subarachnoid space. A spinal anesthetic can be given through this pencil point needle and, after it is withdrawn, the epidural catheter can then be used for multiple dosing. This technique is called a combined spinal epidural (CSE) (Figure 33.4).[26]

The dosages of medications used for labor analgesia are different than for a cerclage or for a cesarean section. The goal is analgesia (i.e., lack of pain) and not anesthesia (i.e., lack of all sensation).

Historically, when labor epidural analgesia was introduced, local anesthetics were the only medications that were available and known to work when administered in the epidural space. Lacking continuous infusion pumps, it was considered desirable to use high concentrations of local anesthetics, so as to effect analgesia for as long as possible. Unfortunately, these high concentrations also frequently caused hypotension, weakness of the lower extremities, and profound numbness, by virtue of blockade of autonomic, motor, and somatic sensory neurons, respectively. It is likely that these high concentrations of local anesthetics also interfered with maternal expulsive efforts during second stage, necessitating operative vaginal deliveries and cesarean sections. Over time, with the introduction of continuous infusion pumps and greater understanding of adjunctive medications that can be administered into the epidural space, it has become possible to reduce the concentration of local anesthetics greatly. It is now possible to combine a very low concentration of local anesthetic with a lipophilic opioid and an alpha-2 adrenergic agonist (most commonly epinephrine) to yield an analgesic solution, which causes minimal hypotension

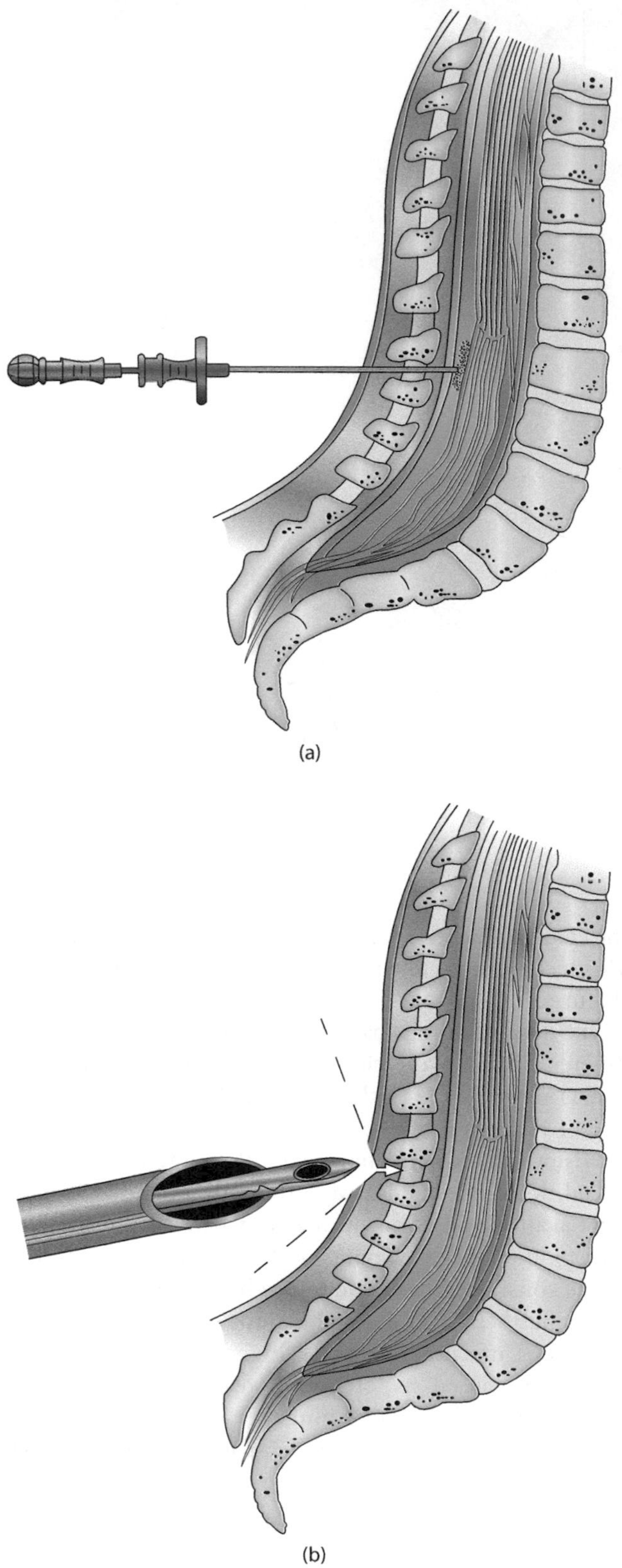

Figure 33.4 (a and b) Combined spinal epidural. (Courtesy of JJ Rudisill.)

and minimal motor and sensory block.[27] Indeed, the degree of motor and sensory block may be so minimal that some of the patients can ambulate short distances while this epidural solution is infusing. Such techniques have been called "walking epidurals," although the authors hasten to note that the principal advantages of these solutions is in the reduced hypotension and the enhanced ability of the patient to perform a Valsalva maneuver, and the possibility of ambulation is more a marketing technique than a clinically significant advantage.[28]

The medications injected as the spinal portion of a labor CSE can also be similarly administered in low dose, so as to minimize hypotension and motor and sensory blocks.[29]

Typically, the epidural is attached to a pump, which automatically gives a constant flow of the very dilute solution for as long as the epidural is needed. The pump can have a patient controlled aspect, which will allow the patient to give occasional small boluses of the very dilute solution to make it over any rough spots (more on the pump later).

Sometimes the pain is not successfully treated as above despite adequate coverage of the corresponding autonomic plane. This may be due to irritation of the body wall adjacent to the visceral structures. Impulses of painful stimuli from these somatic structures are conveyed to the spinal cord via somatic sensory fibers. These are thicker, myelinated fibers, which are less easily blocked and require a more concentrated local anesthetic at the appropriate level. Similarly, pain from manipulation of the uterus may originate from higher segmental levels innervating the peritoneum (T6–T10). From the dorsal horn, the nerve impulse proceeds along ascending pathways to higher centers in the brain where pain is ultimately perceived. These impulses may be altered, usually resulting in attenuation, via descending pathways from the brain.

Different medications and techniques can affect the pathway at various points to modify the perception of pain.[30] Systemic opioids (endogenous or exogenous) decrease painful stimuli indirectly by activating the descending pathways. Nonpharmacologic modes, such as the psychoprophylactic method of Lamaze, also decrease painful stimuli via descending modulation.[31] Conversely, anxiety and emotional distress may block this modulation, thereby increasing the perception of pain. Inhalational agents, such as nitrous oxide and the potent halogenated agents, act by disrupting transmission of stimuli to the spinal cord and between the spinal cord and the brain and by interfering with awareness of the pain at the cerebral cortex.

A self-administered 50/50 combination of oxygen and nitrous oxide used episodically may be a useful adjuvant for labor analgesia. It can be used while waiting for an epidural or CSE. It can also be used to supplement an existing epidural. It does cause a greater incidence of nausea and vomiting, and overuse may theoretically cause problems with the methionine synthetase pathway, but it has been successfully used in some institutions.[32]

Neuraxial (i.e., spinal or epidural) opioids act at opioid receptors located in the dorsal horn itself to inhibit transmission of painful stimuli. Alpha-2 agonists, such as clonidine and epinephrine, also modulate painful stimuli via receptors in the dorsal horn.[33] Thus, opioids and alpha-2 adrenergic agonists added to epidurally administered solutions work by diffusing across the dura and arachnoid, into the CSF, and over to the spinal cord. This epidural combination has proven very efficacious in providing satisfactory analgesia. [34–37]

Contraindications for epidural (and most other regional) blocks include patient refusal, local or widespread infection, coagulopathy, and hypovolemia. If a bleeding tendency is suspected on the basis of history or physical examination, laboratory studies should be obtained before placing the block. If no potential bleeding tendency is suspected, no special laboratory studies have to be obtained.[38] Intravenous access should be established prior to epidural placement. During the onset of an epidural anesthetic, sympathetic blockade and resultant vasodilation and hypotension may occur quickly if the patient is hypovolemic. Since uterine blood flow is not autoregulated, any decrease in systemic blood pressure will cause a decrease in the uterine blood flow. If a large decrease occurs, uteroplacental insufficiency may ensue. This should be treated promptly with vasopressors. Hydration with 0.5–2 l isoosmolar crystalloid without dextrose is suggested before and during the initial dose(s) of epidural local anesthetics to blunt the hypotensive effects from vasodilation. An ultralight labor epidural produces less vasodilation and hypotension. Consequently, fluid preloading may be unnecessary if the local anesthetic concentration is sufficiently low. This would also avoid any potential inhibition of labor that may be seen with rapid infusion of IV fluids.

CESAREAN SECTION

A planned cesarean section can be scheduled electively, hopefully before the patient goes into labor, or can be scheduled expeditiously for failed labor, or emergently when the patient or the fetus or both are in distress. If time permits, a regional anesthetic is generally preferred over a general anesthetic.[39] In emergency circumstances, however, the optimal anesthetic technique will vary from case to case. In a 2003 study,[40] the investigators noted that decision to incision time was a mean of 2.1 minutes faster with general anesthesia than with regional anesthesia. Additionally, the babies born to regionally anesthetized mothers had a pH that was 0.03 lower than the babies born to generally anesthetized mothers, although the investigators allowed that the pH difference may have been a consequence of hypotension management with ephedrine, which has subsequently been demonstrated to lower fetal pH. Whether the harm of the potentially delayed incision is offset by the avoidance of complications associated with general anesthesia is a decision best left to the clinicians at the bedside at the time. Good communication is essential.

Procedure

A spinal or epidural anesthetic for a cesarean section requires a higher dermatomal level and a more pronounced motor and sensory block than a labor analgesic. The standard spinal dose administered into the CSF is usually enough to block all of the motor and sensory innervation to the T6 level, which is adequate for a cesarean section. An epidural anesthetic can achieve the same effect, but generally takes longer and has a higher failure rate due to the risk of an asymmetric or unilateral block.[41] For this reason, the authors generally use epidural anesthetics only for cesarean section patients who already have a preexisting epidural catheter.

General anesthesia may occasionally be necessary and is similar to the general anesthetic described above.[42] Delivery should be as quick as possible to limit transfer of anesthetic drugs to the baby. Other than extreme emergency circumstances, the rapid sequence induction is only started after the patient has been prepped and draped and all teams (anesthetic, obstetric, pediatric) are ready to proceed (i.e., scrubbed and gowned etc.).

If labor is unsuccessful or the fetus or the mother or both are in distress, and an epidural is present, the epidural analgesia can be converted to epidural anesthesia. Converting the analgesic epidural to an epidural anesthetic requires a "top off" dose of a more concentrated solution.[43] There is some controversy as to how long one has to stop the dilute solution before instilling the more concentrated solution.

Procedure

Chloroprocaine, a fast-acting ester local anesthetic, can be used to "top up" the dose. The analgesic dose of local anesthetic is stopped as soon as possible once the need for a cesarean section is suspected. A total of 15–25 cc of 3% chloroprocaine is administered in 5 cc aliquots until a T6 dermatomal level is obtained. Adding a small amount of bicarbonate to the chloroprocaine is generally recommended to hasten the onset of the anesthetic and to also render the injection less painful and safer. It was once believed that chloroprocaine, an ester local anesthetic, would not work well after recent administration of lidocaine or bupivacaine, both amide anesthetics, but that has proven false. Chloroprocaine is metabolized by ester hydrolysis in the plasma with a half-life under 1 minute. Consequently, repeated doses do not accumulate and cause systemic toxicity. Similarly, transfer across the placenta to the fetus is not a concern.

Lidocaine is another viable option for the rapid conversion of a labor epidural analgesic to a surgical anesthetic. Although it features a rapid onset, it is not quite as rapid as choloroprocaine. Additionally, lacking chloroprocaine's rapid metabolism, systemic toxicity and transfer to the fetus are realistic concerns. The sympathetic block seen with anesthetic doses of a local anesthetic agent may cause significant vasodilation and hypotension. Preloading or coloading with IV fluids and early or even prophylactic treatment with vasopressors may be indicated.[44–46]

POSTOPERATIVE PAIN MANAGEMENT AFTER C SECTION

Systemic

There are many ways to provide postoperative pain management after the cesarean section. The goal is to provide analgesia while allowing normal function. The simplest way is to use systemic analgesics. Most obstetricians are familiar with dosing of oral or intramuscular analgesics so we will concentrate on IV administration.

Opioids generally give adequate analgesia in a timely fashion. However, there are sometimes troubling side effects such as pruritis, nausea, vomiting, constipation, etc. Still more troubling is respiratory depression. Respiratory depression can be avoided by titrating the drug. This means giving a small amount of drug every so often and watching and waiting for the analgesic vs. respiratory depressive effect. This can be time consuming and is often impractical. A programmable machine, which allows the patient to safely control his or her own drug administration, is the patient controlled analgesia (PCA) machine. It simply administers small amounts of the selected analgesic every so often upon the patient's request. If the patient starts to get an excessive dose, she will become too sedated to administer more drug before any respiratory depression sets in, especially if the machine is not programmed to administer a continuous infusion of drug. A caveat to using a PCA machine is that it is most effective if the patient starts using it after they have achieved adequate analgesia.

Procedure

The PCA machine can deliver very small volumes (e.g., 1–2 cc/hour) of drug piggy-backed to a working IV. It can deliver a continuous stream of drug or an intermittent bolus of drug or both. The intermittent bolus is triggered by the patient pressing a button and can only be activated every so often (i.e., lockout time). For analgesia, not having a continuous stream of drug prevents possible accumulation when drug is not needed, such as during sleep. The intermittent boluses allow the patient to adjust analgesia during those times of added pain (i.e., walking, moving, etc.). The system only works if there is an adequate amount of drug already present as the small amounts of additional drug is designed to facilitate analgesia while preventing overdose.

Neuraxial

Drugs for analgesia can also be administered neuraxially (i.e., via spinal or epidural) for postoperative pain management. This type of analgesia has the advantage over systemic medication in avoiding some of the side effects, and in placing less of the opioid in the patient's body, which is of particular concern to breastfeeding mothers. The PCA machine can now be used as a patient-controlled epidural analgesia (PCEA).

Procedure

The PCA machine can also deliver slightly larger volumes of drug attached to an epidural catheter. In this instance, a continuous dose of drug is used with additional intermittent boluses as desired.

TAP block

A transversus abdominis plane block (TAP) is a fairly recent technique, which blocks the sensory innervation of the abdominal wall. It is generally used to complement PCA in the immediate postoperative period after a general anesthetic. [47–49] It provides analgesia to the abdominal wall including the intercostal nerves (T7–11), the subcostal nerve (T12) and the iliohypogastric and ilioinguinal nerves (L1). It does not provide analgesia to structures within the peritoneal cavity. Dilute local anesthetic solutions are recommended to avoid systemic toxicity, since the block usually requires a large volume (Figure 33.5).

Procedure

This block is best accomplished by ultrasound guidance but can be performed without it (although it not recommended). The operator stands to the side of the patient and inserts the block needle at the midaxillary line between the lower costal margin and the iliac crest. After visualization, careful aspiration, and test injection, approximately 20 cc of a solution of local anesthetic is injected between the internal oblique and transverse abdominis muscle layers. The block is then repeated on the contralateral side.

CRITICAL CARE

Postdural puncture headache (PDPH) is often an incapacitating situation.[50] The incidence is nearly 100% if there is a puncture of the dura with an epidural needle in a woman of childbearing potential. The incidence is much lower (0–2%) if a small pencil point needle is used for a spinal.[51] The pathophysiology is not fully understood, but it is generally thought that a CSF leak leads to low intracranial pressure, which leads to irritation of the meningeal vessels.[52] The *sine qua non* of this headache is that it is postural in nature. Sitting or standing worsens the headache while lying supine relieves the symptoms almost immediately. Hydration and/or systemic methylxanthines can be used to temporarily relieve symptoms, but placing autologous blood in the epidural space near the presumptive leak (i.e., epidural blood patch) is the definitive solution. This blood seems to stop any further leak and increases pressure in the CSF, which relieves the headache nearly immediately. The timing of the blood patch is somewhat controversial.[53–56] The authors feel that it is best done

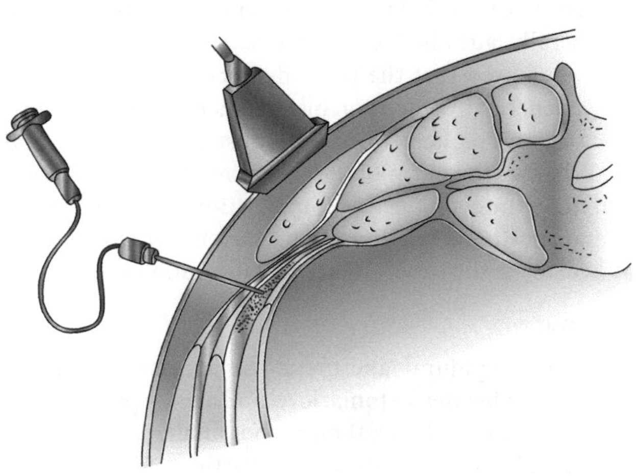

Figure 33.5 TAP block. (Courtesy of JJ Rudisill.)

prophylactically if there is a tear from epidural needle but should be done only if there are symptoms when a fine pencil point spinal needle is used. There is some controversy as to the administration of autologous blood in patients with blood borne pathogens (i.e., bacteremia, AIDS, etc.). An allogeneic blood patch or a patch with other materials such as hetastarch has also been used successfully.[57]

Procedure

An epidural blood patch can be done as a one-person procedure or as a two-person procedure. The patient is placed in the lateral position with her head and lower extremities flexed as much as possible. In the two-person technique, one operator prepares to withdraw autologous blood using strict aseptic technique while the second operator places the epidural needle in a near but different location than the initial insertion; 20 cc of venous blood is sterilely and slowly injected through the epidural needle. In the one-person technique, an epidural catheter is inserted, then the patient is repositioned supine, and the venous blood is aseptically drawn and injected into the epidural catheter. It can be surprisingly difficult to inject blood into an epidural catheter. Sometimes the injection must be terminated before the full 20 cc is injected because the patient experiences an excess of pressure in the spinal column or because the blood has clotted in the syringe. The authors have had success after injecting as little as 11 cc in an epidural blood patch. Finally, care must be taken to avoid injecting the blood into the subarachnoid space, as this is very poorly tolerated by most patients.

In either case, after the blood is injected, the epidural catheter or needle is removed and the patient is placed in semi-Fowler's position for 45 minutes to an hour. If the headache is significantly improved and lower extremity function is normal, the patient may be discharged with instructions to avoid vigorous physical activity for 2 weeks, and to seek emergency care in case of any fever, severe stiff neck, or unusual neurological phenomena.

Critical care for obstetric patients with coexisting diseases usually requires a preoperative assessment of whether any invasive monitoring is warranted and of when or if a regional anesthetic can be given. Preeclampsia is unique to pregnant women and will used as an example of what considerations are necessary to care for a critical care patient.[58]

In preeclampsia, anesthesia personnel are confronted with a hypertensive, intravascularly depleted patient who is very sensitive to cardiovascular insult and who teeters between hypovolemia and congestive heart failure. Painful uterine contractions cause an increase in catecholamine secretion and a decrease in uteroplacental perfusion. This can be magnified in the already tenuous preeclamptic patient. For this and other previously stated reasons, lumbar epidural analgesia is indicated. All preeclamptic patients with normal bleeding and coagulation times should benefit from epidural analgesia for labor and delivery, or anesthesia for cesarean section, unless otherwise contraindicated. Anesthesia personnel must maintain a low threshold for placement of invasive monitoring in the severe preeclamptic patient. Usually, arterial and central venous catheters are sufficient. Placement of a pulmonary artery catheter may occasionally be needed, but is associated with increased morbidity. The benefits of such a procedure must be weighed against its associated risks. If induction of general anesthesia (GA) is planned, short-acting IV antihypertensive drugs may be necessary to prevent excessive increases in blood pressure. Sodium nitroprusside, nitroglycerine, labetalol, or esmolol limited to very short periods of time should have little adverse effect on the newborn.

Magnesium sulfate is the anticonvulsant of choice in the United States for seizure prophylaxis in the preeclamptic patient.[59] An inadvertent overdose may cause severe cardiac and respiratory depression requiring intubation, ventilatory support, and possibly cardiopulmonary resuscitation (CPR). Calcium can be used to competitively antagonize the magnesium.

SUMMARY

The obstetric patient population has become older and more medically complicated over the past several decades. Despite this, maternal morbidity and mortality attributable to obstetric anesthesia have declined, even as more patients require or request anesthetic interventions. This may be attributable to many factors, including a greater understanding of the causes of morbidity, improved monitoring, better medications, a reduction in the use of relatively risky techniques such as GA, and enhancement of the safety and efficacy of epidural analgesia.

Changing attitudes may also have contributed to enhanced patient safety in the labor and delivery suite. As obstetricians and anesthesiologists developed appreciation of, understanding of, and respect for one another's concerns, they have become more effective partners in delivering optimal care for the patients they serve.

ACKNOWLEDGMENT

This chapter contains some figures from the previous edition chapter coauthored by David N. Dhanraj and Michael S. Baggish.

REFERENCES

1. Berghella V, Ludmir J, Simonazzi G, Owen J. Transvaginal cervical cerclage: Evidence for perioperative management strategies. *Am J Obstet Gynecol* 2013; 209: 181–192.
2. Teoh WH, Westphal M, Kampmeier TG. Update on volume therapy in obstetrics. *Best Pract Res Clin Anaesthesiol* 2014; 28: 297–303.
3. Bhattacharyya S, Bisai S, Biswas H, Tiwary MK, Mallik S, Saha SM. Regional anesthesia in transurethral resection of prostate (TURP) surgery: A comparative study between saddle block and subarachnoid block. *Saudi J Anaesth* 2015; 9: 268–271.
4. Yoon HJ, Hong JY, Kim SM. The effect of anesthetic method for prophylactic cervical cerclage on plasma

oxytocin: A randomized trial. *Int J Obstet Anesth* 2008; 17: 26–30.
5. Hebl JR, Niesen AD. Infectious complications of regional anesthesia. *Curr Opin Anaesthesiol* 2011; 24: 573–580.
6. Zaric D, Pace NL. Transient neurologic symptoms (TNS) following spinal anaesthesia with lidocaine versus other local anaesthetics. *Cochrane Database Syst Rev* 2009; 15: CD003006.
7. Gozdemir M, Muslu B, Sert H, et al. Transient neurological symptoms after spinal anaesthesia with levobupivacaine 5 mg/ml or lidocaine 20 mg/ml. *Acta Anaesthesiol Scand* 2010; 54: 59–64.
8. Vassiliadis RM, Taylor PG. Spinal pethidine for elective caesarean section. *Anaesth Intensive Care* 2013; 41: 113–115.
9. Pawlowski J, Orr K, Kim KM, Pappas AL, Sukhani R, Jellish WS. Anesthetic and recovery profiles of lidocaine versus mepivacaine for spinal anesthesia in patients undergoing outpatient orthopedic arthroscopic procedures. *J Clin Anesth* 2012; 24: 109–115.
10. Reina MA, de Leon-Casasola OA, Lopez A, De Andres J, Martin S, Mora M. An in vitro study of dural lesions produced by 25-gauge Quincke and Whitacre needles evaluated by scanning electron microscopy. *Reg Anesth Pain Med* 2000; 25: 393–402.
11. Mercier FJ, Augè M, Hoffmann C, Fischer C, Le Gouez A. Maternal hypotension during spinal anesthesia for caesarean delivery. *Minerva Anestesiol* 2013; 79: 62–73.
12. Roofthooft E. Anesthesia for the morbidly obese parturient. *Curr Opin Anaesthesiol* 2009; 22: 341–346.
13. Lesage S. Cesarean delivery under general anesthesia: Continuing professional development. *Can J Anesth* 2014; 61: 489–503.
14. Hawkins JL. Excess in moderation: General anesthesia for cesarean delivery. *Anesth Analg* 2015; 120: 1175–1177.
15. Quinn AC, Milne DE, Columb M, Gorton H, Knight M. Failed tracheal intubation in obstetric anesthesia: 2 yr national case-control study in the UK. *Br J Anaesth* 2013; 110: 74–80.
16. Warner MW, Salfinger SG, Rao S, Magann EF, Hall JC. Management of trauma during pregnancy. *ANZ J Surg* 2004; 74: 125–128.
17. Van De Velde M, De Buck F. Anesthesia for non-obstetric surgery in the pregnant patient. *Minerva Anestesiol* 2007; 73: 235–240.
18. Djabatey EA, Barclay PM. Difficult and failed intubation in 3430 obstetric general anaesthetics. *Anaesthesia* 2009; 64: 1168.
19. Ni J, Luo L, Wu L, Luo D. The Airtraq™ laryngoscope as a first choice for parturients with an expected difficult airway. *Int J Obstet Anesth* 2014; 1: 94–95.
20. Paolini JB, Donati F, Drolet P. Review article: Video-laryngoscopy: Another tool for difficult intubation or a new paradigm in airway management? *Can J Anaesth* 2013; 60: 184–191.
21. Novikova N, Cluver C. Local anaesthetic nerve block for pain management in labour. *Cochrane Database Syst Rev* 2012; 4: CD009200
22. American Society of Anesthesiology Task Force on Obstetric Anesthesia. Practice guidelines for obstetric anesthesia. *Anesthesiology* 2007; 106: 843–863. [NB: 2015 practice guidelines should be finalized/approved at the Oct 2015 ASA meeting in San Diego]
23. Anderson D. Pudendal nerve block for vaginal birth. *J Midwifery Womens Health* 2014; 59: 651–659.
24. Gizzo S, Noventa M, Fagherazzi S, et al. Update on best available options in obstetrics anaesthesia: Perinatal outcomes, side effects and maternal satisfaction. Fifteen years systematic literature review. *Arch Gynecol Obstet* 2014; 290: 21–34.
25. Antibas PL, do Nascimento Jr P, Braz LG, Vitor Pereira Doles J, Módolo NS, El Dib R. Air versus saline in the loss of resistance technique for identification of the epidural space. *Cochrane Database Syst Rev* 2014; 7: CD008938.
26. Niesen AD, Jacob AK. Combined spinal-epidural versus epidural analgesia for labor and delivery. *Clin Perinatol* 2013; 40: 373–384.
27. Wilson MJ, MacArthur C, Cooper GM, Shennan A; COMET Study Group UK. Ambulation in labour and delivery mode: A randomised controlled trial of high-dose vs mobile epidural analgesia. *Anaesthesia* 2009; 64: 266–272.
28. Stewart A, Fernando R. Maternal ambulation during labor. *Curr Opin Anaesthesiol* 2011; 24: 268–273.
29. Kuczkowski KM. Ambulation with combined spinal-epidural labor analgesia: The technique. *Acta Anaesthesiol Belg* 2004; 55: 29–34.
30. Jones L, Othman M, Dowswell T, et al. Pain management for women in labour: An overview of systematic reviews. *Cochrane Database Syst Rev* 2012; 3: CD009234.
31. Chaillet N, Belaid L, Crochetière C, et al. Nonpharmacologic approaches for pain management during labor compared with usual care: A meta-analysis. *Birth* 2014; 41: 122–137.
32. Klomp T, van Poppel M, Jones L, Lazet J, Di Nisio M, Lagro-Janssen AL. Inhaled analgesia for pain management in labour. *Cochrane Database Syst Rev* 2012; 9: CD009351.
33. Thakur A, Bharadwaj M, Kaur K, Dureja J, Hooda S, Taxak S. Intrathecal clonidine as an adjuvant to hyperbaric bupivacaine in patients undergoing inguinal herniorraphy: A randomised double-blinded study. *J Anaesthesiol Clin Pharmacol* 2013; 29: 66–70.
34. Lv BS, Wang W, Wang ZQ, et al. Efficacy and safety of local anesthetics bupivacaine, ropivacaine and levobupivacaine in combination with sufentanil in epidural anesthesia for labor and delivery: A meta-analysis. *Curr Med Res Opin* 2014; 30: 2279–2289.
35. Sultan P, Murphy C, Halpern S, Carvalho B. The effect of low concentrations versus high concentrations of

local anesthetics for labour analgesia on obstetric and anesthetic outcomes: A meta-analysis. *Can J Anaesth* 2013; 60: 840–854.
36. Genc M, Sahin N, Maral J, et al. Does bupivacaine and fentanyl combination for epidural analgesia shorten the duration of labour? *J Obstet Gynaecol* 2015; 24: 1–4. [Epub ahead of print]
37. Wilson MJ, Moore PA, Shennan A, Lancashire RJ, MacArthur C. Long-term effects of epidural analgesia in labor: A randomized controlled trial comparing high dose with two mobile techniques. *Birth* 2011; 38: 105–110.
38. Goodier CG, Lu JT, Hebbar L, Segal BS, Goetzl L. Neuraxial anesthesia in parturients with thrombocytopenia: A multisite retrospective cohort study. *Anesth Analg* 2015; 121: 988–991.
39. Fassoulaki A, Staikou C, Melemeni A, Kottis G, Petropoulos G. Anaesthesia preference, neuraxial vs general, and outcome after caesarean section. *J Obstet Gynaecol* 2010; 30: 818–821.
40. Dyer RA, Els I, Farbas J, Torr GJ, Schoeman LK, James MF. Prospective, randomized trial comparing general with spinal anesthesia for cesarean delivery in preeclamptic patients with a nonreassuring fetal heart trace. *Anesthesiology* 2003; 99: 561–569.
41. Arendt K, Segal S. Why epidurals do not always work. *Rev Obstet Gynecol* 2008; 1: 49–55.
42. Bauer ME, Kountanis JA, Tsen LC, et al. Risk factors for failed conversion of labor epidural analgesia to cesarean delivery anesthesia: A systematic review and meta-analysis of observational trials. *Int J Obstet Anesth* 2012; 21: 294
43. Depuydt E, Van de Velde M. Unplanned cesarean section in parturients with an epidural catheter in-situ: How to obtain surgical anesthesia? *Acta Anaesthesiol Belg* 2013; 64: 61–74.
44. Banerjee A, Stocche RM, Angle P, Halpern SH. Preload or coload for spinal anesthesia for elective Cesarean delivery: A meta-analysis. *Can J Anaesth* 2010; 57: 24.
45. Tawfik MM, Hayes SM, Jacoub FY, et al. Comparison between colloid preload and crystalloid co-load in cesarean section under spinal anesthesia: A randomized controlled trial. *Int J Obstet Anesth* 2014; 23: 317.
46. Heesen M, Kölhr S, Rossaint R, Straube S. Prophylactic phenylephrine for caesarean section under spinal anaesthesia: Systematic review and meta-analysis. *Anaesthesia* 2014; 69: 143.
47. Baeriswyl, Moira MD, Kirkham, et al. The analgesic efficacy of ultrasound-guided transversus abdominis plane block in adult patients: A meta-analysis. *Anesth Analg* Sep 2015. [Epub ahead of print]
48. Siddiqui MR, Sajid MS, Uncles DR, Cheek L, Baig MK. A meta-analysis on the clinical effectiveness of transversus abdominis plane block. *J Clin Anesth* 2011; 23: 7–14.
49. McDonnell JG, Curley G, Carney J, et al. The analgesic efficacy of transversus abdominis plane block after cesarean delivery: A randomized controlled trial. *Anesth Analg* 2008; 106: 186–191
50. Sachs A, Smiley R. Post-dural puncture headache: The worst common complication in obstetric anesthesia. *Semin Perinatol* 2014; 38: 386–394.
51. Pal A, Acharya A, Pal ND, Dawn S, Biswas J. Do pencil-point spinal needles decrease the incidence of postdural puncture headache in reality? A comparative study between pencil-point 25G Whitacre and cutting-beveled 25G Quincke spinal needles in 320 obstetric patients. *Anesth Essays Res* 2011; 5: 162–166.
52. Harrington BE, Schmitt AM. Meningeal (postdural) puncture headache, unintentional dural puncture, and the epidural blood patch: A national survey of United States practice. *Reg Anesth Pain Med* 2009; 34: 430–437.
53. Agerson AN, Scavone BM. Prophylactic epidural blood patch after unintentional dural puncture for the prevention of postdural puncture headache in parturients. *Anesth Analg* 2012; 115: 133–136.
54. Thew M, Paech MJ. Management of postdural puncture headache in the obstetric patient. *Curr Opin Anaesthesiol* 2008; 21: 288–292.
55. Baysinger CL, Pope JE, Lockhart EM, Mercaldo ND. The management of accidental dural puncture and postdural puncture headache: A North American survey. *Abstract J Clin Anesth* 2011; 23: 349–360.
56. Stein MH, Cohen S, Mohiuddin MA, Dombrovskiy V, Lowenwirt I. Prophylactic vs therapeutic blood patch for obstetric patients with accidental dural puncture—A randomised controlled trial. *Anaesthesia* 2014; 69: 320–326.
57. Vassal O, Baud MC, Bolandard F, et al. Epidural injection of hydroxyethyl starch in the management of postdural puncture headache. *Int J Obstet Anesth* 2013; 22: 153–155.
58. Lambert G, Brichant JF, Hartstein G, Bonhomme V, Dewandre PY. Preeclampsia: An update. *Acta Anaesthesiol Belg* 2014; 65: 137–149.
59. Gambling DR. Magnesium and the obstetric anesthetist. *Int J Obstet Anesth* 2013; 22: 255.

Cardiac monitoring in pregnancy

34

TORRE L. HALSCOTT and ARTHUR JASON VAUGHT

CONTENTS

INTRODUCTION

Cardiac monitoring, invasive or otherwise, has as its goal the reliable ascertainment of the current physiology, as well as any pathology, of the patient's heart. The simplest technique is a thorough auscultation via stethoscope and should be employed regardless of the level of other care that is available. Beyond this initial evaluation, numerous clinical factors may lead to the utilization of the many various methods to gather further insight into the correct diagnosis and ideal management of cardiac lesions in the pregnant patient.

PHYSIOLOGICAL CARDIOVASCULAR CHANGES IN PREGNANCY

The normal increases in cardiac output during pregnancy are predominantly related to increasing heart rate, which progresses throughout gestation. Contrasting with this the stroke volume decreases slightly on average, as a function of the increased basal pulse rate. Additionally, overall blood volume is augmented by 30%–50%, with the peak occurring around 28–32 weeks of pregnancy.[1,2] Dyspnea of pregnancy, lower extremity edema, and some degree of exercise intolerance are all very commonly reported symptoms, particularly in the latter second and third trimesters. These complaints may mimic those of cardiac decompensation, however, and should prompt further investigation if there is clinical suspicion. Assessment for hypertensive disorders germane to pregnancy, such as gestational hypertension and preeclampsia, is an important consideration in such patients as well and may be the first presentation of an otherwise suboptimally treated patient with chronic hypertension. Such cases may portend substantial cardiac strain and must be identified as separate from healthy women with similar initial presentations.

NONINVASIVE CARDIAC MONITORING IN PREGNANCY

Electrocardiogram

Studies originating as early as the 1960s sought to determine if pregnancy status alters the electrocardiogram (EKG) assessment.[3] These, and other investigations, found that common EKG abnormalities are present, such as Q-waves in leads II, III, or aVF, and/or ST segment elevation in inferior leads in one-third of healthy, asymptomatic women during early pregnancy, as well as T-wave inversions in 100% of women in the latter half of gestation (Figure 34.1).[4] Arrhythmias occur frequently in labor also, with over 82% of parturients experiencing some abnormal rhythm during

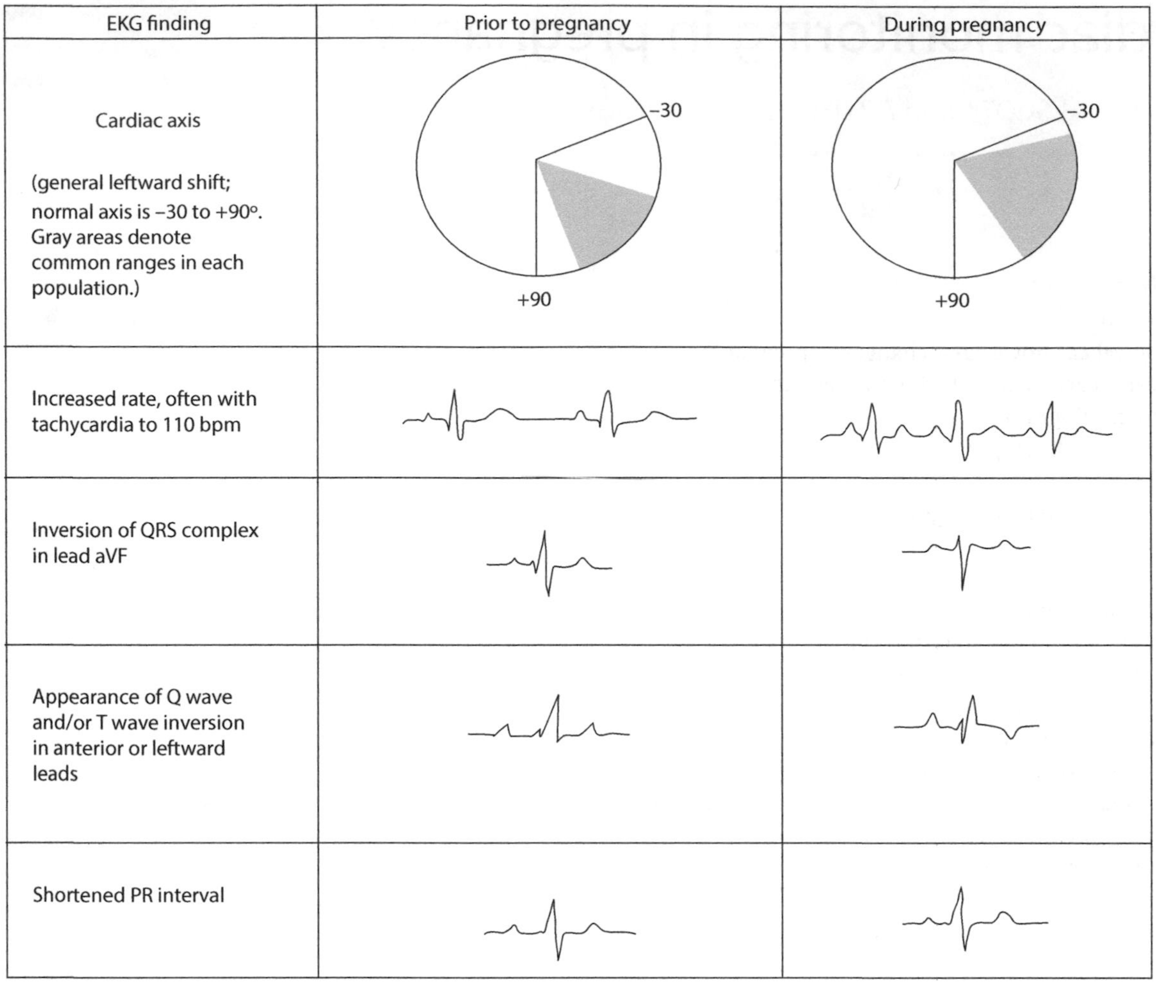

EKG finding
Prior to pregnancy
During pregnancy
Cardiac axis
(general leftward shift; normal axis is −30 to +90°. Gray areas denote common ranges in each population.)
−30
+90
−30
+90
Increased rate, often with tachycardia to 110 bpm
Inversion of QRS complex in lead aVF
Appearance of Q wave and/or T wave inversion in anterior or leftward leads
Shortened PR interval

Figure 34.1 Normal electrocardiogram (EKG) adaptations during pregnancy. EKG changes in normal pregnancy include a reduction in the mean values of PR interval, sinus tachycardia, left axis deviation, inverted or flattened T waves and a Q wave in anterior or leftward leads. BPM denotes beats per minute. (Adapted from Angeli F et al., *Hypertens Res* 37(11), 973–5, 2014.)

this event.[5] In the absence of pathology or symptomatology, however, these are rarely of clinical importance. The EKG remains a cornerstone of evaluation when a potential cardiac concern is present during pregnancy however, and ongoing continuous telemetry is a valuable adjunct in patients with known pathology. An outpatient correlate for assessment of palpitations is the three to seven lead "Holter" monitor worn over the course of one to several days or a newer device that utilizes a one lead cardiac assessment tool that may be employed in a similar manner for up to 2 weeks. These methods appear to function as well in pregnant women as in the nonpregnant population.[6,7]

X-ray and radiography

Chest X-ray

The use of X-ray assessment when a concern for cardiopulmonary disease exists can often further delineate the possible etiologies. Just as in the nonpregnant patient, these tests are readily available, quickly performed, and may provide highly valuable information. How such tests are performed has significance as well. Due to protocol restraints in many institutions, a single X-ray, often obtained portably, in the anterio-posterior (AP) position (the X-ray beam enters the front of the patient's body and exposes the radiograph behind the patient) is the routine radiograph performed. A consequence of this is that the already prominent cardiac silhouette due to normal pregnancy may be exaggerated by the radiographic technique causing concern for cardiomegaly and heart failure. A more accurate manner of evaluation by chest X-ray is to perform imaging from the posterio-anterior (PA) view, as well as laterally when feasible. This better represents the true cardiac size on X-ray with the PA image and additionally provides clearer views of the posterior aspects of the lungs and their bases via the lateral film, as these are often obscured by the hypertrophic breast tissues and/or elevated intra-abdominal contents related to pregnancy itself. Counseling and documentation, for the patient as well as all providers, are beneficial and appropriate given the use of ionizing radiation. Exposures less than 5 rads (0.05 Gray [Gy; 1 rad is equivalent to 0.01 Gy]) have not convincingly been associated with adverse gestational or neonatal/childhood outcomes (Table 34.1).[8,9]

Table 34.1 Radiation exposure to the fetus for common procedures.

Estimated fetal exposure from common radiologic procedures	Amount of radiation in rad
Chest X-ray (two views)	0.02–0.07 mrad
Abdominal X-ray (one view)	100 mrad
Intravenous pyelography	≥1 rad (depending on number of images obtained)
Barium enema or small bowel series	2–4 rad
CT of head or chest	<1 rad
CT of abdomen	3.5 rad

Source: Adapted from the American College of Obstetricians and Gynecologists Committee Opinion number 299, *Obstet Gynecol*, 104(3), 647–51, 2004.
Abbreviation: CT, Computed tomography.

Computed tomography (CT) imaging utilizes ionizing X-ray radiation to manufacture a reconstruction of the portion of the patient's body that is being assessed. The amount of information that may be obtained is substantially increased over individual X-rays in this manner. Unfortunately, pregnant women are at an increased risk of not having this test performed due to fetal concerns. It has been reported that up to 39% of patients may not receive recommended imaging after trauma in pregnancy, and that only 18% receive radiological testing in accordance with guidelines for high-risk traumatic injuries.[10] The radiation dosing is significantly increased with CT compared with X-ray, however, unless multiple studies are repeatedly performed, the total dose should remain below the threshold of 5 rads (0.05 Gy). Therefore, when this test is indicated to evaluate for potentially seriously morbid or lethal conditions, e.g., pulmonary embolism presenting with cardiac decompensation, significant trauma, etc., its use should not be precluded by concerns related to radiation exposure to either the mother or fetus.

Magnetic resonance imaging

The use of magnetic resonance imaging (MRI) has increased in pregnancy, particularly for the evaluation of fetal anomalies or placental abnormalities. Beyond these uses, MRI evaluation of cardiac lesion has become more commonly employed as well. Suspected coronary artery disease, complex congenital cardiac lesions of the mother, pericardial disease, or aortic pathology may be particularly amenable to MRI evaluation.[11] There does not appear to be significant risks associated with MRI in pregnancy.[8] The use of gadolinium contrast is more accepted in Europe, but often avoided in the United States due to the limited available data in humans as well as evidence of harm in very high doses administered within animal studies.[12]

Echocardiography

Ultrasound assessment in real time of the heart, valvular, and cardiac outflow structures is often utilized when there exists concern for abnormalities of these areas. It is employed as an initial evaluation when new symptoms present, as well as an indicator of change in disease for women with known cardiac conditions. Key information may be obtained regarding overall heart anatomy and function, individual atrial and ventricular dynamics, valvular lesions, flow and potentially pressure within the aorta and pulmonary artery, and even the presence of intracardiac thrombi. Most commonly, transthoracic echocardiography (TTE) is the initial test performed. In a majority of patients and situations this modality provides detailed ascertainments for the above-mentioned concerns. Uncommonly, imaging of the desired structures may be suboptimal due to a patient's body habitus, enlarged breast size during pregnancy, or shadowing from prosthetic valves; regardless TTE is almost invariably the most appropriate manner of echocardiogram to obtain first.

The specific application of TTE in pregnancy has shown that the total left ventricular (LV) mass may expand by up to 52%, with concomitant increases in overall ventricular chamber diameter (+13%–22%), specific end-systolic and diastolic diameters (+20% and +12%, respectively), as well as intraventricular septal size (+15%–19%).[13] Doppler insonation as part of the maternal echocardiogram provides information on the velocity of blow flow, relative gradients across valves, and the presence of regurgitant flow if it exists. It appears that the ability to obtain the desired image during gestation is comparable to those that are not pregnant, with 95% of pregnant women having multiple waveforms viewed with Doppler techniques.[14] Additionally, echocardiography has been studied in preeclamptic women compared with normotensive pregnancies, finding higher cardiac output (6.7 L/min versus 5.6 L/min), increased LV diastolic mass (131 g compared with 105 g), and greater total vascular resistance (1397 versus 1205 dyne-second/cm^5) in preeclamptic patients.[15]

Transesophageal echocardiography (TEE) can provide more clear imaging of many structures due to its closer proximity to the heart from the transducer being placed within the esophagus. During this procedure, patients commonly receive conscious sedation, usually with benzodiazepines and/or narcotics. These have been associated with decreased fetal movement and diminished variability on electronic fetal monitoring, though no adverse outcomes have been demonstrated with use in such procedures.[16] General indications for TEE include inability to obtain adequate images with TTE, more definitive assessment of aortic or pulmonic valve lesions, as well as evaluation of aortic pathology, particularly dilation or suspected aneurysm. Pregnancy should not preclude its utilization if such information cannot be gathered in other manners.

INVASIVE CARDIAC MONITORING IN PREGNANCY

In particular situations the use of invasive methods may be deemed warranted. Traditionally this has been most commonly thought of as placement of access into the central vasculature of the body, via either the arterial or venous routes. In practicality though, any inserted device that assesses cardiac function fits within the category of invasive monitoring.

Peripheral arterial access

The most commonly employed, and straightforward, method of invasive monitoring in pregnancy is the use of a peripherally placed arterial catheter, often referred to colloquially as an "arterial line." The catheter is usually placed in the distal radial artery, just proximal to the wrist, though it may also be used in larger arteries, such as the femoral. The rationale for its use is that the blood pressure, with waveform interpretation, may be assessed directly from the artery within which it is inserted. Common indications include the need for repeated arterial blood sampling (e.g., blood gas assessments), as well as in patients where traditional noninvasive sphygmomanometry cannot be reliably obtained, such as in those who are significantly overweight or underweight, have contraindications to pressure cuff use (burns, dialysis fistulae, etc.), or have blood pressures that are too low to be accurately obtained with noninvasive methods. Risks of use include bleeding, infection, nerve injury, compromise of blood supply distal to the artery, and compartment syndrome, though serious harms occur rarely (0.1 to approximately 1% incidences) (Figure 34.2).[17]

Pulmonary artery catheterization

A pulmonary arterial catheter ("Swan-Ganz," named for the physicians who invented the device) can be employed to gain information regarding most of the cardiac chambers and valves, as well as the pressure within the right heart outflow tract. Access to place the catheter is obtained via a distal point of the central venous vasculature, such

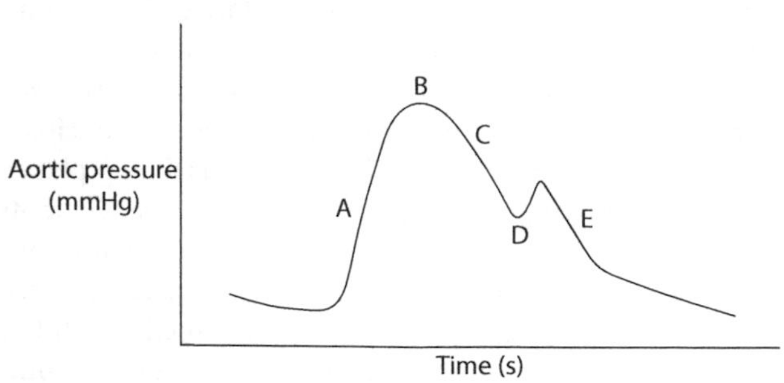

Figure 34.2 An arterial waveform. (A) Upstroke of systole. (B) Peak systole. (C) Decreasing pressure during systole. (D) Incisura. (E) Diastole. (From Esper SA and Pinsky MR, *Best Pract Res Clin Anaesthesiol*, 28(4), 363–80, 2014. With permission.)

as the internal jugular, subclavian, or femoral veins, using sterile technique. As the femoral route is more distant and inferior to the heart than either the jugular or subclavian veins, it is a more challenging option for pulmonary arterial catheterization; due to this, it is often attempted only after failure at the other sites. Furthermore, it may be more difficult to advance the catheter against the pressure of a gravid uterus, therefore more cephalad access points are most appropriate during pregnancy and the immediate postpartum period. After initial access, the catheter is then carefully advanced into the central vasculature via the vena cava until the manometer near the tip reaches the right atrium. Utilizing visual waveform assessment at this time, the placement of the catheter tip though each chamber of the right heart and into the pulmonary artery can be ascertained. Characteristic pressures within each discrete area can aid in determination of the catheter tip location, in conjunction with analysis of the waveforms.

After entering the right heart, then traversing the atrium and ventricle, the catheter is directed through the pulmonary artery and into the subsequent vasculature. It is at this point that the inflated balloon at the tip of the catheter will "wedge" itself into a portion of the distal pulmonary arterial tree. Pressure within the artery ahead of the balloon represents the static pressure exerted backwards from the left side of the heart, transmitted from the left ventricle across the mitral valve, through the left atrium and back toward the balloon via the pulmonary veins. In this manner, left-sided heart pressures can be estimated and utilized to influence management of the patient. In general, the measured parameters derived from pulmonary artery catheterization are similar between pregnant and nonpregnant women, with the significant differences of increased cardiac output and pulse rate, as well as diminished overall systemic and pulmonary vascular resistances during pregnancy (Figure 34.3; Tables 34.2 and 34.3).[18]

In addition to the previously mentioned parameters, these devices can measure the cardiac index, which is the cardiac output in relation to a patient's body surface area (liter/minute/square meter). This measurement provides an individualized representation of heart function as it compares to the size of the respective patient, with a normal range of 2.6–4.2 L/min/m^2, less than 2.2 L/min/m^2 is indicative of cardiac failure. Cardiac index is most commonly ascertained by a thermodilution assessment. This entails injection of a small volume of solution at a known temperature via one port of the pulmonary arterial catheter (any temperature sensitive multiport central catheter may be used as well). The time from injection to a temperature change at the tip of the catheter is used to calculate the cardiac index. Mixed venous oxygen saturation (denoted as SV_O) is another measurement that may be obtained from pulmonary arterial catheterization (and in practicality, any central venous catheter). It is an indicator of perfusion, related to the cardiac output, delivery of oxygen by hemoglobin (related to concentration of hemoglobin, as well as the arterial oxygenation within the lungs), and tissue level oxygen consumption, with a normal range

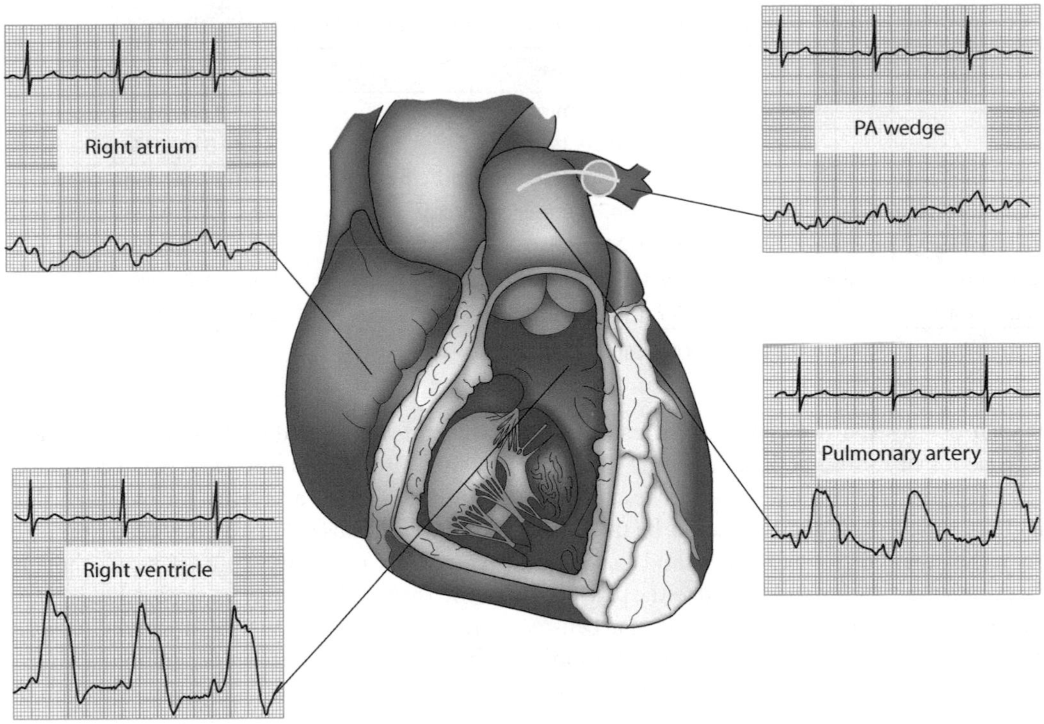

Figure 34.3 Representation of each pressure waveform as the pulmonary artery (PA) catheter moves through the right-sided cardiac chambers to its desired location in the pulmonary artery. (From Whitener S et al., *Best Pract Res Clin Anaesthesiol*, 28(4): 323–335, 2004. With permission.)

Table 34.2 Normal intracardiac pressures derived from pulmonary artery catheterization.

Parameter	Range (mean) in mmHg
Central venous pressure	1–8 (3)
Right ventricular systolic pressure	15–30 (25)
Right ventricular diastolic pressure	1–7 (6)
Pulmonary artery systolic pressure	15–30 (25)
Pulmonary artery diastolic pressure	4–12 (9)
Pulmonary artery mean pressure	9–19 (15)
Pulmonary artery wedge pressure	4–12 (9)
Mixed venous oxygen saturation	65%–75%
Cardiac output	4–8 L/min
Cardiac index	2.5–4 L/min/m^2

Source: Adapted from Whitener S et al., *Best Pract Res Clin Anaesthesiol*, 28(4), 323–335, 2004. With permission.

of 65%–75%. If any of the preceding factors decrease significantly, (or increase in the case of oxygen consumption by organs and tissues), SV_O will be negatively affected, and the oxygen needs of the patient will not be met by the current intrinsic supply. SV_O appears to have good sensitivity as an early indicator of hemodynamic instability, although management guided by this parameter has not been consistently correlated with a survival benefit in the general intensive care unit (ICU) patient population.[19]

While the use of pulmonary artery catheters gained widespread adoption within the decades after its introduction, more recently further examination of the clinical benefit of their use has been undertaken. Early studies of general ICU patients demonstrated increased mortality, length of stays, and costs with the use of pulmonary artery catheters, though these were nonrandomized or retrospective in nature.[20] Later randomized trials did not routinely find these excess risks with the use of a catheter, however, neither was a benefit consistently demonstrated. Use in pregnancy is limited to nonrandomized small cohort studies or anecdotal evidence and has not demonstrated convincing influence on management.[21,22] The Cochrane Collaboration performed a systematic review and meta-analysis for outcomes related to pulmonary artery catheter guided management in studies of high-risk surgical as well as ICU patients. This analysis included 13 trials with over 5600 patients, and concluded

Table 34.3 Comparative hemodynamic parameters in healthy nonpregnant and pregnant patients.

Parameter	Nonpregnant	Pregnant
Cardiac output	4.3 ± 0.9 L/min	6.2 ± 1.0 L/min
Pulse rate	71 ± 10 beats/min	83 ± 10 beats/min
Systemic vascular resistance	1530 ± 520 dyne-second/cm^5	1210 ± 266 dyne-second/cm^5
Pulmonary vascular resistance	119 ± 47 dyne-second/cm^5	78 ± 22 dyne-second/cm^5
Pulmonary capillary wedge pressure	6.3 ± 2.1 mmHg	7.5 ± 1.8 mmHg
Mean arterial pressure	86.4 ± 7.5 mmHg	90.3 ± 5.8 mmHg
Central venous pressure	3.7 ± 2.6 mmHg	3.6 ± 2.5 mmHg

Source: Adapted from Clark SL et al., *Am J Obstet Gynecol*, 161(6 Pt 1), 1439–42, 1989.

that the use of such devices did not confer an overall benefit, nor harm, in terms of mortality, length of stay (in the ICU as well as overall), and costs related to care.[2] The authors concluded that these monitoring devices should be used as diagnostic tools rather than therapeutic ones, and that the decision to utilize one should be individualized to the patient. Therefore, given possible harms without evidence for benefit in well-designed trials, pulmonary artery catheterization should be used extremely rarely, if at all, in pregnant women.

Central venous pressure assessment

Any centrally placed venous catheter equipped with a manometer, such as a pulmonary artery catheter, may also be employed to assess the static pressure within the central venous vasculature. In practice, such a catheter may only be advanced to the level of the vena cava (superior or inferior depending on access point, e.g., the jugular vein or the femoral), with the goal of ascertaining this specific parameter to aid in management. Central venous pressure corresponds to the cardiac preload, with the normal range being 1–8 mmHg. Values above 12 mmHg are generally considered to be correlated with cardiac pump failure, fluid overload, or both. Initially assessment of central venous pressure was thought to be a specific indicator of fluid status and useful guide to management. Studies that have critically evaluated this tool have found that the correlation with fluid status, and responsiveness to fluid resuscitation, is poor when central venous pressure measurements are the key factor to guide management.[24] Similar to pulmonary arterial catheter use, if central venous pressure monitoring is employed, it should be used as an adjunct to diagnosis rather than as an essential tool.

Cardiac catheterization

In rare occasions during pregnancy and the postpartum period, more direct information regarding left ventricular function is desired. When this occurs, traditional cardiac catheterization may be utilized. Additionally, assessment of the coronary arteries, such as in the case of suspected myocardial infarction, can only be obtained in this manner. Definitive diagnosis and percutaneous coronary intervention, i.e., coronary angiography and placement of an intraluminal stent if indicated, should be undertaken in the pregnant patient for the same indications as in the nonpregnant. Furthermore, if coronary artery bypass graft surgery is warranted, it should not be delayed by a patient's gestational status. The risks of untreated acute coronary syndromes, to both the mother and fetus, far outweigh the potential risks of interventions.[25] Fluoroscopy is commonly utilized in percutaneous intervention procedures, though the radiation dose that the fetus may be exposed to is substantially below the threshold for concern of 5 rads (0.05 Gy), with ranges from 0.0002 to 0.001 rad per minute with electrophysiology studies, and up to 0.02 rad per minute with traditional coronary angiography.[26] Cardiopulmonary bypass is necessary if bypass graft surgery is performed and concern exists for uterine perfusion in these circumstances. Increased pump flow rates (>2.5 L/min/m^2) and perfusion pressures (>70 mmHg) may be employed to augment uterine blood flow during cardiac surgery.[27] Normothermic bypass may have a fetal survival benefit as compared with hypothermic surgery as well.[28] In the case of such cardiac procedures and surgeries, an obstetrician and maternal–fetal medicine subspecialist should be immediately available to monitor and intervene if an obstetrical indication warrants.

Nuclear medicine testing

Except in exceedingly rare instances where the potential information cannot be gathered in another manner, nuclear medicine investigations are not usually performed during pregnancy. This is due to the unknown long-term effects on the fetus of the commonly utilized radiopharmaceuticals, although the theoretical risks are believed to be low.[29,30] Consultation with a dosimetrist to assess the potential fetal exposure to radioactive isotopes is advised if this testing is to be employed, as well as thorough counseling with the patient.

SPECIFIC CONDITIONS AND HEMODYNAMIC ASSESSMENT

Hypertensive disorders, preeclampsia, and pulmonary edema

Hypertension conditions, both those preexistent to pregnancy and those arising during gestation, are relatively common occurrences. Current incidences of all hypertensive disorders that may coexist with pregnancy range from 5% to 10%, and the frequency of preeclampsia has increased 25% in recent decades.[31] The vast majority of these patients are able to be managed without a need for intensive interventions, though the risks for significant clinical deterioration are substantially higher in this population than in healthy parturients.[32] The patients that are most apt to be candidates for invasive monitoring related to hypertensive disease are those that are refractory to intravenous antihypertensive therapy, develop pulmonary edema, are significantly oliguric, or demonstrate evidence of other end-organ harm related to their elevated blood pressure (renal failure, cerebral complications, etc.).[33] In these settings, the use of invasive cardiac monitoring may inform cardiac function and its relation to the clinical presentation, as well as progress in recovery. These disorders have increased systemic vascular resistance in common, which can be evaluated with invasive monitoring, though it is unlikely to change significantly in the immediate time of treatment. A more variable parameter that can be evaluated via this method is the intravascular fluid status of the patient, the response to diuretic use and intravenous hydration. Regardless, the diagnosis and treatment of pulmonary edema can be done without invasive monitoring, though in complex cases this technique may further inform etiology, particularly with pulmonary capillary wedge pressure measurements (risk for adverse outcomes increases with pressures above 18–20 mmHg).[22] The goal of treatment for pulmonary edema, regardless of etiology (cardiac dysfunction, preeclampsia, iatrogenic, etc.) is to mobilize fluid from the lung parenchyma and reestablish proper oxygenation. This condition occurs in up to 0.5% of all gestations and if not properly identified and combatted, may lead to cardiovascular collapse.[22] Data are limited in the use of invasive monitoring as it correlates with clinical outcomes in such settings, therefore its implementation should be individualized to each case. Echocardiography has been evaluated as a noninvasive alternative to central access in hypertensive disorders concomitant with pregnancy. Early case series demonstrated that echocardiography was felt to be an adequate tool to guide management of such patients.[34] The correlation of echocardiographic data with that of pulmonary arterial catheter derived measurements has been evaluated as well, finding agreement between the two modalities of 79%–98% for cardiac output and estimated index, stroke volume, left ventricular filling pressure, pulmonary arterial systolic pressure, and right atrial pressure.[35] The ability to obtain proper images and measurement in pregnancy appears to be very successful, with rates ranging from 91% to 99% in cohorts across multiple trimesters and body mass indexes.[36] Of paramount importance to the management of these patients is very strict, accurate monitoring of fluid status, even if invasive monitoring is not utilized.

Cardiac failure and structural disease

Overt cardiac failure or purely cardiogenic dysfunction necessitating intervention in pregnancy and the postpartum period is rare, occurring in at most, 1 per 1000 gestations, with the greatest frequency in patients of African descent.[37] The diagnosis of peripartum cardiomyopathy may be entertained during the latter half of pregnancy and extending to 6 months after delivery, and requires new onset depressed ejection fraction of <45% (or fractional shortening of <30%) with an end-diastolic left ventricular diameter of >2.7 cm/m^2 of body surface area, no prior cardiac history, and the absence of a separate likely causative factor.[38] More common than this diagnosis are patients with known cardiac dysfunction or a history of cardiac surgery, however.[39] Regardless of etiology, these patients warrant thorough evaluation and often complex plans of care. Examination of how patients with preexistent structural cardiac disease, e.g., congenital lesions that have been repaired, adapt to pregnancy demonstrates that the physiologic responses are attenuated compared with uncomplicated parturients, with lower systolic and diastolic function overall.[40] This should be borne in mind when performing surveillance or diagnosis in such patients as their gestations progress. Additionally, such patients may require endocarditis prophylaxis if invasive monitoring is considered, specifically those with prosthetic valves, prior endocarditis, transplant recipients, those with implanted devices (shunts and conduits), and patients that have had corrective cardiac surgery of a congenital anomaly within 6 months.[41] The use of echocardiography to evaluate parameters that may otherwise be obtained through invasive monitoring, i.e., via a pulmonary artery catheter, in these patients has demonstrated success and acceptability, including utilizing ultrasound during other invasive procedures to preclude the use of fluoroscopy.[42] In those in whom the diagnosis of new-onset cardiomyopathy is made, the goal of treatment is predominantly supportive in nature, until recovery occurs or other definitive therapies can be instituted. Spontaneous resolution may take several months to a year, and patients may require bridging therapy, such as ventricular assist devices, during a prolonged convalescence or toward a cardiac transplant. Very few patients have been managed in pregnancy or the postpartum period with these devices, though successful outcomes have been reported; if indicated they should be employed.[43]

A special subset of this population is patients who have undergone heart and/or lung transplants. From an anatomical and functional stand point, these patients often do well, as healthy organs were transplanted to them. The largest concerns are related to rejection of the transplanted organs during pregnancy, though this does not appear to be increased above the baseline general population rate of rejection for thoracic transplants, and may be further attenuated by the relative immunosuppression during pregnancy.[44] Invasive monitoring should be individualized for these patients, and a history of a cardiopulmonary transplant should not, in itself, be an indication for its use.[45]

Pulmonary hypertension

Perhaps the diagnosis that most consistently bears the use of invasive cardiac monitoring in pregnancy is pulmonary hypertension. If this diagnosis is initially made during pregnancy, it is most commonly by echocardiography, though overestimation of pulmonary arterial pressure by this technique has been described in approximately one-third of patients, with similar findings in the pregnant population.[46] Furthermore, the correlation between echocardiography and definitive diagnosis by right heart catheterization (made by direct ascertainment of a mean pulmonary artery pressure >25 mmHg) has been found to be poor, ranging from 52% to 76% agreement in either initial diagnosis or serial assessments.[47] If the condition is reasonably suspected, detailed investigation should be undertaken, including right heart catheterization, as this condition carries a significant risk of maternal mortality. It has been reported to range from 10% to 50% depending on disease severity, with the worst prognosis in those with Eisenmenger syndrome (development of a right to left cardiac shunt due to excessive right ventricular hypertrophy arising from persistent exposure to elevated pulmonary artery pressure).[48] With cardiac catheterization, the accurate disease burden can be evaluated, as well as reassessment if clinical deterioration occurs. The scenario where an echocardiographic diagnosis of pulmonary hypertension is made, though clinically the patient appears well, poses a diagnostic and management challenge, therefore multidisciplinary discussion as to how to proceed, along with extensive counseling for the patient, should be undertaken. If invasive monitoring is utilized, the goal of monitoring should be to maintain intracardiac and pulmonary pressure in the range that the patient usually bears. Substantial decreases via medical interventions (untreated hypovolemia, vasodilatory medications, etc.) may precipitate cardiovascular collapse via reduced preload to an already compromised right heart. Obstetrical hemorrhage may also pose an exaggerated risk to parturients with pulmonary hypertension, as it equates to a rapid decrease in preload as well due to volume loss. Regional anesthesia use as opposed to general anesthesia is preferred, due to the vasodilatory effects of the latter, and has demonstrated successful use in many cases of pulmonary hypertension in pregnancy.[49]

Valvular lesions

Abnormalities of cardiac valves during gestation comprise a heterogeneous group of lesions and prognoses. Regurgitant valvulopathies (most commonly mitral, aortic, or tricuspid regurgitation) tend to tolerate pregnancy particularly well, and many actually improve in function during gestation, due to the relatively increased pulse rate and diminished systemic vascular resistance overall.[50] Stenotic lesions, such as mitral, aortic, or pulmonic stenosis (tricuspid stenosis is quite rare, particularly during pregnancy), present greater risks to the mother, especially as gestation progresses. This is further modulated by disease severity, which tends to remain constant anatomically over the months of gestation.

Mitral stenosis is unique among valvular lesions in that the obstruction presents the first obstacle to forward flow of oxygenated blood returning from the lungs. Due to this, excess fluid retention or administration can rapidly lead to pulmonary edema in such patients. Invasive monitoring has been utilized in these cases to evaluate the pulmonary capillary wedge pressure, and by proxy the left ventricular pressure, to assess the response to the intravascular changes associated with labor and delivery. The greatest risk appears to be in the immediate postpartum period, concomitant with the "auto-transfusion" of blood and increased systemic vascular resistance that occurs with loss of the low resistance uteroplacental vascular bed at delivery.[51] Due to this, the goal of fluid management for mitral stenosis during pregnancy, labor, delivery, and the immediate postpartum hospitalization is to limit the fluid burden, both intrinsically and iatrogenically, with strict attention to input and output. If warranted, balloon valvuloplasty may be performed during pregnancy to alleviate symptoms and theoretically decrease the incidence of pulmonary edema; it is a lower risk (1% for major complications) and preferred intervention as compared with traditional surgical valvotomy, which has been reported with a maternal mortality risk of as much as 5%, and fetal mortality of 5%–30%.[51]

Aortic stenosis, and the very similar condition of subaortic (nonvalvular) stenosis, also represent outflow obstructions, though due to the increased resistance across the reduced valve area, adequate stroke volume and pulsatile flow are required to maintain cardiac output. Cardiac output increases substantially during pregnancy, as does overall blood volume therefore, mild-to-moderate lesions tend to have uneventful courses. In cases of severe stenosis, however, forward flow from the left heart to the systemic vasculature may be compromised, particularly in the instance of substantial blood loss or peripheral vasodilation. Valvuloplasty for aortic lesions has been described during pregnancy as well, with similarly good outcomes as those for mitral stenosis, and it is the preferred method if indicated during gestation compared with open cardiac surgical intervention.[52] If a prosthetic valve is in the aortic position, those with bioprostheses tend to have a lower rate of complications overall than those with mechanical valves, and as such, this should be a part of the counseling for women of childbearing age that are candidates for valve replacement.[53] The use of anticoagulation with mechanical valves theoretically increases the risk of postpartum bleeding, though consistent evidence to demonstrate this is limited.[54] Regardless, resources should be readily available to rapidly correct any significant blood loss if it occurs.

Stenosis of the pulmonary valve is tremendously rare, both apart from as well as within pregnancy. Management should be thought of similarly to the principles governing outflow obstructions such as aortic stenosis. Intervention during pregnancy should be undertaken only when the benefits are thought to significantly outweigh the potential risks due to the limited knowledge of this condition during gestation. An important distinction to be made is the presence of absence of pulmonary hypertension in patients that present with symptoms related to a pulmonary outflow lesion, as the prognoses and management may be significantly different.

Similarly to other cardiac conditions discussed previously, regional anesthesia is the preferred, lower risk method for pain relief during labor and delivery. The goal of management is to assist the patient through the physiologic changes of pregnancy and childbirth in a similar fashion to how each individual has adapted with their unique pathology during gestation (Tables 34.4 and 34.5).[55,56]

Table 34.4 Classification of maternal risk related to cardiac valve disease according to the American College of Cardiology, American Heart Association, and European Society of Cardiology.

Low-risk conditions	High-risk conditions
• Asymptomatic, or mildly symptomatic aortic or mitral regurgitation • Mitral valve prolapse with mild or moderate regurgitation, ejection fraction >50% • Mild mitral stenosis without pulmonary hypertension • Mild-to-moderate pulmonary valve stenosis • Asymptomatic aortic stenosis with ejection fraction >50% and mean gradient <25 mmHg	• Aortic or mitral regurgitation in patients with NYHA class III or IV functional status (symptoms with minimal exertion or at rest) • Mitral stenosis in patients with NYHA class II–IV (symptoms with exertion above normal, or greater) • Ejection fraction <40% • Marfan syndrome, particularly with a dilated aortic root >4.0 cm • Mechanical valves • Severe aortic stenosis, regardless of symptoms • Severe pulmonary hypertension (pulmonary artery pressure > 75% of systemic pressure)

Source: Adapted from Pessel C and Bonanno C, *Semin Perinatol*, 38(5), 273–84, 2014.
Abbreviation: NYHA, New York Heart Association.

Table 34.5 Classification of severity for left-sided heart lesions in adults.

	Disease severity		
Parameter	**Mild**	**Moderate**	**Severe**
Mitral stenosis			
Mean gradient	<5 mmHg	5–10 mmHg	>10 mmHg
Valve area	1.2–2.0 cm^2	1–1.5 cm^2	<1 cm^2
Aortic stenosis			
Mean gradient	<25 mmHg	25–40 mmHg	>40 mmHg
Valve area	1.5–2.0 cm^2	1–1.5 cm^2	<1 cm^2

Source: Adapted from Pessel C and Bonanno C, *Semin Perinatol*, 38(5), 273–84, 2014.

Shock, trauma, and massive transfusion

Shock is the state of insufficient tissue perfusion related to inadequate supply of oxygen via the vascular system to meet the demands of the body. Five main classifications exist; hypovolemic, cardiogenic, distributive (vasodilatory, commonly related to sepsis, overdose, anaphylaxis, or neurological injury), obstructive (massive pulmonary embolism, vena cava obstruction, etc.), and dissociative (mismatched perfusion states, often related to metabolic disorders, poisoning, etc.). The most commonly encountered shock conditions in the parturient are hypovolemic and distributive related to sepsis.[57,58] Blood loss related shock may occur prior to a patient's presentation, such as with placental abruption, at the time of delivery, in the case of intraoperative blood loss, or after delivery, in postpartum hemorrhage. Regardless of etiology, careful assessment of vital signs and estimation of blood loss, even if unwitnessed by a provider, are of paramount importance. Prompt diagnosis and institution of therapy are the goal of care. Central access, with or without invasive monitoring, will allow for the rapid repletion of lost blood, coagulation factors, and platelets, if indicated. In the patient with a clear hypovolemic etiology, the utility of invasive monitoring is not readily apparent, though these patients may often require admission to an intensive care unit. It is important to understand the appropriate use of each blood product, both from an individual patient care perspective and a resource utilization one. Each unit of packed red blood cells should increase hemoglobin by 1 g/dL and hematocrit by 3%–5% (with usual goals to maintain these above 7 g/dL and 22%, respectively), and is approximately 300–400 mL. Fresh frozen plasma contains all clotting factors and approximately 500 mg of fibrinogen, in 200–300 mL of fluid. These two products are the mainstay of therapy in hypovolemic shock due to hemorrhage, and comprise the elements of published protocols for massive transfusion.[59] If concerns for ongoing coagulopathy exists, though the patient is already volume overloaded, consideration can be made to administer cryoprecipitate (a distillate of fresh frozen plasma that contains 250 mg of fibrinogen and clotting factors VIII and XIII, along with von Willebrand factor). The benefit of this product is the delivery of a substantial amount of fibrinogen in a small amount of fluid (usually 20–30 mL); it is not meant to be a more efficacious alternative or additive to fresh frozen plasma, but rather only for instances where total fluid administration is of concern. The same is true of specialized solutions of recombinant factors, such as VII and VIII. The use of these agents should be reserved for those with specifically diagnosed disorders of these factors. Additionally, uterotonic drugs should be employed as needed, with care to ensure that the patient's volume status and cardiac output provide for adequate delivery to the uterus. More recently, the use of tranexamic acid (doses of 0.5–1 g, intravenously) has shown lower rates of obstetrical bleeding related to cesarean delivery and postpartum hemorrhage.[60] Compression methods, such as intrauterine balloon tamponade and external extremity compressive devices, should be utilized as appropriate as well (Table 34.6).

Septic shock may be precipitated by any infection, with unique concerns in pregnancy due to chorioamnionitis/endometritis, pyelonephritis, and pulmonary etiologies. If an infectious etiology is suspected during pregnancy or postpartum that requires intensive care, immediate broad-spectrum antimicrobial and/or antiviral therapy should be instituted. Once a clear cause is isolated, treatment can be directed at that specific agent. While this aspect of care is ongoing, further circulatory support may be warranted. In such cases, pressor medications may be utilized. Central access is desirable for these and invasive monitoring may be employed also. "Early goal directed therapy" has become the standard of care for septic shock in intensive care units and demonstrated a significant survival benefit.[61] This protocol utilizes assessment of venous oxygen saturation (traditionally with central venous access) with the target of maintaining this value above 65%–70%, with a central venous pressure of 8–12 mmHg. Additionally, this idea has evolved into the Surviving Sepsis Campaign Guidelines, which codified a plan of care to include administration of antibiotics ideally within the first hour of admission to an intensive care unit, serial serum lactate assessments (with fluid and/or pressor resuscitation if >4 mmol/L), urine output ≥5 mL/kg/h, and maintenance of mean arterial pressure (MAP) above 65 mmHg.[62] These principles have not been studied in pregnant patients, though they should generally be applied to this population, given the likely benefits.[63,64] While a pulmonary arterial catheter is not routinely part of such therapies, in cases of severe pulmonary infections with persistent edema, they may be desired on an individualized basis (Table 34.7).

Trauma is a relatively common occurrence in pregnancy, with up to 8% of women experiencing some form during gestation.[65] Fortunately, the vast majority of these are minor and do not result in harm to the mother or fetus.[65] In cases of significant trauma patients should be seen in a referral center and undergo a routine trauma assessment. Concomitant with this should be evaluation by the obstetrics team, as both the mother and fetus are at risk from the same potential injury. Specific injuries, such as penetrating trauma from knives or projectiles, should be treated in the usual manner, in consultation with a high-risk pregnancy specialist as well. Blunt trauma may bear a risk of up to 40% of placental abruption, depending on the severity of the incident, and warrants prolonged surveillance via electronic fetal monitoring.[66] If reassuring monitoring is present for 4 hours after the trauma, the risk of abruption is <1%.[65] Ultrasonography is often employed in such settings as well, though the ability of it to detect an abruption, even when its presence is confirmed at delivery, is poor, ranging from 25% to 50% at best.[67] Additionally, the utility of testing for fetomaternal hemorrhage remains of unproven benefit.[68] Invasive monitoring generally does not have a role in care due to trauma alone, though the potentially coexistent conditions of blood loss hypovolemia, neurological injury mediated shock, or sepsis, may lead to consideration of its use. Any trauma during pregnancy should prompt a discussion of the possibility of partner violence, as this presents an unfortunately common and dangerous ongoing situation for women.

RISKS OF INVASIVE MONITORING USE

As with any procedure the potential benefits and risks associated with it must be assessed and discussed amongst the care team and patient. Central catheter access and invasive monitoring techniques also bear unique complications. Major complications occur in up to 5% of pulmonary artery catheter placements, largely comprised of pneumothorax, venous embolism, arrhythmias requiring medical treatment, infection, and significant bleeding.[33] Central catheters have similar concerns, except a lower incidence for generation of arrhythmias as their placement does not traverse the cardiac chambers with proper technique. Data in pregnant patients are much more limited

Table 34.6 Classification of hypovolemic shock due to blood loss.

Parameter	Class I	Class II	Class III	Class IV
Blood loss (mL)	Up to 750	750–1500	1500–2000	>2000
Blood loss (% of total volume)	Up to 15	15–30	30–40	>40
Pulse (per minute)	<100	>100	>120	>140
Blood pressure	Normal	Normal	Decreased	Decreased
Pulse pressure	Normal or increased	Decreased	Decreased	Decreased
Respiratory rate (per minute)	14–20	20–30	30–40	>40
Urine output (mL/h)	>30	20–30	5–15	Minimal
Recommended fluid replacement	Crystalloid	Crystalloid	Crystalloid and blood products	Crystalloid and blood products

Source: Adapted from *Goldman's Cecil Medicine*, 24th edition, Goldman L and Schafer AI (eds.), Rivers EP, Approach to the Patient with Shock, pp. 645–53, Copyright 2012, with permission from Elsevier.

Table 34.7 Vasopressor medications.

Medication	Dose range	Vascular effects	Cardiac effects	Typical use
Phenylephrine	20–200 μg/min	Moderate to significant vasoconstriction	No effect on rate and contractility	General pressor support, supraventricular arrhythmias
Norepinephrine	1–20 μg/min	Moderate to significant vasoconstriction	Moderately increased rate and contractility	Septic shock (first line agent)
Epinephrine	1–20 μg/min	Moderate to significant vasoconstriction	Significantly increased rate and contractility	Refractory shock, anaphylaxis, bradycardia
Vasopressin	0.04–0.1 units/min	Moderate to significant vasoconstriction	No effect on rate and contractility	Septic shock, postcardiac surgery
Dopamine	1–20 μg/kg/min	Vasodilation at low doses, mild-to-moderate vasoconstriction at higher doses	Mild-to-moderate increase in rate and contractility	General pressor support, renal perfusion
Dobutamine	1–20 μg/kg/min	Mild vasodilation	Mild to significant increase in rate and contractility	Septic and cardiogenic shock
Milrinone	37.5–75 μg/kg bolus; 0.375–0.75 μg/min	Mild vasodilation	Mild increase in rate, moderate to significant increase in contractility	Cardiogenic shock, use caution with renal insufficiency

Source: Adapted from *Goldman's Cecil Medicine*, 24th edition, Goldman L and Schafer AI (eds.), Rivers EP, Approach to the Patient with Shock, pp. 645–53, Copyright 2012, with permission from Elsevier.

than in the general intensive care population though similar rates of complications have been found. Case series and cohort studies have demonstrated adverse events to occur in as much as 50% of pregnant or postpartum patients, with substantial risks of infection or cellulitis, both of which necessitate line removal and may precipitate severe illness in the patient.[69,70] The decision to use invasive monitoring or not should be made in a collaborative manner with all care teams as well as the patient (including family if desired) and tailored to the specific clinical scenario.

EMERGING MONITORING MODALITIES

Given that invasive cardiac monitoring use has declined overall in the past decade, largely due to the previously discussed findings, it has also likely decreased in the pregnant and postpartum population. This trend will probably continue in the foreseeable future, as the benefit of obtaining similar information without the need to place a central catheter is desirable. Within this current clinical environment newer monitoring devices to assess cardiac function in a noninvasive manner have begun to gain wider implementation. Bioimpedence refers to assessment of electrical currents generated by the heart as a function of the cardiac cycle and fluid content of the body. It has been studied in pregnant women against echocardiographic measures and found to have good agreement between the two methods for cardiac output, stoke volume, and systemic vascular resistance.[71] A related technique, bioreactance, uses a device generating mild electrical current through the patient's thorax which is then used to calculate various parameters based on frequency and phase changes in that current. An investigation of this device's utility in pregnant women with and without preeclampsia compared with nonpregnant women demonstrated the ability to obtain cardiac output, stroke volume, systemic vascular resistance, and other measurements in these patients. Additionally, findings were in correlate with the expectations that preeclamptic women would have higher mean arterial pressures as well as systemic resistances.[72] Minimally invasive monitoring devices have become available as well, including a modality that uses peripherally inserted arterial access to derive similar measures as the preceding methods, such as the central venous pressure and cardiac index. An observational study of women undergoing cesarean delivery demonstrated that this device was able to obtain reasonable measurements of these parameters.[73] It should be borne in mind that the studies of these monitoring techniques in pregnant women are few, with small sample sizes. In larger comparative investigations in the general population, these modalities have demonstrated relatively good agreement with invasive monitoring derived values, particularly for bioimpedence and bioreactance devices, though the peripheral arterial access device appears to have significant discrepancies in cases of low systemic vascular resistance, e.g., shock.[74,75] Further studies are needed in both the pregnant and general populations to determine how these devices may impact clinical outcomes.[75]

COMMUNICATION WITH OTHER CARE TEAMS

Of paramount importance in the care of all patients, though especially critically ill ones, is open, thorough, and collegial communication. Due to the demands placed on clinicians and the health care system currently, this can sometimes be challenging, and perhaps it is even more so for teams caring for a patient with an unfamiliar condition. Obstetricians and high-risk pregnancy specialists have some experience with critically ill parturients, though it is not a common occurrence. Intensivists, cardiologists, pulmonologists, anesthesiologists, and other critical care specialists have knowledge and expertise in such settings, though the unique aspects of the pregnant or postpartum patient's physiology and potential pathologies are not routinely part of their practice. It is for these reasons that the woman requiring intensive care related to her gestation must be approached from a multidisciplinary viewpoint. There exists a wealth of literature to demonstrate improved outcomes, less need for interventions, greater patient and family satisfaction, and improved care team functioning with the use of protocols to promote greater and more clear, consistent communication in critical care.[76–79] This mentality should be applied to the seriously ill parturient as well. The Obstetrics team should personally apprise the critical care providers about the patient upon admission to the intensive care unit, as well as have at least one member present and participative in the daily rounds discussion for the patient along with the intensivist team. In this way any questions or concerns outside of the usual scope of either team can be addressed in a timely manner and all appropriate care instituted. The American College of Obstetricians and Gynecologists, along with the Society for Maternal-Fetal Medicine, has recently put forth recommendations for levels of maternal care. The highest level calls for well-implemented collaboration between the Obstetrics and critical care teams, as well as the presence of a high-risk pregnancy specialist with expertise in critical care.[80] Currently, there are few such providers, though a greater interest in the management of complex maternal conditions has prompted more trainees to gain this expertise, and as pregnant patients continue to experience the need for intensive treatment, these individuals will lead in such care.

REFERENCES

1. Angeli F, Angeli E, Verdecchia P. Electrocardiographic changes in hypertensive disorders of pregnancy. *Hypertens Res* 2014; 37(11): 973–5.
2. Carlin A, Alfirevic Z. Physiological changes of pregnancy and monitoring. *Best Pract Res Clin Obstet Gynaecol* 2008; 22(5): 801–23.
3. Wenger NK, Hurst JW, Strozier VN. Electrocardiographic changes in pregnancy. *Am J Cardiol* 1964; 13: 774–8.
4. Veille JC, Kitzman DW, Bacevice AE. Effects of pregnancy on the electrocardiogram in healthy subjects during strenuous exercise. *Am J Obstet Gynecol* 1996; 175(5): 1360–4.
5. Köşüş A, Köşüş N, Açikgöz N et al. Maternal arrhythmias detected with electrocardiography during labour: Are they significant clinically? *J Obstet Gynaecol* 2011; 31(5): 396–9.
6. Cruz MO, Hibbard JU, Alexander T, Briller J. Ambulatory arrhythmia monitoring in pregnant patients with palpitations. *Am J Perinatol* 2013; 30(1): 53–8.
7. Knotts RJ, Garan H. Cardiac arrhythmias in pregnancy. *Semin Perinatol* 2014; 38(5): 285–8.
8. ACOG Committee on Obstetric Practice. ACOG Committee Opinion Number 299, September 2004. Guidelines for diagnostic imaging during pregnancy. *Obstet Gynecol* 2004; 104(3): 647–51.
9. Rajaraman P, Simpson J, Neta G et al. Early life exposure to diagnostic radiation and ultrasound scans and risk of childhood cancer: Case-control study. *BMJ* 2011; 342: d472.
10. Shakerian R, Thomson BN, Judson R, Skandarajah AR. Radiation fear: Impact on compliance with trauma imaging guidelines in the pregnant patient. *J Trauma Acute Care Surg* 2015; 78(1): 88–93.
11. Ain DL, Narula J, Sengupta PP. Cardiovascular imaging and diagnostic procedures in pregnancy. *Cardiol Clin* 2012; 30(3): 331–41.
12. Litmanovich DE, Tack D, Lee KS, Shahrzad M, Bankier AA. Cardiothoracic imaging in the pregnant patient. *J Thorac Imaging* 2014; 29(1): 38–49.
13. Keser N. Echocardiography in pregnant women. *Anadolu Kardiyol Derg* 2006; 6(2): 169–73.
14. Vogt M, Müller J, Kühn A et al. Cardiac adaptation of the maternal heart during pregnancy: A color-coded tissue Doppler imaging study—Feasibility, reproducibility and course during pregnancy. *Ultraschall Med* 2015; 36(3): 270–5.
15. Rizwana S, Nandita M. Echocardiographic assessment of cardiovascular hemodynamic in preeclampsia. *J Obstet Gynaecol India* 2011; 61(5): 519–22.
16. Neuman G, Koren G. Safety of procedural sedation in pregnancy. *J Obstet Gynaecol Can* 2013; 35(2): 168–73.
17. Scheer B, Perel A, Pfeiffer UJ. Clinical review: Complications and risk factors of peripheral arterial catheters used for haemodynamic monitoring in anaesthesia and intensive care medicine. *Crit Care* 2002; 6(3): 199–204.
18. Clark SL, Cotton DB, Lee W et al. Central hemodynamic assessment of normal term pregnancy. *Am J Obstet Gynecol* 1989; 161(6 Pt 1): 1439–42.
19. Hartog C, Bloos F. Venous oxygen saturation. *Best Pract Res Clin Anaesthesiol* 2014; 28(4): 419–28.
20. Connors AF, Speroff T, Dawson NV et al. The effectiveness of right heart catheterization in the initial care of critically ill patients. *JAMA* 1996; 276: 889–97.
21. Gilbert WM, Towner DR, Field NT, Anthony J. The safety and utility of pulmonary artery catheterization in severe preeclampsia and eclampsia. *Am J Obstet Gynecol* 2000; 182(6): 1397–403.
22. Dennis AT, Solnordal CB. Acute pulmonary oedema in pregnant women. *Anaesthesia* 2012; 67(6): 646–59.
23. Rajaram SS, Desai NK, Kalra A et al. Pulmonary artery catheters for adult patients in intensive care. *Cochrane Database Syst Rev* 2013; (2): CD003408.

24. Busse L, Davison DL, Junker C, Chawla LS. Hemodynamic monitoring in the critical care environment. *Adv Chronic Kidney Dis* 2013; 20(1): 21–9.
25. Ruys TP, Cornette J, Roos-Hesselink JW. Pregnancy and delivery in cardiac disease. *J Cardiol* 2013; 61(2): 107–12.
26. Colletti PM, Lee KH, Elkayam U. Cardiovascular imaging of the pregnant patient. *AJR Am J Roentgenol* 2013; 200(3): 515–21.
27. Chandrasekhar S, Cook CR, Collard CD. Cardiac surgery in the parturient. *Anesth Analg* 2009; 108: 777–85.
28. Barth WH Jr. Cardiac surgery in pregnancy. *Clin Obstet Gynecol* 2009; 52(4): 630–46.
29. Waksmonski CA. Cardiac imaging and functional assessment in pregnancy. *Semin Perinatol* 2014; 38(5): 240–4.
30. Bural GG, Laymon CM, Mountz JM. Nuclear imaging of a pregnant patient: Should we perform nuclear medicine procedures during pregnancy? *Mol Imaging Radionucl Ther* 2012; 21(1): 1–5.
31. Moussa HN, Arian SE, Sibai BM. Management of hypertensive disorders in pregnancy. *Womens Health (Lond Engl)* 2014; 10(4): 385–404.
32. Callaghan WM, Creanga AA, Kuklina EV. Severe maternal morbidity among delivery and postpartum hospitalizations in the United States. *Obstet Gynecol* 2012; 120(5): 1029–36.
33. Young P, Johanson R. Haemodynamic, invasive and echocardiographic monitoring in the hypertensive parturient. *Best Pract Res Clin Obstet Gynaecol* 2001; 15(4): 605–22.
34. Belfort MA, Mares A, Saade G et al. Two-dimensional echocardiography and Doppler ultrasound in managing obstetric patients. *Obstet Gynecol* 1997; 90(3): 326–30.
35. Belfort MA, Rokey R, Saade GR, Moise KJ Jr. Rapid echocardiographic assessment of left and right heart hemodynamics in critically ill obstetric patients. *Am J Obstet Gynecol* 1994; 171(4): 884–92.
36. Dennis AT. Transthoracic echocardiography in obstetric anaesthesia and obstetric critical illness. *Int J Obstet Anesth* 2011; 20(2): 160–8.
37. Tibazarwa K, Lee G, Mayosi B et al. The 12-lead ECG in peripartum cardiomyopathy. *Cardiovasc J Afr* 2012; 23(6): 322–9.
38. Rutherford JD. Heart failure in pregnancy. *Curr Heart Fail Rep* 2012; 9(4): 277–81.
39. Ray P, Murphy GJ, Shutt LE. Recognition and management of maternal cardiac disease in pregnancy. *Br J Anaesth* 2004; 93(3): 428–39.
40. Cornette J, Ruys TP, Rossi A et al. Hemodynamic adaptation to pregnancy in women with structural heart disease. *Int J Cardiol* 2013; 168(2): 825–31.
41. Thanavaro KL, Nixon JV. Endocarditis 2014: An update. *Heart Lung* 2014; 43(4): 334–7.
42. Vitarelli A, Capotosto L. Role of echocardiography in the assessment and management of adult congenital heart disease in pregnancy. *Int J Cardiovasc Imaging* 2011; 27(6): 843–57.
43. LaRue S, Shanks A, Wang IW et al. Left ventricular assist device in pregnancy. *Obstet Gynecol* 2011; 118(2 Pt 2): 426–8.
44. Vos R, Ruttens D2, Verleden SE2 et al. Pregnancy after heart and lung transplantation. *Best Pract Res Clin Obstet Gynaecol* 2014; 28(8): 1146–62.
45. Wu DW, Wilt J, Restaino S. Pregnancy after thoracic organ transplantation. *Semin Perinatol* 2007; 31(6): 354–62.
46. Rich JD, Shah SJ, Swamy RS et al. Inaccuracy of Doppler echocardiographic estimates of pulmonary artery pressures in patients with pulmonary hypertension: Implications for clinical practice. *Chest* 2011; 139(5): 988–93.
47. Farber HW, Foreman AJ, Miller DP, McGoon MD. REVEAL Registry: Correlation of right heart catheterization and echocardiography in patients with pulmonary arterial hypertension. *Congest Heart Fail* 2011; 17(2): 56–64.
48. Connolly HM. Pregnancy in women with congenital heart disease. *Curr Cardiol Rep* 2005; 7(4): 305–9.
49. Maxwell BG, El-Sayed YY,Riley ET, Carvalho B. Peripartum outcomes and anaesthetic management of parturients with moderate to complex congenital heart disease or pulmonary hypertension. *Anaesthesia* 2013; 68(1): 52–9.
50. Pessel C, Bonanno C. Valve disease in pregnancy. *Semin Perinatol* 2014; 38(5): 273–84.
51. Nelson-Piercy C, Chakravarti S. Cardiac disease and pregnancy. *Anaesth Intens Care Med* 2007; 8: 312–6.
52. Traill TA. Valvular heart disease and pregnancy. *Cardiol Clin* 2012; 30(3): 369–81.
53. Heuvelman HJ, Arabkhani B, Cornette JM et al. Pregnancy outcomes in women with aortic valve substitutes. *Am J Cardiol* 2013; 111(3): 382–7.
54. Stout KK, Otto CM. Pregnancy in women with valvular heart disease. *Heart* 2007; 93(5): 552–8.
55. Ioscovich AM, Goldszmidt E, Fadeev AV et al. Peripartum anesthetic management of patients with aortic valve stenosis: A retrospective study and literature review. *Int J Obstet Anesth* 2009; 18(4): 379–86.
56. Sachs A, Aaronson J, Smiley R. The role of the anesthesiologist in the care of the parturient with cardiac disease. *Semin Perinatol* 2014; 38(5): 252–9.
57. Cohen WR. Hemorrhagic shock in obstetrics. *J Perinat Med* 2006; 34(4): 263–71.
58. Martin SR, Foley MR. Intensive care in obstetrics: An evidence-based review. *Am J Obstet Gynecol* 2006; 195(3): 673–89.
59. Pacheco LD, Saade GR, Costantine MM, Clark SL, Hankins GD. The role of massive transfusion protocols in obstetrics. *Am J Perinatol* 2013; 30(1): 1–4.
60. Sentilhes L, Lasocki S, Ducloy-Bouthors AS et al. Tranexamic acid for the prevention and treatment of postpartum haemorrhage. *Br J Anaesth* 2015; 114(4): 576–87.

61. Chelkeba L, Ahmadi A, Abdollahi M, Najafi A, Mojtahedzadeh M. Early goal-directed therapy reduces mortality in adult patients with severe sepsis and septic shock: Systematic review and meta-analysis. *Indian J Crit Care Med* 2015; 19(7): 401–11.
62. Dellinger RP, Levy MM, Rhodes A et al. Surviving Sepsis Campaign Guidelines Committee including the Pediatric Subgroup. Surviving sepsis campaign: International guidelines for management of severe sepsis and septic shock: 2012. *Crit Care Med* 2013; 41(2): 580–637.
63. Pacheco LD, Saade GR, Hankins GD. Severe sepsis during pregnancy. *Clin Obstet Gynecol* 2014; 57: 827–834.
64. Price LC, Slack A, Nelson-Piercy C. Aims of obstetric critical care management. *Best Pract Res Clin Obstet Gynaecol* 2008; 22(5): 775–99.
65. Warner MW, Salfinger SG, Rao S, Magann EF, Hall JC. Management of trauma during pregnancy. *ANZ J Surg* 2004; 74(3): 125–8.
66. Williams J, Mozurkewich E, Chilimigras J, Van De Ven C. Critical care in obstetrics: Pregnancy-specific conditions. *Best Pract Res Clin Obstet Gynaecol* 2008; 22(5): 825–46.
67. Mirza FG, Devine PC, Gaddipati S. Trauma in pregnancy: A systematic approach. *Am J Perinatol* 2010; 27(7): 579–86.
68. Murphy NJ, Quinlan JD. Trauma in pregnancy: Assessment, management, and prevention. *Am Fam Physician* 2014; 90(10): 717–722.
69. Ogura JM, Francois KE, Perlow JH, Elliott JP. Complications associated with peripherally inserted central catheter use during pregnancy. *Am J Obstet Gynecol* 2003; 188(5): 1223–5.
70. Nuthalapaty FS, Beck MM, Mabie WC. Complications of central venous catheters during pregnancy and postpartum: A case series. *Am J Obstet Gynecol* 2009; 201(3): 311.e1–5.
71. Burlingame J, Ohana P, Aaronoff M, Seto T. Noninvasive cardiac monitoring in pregnancy: Impedance cardiography versus echocardiography. *J Perinatol* 2013; 33(9): 675–80.
72. Ohashi Y, Ibrahim H, Furtado L et al. Non-invasive hemodynamic assessment of non-pregnant, healthy pregnant and preeclamptic women using bioreactance. *Rev Bras Anestesiol* 2010; 60(6): 335–40, 603–13.
73. Auler JO Jr, Torres ML, Cardoso MM et al. Clinical evaluation of the flotrac/Vigileo system for continuous cardiac output monitoring in patients undergoing regional anesthesia for elective cesarean section: A pilot study. *Clinics (Sao Paulo)* 2010; 65(8): 793–8.
74. Marik PE. Noninvasive cardiac output monitors: A state-of the-art review. *J Cardiothorac Vasc Anesth* 2013; 27(1): 121–34.
75. Armstrong S, Fernando R, Columb M. Minimally- and non-invasive assessment of maternal cardiac output: Go with the flow! *Int J Obstet Anesth* 2011; 20(4): 330–40.
76. Vergales J, Addison N, Vendittelli A et al. Face-to-face handoff: Improving transfer to the pediatric intensive care unit after cardiac surgery. *Am J Med Qual* 2015; 30: 119–25.
77. Lane D, Ferri M, Lemaire J, McLaughlin K, Stelfox HT. A systematic review of evidence-informed practices for patient care rounds in the ICU. *Crit Care Med* 2013; 41(8): 2015–29.
78. Segall N, Bonifacio AS, Schroeder RA et al. Durham VA Patient Safety Center of Inquiry. Can we make postoperative patient handovers safer? A systematic review of the literature. *Anesth Analg* 2012; 115(1): 102–15.
79. Scheunemann LP, McDevitt M, Carson SS, Hanson LC. Randomized, controlled trials of interventions to improve communication in intensive care: A systematic review. *Chest* 2011; 139(3): 543–54.
80. American College of Obstetricians and Gynecologists and Society for Maternal–Fetal Medicine, Menard MK, Kilpatrick S et al. Levels of maternal care. *Am J Obstet Gynecol* 2015; 212(3): 259–71.

Trauma in pregnancy

35

RAVI CHOKSHI, RUOFAN YAO, and LAUREN A. PLANTE

CONTENTS

INTRODUCTION

Few emergencies are as complex and anxiety inducing as a major trauma case involving a pregnant woman, where the safety and well-being of both the gravid woman and her developing fetus must be assessed and safeguarded simultaneously. Alterations in both anatomy and physiology during pregnancy must be kept in mind even in the chaos of the trauma room. Input will be required from emergency medicine, surgery, and obstetrics, with involvement as needed from other specialties such as anesthesiology, radiology, pediatrics, and critical care medicine.

EPIDEMIOLOGY

In the United States, up to 8% of women will experience a traumatic injury during pregnancy,[1] though figures are not well sourced or supported. Fortunately, the great majority of these injuries are minor. However, trauma remains a leading cause of nonpregnancy-related maternal death, accounting for more than 25% of maternal deaths reported to the (voluntary) Pregnancy Mortality Surveillance System.[2] The maternal mortality rate from trauma during pregnancy was 1.4% in the U.S. National Trauma Data Bank[3] and 5.1% in a national registry from the United Kingdom[4]; U.K. figures, however, show a much lower incidence of trauma during pregnancy than American data. Pregnancy does not make injury more lethal: In fact, in the National Trauma Data Bank, pregnant women had a 40% lower risk of death than age-matched nonpregnant women who sustained trauma,[5] though mortality rates in the U.K. were much the same between pregnant and nonpregnant women after trauma.[4]

Trauma may be blunt or penetrating. About 90% of abdominal trauma during pregnancy is due to blunt injury,[6] the major contributors being motor vehicle accidents (MVA), assault, and fall. Penetrating trauma is more dangerous to both mothers and fetuses: Maternal mortality rates in a large case series were 2% for blunt versus 7% for penetrating abdominal trauma, while fetal mortality was 10% versus 73%.[6] Because MVA contribute so greatly to trauma incidence in the U.S., attention has been paid to ways to reduce mortality, specifically with use of restraints and airbags. The National Automotive Sampling System/Crashworthiness Data System (NASS/CDS) database reports there are approximately 160,000 MVAs annually which involve pregnant women, resulting in an estimated 160 maternal deaths and an additional 600–2600 fetal losses[7] even when the mother survives. The NASS/CDS database showed that nearly 25% of pregnant crash victims were unrestrained. The degree of severity is shown by the fact that airbags deployed only 33% of the time, and 99% of injuries were deemed minor.[7]

Interpersonal violence accounts for 10%–12% of blunt trauma cases from U.S. case series.[3,6,8] Of these, a disturbing 43% are related to domestic violence (DV) (Aboutanos et al. 2007), also known as intimate partner violence (IPV). The incidence of DV is almost certainly underreported. Assault during pregnancy triples the risk of preterm labor and of stillbirth, quadruples the risk of abruption, and increases nearly fourfold the risk of maternal death.[9] In a series from a metropolitan trauma center in South Africa, more than half of pregnant women admitted after trauma had been subjected to deliberate assault.[10]

Falls contributed 14% of trauma admissions in a large database series from California[8] and 48% in a single-center case series limited to minor trauma.[11] A cross-sectional study of pregnant women in Nigeria found that 32% reported having fallen during pregnancy, with the highest number of falls occurring in the third trimester[12]; not all were taken to hospital. A linked data set from Washington State calculated 49 fall hospitalizations per 100,000 deliveries, of whom 79% were in the third trimester; most suffered no more than minor injuries[13] but the rate of adverse pregnancy outcomes nevertheless was increased. Postural stability worsens during pregnancy, and objective measures of fall risk are highest in the third trimester.[14]

Other causes of trauma include thermal injury. No reliable estimates of burn injury during pregnancy have been generated for North America, though El Kady, dividing number of burn admissions by total number of deliveries in California during the time period studied, calculated 0.06 burn admissions per 1000 deliveries.[8] Case series from the developing world (India, Iran), where burns are much more common, probably have limited applicability here, but do link the probability of maternal survival to the total body surface area burned.[15,16] Fetal survival depends on maternal survival and gestational age achieved.

Among pregnant women admitted to California hospitals following trauma, fractures, dislocation, or sprains were the most common injuries, affecting 36%; 6% sustained intracranial injuries, 6% internal injuries (chest, abdomen, pelvis), 2% nerve and spinal cord injuries, and 2% were admitted with burns.[8] Women who delivered during the admission for trauma had worse outcomes than a control group without injury: Odds ratios of 42 for uterine rupture, 9.2 for abruption, 7.8 for cesarean hysterectomy, and 69.5 for maternal death were reported. Women who had been hospitalized for injury but discharged undelivered had better outcomes than those delivered during the trauma hospitalization, but still worse than the control group who had had no trauma. Fetal outcomes were also worse among the group delivered during trauma hospitalization, if less dramatic: Odds ratio was 4.7 for fetal death, 3.1 neonatal death, and 2.1 for preterm delivery.[8] It is obvious, however, that severity of injury was related to the probability that delivery would occur during the admission for trauma, while women with less severe injuries could be discharged home undelivered.

ASSESSMENT AND MANAGEMENT OF THE ACUTELY INJURED GRAVIDA

Trauma survey

"The best initial treatment for the fetus is the provision of optimal resuscitation of the mother"—*ATLS*, 9th edition.[17]

The primary survey remains the foundation of trauma triage, regardless of pregnancy. Abiding by Advanced Trauma Life Support (ATLS®) guidelines for assessment and management of the injured patient has been shown to improve patient outcomes[17] and this remains true in the obstetric patient. As a rule, maternal resuscitation and stabilization directly improve fetal outcomes.

The primary survey in the obstetric patient closely follows nonpregnant guidelines with a few caveats we will discuss below.

PREHOSPITAL PHASE

Assuming the pregnancy is known to the patient herself, awareness and reporting of pregnancy by the prehospital triage team allows for mobilization of the obstetric team so they can be present and ready for arrival of the patient in the trauma bay. Knowledge of the approximate gestational age will also allow for fetal assessment as indicated during the secondary survey. Field triage recommendations from the Centers for Disease Control (CDC) cite pregnancy (>20 weeks) as a reason for EMS to contact medical control and transport to a trauma center or to a hospital with specific resources, i.e., obstetrical services.[18] Hospitals may also use the presence of pregnancy as a criterion for trauma team activation and hospital admission,[19] though others decry the practice[20] as it represents overtriage: Pregnant patients are no more likely to have major injury, and routine trauma team activation in these cases is probably not cost effective.

PRIMARY SURVEY

The underlying principles behind ATLS[17] remain valid in the obstetric patient.

- **Treat the greatest threat to life first.**
  - **That is, in order of danger: Loss of airway is more emergent than loss of ability to breathe, which is more important than loss of blood volume, which is much more important than fetal "distress."**
- **Lack of definitive diagnosis should not delay indicated treatment.**
  - **Presence of a fetus should not distract the trauma team from initiating life-saving maneuvers.**
- **Detailed history is not essential to evaluation of a patient with acute life-threatening injuries.**
  - **Obstetric history and assessment can follow during the secondary survey, after initial resuscitation has been conducted. Obstetric history taking should not trump the primary survey.**

The primary survey is generally performed by the emergency medicine or trauma team. The mnemonic ABCDE as prescribed by ATLS should be followed for the primary survey.

A—Airway (with cervical spine protection)
B—Breathing
C—Circulation: Identify and stop bleeding
D—Disability or neurologic status
E—Exposure (undress the patient) and Environment (prevent hypothermia)

Only after these have been addressed is attention turned to F—fetus.

Any woman of childbearing age should be assessed for pregnancy via clinical history, physical examination, urine, or serum testing. This evaluation can be performed concurrently with the primary survey, as long as it does not interfere, or await the secondary survey if pregnancy is not initially evident. Determination of gestational age is important during the secondary survey, as it may influence the nature of interventions required.

AIRWAY AND BREATHING

Pregnant patients exhibit an increase in oxygen consumption, an increase in tidal volume, and a decrease in functional residual capacity (FRC). Patients in the second trimester and beyond are usually hypocapnic ($PaCO_2 = 30$ mmHg) and therefore a "normal" $PaCO_2$ of 35–40 may be falsely reassuring as it may in fact reflect impending respiratory failure.[17] Early ventilatory support, including intubation if needed, is prudent to ensure adequate oxygenation.

Pregnancy increases risk for airway complications because of weight gain, airway mucosal edema, and delayed gastric emptying. Failed intubation is four to eight times more likely in the obstetric patient than the general population,[19,21] and even in current practice[22] a rate of 1:224 is seen. Failed intubation in a pregnant patient is associated with more extreme hypoxemia because of alterations in oxygen demand, minute ventilation, and FRC: In a case–control study of obstetric anesthesia cases, oxygen saturations as low as 40% were reached.[22] Availability of experienced anesthesia staff is vital to the safety of the obstetric patient.

Given the possibility of a full stomach in every trauma patient, definitive airway management often includes rapid sequence intubation (RSI) with cricoid pressure. This involves an agent for induction of anesthesia and another for muscle relaxation. Propofol and ketamine are commonly utilized in trauma cases; like all induction agents, they cross the placenta and therefore will depress fetal neurobehavior. If delivery occurs soon afterward, there is no opportunity for maternal metabolization and excretion, so neonatal depression may ensue and the pediatrician should be prepared to address it. Muscle relaxants, both depolarizing and nondepolarizing agents, *do not* cross the placenta.

Because of the higher minute ventilation and decreased FRC common to pregnancy, there is more potential for desaturation: The threshold for giving supplemental oxygen should be low even if definitive airway management is not required.

Given the elevation of the diaphragm with the enlarged uterus, if a thoracostomy tube is required, it should be placed one to two intercostal spaces higher than the usually accessed fifth intercostal space to avoid intra-abdominal injury.[1,23]

CIRCULATION

Pregnant patients exhibit the physiologic differences seen in Table 35.1.

Given the increased plasma volume and cardiac output, a pregnant patient can hemorrhage 1200–1500 mL of blood before exhibiting signs and symptoms of hypovolemia. However, the resulting catecholamine release and vasoconstriction may reduce placental perfusion and produce fetal distress prior to signs of maternal distress. The therapy remains maternal stabilization, as pregnant patients do respond appropriately to volume resuscitation. It should be mentioned that a pregnant patient is expected to have a slightly elevated resting heart rate and relative hypotension, both signs that may falsely raise concern for hemorrhage. A good clinical sense and experience treating obstetric patients will come useful.

Transfusion of blood products is indicated as needed to maintain maternal physiologic needs. If cross-matched blood is not available or there is not enough time for cross-matching, O-negative blood should be transfused to avoid Rh sensitization in Rh-negative women. Maternal hematocrit does not correspond in any way with fetal hematocrit.

It is important to bear in mind the influence of the gravid uterus in compressing the inferior vena cava when a patient is in the supine position. The decrease in venous return and preload can lead to a 30% reduction in cardiac output and possibly dampen resuscitative efforts. Every effort should be made to either place the patient in a left lateral position or manually displace the uterus to the left side to relieve compression of the inferior vena cava (IVC). The venous congestion caused by uterine compression may also impede medication delivery via intravenous access below the diaphragm: Femoral access should be avoided. If the pneumatic antishock garment (PASG, also known as military or medical antishock trousers, MAST) is used, the abdominal section should not be inflated because of concern it may interfere with placental perfusion,[23] but this is a largely obsolete technology.

DISABILITY

Altered sensorium in the pregnant patient mandates including eclampsia and the posteclamptic (post-ictal) state in the differential. Evidence of hypertension,

Table 35.1 Physiologic differences in pregnant patients.

Increased plasma volume	**Up to 45%**
Increased cardiac output	By 1–1.5 L/min ; 20% of cardiac output distributed to uterus and placenta in 3rd trimester
Decreased hematocrit	31%–35%
Elevated resting heart rate	By 10–15 beats/min
Decreased systolic and diastolic blood pressure	By 5–15 mmHg

hyperreflexia and proteinuria further support eclampsia, but in the setting of hemorrhage from trauma, hypertension may be absent.

Active seizures in a pregnant patient, absent head trauma, can be presumed to be eclampsia and managed by intravenous magnesium sulfate (6 g bolus + 2 g/hour) while obstetrical or neurological consultation is requested.

EXPOSURE

Evaluation should include a pelvic examination for vaginal bleeding as a source of hemorrhage. However, if vaginal bleeding is identified, digital examination should be deferred until placenta previa is excluded.

SECONDARY SURVEY

After completion of the primary survey, the establishment of resuscitative efforts as needed, and restoration of normal vital signs, the obstetrician has a role in the secondary survey:

- Assessment of gestational age and viability
- Evaluate specific obstetric emergencies such as uterine rupture or placental abruption
- Check cervical dilation and rupture of membranes (screen for preterm labor)
- Begin the process of fetal assessment

This is the time to obtain a history, whether from the patient herself or from family members or other sources. This is also the time to obtain needed imaging studies (Figure 35.1).

Blunt injury accounts for the majority of trauma in pregnancy (see section "Epidemiology"). The mechanism of injury may be useful in directing evaluation toward commonly associated injury patterns: For example, thoracic injury after head-on motor vehicle collision, head injury or aortic trauma after auto-versus-pedestrian accidents, etc.[17] The presence of a space-occupying gravid uterus affects these patterns.

In the first trimester, the uterus remains in the bony pelvis, making direct fetal injury rare (<1%). In later gestation, while the fetus remains somewhat protected by the presence of multiple layers (amniotic fluid, uterine myometrium, and the maternal abdominal wall) the risk of direct fetal injury from blunt trauma does increase. The same layers serve to shield maternal viscera. At any gestational age, the trajectory of ballistic wounding (bullets, shrapnel) is unpredictable.

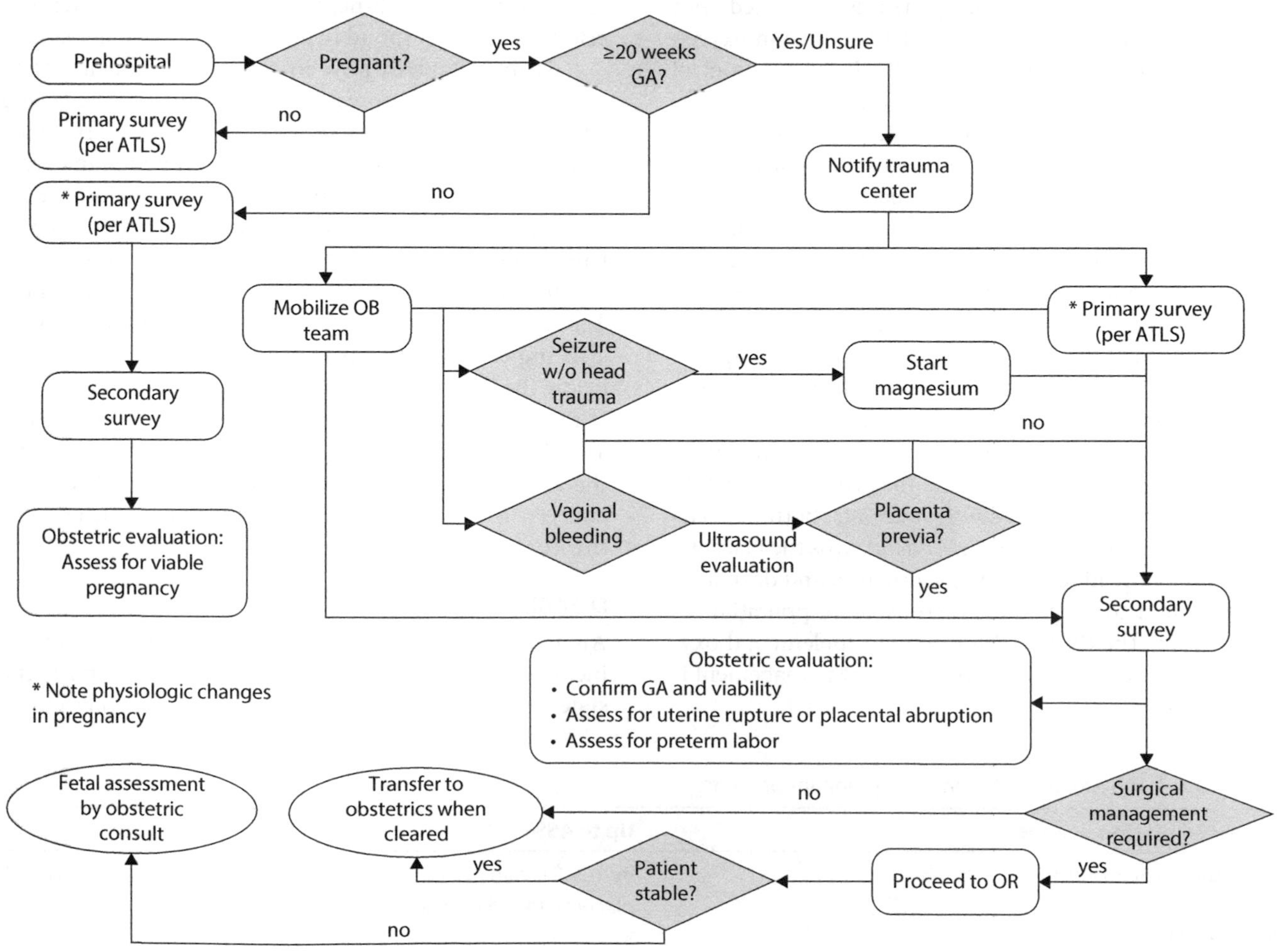

Figure 35.1 Mechanisms of injury—changes in anatomy.

Fetal injury is more commonly a result of indirect factors after blunt trauma, however: The uterus is deformable with high pressures, but as the placental attachment site is not, shear forces may result in placental abruption. Abruption has been reported to follow both major and minor degrees of maternal abdominal trauma. Though placental abruption is more likely at the time of admission for trauma, rates are also higher even among women who were discharged undelivered after trauma.[8]

Restraints (seat belts), properly worn, are protective to the pregnant patient (and therefore her fetus) involved in an MVA. Unrestrained pregnant women experience a higher risk of complications including premature delivery and fetal death. Proper placement involves a shoulder restraint above and a lap belt below the uterus. Airbags and their deployment have not been proven to increase fetal risks in pregnancy and, in fact, would be expected to save fetal lives by the simple expedient of saving maternal lives.

Penetrating injury is less common in pregnancy than blunt trauma but increases the likelihood of direct fetal injury. The uterus and its contents protect the patient's viscera, but the fetus generally does poorly.

As gestational age increases, the uterus displaces the bowel cephalad, so bowel injury becomes less likely with advancing gestation. The gravid uterus also displaces the bladder out of the bony pelvis, making it more susceptible to injury. Hematuria warrants prompt investigation. If maternal urine is contaminated with meconium or vernix, it is especially concerning for vesicouterine rupture.

The gravid uterus receives up to 600 mL/min of blood supply in the third trimester (20% of the cardiac output) and in the event of uterine rupture can be a major source of blood loss. It is possible for the uterus to distend enough to accommodate the entire circulating blood volume, thereby providing a large potential space for blood loss.

Pelvic fractures, which may result from blunt trauma, can be a source of significant retroperitoneal blood loss, especially because of the engorgement of pelvic vessels in pregnancy. A stable maternal pelvic fracture does not exclude vaginal delivery but consultation with an orthopedic surgeon would be indicated for safe patient positioning, since a standard lithotomy position may be imprudent under the circumstances.

EVALUATION OF FETO-MATERNAL HEMORRHAGE

The presence and degree of feto-maternal hemorrhage (FMH) has been studied as an indicator of the severity of obstetric trauma.[24] The inelastic placenta attached to the more elastic myometrium is prone to injury, and any disruption can result in fetal blood being spilled into the maternal circulation. FMH has been noted to occur in 10%–30% of traumas, with increasing incidence with advancing gestation. This is particularly important in Rh negative patients that have the potential for Rh alloimmunization. Even minor trauma has the potential for causing an Rh sensitization event in the mother, and all Rh-negative patients should receive anti-D immune globulin G within 72 hours of the event.[23]

While even 0.001 mL of fetal blood can result in alloimmunization, the routine dose of 300 μg Rh immune globulin will provide prophylaxis against 30 mL of fetal blood (15 mL of fetal RBC). If there is concern for larger FMH, the Kleihauer–Betke (KB) test can quantify the amount of fetal blood cells in maternal circulation so as to calculate the needed dose of Rh immune globulin.

Muench et al.[24] studied the utility of KB testing in all cases of maternal trauma regardless of Rh status and reported that a positive KB correlated with presence of contractions and progression to preterm labor. These authors have advocated routine KB testing in all trauma cases, but others recommend routine testing only in Rh-negative patients[23] since tocodynamometry is likely to be performed in all patients regardless.

COAGULOPATHY AND TRAUMA

Nonobstetric bleeding in a pregnant trauma patient should follow standard trauma protocols. Site-specific bleeding from a major injury can be life-threatening and should be stabilized emergently with either temporary (compression) or definitive (surgical or interventional) management. While anatomical bleeding can be corrected surgically, diffuse microvascular bleeding from a deranged coagulation system cannot, and may vitiate lifesaving interventions.

Recent literature from trauma and critical care sources shows that coagulopathy is present in one-third of bleeding trauma patients upon initial presentation to the hospital.[25] These patients require more transfusions and have longer stays in the intensive care unit (ICU), higher incidence of multiorgan dysfunction and a fourfold increase in mortality, compared with patients with a functional coagulation system. Especially pertinent in obstetrics is the role of placental abruption, overt or concealed, and its potential to trigger coagulopathy.

Post-traumatic coagulopathy has been mainly attributed to either widespread activation of the clotting cascade, leading to consumptive coagulopathy, or dilutional coagulopathy secondary to large-volume crystalloid resuscitation. While intravenous fluids can be lifesaving, large-volume infusions may worsen bleeding by increasing intravascular hydrostatic pressures and washing away clots that are being formed.[25,26] Strategies of hypotensive or hemostatic resuscitation are directed not at maintaining normal blood pressure but at maintaining only the minimal cardiac output required to sustain organ function while preserving normal coagulation. This typically requires limiting crystalloids, accepting lower blood pressures, administering antifibrinolytic agents such as tranexamic acid, and transfusing plasma and platelets early, rather than red blood cells (RBC) only.[26] Operative control of bleeding is achieved quickly, even if this means damage control rather than definitive surgery. It must be pointed out that hypotensive resuscitation has not been studied in pregnancy, though it has been proposed as an adjunct to surgical control of postpartum hemorrhage.[27] Hypothermia and acidosis are known to hinder clotting factor function and worsen coagulopathy: Thus, precautions must be taken to avoid them.

Although the degree of coagulopathy is related to severity of injury, hemodynamically stable patients may, rarely, present with clotting dysfunction. A distinct coagulopathy of trauma seems to be directly related to the degree of tissue hypoperfusion precipitated by the shock state. Acute coagulopathy of trauma-shock (ACoTS), characterized by systemic anticoagulation and hyperfibrinolysis, has not been specifically studied in pregnancy trauma and is beyond the scope of this chapter.

Pacheco et al., after a thorough review of current trauma literature, advocate changes in resuscitation protocols for obstetric hemorrhage,[28] which may be considered in case of severe trauma complicating pregnancy. They recommend hemostatic resuscitation that involves the following:

- Limitation of aggressive crystalloid use early in resuscitation, and perhaps permissive hypotension; permissive hypotension has not been studied during pregnancy, however, and the fetoplacental effects are unknown.
- Early administration of fresh frozen plasma (FFP) and platelets along with packed RBC, aiming for a ratio of 1:1:1 without waiting for coagulation laboratory tests.
- Early use of recombinant factor VII (rFVIIa).

Trauma literature now strongly advocates a 1:1:1 ratio of transfusing FFP and platelets with RBC to reduce the development of coagulopathy. Combat injury data has shown significant improvement in survival outcomes with higher plasma to packed RBC (PRBC) transfusion ratio,[29] as have subsequent trials in a civilian trauma population,[30] and a policy of high plasma-to-RBC ratios has subsequently been adopted into many massive hemorrhage protocols, including obstetric hemorrhage. However, as Pacheco et al. point out, trauma studies are significantly weakened by the possibility of survival bias: FFP takes time to thaw and thus the patient who receives it has already survived longer. The few studies attempting to address this bias have shown no benefit from higher plasma transfusion ratios. More prospective studies are needed to provide guidance, but at the time of this writing, early FFP and platelet transfusion is recommended.

In case of a planned (nonemergent) trip to the operating room, intraoperative cell salvage is a viable option for obstetric patients and can reduce the need for allogenic blood products. The theoretical concern for an amniotic fluid embolism caused by unfiltered amniotic fluid in salvaged blood has not been seen in clinical practice in over 400 obstetric patients.[1]

DIAGNOSTIC IMAGING MODALITIES AND SPECIAL CONSIDERATIONS DURING PREGNANCY

After maternal resuscitation and stabilization, focus is shifted to the diagnosis of nonobvious injuries and evaluation and management of the fetus. This constitutes the secondary survey.

Diagnostic imaging is often important to determine the extent of intra-abdominal or other internal injury and to confirm whether there is a need for nonobstetric laparotomy or other surgery.

Focused assessment with sonography in trauma (FAST) is typically used during the secondary survey to look for free intraperitoneal fluid. During this examination one visualizes the pericardium, the right upper quadrant, left upper quadrant and the suprapubic area in a search for free fluid.[17,23] In pregnant patients, FAST performs well: Sensitivity was 83% and specificity 98% in a group of 127 who had sustained blunt abdominal trauma.[31] It does depend to a certain extent on the sonographer's skill and the acoustic attenuation of the abdominal wall, being less satisfactory in obesity.

Bedside ultrasonography (US) can also be utilized to determine the approximate gestational age (GA) of the fetus and presence (or absence) of fetal cardiac activity. The location of the placenta, presence of a retroplacental clot, and position of the fetus can be determined, but sensitivity of ultrasound for placental abruption is inadequate. As an adjunct to the secondary survey, continuous electronic fetal heart rate monitoring may be appropriate, depending on gestational age, severity of maternal injury and potential for fetal decompensation. Presence of fetal well-being can also be utilized as an additional marker of maternal physiologic stability. Fetal concerns cannot, of course, be allowed to override maternal concerns.

Computed tomography (CT) scanning is a crucial element of trauma imaging. The concern for CT in a pregnant patient revolves around the radiation exposure to the developing fetus. The potential for harm from radiation exposure depends on the gestational age. Immediately after conception (<2 weeks), there may be blastocyst failure, with harm being an all-or-nothing event. Between 2 and 10 weeks the embryo or fetus is vulnerable to teratogenesis with the threshold thought to be from 50 to 150 mGy; after 10 weeks, the major concerns with high exposures would be fetal growth restriction or effects on brain development.[23]

Fetal exposure from background radiation ranges from 0.5 to 1.0 mGy in a normal pregnancy. A single CT of the chest has an estimated exposure of 0.2 mGy.[32] In contrast, a CT of the abdomen and pelvis with the fetus in direct view can approach 50 mGy but, unless repeated, usually still remains below the threshold. Techniques to reduce the fetal radiation dose may be employed if the radiologist deems they will not compromise image quality.

Reaching 50 mGy of exposure increases the overall lifetime cancer risk by 2% in the perinate and doubles the risk of fatal childhood cancer (new risk: 1 in 1000).[32]

NONOBSTETRIC SURGERY DURING PREGNANCY

Maternal injury during pregnancy may require surgical intervention. Craniotomy, thoracotomy, laparotomy, or surgery of the extremities may be required. Nonemergent procedures may be deferred for hours or, more rarely, even days in some cases, such as extremity fractures, in order to optimize presurgical and preanesthetic circumstances. In some cases, the surgical technique may be altered by the fact of pregnancy, as when the orthopedist chooses an open plating technique for repair of long bone fracture rather than percutaneous plating or an intramedullary nail, so as to reduce total radiation exposure intraoperatively.[33]

If emergency laparotomy is indicated for trauma, the goals for surgery should be clearly elucidated. Gunshot wounds to the maternal abdomen will typically require exploration, but typically will be associated with fetal death. Penetrating abdominal trauma from stab wounds may injure the uterus and thereby injure the fetus, but if the uterus is large enough, will not usually have injured other maternal viscera. The enlarging uterus will have pushed bowel cephalad, however, so upper abdominal injuries may well be associated with bowel trauma.

In recent years, the concept of selective nonoperative management (SNOM) of abdominal trauma has come to the fore, first for blunt trauma and then for penetrating trauma.[34,35] Candidates for this type of management must be hemodynamically stable, have no evidence of peritonitis, and have no hollow viscus injury on CT scan; solid-organ injury does not rule out SNOM. This approach has been successful in reducing exploratory laparotomy among adult (nonpregnant) patients after abdominal trauma, though 15%–20% will fail SNOM and require laparotomy.[34] Evaluation of selective nonoperative management among pregnant patients after abdominal trauma remains limited, however. A small series from Lebanon reported on 14 pregnant patients injured by high-velocity bullets or shrapnel, among whom three were managed expectantly, at 25, 32, and 34 weeks: All three fetuses survived and eventually delivered vaginally.[36] The authors note that expectant management in these cases was predicated on the absence of major fetal injuries as shown by x-ray or ultrasound imaging. Outcomes were better than those in which immediate cesarean was undertaken, though the decision to take the patient to surgery was confounded by indication: That is, there was "fetal distress" in two cases, bullet-induced fetal fractures in two, two traumatic uterine ruptures, and in two cases the uterus had to be emptied to get surgical access to a maternal injury in the liver or retroperitoneum. Three other cases in which cesarean was undertaken without either a fetal indication for cesarean or a clear maternal indication for laparotomy all resulted in stillbirth.

Intraoperative fetal monitoring is sometimes used during nonobstetric surgery but cannot be routinely recommended. Not only is it technically and logistically difficult to perform during abdominal surgery, but it raises the possibility that concerns about fetal well-being may trump concerns about maternal stability. The Committee on Obstetric Practice of the American College of Obstetricians and Gynecologists states, "The decision to use fetal monitoring should be individualized," and points out that all the following must apply if it is to be undertaken: "The fetus is viable; it is physically possible to perform intraoperative fetal monitoring; a health care provider with obstetric surgery privileges is available and willing to intervene during the surgical procedure for fetal indications; when possible, the woman has given informed consent to emergency cesarean delivery; the nature of the planned surgery will allow the safe interruption or alteration of the procedure to provide access to perform emergency delivery."[37]

CARDIAC ARREST

In the event of cardiopulmonary arrest of a patient past mid-pregnancy, effective cardiopulmonary resuscitation is difficult to achieve. Aortocaval compression by the uterus interferes with return to the heart when the patient is supine. Left uterine displacement has been advocated, with a wedge under the right hip, but manual uterine displacement from above is more effective.[38] Chest compressions and ventilations should be delivered according to standard protocols.

There is good evidence to recommend expedited delivery of the fetus within 4 minutes of arrest for *both maternal and fetal benefit*, especially after the threshold for neonatal viability (>24 weeks) or in the case of a potentially reversible cause of maternal arrest. Recent clinical practice guidelines from the SOGC[23] and from the American Heart Association[38] emphasize the role of perimortem cesarean delivery in improving the chances for return of spontaneous circulation in the mother as well as the outcome for the perinate.

The push for perimortem cesarean delivery (PMCD) within 4 minutes of maternal cardiac arrest originated from a seminal paper published 30 years ago.[39] The authors outlined the potential maternal and fetal benefits and targeted a time of 4 minutes to begin the procedure, 5 minutes to effect delivery. This target reflected the difficulty of performing effective cardiopulmonary resuscitation (CPR) in a gravid patient past midpregnancy and the time threshold believed to apply for maternal and fetal oxygen reserve. Subsequent case series have reported return of spontaneous circulation after aortocaval compression is relieved with delivery of the fetus. Katz[40] reviewed more than 200 cases of maternal cardiac arrest and found only three cases in which effective CPR was achieved prior to delivery of the fetus.

As far as the fetus is concerned, ischemic brain injury occurs 4–5 minutes after cessation of blood flow, and the hope is that neurologic injury to the fetus may be prevented if it is delivered within that time frame.[39] Neonatal survival with normal neurological development has been documented, however, even 30 minutes after maternal arrest,[41] so delivery should not be considered futile if more than 5 minutes have passed.

In nonresuscitatable causes of maternal cardiopulmonary arrest (e.g., massive trauma), perimortem cesarean section should be performed immediately for the benefit of the fetus. Nonobstetric providers can employ a "two fingerbreadth" rule if they need to estimate viability: Palpation of the uterine fundus two fingerbreadths above the umbilicus approximates 24 weeks gestation, at which time extrauterine survival is possible.

Once the decision is made to proceed with PMCD, no delay should be made to check fetal heart rate or move the patient to the operating room. Ultrasonography is difficult to perform in such a setting and only wastes crucial time. Neither sterile technique nor anesthesia is required, and the consent of the mother will, obviously, be impossible. Neonatology providers should be informed and urgently available, but the procedure should not wait for them to arrive. CPR should be continued during the procedure and the obstetrician or delivering physician should perform laparotomy in a manner they are most comfortable with.[38]

Either midline vertical or Pfannenstiel (transverse) incision can be utilized, according to the operator's preference, as long as speed can be achieved. After delivery of the fetus, the placenta should be delivered and the uterus closed with care to prevent bladder and bowel injury in potentially resuscitable cases. While there will be no bleeding during the surgery, because there will have been no circulation, hemorrhage is possible after return of spontaneous circulation.[42] The surgeon should be prepared to treat both uterine atony and coagulopathy.

The ethics and legality of PMCD have been addressed by others[40,42] and will be mentioned here briefly. In cases of fatal nonresuscitatable maternal trauma, the medical provider's obligation to the fetus should be obvious and would require immediate action. In cases where maternal resuscitation is possible, though PMCD may appear morbid and even barbaric, the evidence is clear on its potential both as an aid to maternal resuscitation and as a tool to deliver a liveborn baby. In terms of legality and consent, as of 2012 no instances of legal action (either civil or criminal) have been entered against a physician for performing PMCD. However, there are cases in which physicians have been sued either for not performing PMCD or not doing so in a timely manner.[40]

REFERENCES

1. Mendez-Figueroa H, Dahlke JD, Vrees RA, Rouse DJ. Trauma in pregnancy: An updated systematic review. *Am J Obstet Gynecol* 2013; 209: 1–10.
2. Chang J, Berg CJ, Saltzman LE, Herndon J. Homicide: A leading cause of injury deaths among pregnant and postpartum women in the United States, 1991–1999. *Am J Public Health* 2005; 95: 471–7.
3. Ikossi DG, Lazar AA, Morabito D, Fildes J, Knudson MM. Profile of mothers at risk: An analysis of injury and pregnancy loss in 1,195 trauma patients. *J Am Coll Surg* 2005; 200: 49–56.
4. Battaloglu E, McDonnell D, Chu J, Lecky F, Porter K. Epidemiology and outcomes of pregnancy and obstetric complications in trauma in the United Kingdom. *Injury* 2016; 47: 184–7.
5. John PR, Shiozawa A, Haut ER, et al. An assessment of the impact of pregnancy on trauma mortality. *Surgery* 2011; 149: 94–8.
6. Petrone P, Talving P, Browder T, et al. Abdominal injuries in pregnancy: A 155-month study at two level 1 trauma centers. *Injury* 2011; 42: 47–9.
7. Manoogian S. Comparison of pregnant and non-pregnant occupant crash and injury characteristics based on national crash data. *Accident Analysis Prevention* 2015; 74: 69–76.
8. El Kady D, Gilbert WM, Anderson J, Danielsen B, Towner D, Smith LH. Trauma during pregnancy: An analysis of maternal and fetal outcomes in a large population. *Am J Obstet Gynecol* 2004; 190: 1661–8.
9. Gulliver PJ, Dixon RS. Immediate and long-term outcomes of assault in pregnancy. *Austr NZ J Obstet Gynaecol* 2014; 54: 256–62.
10. Wall SL, Figuerido F, Laing GL, Clarke DL. The spectrum and outcome of pregnant trauma patients in a metropolitan trauma service in South Africa. *Injury* 2014; 45: 1220–3.
11. Cahill AG, Bastek JA, Stamilio DM, Odibo AO, Stevens E, Macones GA. Minor trauma in pregnancy—is the evaluation unwarranted? *Am J Obstet Gynecol* 2008; 198: 208.e1–208.e5.
12. Okeke T, Ugwu E, Ikeako L, et al. Falls among pregnant women in Enugu, southeast Nigeria. *Nigerian J Clin Pract* 2014; 17: 292–5.
13. Schiff MA. Pregnancy outcomes following hospitalization for a fall in Washington State from 1987 to 2004. *BJOG* 2008; 115: 1648–54.
14. Inanir A, Cakmak B, Hisim Y, Demirturk F. Evaluation of postural equilibrium and fall risk during pregnancy. *Gait & Posture* 2014; 39: 1122–5.
15. Subrahmanyam M. Burns during pregnancy—effect on maternal and foetal outcomes. *Ann Burns Fire Disasters* 2006; 19:177–9.
16. Maghsoudi H, Samnia R, Garadaghi A, Kianvar H. Burns in pregnancy. *Burns* 2006: 32: 246–50.
17. American College of Surgeons. *Advanced Trauma Life Support Student Course Manual.* 9th edition, 2012. American College of Surgeons. Chicago IL.
18. Sasser SM, Hunt RC, Faul M, et al. Guidelines for field triage of injured patients: Recommendations of the National Expert Panel on Field Triage, 2011. *MMWR Recomm Rep.* 2012; 61: 1–20.
19. Einav S, Sela HY, Weiniger CF. Management and outcomes of trauma during pregnancy. *Anesthesiol Clin* 2013; 31: 141–56.
20. Greene W, Robinson L, Rizzo AG, et al. Pregnancy is not a sufficient indicator for trauma team activation. *J Trauma* 2007; 63: 550–5.
21. Samsoon GLT, Young JRB. Difficult tracheal intubation: A retrospective study. *Anaesthesia* 1987; 42: 487–90.
22. Quinn AC, Milne D, Columb M, Gorton H, Knight M. Failed tracheal intubation in obstetric anaesthesia: 2 yr national case-control study in the UK. *Br J Anaesthesia* 2013; 11: 74–80.
23. Jain V, Chari R, Maslovitz S, et al. for the Society of Obstetricians and Gynaecologists of Canada. SOGC Clinical Practice Guideline no. 325, June 2015. Guidelines for the management of a pregnant trauma patient. *J Obstet Gynaecol* 2015; 37: 553–71.

24. Muench MV, Baschat AA, Reddy UM, et al. Kleihauer-Betke testing is important in all cases of maternal trauma. *J Trauma* 2004; 57: 1094–98.
25. Spahn DR, Bouillon B, Cerny V, et al. *Management of Bleeding and Coagulopathy Following Major Trauma: An Updated European Guideline.* Crit Care 2013;17:R76.
26. Dutton RP. Haemostatic resuscitation. *Br J Anaesthesia* 2012: i39–46.
27. Ekelund K, Hanke G, Stensballe J, Wikkelsøe A, Krebs Albrechtsen C, Afshari A. Hemostatic resuscitation in postpartum hemorrhage: A supplement to surgery. *Acta Obstet Gynecol Scand* 2015; 94: 680–92.
28. Pacheco LD, Saade GR, Gei AF, Hankins GDV. Cutting-edge advances in the medical management of obstetrical hemorrhage. *Am J Obstet Gynecol* 2011; 205: 526–531.
29. Borgman MA, Spinella PC, Perkins JG, et al. The ratio of blood products transfused affects mortality in patients receiving massive transfusions at a combat support hospital. *J Trauma* 2007; 63: 805–13.
30. Holcomb JB, Wade CE, Michalek JE, et al. Increased plasma and platelet to red blood cell ratios improves outcome in 466 massively transfused civilian trauma patients. *Ann Surg* 2008; 248: 447–58.
31. Goodwin H, Homes JF, Wisner DH. Abdominal ultrasound examination in pregnant blunt trauma patients. *J Trauma* 2001; 50: 689–94.
32. American College of Obstetricians and Gynecologists. In: *Committee on Obstetric Practice.* Practice Bulletin no. 299, September 2004 (reaffirmed 2014.) Guidelines for diagnostic imaging during pregnancy.
33. Flik K, Kloen P, Toro JB, Urmey W, Nijhuis JG, Helfet DL. Orthopaedic trauma in the pregnant patient. *J Am Acad Orthop Surg* 2006; 14: 175–82.
34. Nabeel Zafar S, Rushing A, Haut ER, et al. Outcome of selective non-operative management of penetrating abdominal injuries from the North American National Trauma Database. *Br J Surgery* 2011; 99: 155–65.
35. Lamb CM, Garner JP. Selective non-operative management of civilian gunshot wounds to the abdomen: A systematic review of the evidence. *Injury* 2013; 45: 659–66.
36. Awwad JT, Azar GB, Seoud MA, Mroueh AM, Karam KS. High-velocity penetrating wounds of the gravid uterus: Review of 16 years of civil war. *Obstet Gynecol* 1994; 83: 259–64.
37. American College of Obstetricians and Gynecologists. Committee on Obstetric Practice. Practice Bulletin no. 474, Feb 2011. Nonobstetric surgery during pregnancy.
38. Jeejeebhoy FM, Zelop CM, Lipman S, et al, on behalf pf the American Heart Association Emergency Cardiovascular Care Committee, Council on Cardiopulmonary, Critical Care, Perioperative and Resuscitation, Council on Cardiovascular Diseases in the Young, and Council on Clinical Cardiology. Cardiac arrest in pregnancy: A scientific statement from the American Heart Association. *Circulation* 2015;132:00–00.doi10.1161/CIR.0000000000000300.
39. Katz VL, Dotters DJ, Droegemueller W. Perimortem cesarean delivery. *Obstet Gynecol* 1986; 68: 571–6.
40. Katz VL. Perimortem cesarean delivery: Its role in maternal mortality. *Semin Perinatol* 2012; 36: 68–72.
41. Capobianco G, Balata A, Mannazzu MC, et al. Perimortem cesarean delivery 30 minutes after a laboring patient jumped from a fourth-floor window: Baby survives and is normal at age 4 years. *Am J Obstet Gynecol* 2008; 198: e15–e16.
42. Drukker L, Hants Y, Sharon E, Sela HY, Grisaru-Granovsky S. Perimortem cesarean section for maternal and fetal salvage: Concise review and protocol. *Acta Obstet Gynecol Scand* 2014; 93: 965–72.

Surgery during pregnancy

36

GEORGE A. MAZPULE, GREGORY GRIMBERG, TOGHRUL TALISHINSKIY, and DONALD A. MCCAIN

CONTENTS

Approximately 0.75–2% of pregnant women need nonobstetric surgery. This chapter's objective is to provide a concise yet broad overview of the most common nonobstetric surgical issues in the pregnant patient. The topics covered in this chapter range from the most common causes of abdominal pain, such as appendicitis, biliary tract disease, and bowel obstruction to the management of certain malignancies. Making an early diagnosis and implementing timely treatment of these conditions is paramount in minimizing both fetal and maternal morbidity. However, physiological changes during pregnancy may confound the etiology and lead to difficulty in diagnosis (Table 36.1). Having knowledge of these changes that occur during pregnancy may lead to earlier diagnosis and more appropriate management plan.

APPENDICITIS

Acute appendicitis is the most common nonobstetric surgical disease during pregnancy. Approximately 1 out of 1250 pregnant females is diagnosed with appendicitis with about half of these cases occurring during the second trimester. Anatomical changes in the size of the gravid uterus and normal physiologic leukocytosis during pregnancy may make the diagnosis challenging. The presence of nausea and vomiting is nonspecific and may occur in a normal pregnant patient, especially during the first trimester.

The most consistent presenting symptom is right lower quadrant pain.[1] However, the presence of this pain is not specific to appendicitis. Anorexia, nausea, and vomiting usually occur within 24 hours of the onset of pain. The patient may develop right upper quadrant pain as the appendix is displaced medially and cephalad by the enlarging uterus. An increase in the normally elevated white blood cell count with a left shift may be seen.

An abdominal ultrasound examination is usually the first diagnostic test of choice. It poses no known risks to the fetus and has good diagnostic sensitivity. If the ultrasound examination is not diagnostic, the next choice of imaging study remains controversial. Both computed tomography (CT) and magnetic resonance imaging (MRI) have greater than 95% sensitivity and specificity in the diagnosis of appendicitis. Low-dose CT can be used after the second week of embryonic age.[7] MRI is generally considered safe in the second and third trimesters of pregnancy,

Table 36.1 Maternal physiologic changes during pregnancy.

Clinical
Dyspnea
Peripheral edema
Systolic ejection murmur
Nausea
Cardiovascular
Increased heart rate (to about 90)
Decreased blood pressure (by about 5–10 mmHg)
Increased cardiac output (by 30–50%)
Decreased systemic vascular resistance (SVR)
Increased blood volume and plasma volume (by 1–1.5 L)
Decreased venous return of blood to the heart
Decreased iliac artery flow
Respiratory
Elevated diaphragm
Functional residual capacity (FRC) decrease by 15–20%
Increased minute ventilation
Pa_{O_2} increase (to approximately 105 mmHg)
Pa_{CO_2} decrease (to approximately 30 mmHg)
pH increase (to approximately 7.44)
Gastrointestinal
Decreased gastric motility
Mild elevation in alkaline phosphatase
Hematologic
Hypercoagulability
Decreased plasma total protein and albumin levels
Renal
Dilation of collection systems
Relaxation of bladder with increased capacity
Increased glomerular filtration rate (GFR) by 30–50%

regarding safety in the first trimester is limited. However, it remains a useful imaging tool due to its lack of ionizing radiation. Because of this, some clinicians choose MRI before CT if both are readily available. Regardless of which imaging modality is utilized, prompt diagnosis of appendicitis is important, since fetal morbidity increases from 2% to 8.5% in simple appendicitis to as high as 35% in perforated appendicitis.

The treatment of simple acute appendicitis is appendectomy. However, if advanced appendicitis is seen, involving a phlegmon, abscess or perforation, nonoperative management is preferred. The patient is prescribed broad spectrum antimicrobials. Percutaneous drainage of fluid (abscess) collections with radiological guidance can be performed if needed. The role for interval appendectomy is still unclear, but should be considered.

BILIARY TRACT DISEASE

About 1–8 of every 10,000 pregnant women are affected by biliary tract disease.[3] The symptomatology is similar to nonpregnant patients and includes nausea, vomiting, and right upper quadrant pain associated with the ingestion of a fatty meal. Abdominal pain that persists is often seen in those with acute cholecystitis. The diagnostic test of choice is an abdominal ultrasound examination. Ultrasound findings may include pericholecystic fluid, a thickened gallbladder wall, and a sonographic Murphy's sign.

Biliary colic is treated with analgesia and usually does not require cholecystectomy unless the patient has persistent vomiting. Elective cholecystectomy can be done after delivery, since over 90% of pregnant females with biliary colic have resolution of their symptoms with conservative management. However, cholecystectomy is safe in the first or second trimesters if clinically indicated. The laparoscopic approach has been proven to be safe during pregnancy and may be superior to open cholecystectomy.[2] However, laparoscopy may be technically difficult during the third trimester due to the size of the uterus.[3] Percutaneous cholecystostomy is also a viable option in unstable patients.

PANCREATITIS

Pancreatitis occurs in about 1 in 1,000–12,000 pregnancies. Maternal mortality may range from 0% to 18%, depending on severity. Preterm delivery is seen from 15% to 32%. About 65% of acute pancreatitis is caused by gallstones, followed by hyperlipidemia.[4] An elevated amylase and lipase are seen, along with a disproportionate elevation in alkaline phosphatase.

Aggressive resuscitation and nutrition are crucial in patients with pancreatitis. An abdominal ultrasound should be done to evaluate for cholelithiasis. If the pancreatitis is severe as determined by Ransom's criteria or the Acute Physiology and Chronic Health Evaluation (APACHE) score, a CT scan with IV contrast is performed to assess the presence of pancreatic necrosis.

The management of gallstone pancreatitis may include cholecystectomy, most commonly done during the second trimester if possible. Endoscopic retrograde cholangiopancreatography can be safely utilized if indicated by the presence of biliary obstruction.[5] If used within 48 hours of presentation in indicated patients, morbidity and mortality are decreased. Pelvic shielding should be utilized. In case of severe pancreatitis, the patient should be admitted to the intensive care unit (ICU) due to their high risk of cardiovascular and respiratory failure. Parental nutrition is safe to use during pregnancy and should be implemented when adequate oral nutrition is not possible. However, enteral feeding is preferred if possible to prevent gut permeability and bacterial translocation. Antimicrobials may be indicated if >30% of the pancreas is necrotic. If so, the drug of choice is imipenem–cilestatin. If the patient shows no improvement after medical management for 10–14 days and has pancreatic necrosis, pancreatic debridement is necessary if infection is proven by a fine needle aspiration of the pancreatic fluid. If the necrosis is sterile, up to 3 weeks of nonoperative medical management may be needed.

INTESTINAL OBSTRUCTION

Intestinal obstruction is uncommon during pregnancy, occurring from 1 in 1,500 to 66,500 pregnancies. As in the nonobstetric patient, the most common etiology of obstruction is adhesions due to previous surgery, followed by volvulus, intussusception, malignancy, hernias, and diverticular disease.[6] Up to 25% of cases are due to cecal volvulus due to its displacement by the enlarging gravid uterus.

The presenting symptoms of intestinal obstruction include pain, nausea, vomiting, and distension. Patients may be obstipated, but some may still have bowel movements due to evacuation of stool distal to the point of obstruction. Physical examination should focus on evaluation for abdominal tenderness and the presence of hernias. Bowel ischemia should be suspected if the patient shows signs of peritonitis with or without fever and leukocytosis. The first imaging study of choice is abdominal plain films. Radiologic signs of obstruction include small bowel distension with air fluid levels and a paucity of air in the large colon. If these images are inconclusive, further imaging studies, such as CT or MRI, may be appropriate.

The management of obstruction includes placement of a nasogastric tube, aggressive fluid resuscitation, electrolyte replacement, and the placement of a Foley catheter to adequately measure urine output. If the patient does not show signs of bowel ischemia or complete obstruction, nonoperative medical management can be successful in up to 80% of patients. However, if there are signs of bowel ischemia or a complete obstruction, an urgent laparotomy is required. Untreated bowel ischemia may lead to preterm labor in over 50% of patients with fetal mortality approaching 50% if septic shock develops. Thus early surgical intervention is critical.

INTRA-ABDOMINAL BLEEDING

Sudden hypotension with abdominal pain may be caused by a ruptured hepatic adenoma during pregnancy. Due to high circulating estrogen levels, adenomas can increase in size leading to a higher chance of rupture. Due to the lethality of massive intraabdominal hemorrhage from a ruptured adenoma, nonpregnant women with a known hepatic adenoma are advised not to take oral contraceptives as well as avoid pregnancy until the adenoma regresses in size. Prophylactic resection may play a role if pregnancy is planned. If a hepatic adenoma rupture is suspected, management involves aggressive fluid resuscitation and blood transfusion if needed. Bleeding may be controlled via hepatic artery embolization or hepatic artery ligation.

Splenic artery aneurysms may also cause intra-abdominal bleeding in pregnant patients. Management includes splenic artery embolization or surgery. If the aneurysm is proximal, it may be amenable to aneurysmectomy and reanastomosis of the splenic artery. If it is located near the spleen, then splenectomy may be the only option to control the hemorrhage. Although rare, splenic artery aneurysm rupture may have a maternal mortality of 75% and fetal mortality of 95%.[7]

INFLAMMATORY BOWEL DISEASE

Pregnant females with inflammatory bowel disease (IBD) do not have an increased risk of relapse compared to nonpregnant females. However, there is an increased risk in adverse pregnancy outcomes. The most common complications are preterm delivery and low birth weight. If maternal IBD is active there may include a higher rate of miscarriage, and risks to the fetus may be increased at delivery. However, if the pregnancy is carried to term, fetal morbidity and mortality may be low.

Acute exacerbations during pregnancy increase the rate of adverse maternal and fetal outcomes. Urgent and appropriate treatment may prevent these complications. While most medications for IBD carry a low risk for the fetus, some such as methotrexate are contraindicated. 5-aminosalicylic acid (5-ASA) and corticosteroids are the preferred drugs used to treat relapses. Infliximab may be given up until gestational weeks 24–26, due to it being able to cross the placenta. Ciprofloxacin and metronidazole should be avoided in the first trimester. Medications should not be stopped during pregnancy, as discontinuation of maintenance therapy may lead to a higher chance of relapse and fetal morbidity. The indications for surgery are the same as in the nonpregnant female. The risk to the fetus of continued illness due to IBD is greater than the risks of surgery.[8]

DEEP VENOUS THROMBOSIS

Deep venous thrombosis (DVT) occurs in 12.1 per 10,000 pregnant females with the highest risk later in gestation and until 3 weeks postpartum. Pulmonary embolism occurs at a rate of 5.4 per 10,000 pregnancies. Pregnant women are 6–10 times more likely to develop a DVT than nonpregnant women. Numerous factors contribute to this increased risk. Venous stasis of the lower extremities is caused by compression of the inferior vena cava by the gravid uterus. The levels of coagulation factors II, III, and X are increased and protein S is decreased, leading to a hypercoagulable state. Fibrin also becomes elevated in pregnancy due to an inhibited fibrinolysis. DVTs usually present in the left leg about 70% of the time.

DVT can usually be diagnosed via a venous Doppler ultrasound examination and is the diagnostic test of choice. In some cases, repeat Doppler ultrasound imaging or MRI may be required if the initial test fails to show a DVT in a patient with high suspicion. If pulmonary embolism (PE) is suspected, a ventilation perfusion (VQ) scan or CT angiography of the chest may be done with low risk to the fetus. Due to potential counfounding by the normal physiologic changes of pregnancy, a hypercoagulable workup should be postponed until at least 6 weeks postpartum. Molecular genetic testing may be done for prothrombin and Factor V Leiden mutations, as these are not affected by pregnancy. Once diagnosed, patients should be hospitalized for medical management with low molecular weight heparin (LMWH) or unfractionated heparin (UH). However, LMWH is often preferred because of its ease of dosing and lower side effect profile.[9] Therapy should be continued at a therapeutic dose for 3 months, and then continued at prophylactic doses until 3 weeks postpartum. LMWH and UH do not cross the placenta and are safe to use during pregnancy. Antifactor Xa levels should be followed to ensure that the dose of LMWH is therapeutic.

If heparin is prescribed and heparin-induced thrombocytopenia (HIT) develops, danaparoid and fondaparinux can be used. They are heparinoid molecules and do not cross-react with antibodies found in HIT. Direct thrombin inhibitors and factor Xa inhibitors are currently not recommended to be used due to lack of safety data during pregnancy. Vitamin K antagonists, such as warfarin, are relatively contraindicated due to their ability to cross the placenta and cause teratogenicity. [10]

DIAGNOSTIC IMAGING IN PREGNANT PATIENTS

Maternal and fetal radiation exposure from diagnostic imaging during pregnancy is affected by several factors such as the gestational age, anatomic site being imaged, imaging modality, and imaging technique. The effects of ionizing radiation include teratogenic and sometimes carcinogenic risks. Therefore, the benefit of the imaging study chosen in the workup of a pregnant female should outweigh its risks.

There is negligible effect of radiation on the fetus when it is exposed to less than 50 mGy, and pelvic shielding should be used when possible. Specific radiation risks are seen in Table 36.2.

If a CT is to be used, low-dose radiation modes should be used. While the safety of MRI has not yet been established, no adverse effects to the fetus have been found. MRI is sometimes used in lieu of CT due to its lack of ionizing radiation, such as the evaluation of a pregnant patient with suspected appendicitis who has had an inconclusive ultrasound. Regardless of the imaging test used, a thorough discussion about its risks and benefits should be had with the patient. It is important to note that a delay in diagnosis may increase maternal and fetal morbidity and mortality. Therefore, if an imaging test is clinically indicated, it should be done in order to make a diagnosis and to implement appropriate therapy.[11,12]

PREGNANCY-ASSOCIATED NEOPLASIA AND RELATED ENDOCRINE ISSUES

Cancer is the second most common cause of death in reproductive-aged females after accidental injury.[13] Recent data indicate that the overall risk of malignancy during pregnancy has nearly doubled from 1 in 2000 in 1964[14] up to 1 per 1000 pregnant women in 1995 (Table 36.3),[15] which is expected to increase as maternal age increases. The median age of pregnancy in the United States has been steadily increasing over the past 40 years to greater than 26 years,[16] up from 21 in 1970.[17] A survey of the California State Cancer Registry demonstrated that the most common nongynecological cancers associated with pregnancy were breast, thyroid, melanoma, and Hodgkin's lymphoma.[18] This section will focus on the most common nongynecologic neoplasms and related diseases of general surgical importance in the pregnant patient.

Table 36.2 Estimated radiation exposure from radiography.

Radiographic test	Estimated ionizing radiation exposure (mGy)
Chest radiograph	<0.01 mGy
Abdominal CT	29–42 mGy
Pelvic CT	20–80 mGy
Barium enema	10–20 mGy
Nuclear study	<10 mGy
Fluoroscopy	10 mGy per minute
Ultrasound	None
MRI	None

Note: 1 rad = 10 mGy.

Table 36.3 Risks of malignany in pregnancy.

Tumor type	Incidence
Breast cancer	1:3,000–10,000
Hodgkin's lymphoma	1:1000–6000
Melanoma	2–5:100,000
Thyroid cancer	14:100,000

Source: Reproduced from Pavlidis NA, *Oncologist*, 7(4), 279–287, 2002. With permission.

DIAGNOSIS AND MANAGEMENT OF PUERPERAL BREAST MASSES

During pregnancy and lactation, examination of the breast is more difficult due to the changing hormonal milieu, alterations in breast texture, size, volume, water content, density, and tenderness. A careful breast examination is recommended to establish a baseline as soon as pregnancy is diagnosed since small masses can be missed as gestation progresses.[19]

Pregnancy-associated breast cancer (PABC) is defined as any breast cancer that occurs during pregnancy or within a year of childbirth. These breast cancers are usually infiltrating ductal adenocarcinomas, poorly differentiated, associated with a poor prognosis, tend to present in an advanced stage, are hormonal receptor negative, HER-2/neu positive and may be associated with a delay in diagnosis.[20] Ultrasound, mammography, and MRI examinations are the usual imaging modalities that are available to evaluate breast masses.[21]

It is recommended that all patients with a palpable breast mass that persists for longer than 2 weeks should be evaluated with an ultrasound examination. Ultrasound is the first-line imaging study of a palpable breast mass in pregnant patients due to a number of unique factors: safety (lack of ionizing radiation), distinguishing characteristics between benign and malignant lesions, high sensitivity and specificity, and ability to perform a guided core needle biopsy at the same time.

Differential diagnosis of breast masses includes cystic lesions such as abscesses and galactoceles, benign solid masses including fibroadenomas, lactating adenomas, hamartomas, and rarely malignant solid masses such as lymphoma, leukemia, and sarcoma. For galactoceles, the diagnosis and treatment are by aspiration. For abscesses, treatment with incision and drainage or aspiration is acceptable, although for suspicious masses a biopsy including the abscess wall is important to rule out a necrotic breast cancer. Some benign solid masses can grow in size throughout the pregnancy, sometimes rapidly as pregnancy progresses.

Mammography is often perceived to have a high radiation dose although it has been shown to be safe during pregnancy.[22] The radiation dose of standard mammography is less than 3 mGy to the mother; the dose to the uterus is less than 0.03 μGy,[23] which is less than the 50 mGy threshold below which no teratogenic effects on the fetus have been reported.[24] However, even with its relative safety and with the sensitivity and specificity of mammography in PABC between 78% and 90%, mammography is usually reserved for specific circumstances.[25] It detects suspicious microcalcifications not picked up by ultrasound examination, and in multifocal, multicentric, and contralateral disease. In addition, bilateral mammography is recommended for any patient with a highly suspicious mass found on physical examination or on ultrasound imaging and any patient found to have a newly diagnosed PABC.[26] In women over the age of 40 who are pregnant routine screening mammography should not be done until after delivery and preferably after cessation of lactation.

Although more sensitive in diagnosing breast cancer than mammography, contrast-enhanced MRI is usually not used in the evaluation/screening in pregnant patients as gadolinium ions can cross the placenta and can also dissociate into toxic-free ions.[27] Gadolinium ions can cross the placenta and can also dissociate into toxic-free ions,[27] which limits it routine use.

A suspicious breast mass (palpable solid and complex cystic mass) identified on ultrasound should be biopsied using ultrasound guided core needle biopsy technique. Benign lesions such as fibroadenoma, lactating adenoma, or hamartoma can be followed until the postpartum period and then be subsequently excised. Excisional biopsy is needed for clinically and radiologically suspicious masses that even have an equivocal or benign core needle biopsy. A rare complication of core needle biopsy is a milk fistula formation,[28] a benign entity which can be treated by suppression of lactation. A management algorithm for puerperal breast masses is shown in Figure 36.1.

DIAGNOSIS

PABC affects up to 1 in 3000 pregnant women, with breast cancer representing the second most common malignancy during pregnancy after cervical cancer.[29] A high index of suspicion is needed to make the diagnosis of puerperal breast cancer. Delay in the diagnosis of PABC increases the risk of axillary metastasis. It has been reported that a 1-month delay in treatment in early-stage breast cancer increases the risk of axillary lymph node involvement by 0.9–1.8%, a 3-month delay by 2.6–5.2%, and a 6 month delay by 5.1–10.2% depending on doubling time of 130 vs. 65 days.[30] A recent meta-analysis has shown a less favorable outcome for those diagnosed postpartum than during pregnancy. This may be due to the difficulty in making the diagnosis during pregnancy.[31]

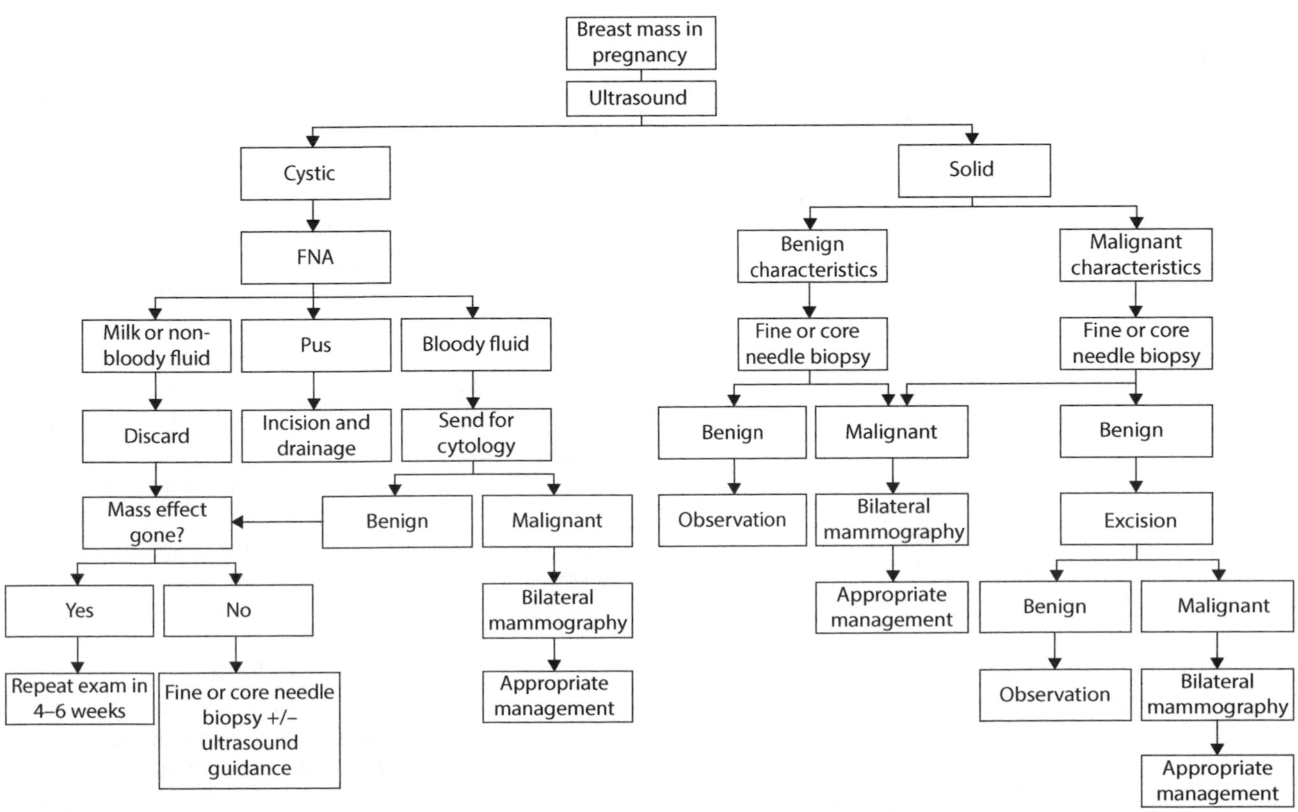

Figure 36.1 Management algorithm for breast masses in pregnancy. FNA: Fine needle aspiration.

Since ultrasound is often used as the primary imaging modality for the evaluation of breast masses during pregnancy, it is important to note that the imaging features of suspicious masses include an increased posterior acoustic enhancement and large cystic components.[32] Other suspicious ultrasound findings include spiculated masses with heterogeneous internal echoes.

PRETHERAPEUTIC STAGING

Preoperative staging begins with a complete physical examination, which includes the size of the lesion, presence of palpable axillary, and/or supraclavicular lymph nodes. Axillary lymph nodes are the most important prognostic determinant for survival in breast cancer. The presence of a palpable supraclavicular lymph node requires a core needle biopsy or open biopsy since that is at the minimum a stage IIIC breast cancer. By using the clinical tumor, node, metastasis (TNM) staging system (Tables 36.4 and 36.5), appropriate workup for breast cancer can be ordered for a metastatic workup. The workup for PABC is the same as for nonpregnant patients, for clinical stage I or II; the only studies required besides the clinical examination are a chest X-ray and liver function tests. For clinical stage III, an MRI examination may be needed as the incidence of metastasis justifies its risk.

Table 36.4 Clinical TNM staging of breast cancer.

Tis: carcinoma in situ
T1: tumor ≤ 2 cm
T2: tumor > 2 cm but ≤ 5 cm
T3: tumor > 5 cm
T4: tumor of any size with skin or chest wall involvement
N0: no palpable axillary lymph nodes
N1: palpable mobile axillary lymph nodes
N2: palpable fixed axillary lymph nodes
N3: palpable supraclavicular lymph nodes
M0: no metastasis
M1: metastatic disease present

Source: NCCN Clinical Practice Guidelines in Oncology: Breast Cancer. V 1.2016. National Comprehensive Cancer Network. With permission

Abbreviations: T: tumor; N: nodes; M: metastasis.

Table 36.5 Clinical stage grouping of breast cancer.

T	N	M	Stage
1	0	0	I
1	1	0	IIA
2	0	0	
2	1	0	IIB
3	0	0	
1	2	0	IIIA
2	2	0	
3	1	0	
3	2	0	
3	0–2	0	IIIB
Any	3	0	IIIC
Any	Any	1	IV

Source: NCCN Clinical Practice Guidelines in Oncology: Breast Cancer. V 1.2016. National Comprehensive Cancer Network. With permission.

TREATMENT

The treatment goals of PABC are different than in the nonpregnant patient because exposure to radiation therapy and endocrine therapy is usually contraindicated during pregnancy. Selective chemotherapy may be permitted after the first trimester.[33] A subsequent pregnancy should be avoided for 2 years after completion of chemotherapy. Therefore, the primary treatment for resectable breast cancer is surgical removal. The goals of surgery include the removal of the lesion with mastectomy or lumpectomy followed by radiation therapy (generally reserved for patients with findings of breast cancer in mid to late third trimester); lymph node staging must be performed at the time of the initial operation for appropriate TNM clinical staging. Lymph node staging can be performed by sentinel lymph node biopsy (SLNB), with radioactive tracer injection and/or blue dye. Isosulfan blue has a small, ~1%, severe risk of maternal allergic reaction and it is not used frequently. SLNB while once thought to be contraindicated during pregnancy has been demonstrated to be relatively safe with low prenatal doses of radiation and does not increase the risk of prenatal malformation or death.[34] Positive SLNB or palpable axillary nodes require level I and II axillary node dissection.

Chemotherapy during pregnancy requires the understanding that there are several critical periods during gestation: days 8–14 from conception correspond to the all-or-none phenomenon during which survival from exposure during this period does not result in congenital defects. During the organogenesis period (weeks 2–8 from conception) fetal exposure to potentially toxic compounds may have teratogenic effects. From week 8 onward is the fetal phase, during which selective chemotherapy is generally considered safe but may be associated with an increased risk of intrauterine growth restriction, prematurity, low birth weight, and bone marrow toxicity.[35] Indications for the use of chemotherapy in PABC patients are similar to those of nonpregnant patients (those with tumor size over 1 cm with poorly differentiated or hormone receptor negative and or those with lymph node metastasis). As most PABC are hormone receptor negative, chemotherapy is used more frequently than hormonal therapy. The most common chemotherapy agents used are 5-fluorauracil, doxorubicin, and cyclophosphamide. In an attempt to devise a standardized protocol for the management of breast cancer during pregnancy (Figure 36.2), one study demonstrated no congenital malformations or immediate postpartum deficits.[36] Subsequent pregnancy should be allowed 2 years after the completion of chemotherapy.

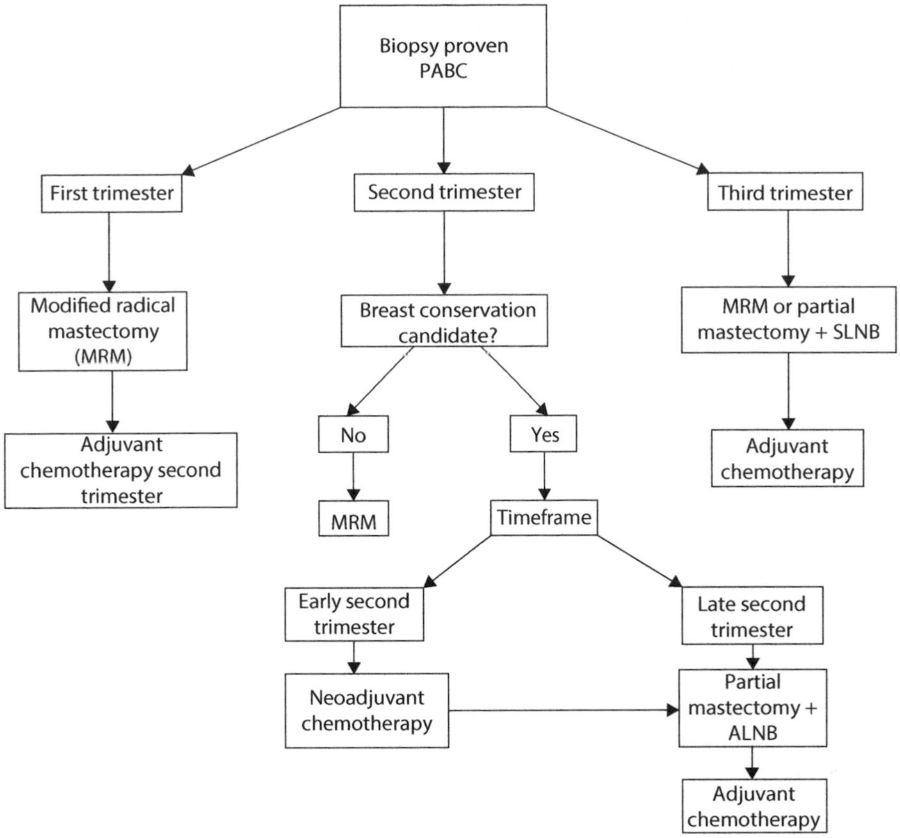

Figure 36.2 Management of breast cancer during pregnancy.

FUTURE PREGNANCY IN BREAST CANCER SURVIVORS

The issue of childbearing ability becomes an important issue to discuss with PABC patients. Factors including chemotherapy agents used, total dose of agent given, and patient's age are the most significant risk factors for ovarian dysfunction. For example, amenorrhea decreases with anthracycline-based adjuvant chemotherapy, whereas cyclophosphamide/methotrexate/5-fluorauracil combination regimen has an increased risk of amenorrhea. In some patients over the age of 40, amenorrhea was found to be irreversible.[37] More importantly, multiple studies have demonstrated that subsequent pregnancies do not increase the risk of recurrence to the mother and the risk of mortality is not increased in the mother or the offspring.

MELANOMA

The workup and management for malignant melanoma are the same during pregnancy as in nonpregnant females. Suspicious lesions often follow the "ABCDE rule": Asymmetry, border irregularity, color variation throughout, diameter greater than 1 cm, and evolution of the lesion over time. With smaller lesions an excisional biopsy is usually performed; with larger lesions, a full-thickness punch biopsy will provide the most information. The strongest predictive factor for survival with melanoma is tumor thickness, since it is correlated with lymph node metastasis. The Breslow thickness of the melanoma suggests the size of the margins to be taken as 0.5 cm for in situ lesions, 1 cm for less than 1 mm thickness, and 2 cm margins for tumors greater than 1 mm in thickness. Examination of lymph nodes should occur; patients with palpable lymph nodes should undergo lymphadenectomy. Tumors with a thickness size larger than 1 mm with no palpable nodes require a SLNB (as discussed in the section on PABC). SLNB is a safe procedure needed for staging. Clinical staging by Breslow thickness, presence of ulceration, nodal metastasis, and metastasis of melanoma is via TNM system (Tables 36.6 and 36.7).[38]

In a large study, the overall occurrence rate of cutaneous malignant melanoma was 8.5 per 100,000 pregnant women. Overall, there were no statistical differences between pregnancy-associated malignant melanoma and melanoma in a nonpregnant control as to incidence, tumor thickness, metastasis rate, to lymph nodes.[39]

Epidemiologic evidence points to a decreased risk of melanoma in women with earlier age at first birth and multiparous vs. nulliparous and the time since the most recent birth as unrelated to the risk of cutaneous malignant melanoma.[40] Of note, pregnant patients with stage IV disease should have a pathologic evaluation of the placenta because metastasis occurs in 31% of malignant melanomas. In those with placental involvement, the risk of fetal involvement is 22%.[41]

LYMPHOMA

The signs and symptoms of lymphoma during pregnancy are similar to those in nonpregnant females. The diagnosis of lymphoma requires a lymph node biopsy for

Table 36.6 TNM staging categories for cutaneous melanoma.

Classification	Thickness (mm)	Ulceration status/mitoses
T		
Tis	NA	NA
T1	≤1.00	a: Without ulceration and mitosis <1/mm^2 b: With ulceration or mitoses ≥1/mm^2
T2	1.01–2.00	a: Without ulceration b: With ulceration
T3	2.01–4.00	a: Without ulceration b: With ulceration
T4	>4.00	a: Without ulceration b: With ulceration
N	**No. of Metastatic Nodes**	**Nodal Metastatic Burden**
N0	0	NA
N1	1	a: Micrometastasis[a] b: Macrometastasis[b]
N2	2–3	a: Micrometastasis[a] b: Macrometastasis[b] c: In transit metastases/satellites without metastatic nodes
N3	4+ metastatic nodes, or matted nodes, or in transit metastases/satellites with metastatic nodes	
M	**Site**	**Serum LDH**
M0	No distant metastases	NA
M1a	Distant skin, subcutaneous, or nodal metastases	Normal
M1b	Lung metastases	Normal
M1c	All other visceral metastases	Normal
	Any distant metastases	Elevated

Source: Balch CM et al., *J Clin Oncol*, 27/36, 6199–6206, 2009. With permission.
Abbreviations: NA, not applicable; LDH, lactate dehydrogenase; T, tumor; N, nodes; M, metastasis.
[a] Micrometastases are diagnosed after sentinel lymph node biopsy.
[b] Macrometastases are defined as clinically detectable nodal metastases confirmed pathologically.

pathologic analysis. Staging of the disease includes imaging studies, a CT scan, and positron emission tomography (PET)-CT. The radiation exposure for the mother/fetus is a considerable amount but even if under the 50 mGy limit, it is still a cause of concern and a topic of discussion for both the practitioner and the patient. The prognosis for the patient depends on type and then subtype: Hodgkin's lymphoma (HL) vs. non-Hodgkin's lymphoma (NHL). There are two factors to balance in pregnant patients with lymphoma: chance of cure for the mother and risk to the offspring.

HL increases in frequency during the third decade of life and is the most common form of lymphoma during pregnancy.[42] The current treatment for HL is the four-drug regimen: adriamycin, bleomycin, vinblastine, and dacarbazine. Radiation therapy is limited to women with early stage HL, it is limited to the neck region and it involves proper shielding to the abdomen.[42] Chemotherapy is the mainstay treatment for lymphoma, with the timing of initiation of chemotherapy based on the trimester of pregnancy. Patients are usually not given chemotherapy during the first trimester since the period of organogenesis leads to high teratogenicity rates. Use of chemotherapy agents during the first trimester is associated with spontaneous abortions and fetal death. Treatment with chemotherapeutic agents during the second and third trimester is associated with preterm delivery, low birth weight, intrauterine growth restriction, and fetal death. However, with advanced stage disease and more aggressive subtypes of HL, delaying chemotherapy until after the first trimester is associated with lower maternal survival. Therefore, the option of elective termination of pregnancy and early initiation of chemotherapy may be advised. Overall, the prognosis of HL during pregnancy is similar compared to that in non-pregnant controls[43] (see Figure 36.3).

NHL is a group of malignancies whose treatment depends on the subtype: indolent, aggressive, and very aggressive. Indolent NHL includes follicular lymphoma, chronic lymphocytic leukemia, and marginal

Table 36.7 Anatomic group stagings for cutaneous melanoma.

	Clinical staging[a]				Pathologic staging[b]		
	T	N	M		T	N	M
0	Tis	N0	M0	0	Tis	N0	M0
IA	T1a	N0	M0	IA	T1a	N0	M0
IB	T1b	N0	M0	IB	T1b	N0	M0
	T2a	N0	M0		T2a	N0	M0
IIA	T2b	N0	M0	IIA	T2b	N0	M0
	T3a	N0	M0		T3a	N0	M0
IIB	T3b	N0	M0	IIB	T3b	N0	M0
	T4a	N0	M0		T4a	N0	M0
IIC	T4b	N0	M0	IIC	T4b	N0	M0
III	Any T	N > N0	M0	IIIA	T1-4a	N1a	M0
					T1-4a	N2a	M0
				IIIB	T1-4b	N1a	M0
					T1-4b	N2a	M0
					T1-4a	N1b	M0
					T1-4a	N2b	M0
					T1-4a	N2c	M0
				IIIC	T1-4b	N1b	M0
					T1-4b	N2b	M0
					T1-4b	N2c	M0
					Any T	N3	M0
IV	Any T	Any N	M1	IV	Any T	Any N	M1

Source: Balch CM et al., *J Clin Oncol* 27/36, 6199–6206, 2009. With permission

[a] Clinical staging includes microstaging of the primary melanoma and clinical/radiologic evaluation for metastases. By convention, it should be used after complete excision of the primary melanoma with clinical assessment for regional and distant metastases.

[b] Pathologic staging includes microstaging of the primary melanoma and pathologic information about the regional lymph nodes after partial (i.e., sentinel node biopsy) or complete lymphadenectomy. Pathologic stage 0 or stage 1A patients are the exception; they do not require pathologic evaluation of their lymph nodes.

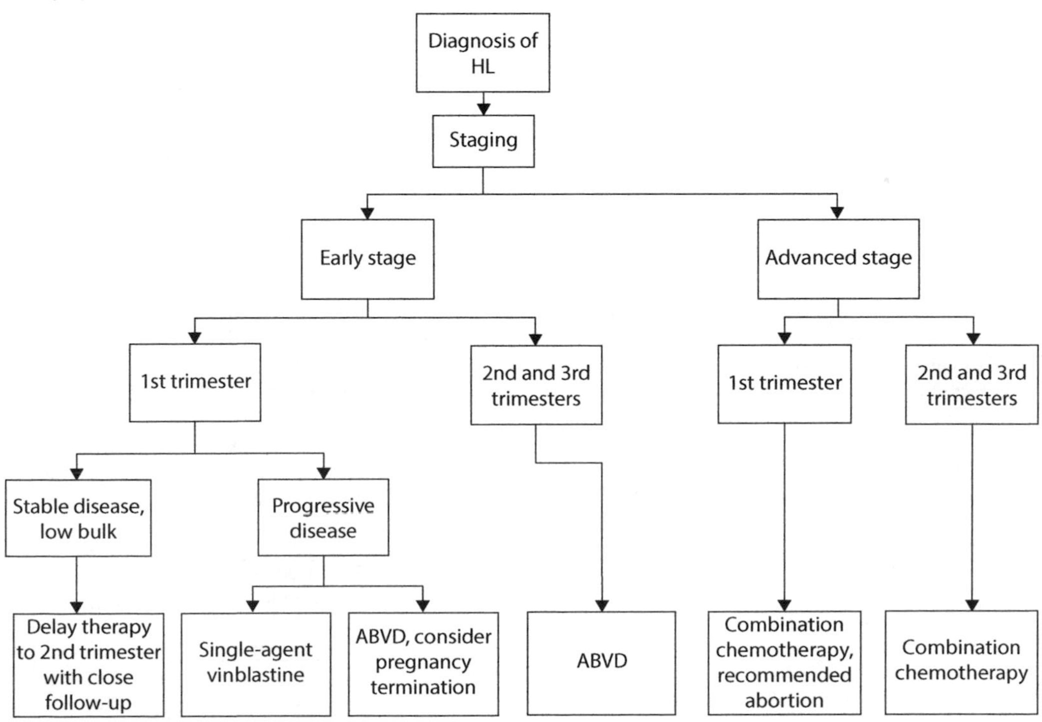

Figure 36.3 Suggested algorithm for HL management during pregnancy. (From Abadi U, Koren G, Lishner M, *Hematology Oncol Clin North Am,* 25(2), 277–291, 2011. With permission.)

zone lymphoma, which is usually diagnosed at an older age and is thus uncommon in pregnancy; it progresses slowly and treatment is dependent upon whether the patient is asymptomatic (watchful waiting is recommended) or symptomatic (a variety of chemotherapy agents are used). Aggressive NHL is the most common subtype and it includes mantle cell lymphoma and diffuse large B-cell lymphoma. Combination chemotherapy with cyclophosphamide, doxorubicin, vincristine, and prednisone (CHOP) is typically used with rituximab added for CD 20-positive tumors. CHOP combination chemotherapy has not been well studied in literature and studies often have contradicting results as to the safety during first and subsequent trimesters. One study found no birth defects in children of pregnant patients given CHOP even during the first trimester[44] and another study found no birth defects with the use of rituximab throughout all trimesters.[45] Very aggressive NHL includes Burkett's lymphoma and B/T-cell lymphoblastic lymphoma, all of which are best described by rapid tumor growth, CNS involvement, risk for tumor lysis syndrome, and relapse. Due to the aggressive and rapidly progressive nature, this subtype of NHL must be treated immediately with diagnosis, the toxicity of agents used especially the teratogenicity of methotrexate may require the option of abortion at early stages of pregnancy (see Figure 36.4).

ENDOCRINE TUMORS

Thyroid masses/differentiated thyroid cancer

Thyroid cancer is the most common endocrine malignancy associated with pregnancy. Survival outcomes, recurrence rates, and thyroid cancer subtypes are similar between pregnant and nonpregnant females.[46] The greatest risk factor for thyroid cancer appears to be ionizing radiation.[47] Increased estrogen production during pregnancy increases the size of the thyroid gland, T3, T4, Thyroid Stimulating Hormone (TSH), and is a risk factor for the development of thyroid nodules both benign and malignant.[48] A family history of thyroid cancer and suspicion for multiple endocrine neoplasia based on multiple malignancies are important in obtaining a history for medullary thyroid cancer.

The workup of thyroid masses during pregnant patients includes a thorough history and physical examination, serum thyroid function testing, and an ultrasound examination of the neck. Fine needle aspiration of the thyroid gland is used for suspicious findings. Ultrasound findings of differentiated thyroid cancer may be hypoechoic areas, irregular margins of the lesion, and fine punctate calcifications. Stable tumors without metastatic nodes or capsular invasion may be followed with serial thyroid ultrasound examinations every trimester[49] and with thyroid function testing every 4 weeks. Indications for surgery include an increase in size of the tumor diameter

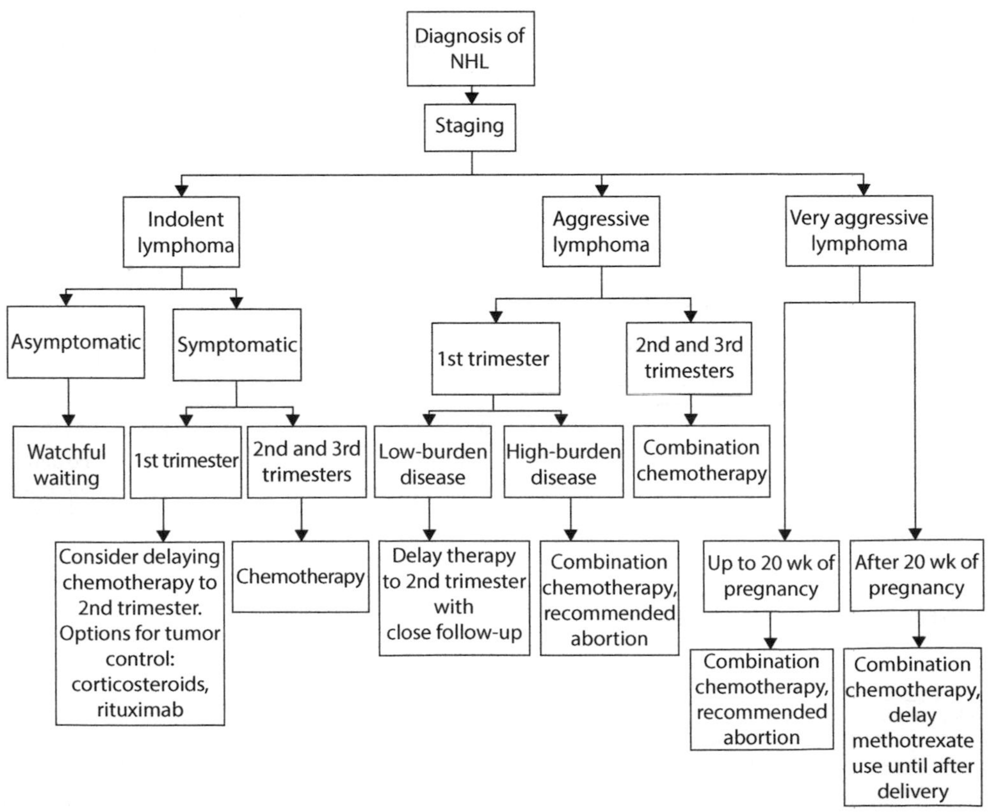

Figure 36.4 Suggested algorithm for NHL management during pregnancy. (From Abadi U, Koren G, Lishner M, *Hematology Oncol Clin North Am,* 25(2), 277–291, 2011. With permission.)

by 20% and volume by 50%, and evidence of metastasis.[50] Most recommendations for the treatment of differentiated thyroid cancer in pregnancy are to postpone treatment until after delivery because the prognosis in pregnant vs. nonpregnant patients is the same and outcomes of surgery during pregnancy and afterwards were similar.[51] However, in patients with medullary cancer, radical surgery including total thyroidectomy, central neck dissection with modified radical neck dissection with palpable nodes should be considered.[52]

Thyroid hormones

Due to the increased serum levels of hormones during pregnancy, the thyroid gland size and hormone levels vary throughout the course of pregnancy than in age-matched nonpregnant controls. Maternal total thyroid hormone levels increase, however, TSH decreases in early pregnancy due to the weak stimulation of TSH receptors by increasing concentrations of human chorionic gonadotropin (hCG) during the first trimester. This decrease in TSH causes secretion of thyroid hormone and increases free T4 levels, causing even further TSH suppression by acting on thyroid releasing hormone (TRH) centrally. However, after the first trimester of pregnancy, TSH levels begin to return to a baseline level and then even increase during the third trimester.[53]

Thyroid hormones have a significant effect on fetal brain development. Maternal thyroxine (T4) crosses the placenta to the fetus throughout gestation[54]; maternal thyroid hormone levels are especially important during the first trimester when the fetal thyroid gland can synthesize thyroid hormone after the 12th week.[55] Both hypothyroidism and hyperthyroidism may have a negative effect on maternal and fetal outcomes.

Hypothyroidism

Studies on dietary iodine deficiency in pregnancy demonstrate that severe maternal and fetal hypothyroidism result in mental retardation and the neurologic defects of spasticity, ataxia, and deaf-mutism; with less severe hypothyroidism only mental retardation resulted.[56] Pregnancies in patients with subclinical hypothyroidism were associated with increasing risk for preterm birth and placental abruption[57] compared to euthyroid patients.

Symptomatic hypothyroidism has nonspecific symptoms that can be difficult to distinguish from some of the usual complaints during pregnancy such as fatigue, cold intolerance, weight gain, and constipation. It is estimated overt hypothyroidism affects up to 3 in 1000 pregnancies.[58] The diagnosis is established by TSH and free T4 serum levels. The goal of treatment is return to euthyroid usually with the prescription of levothyroxine. The TSH level should be measured at 6- to 8-week intervals. While there is no recommendation for routine screening of thyroid levels during pregnancy, it is suggested that women with symptomatology consistent with hypothyroidism undergo testing for TSH and free T3, T4 levels to allow for earlier diagnosis and treatment. Females with a history of hypothyroidism prior to pregnancy should have a serum TSH analysis during their first prenatal visit. In general, levothyroxine requirements increase during early pregnancy and therefore patients on levothyroxine supplementation should have their doses adjusted during pregnancy by having periodic serum TSH monitoring and clinical symptomatology.[59]

Hyperthyroidism

Overt hypothyroidism has an incidence of 1 in 2000 pregnancies. The majority of symptomatic hyperthyroidism during pregnancy is due to Graves' disease. Propylthiouracil or methimizole is the treatment of choice depending on gestational age. The symptoms of hyperthyroidism during pregnancy, much like the symptoms of hypothyroidism may be masked by "normal" symptoms of pregnancy. Hyperthyroidism is associated with heat intolerance, palpitations, nervousness, hyperemesis gravidum, and weight loss/poor weight gain. The diagnosis is established by measurement of serum TSH and free T4 levels. Treatment of hyperthyroidism during pregnancy is associated with improved maternal and fetal outcomes. Thioamides such as propylthiouracil and methimazole are used during pregnancy and each has its risks and benefits; however, both were demonstrated to be equally effective and safe in treating hyperthyroidism during pregnancy.[60]

Radioactive iodine should not be prescribed during pregnancy since it can cross the placenta and permanently damage the fetal thyroid. A large study has demonstrated that euthyroid mothers had better outcomes than those who were still hyperthyroid. Those still hyperthyroid were at increased risk for preterm birth, preeclampsia, fetal growth restriction, maternal heart failure, and pregnancy loss.[61]

Pheochromocytoma

Pheochromocytoma during pregnancy is a rare but potentially fatal condition. The medical literature on the topic is sparse and mostly consists of case reports. Careful assessment of family history is important in pregnant patients with new onset hypertension, multiple endocrine neoplasias IIA, and von Hippel–Lindau and other genetic tumors contributing up to 25% of pheochromocytomas in puerperium. Symptoms and signs are often similar to symptomatology of other medical complications of pregnancy including hypertension, palpitations, headaches, vomiting. Pheochromocytoma is often mistaken for preeclampsia.

Urinary catecholamine levels are not altered by pregnancy but pheochromcytoma can be confirmed by measuring a 24-hour urine vanylmandelic acid (VMA) or catecholamines.[62] Abdominal ultrasound findings may include large, sharp margins, of a solid tumor with or without central necrosis, or hemorrhage in adrenal pheochromocytomas.[63]

Medical therapy is the first choice. It is important to start alpha adrenergic blockade in order to decrease hypertension and reduce mortality. Phenoxybenzamine or prazosin is typically used and safe in pregnancy with beta blockade started once alpha blockers are effective.[64] Surgical treatment depends on the timing of discovery and gestational age. In early pregnancy, an exploratory laparotomy can be performed. Cases discovered in the second trimester can undergo resection once alpha and beta blockade are achieved. In late pregnancy, an exploratory laparotomy and cesarean section can be performed at the same time when fetal maturity is reached. Alternatively, if hypertension is well controlled, vaginal delivery with postpartum resection is possible.

REFERENCES

1. Brown JJ, Wilson C, Coleman S, Joypaul BV. Appendicitis in pregnancy: An ongoing diagnostic dilemma. *Colorectal Dis* 2009; 18: 116–22.
2. Sadot E, Telem DA, Arora M, et al. Laparoscopy: A safe approach during pregnancy. *Surg Endosc* 2010; 24: 383–9.
3. Jelin EB, Smink DS, Vernon AH, Brooks DC, et al. Management of biliary tract disease during pregnancy: A decision analysis. *Surg Endosc* 2008; 22: 54–60.
4. Eddy JJ, Gideonsen MD, Song JY, et al. Pancreatitis in pregnancy: A 10 year retrospective of 15 midwest hospitals. *Obstet Gynecol* 2008; 112: 1075–81.
5. Tang SJ, Mayo MJ, Rodriguez-Frias E, et al. Safety and utility of ERCP during pregnancy. *Gastrointest Endosc* 2009; 69: 453–61.
6. Connolly MM, Unti JA, Nora PF. Bowel obstruction in pregnancy. *Surg Clin North Am* 1995 Feb; 75(1): 101–13.
7. Sadat U, Dar O, Walsh S, Varty K. Splenic artery aneurysms in pregnancy: A systematic review. *Int J Surg* 2008; 6: 261–5.
8. Van der Woude CJ, Ardizzone S, Bengtson MB, et al. The second European evidenced-based consensus on reproduction and pregnancy in inflammatory bowel disease. *J Crohn's Colitis* 2015: 1–15.
9. Chan WS, Rey E, Kent NE. Venous thromboembolism and antithrombotic therapy in pregnancy: SOGC. *Clin Pract Guideline* 2014; 26: 527–53.
10. Greer, I. Thrombosis in pregnancy: Updates in diagnosis and management. *Am Soc Hematol* 2012; 1: 203–7.
11. Wang P, Chong ST, Kielar AZ, et al. Imaging of pregnant and lactating patients. Part I, evidence-based review and recommendations. *AJR* 2012; 198: 778–84.
12. Chen MM, Coakley FV, Kaimal A, Laros RK Jr. Guidelines for computed topography and magnetic resonance imaging use during pregnancy and lactation. *Obstet Gynecol* 2008; 112: 333–40.
13. Jemal A, Siegel R, Xu J, Ward E. Cancer statistics, 2010. *CA Cancer J Clin* 2010; 60: 277–300.
14. Williams, TJ. Turnbull, K. Carcinoma in situ and pregnancy. *Obstet Gynecol* 1964; 24(6): 857–64.
15. Pavlidis NA. Coexistence of pregnancy and malignancy. *Oncologist* 2002; 7(4): 279–87.
16. Hamilton BE, Martin JA, Osterman MJK, et al. Births: Final data for 2014. National vital statistics reports; vol 64 no 12. Hyattsville, MD: National Center for Health Statistics, 2015.
17. Mathews TJ, Hamilton BE. Mean age of mother, 1970–2000. National vital statistics reports; vol 51 no 1. Hyattsville, MD: National Center for Health Statistics, 2002.
18. Smith LH, Danielsen B, Allen ME, Cress R. Cancer associated with obstetric delivery: Results of linkage with the California cancer registry. *Am J Obstet Gynecol* 2003; 189(4): 1128–35.
19. Woo JC, Yu T, Hurd TC. Breast cancer in pregnancy: A literature review. *Archives of Surgery* 2003; 138(1): 91–8.
20. Viswanathan S, Ramaswamy B. Pregnancy-associated breast cancer. *Clin Obstet Gynecol* 2011; 54(4): 546–55.
21. Vashi R, Hooley R, Butler R, Geisel J, Philpotts L. Breast imaging of the pregnant and lactating patient: Imaging modalities and pregnancy-associated breast cancer. *Am J Roentgenol* 2013; 200(2): 321–8.
22. Wang PI, Chong ST, Kielar AZ, et al. Imaging of pregnant and lactating patients: Part 2, evidence-based review and recommendations. *Am J Roentgenol* 2012; 198(4): 785–792.
23. Sechopoulos I, Vedantham S, Suryanarayanan S, D'Orsi CJ, Karellas A. Radiation dose to organs and tissues from mammography: Monte Carlo and phantom study 1. *Radiology* 2008; 246(2): 434–43.
24. American College of Radiology. *ACR Practice Guideline for Imaging Pregnant or Potentially Pregnant Adolescents and Women with Ionizing Radiation.* Reston, VA: American College of Radiology, 2008.
25. Robbins J, Jeffries D, Roubidoux M, Helvie M. Accuracy of diagnostic mammography and breast ultrasound during pregnancy and lactation. *Am J Roentgenol* 2011; 196(3): 716–22.
26. Yang WT, Dryden MJ, Gwyn K, et al. Imaging of breast cancer diagnosed and treated with chemotherapy during pregnancy 1. *Radiology* 2006; 239(1): 52–60.
27. Webb JAW, Thomsen HS. Gadolinium contrast media during pregnancy and lactation. *Acta Radiol* 2013; 54(6): 599–600.
28. Schackmuth EM, Harlow CL, Norton LW. Milk fistula: A complication after core breast biopsy. *AJR. Am J Roentgenol* 1993; 161(5): 961–2.
29. Antonelli NM, Dotters DJ, Katz VL, Kuller JA. Cancer in pregnancy: A review of the literature. Part I. *Obstet Gynecol Surv* 1996; 51(2): 125–34.
30. Nettleton J, Long J, Kuban D, et al. Breast cancer during pregnancy: Quantifying the risk of treatment delay. *Obstet Gynecol*; 87(3): 414–8.
31. Azim HA, Santoro L, Russel-Edu W, et al. Prognosis of pregnancy-associated breast cancer: A meta-analysis of 30 studies. *Cancer Treat Rev* 2012; 38(7): 834–42.

32. Ahn BY, Kim HH, Moon Wk, et al. Pregnancy- and lactation-associated breast cancer mammographic and sonographic findings. *J ultrasound Med* 2003; 22(5): 491–7.
33. Navrozoglou I, Vrekoussis T, Kontostolis E, et al. Breast cancer during pregnancy: A mini-review. *Eur J Surg Oncol (EJSO)* 2008; 34(8): 837–43.
34. Gentilini O, Cremonesi M, Trifirò G, et al. Safety of sentinel node biopsy in pregnant patients with breast cancer. *Ann oncol* 2004; 15(9): 1348–51.
35. Brewer M, Kueck A, Runowicz CD. Chemotherapy in pregnancy. *Clin Obstet Gynecol* 2011; 54(4): 602–18.
36. Berry DL, Theriault RL, Holmes FA, et al. Management of breast cancer during pregnancy using a standardized protocol. *J Clin Oncol* 1999; 17(3): 855–61.
37. Gadducci A, Cosio S, Genazzani AR. Ovarian function and childbearing issues in breast cancer survivors. *Gynecol endocrinol* 2007; 23(11): 625–31.
38. Balch CM, Gershenwald JE, Soong SJ, et al. Final version of 2009 AJCC melanoma staging and classification. *J Clin Oncol* 2009; 27(36): 6199–206.
39. O'Meara AT, Cress R, Xing G, et al. Malignant melanoma in pregnancy. *Cancer* 2005; 1036: 1217–26.
40. Lambe M, Thörn M, Sparén P, et al. Malignant melanoma: Reduced risk associated with early childbearing and multiparity. *Melanoma Res* 1996; 6(2): 147–54.
41. Alexander A, Samlowski WE, Grossman D, et al. Metastatic melanoma in pregnancy: Risk of transplacental metastases in the infant. *J Clin Oncol* 2003; 21(11): 2179–86.
42. Abadi U, Koren G, Lishner M. Leukemia and lymphoma in pregnancy. *Hematology Oncol Clin North Am* 2011; 25(2): 277–91.
43. Lishner M, Zemlickis D, Degendorfer P, et al. Maternal and foetal outcome following Hodgkin's disease in pregnancy. *Br J Cancer* 1992; 65: 114–7.
44. Avilés A, Neri N. Hematological malignancies and pregnancy: A final report of 84 children who received chemotherapy in utero. *Clin Lymphoma* 2001; 2(3): 173–7.
45. Kimby E, Sverrisdottir A, Elinder G. Safety of rituximab therapy during the first trimester of pregnancy: A case history. *Eur J Haematol* 2004; 72(4): 292–5.
46. Herzon FS, Morris DM, Segal MN, et al. Coexistent thyroid cancer and pregnancy. *Arch Otolaryngol Head Neck Surg* 1994; 120(11): 1191–3.
47. Paoff K, Preston-Martin S, Mack WJ, Monroe K. A case-control study of maternal risk factors for thyroid cancer in young women (California, United States). *Cancer Causes Control* 1995; 6(5): 389–97.
48. Derwahl M, Nicula D. Estrogen and its role in thyroid cancer. *Endocr Relat Cancer* 2014; 21(5): T273–83.
49. Stagnaro-Green A, Abalovich M, Alexander E, et al. Guidelines of the American Thyroid Association for the diagnosis and management of thyroid disease during pregnancy and postpartum. *Thyroid* 2011; 21(10): 1081–125.
50. Mazzaferri EL. Approach to the pregnant patient with thyroid cancer. *J Clin Endocrinol Metab* 2011; 96(2): 265–72.
51. Moosa M, Mazzaferri EL. Outcome of differentiated thyroid cancer diagnosed in pregnant women. *J Clin Endocrinol Metab* 1997; 82(9): 2862–6.
52. Massoll N, Mazzaferri EL. Diagnosis and management of medullary thyroid carcinoma. *Clin Lab Med* 2004; 24: 49–83.
53. Kilpatrick SJ. *ACOG Guidelines at a Glance Thyroid Disease in Pregnancy.* San Francisco, CA: American Congress of Obstetricians and Gynecologists, 2015.
54. Bernal J. Thyroid hormone receptors in brain development and function. *Nat Clin Pract Endocrinol Metab* 2007; 3(3): 249–59.
55. Calvo RM, Jauniaux E, Gulbis B, et al. Fetal tissues are exposed to biologically relevant free thyroxine concentrations during early phases of development. *J Clin Endocrinol Metab* 2002; 87(4): 1768–77.
56. Delange F. The disorders induced by iodine deficiency. *Thyroid* 1994; 4(1): 107–28.
57. Casey BM, Dashe JS, Wells CE, et al. Subclinical hypothyroidism and pregnancy outcomes. *Obstet Gynecol* 2005; 105(2): 239–45.
58. Casey BM, Leveno KJ. Thyroid disease in pregnancy. *Obstet Gynecol* 2006; 108(5): 1283–92.
59. Alexander EK, Marqusee E, Lawrence J, et al. Timing and magnitude of increases in levothyroxine requirements during pregnancy in women with hypothyroidism. *N Engl J Med* 2004; 351(3): 241–9.
60. Wing DA, Millar LK, Koonings PP, et al. A comparison of propylthiouracil versus methimazole in the treatment of hyperthyroidism in pregnancy. *Am J Obstet Gynecol* 1994; 170(1): 90–5.
61. Davis LE, Lucas MJ, Hankins GD, et al. Thyrotoxicosis complicating pregnancy. *Am J Obstet Gynecol* 1989; 160(1): 63–70.
62. Ahlawat SK, Jain S, Kumari S, et al. Pheochromocytoma associated with pregnancy: Case report and review of the literature. *Obstet Gynecol Sur*1999; 54(11): 728.
63. Bowerman RA, Silver TM, Jaffe MH, et al. Sonography of adrenal pheochromocytomas. *Am J Roentgenol* 1981; 137(6): 1227–31.
64. Burgess III GE. Alpha blockade and surgical intervention of pheochromocytoma in pregnancy. *Obstet Gynecol* 1979; 53(2): 266–70.

Urologic complications during pregnancy

37

CHARBEL SALAMON

CONTENTS

Pregnancy affects most maternal organ systems and the urinary tract is no exception. The physiologic changes of pregnancy may alter the presentation of many pathologic conditions ranging from urinary tract infections and nephrolithiasis to serious trauma.

Knowledge of the physiologic changes and their effect on the urinary tract is paramount to avoiding under-or overdiagnosis of pregnant women presenting with a urinary tract related complaint. A high index of suspicion is often required to avoid a delay in diagnosis and treatment. The evaluation and management of the pregnant patient may differ significantly from patients experiencing similar urologic complaints in a nonobstetric setting. Thus, a thorough understanding of potential urologic problems encountered during pregnancy is crucial in order to minimize morbidity to the mother and fetus through early recognition and intervention. This chapter will provide a comprehensive review of urologic complications and issues related to pregnancy.

PHYSIOLOGIC CHANGES OF PREGNANCY

Pregnancy affects the entire urinary tract from the kidneys to the urethra.

Renal changes

Both kidneys increase in size and volume during pregnancy. Kidney volume increases by up to 30% due to an increase in renal vascular and interstitial size leading to increase in glomerular filtration without any histological changes in the number of nephrons. Renal adaptations associated with pregnancy include a 30–50% increase in glomerular filtration rate and renal plasma flow.[5] These changes lead to a 25% reduction in serum creatinine and blood urea nitrogen levels. Serum levels of 1,25-dihydroxyvitamin D are found to be elevated during pregnancy, promoting a hypercalciuric state by increasing intestinal absorption of calcium and stimulating urinary calcium excretion.[6] Dilation of the renal pelvis and ureters, which begins by the end of the first trimester and is present in about 90% of women by the third trimester, has been recognized as a physiologic response to mechanical and hormonal changes of pregnancy.

Ureters

This physiologic dilation of the ureters and renal pelvises (pyelouretectasis) occurs only above the pelvic brim. The lower third of the ureters retain a normal caliber despite the fact that they must course around the rapidly enlarging gravid uterus. Hypertrophy of Waldeyer's sheath may prevent hormone-induced dilatation below the pelvic brim. The right ureter is more often affected than the left. In a review of 220 excretory urograms during pregnancy, Schulman and Herlinger reported greater dilation of the right side in 86% of the cases.[1] This is attributed to mechanical pressure at the pelvic brim by the dextrorotation of the pregnant uterus as it rises out of the pelvis, whereas the left ureter is protected by the sigmoid colon.[2] Hormonal changes (high concentrations of progesterone) leading to increased urinary tract compliance and reduced ureteral muscle tone are believed to be primarily responsible for dilation of the upper urinary system during the first trimester.[3,4]

Bladder

The bladder mucosa becomes edematous and hyperemic in pregnancy. The enlarging uterus displaces the bladder superiorly and anteriorly and flattens it. Progesterone-induced bladder flaccidity may cause incompetence of the vesicoureteral valve. This change, combined with increased intravesical and decreased intraureteral pressure, appears to result in intermittent vesicoureteral reflux.

Urinary frequency and nocturia

Urinary frequency (voiding >7 times per day) and nocturia (night time voiding) are among the most common pregnancy-related complaints, affecting over 80% of women at some point during gestation. Frequency appears to be multifactorial, which is in part due to changes in bladder function and in part to an increase in urine output and begins in the first trimester. Nocturia is common and increases with advancing gestation. In a survey of 256 pregnant women, 86% reported nocturia by the third trimester, with 20% of women indicating they voided three or more times at night. The major cause of nocturia appears to be that pregnant women excrete larger amounts of sodium and water during the night than nonpregnant women. In the latter stages of pregnancy, this may be partially attributable to nocturnal mobilization of dependent edema in the lateral position.

Urgency and incontinence—Several studies have described an increase in urgency and urinary incontinence during pregnancy, which may be due to uterine pressure on the bladder, hormonal effects on the suspensory ligaments of the urethra, and/or altered neuromuscular function of the urethral striated sphincter. Urinary incontinence during pregnancy is associated with an increased risk of persistent incontinence 6 months postpartum.

URINARY TRACT INFECTION AND PYELONEPHRITIS

Asymptomatic bacteriuria

Asymptomatic bacteriuria affects 2–7% of all pregnant women.[5,6] Although pregnancy itself is not believed to predispose women to urinary tract infections, approximately 25% of pregnant women with documented asymptomatic bacteriuria without treatment progress to pyelonephritis. Antimicrobial treatment of asymptomatic bacteriuria has been shown to reduce the incidence of pyelonephritis to 3–4%.[8] Prematurity, maternal hypertension, and maternal anemia have been associated with pyelonephritis during pregnancy.[7,8] The guidelines from the Infectious Diseases Society of America and The American College of Obstetricians and Gynecologist recommend routine screening early in pregnancy for asymptomatic bacteriuria. The screening should be through a clean catch urine culture with sensitivities.

A test of cure about 1 week after the completion of therapy is recommended given that up to 30% of women fail to clear asymptomatic bacteriuria. Women with persistent bacteriuria should receive a second course of antibiotics. Consideration should be given for repeat urine cultures at regular intervals throughout the pregnancy in women with persistent or recurrent asymptomatic bacteriuria. Persistent bacteriuria (with the same organism) despite two courses of appropriate antimicrobials might warrant suppressive therapy.

Acute cystitis

Acute cystitis should be suspected in pregnant women with dysuria. Urinary frequency and urgency are frequently present in normal pregnancy and are less reliable although any acute change in symptoms should warrant a culture. The presence of fever and chills, flank pain, and costovertebral angle tenderness should raise suspicion for pyelonephritis. The diagnosis of acute cystitis is confirmed by finding of bacterial growth on urine culture. Prior to confirming the diagnosis, empiric treatment is typically initiated in a patient with consistent symptoms and pyuria on urinalysis. Pyuria is usually present in almost all pregnant women with symptomatic urinary tract infection, and its absence strongly suggests an alternative diagnosis. As with asymptomatic bacteriuria, a follow-up culture should be obtained as a test of cure. In women who have recurrent cystitis during pregnancy, antimicrobial prophylaxis for the duration of pregnancy is a reasonable strategy to prevent additional episodes. Prophylaxis can be postcoital or continuous. In the setting of other conditions that potentially increase the risk of urinary complications during episodes of cystitis (e.g., diabetes or sickle cell trait), prophylaxis following the first episode of cystitis during pregnancy is also reasonable. Daily or postcoital prophylaxis with low dose nitrofurantoin (50–100 mg PO postcoitally or at bedtime) or cephalexin (250–500 mg PO postcoitally or at bedtime) can be used.

An awareness of potential drug toxicities to the mother and fetus is important prior to antibiotic administration (Table 37.1).[9] Recurrent or persistent bacteriuria episodes are associated with an increased risk of structural abnormalities of the urinary tract,[9] and these patients might benefit from further postpartum, urologic workup.

Acute pyelonephritis

Acute pyelonephritis is a manifestation of infection of the upper urinary tract and kidneys. The typical symptoms of acute pyelonephritis include fever (>38°C or 100.4°F), flank pain, nausea, vomiting, and/or costovertebral angle tenderness. Given that pyelonephritis could develop following asymptomatic bacteriuria. Symptoms of cystitis such as dysuria are not always present.

Pregnant women may become quite ill and are at risk for both medical and obstetrical complications from pyelonephritis. It has been estimated that as many as 20% of women with severe pyelonephritis develop complications that include septic shock syndrome or its variants, such as acute respiratory distress syndrome (ARDS).

For pregnant women who present with such symptoms, a urinalysis and urine culture should be obtained. Pyuria is present in the majority of women with pyelonephritis, and its absence suggests an alternative diagnosis or complete obstruction. It is reasonable to obtain blood cultures in those with signs of sepsis or serious underlying medical conditions such as diabetes.

Imaging is not routinely used to diagnose pyelonephritis. However, in patients with pyelonephritis who are severely ill or who also have symptoms of renal colic or history of renal stones, diabetes, history of prior urologic surgery, immunosuppression, repeated episodes of pyelonephritis, or urosepsis, imaging of the kidneys can be helpful to evaluate for complications. In pregnant women, renal ultrasound is the preferred imaging modality in order to avoid contrast or radiation exposure.

Management of acute pyelonephritis in pregnant women includes hospital admission for parenteral antibiotics. Antibiotic therapy can be converted to an oral regimen tailored to the susceptibility profile of the isolated organism following clinical improvement. Following the treatment course, suppressive antibiotics are typically used for the remainder of the pregnancy to prevent recurrence.

NEPHROLITHIASIS DURING PREGNANCY

The overall incidence of urolithiasis during pregnancy is estimated to be one in 1500 pregnancies,[17] which approximates the incidence in nonpregnant women of childbearing age.[22] Although 50–80% of stones in pregnant women pass spontaneously, 23 urinary calculi must be taken seriously, as they have been associated with premature labor.[21,20] Although right-sided hydronephrosis is more commonly identified during pregnancy, multiple investigators report equivalent stone rates bilaterally.[21] Approximately 90% of urinary stones occur during the second and third trimesters, making it a rare occurrence in the first trimester.

Clinical presentation

There is little difference in the presentation of urinary colic between the pregnant and nonpregnant females. Complaints of flank or abdominal pain, nausea, vomiting, dysuria, frequency, urgency, or any combination of the above are customary. In the setting of calculi, the incidence of hematuria is 50–75%. Mechanical and hormonal changes have both been found to cause vascular dilation of the ureter and renal pelvis, leading to bleeding. Therefore, hematuria alone is not enough to make the diagnosis. A thorough past medical history is vital to an accurate and timely diagnosis. Some 35–40% of patients were found to have prior urologic procedures or a history of stone disease.[21,22] Fever is not infrequent, but it is a more ominous sign and must be monitored closely. Physicians should maintain a high index of suspicion for obstructing urinary calculi, especially in patients diagnosed with pyelonephritis who fail to defervesce after at least 48 hours

Table 37.1 Potential toxicity of antibiotics during pregnancy

Drug	Fetal	Maternal
Aminoglycosides	CNS toxicity, ototoxicity	Ototoxicity, nephrotoxicity
Cephalosporins	–	–
Chloramphenicol	Gray syndrome	Bone marrow toxicity
Clindamycin	–	Pseudomembranous colitis
Erythromycins	–	–
Isoniazide	Neuropathy, seizures	Hepatotoxicity
Metronidazole	–	Blood dyscrasia
Nitrofurantoin	G6PD hemolysis	Neuropathy, interstitial pneumonia
Penicillin	–	–
Quinolones	Bone growth malformation	–
Sulfonamides	G6PD hemolysis, kernicterus	–
Tetracycline	Tooth dysplasia, bone growth inhibition	Hepatotoxicity, renal failure
Trimethoprim/sulfamethoxazole	Folate depletion	Vasculitis

of intravenous antibiotic therapy. Peritoneal signs found on abdominal examination should raise suspicion of non-urologic etiology; differential diagnoses include appendicitis, pyelonephritis, cholecystitis, small and large bowel disease, and ovarian and uterine etiology.

Diagnosis

Numerous diagnostic tests, including standard radiography, ultrasound, computed tomography (CT), and magnetic resonance imaging (MRI), have been used to help identify stones during pregnancy.

Ultrasound appears particularly attractive as a first-line intervention because of the avoidance of radiation. With hydronephrosis of pregnancy being extremely common, ultrasound is nonspecific for obstruction when calculi are not clearly identified.[21] Using color Doppler, some have associated the lack of ureteral jets,[24] or the presence of a dilated ureter below the iliac artery with obstruction.[32] Shokeir et al. reported on 22 pregnant patients, using elevated renal resistive index to diagnose unilateral obstruction with sensitivity and specificity of 45% and 91%, respectively.[25] Transvaginal ultrasound may aid in identifying calculi in the distal ureter or in the ureterovesical junction.

Magnetic resonance (MR) urography has also been used to differentiate the physiologic hydronephrosis of pregnancy from pathologic obstruction with good results.[26] MRI has not been found to cause cellular mutagenesis and is believed to be safe during pregnancy.

Low-dose computed tomography (CT) can be used in the second and third trimester but not in the first trimester, when the fetus is most susceptible to radiation-induced injury. Some evidence suggests that low-dose CT is highly sensitive and specific for the detection of renal and ureteral calculi in pregnant women and confers a low risk of fetal harm.

Treatment

Given the high rates of spontaneous stone passage, the initial management should be conservative with hydration, antiemetics, and adequate pain control. The use of nonsteroidal anti-inflammatories (NSAIDs) may cause constriction of the fetal ductus arteriosus and should be restricted especially after 32 weeks' gestation. Alternative pain management medications include acetaminophen and opioids.

Immediate surgical intervention is warranted in cases complicated by sepsis, intractable pain, renoureteral colic precipitating premature labor, a solitary kidney, or bilateral ureteral obstruction. Endoscopic ureteral stenting is part of the urologist's routine stone management armamentarium. Local or intravenous sedation is usually sufficient. Ultrasound has replaced fluoroscopy in many institutions to confirm accurate stent placement.[27] Hyperuricosuria and absorptive hypercalciuria found during pregnancy may cause accelerated encrustation, requiring more frequent stent exchanges every 4–6 weeks until delivery.[28]

There are few studies evaluating extracorporeal shock wave lithotripsy (ESWL) during pregnancy. More studies are required, but the present literature raises serious concerns about ESWL treatment during pregnancy and should be considered experimental.

Innovative techniques and technological advances have made an astounding impact on the field of endourology in recent years. Originally, some believed that the ureter of the pregnant female would be difficult to navigate secondary to distortion.[29] In reality, physiologic hydroureteronephrosis may make ureteroscopy easier. Over the past decade, a number of reports have supported the use of rigid and flexible ureteroscopy to treat pregnant women with calculi.[19,22,25,27,30,30–34] Modern ureteroscopes are less traumatic, and ureteroscopy may often be performed without fluoroscopy[35] or dilation of the ureteral orifice.[30] The majority of urologists maintain a temporary ureteral stent in place for 1–4 days after ureteroscopy. Some authorities prefer holmium:YAG laser lithotripsy to electrohydraulic lithotripsy for its low peak pressures.[36] Furthermore, some avoid using ultrasonic lithotripsy for fear of causing hearing injury to the fetus.[33] Continuous fetal monitoring may be maintained at all times throughout the operative procedure. Ureteroscopy may also assist in differentiating ureteral colic from pain related to physiologic hydronephrosis. Ulvik et al. detailed ureteroscopy in 24 pregnant patients.[33] In 48% of those cases, urinary calculi were not identified. Without undergoing ureteroscopy, these patients might have suffered from a stent or nephrostomy tube for the remainder of their pregnancy without justification. To date, no major complications from ureteroscopy have been reported. Minor complications include fever in three patients (two had preoperative urinary tract infections) and one ureteral perforation managed with a ureteral stent.[33] Relative contraindications to ureteroscopy include an inexperienced ureteroscopist, inadequate endoscopic instruments, stone burden greater than 1 cm, multiple calculi, transplanted kidney, sepsis, and a solitary kidney.[37] Overall, ureteroscopy has been shown to be a safe and effective procedure for the diagnosis and treatment of urinary calculi in the pregnant patient.

HYDROURETERONEPHROSIS AND SPONTANEOUS RENAL RUPTURE

Mechanical obstructive uropathy may cause acute pain, hypertension, or even acute renal failure.[8–10] Spontaneous rupture of the kidney or collecting system is a rare event, often presenting with flank pain, hematuria, hypotension, an expanding flank mass, or signs of an acute abdomen.[11] If unrecognized, rupture may lead to catastrophic consequences, including maternal shock and intrauterine fetal demise. Rupture associated with hydronephrosis of pregnancy is often preceded by abnormally massive dilation, repeated episodes of pyelonephritis, or a history of prior renal disease causing inelastic or scarred renal parenchyma. Oesterling et al. described 16 cases of spontaneous rupture during pregnancy: 10 cases of collecting system rupture and six cases of renal parenchymal rupture.[12] Five cases occurred in the second trimester and 11 were diagnosed during the third trimester or immediately postpartum. Only three cases involved the left kidney, all of which had preexisting renal disease. Of the six cases with parenchymal rupture, five were managed with a nephrectomy and one patient died prior to surgery. In contrast, only 4 of the 10 patients with renal pelvic rupture underwent nephrectomy. The remainder of patients were managed conservatively with successful renal salvage and appropriate internal (five) or external (one) drainage.

The greatest risk of renal rupture occurs between week 18 of gestation and the immediate postpartum period. A conservative approach with bed rest in the contralateral decubitus position should be attempted in cases recognized early. Symptomatic hydronephrosis can be managed with early urinary diversion, utilizing a percutaneous nephrostomy or internal ureteral stent. Since renal cell carcinoma is the most common renal neoplasm during pregnancy, and spontaneous rupture is possible, postpartum radiographic studies are important in those treated with successful renal salvage. Asymptomatic angiomyolipomas have the propensity to grow rapidly during pregnancy.[15] Therefore, to avoid the risk of spontaneous rupture, some have suggested that women who intend to conceive should undergo prophylactic angioembolization for tumors greater than 4 cm.[16]

PREVIOUS BLADDER AUGMENTATION OR URINARY DIVERSION

There is limited experience regarding pregnancy in patients with urinary diversion or bladder augmentation. Chronic bacteriuria and recurring urinary tract infections are common in this patient population. Hill and Kramer found that urinary tract infections or pyelonephritis developed in 9 of out 15 pregnancies.[38] Therefore, some recommend antibiotic prophylaxis with routine urine cultures to decrease the risk of serious infectious episodes.[39–41] Close monitoring of renal function with routine blood work and monthly renal ultrasounds is important.

Obstetric indications should determine the preferred route of delivery. However, cesarean section should be considered in cases with artificial sphincter placement or bladder neck reconstruction.[32,38] However, during cesarean section, injury to the vascular pedicle of the cystoplasty is possible. To avoid this complication, a high uterine incision rather than a low transverse incision should be used. Urologic consultation may prove invaluable in complicated cases.

UROLOGIC MALIGNANCY

Malignancy during pregnancy is an uncommon occurrence with an estimated incidence of approximately one per 1000 gestations.[42] Although the pregnant female undergoes immunologic changes that enable the fetus to survive, there is little evidence that pregnancy exacerbates the malignant course.[23]

Renal malignancy

Renal cell carcinoma, followed by angiomyolipoma, is the most common renal lesion discovered during pregnancy. Flank mass or hematuria is the presenting symptom in 88% and 47% of pregnant patients with renal tumors, respectively.[43] Diagnostic evaluations of renal lesions during pregnancy are similar to nephrolithiasis and include ultrasound or MRI. Management strategies for suspicious renal tumors are usually based upon the stage of pregnancy, but cases must be individualized according to the wishes of the mother. Most agree that a nephrectomy is warranted if renal malignancy is discovered in the first trimester and that surgery should be postponed until after delivery if the diagnosis is made in the third trimester.[44] Differences of opinion exist regarding second-trimester treatment. Some hold that one should postpone surgery until the third trimester,[45] while others advocate waiting until later gestation with testing for fetal lung maturity, and then proceeding with nephrectomy.[44] In this way, the morbidity of premature delivery is reduced.

Bladder malignancy

Fewer than 30 cases of bladder cancer diagnosed during pregnancy have been reported in the literature. Therefore, physicians must be diligent to workup hematuria not explained by other benign causes with cystoscopy and renal ultrasound. Cystoscopy may be performed throughout pregnancy. Some have even suggested that a well-performed bladder ultrasound can replace cystoscopy.[44] If present bladder tumors should be resected transurethrally. Low-grade lesions may be followed, while high-grade lesions with muscle involvement may require cystectomy.

URINARY TRACT INJURY

Obstetrical injuries to the urinary tract are usually related to the delivery process.

Urethral injury

Urethral injuries during pregnancy are almost exclusively related to vaginal delivery. In the developing world, obstructed labor leads to ischemia and subsequent fistulization. These injuries are almost never seen in developed countries with attended hospital deliveries. Precipitous deliveries and operative vaginal deliveries might be associated in rare instances with urethral lacerations that require significant repair.

Bladder injury

About a third of all deliveries in the United States are performed by cesarean section,[47] the overwhelming majority of obstetric urinary tract injuries occur during this procedure. The most important concept pertaining to urinary tract injury occurring during surgery is to maintain a high index of suspicion. Injuries discovered intraoperatively may be repaired immediately to minimize morbidity, while injuries identified in a delayed fashion may have devastating consequences, such as fistula formation.

The reported incidence of bladder injury during cesarean section ranges from 0.0016% to 0.94%.[47] Eisenkop et al.

reported a higher incidence of cystotomies during repeat than primary cesarean section: 0.6% and 0.19%, respectively. In that review of 52 bladder injuries, prior cesarean section with "dense bladder adhesions" was cited as the most common factor associated with bladder injury.[48] In one large study, 75% (12/16) of cystotomies took place during emergent cesarean section.[46]

In performing a cesarean section, all of the aforementioned risk factors should be considered. The peritoneal cavity should be entered at the superior most portion of the incision, particularly in patients with prior surgery. Even in emergent conditions, a disciplined approach should be followed. Bladder drainage with an indwelling catheter is valuable. By preventing the gravid uterus from displacing the bladder superiorly, a urethral catheter may help avoid bladder injury upon entering the abdomen. In obtaining hemostasis, blind suturing or clamping should be strictly discouraged. Rather, the bleeding area should be compressed until identification of bleeding vessels and their anatomic relationship to the bladder and ureters is determined. If significant dissection occurs in the vicinity of the bladder, a thorough evaluation of bladder integrity must be performed.

The instillation of sterile dye such as methylene blue or indigo carmine into the bladder through a urethral catheter is the easiest method to detect bladder injuries. Once the diagnosis of a bladder injury is made, the limits of the defect should be clearly defined and all devitalized tissue debrided.

Ureteral injury

The incidence of ureteral injury during cesarean section ranges from 0.027% to 0.09%.[46,48] Both of these major studies reported equal injury rates in comparing the left and right ureters; however, others have found the left ureter to be more vulnerable.[49,50] Fortunately, the overall incidence of ureteral injuries is decreasing.[51] Intraoperative diagnosis of ureteral injury during cesarean section ranges from 25% to 71%. Injuries initially missed were usually diagnosed within 14 days. The predominant belief is that ureteral injuries result from hemostatic attempts at uterine incisions that extend into the broad ligament.[51] In a study evaluating 21 iatrogenic ureteral injuries from obstetric and gynecologic etiologies, Meirow et al. associated enlarged uteri, adhesions in the pelvis, and significant haemorrhage with ureteral damage.[50] A complete understanding of pelvic anatomy and the course of the ureter is essential in the prevention of operative ureteral injury. As with bladder injuries, any suspicion of a ureteral injury requires a thorough evaluation.

Intraoperative recognition

Several modalities have been described to assess ureteral integrity intraoperatively. A diagnostic cystoscopy followed by intravenous injection of methylene blue has been used to identify ureteral injuries. One should observe equal efflux of urine bilaterally. Urine flow asymmetry may suggest partial obstruction, and further evaluation by performing a retrograde ureterogram and passing ureteral catheters in a retrograde fashion may be performed. Time should also be taken to look for blue dye in the retroperitoneal space.

Delayed postoperative recognition

The most critical principle of making the postoperative diagnosis of urinary tract injury is to have a high index of suspicion, since early symptoms and signs may be subtle. Any suspicion of injury should be promptly investigated. Early diagnosis facilitates management of the injury and speeds recovery. Some signs and symptoms may alert the clinician to the possibility of a missed injury. Bladder injuries may present with oliguria, fever, suprapubic pain, abdominal distention, ileus, gross hematuria, or vaginal watery secretions. In addition to these findings, ureteral injuries may also present with flank tenderness and hydronephrosis. Numerous types of genitourinary fistulas are common with bladder and ureteral defects. Neuman et al. reviewed 30 years of experience with ureteral injuries and found urinary leakage (44%), pain (33%), fever (5%), and urosepsis (12%) to be the most common presenting symptoms.[51]

Bladder repair

Depending upon the experience and comfort level of the obstetrician, urology involvement may not be necessary for simple cystotomies. For more complicated repairs, intraoperative urology consultation is recommended. Fortunately, most cystotomies do not involve the ureteral orifices or trigone and a simple closure is satisfactory.

For simple cystotomies, a running or interrupted closure of the mucosa with 3–0 Vicryl suture followed by a running, imbricating stitch of the muscularis with 2–0 Vicryl suture can be used. A running third layer to reapproximate the serosa could be performed as well. Suturing the mucosa layer separately appears to minimize bleeding from mucosal edges. Use of nonabsorbable suture is contraindicated, as it may function as a nidus for calculi or infection. Filling the bladder dye such as methylene blue allows the closure to be evaluated to determine whether additional sutures are needed. For simple cystotomies a urethral catheter remains for approximately 7 days. A voiding cystourethrogram prior to catheter removal is not required. No further antibiotic prophylaxis is needed beyond the preoperative ones.

Complicated bladder injuries that involve the ureteral orifices or bladder trigone should be closely evaluated for ureteral injury, a diagnostic cystoscopy with confirmation of bladder and ureteral integrity should be performed at the conclusion of the bladder repair.

Ureteral repair

Like bladder injuries, management of ureteral injuries depends upon the time of diagnosis, location, and extent of injury. Intraoperative discovery and repair are almost always preferred to delayed correction to avert the cost and morbidity of subsequent procedures.

Distal ureteral injuries may occur secondary to improperly placed sutures. If the tissue has not been devitalized, they may be managed simply by removal of the offending agent and retrograde placement of an 8F double-J stent.

The Foley catheter and stent are usually removed at 1 and 2 weeks, respectively.

Transection or "crush" injuries of the ureter within 5 cm of the bladder are most definitively managed with ureteroneocystotomy. Lead better Politano is an intravesical technique that involves creating a submucosal tunnel to create a "flap valve" and prevent reflux. The ureter enters the bladder superiorly for a distance of 2–3 cm, is tunneled under the mucosa, and anastomosed directly to the bladder mucosa with interrupted absorbable sutures. Extravesical approaches, such as the Lich-Gregoire, involve incision of the detrusor muscle to create a trough for the ureter, followed by mucosal anastomosis and subsequent closure of the trough to create an antirefluxing mechanism. Regardless of the reimplantation technique anastamosis of bladder mucosa to ureteral mucosa and a tension-free anastamosis must be performed and a temporary ureteral stent is usually placed.

Ureteral injuries 5–10 cm above the bladder can still be managed with a ureteroneocystotomy; however, a psoas hitch is often required to allow the ureter sufficient length for a tension-free anastamosis.[52] This procedure mobilizes the bladder upward and secures it to the psoas fascia with absorbable suture. In some circumstances when additional length is needed, a Boari flap may be used. This technique, as shown in Figure 37.1, swings a flap of ipsilateral bladder cranially to meet the distal portion of ureter. Very rarely, when none of the above procedures are possible, transureteroureterostomy may be performed, as shown in Figure 37.2. In all cases of ureteral reimplantation, an abdominal drain, ureteral stent, and urethral catheter are left in place.

Proximal ureteral injuries are extremely rare during cesarean section. In such cases, ureteroureterostomy is often the procedure of choice. The ureteral edges are debrided, spatulated obliquely with Pott's scissors on opposite sides, and then reattached in an interrupted fashion, using 4-0 or 5-0 chromic suture (Figure 37.3). An abdominal drain, stent, and catheter are left in place. Other options for managing proximal ureteral injuries include autotransplantation or interposition of a segment of ileum.

Delayed repair

The management of ureteral injuries discovered postoperatively is more controversial.

A defect discovered within 7–10 days of delivery in an otherwise uncomplicated patient may still undergo

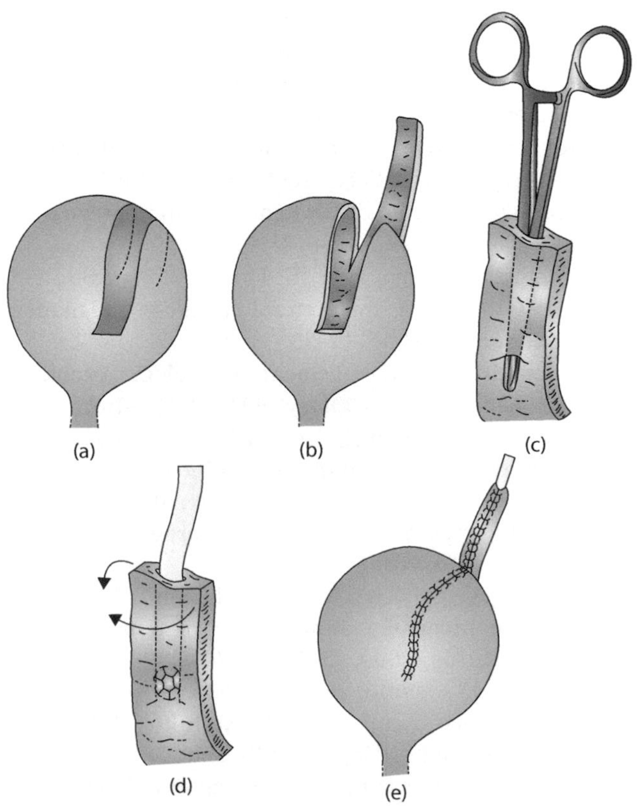

Figure 37.1 Ureteroneocystotomy utilizing a Boari flap.

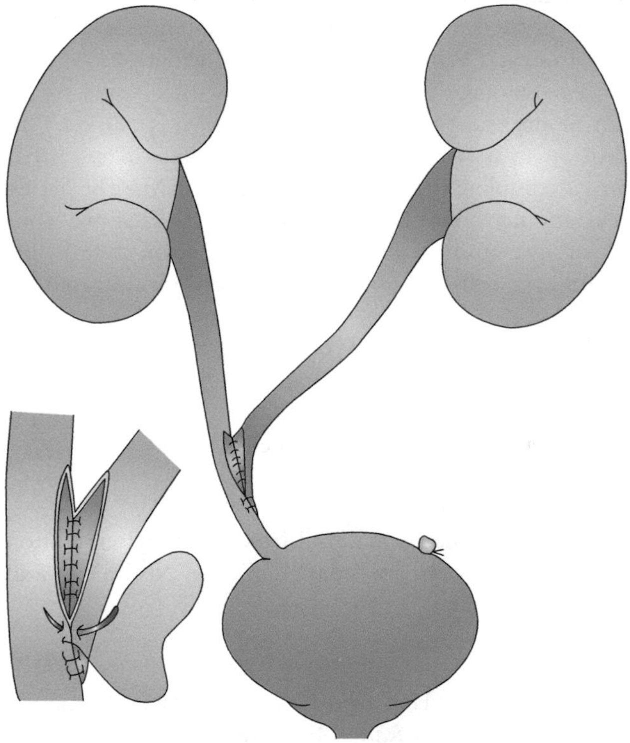

Figure 37.2 Transureteroureterostomy.

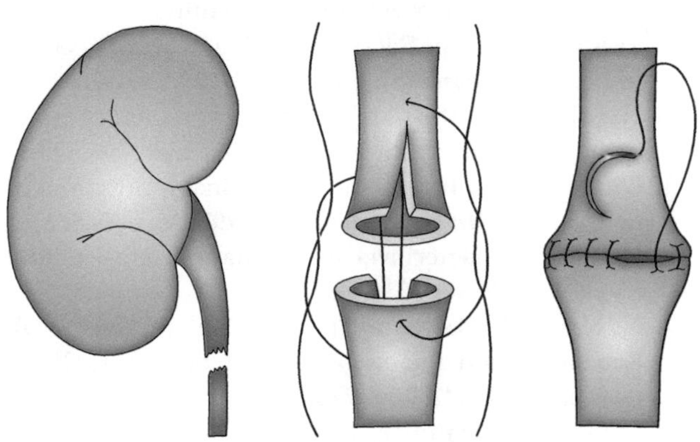

Figure 37.3 Ureteroureterostomy.

immediate repair at that time.[47] Early immediate intervention may save the patient significant morbidity that is associated with delayed repair. One cannot stress enough the value of intraoperative discovery and repair of the injury. A high index of suspicion is paramount to early diagnosis and immediate repair, if not intraoperative, at least within a couple of days and prior to discharge.

Others support urinary diversion with a percutaneous nephrostomy tube followed by future definitive repair. In a review of over 300 genitourinary fistulas from 1970 to 1985, Lee et al. stated that definitive repair should be delayed for 8–12 weeks.[53] This allows edema and inflammation to subside, tissue to regain its blood supply, prior suture material to disintegrate, and tissue planes to be more easily dissected. Time may even prove to be therapeutic, as one study found that 4 out of 21 cases of ureteral obstruction spontaneously resolved after urinary diversion because of absorbed suture material.[50]

One of the most devastating consequences of urinary tract injury is genitourinary fistula formation. While a small percentage of fistulas resolve with urinary diversion alone, the vast majority requires reoperation.[53] In addition to a thorough history and physical examination, a complete diagnostic workup to define the fistula location and characteristics is necessary. This may consist of dye studies, cystography, CT scan, endoscopic evaluation, retrograde pyelogram, and/or intravenous pyelogram.

A comprehensive review of genitourinary fistula repair is beyond the scope of this chapter; however, we strongly encourage a team approach with involvement of multiple specialties to confront these challenging issues.

ACKNOWLEDGMENT

This chapter contains material from the previous edition chapter co-authored by Stuart S. Kesler, Neel Shah, and Jonathan J. Hwang.

REFERENCES

1. Schulman A, Herlinger H. Urinary tract dilatation in pregnancy. *Br J Radiol* 1975; 48: 638–645.
2. Waltzer WC. The urinary tract in pregnancy. *J Urol* 1981; 125: 271–276.
3. Klarskov P, Gerstenberg T, Ramirez D et al. Prostaglandin type E activity dominates in urinary tract smooth muscle in vitro. *J Urol* 1983; 129: 1071–1074.
4. Hsia TY, Shortliffe LM. The effect of pregnancy on rat urinary tract dynamics. *J Urol* 1995; 154: 684–689.
5. Lucas MJ, Cunningham FG. Urinary infection in pregnancy. *Clin Obstet Gynecol* 1993; 36: 855–868.
6. Whalley P. Bacteriuria of pregnancy. *Am J Obstet Gynecol* 1967; 97: 723–738.
7. Gilstrap LC, Leveno KJ, Cunningham FG et al. Renal infection and pregnancy outcome. *Am J Obstet Gynecol* 1981; 141: 709–716.
8. Schieve LA, Handler A, Hershow R et al. Urinary tract infection during pregnancy: Its association with maternal morbidity and perinatal outcome. *Am J Public Health* 1994; 84: 405–410.
9. Zinner SH, Kass EH. Long-term (10 to 14 years) follow-up of bacteriuria of pregnancy. *N Engl J Med* 1971; 285: 820–824.
10. Quinn AD, Kusuda L, Amar AD, Das S. Percutaneous nephrostomy for treatment of hydronephrosis of pregnancy. *J Urol* 1988; 139: 1037–1038.
11. Laverson PL, Hankins GD, Quirk JG Jr. Ureteral obstruction during pregnancy. *J Urol* 1984; 131: 327–329.
12. Homans DC, Blake GD, Harrington JT, Cetrulo CL. Acute renal failure caused by ureteral obstruction by a gravid uterus. *JAMA* 1981; 246: 1230–1231.
13. Meyers SJ, Lee RV, Munschauer RW. Dilatation and nontraumatic rupture of the urinary tract during pregnancy: A review. *Obstet Gynecol* 1985; 66: 809–815.
14. Oesterling JE, Besinger RE, Brendler CB. Spontaneous rupture of the renal collecting system during pregnancy: Successful management with a temporary ureteral catheter. *J Urol* 1988; 140: 588–590.
15. Fernandez AM, Minguez R, Serrano P et al. [Rapidly-growing renal angiomyolipoma associated with pregnancy]. *Actas Urol Esp* 1994; 18: 755.
16. Yanai H, Sasagawa I, Kubota Y et al. Spontaneous haemorrhage during pregnancy secondary to renal angiomyolipoma. *Urol Int* 1996; 56: 188–191.
17. Drago JR, Rohner TJ, Jr, Chez RA. Management of urinary calculi in pregnancy. *Urology* 1982; 20: 578–581.
18. Coe FL, Parks JH, Lindheimer MD. Nephrolithiasis during pregnancy. *N Engl J Med* 1978; 298: 324–326.
19. Denstedt JD, Razvi H. Management of urinary calculi during pregnancy. *J Urol* 1992; 148: 1072–1074.
20. Loughlin KR, Bailey RB, Jr. Internal ureteral stents for conservative management of ureteral calculi during pregnancy. *N Engl J Med* 1986; 315: 1647–1649.
21. Horowitz E, Schmidt JD. Renal calculi in pregnancy. *Clin Obstet Gynecol* 1985; 28: 324–338.
22. Lifshitz DA, Lingeman JE. Ureteroscopy as a first-line intervention for ureteral calculi in pregnancy. *J Endourol* 2002; 16: 19–22.
23. Loughlin KR. Management of urologic problems during pregnancy. *Urology* 1994; 44: 159–169.
24. Deyoe LA, Cronan JJ, Breslaw BH, Ridlen MS. New techniques of ultrasound and color Doppler in the prospective evaluation of acute renal obstruction. Do they replace the intravenous urogram? *Abdom Imaging* 1995; 20: 58–63.
25. Shokeir AA, Mahran MR, Abdulmaaboud M. Renal colic in pregnant women: Role of renal resistive index. *Urology* 2000; 55: 344–347.
26. Spencer JA, Tomlinson AJ, Weston MJ, Lloyd SN. Early report: Comparison of breath-hold MR excretory urography, Doppler ultrasound and isotope renography in evaluation of symptomatic hydronephrosis in pregnancy. *Clin Radiol* 2000; 55: 446–453.

27. Scarpa RM, De Lisa A, Usai E. Diagnosis and treatment of ureteral calculi during pregnancy with rigid ureteroscopes. *J Urol* 1996; 155: 875–877.
28. Borboroglu PG, Kane CJ. Current management of severely encrusted ureteral stents with a large associated stone burden. *J Urol* 2000; 164: 648–650.
29. Kroovand RL. Stones in pregnancy and in children. *J Urol* 1992; 148: 1076–8.
30. Watterson JD, Girvan AR, Beiko DT et al. Ureteroscopy and holmium: YAG laser lithotripsy: An emerging definitive management strategy for symptomatic ureteral calculi in pregnancy. *Urology* 2002; 60: 383–387.
31. Rittenberg MH, Bagley DH. Ureteroscopic diagnosis and treatment of urinary calculi during pregnancy. *Urology* 1988; 32: 427.
32. Harmon WJ, Sershon PD, Blute ML et al. Ureteroscopy: Current practice and long-term complications. *J Urol* 1997; 157: 28–32.
33. Ulvik NM, Bakke A, Hoisaeter PA. Ureteroscopy in pregnancy. *J Urol* 1995; 154: 1660–1663.
34. Vest JM, Warden SS. Ureteroscopic stone manipulation during pregnancy. *Urology* 1990; 35: 250–252.
35. Shokeir AA, Mutabagani H. Rigid ureteroscopy in pregnant women. *Br J Urol* 1998; 81: 678–681.
36. Vorreuther R. New tip design and shock wave pattern of electrohydraulic probes for endoureteral lithotripsy. *J Endourol* 1993; 7: 35–43.
37. Biyani CS, Joyce AD. Urolithiasis in pregnancy. II. Management. *BJU Int* 2002; 89: 819–823.
38. Hill DE, Kramer SA. Management of pregnancy after augmentation cystoplasty. *J Urol* 1990; 144: 457–459.
39. Hensle TW, Bingham JB, Reiley EA et al. The urological care and outcome of pregnancy after urinary tract reconstruction. *BJU Int* 2004; 93: 588–590.
40. Volkmer BG, Seidl EM, Gschwend JE et al. Pregnancy in women with ureterosigmoidostomy. *Urology* 2002; 60: 979–982.
41. Creagh TA, McInerney PD, Thomas PJ, Mundy AR. Pregnancy after lower urinary tract reconstruction in women. *J Urol* 1995; 154: 1323–1324.
42. Williams SF, Bitran JD. Cancer and pregnancy. *Clin Perinatol* 1985; 12: 609–623.
43. Walker JL, Knight EL. Renal cell carcinoma in pregnancy. *Cancer* 1986; 58: 2343–2347.
44. Loughlin KR. The management of urological malignancies during pregnancy. *Br J Urol* 1995; 76: 639–644.
45. Hendry WF. Management of urological tumours in pregnancy. *Br J Urol* 1997; 80 (Suppl 1): 24.
46. Rajasekar D, Hall M. Urinary tract injuries during obstetric intervention. *Br J Obstet Gynaecol* 1997; 104: 731–734.
47. Davis JD. Management of injuries to the urinary and gastrointestinal tract during cesarean section. *Obstet Gynecol Clin North Am* 1999; 26: 469–480.
48. Eisenkop SM, Richman R, Platt LD, Paul RH. Urinary tract injury during cesarean section. *Obstet Gynecol* 1982; 60: 591–596.
49. Thomas DP, Burgess NA, Gower RL, Peeling WB. Ureteric injury at caesarean section. *Br J Urol* 1994; 74: 122–123.
50. Meirow D, Moriel EZ, Zilberman M, Farhas A. Evaluation and treatment of iatrogenic ureteral injuries during obstetric and gynecologic operations for nonmalignant conditions. *J Am Coll Surg* 1994; 178: 144–148.
51. Neuman M, Eidelman A, Langer R et al. Iatrogenic injuries to the ureter during gynecologic and obstetric operations. *Surg Gynecol Obstet* 1991; 173: 268–272.
52. Ehrlich RM, Melman A, Skinner DG. The use of vesico-psoas hitch in urologic surgery. *J Urol* 1978; 119: 322–325.
53. Lee RA, Symmonds RE, Williams TJ. Current status of genitourinary fistula. *Obstet Gynecol* 1988; 72: 313–319.

38 Management of malignant and premalignant lesions of the female genital tract during pregnancy

VANCE BROACH and MARIO M. LEITAO

CONTENTS

Approximately 1 in 1000 women will be diagnosed with cancer while pregnant.[1–3] While this rate seems quite low, the incidence of cancer in pregnancy is increasing, in part due to the increasing age at which women are becoming pregnant.[4] Cervical cancer is the most common malignancy diagnosed in the pregnant patient, with an estimated incidence of approximately 1 in 2200,[5] followed by breast cancer, melanoma, ovarian cancer, thyroid cancer, and other malignancies.

Treatment of premalignant and malignant lesions in the pregnant patient presents a unique challenge. The impact of treatment on the mother and developing fetus needs to be considered, and there is a paucity of prospective literature available to guide treatment decisions. Randomized trials are sparse due to the unique ethical considerations of conducting clinical trials involving pregnant patients. Given these challenges, clinicians are often reluctant to treat pregnant women who have been diagnosed with cancer. This reluctance was demonstrated in the results of a physician survey published in 2011. Physicians indicated a preference toward pregnancy termination, delay of treatment, or preterm delivery even when these were not indicated. This underscores the challenges of treating pregnant patients, as well as the importance and need for clinicians to familiarize themselves with all available data in this area.[6]

This chapter will discuss the diagnosis and management of preinvasive and invasive cervical cancer, adnexal masses, and ovarian cancer in the pregnant patient. Vulvar and vaginal cancers are diagnosed with exceeding rarity in pregnant patients and will not be discussed in detail here. We will specifically highlight deviations from standard practice due to considerations of physiology of pregnancy and fetal development.

PREINVASIVE CERVICAL LESIONS

Cervical dysplasia is the result of human papilloma virus (HPV) infection in greater than 99% of squamous cell dysplasia cases.[7–9] HPV prevalence among pregnant patients is reported to be up to 42%.[10] There are more than 100 subtypes of HPV; however, HPV types 16 and 18 are found in approximately 50% of preinvasive cervical lesions and approximately 70% of invasive cervical cancers. Five additional HPV types (31, 33, 45, 52, and 58) account for 19% of invasive cervical cancers.[11]

HPV vaccination

Currently, three different HPV vaccines are available in the United States and vary by the number and type of HPV they immunize against. Cervarix® (GlaxoSmithKline), a bivalent vaccine, targets HPV 16 and 18.[12] Gardasil® (Merck & Co, Inc), a quadrivalent vaccine targets HPV types 16, 18, 6, and 11.[13,14] Gardasil® 9, a nine-valent vaccine, targets HPV types 16, 18, 6, 11, 31, 33, 45, 52, and 58.[15] Gardasil® 9 is currently the most widely used HPV vaccine worldwide.

None of these vaccines are U.S. Food and Drug Administration (FDA)–approved for use in pregnant women due to the lack of safety data. However, none of these vaccines contain a live virus and have little theoretical potential to harm the developing fetus. Women who receive the vaccine while unknowingly pregnant should be assured by their care provider that there is no evidence of adverse effects to the fetus. However, given the lack of safety data, women who begin the vaccine and become pregnant are recommended to complete the course postpartum. The optimal time for HPV vaccination is before the initiation of sexual activity.

Cervical cancer screening

Guidelines for the management of abnormal cervical cytology have been published in the 2006 Bethesda consensus guidelines and were revised and updated most recently in September 2012. Management of abnormal cytology per the Bethesda consensus guidelines in the pregnant patient is summarized below.[16]

Atypical squamous cells of undetermined significance (ASCUS) and low-grade squamous intraepithelial lesions (LSILs)

In women with ASCUS or LSILs, colposcopy is the preferred next step in management. However, it is acceptable to defer colposcopy until at least 6 weeks postpartum. HPV status in the setting of ASCUS cytology will provide useful information. If HPV testing is negative in the setting of ASCUS, the patient will not require colposcopy but merely should resume routine screening.

Atypical squamous cells, high-grade lesions (ASC-H), high-grade squamous intraepithelial lesions (HSIL), and atypical glandular cells (AGC)

Women with atypical squamous cells, high-grade lesions (ASC-H), high-grade squamous intraepithelial lesions (HSIL), and atypical glandular cells (AGC) cannot be excluded and should be offered colposcopy as in the nonpregnant patients.

Colposcopy in the pregnant patient

The goal of colposcopy in the pregnant patient is to identify any lesions suspicious for cervical intraepithelial neoplasia (CIN) 2/3 or invasive cancer. Colposcopy can be facilitated in the pregnant patient, particularly in patients who are at >20 weeks gestation, due to the frequency with which cervical ectropion is more pronounced in the gravid patient, thus increasing the ease with which the transition zone can be identified.[17] However, physiologic changes of the cervix in pregnancy can also make identifying dysplastic lesions more challenging. Increased vascularity, cervical edema, and softening of the cervix can obscure dysplastic lesions or make normal cervical tissue appear malignant. When performing colposcopy during pregnancy, cervical biopsy can be performed safely and has not been shown to be associated with increased risk of complication.[18] As in the nonpregnant patient, bleeding can be encountered at the time of biopsy and may be controlled with suture or hemostatic agents, including but not limited to ferric subsulfate solution, silver nitrate, oxidized cellulose polymer (Surgicel), and others. Endocervical curettage (ECC) is not recommended in pregnant patients due to the theoretical risk of affecting cervical competency, although this has not been proven.

The reliability of identifying dysplastic lesions by colposcopy in the gravid patient has been evaluated in several studies. Fader et al. reported the outcomes of 1079 patients who had an abnormal Pap smear while pregnant. Final pathology was equal to or less than impression on colposcopic examination in all 89 patients who underwent cervical biopsies. Additionally, no patients had progression of dysplastic lesions to cancer while pregnant.[19] In another report, Economos et al. evaluated 612 patients over a 17-year period who had abnormal cytologic screening.[17] In these patients, no carcinoma was missed on colposcopic evaluation. Another study by Baldauf et al. noted that the colposcopic impression underestimated the severity of cervical dysplasia in 9.8% of cases; however, discordance was not related to pregnancy.[18] While colposcopic evaluation is accurate in the pregnant patient, dysplastic lesions frequently persist into the postpartum period.[20] For this reason, if treatment is delayed until after delivery, patients are advised to have repeat colposcopy in the postpartum period.

Cervical conization in pregnancy

Cervical conization is indicated in the nonpregnant patient for carcinoma in situ (CIS) or invasive cancer on biopsy, moderate or severe dysplasia either on cervical biopsy or ECC, discrepancy between Pap and colposcopic-guided biopsy, or inadequate colposcopy. In gravid patients, these indications do not apply. Conization should only be performed in the gravid patient if the diagnosis of invasive cancer will alter the timing or mode of delivery. This is due to the increased risk of complications associated with cone biopsy in pregnancy. Complications include bleeding, premature rupture of membranes, miscarriage, preterm labor, and chorioamnionitis. Hannigan et al. reviewed their experience in treating 82 pregnant patients with cervical conization,[21] and found that bleeding was the most common complication. Ten patients (12.4%) had an estimated blood loss greater than 500 mL, two patients required blood transfusion, three required readmission for bleeding, and one patient required multiple trips to the operating room in order to obtain hemostasis. Three patients had miscarriage following the procedure.[21] Averette et al. published a series of 180 patients who had cone biopsy during pregnancy in 1970. They found that the risk of bleeding increased with conization further along the pregnancy. In the series, fetal loss was likely associated with conization in eight pregnancies (4.5%).[22]

Cerclage at the time of conization has been reported; however, it is not clear whether or not cerclage abrogates the potential complications of conization. Goldberg et al. published their experience of 17 patients who had cerclage placed at the time of conization in 1991.[23] The authors reported no complications from bleeding or pregnancy loss.

As with colposcopy, physiologic changes of pregnancy, specifically the eversion of the squamo-columnar junction, often make conization easier in the gravid patient. If conization is required, these anatomic changes allow for minimal tissue to be removed, theoretically limiting disruption of the internal cervical os and bleeding.

The loop electrosurgical excision procedure (LEEP) has been evaluated as an alternative to cold knife conization, with the benefit of LEEP being decreased blood loss with the use of electrocautery. The potential drawback of LEEP classically is the cauterized edge leading to difficulty in assessing dysplastic involvement of the margin. Robinson et al. reported their experience on 20 patients undergoing LEEP while pregnant. Two patients (10%) required blood transfusion due to bleeding. Of the patients with dysplasia, 57% were found to have positive margins.[24] Mitsuhashi and Sekiya reported their experience with nine patients undergoing LEEP in patients at less than 14 weeks gestation. No bleeding complications were reported, and two patients required additional treatment postpartum.[25] While the use of LEEP in pregnant patients is infrequently reported in the literature, case reports have indicated that it is as safe as cold knife conization. Given that the goal of conization in pregnancy is for diagnosis of invasive cancer, LEEP may be appropriate in select pregnant patients.

Management of preinvasive cervical lesions

The risk of progression of even high-grade lesions to invasive cervical cancer during pregnancy is minimal.[26] For this reason, treatment of cervical dysplasia should be deferred until 6–8 weeks following delivery. At that time, reevaluation of the cervix via colposcopy should be performed. In some cases, regression of high-grade lesions may be seen and treatment should be guided by postpartum colposcopy and biopsy results.[27]

The mode of delivery does not appear to have a definitive effect on the rate of regression of cervical dysplasia. Adhoot et al. reviewed their experience with 138 patients with cervical dysplasia in 1998. Among the women with high-grade dysplasia, 60% who delivered vaginally had regression of the lesion versus 0% who delivered via cesarean section. More recently, Kaneshiro et al. reviewed their experience with 201 patients with cervical dysplasia in pregnancy in 2005. They found no difference in rate of regression for dysplasia of any severity between patients who underwent vaginal and cesarean delivery.[28–30] Recommendations for route of delivery should not be based on presence of cervical dysplasia, but should be based on obstetric indications.

INVASIVE CERVICAL LESIONS

Cervical cancer is the most common cancer of the female genital tract diagnosed during pregnancy. One to two of 10,000 women will be diagnosed with cervical cancer while pregnant, accounting for 1–3% of all cervical cancers.[31–33]

Staging

Staging for cervical cancer is performed clinically irrespective of pregnancy status. Staging follows the guidelines of the International Federation of Gynecology and Obstetrics (FIGO) classification system, which was updated most recently in 2009 and is summarized in Table 38.1[34]. Physical examination is the cornerstone of the staging assessment. Examination of the cervix with tumor, uterus, vulva and vagina, parametria, groins, and supraclavicular regions is essential. If needed to adequately assess these areas, examination under anesthesia can be considered. Anatomic changes of pregnancy can make designating the stage more difficult, particularly when assessing for involvement of the parametria, bladder, and rectum. In patients who are not pregnant, staging can be further aided by intravenous (IV) pyelogram to assess for hydronephrosis and barium enema, as well as plain film X-rays. However, these staging modalities are rarely used in developed countries. Computed tomography (CT), magnetic resonance imaging (MRI), and positron emission tomography (PET) can be used for pretreatment planning but are not permitted for staging. Many now routinely use clinical examination in the office and MRI information *in lieu* of exams under anesthesia.

Table 38.1 International federation of gynecology and obstetrics (FIGO) cervical cancer staging.

FIGO stage	Definition
IA1	Invasive carcinoma diagnosed only by microscopy; stromal invasion with a maximum depth of 5.0 mm measured from the base of the epithelium and a horizontal spread of 7.0 mm or less; vascular space involvement, venous or lymphatic, does not affect classification
IA2	Measured stromal invasion ≤3.0 mm in depth and ≤7.0 mm in horizontal spread
IB	Measured stromal invasion >3.0 mm and ≤5.0 mm with a horizontal spread ≤7.0 mm
IB1	Clinically visible lesion confined to the cervix or microscopic lesion greater than T1a/IA2
IB2	Clinically visible lesion ≤4.0 cm in greatest dimension
II	Clinically visible lesion >4.0 cm in greatest dimension
IIA	Cervical carcinoma invades beyond uterus but not to pelvic wall or to lower third of vagina
IIA1	Tumor without parametrial invasion
IIA2	Clinically visible lesion ≤4.0 cm in greatest dimension
IIB	Clinically visible lesion >4.0 cm in greatest dimension
III	Tumor with parametrial invasion
IIIA	Tumor extends to pelvic wall and/or involves lower third of vagina and/or causes hydronephrosis or nonfunctional kidney
IIIB	Tumor involves lower third of vagina, no extension to pelvic wall
IV	Tumor extends to pelvic wall and/or causes hydronephrosis or nonfunctional kidney
IVA	Tumor invades mucosa of bladder or rectum and/or extends beyond true pelvis (bullous edema is not sufficient to classify a tumor as T4)
IVB	Tumor invades mucosa of bladder or rectum (bullous edema is not sufficient to classify a tumor as T4) Tumor extends beyond true pelvis

Source: Pecorelli S, *Int J Gynaecol Obstet,* 105(2), 103–4, 2009.

In the gravid patient, radiation should be limited and imaging should be obtained only when necessary for treatment planning. Therefore, abdominal X-rays and CT imaging should be avoided in pregnant patients if possible. In patients who have microscopic disease, routine imaging is actually not necessary. Plain film imaging of the chest with abdominal shielding is useful for identifying metastases in patients with grossly visible lesions. Imaging of the urinary tract by MRI or ultrasound to assess for local spread should be considered in patients with stage IB1 and higher lesions. MRI has been established as a useful modality for assessing regional spread in the nongravid patient with cervical cancer. In the nongravid patient, MRI accuracy of predicting parametrial involvement is 97%, with a negative predictive value rate approaching 100%. MRI is not as beneficial when used to identify nodal disease, particularly when the volume of disease is low.[35] MRI is considered safe in pregnancy based on somewhat limited data and should be used when clinically appropriate.[36]

Management of invasive cervical cancer

Management of cervical cancer in pregnant patients requires a multidisciplinary approach. Treatment must be individualized and take into account the patient's gestational age, stage of disease, and desire to preserve the pregnancy. Surgical and chemotherapeutic treatment modalities have been used in pregnant patients; however, radiation therapy should be avoided in patients who wish to continue their pregnancy, as it is associated with fetal death and injury.[37]

Some patients may elect to terminate pregnancy. After termination, treatment may proceed as in the nonpregnant patient. In patients at less than 20 weeks gestation with early-stage disease (FIGO stage IB1 or less), either a simple or radical hysterectomy (depending on substage) may be performed with the fetus in situ provided the patient does not wish to preserve fertility (Figure 38.1). The ovaries should be preserved, if feasible, as in nonpregnant patients. In patients who desire termination and who receive nonsurgical management for advanced disease, spontaneous abortion may result from chemoradiation. However, uterine evacuation should be considered in patients who desire termination of pregnancy and who have either locally advanced and/or metastatic disease given the possibility the pregnancy may persevere despite the side effects of chemoradiation.[38] If patients receive chemoradiation for definitive treatment during the first trimester, the mean reported time to spontaneous abortion is 33 days (range, 27–50 days). For patients who receive chemoradiation during the second trimester, the mean reported time to spontaneous abortion is 44 days (range, 33–66 days).[39] It is extremely rare to diagnose locally advanced disease in patients who are in their third trimester. Delay of treatment until fetal maturity may be considered in this rare situation. It would be prudent to consider cesarean delivery prior to onset of labor to minimize excessive bleeding from the cervical disease. It would also be prudent to have

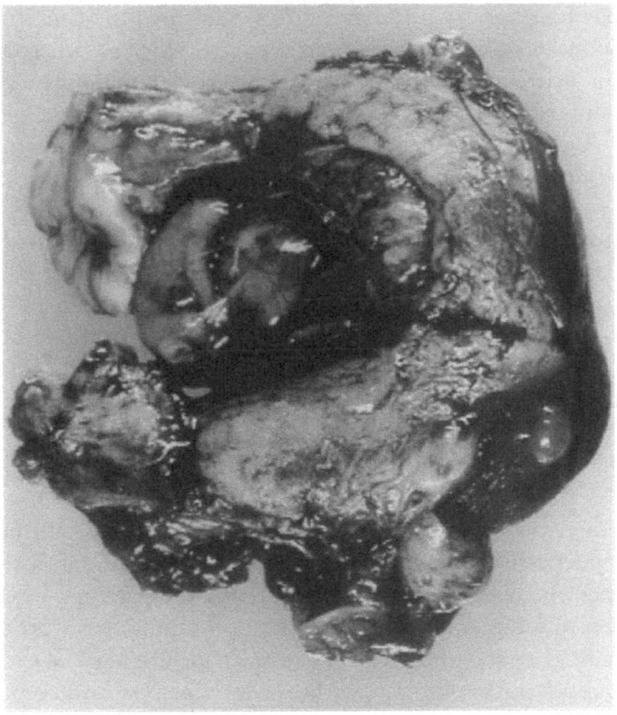

Figure 38.1 Radical hysterectomy specimen with a 14-week fetus in utero. (From Gibbon DG, Nieves-Neira W, Wagreich A et al., *Operative Obstetrics*, Boca Raton, FL: Taylor & Francis, 2006. With permission.)

a surgeon available who could assist in case of intraoperative difficulties and/or bleeding.

Gestational age less than 25 weeks

In women with previable pregnancies diagnosed with cervical cancer, lymph node assessment should be offered (Figure 38.2).

Lymph node assessment

Lymph node involvement is an indication of advanced disease and patients with previable pregnancies who desire an opportunity to retain their pregnancy should receive neoadjuvant chemotherapy. If lymph nodes are not involved, patients should receive treatment based on the local extent of disease. Lymphadenectomy has been evaluated in the pregnant patient. Vercellino et al. published their experience with minimally invasive lymphadenectomy in 32 pregnant patients. The authors reported no intraoperative complications, a mean blood loss of 5.3 mL, and a mean nodal count of 14.[40] Additional case reports have also demonstrated the safety and successful use of pelvic lymphadenectomy using conventional laparoscopy and robotic-assisted laparoscopy.[41,42]

Sentinel lymph node evaluation

In nongravid patients, sentinel lymph node (SLN) evaluation is becoming more widely used for gynecologic cancers. In pregnant patients, data regarding its use are

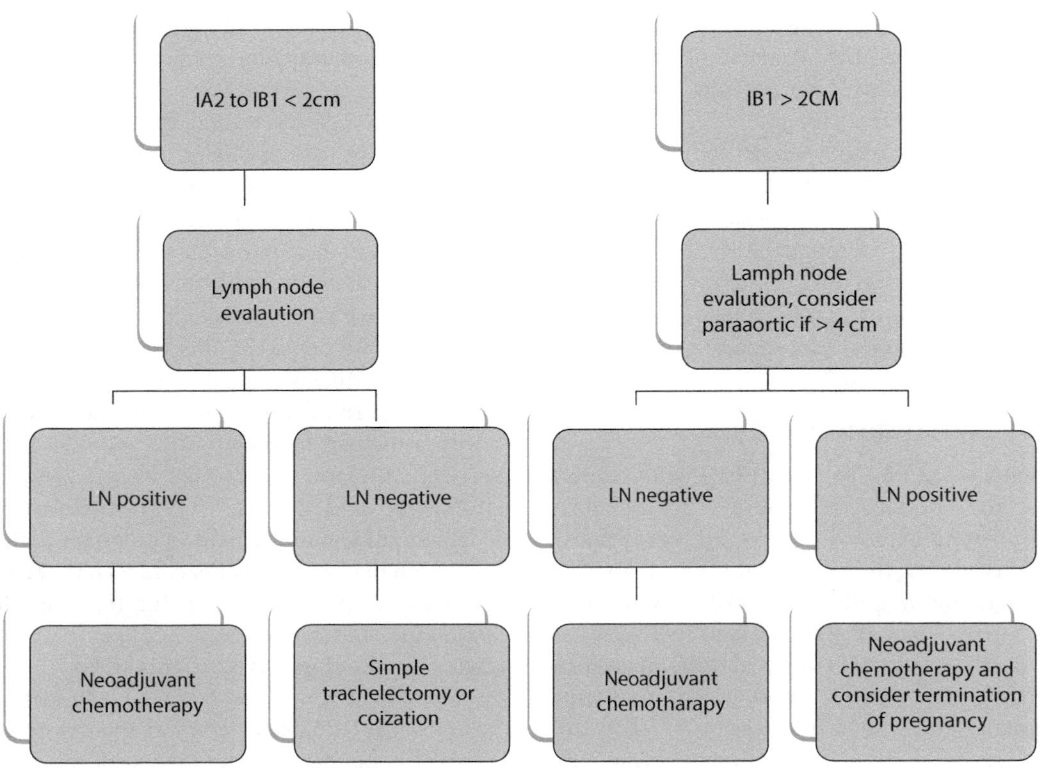

Figure 38.2 Gestational age <25 weeks. (Adapted from Amant F, Halaska MJ, Fumagalli M et al., *Int J Gynecol Cancer,* 24(3), 394–403, 2014.)

limited to case reports and series. Papadia et al. reported the experience of two cases of SLN mapping using indocyanine green (ICG). In both cases, bilateral mapping was successful and no adverse events related to ICG were reported.[43] ICG is an FDA pregnancy category C medication. Silva et al. reported their experience of successful SLN identification using radiolabeled colloid injection in a pregnant patient.[44] No definitive conclusions regarding safety and appropriateness of use can be made regarding SLN mapping in pregnant patients, but as the technique becomes more widely used, its utility in pregnant patients will become clearer. SLN mapping may help pregnant patients avoid the increased complexity and morbidity of comprehensive pelvic lymphadenectomy. Considering there will likely never be a randomized or a safety trial in the use of ICG in the pregnant patient, it may still be something to consider as an alternative to lymphadenectomy after thorough discussion with the patient.

Stage IA1 disease

For patients with stage IA1 disease at less than 25 weeks gestation, treatment with conization is appropriate. Takushi et al. published their experience treating eight patients with stage IA1 cervical cancer diagnosed by cone biopsy. Patients were treated expectantly and underwent definitive management after delivery by either repeat conization or hysterectomy, and no patients were found to have progression of disease during that time.[45] Yahata et al. reported their experience in treating four patients with stage IA1 cervical adenocarcinoma with laser conization in pregnancy. Two of these patients were found to have positive margins; one underwent repeat cone at 20 weeks gestation while the other underwent repeat cone biopsy at 5 weeks postpartum. No patients had residual tumor on repeat biopsy or recurrence.[46]

After delivery, women who wish to maintain future fertility do not require further treatment. They should undergo surveillance per the American Society for Colposcopy & Cervical Pathology (ASCCP) consensus guidelines. In women who do not wish to maintain future fertility, simple hysterectomy can be considered either at the time of cesarean section or as a separate procedure at a later date.

Stage IA2 to IB1 disease with tumor <2 cm

For patients with stage IA2 to IB1 disease with tumors smaller than 2 cm in dimension, nongravid patients have classically been treated with radical procedures to remove the parametria. However, the risk of parametrial involvement in these patients is quite low (<1%). Covens et al. reported their experience of 842 patients with radical surgery for early-stage cervical cancer and found an incidence of 0.6% in patients with tumors <2 cm, no lymph node involvement, and <10 mm invasion.[47,48] For this reason, conization or simple trachelectomy is being considered after lymph node evaluation. Radical procedures have been reported with both successful oncologic and obstetric outcomes.[49,50] However, radical trachelectomy has been reported to have a 32% associated incidence of spontaneous abortion. Given the low risk of parametrial involvement, radical surgery can be avoided in these pregnant patients.[37]

Women who wish to preserve fertility should be counseled regarding possible radical trachelectomy 6–8 weeks postpartum. Increasingly, stage IA2 to IB1 lesions smaller than 2 cm are being treated with conization and lymphadenectomy; the decision for radical trachelectomy should be made after a discussion with the patient regarding the risks and benefits, as in nongravid patients. Women who do not wish to preserve fertility should undergo definitive treatment with radical hysterectomy either at the time of cesarean section or as a second procedure.

Stage IB1 disease with tumor ≥2 cm

For patients with stage IB1 tumors ≥2 cm and with no evidence of lymph node involvement, the preferred treatment is neoadjuvant chemotherapy if the patient wishes to continue with the pregnancy. Additionally, in pregnant patients who have IB1 tumors measuring 2–4 cm, radical trachelectomy has been described as an acceptable treatment. As discussed above, radical trachelectomy has been performed successfully in the pregnant patient; however, the procedure can carry an increased risk of miscarriage.[49,50] The decision to proceed with radical trachelectomy versus chemotherapy needs to be discussed on a case-by-case basis and treatment should be individualized. The goal of neoadjuvant chemotherapy is to stabilize tumor growth until definitive management can be administered postpartum. Amant et al. reviewed their experience with 50 women who received neoadjuvant chemotherapy for cervical cancer during pregnancy. The average gestational age at diagnosis was 19.2 weeks, and the average gestational age at delivery was 33.2 weeks. Only 3.1% of patients had progression of disease while on treatment. The chemotherapeutic regimen was platinum based and administered at 3-week intervals either alone or in combination with paclitaxel, vincristine, 5-flurouracil, cyclophosphamide, or bleomycin. The overall survival rate was 79%, with a median follow-up of 24 months. Among patients with stage IB1 disease, the overall survival rate was 94%, with a median follow-up of 12 months. For those with stage IB2 disease, the overall survival rate was 70%, with a median follow-up of 27 months. For higher-stage disease, the overall survival rate was 70%, with a median follow-up of 14 months.[37,51] While there are no prospective data to guide management in pregnant patients, the combination of cisplatin and paclitaxel has been reviewed in a series of 27 patients undergoing treatment for breast and ovarian cancers, and the use of taxane was not associated with increased fetal risks in this series.[52]

Chemotherapy should not be administered within 3 weeks of anticipated delivery in an attempt to decrease the risk of bone marrow suppression of the fetus. Other chemotherapeutic agents that may be used for treatment in nongravid patients, such as gemcitabine, vinorelbine, and topotecan, as well as biologic agents, such as bevacizumab, are not recommended for use in pregnant patients as data regarding their safety are lacking.

Gestational age greater than 25 weeks

Lymph node sampling in patients of gestational age greater than 25 weeks is difficult to perform due to the size and location of the uterus. For this reason, the treatment decision is often not affected by nodal status in these patients.

Stage IA2 to IB1 with tumor <2 cm

In patients with stage IA2 to IB1 disease with tumor <2 cm, treatment can be delayed until after delivery. Women should undergo routine pelvic examination and should be considered for repeat imaging studies to ensure no progression of disease during this time. If during this time, progression of disease is observed, treatment with neoadjuvant chemotherapy or delivery followed by definitive treatment should be considered. A number of case reports and series have been published showing outcomes in cases of delayed treatment of invasive cervical cancer in order to allow for further fetal development. For example, Takushi et al. published a series of 12 patients with stage IA1 to IB2 cervical cancer and delayed treatment for 6–25 weeks. No progression of disease was noted, and all patients were alive with no evidence of disease at last follow-up.[45] Germann et al. published their experience treating 21 patients, 9 of whom delayed therapy for stage IB1 cervical cancer. No difference was seen in outcomes of patients who delayed their treatment versus those who did not.[53]

Stage IB1 ≥2 cm

There are minimal retrospective data to help guide the treatment of women diagnosed at greater than 25 weeks gestation with stage IB1 disease and tumors ≥2 cm or higher stage. Options for therapy include delayed treatment to allow for fetal maturity versus neoadjuvant chemotherapy. Outcome data are lacking for these patients, and treatment should be individualized with multidisciplinary input. Delayed treatment may be preferred in these cases.

Metastatic disease

In women with evidence of metastatic disease (stage IV), curative treatment is not an option. Chemotherapy should be offered as in the nonpregnant patient. The mainstay of chemotherapy for advanced or metastatic cervical cancer is a combination of cisplatin and paclitaxel. These agents are administered every 3 weeks for a total of six cycles. Chemotherapy should be stopped approximately 3 weeks before delivery is expected in an attempt to decrease potential complications of bone marrow suppression in the fetus at the time of birth. Chemotherapy can generally be administered safely and with relatively low risk of harm to the developing fetus. Chemotherapy is ideally administered after the first trimester when the risk of early miscarriage is lower and organogenesis has completed.[54] Zagouri et al. published their review of the use of platinum-based chemotherapy for the treatment of cervical cancer in 2013. They reviewed outcomes of 48 pregnancies and found that the majority of complications were related to prematurity rather than the direct effect of chemotherapy.[55]

Recently, the results of the Gynecologic Oncology Group (GOG) 240 trial were published and showed a 4-month survival benefit in women with advanced cervical cancer when bevacizumab, an antiangiogenic biologic agent, was added to cisplatin and paclitaxel.[56] However, given the lack of safety data available for biologic agents such as bevacizumab, they are not currently recommended for use in pregnant patients.

Conclusions

Cervical cancer is the most common cancer diagnosed in the pregnant patient, and treatment varies depending on the patient's wish to continue with the pregnancy, desire for future fertility, stage of disease, and gestational age. Oncologic outcomes do not appear to be affected by the diagnosis and treatment of cervical cancer during pregnancy.[57–59] Fetal outcomes also appear to be similar to those of babies of similar gestational age,[60] although the diagnosis of cervical cancer in pregnancy has been linked to higher rates of iatrogenic prematurity and low birth weights as demonstrated in the study by Dalrymple et al., who evaluated 434 cases of cervical cancer diagnosed in or around pregnancy through California registry records.[57] Treatment for cervical cancer requires a multidisciplinary approach and should be individualized.

ADNEXAL MASSES AND OVARIAN CANCER

Adnexal masses are infrequently encountered in the pregnant patient, with incidence rates ranging from 1 in 2200 to 2 in 100. One percent to 7.9% of these masses will be malignant.[61–65] Smith et al. published an observational study of 9375 patients with ovarian masses; 0.93% of the masses were found to be malignant and 1.2% of these masses were found to be borderline tumors.[3] A review of epithelial ovarian cancers by Palmer et al. showed that the majority of epithelial ovarian malignancies diagnosed in pregnancy are stage I (59%); 5% are stage II, 26% are stage III, and 10% are stage IV.[66] This section will discuss the diagnosis and management of both benign and malignant ovarian masses in the pregnant patient. (Figure 38.3)

Benign ovarian masses

Ovarian masses in pregnant patients are often asymptomatic but may present with nonspecific symptoms such as constipation, abdominal pain, urinary symptoms, and bloating, as in nonpregnant patients.[67] Patients may also have an adnexal mass identified at the time of obstetric ultrasound or with acute onset of abdominal pain related to torsion or cyst rupture. Ovarian torsion is a rare event, particularly when adnexal masses are 5 cm or smaller. Ovarian torsion is similarly rare in the second and third trimesters, presumably due to the physical obstruction to twisting of the ovary around its pedicle provided by the growing uterus.[68] Torsion appears to be most common in the late first trimester and early second trimester among

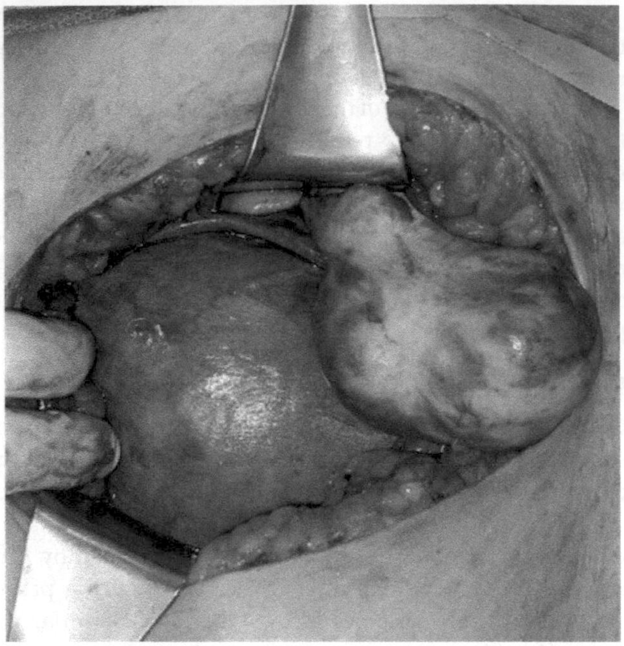

Figure 38.3 Large ovarian cyst and gravid uterus. (From Gibbon DG, Nieves-Neira W, Wagreich A et al., *Operative Obstetrics*, Boca Raton, FL: Taylor & Francis, 2006. With permission.)

adnexal masses measuring 6–8 cm. In their review, Yen et al. found a 22% increased risk of torsion for masses 6–8 cm in diameter compared with masses either smaller or larger.[69]

In the first trimester, the majority of adnexal masses less than 5 cm in diameter are functional cysts, and 70% of these masses will resolve spontaneously.[70] For this reason, removal of ovarian masses in the first trimester should be avoided. Additionally, the corpus luteum supplies the majority of progesterone support during the first 8 weeks of gestation.[71] If the corpus luteum is removed prior to this time, consideration should be made for progesterone supplementation until the placenta begins providing progesterone support for the pregnancy.

Simple ovarian masses of any size are most often functional, although they may represent cystadenoma or hydrosalpinx. Complex ovarian masses larger than 5 cm in diameter are most often mature teratomas, although theca lutein cysts, endometrioma, and extrauterine pregnancies remain on the differential.[64,72]

Borderline tumors, or tumors of low-malignant potential, are associated with excellent outcomes in the nongravid patient as well as the gravid patient. However, patients who are found to have borderline tumors should continue to be followed long term after their pregnancy despite the relatively benign course of their disease. Gershenson et al. published on their experience with serous borderline tumors and found that 44% of patients with serous borderline tumors with noninvasive implants will have a recurrence within 20 years, and 80% of those patients will have low-grade invasive serous carcinoma.[73]

Suspected benign ovarian masses should be managed conservatively in the first trimester due to the risk of miscarriage associated with surgical management, the possibility of spontaneous resolution without surgical intervention, and the minimization of potential teratogenic effects of perisurgical medication administration.[74]

Similarly, surgical intervention appears to be associated with increased morbidity such as fetal stress and preterm labor in patients during the third trimester.[75] If surgical management is indicated either due to concern for torsion or malignancy, the optimal timing is in the second trimester between 16 and 20 weeks.

Selection of surgical approach is based on gestational age, the size of the adnexal mass, and suspicion of malignancy. Minimally invasive surgery for adnexal masses in the nonpregnant patient, whether via conventional laparoscopy or robotically assisted laparoscopy, has been shown to be of considerable benefit over laparotomy and is associated with a reduction in fever, urinary tract infection, postoperative complications, postoperative pain, duration of hospital stay, and total cost.[76] Adverse events appear to be related to the underlying indication for surgery and not the minimally invasive surgical modality.[77]

Imaging adnexal masses in pregnancy

The benefit of ultrasound in characterizing adnexal masses has been well established in the nongravid patient and is the primary imaging method of choice in the pregnant patient as well. If further imaging is required, MRI is preferred in the pregnant patient, as there is no risk of radiation to the developing fetus. The safety of MRI has been established in the pregnant patient and can help characterize adnexal masses that are not fully visualized by ultrasonography.[78,79] CT should be avoided in the pregnant patient unless all other imaging modalities are not able to provide essential information regarding treatment planning. While the radiation exposure of an abdominal CT is less than the amount associated with fetal anomalies, long-term outcome data for these exposed infants are not available, and cases of secondary cancers have been reported.[80]

Tumor markers

In distinguishing benign from malignant lesions and for assessing response to therapy in the nongravid patient, tumor markers are often of considerable benefit. However, some of these serologic tests used in the nongravid patient are physiologically elevated in pregnancy, and their usefulness is therefore limited in some instances. Cancer antigen 125 (CA125) has been established as a useful biomarker in the nonpregnant patient for epithelial ovarian cancer.[81] However, CA125 can be physiologically elevated in pregnancy, potentially limiting its usefulness in some cases.[82] Another marker of epithelial ovarian cancer, human epididymis protein 4 (HE4), has more recently emerged as a marker for epithelial ovarian cancer.[83] HE4 expression is, however, physiologically lower in pregnant patients compared with nonpregnant controls, thus also potentially limiting its usefulness.[84] Lactate dehydrogenase is a useful marker for ovarian dysgerminoma in the nongravid patient. Its expression has not been shown to be affected by pregnancy, except in cases of hypertensive disorders such as **H**emolysis, **EL**evated liver enzymes, and **L**ow **P**latelet (HELLP) syndrome.[85] Alpha-fetoprotein (AFP) is used in the nonpregnant patient as a marker of germ cell tumors. Maternal serum AFP levels are normally elevated in pregnancy and are used as a marker of aneuploidy. AFP levels should be correlated with clinical and radiographic findings when being used as a marker of germ cell tumors in the pregnant patient.[86] Inhibin A is useful in monitoring treatment for ovarian granulosa cell tumors in the nonpregnant patient; however, its levels are physiologically elevated in the pregnant patient and interpretation is, therefore, not reliable in the gravid patient.[87]

Surgical and chemotherapeutic management of ovarian cancers

As stated earlier, the majority of ovarian malignancies are diagnosed at an early stage during pregnancy. The mainstay of management is surgical resection followed by chemotherapy. In patients in whom an adnexal mass is suspected, surgical resection of the mass with frozen section analysis should be performed by a gynecologic oncologist or with a gynecologic oncologist present should malignancy be identified. If malignancy is suspected on intraoperative frozen section, surgical staging should be performed. The surgical staging procedure for ovarian cancer should be performed with the exception of omitting hysterectomy and removal of contralateral ovary depending on the wishes of the patient for maintenance of the current pregnancy and for future fertility. This staging procedure is summarized in Table 38.2. In the pregnant patient, the contralateral ovary may be retained unless grossly involved with disease. Traditionally, this procedure has been performed through a vertical midline incision. However, in the nonpregnant and pregnant patient, a minimally invasive approach to staging has gained popularity. Reports of conventional laparoscopy and robotic-assisted laparoscopic staging for ovarian cancer have been published, with good oncologic and maternal–fetal outcomes, and can be considered in select patients.[88]

In patients who have metastatic disease noted at the time of surgical exploration, the goal of surgery should be the removal of all visible disease, as in the nonpregnant patient. In nonpregnant patients, complete gross resection of all visible disease has been associated with the longest overall survival.[89] Individualization of the extent of surgical effort and debulking should be considered on a case-by-case basis. In some instances, it may be most appropriate to delay surgical debulking and give neoadjuvant chemotherapy, delaying surgical cytoreduction until after delivery. Cases with this approach have been published, with acceptable oncologic and maternal–fetal outcomes.[90–93]

Table 38.2 Surgical staging for ovarian carcinoma.

Peritoneal washings
Intact tumor removal
Abdominal exploration to identify visible metastatic disease
Removal of uterus, remaining tube and ovary. This may be omitted in the pregnant patient depending on the desire of the patient to maintain current pregnancy and future fertility.
Omentectomy
Lymph node sampling
Random peritoneal biopsies

In women with epithelial ovarian cancer, patients with early-stage disease and high-risk features (serous or clear cell histology, high grade, stage IC or II) and those with advanced-stage disease should be offered chemotherapy either in the neoadjuvant setting or adjuvant setting following surgical cytoreduction. For newly diagnosed ovarian cancer, the optimal treatment approach is a combination of a platinum and taxane-based therapy. The safety of platinum chemotherapy in the gravid patient was reviewed by Mir et al. in 2008. They reviewed 43 patients who underwent platinum administration, 36 with cisplatin, 6 with carboplatin, and 1 with both agents. In the patients who received cisplatin, three infants were found to have intrauterine growth restriction (IUGR), two had oligohydramnios, and one each had polyhydramnios and ventriculomegaly. No fetal toxicities were seen in the patients who received carboplatin.[94] The use of taxanes is less well studied in pregnancy. The available case reports show no fetal anomalies or toxicities associated with taxane administration.[94–97]

For the nongravid patient in whom an optimal cytoreduction is achieved (<1 cm gross residual disease at the time of surgical debulking), a combination of intraperitoneal (IP) and IV chemotherapy has been associated with the longest overall survival, as demonstrated by the long-term follow-up results of the GOG 172 study.[98,99] In the gravid patient, however, there are minimally published data on the side effects of IP therapy. Smith et al. published a case report of a patient diagnosed at 12 weeks gestation who received four cycles of IP/IV therapy and at 37 weeks delivered a male infant weighing 4 pounds 11 ounces with bilateral congenital talipes equinovarus.[100] Given the paucity of data regarding IP chemotherapy use, IV paclitaxel and carboplatin are considered the standard regimen for women receiving chemotherapy for epithelial ovarian cancer.

Chemotherapy should be delayed until after the first trimester as rates of miscarriage, fetal toxicity, and congenital malformations are high with chemotherapy use during organogenesis.[101] Considerations of dose and cycle number and cycle frequency are the same as for the nongravid patient.

For germ cell tumors, the most common chemotherapeutic regimen consists of bleomycin, etoposide, and cisplatin (BEP). Chemotherapy is recommended for all patients, except those with stage IA dysgerminomas or stage I, grade 1 immature teratomas. As with epithelial ovarian cancer, therapy should be delayed until after the first trimester and may be delayed until after delivery. Few case reports are available to guide the decision as to timing of therapy, but delay until after delivery has been described.[102] In one case published by Aoki et al., a patient was diagnosed with a yolk sac tumor at 22 weeks gestation, and chemotherapy was delayed until after delivery. Recurrence was diagnosed at 34 weeks gestation and the patient underwent delivery along with secondary cytoreductive surgery followed by BEP chemotherapy. She was alive with no evidence of disease 39 months following treatment.[103]

CONCLUSIONS

Management of malignancy in the pregnant patient requires a multidisciplinary approach. The developing fetus and unique physiology of the expectant mother can present challenges to treatment requiring deviations from standard practice. Knowledge of the physiology of pregnancy and the effect of therapies on both the mother and the fetus is paramount in order to provide safe and effective therapy.

REFERENCES

1. Oduncu FS, Kimmig R, Hepp H, Emmerich B. Cancer in pregnancy: Maternal–fetal conflict. *J Cancer Res Clin Oncol* 2003; 129(3): 133–46.
2. Smith, LH, Danielsen B, Allen ME, Cress R. Cancer associated with obstetric delivery: Results of linkage with the California cancer registry. *Am J Obstet Gynecol* 2003; 189(4): 1128–35.
3. Smith LH, Dalrymple JL, Leiserowiz GS, et al. Obstetrical deliveries associated with maternal malignancy in California, 1992 through 1997. *Am J Obstet Gynecol* 2001; 184(7): 1504–12; discussion 1512–3.
4. Matthews TJ, Hamilton BE. Delayed childbearing: More women are having their first child later in life. *NCHS Data Brief* 2009; (21): 1–8.
5. Jolles CJ. Gynecologic cancer associated with pregnancy. *Semin Oncol* 1989; 16(5): 417–24.
6. Han SN, Kesic VI, Van Calsteren K, et al. Cancer in pregnancy: A survey of current clinical practice. *Eur J Obstet Gynecol Reprod Biol* 2013; 167(1): 18–23.
7. Walboomers JM, Jacobs MV, Manos MM, et al. Human papillomavirus is a necessary cause of invasive cervical cancer worldwide. *J Pathol* 1999; 189(1): 12–9.
8. zur Hausen H., Papillomaviruses in the causation of human cancers—A brief historical account. *Virology* 2009; 384(2): 260–5.
9. Forman D, de Martel C, Lacey Cj, et al. Global burden of human papillomavirus and related diseases. *Vaccine* 2012; 30(suppl 5): F12–23.
10. Kemp EA, Hakenewerth AM, Laurent SL, et al. Human papillomavirus prevalence in pregnancy. *Obstet Gynecol* 1992; 79(5(Pt 1)): 649–56.
11. Serrano, B, Alemany L, Tous S, et al. Potential impact of a nine-valent vaccine in human papillomavirus related cervical disease. *Infect Agent Cancer* 2012; 7(1): 38.
12. Cervarix—A second HPV vaccine. *Med Lett Drugs Ther* 2010; 52(1338): 37–8.
13. FUTURE II Study Group. Quadrivalent vaccine against human papillomavirus to prevent high-grade cervical lesions. *N Engl J Med* 2007; 356(19): 1915–27.
14. Munoz N, Kjaer SK, Sigurdsson K, et al. Impact of human papillomavirus (HPV)-6/11/16/18 vaccine on all HPV-associated genital diseases in young women. *J Natl Cancer Inst* 2010; 102(5): 325–39.
15. Joura EA, Giuliano AR, Iversen OE, et al. A 9-valent HPV vaccine against infection and intraepithelial neoplasia in women. *N Engl J Med* 2015; 372(8): 711–23.
16. Massad LS, Einstein MH, Huh WK, et al. 2012 updated consensus guidelines for the management of abnormal cervical cancer screening tests and cancer precursors. *Obstet Gynecol* 2013; 121(4): 829–46.
17. Economos K, Perez Veridiano N, Delke I, et al. Abnormal cervical cytology in pregnancy: A 17-year experience. *Obstet Gynecol* 1993; 81(6): 915–8.
18. Baldauf JJ, Dreyfus M, Ritter J, Philippe E. Colposcopy and directed biopsy reliability during pregnancy: A cohort study. *Eur J Obstet Gynecol Reprod Biol* 1995; 62(1): 31–6.
19. Fader AN, Alward EK, Niederhauser A, et al. Cervical dysplasia in pregnancy: A multi-institutional evaluation. *Am J Obstet Gynecol* 2010; 203(2): 113.e1–6.
20. Kaplan KJ, Dainty LA, Dolinsky B, et al. Prognosis and recurrence risk for patients with cervical squamous intraepithelial lesions diagnosed during pregnancy. *Cancer* 2004; 102(4): 228–32.
21. Hannigan EV, Whitehouse HH 3rd, Atkinson WD, Becker SN. Cone biopsy during pregnancy. *Obstet Gynecol* 1982; 60(4): 450–5.
22. Averette HE, Nasser N, Yankow SL, Little WA. Cervical conization in pregnancy. Analysis of 180 operations. *Am J Obstet Gynecol* 1970; 106(4): 543–9.
23. Goldberg GL, Altaras MM, Block B. Cone cerclage in pregnancy. *Obstet Gynecol* 1991; 77(2): 315–7.
24. Robinson WR, Webbb S, Tirpack J, et al. Management of cervical intraepithelial neoplasia during pregnancy with LOOP excision. *Gynecol Oncol* 1997; 64(1): 153–5.
25. Mitsuhashi A, Sekiya S. Loop electrosurgical excision procedure (LEEP) during first trimester of pregnancy. *Int J Gynaecol Obstet* 2000; 71(3): 237–9.
26. Serati M, Uccella S, Laterza RM, et al. Natural history of cervical intraepithelial neoplasia during pregnancy. *Acta Obstet Gynecol Scand* 2008; 87(12): 1296–300.
27. Paraskevaidis E, Koliopoulos G, Kalantaridou S, et al. Management and evolution of cervical intraepithelial neoplasia during pregnancy and postpartum. *Eur J Obstet Gynecol Reprod Biol* 2002; 104(1): 67–9.
28. Kaneshiro BE, Acoba JD, Holzman J, et al. Effect of delivery route on natural history of cervical dysplasia. *Am J Obstet Gynecol* 2005; 192(5): 1452–4.
29. Ahdoot D, Van Nostrand KM, Nguyen NJ, et al. The effect of route of delivery on regression of abnormal cervical cytologic findings in the postpartum period. *Am J Obstet Gynecol* 1998; 178(6): 1116–20.

30. Siristatidis C, Vitoratos N, Michailidis E, et al. The role of the mode of delivery in the alteration of intrapartum pathological cervical cytologic findings during the postpartum period. *Eur J Gynaecol Oncol* 2002; 23(4): 358–60.
31. Barber HR, Brunschwig A. Gynecologic cancer complicating pregnancy. *Am J Obstet Gynecol* 1963; 85: 156–64.
32. Nguyen C, Montz FJ, Bristow RE. Management of stage I cervical cancer in pregnancy. *Obstet Gynecol Surv* 2000; 55(10): 633–43.
33. Creasman WT. Cancer and pregnancy. *Ann N Y Acad Sci* 2001; 943: 281–6.
34. Pecorelli S. Revised FIGO staging for carcinoma of the vulva, cervix, and endometrium. *Int J Gynaecol Obstet* 2009: 105(2): 103–4.
35. Sahdev A, Sohaib SA, Wenaden AE, et al. The performance of magnetic resonance imaging in early cervical carcinoma: A long-term experience. *Int J Gynecol Cancer* 2007; 17(3): 629–36.
36. Chen MM, Coakley FV, Kaimai A, Laros RK Jr. Guidelines for computed tomography and magnetic resonance imaging use during pregnancy and lactation. *Obstet Gynecol* 2008; 112(2 Pt 1): 333–40.
37. Amant F, Halaska MJ, Fumagalli M, et al. Gynecologic cancers in pregnancy: Guidelines of a second international consensus meeting. *Int J Gynecol Cancer* 2014; 24(3): 394–403.
38. Sood AK, Sorosky JI, Mayr N, et al. Radiotherapeutic management of cervical carcinoma that complicates pregnancy. *Cancer* 1997; 80(6): 1073–8.
39. Prem KA, Makowski EL, McKelvey JL. Carcinoma of the cervix associated with pregnancy. *Am J Obstet Gynecol* 1966; 95(1): 99–108.
40. Vercellino GF, Koehler C, Erdemoglu E, et al. Laparoscopic pelvic lymphadenectomy in 32 pregnant patients with cervical cancer: Rationale, description of the technique, and outcome. *Int J Gynecol Cancer* 2014; 24(2): 364–71.
41. Rojas C, Moroney JW. Robotic surgical staging for cervical cancer diagnosed during pregnancy: Immediate versus delayed definitive treatment. *Gynecol Oncol Case Rep* 2013; 5: 40–2.
42. Favero G, Lanowska M, Schneider A, et al. Laparoscopic pelvic lymphadenectomy in a patient with cervical cancer stage Ib1 complicated by a twin pregnancy. *J Minim Invasive Gynecol* 2010; 17(1): 118–20.
43. Papadia A, Mohr S, Imboden S, et al. Laparoscopic ICG sentinel lymph node mapping in pregnant cervical cancer patients. *J Minim Invasive Gynecol* 2015; 23(2): 270–3.
44. Silva LB, Silva-Filho AL, Traiman P, et al. Sentinel node mapping in a pregnant woman with cervical cancer: A case report. *Int J Gynecol Cancer* 2006; 16(3): 1454–7.
45. Takushi M, Moromizato H, Sakumoto K, Kanazawa K. Management of invasive carcinoma of the uterine cervix associated with pregnancy: Outcome of intentional delay in treatment. *Gynecol Oncol* 2002; 87(2): 185–9.
46. Yahata T, Numata M, Kashima K, et al. Conservative treatment of stage IA1 adenocarcinoma of the cervix during pregnancy. *Gynecol Oncol* 2008; 109(1): 49–52.
47. Covens A, Rosen B, Murphy J, et al. How important is removal of the parametrium at surgery for carcinoma of the cervix? *Gynecol Oncol* 2002; 84(1): 145–9.
48. Herod JJ, Decruze SB, Patel RD. A report of two cases of the management of cervical cancer in pregnancy by cone biopsy and laparoscopic pelvic node dissection. *BJOG* 2010; 117(12): 1558–61.
49. Abu-Rustum NR, Tal MN, DeLair D, et al. Radical abdominal trachelectomy for stage IB1 cervical cancer at 15-week gestation. *Gynecol Oncol* 2010; 116(1): 151–2.
50. Kyrgiou M, Horwell DH, Farthing A. Laparoscopic radical abdominal trachelectomy for the management of stage IB1 cervical cancer at 14 weeks' gestation: Case report and review of the literature. *BJOG* 2015; 122(8): 1138–43.
51. Rydzewska L, Tiernay J, Vale CL, Symonds PR. Neoadjuvant chemotherapy plus surgery versus surgery for cervical cancer. *Cochrane Database Syst Rev* 2012; 12: Cd007406.
52. Cardonick E, Bhat A, Gilmandyar D, Somer R. Maternal and fetal outcomes of taxane chemotherapy in breast and ovarian cancer during pregnancy: Case series and review of the literature. *Ann Oncol* 2012; 23(12): 3016–23.
53. Germann N, Haie-Meder C, Morice P, et al. Management and clinical outcomes of pregnant patients with invasive cervical cancer. *Ann Oncol* 2005; 16(3): 397–402.
54. Cardonick E, Iacobucci A. Use of chemotherapy during human pregnancy. *Lancet Oncol* 2004; 5(5): 283–91.
55. Zagouri F, Sergentanis TN, Chrysikos D, Bartsch R. Platinum derivatives during pregnancy in cervical cancer: A systematic review and meta-analysis. *Obstet Gynecol* 2013; 121(2 Pt 1): 337–43.
56. Tewari KS, Sill MW, Long HJ 3rd, et al. Improved survival with bevacizumab in advanced cervical cancer. *N Engl J Med* 2014; 370(8): 734–43.
57. Dalrymple JL, Gilbert WM, Leiserowitz GS, et al. Pregnancy-associated cervical cancer: Obstetric outcomes. *J Matern Fetal Neonatal Med* 2005; 17(4): 269–76.
58. Stensheim H, Møller B, van Dijk T, Fosså SD. Cause-specific survival for women diagnosed with cancer during pregnancy or lactation: A registry-based cohort study. *J Clin Oncol* 2009; 27(1): 45–51.
59. Pettersson BF, Andersson S, Hellman K, Hellström AC. Invasive carcinoma of the uterine cervix associated with pregnancy: 90 years of experience. *Cancer* 2010; 116(10): 2343–9.
60. Zemlickis D, Lishner M, Degendorfer P, et al. Maternal and fetal outcome after invasive cervical cancer in pregnancy. *J Clin Oncol* 1991; 9(11): 1956–61.

61. Beischer NA, Buttery BW, Fortune DW, Macafee CA. Growth and malignancy of ovarian tumours in pregnancy. *Aust N Z J Obstet Gynaecol* 1971; 11(4): 208–20.
62. Hess LW, Peaceman A, O'Brein WF, et al. Adnexal mass occurring with intrauterine pregnancy: Report of fifty-four patients requiring laparotomy for definitive management. *Am J Obstet Gynecol* 1988; 158(5): 1029–34.
63. Koonings PP, Platt LD, Wallace R, Incidental adnexal neoplasms at cesarean section. *Obstet Gynecol* 1988; 72(5): 767–9.
64. Schmeler KM, Mayo-Smith WW, Peipert JF, et al. Adnexal masses in pregnancy: Surgery compared with observation. *Obstet Gynecol* 2005; 105(5 Pt 1): 1098–103.
65. Leiserowitz GS. Managing ovarian masses during pregnancy. *Obstet Gynecol Surv* 2006; 61(7): 463–70.
66. Palmer J, Vatish M, Tidy J. Epithelial ovarian cancer in pregnancy: A review of the literature. *BJOG* 2009; 116(4): 480–91.
67. Goff BA, Mandel LS, Melancon CH, Muntz HG. Frequency of symptoms of ovarian cancer in women presenting to primary care clinics. *JAMA* 2004; 291(22): 2705–12.
68. Bernhard LM, Klebba PK, Gray DL, Mutch DG. Predictors of persistence of adnexal masses in pregnancy. *Obstet Gynecol* 1999; 93(4): 585–9.
69. Yen CF, Lin SL, Murk W, et al. Risk analysis of torsion and malignancy for adnexal masses during pregnancy. *Fertil Steril* 2009; 91(5): 1895–902.
70. Giuntoli RL, 2nd, Vang RS, Bristow RE. Evaluation and management of adnexal masses during pregnancy. *Clin Obstet Gynecol* 2006; 49(3): 492–505.
71. Csapo AI, Pulkkinen MO, Wiest WG. Effects of luteectomy and progesterone replacement therapy in early pregnant patients. *Am J Obstet Gynecol* 1973; 115(6): 759–65.
72. Chiang G, Levine D. Imaging of adnexal masses in pregnancy. *J Ultrasound Med* 2004; 23(6): 805–19.
73. Gershenson DM, Silva EG, Tortolero-Luna G, et al. Serous borderline tumors of the ovary with noninvasive peritoneal implants. *Cancer* 1998; 83(10): 2157–63.
74. Novak ER, Lambrou CD, Woodruff JD. Ovarian tumors in pregnancy. An ovarian tumor registry review. *Obstet Gynecol* 1975; 46(4): 401–6.
75. Whitecar MP, Turner S, Higby MK. Adnexal masses in pregnancy: A review of 130 cases undergoing surgical management. *Am J Obstet Gynecol* 1999; 181(1): 19–24.
76. Medeiros LR, Rosa DD, Bozzetti MC, et al. Laparoscopy versus laparotomy for benign ovarian tumour. *Cochrane Database Syst Rev* 2009; (2): Cd004751.
77. Al-Fozan, H, Tulandi T. Safety and risks of laparoscopy in pregnancy. *Curr Opin Obstet Gynecol* 2002; 14(4): 375–9.
78. Telischak NA, Yeh BM, Joe BN, et al. MRI of adnexal masses in pregnancy. *AJR Am J Roentgenol* 2008; 191(2): 364–70.
79. Brown MA, Birchard KR, Semelka RC. Magnetic resonance evaluation of pregnant patients with acute abdominal pain. *Semin Ultrasound CT MR* 2005; 26(4): 206–11.
80. Prenatal X-ray exposure and childhood cancer in twins. *N Engl J Med* 1985; 312(24): 1574–5.
81. Bast RC, Jr, Klug TL, St John E, et al. A radioimmunoassay using a monoclonal antibody to monitor the course of epithelial ovarian cancer. *N Engl J Med* 1983; 309(15): 883–7.
82. Sarandakou A, Protonotariou E, Rizos D. Tumor markers in biological fluids associated with pregnancy. *Crit Rev Clin Lab Sci* 2007; 44(2): 151–78.
83. Molina R, Escudero JM, Augé, et al. HE4 a novel tumour marker for ovarian cancer: Comparison with CA 125 and ROMA algorithm in patients with gynaecological diseases. *Tumour Biol* 2011; 32(6): 1087–95.
84. Moore RG, Miller MC, Eklund EE, et al. Serum levels of the ovarian cancer biomarker HE4 are decreased in pregnancy and increase with age. *Am J Obstet Gynecol* 2012; 206(4): 349.e1–7.
85. Demir SC, Evruke C Ozgunen FT, et al. Factors that influence morbidity and mortality in severe preeclampsia, eclampsia and hemolysis, elevated liver enzymes, and low platelet count syndrome. *Saudi Med J* 2006; 27(7): 1015–8.
86. Elit L, Bocking A, Kenyon C, Natale R. An endodermal sinus tumor diagnosed in pregnancy: Case report and review of the literature. *Gynecol Oncol* 1999; 72(1): 123–7.
87. Luisi S, Florio P, Reis FM, Petraglia F. Inhibins in female and male reproductive physiology: Role in gametogenesis, conception, implantation and early pregnancy. *Hum Reprod Update* 2005; 11(2): 123–35.
88. Chen CH, Chiu LH, Chan C, Liu WM. Management of ovarian cancer in 14th gestational week of pregnancy by robotic approach with preservation of the fetus. *Gynecol Obstet Invest* 2015; 80(2): 139–44.
89. Shih KK, Chi DS. Maximal cytoreductive effort in epithelial ovarian cancer surgery. *J Gynecol Oncol* 2010; 21(2): 75–80.
90. Sood AK, Shahin MS, Sorosky JI. Paclitaxel and platinum chemotherapy for ovarian carcinoma during pregnancy. *Gynecol Oncol* 2001; 83(3): 599–600.
91. Picone O, Lhommé C, Tournaire M, et al. Preservation of pregnancy in a patient with a stage IIIB ovarian epithelial carcinoma diagnosed at 22 weeks of gestation and treated with initial chemotherapy: Case report and literature review. *Gynecol Oncol* 2004; 94(2): 600–4.
92. Ferrandina G, Distefano M, Testa A, et al. Management of an advanced ovarian cancer at 15 weeks of gestation: Case report and literature review. *Gynecol Oncol* 2005; 97(2): 693–6.
93. Mendez LE, Mueller A, Salom E, et al. Paclitaxel and carboplatin chemotherapy administered during pregnancy for advanced epithelial ovarian cancer. *Obstet Gynecol* 2003; 102(5 Pt 2): 1200–2.

94. Mir O, Berveiller P, Ropert S, et al. Use of platinum derivatives during pregnancy. *Cancer* 2008; 113(11): 3069–74.
95. Zagouri F, Sergentanis TN, Chrysikos D, et al. Taxanes for ovarian cancer during pregnancy: A systematic review. *Oncology* 2012; 83(4): 234–8.
96. Zagouri F, Sergentanis TN, Chrysikos D, et al. Taxanes for breast cancer during pregnancy: A systematic review. *Clin Breast Cancer* 2013; 13(1): 16–23.
97. Mir O, Berveiller P, Goffinet F, et al. Taxanes for breast cancer during pregnancy: A systematic review. *Ann Oncol* 2010; 21(2): 425–6.
98. Barlin JN, Dao F, Bou Zgheib, et al. Progression-free and overall survival of a modified outpatient regimen of primary intravenous/intraperitoneal paclitaxel and intraperitoneal cisplatin in ovarian, fallopian tube, and primary peritoneal cancer. *Gynecol Oncol* 2012; 125(3): 621–4.
99. Tewari D, Java JJ, Salani R, et al. Long-term survival advantage and prognostic factors associated with intraperitoneal chemotherapy treatment in advanced ovarian cancer: A gynecologic oncology group study. *J Clin Oncol* 2015; 33(13): 1460–6.
100. Smith ER, Borowsky ME, Jain VD, Intraperitoneal chemotherapy in a pregnant woman with ovarian cancer. *Obstet Gynecol* 2013; 122(2 Pt 2): 481–3.
101. Selig BP, Furr JR Huey RW, et al. Cancer chemotherapeutic agents as human teratogens. *Birth Defects Res A Clin Mol Teratol* 2012; 94(8): 626–50.
102. Shimizu Y, Komiyama S, Kobayashi T, et al. Successful management of endodermal sinus tumor of the ovary associated with pregnancy. *Gynecol Oncol* 2003; 88(3): 447–50.
103. Aoki Y, Higashino M, Ishii S, Tanaka K. Yolk sac tumor of the ovary during pregnancy: A case report. *Gynecol Oncol* 2005; 99(2): 497–9.

Gestational trophoblastic disease

39

BABAK LITKOUHI and ABDULLA AL-KHAN

CONTENTS

Gestational trophoblastic diseases (GTD) are a number of related benign and malignant disorders characterized by trophoblastic proliferation. Complete (CHM) and partial (PHM) hydatidiform moles are benign gestational events that most often resolve after uterine evacuation. In a minority of patients, moles may persist or transform, resulting in malignant disease (gestational trophoblastic neoplasia [GTN]). Rarely, GTN may follow nonmolar gestations, including normal, aborted, or ectopic pregnancies. GTN comprises of invasive mole, choriocarcinoma, placental site trophoblastic tumor (PSTT), and epithelioid trophoblastic tumor (ETT), although most commonly the histology is unknown unless surgery is performed.

Although much of our knowledge of the etiology of GTD is incomplete, they are among the most curable types of gynecologic malignancy, even in the case of widely metastatic disease. The diagnosis, management, and follow-up of GTD are a multidisciplinary endeavor. This chapter will discuss the epidemiology, pathology, diagnosis, and management of GTD, as well as the future reproductive outcomes of women affected by these diseases.

EPIDEMIOLOGY

Hydatidiform mole is a rare complication of pregnancy, and as such, its epidemiology is not completely understood. Its incidence appears to vary among different ethnic groups and geographic areas. Most reports suggest the incidence of hydatidiform mole is greater in Southeast Asia than in the Western Hemisphere. The reported incidence of this disease in the Western countries is estimated to be 1/2000 pregnancies, versus 1/77 for some countries in Asia such as Indonesia, China, and the Philippines. It is estimated that in the United States, one in 1000–1500 pregnancies is complicated by trophoblastic disease. The reason for this difference in the rates of hydatidiform mole between the United States and Asian countries is uncertain. It may involve genetic, nutritional, immunologic, or environmental factors.[1–3]

An increased incidence of hydatidiform mole has been noted among women at the extremes of reproductive age.[3] The incidence seems to be higher[4,5] among women over 45 years of age and those under 15. Spontaneous or induced abortions and infertility have also been associated with an increased risk of mole, while term pregnancies seem to be protective.[1,6] It has been hypothesized that altered nutrition and low socioeconomic status may contribute to the high incidence of hydatidiform mole in Asia. Low consumption of vitamin A (carotene) and animal protein has been associated with a higher incidence of molar pregnancy.[7,8]

It should be noted that not all studies agree with these observations.[1,9] More so, these findings are more consistently associated with CHM rather than PHM, as the epidemiology of PHM is less well understood and may be more related to reproductive risk factors such as oral contraceptive use and irregular menstrual cycles.[10]

A consistent finding has been that patients with a history of hydatidiform mole have an approximately 10- to 20-fold increased risk of a future molar pregnancy.[11,12] There are also reports of cases of familial recurrent hydatidiform mole.[13] These observations suggest that there may be genetic susceptibility to this disease, but do not rule out a common environmental factor.

PATHOGENESIS AND CLASSIFICATION OF HYDATIDIFORM MOLES

Hydatidiform mole is an abnormal gestational event characterized by abnormal fetal development and placental (trophoblastic) overgrowth. Vassilakos and Kajii[14] proposed a classification scheme for molar gestations in 1976. Their work was later supported by investigators such as Szulman and Surti,[15] and is still the classification that is used. These investigators classified molar gestations as complete or partial based on morphologic and cytogenetic characteristics. Table 39.1 shows the current World Health Organization (WHO) classification of GTD.

Table 39.1 WHO classification of GTD.

Molar pregnancies	
	Complete hydatidiform mole
	Partial hydatidiform mole
	Invasive mole
Neoplasms	
	Gestational choriocarcinoma
	Placental site trophoblastic tumor
	Epithelioid trophoblastic tumor
Nonneosplastic lesions	
	Exaggerated placental site
	Placental site nodule

A CHM is characterized by (1) absent fetal or embryonic tissue (except in the rare case of a CHM with coexistent normal twin); (2) the absence of normal chorionic villi; (3) diffuse vesicular swelling of the villi; (4) diffuse trophoblastic hyperplasia and atypia. Macroscopically, CHM are classically clinically described as appearing as a "bunch of grapes." Approximately 90% of the complete moles have a 46,XX chromosomal complement; the other 10% have a 46,XY karyotype. Almost all CHM are of androgenic origin, and chromosome-banding techniques, enzyme markers, and HLA antigen typing can confirm the diploid chromosomal complement of paternal origin. CHM typically originates by the fertilization of an empty egg, or "blighted ovum," by a haploid sperm, which later duplicates to give the 46,XX complement. The 46,XY mole originates by dispermy or the fertilization of a "blighted ovum" by two spermatozoa. The mechanisms involved in this abnormal fertilization pattern remain uncertain. The potential for subsequent malignancy (i.e., GTN) is greater with CHM than with PHM.

A partial mole is defined by the coexistence of a hydatidiform mole with fetal or embryonic tissues. Histologically, PHMs contain (1) focal hydropic swelling and cavitation of the villi; (2) focal trophoblastic hyperplasia with or without atypia; (3) scalloping of the outline of the villi; (4) trophoblastic inclusions; and (5) identifiable fetal or embryonic tissues (Figures 39.1 and 39.2). The fetus typically demonstrates the gross stigmata of triploidy.[16] Cytogenetically, PHMs contain a triploid karyotype, with an extra set of chromosomes of paternal origin, again either from reduplication or, less commonly, from dispermic fertilization. Rarely, a chromosomally normal fetus may coexist as a twin PHM, and extremely rarely, as a singleton normal diploid fetus may coexist with a partial molar placenta.[17,18] Although some investigators have suggested the existence of diploid PHM, this is most likely due to misclassification rather than the true existence of such an entity.[19] Although the malignant potential of a PHM is less than that of a CHM, these pregnancies should be similarly managed with close follow-up with human chorionic gonadotropin (HCG) titers after evacuation.[16]

With more widespread use ultrasound and early first termination of abnormal gestations, difficulties have arisen with pathology diagnosis of molar gestations, as there may be overlapping features to early first trimester CHM, PHM, and hydropic spontaneous abortion. Nonetheless, accurate diagnosis remains important as the clinical consequences, management, and prognosis of these entities differ significantly.[20,21] This scenario may be seen when (1) most of the products of conception are passed before presentation, (2) tissue is inadvertently discarded during the evacuation procedure or during its handling in the laboratory, and (3) overlapping morphologic features are present. In these circumstances, an accurate diagnosis may be facilitated by flow cytometry to assess the DNA ploidy. Moreover, immunohistochemical staining for *p57* gene products may aid in the diagnosis. *P57*, as well as *PHLDA2*, is maternally expressed, paternally imprinted. As such, CHM would be recognized by diploidy and absent p57 staining, PHM by triploidy and positive p57 staining, and hydropic abortions by diploidy and positive p57 staining.[19]

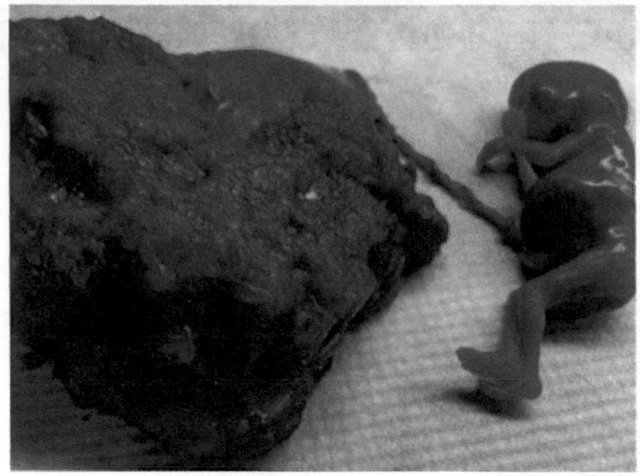

Figure 39.1 Partial hydatiform mole with hydropic swelling of the villi.

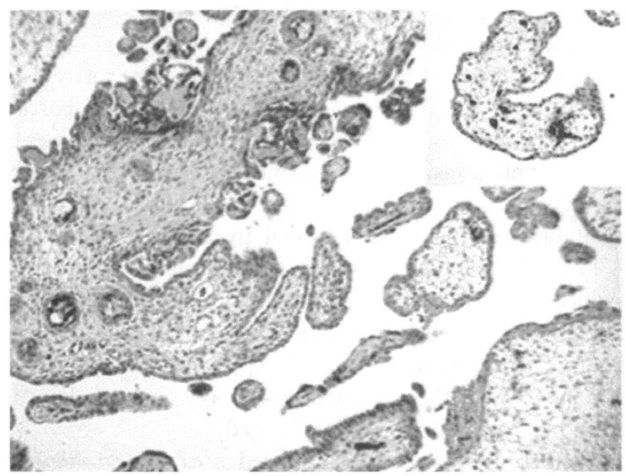

Figure 39.2 Histopathology slide of partial hydatidiform mole showing hydropic villi and trophoblastic proliferation.

CLINICAL PRESENTATION

The clinical presentation of a gravida with a molar gestation has changed over the last several decades with diagnosis by ultrasound and HCG testing.[22,23] Presenting signs and symptoms will vary greatly depending on the gestational age at diagnosis, the HCG titer, and whether the gestation is a CHM or PHM.

HCG is generally higher in a molar gestation than in a normal pregnancy. During normal pregnancies, HCG typically peaks around 8–11 weeks at about 100,000 mIU/mL. In contrast, titers in excess of 100,000 mIU/mL may be noted in up to half of CHM. PHMs, on the other hand, typically demonstrate[19] lower titers that are rarely >100,000 mIU/mL.[8] However, a single titer cannot be used as the only criterion for diagnosis, as the differential diagnosis for abnormally high HCG includes normal twin gestations, conditions that increase placenta mass, as well nongestational malignant tumors.

Excessive uterine size and vaginal bleeding are the two most commonly reported signs and symptoms. Historically, clinical examination may reveal a discrepancy between uterine size and dates in up to 50% of the cases. The uterus can be enlarged by tissue as well as blood. Vaginal bleeding is a nearly universal symptom of hydatidiform mole. Although some cases present with severe bleeding and/or anemia, these sequela are less likely with earlier diagnosis and intervention.[22]

Theca lutein cysts may be observed in a quarter of molar pregnancies (Figures 39.3 and 39.4).[24] These cysts are formed secondary to hyperstimulation of the ovaries by HCG secreted from trophoblastic tissue. The diagnosis can be made clinically by palpation of an adnexal mass, or sonographically. The management is conservative, as these cysts regress after evacuation of the mole and normalization of the HCG. Rarely, they may result in acute ovarian torsion requiring surgery. In these cases, the cysts may be drained intraoperatively—oophorectomy is unnecessary, unless the ovary is found to be nonviable.

Approximately one quarter of molar pregnancies present with hyperemesis gravidarum. The occurrence of pregnancy-induced hypertension (PIH) before 24 weeks' gestation has been regarded as a *sine qua non* of molar pregnancy. Rarely, subclinical or acute thyrotoxicosis can be seen in these patients due to high levels of serum HCG. Trophoblastic embolization resulting is respiratory distress and compromise occurs even more rarely, most commonly after evacuation of an advanced molar gestation with a high HCG titer.[22] These severe sequela are discussed in more detail below.

As noted above, with earlier diagnosis and management, many of the above-noted presenting signs and symptoms have become more rare. Most correlate with the HCG titer and trophoblastic tumor burden at diagnosis, and are accordingly less commonly seen with PHM than CHM. A recent report on CHMs from a large regional trophoblastic center reported vaginal bleeding and size greater than dates as the most common presenting signs (~50%, ~25% respectively). Over half of patients presenting in the last two decades presented at <11 weeks' gestation. Severe anemia, PIH, clinical hyperthyroidism, and respiratory distress/trophoblastic embolization occurred in less than 5% of patients, while hyperemesis was present in about 15%.[23]

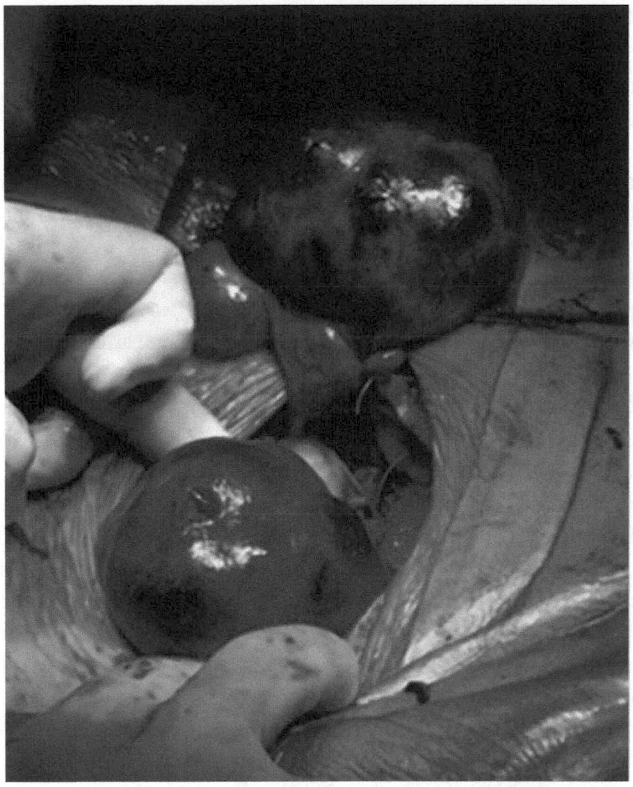

Figure 39.3 Theca-lutein cysts noted at the time of surgery.

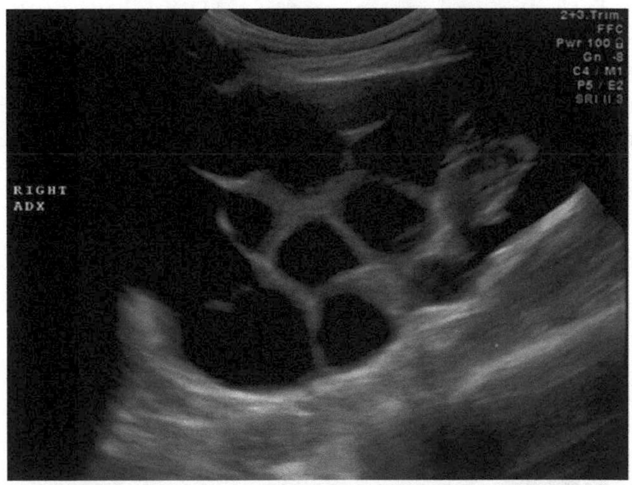

Figure 39.4 Ultrasound demonstrating theca-lutein cysts.

The majority of patients with PHM present with vaginal bleeding and absence of fetal heart activity. Missed or incomplete abortion is the most common diagnosis, and PHM is commonly not suspected prior to its identification on final pathology.[8]

DIAGNOSIS

Several diagnostic modalities have been used to identify molar pregnancy, including histologic evaluation, amniography, sonography, and HCG titers.

Diagnosis ultimately depends on histologic examination. Such an evaluation is required for all cases of missed or incomplete abortions, and in elective terminations of pregnancy. Histologic features of molar gestations are described above. Amniography is no longer used, as it requires the pregnancy to be over 14 weeks to permit access to an abdominal uterus, and involves exposure to ionizing radiation.

Sonographic examination is the principal diagnostic tool for the diagnosis of molar pregnancy. Its advantages include the absence of ionizing radiation, the ability to identify the morphologic features of the placenta and the presence or absence of a normal fetus, and to correlate these findings to HCG levels. The introduction of vaginal sonography has facilitated the diagnosis of hydatidiform mole during the first trimester and in obese patients where the abdominal approach might be inconclusive.[25] Molar changes can be detected around 8 weeks of gestation by ultrasonography. The classical "snowstorm pattern" was seen with older low-frequency ultrasound, while modern high-frequency ultrasound can show clearly defined cystic spaces representing hydropic villi. Computed tomography (CT) scan and magnetic resonance imaging (MRI) may be used selectively when there is a concern for concurrent metastatic disease or unclear uterine/fetal anatomy (Figure 39.5).[26]

Evaluation and management of GTD has been greatly aided by the availability of a reliable and highly sensitive tumor marker, HCG. Trophoblastic tissue produces HCG when viable tissue is present. This glycoprotein is composed of two polypeptide subunits (α and β). The structures of the

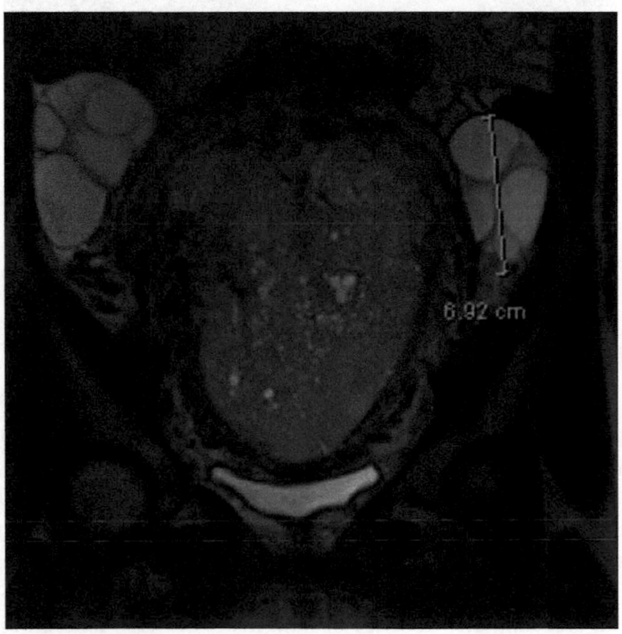

Figure 39.5 MRI showing a complete hydatidiform mole with theca-lutein cysts.

α-subunits of HCG and the pituitary hormones TSH (thyroid stimulating hormone), FSH (follicular stimulating hormone, LH (luteinizing hormone) are similar. The β-subunits have a unique amino acid content and sequence, which confer the immunologic and biologic specificity of each hormone. Importantly, circulating HCG is not only secreted by cells, but also exists as HCG degradation fragments. These HCG fragments are not biologically active, yet can function as tumor markers. Two types of HCG tests are commonly available, those that detect the intact HCG dimer only, and those that detect total HCG, including intact HCG dimer, free β-HCG, and other the variants/fragments. These total HCG assays are commonly known as "β-HCG tests." More so, it is important to select an appropriate "HCG tumor marker" assay during the evaluation of GTD to assure appropriate sensitivity of the assay, especially as HCG levels drop to normal or near normal levels. At these levels, false-negative testing has been reported in patients with active trophoblastic tumors, and omission of timely therapy in this setting has resulted in disastrous clinical consequences. Importantly, HCG testing may also result in false-positive test as a result of "phantom-HCG," quiescent GTD, pituitary HCG, and nontrophoblastic neoplasms. Physicians evaluating patients presenting with atypical or low HCG levels are urged to consultant with a clinician with expertise in these matters. While beyond the scope of this text, in depth reviews of HCG testing can be found elsewhere.[27–29]

MEDICAL COMPLICATIONS OF GESTATIONAL TROPHOBLASTIC DISEASE

As outlined above, the severity and clinical presentation of molar gestations vary and depend to a large extent on the absolute HCG titer, and the presence of CHM vs. PHM. Some of the severe sequela may require a significant degree of clinical expertise during management.

Although rare, clinical hyperthyroidism may present with tremor, warm skin, tachycardia, weight loss, and a palpable goiter. The laboratory findings include normal or suppressed TSH levels, increased thyroxine (T4), and triiodothyronine (T3), and a suppressed response to thyroid-releasing hormone (TRH). There is a degree of homology between HCG and TSH, and it is thought that HCG has a weak thyrotropin-stimulating effect on the thyroid gland when present at high concentrations, although the exact mechanism for this effect has not been clarified. Hydatidiform mole-induced thyrotoxicosis may present as a medical emergency. In this setting, any significant stress may precipitate thyroid storm. These patients require medical stabilization with beta-blockers and antithyroid drugs (e.g., PTU) prior to induction of anesthesia and surgery.

Some degree of anemia from vaginal bleeding is common with hydatiform moles. Rarely, major blood loss may precipitate the development of disseminated intravascular coagulation (DIC). DIC may also be precipitated by release of thromboplastic substances from the molar tissue into the maternal circulation. The treatment consists of evacuation of the molar tissue and supportive care with correction of the fibrinogen and platelet depletion as needed.

Respiratory complications can be the sequelae of metastatic disease, pulmonary edema from fluid overload, trophoblastic embolization, or other perioperative complications (e.g., adult respiratory distress syndrome). Historically, this phenomenon occurred in 2% of molar gestations and correlates with HCG burden and uterine size (more common >14–16 weeks). Most often this occurs in the immediate postoperative period, and usually resolves within 48–72 hours. Patients may be asymptomatic or have minimal symptoms, while others may require oxygen support, sedation, steroids, and positive-pressure ventilation for their respiratory compromise.[30] Clinical evaluation may reveal diffuse rales and pulmonary infiltrates, which should not be confused with metastatic disease. The occurrence of subclinical trophoblastic embolization has been well documented by the finding of trophoblastic tissue in the lungs during autopsy,[31] and by the recovery of multinucleated giant cells and large mononuclear cells from pulmonary artery blood specimens.[32] Hankins studied the hemodynamic profile in six pregnancies with the diagnosis of mole prior to, during, and after evacuation, to assess the degree of thromboplastic embolization associated with pulmonary distress. Minimal thromboplastic embolization did not appear to alter systemic or pulmonary hemodynamic parameters. Although the pulmonary vascular reaction did not appear to be anaphylactoid in nature, the phenomenon did appear to be dose related. Nonetheless, embolization sufficient to cause pulmonary compromise was rare.

All patients with pulmonary dysfunction require a thorough workup, including physical examination with close attention to the respiratory system, chest radiography, arterial blood-gas determination, and in rare cases, placement of a pulmonary artery catheter. The finding of severe hypoxemia and/or pulmonary edema requires access to intensive care and consultation with a pulmonary specialist. If respiratory compromise occurs prior to evacuation of the mole, the procedure should still be performed after supportive measurements have been established.[30,31]

Very rarely, a molar gestation may coexist with a normal twin pregnancy. Initial management includes ultrasonography, amniocentesis and chromosomal evaluation, HCG titers, chest imaging to assess for metastases, and additional laboratory studies (see below) to assess for maternal complications (e.g., thyrotoxicosis). MRI may yield additional information regarding fetal–placental anatomy and biopsy of the placenta maybe considered in select cases as well (e.g., to assess for mosaicism). Management commonly entails termination of pregnancy. There are, however, numerous case reports of successful conservative management of these twin pregnancies to term or near term,[33,34] although large case series are lacking. A series from Charing Cross Hospital in London reported on 77 pregnancies with CHM and a normal twin; 24 terminated pregnancy, while 53 were managed conservatively. Of these, about half the pregnancies reached 24 weeks, and 20 live births occurred. The risk of postmole GTN requiring chemotherapy did not appear to be different between those managed conservatively and those managed with termination.[35] In contrast, most other studies have also suggested an increased risk of postmole malignancy (GTN) and maternal complications such as PIH and thyrotoxicosis.[31,36] Management of these complex cases should be done in a multidisciplinary manner, with specialists in maternal fetal medicine and gynecologic oncology.

TREATMENT AND FOLLOW-UP OF MOLAR GESTATIONS

Prior to the termination of a molar pregnancy, a complete history, physical examination, baseline laboratory studies are typically obtained (Table 39.2). Chest imaging (x-ray) should be obtained in the case of pulmonary symptoms. Chest imaging, along with liver, renal, and thyroid function test, should also be obtained with advanced presentations and/or very high HCG levels. In otherwise healthy individuals, it is rare that these studies will disclose clinically significant sequela prior to the second trimester. Rh(D) antigen is expressed on trophoblasts and accordingly, Rh(D)-negative women should receive anti-D immunoglobulin after evacuation to prevent maternal alloimmunization.

The preferred method for treatment of a molar gestation is suction curettage. The uterus can be completely evacuated transvaginally with minimal danger of hemorrhage, even in cases of enlarged uterus. The patient should be typed and cross-matched for blood prior to the procedure. Either general or conduction anesthesia can be used. In rare emergencies, paracervical block combined with intravenous narcotic analgesia can be used. The patient is placed in lithotomy, and the cervix is serially and gently dilated to allow the introduction of a 9- to 12-mm plastic cannula into the uterine cavity in the standard manner. An oxytocin drip is initiated simultaneously with the activation of the suction pump. The curette is rotated in place until the molar tissue is evacuated. This should be associated with a decrease in the uterine size. The suction curette can then be removed and the remaining products removed by gentle sharp curettage. This last specimen should be submitted for histologic investigation separately. The physician should exercise caution during the performance of the sharp curettage in order to avoid perforation or subsequent Asherman syndrome.[37]

Table 39.2 Laboratory workup for molar gestations.

Complete blood count with differential
Serum HCG titer
Blood type and cross-match
PT, PPT, ±fibrinogen
Liver function tests
Renal function tests
Thyroid function tests
Chest x-ray

Abbreviations: PT, prothrombin time; PTT, partial thromboplastin time.

There is minimal data on the use of medical abortifacients for nonsurgical evacuation of molar gestations. There is a theoretical concern that inducing uterine contractions may increase the risk of trophoblastic embolization or metastatic disease, in addition to increasing the risk of bleeding and retained trophoblastic tissue.[37] Accordingly, their use for this purpose is not encouraged.

After evacuation of a molar gestation, a minority of patients will develop postmole malignant disease (GTN) and require further therapy. This occurs in approximately 15–20% of patients with CHM.[23,38] For patients with PHM, the risk of postmole GTN appears to be much lower, 1–6%.[38–40] Interestingly, the lower numbers within these reported ranges tend to be from larger series with central pathology review and uniform HCG testing and follow-up. Consequently, they may represent a more accurate estimate of the true likelihood of post-mole GTN. For CHM, three quarters of postmole GTN will be confined to the uterus, while metastases, most commonly to the lungs, will occur in approximately one quarter of patients (see below). In PHM, almost all cases of postmole GTN are confined to the uterus. In CHM, both age >40 and signs of marked trophoblastic proliferation (excessive uterine size, theca-lutein cysts, preevacuation HCG >100,000) are prognostic factors for the development of postmole GTN.[41,42] In fact, in patients with these features, 31% and 9% developed nonmetastatic and metastatic GTN, respectively. For patients lacking these features, the risks of nonmetastatic and metastatic GTN were 3.4% and 0.6%, respectively.[42] A recent study suggested the rate of HCG decline after evacuation may be a better predictor of the subsequent risk of GTN.[43] Risk factors for the development of postmole GTN with PHM are not as well defined. Histologically, invasive mole occurs more commonly than choriocarcinoma, although most often the histology will be unknown unless surgery occurs.

Given the risk of postmole GTN, all patients must be followed with a sensitive HCG assay in a serial fashion to document remission. This should be done on a weekly or biweekly basis until the HCG levels are normal for three consecutive measurements. Thereafter, the American College of Obstetricians and Gynecologists suggests HGG levels be followed monthly until levels are normal for 6 months. This duration of follow-up has recently been called into question, with studies suggesting a more abbreviated period of surveillance may be appropriate, especially with use of a modern sensitive HCG assay and after evacuation of a PHM.[44,38]

Documentation of a rise or plateau in the HCG titer, a prolonged HCG normalization time (>6 months), or histopathologic diagnosis of choriocarcinoma is considered diagnostic of GTN (Table 39.3) (FIGO). A rise is commonly regarded as occurring when sequential HCG titers increase greater than 10%. Although not part of the formal FIGO criteria, the development of metastases is also commonly used to define GTN. Patients diagnosed with GTN require evaluation and management with a gynecologic oncologist or medical oncologist with expertise in their management. With a rare exception, these patients

Table 39.3 Criteria for the diagnosis of GTN (FIGO).

1. Plateau of HCG lasts for four measurements over the period of 3 weeks or longer; i.e., days 1, 7, 14, 21
2. Rise in HCG on 3 weekly consecutive measurements over 2 weeks or longer; i.e., days 1, 7, 14
3. HCG remains elevated 6 months or longer
4. Histologic diagnosis of choriocarcinoma

Source: FIGO Oncology Committee, FIGO staging for gestational trophoblastic neoplasia 2000, FIGO Committee Report, *Int J Gynaecol Obstet*, 2002, 77, 285–287.

(diagnosed either postmole or otherwise) require chemotherapy for cure. Imaging studies used during this evaluation process may include pelvic ultrasound, chest x-ray, CT of the chest, abdomen, pelvis, and head MRI.

Controversy exists regarding the benefit of repeat curettage for a plateauing or rising HCG after evacuation of a mole. Most studies suggest this procedure may result in avoidance of chemotherapy for postmole GTN in 10–20% of patients.[45,46] The risk of perforation at the time of repeat curettage has been reported as high as 8%. Repeat curettage is rarely therefore indicated, but may have a role for patients with retained intracavitary molar contents and moderate or severe vaginal bleeding, or in the rare case of persistent disease that appears to be confined to the endometrium when the HCG is low. It should not be used during management of high-risk GTN or metastatic disease. A prospective trial investigating this issue has recently closed to accrual (GOG 242).

It is important to determine the patient's reproductive desires before a management plan is initiated. In patients who have completed families, hysterectomy (without chemotherapy) may be considered as an alternative to uterine evacuation. As noted above, 15–20% of patients with CHM and up to 5% of patients with PHM will develop postmole GTN and require subsequent therapy. In patients with CHM, three-quarters of these cases are confined to the uterus, while in PHM, extra-uterine disease is quite unlikely. For these patients, hysterectomy may be definitive and avoid the need for chemotherapy due to postmole GTN. Importantly, while the risk of invasive disease confined to the uterus is eliminated with primary hysterectomy, there is still a risk of metastatic GTN, and thus these patients should still be followed closely with HCG titers until normalization occurs as outlined above.

Prophylactic chemotherapy after molar evacuation has been suggested to decrease the incidence of postmole GTN. A prospective, randomized study to assess this was performed in South Korea.[47] The authors reported a significant decrease in the risk of postmole GTN in high-risk patients. A similar conclusion was reached by the authors of a 2012 meta-analysis. Although there were concerns regarding the methodological quality of the included studies, these authors noted prophylactic chemotherapy decreased the risk of postmole GTN. Yet, they also noted that in patients who received prophylactic chemotherapy and nevertheless developed GTN, the time interval to diagnosis was delayed, and the overall number of cycles of chemotherapy necessary to achieve remission was increased.[48] Furthermore, there is concern about exposing patients to a potentially toxic treatment when only 15–20% are at risk of developing GTN. Accordingly, routine prophylactic chemotherapy is not recommended, but its use may be considered selectively in woman at high risk of postmole GTN. This includes women over the age of 40 with a high trophoblastic burden (HCG titer >100,000 mIU/mL),[41] especially when there is concern that clinical or HCG follow-up is impractical or unlikely.

A patient may ovulate as early as 2–4 weeks after uterine evacuation.[49] Therefore, effective contraception should be started early, and continued throughout the duration of HCG surveillance. The preferred method of contraception is debatable, as some earlier studies suggested an increased risk of postmole GTN in patients using oral contraception.[50] More contemporary studies performed in the era of modern low(er) dose oral contraceptives, suggest otherwise. Studies from both the Gynecologic Oncology Group in the United States[51] and from The Charing Cross Hospital in London have shown no increased risk of postmole GTN with oral contraceptives.[52] Barrier contraception is an alternative when oral contraception is contraindicated, but there is a higher overall failure rate with this technique.[51] Intrauterine device is not recommended due to the risk of infection and perforation.

Patients undergoing treatment for a molar gestation can largely anticipate normal subsequent pregnancy outcomes. Although the likelihood of most reproductive outcomes, such as live term and preterm birth, is unchanged, the risk of subsequent molar gestation increases 10- to 20-fold, with repeat mole occurring in 1–2% of patients.[11,12] Molar pregnancy also appears to be associated with an increased risk of postmole GTN,[11] and this may occur after a normal term or normal intervening pregnancy. Subsequent pregnancies should therefore be approached with this in mind. An early first trimester ultrasound should document the absence of molar changes. After delivery, the placenta should be sent for evaluation, and an HCG titer should be obtained at 6–8 weeks postpartum. Some patients might present during the postpartum period with abnormal uterine bleeding or an enlarged uterus. Such abnormalities during a seemingly normal puerperium should prompt a careful evaluation for GTN.

TREATMENT OF GTN

Histologically, malignant GTNs are categorized as outlined in Table 39.1. Although different staging systems have been used in the past, the FIGO staging system adopted in 2000 has been widely used and accepted and is the current favored international staging system. FIGO assigns an anatomic numerical stage (I–IV), as well as a modified WHO risk score based on multiple prognostic features (Tables 39.4 and 39.5). Scores of 0–6 are considered *low risk*, while those ≥7 are considered *high risk*.

A number of imaging modalities can be used during the clinical evaluation of the patient. These include chest x-ray, pelvic ultrasound, CT of the chest, abdomen, and pelvis, MRI of the head, and, at times, PET scan. While CT scan will identify pulmonary metastases in 40% of patients with negative chest x-ray,[53] chest x-ray should be used when counting metastases during staging and calculating a FIGO risk score.

As outlined above, most cases of postmole GTN will present with either a risk or plateau in HCG titers. Often, patients will have continued bleeding from the uterus,

Table 39.4 FIGO anatomic staging of GTN (FIGO).

Stage 1	GTN confined to the uterus
Stage 2	GTN extends outside of uterus, but limited to genital structures (vagina, adnexa, broad ligament)
Stage 3	GTN extends to lung, with or without genital tract involvement
Stage 4	All other metastatic sites (liver, GI, brain)

Source: FIGO Oncology Committee, FIGO staging for gestational trophoblastic neoplasia 2000, FIGO Committee Report, *Int J Gynaecol Obstet*, 2002, 77, 285–287.

Table 39.5 Modified WHO prognostic scoring system adapted by FIGO.

Scores	0	1	2	4
Age	<40	≥40	–	–
Antecedent pregnancy	Mole	Abortion	Term	–
Interval from index pregnancy (months)	<4	4–<7	7–<13	≥13
Pretreatment serum HCG (mIU/mL)	$<10^3$	10^3–$<10^4$	10^4–$<10^5$	$\geq 10^5$
Largest tumor size (including uterus)	–	3–<5 cm	≥5 cm	–
Site of metastases	Lung	Spleen, kidney	GI	Liver, brain
Number of metastases	–	1–4	5–8	>8
Previous failed chemotherapy	–	–	Single drug	2 or more drugs

and may exhibit other signs of trophoblastic proliferation such as persistent theca-lutein cysts. GTN developing after nonmolar gestations presents with signs and symptoms related to the affected organ, along with an elevated HCG. Clinicians should consider GTN in a premenopausal female presenting with a metastatic malignancy of unknown origin, as a positive HCG titer in the absence of pregnancy often confirms the diagnosis.

As noted above, three-quarters of patients with post-mole GTN will have disease confined to the uterus. When present, metastatic disease most commonly occurs in the lungs (80% of cases) and vagina (30% of cases). Pulmonary metastases may be asymptomatic, or may present with cough, dyspnea, or hemoptysis. Imaging may show an alveolar "snowstorm" pattern or discrete rounded lesions. Vaginal metastases are highly vascular as may appear reddish-purple, most commonly being located in the vagina fornices or suburethrally. Biopsy of these lesions should be avoided as it may cause rapid exsanguination. Metastases to other sites, such as brain and liver, are rare in the absence of pulmonary metastases. Their prognosis, however, is much poorer, as reflected in the FIGO staging system; yet even in these patients a large majority will be cured with multiagent chemotherapy. Rarely, surgery is required secondary to complications such as bleeding, or to resect resistant disease sites that are not responding to chemotherapy.

Most patients developing GTN can anticipate cure with single-agent or multiagent chemotherapy, even in the setting of widely metastatic disease. Patients whom are stage I–III, with a *low-risk* score (0–6) can be managed by single-agent chemotherapy. In cases of resistance, they should be switched to multiagent chemotherapy. *High-risk* patients (score ≥ 7), on the other hand, should be managed with multiagent chemotherapy at the onset, as failure to do so may result in the development of chemoresistance and a lower likelihood of cure.

Placental site trophoblastic tumor and epitheliod trophoblastic tumor are rare forms of GTD that typically have a poor prognosis. The evaluation and management of these diseases are beyond the scope of this text.

CHEMOTHERAPY

Out outlined above, almost all patients with GTN require chemotherapy. Exceptions to this may be patients cured with a second curettage after primary uterine evacuation of a hydatiform mole, or patients with small vaginal or pulmonary metastases after molar evacuation with a spontaneously dropping HCG. Chemotherapy should be given by a gynecologic oncologist or a medical oncologist with expertise dealing with this condition. Patients with nonmetastatic or stage II–III *low-risk* scores (0–6) can be managed by single-agent chemotherapy and switched to multiagent chemotherapy if resistance ensues. *High-risk* patients (score ≥7), on the other hand, should be managed with multiagent chemotherapy at the onset. Failure to initiate multiagent chemotherapy in high-risk patients is associated with a lower likelihood of cure.

Patients are followed with weekly HCG measurements during chemotherapy. An HCG rise or plateau is suggestive of resistant disease, and patients should be switched to an alternative single- or multiagent regimen as appropriate. Imaging should be repeated in this setting, as focal sites of resistant disease are often amenable to surgical resection. Chemotherapy is administered in a dose-intensive manner, and continues for two or three consolidation cycles after normalization of HCG (it is estimated that 10^5 malignant cells still exist in vivo at the time of initial HCG normalization). Patients are encouraged to stay on oral contraceptive pills during chemotherapy and during the posttreatment period of surveillance (typically 1 year).

A number of single-agent methotrexate or actinomycin-D protocols have been described (Table 39.6).[54] These are usually administered every 2 weeks. There is no definitive evidence of the superiority of one regimen over another, yet most series suggest that daily treatment protocols are more effective than pulsed weekly or biweekly therapy. The use of multiagent chemotherapy with etoposide, methotrexate, actinomycin-D alternating with cyclophosphamide and vincristine (EMA-CO) over the last three decades has led to a significant improvement in the outcome of high-risk and low-risk resistant patients. Modifications of this regimen include the use of high-dose methotrexate (HD EMA-CO), the substitution of cisplatin and etoposide for cyclophosphamide and vincristine (EMA-EP). Paclitaxel/etoposide alternating with paclitaxel/cisplatin (TE/TP) can be used for resistant disease. Central nervous system (CNS) metastases may be treated with concurrent intrathecal methotrexate or brain irradiation. Survival after treatment for low-risk disease approaches 100%.[55] Patients with high-risk disease can expect survival rates of greater than 90% with expert care and multiagent chemotherapy, combined with selective use of surgery for resistant disease.[56]

The major side effects of chemotherapy are alopecia, myelosuppression, neuropathy, nausea, vomiting, mucositis/stomatitis, and end-organ damage (renal or hepatic toxicity). The common toxicities for a number of chemotherapeutic drugs used for the treatment of GTN are summarized in Table 39.7.

Table 39.6 Chemotherapy for low-risk GTN.

Methotrexate 0.4 mg/kg daily for 5 days IV or IM, given every 2 weeks
Methotrexate 1 mg/kg IM days 1, 3, 5, 7; alternating with folinic acid 0.1 mg/kg IM days 2, 4, 6, 8, given every 2 weeks
Methotrexate 50mg/m2 given weekly IM
Actinomycin-D 12 µg/kg daily for 5 days IV, given every 2 weeks
Actinomycin D 1.25 mg/m2 IV, given every 2 weeks
Methotrexate 300 mg/m2 infusion over 12 hours, followed by folinic acid rescue, given every 18 days

Source: Ngan HY et al., *Int J Gynaecol Obstet*, 2012 Oct, 119 (Suppl 2), S130–S136.

Table 39.7 Chemotherapy used in the treatment of GTN.

Drug	Common side effect
Methotrexate	Myelosuppression, mucositis, nephrotoxicity, transaminitis
Actinomycin-D	Myelosuppression, nausea/ vomiting, mucositis, alopecia
Etoposide	Myelosuppression, nausea/ vomiting, alopecia
Cyclophosphamide	Myelosuppression, hemorrhagic cystitis, nausea/vomiting, alopecia, amenorrhea
Vincristine	Neurotoxicity, alopecia, constipation
Cisplatin	Nephrotoxicity, nausea/vomiting, myelosuppression, neuropathy, ototoxicity
Paclitaxel	Myelosuppression, allergic reactions, alopecia, neuropathy

The majority of women undergoing chemotherapy for GTN will resume normal menses, although menopause seems to occur at a slightly earlier age.[57,58] Administration of a gonadotropin-releasing hormone agonist during chemotherapy appears to prevent ovarian failure and increases the likelihood of future pregnancy.[59,60] Patients whom become pregnant after treatment of GTN can generally expect normal pregnancy outcomes,[11] although many will express anxiety and fear of disease recurrence.[61] Patients treated with chemotherapy do not appear to be at an increased risk of having offspring with congenital anomalies.[62]

REFERENCES

1. Brinton LA, Wu B, Wang W, Ershow AG. Gestational trophoblastic disease: Case-control study from the People's Republic of China. *Am J Obstet Gynecol* 1989; 161: 121–127.
2. Berkowitz RS, Goldstein DP, Bernstein MR. Natural history of partial molar pregnancy. *Obstet Gynecol* 1983; 66: 677.
3. Pratola D, Wilkins P. The placenta, umbilical cord and amnio sac. In: Gompel C, Silvergery SG (eds), *Pathology in Gynecology and Obstetrics*, pp. 481–491. Lippincott, JB: Philadelphia, 1985.
4. Sebire NJ, Foskett M, Fisher RA, et al. Risk of partial and complete hydatidiform molar pregnancy in relation to maternal age. *Br J Obstet Gynaecol* 2002; 109: 99–102.
5. Parazzini F, LaVecchia C, Pampallona S. Parental age and risk of complete and partial hydatidiform mole. *Br J Obstet Gynaecol* 1986; 93: 582–585.
6. Acaia B, Parazzini F, LaVecchia C, et al. Increased frequency of complete hydatidiform mole in women with repeated abortion. *Gynecol Oncol* 1988; 31: 310–314.
7. Parazzini F, LaVecchia C, Mangili G., et al. Dietary factors and risk of trophoblastic disease. *Am J Obstet Gynecol* 1988; 158: 93–99.
8. Berkowitz RS, Cramer DW, Bernstein MR, et al. Risk factors for complete molar pregnancy from a case-control study. *Am J Obstet Gynecol.* 1985; 152: 1016–1020.
9. Parazzini F, Mangili G, LaVecchia C., et al. Risk factors for gestational trophoblastic disease: a separate analysis of complete and partial hydatidiform moles. *Obstet Gynecol.* 1991; 78: 1039–1045.
10. Berkowitz RS, Marilyn R, Bernstein MR, et al. Case-control study of risk factors for partial molar pregnancy. *Am J Obstet Gynecol* 1995; 173: 788–794.
11. Vargas R, Barroilhet LM, Esselen K, et al. Subsequent pregnancy outcomes after complete and partial molar pregnancy, recurrent molar pregnancy, and gestational trophoblastic neoplasia: an update from the New England Trophoblastic Disease Center. *J Reprod Med* 2014 May–Jun; 59(5–6): 188–194.
12. Eagles N, Sebire NJ, Short D, et al. Risk of recurrent molar pregnancies following complete and partial hydatidiform moles. *Hum Reprod* 2015 Sep; 30(9): 2055–2063.
13. Fisher RA, Hodges MD, Newlands ES. Familial recurrent hydatidiform mole: A review. *J Reprod Med* 2004; 49(8): 595–601.
14. Vassilakos P, Kajii T. Letter: Hydatidiform mole: two entities. *Lancet* 1976 Jan 31; 1(7953): 259.
15. Szulman AE, Surti U. The syndromes of partial and complete molar gestation. *Clin Obstet Gynecol* 1984; 27: 172–180.
16. Watson EJ, Hernandez E, Miyazawa K. Partial hydatidiform moles. A review. *Obstet Gynecol Surv* 1987; 42: 540–544.
17. Hsieh CC, Hsieh TT, Hsueh C, et al. Delivery of a severely anaemic fetus after partial molar pregnancy: Clinical and ultrasonographic findings. *Hum Reprod* 1999 Apr; 14(4): 1122–1126.
18. Dhingra KK, Gupta P, Saroha V, et al. Partial hydatidiform mole with a full-term infant. *Indian J Pathol Microbiol* 2009; 52(4): 590–591.
19. Genest DR, Ruiz RE, Weremowicz S. et al. Do non-triploid partial hydatidiform moles exist? A histologic and flow cytometric reevaluation of nontriploid specimens. *J Reprod Med* 2002; 47: 363–368.
20. Berkowitz RS, Goldstein DP. Gestational trophoblastic disease. *Cancer* 1995; 76: 2079–2085.
21. Sebire NJ, Fisher RA, Foskett M, et al. Risk of recurrent hydatiform mole and subsequent pregnancy outcome following complete or partial hydatiform molar pregnancy. *Br J Obstet Gynaecol* 2003; 110: 22–26.
22. Soto-Wright V, Bernstein M, Goldstein DP, et al. The changing clinical presentation of complete molar pregnancy. *Obstet Gynecol* 1995 Nov; 86(5): 775–779.
23. Sun SY, Melamed A, Goldstein DP, et al. Changing presentation of complete hydatidiform mole at the New England Trophoblastic Disease Center over the past three decades: does early diagnosis alter risk for gestational trophoblastic neoplasia? *Gynecol Oncol* 2015; 138(1): 46–49.

24. Montz FJ, Schlaerth JB, Morrow CP. The natural history of theca lutein cysts. *Obstet Gynecol* 1988 Aug; 72(2): 247–251.
25. Trimor-Tritsch IE, Rottem S, Blumenfeld Z. Pathology of the early intrauterine pregnancy. In: Timor-Tritsch IE, Rottem S (eds.), *Transvaginal Sonography*, pp. 109–124. Elsevier: New York, 1988.
26. Powell MC, Buckely J, Worthington BS, Symonds EM. Magnetic resonance imaging and hydatidiform mole. *Br J Radiol* 1986; 59: 561–564.
27. Olsen TG, Barnes AA, King JA. Elevated HCG outside of pregnancy—Diagnostic considerations and laboratory evaluation. *Obstet Gynecol Surv* 2007; 62(10): 669–674.
28. Muller CY, Cole LA. The quagmire of hCG and hCG testing in gynecologic oncology. *Gynecol Oncol* 2009; 112: 663–672.
29. Cole LA. Human chorionic gonadotropin tests. *Expert Rev Mol Diagn* 2009; 9(7): 721–747.
30. Kohorn EI. Molar pregnancy. Presentation and diagnosis. *Clin Obstet Gynecol* 1984; 27: 181–191.
31. Vejerslev L, Sunde L, Hansen B, et al. Hydatidiform mole and fetus with normal karyotype: Support of a separate entity. *Obstet Gynecol* 1991; 77: 868.
32. Hankins GD, Wendel GD, Snyder RR, Cunningham EG. Trophoblastic embolization during molar evacuation. Central hemodynamic observations. *Obstet Gynecol* 1987; 69: 368–372.
33. Feinberg FR, Lockwood CJ, Salafia C, Hobbins JC. Sonographic diagnosis of a pregnancy with a diffuse hydatidiform mole and coexistent 46,XX fetus. A case report. *Obstet Gynecol* 1988; 72: 485–488.
34. Thomas EJ, Pryce WI, Maltby EL, Duncan SLB. The prospective management of a coexisting hydatidiform mole and fetus. *Aust N Z J Obstet Gynaecol* 1987; 27: 343–345.
35. Sebir NJ, Foskett M, Paradinas FJ. Outcome of twin pregnancies with complete hydatidiform mole and healthy co-twin. *Lancet* 2002; 359: 2165–2166.
36. Steller MA, Genest DR, Bernstein MR, Lage JM, Goldstein DP, Berkowitz RS. Natural history of twin pregnancy with complete hydatidiform mole and coexisting fetus. *Obstet Gynecol* 1994; 83(1): 35–42.
37. Schlaerth JB. Methodology of molar pregnancy termination. *Clin Obstet Gynecol* 1984; 27: 192–198.
38. Schmitt C, Doret M, Massardier J, et al. Risk of gestational trophoblastic neoplasia after hCG normalisation according to hydatidiform mole type. *Gynecol Oncol* 2013; 130(1): 86–89.
39. Hancock BW, Nazir K, Everard JE. Persistent gestational trophoblastic neoplasia after partial hydatidiform mole incidence and outcome. *J Reprod Med* 2006; 51(10): 764–766.
40. Wolfberg AJ, Feltmate C, Goldstein DP, et al. Low risk of relapse after achieving undetectable HCG levels in women with partial molar pregnancy. *Obstet Gynecol* 2006; 108(2): 393–396.
41. Elias KM, Shoni M, Bernstein M, et al. Complete hydatidiform mole in women aged 40 to 49 years. *J Reprod Med* 2012 May–Jun; 57(5–6): 254–258.
42. Berkowitz RS, Goldstein DP. Presentation and management of molar pregnancy. In Hancock, Newland, Berkowitz (eds.), *Gestational Trophoblastic Disease*. 1997, Chapman and Hall.
43. Wolfberg AJ, Berkowitz RS, Goldstein DP, et al. Postevacuation hCG levels and risk of gestational trophoblastic neoplasia in women with complete molar pregnancy. *Obstet Gynecol* 2005 Sep; 106(3): 548–552.
44. Wolfberg AJ, Feltmate C, Goldstein DP, et al. Low risk of relapse after achieving undetectable HCG levels in women with complete molar pregnancy. *Obstet Gynecol* 2004 Sep; 104(3): 551–554.
45. Schlaerth JB, Morrow CP, Rodriguez M. Diagnostic and therapeutic curettage in gestational trophoblastic disease. *Am J Obstet Gynecol* 1990 Jun; 162(6): 1465–1470.
46. Lao TTH, Lee FHC, Yeung SSL. Repeat curettage after evacuation of hydatidiform mole. *Acta Obstet Gynecol Scand* 1987; 66: 305–307.
47. Kim DS, Moon H, Kim KT, et al. Effects of prophylactic chemotherapy for persistent trophoblastic disease in patients with complete hydatidiform mole. *Obstet Gynecol* 1986; 67: 690–694.
48. Fu J, Fang F, Xie L, et al. 2012. Prophylactic chemotherapy for hydatidiform mole to prevent gestational trophoblastic neoplasia. *Cochrane Database Syst Rev* 2012 Oct 17; 10.
49. Pak-Chung H, Wong L, Ho-Kei M. Return of ovulation after evacuation of hydatidiform moles. *Am J Obstet Gynecol* 1985; 153: 638.
50. Stone M, Dent J, Kardana A, Bagshawe KD. Relationship of oral contraception to development of trophoblastic tumour after evacuation of a hydatidiform mole. *Br J Obstet Gynaecol* 1976 Dec; 83(12): 913–916.
51. Curry SL, Schlaerth JB, Kohorn EL, et al. Hormonal contraception and trophoblastic sequelae after hydatidiform mole (a Gynecology Oncology Group Study). *Am J Obstet Gynecol* 1989; 160: 805–809.
52. Braga A, Maestá I, Short D, et al. Hormonal contraceptive use before hCG remission does not increase the risk of gestational trophoblastic neoplasia following complete hydatidiform mole: a historical database review. *Br J Obstet Gynaecol* 2015 Oct 7.
53. Mutch DG, Soper JT, Baker ME, et al. Role of computed axial tomography of the chest in staging patients with nonmetastatic gestational trophoblastic disease. *Obstet Gynecol* 1986 Sep; 68(3): 348–352.
54. Ngan HY, Bender H, Benedet JL, et al. Trophoblastic disease. *Int J Gynaecol Obstet* 2012 Oct; 119(Suppl 2): S130–S136.
55. McNeish IA, Strickland S, Holden L, et al. Low-risk persistent gestational trophoblastic disease: outcome after initial treatment with low-dose methotrexate and folinic acid from 1992 to 2000. *J Clin Oncol* 2002 Apr 1; 20(7): 1838–1844.

56. Agarwal R, Alifrangis C, Everard J, et al. Management and survival of patients with FIGO high-risk gestational trophoblastic neoplasia: the U.K. experience, 1995–2010. *J Reprod Med* 2014 Jan–Feb; 59(1–2): 7–12.
57. Wong JM, Liu D, Lurain JR. Reproductive outcomes after multiagent chemotherapy for high-risk gestational trophoblastic neoplasia. *J Reprod Med* 2014 May–Jun; 59(5–6): 204–208.
58. Bower M, Rustin GJ, Newlands ES, et al. Chemotherapy for gestational trophoblastic tumours hastens menopause by 3 years. *Eur J Cancer* 1998 Jul; 34(8): 1204–1207.
59. Blumenfeld Z, Avivi I, Linn S, et al. Prevention of irreversible chemotherapy-induced ovarian damage in young women with lymphoma by a gonadotropin-releasing hormone agonist in parallel to chemotherapy. *Human Reprod* 1996; 11: 1620–1626.
60. Moore HC, Unger JM, Phillips KA, et al. Goserelin for ovarian protection during breast-cancer adjuvant chemotherapy. *N Engl J Med* 2015 Mar 5; 372(10): 923–932.
61. Garner E, Goldstein DP, Berkowitz RS, et al. Psychosocial and reproductive outcomes of gestational trophoblastic diseases. *Best Pract Res Clin Obstet Gynaecol* 2003 Dec; 17(6): 959–968.
62. Green DM, Zevon MA, Lowrie G, et al. Congenital anomalies in children of patients who received chemotherapy for cancer in childhood and adolescence. *N Engl J Med* 1991; 325: 141–146.

Patient safety

40

MARIA LYN QUINTOS-ALAGHEBAND and GENEVIEVE B. SICURANZA

CONTENTS

> "The patient safety movement has changed the way we practice medicine."
>
> —Anonymous

INTRODUCTION

Patient safety as defined by the Agency for Healthcare Research and Quality (AHRQ) is a discipline in the health care profession that applies safety science methods toward the goal of achieving a trustworthy system of health care delivery.[1] Using key words such as *discipline, safety science,* and *achieving trustworthiness,* patient safety is conceptualized. There is a growing body of safety science knowledge applicable to the health care environment. Now, more than ever, there is increasing recognition that safety must be an integral part of the practice of medicine. As a matter of fact, we are already seeing this type of transformation in our health care system.

The Institute of Medicine (IOM) in its landmark publication *To Err is Human: Building a Safer Healthcare System,* in 2000, called to public attention the fact that delivery of health care is not error free and estimated that 98,000 deaths annually might be attributed to preventable medical errors. The report cited that this epidemic of medical errors arises from a decentralized and fragmented health care delivery model or "nonsystem"[2] and not particularly a result of individual recklessness or "bad apple problem." This report calls for a comprehensive strategy to redesign the health care system toward a *culture of safety.* In order for this to happen, multiple stakeholders need to work together.

Some of the main strategies outlined include the creation of national leadership, i.e., an organization that will set national safety goals and monitor progress toward meeting them. Other strategies include increased funding for research, tools, and protocols to advance the application of the science of safety to health care and also the creation of mandatory public reporting and voluntary reporting systems. These systems will provide opportunities for shared learning and will foster accountability to the consumer.

After the year 2000 IOM report, there was another publication, in 2001, *Crossing the Quality Chasm*,[3] which embodied the report issued by the Committee on Quality of Health Care in America. This report, a product of comprehensive literature review and expert opinion, highlights the gap between the current health care system and the one we should have. It describes needed changes in four key areas: (a) the use of information technology; (b) payment reforms; (c) development of best practices, decision support tools and accountability; and (d) professional education and training.[3] The committee presented an agenda that calls for quality improvements in six areas of patient care: Safety, timeliness, effectiveness, efficiency, equitability, and patient-centeredness.

Since the year 2000 IOM report, the American College of Obstetricians and Gynecologist (ACOG) and other health care organizations have responded by focusing on key patient safety principles which include development of a culture of safety, implementation of safe medication practices; reduction of surgical errors; improvement of communication among healthcare providers; improvement of communication with patients; creation of partnership with patients; and safety as a priority in every aspect of medical practice.[4,5] In the United States today, the most frequent reason for hospital admission is obstetrics, with approximately four million hospitalizations per year.[6] It is clear that the obstetrician has a large responsibility to the patient, society, and the health care industry in providing safe and quality care. Adverse obstetrical outcomes are difficult to estimate. One study over the course of 7 years estimated that near miss morbidities involved 45.5% of all deliveries, 16% of all deliveries were complicated by a severe morbidity and 40% of maternal deaths were preventable.[6]

MEDICAL ERRORS

Definition

The safety literature defines an error as "an act of commission (doing something wrong) or omission (failing to do the right thing) leading to an undesirable outcome or significant potential for such an outcome."[7] When an error reaches the patient, it can lead to an adverse event. The IOM defines a preventable adverse event as an injury caused by medical management, rather than the underlying condition of the patient, which is attributable to medical error. Not all adverse events are created equal. Adverse events that lead to death or major disability are considered sentinel events. Errors that do not reach the patient or reach the patient but did not lead to harm are called "near misses." Near misses can illustrate important systems vulnerabilities and offer tremendous learning opportunities to the organization. The different types of medical errors are shown in Table 40.1.[2,8]

Table 40.1 Classification of medical errors (Institute of Medicine approach).

Classification of medical errors
Diagnostic errors
• Error or delay in diagnosis
• Failure to employ indicated tests
• Use of outmoded tests or therapy
• Failure to act on results of monitoring or testing
• Failure to rescue
Treatment errors
• Errors in the performance of an operation, procedure or test
• Error in administering the treatment
• Error in the dose or method of using a drug
• Avoidable delay in treatment or responding to an abnormal test
• Inappropriate (not indicated) care
Prevention errors
• Failure to provide prophylactic treatment
• Inadequate monitoring or follow-up treatment
Other systems' errors due to human or nonhuman factors
• Failure of communication
• Equipment failure

Sources: Kohn L, Corigan JM, Donaldson, MS, Institute of Medicine. *To Err Is Human: Building a Safer Health System*. Washington, DC: National Academy Press, 2000; Leape L, *Qual Rev Bull*, 19: 144–149, 1993.

Theories of error causation

One way of understanding the etiology of medical errors or systems' accidents is the *Swiss cheese* model popularized by James Reason.[9] Defences, barriers, and safeguards are portrayed as cheese slices. In an ideal world, all of these layers are intact. In reality, however, they are more like slices of Swiss cheese with each layer having many holes or gaps. These gaps are created by either active failures or latent conditions.[9] Active failures are the unsafe actions of humans in contact with the system. They include slips, lapses, and procedural violations. Latent conditions are defects residing in the system. The majority of adverse events arise from a combination of these two factors.

Root cause analysis (RCA)

RCA is a detailed retrospective analysis of sequence of events and underlying causes after an adverse event has occurred. It seeks to define systems' failures and identify all the contributing factors that lead to the adverse event. A root cause is defined as the most basic causal factor that if corrected will prevent recurrence of a similar adverse event. Thus, identifying the real root cause is critical to system redesign.

The RCA process needs a standardized approach that should start with timely and thorough data collection to map out the systems' events leading to the error. Then, it requires a detailed analysis of underlying problems to determine all contributing causes. One practical approach is to ask the five "whys" or a more extensive series of "whys" until the root cause is identified. The fishbone or cause-and-effects diagram is a useful visual tool to plot the possible causes and subcauses. In order to be successful in preventing recurrences, corrective actions should directly target the root cause or causes. The RCA should produce a corrective action plan. The subsequent outcomes following the corrective action plan should be tracked and measured. The RCA focuses on systems and processes starting at the bedside and spreading throughout the organization. The goal is to construct an action plan that will reduce the chance of similar adverse events occurring in the future.

RCA follows the five rules of causation. *Rule #1* is to demonstrate the cause and the effect, i.e., there should be a clear link between the root cause and the adverse outcome. *Rule #2* is to avoid negative terms and use clear, positive, and proactive language. *Rule #3*. If there is evidence of human error, the exact underlying cause should be identified (e.g., double shift). *Rule #4*. In the event of a procedural deviation, the exact deviation should be identified. *Rule #5*: There is no failure in not doing something that was not explicitly known to be a duty. As Meltzoff argued, proximal events are not necessarily the cause of anything (*post hoc ergo propter hoc*).[10]

The RCA does acknowledge the plurality of causes (levers) in adverse outcomes. The Joint Commission database indicates an average of four to six root causes for each sentinel event. RCA's aim is to identify the causality–comparative interactions where the addition of one or more variables results in a distinct adverse outcome. The Joint Commission has identified common root cause categories including human factors (staffing, resident supervision), communication (staff, administration, patient or family), assessment (adequate, timely), and leadership (prioritization, resource allocation, performance improvement).[11]

Failure modes and effect analysis (FMEA)

FMEA is prospective. FMEA was initially developed by reliability engineers to address potential problems that may arise in the military. It is used to define every aspect of the system's design and interactions and identify resultant effects on systems operations. Its primary benefit is early identification of systems failure before a catastrophic event occurs.

FMEA is process focused.[12] FMEA approach maps out the process and subprocesses to determine what can go wrong and how it can go wrong (failure mode). It then analyzes the probability, i.e., how many times it is likely to occur and the severity or impact, i.e., what can happen when it occurs. Targeted high-risk processes prevent adverse events from occurring. Thus, FMEA is a proactive approach to manage the system's vulnerabilities.

FOCUSED PATIENT SAFETY INITIATIVES

Improving communication

The Joint Commission reports that in 2010, of all perinatal adverse events, 70% were associated with communication breakdown.[11] The Joint Commission identified communication failure to be responsible for 60% of sentinel events and 50% of adverse anesthesia events. Formal communication strategies used by multidisciplinary teams caring for patients have proven to decrease medical errors, thus improving patient safety and quality. Communications aids such as situation, background, assessment, recommendation (SBAR) and "I Pass the Baton" in TeamStepps have both been proven to be effective.[12,13]

"Hand offs" and "sign outs" present some of the most critical events in medicine. The Joint Commission advises that a well-defined and specific process for hand offs be utilized between providers to ensure effective communication. Care should be taken to ensure that hand offs are performed in a standardized, multidisciplinary, confidential, and secure fashion and are free of interruptions or distractions. In Labor and Delivery units, the standardization of the nomenclature used to describe electronic fetal heart rate patterns has improved communication between providers and has minimized misinterpretation during fetal assessment.[14]

"Huddles" during patient care allow the team to come together, review the care of the patient, and give the opportunity for individual members of the team to express concerns. It has been demonstrated that huddles result in a decrease in the number of errors, identification of near misses, and strengthening of the interdisciplinary working relationships.[15] Staff members become empowered and there is a greater sense of responsibility and accountability. High reliability organizations encourage huddles as a means of "flattening" the hierarchy and recognizing the team member who has the most information regarding a particular patient. Huddles foster a community of collaboration, mutual respect among all team members, and improved collegiality. Huddles between obstetricians and neonatalologists have demonstrated improved neonatal resuscitation outcomes.[14]

Communication with patients and families is critical. The goal of patient safety, patient focused care, and communication are all an integral part of the practice of medicine. According to ACOG, communication with patients et al. is a "moral obligation" of the physician.[15] Adverse events should be communicated or disclosed to the patient and family, as soon as possible, in a clear and concise manner. The relationship with the patient should be one of partnership. This results in patients being included as members of the health care team and, as such, they should be advised and consulted regarding all possible treatment options.

Safe medication practice

Errors can occur at any point in the medication delivery process including prescription, transcription, dispensing, and administration. Because the process is complex it is important to analyze all the risk points in the pathway and design processes to reduce potential for errors (Table 40.2; see also Table 40.3).[16,17] The use of computerized provider order entry systems (CPOE) and built-in clinical decision support systems can reduce the incidence of medication errors. Clinical decision support systems can help with correct dosage calculations and flag alerts for drug-to-drug interactions or dosages that fall out of usual ranges.

Table 40.2 Strategies to decrease medication errors.

Observe the Joint Commission "Do Not Use" list (Table 40.3)
Use of the "five rights" of medication administration: right patient, right route, right dose, right time and right drug.
Double checking for high-risk medications.
Prevention of interruptions and avoidance of verbal orders.
Medication reconciliation.

Source: Wachter R, *Understanding Patient Safety* (2nd edition), New York, NY: McGraw Hill Medical, 2012.

The pharmaceutical industry has just begun to address some of these issues to some extent by ensuring that labels are distinctive for different concentrations of the same drug. At the institutional level, a multidisciplinary medication safety workgroup should be established to monitor adverse drug events. Medication errors and near-miss reporting ensures safe medication practices. In addition, education and partnership with patients can greatly improve medication safety.

Checklist

Successful use of checklists is possible when applied to processes that are simple, intuitive, stardardized, and time sensitive. Checklists are considered to be the essential resource for any High Reliability Organization (i.e., airline, nuclear submarines). However, equity is not readily apparent across all industries due to the vastly different cultures. The adoption of checklists in medicine is a complex matter. Checklists will not replace the high level of cognitive function that is required when practicing medicine but they can play a powerful role in preventing errors.[17,18]

In 2010, The Joint Commission and the Society for Maternal Fetal Medicine advised adoption of protocols to decrease maternal mortality and morbidity due to hemorrhage.[19] Adoption of these protocols by large health care systems demonstrated a reduction in the severity of maternal hemorrhage, the number of blood products transfused, and the frequency of disseminated intravascular coagulation.[19] Checklists for obstetrical hemorrhage that support protocol adherence include hemorrhage risk assessment, blood bank request, blood and clots quantified by weighing, laboratory results during the various stages of hemorrhage, uterotonic use under direct physician supervision, blood products administered as per protocol, quantity and type of blood products administered, and number of peripartum hysterectomies.[19]

The World Health Organization's *safe surgery saves* has been embraced by Federation of International Gynecological Oncologists (FIGO). This involves a 19-item checklist to be followed prior to the induction of anesthesia, incision, and sign out prior to leaving the operating room for the recovery room. Through the use of a "time out" prior to any surgical or invasive procedure, the correct nature of the procedure is reviewed along with the patient's identity. The Joint Commission Universal protocol is designed to ensure correct person, site, and procedure.[20]

Bundles

The National Partnership for Maternal Safety Council on Patient Safety in Women's Healthcare established a Consensus Bundle on obstetric hemorrhage.[21] A bundle of evidence-based practices when performed together have been shown to improve patient outcomes. The items included in the consensus hemorrhage bundle are shown in Table 40.4.[22]

This bundle was crafted with input from multiple authoritive groups including the American Association of Blood Banks, The American Academy of Family Physicians, the American College of Nurse–Midwives, and the American College of Obstetrics and Gynecology. The ultimate goal is that each institution should standardize the bundle as fits their institution and utilize it at *every* hemorrhage event.[22]

Electronic health records (EHR)

The EHR provides a platform enabling providers to communicate with each other efficiently, thus providing better patient care. The ideal EHR should support safe prescribing and administration of medications while tracking and reporting adverse events. The EHR should also foster

Table 40.3 Official Joint Commission "do not use" list.

Do not use	Potential problem	Use instead
U, u (unit)	Mistaken for "0" (zero), the number "4" (four) or "cc"	Write "unit"
IU (International Unit)	Mistaken for IV (intravenous) or the number 10 (ten)	Write "International Unit"
Q.D., QD, q.d., qd (daily)	Mistaken for each other	Write "daily"
Q.O.D., QOD, q.o.d, qod (every other day)	Period after the Q mistaken for "I" and the "O" mistaken for "I	Write "every other day"
Trailing zero (X.0 mg)	Decimal point is missed	Write X mg
Lack of leading zero (.X mg)		Write 0.X mg
MS	Can mean morphine sulfate or magnesium sulfate	Write "morphine sulfate"
MSO_4 and $MgSO_4$	Confused for one another	Write "magnesium sulfate"

Exception: A "trailing zero" may be used only where required to demonstrate the level of precision of the value being reported, such as for laboratory results, imaging studies that report size of lesions, or catheter/tube sizes. It may not be used in medication orders or other medication-related documentation.

Source: The Joint Commission, Facts about the Official "Do Not Use" List of Abbreviations, http://www.jointcommission.org/facts_about_do_not_use_list/. Accessed October 28, 2016.

Table 40.4 Consensus bundle on obstetric hemorrhage.

Readiness

- Hemorrhage cart on every unit complete with supplies, checklists and instruction cards on the use of intrauterine balloons and compression sutures
- Accessible uterotonics
- Hemorrhage response team delineation (bloodbank, gyn-oncology, etc.)
- Emergency release of blood products
- Unit education on protocols and simulations

Recognition and prevention

- Risk assessment prenatally, on admission and during labor/section
- Quantitative measurement of blood loss
- Active management of third stage of labor

Response

- Stage based hemorrhage management plan with checklists
- Support program for patient, families, and staff

Reporting

- Establish culture of huddles and debriefs
- Multidisciplinary review of serious hemorrhage for system issues
- Monitor outcomes and process metrics in perinatal quality improvement committee

Source: Modified from Council on Patient Safety in Women's Health Care, http://www.safehealthcareforeverywoman.org/. Accessed October 28, 2016.

prescriber compliance with guidelines. The obstacles to the EHR have been numerous including cost, poor design, alteration in workflow, time, and resource consuming. Successful implementation requires physician champions to get involved with the creation of a design suitable to the needs of the patients and providers. In addition, universal use of one program within one organization would foster provider communication and efficient and quality medical care for patients. Future studies should be designed to demonstrate the benefits for both the provider and the patient.[16]

Emergency preparedness

Rapid response teams (RRT) are designated emergency response teams that bring critical care expertise to the patient's bedside. Any member of the health care staff, or family member or patient, should be able to activate a rapid response team. Each institution and department should establish their own criteria and the key staff of the RRT should be immediately available 24/7. Each member of the team should have a well-defined and specific role. The team should use standard communication tools such as situation, background, assessment, recommendation (SBAR) to ensure rapid and effective communication. Debriefing after every RRT event assures quality and process improvement. The hospital's administration involvement is an integral part of this process in order to make sure that the appropriate resources are provided. If the condition of the patient requires an increase in the level of care, the RRT should facilitate this process by locating an available bed and facilitating the patient transfer. Some examples of Ob/Gyn scenarios requiring an RRT action are hypertensive crisis, hemorrhage, eclampsia, or respiratory distress.[23]

Partnership with patients

Engaging patients in a partnership will improve patient care, patient and provider satisfaction, and may ward off medical professional liability action. Informed consent needs to be regarded as a contract, which ensures that the patient understands the diagnosis, treatment, possible complications, as well as other available treatment options. Ideally, a friend or a family member should accompany a patient during this discussion.[21]

CULTURE OF SAFETY

The American Congress of Obstetrics and Gynecology is committed to patient safety and quality. The congress has suggested that the OB/Gyn community establishes practices, which will support the safe care of patients and promote the practice of high-quality medicine.[5] To that end, developing a "*culture of patient safety*" is essential. A culture of safety recognizes the need to avoid medical errors. This culture extends across all levels of an organization, from the bedside (provider and staff) to the boardroom of the organization. A culture of safety requires a "*just culture*".

Just culture

Dr. Lucian Leape in his testimony to congress in 1997 stated that the single greatest impediment to error prevention is that "we punish people for making mistakes."[24] The traditional thinking of equating error with incompetence, and attributing blame and shame, as effective means to modify behavior pose barriers to reporting and opportunities for identifying the system's failures to prevent recurrence.

In his book *Whack-a-Mole,* David Marx, an expert in human error and champion of the *Just Culture* philosophy, writes: "Just as tornados and lightning strikes are unavoidable, predictable components of the weather, I know that human fallibility, my own included, is an unavoidable, predictable component of being human."[25]

Because humans will make mistakes one of the major attributes of *Just Culture* is the design of safe systems. Safe systems help humans with correct and safe choices and ensure that when an error occurs it can be detected early and mitigate harm to the patient.[24]

Just culture creates an environment where the individuals feel safe to report errors, are encouraged to continuously learning from mistakes, and supports safe behavior choices. It analyzes behavioral choices along four concepts: human error, negligence, intentional rule violations, and reckless conduct.[26]*Just culture* holds the organization accountable to respond to staff behaviors fairly and justly and it is not to be construed for total amnesty; just culture supports disciplined behavioral choices and shared accountability.

A *just culture* recognizes that errors are inevitable. How an organization responds to an error will determine if a *just culture* exists. A *just culture* examines the error in order to determine if the error is secondary to a process or system failure or due to reckless behavior of the staff or provider. The investigation requires cool heads, transparency, and a reproducible resolution. Staff involved may be consoled, counseled, or punished, all depending on the type of error.

Disruptive behavior affects both the staff and the patient negatively. Disruption can range from verbal tantrums and physical assaults to sarcasm, humiliation, and passive-aggressive behavior. Organizations must have processes in place in order to deal with such individuals ensuring that such behaviors are stopped. Recognition, education, reporting, and training of all care givers ensure that such behavior does not occur or recur.[27]

Medical disclosure and apologies

Full disclosure to the patient and/or family of what caused the adverse event is one of the most important conversations that the physician or hospital staff can have with the patient and their family.[28] Full disclosure protects the existing trust between the patient and physician or hospital staff, thus allowing continuation of the therapeutic relationship. Full disclosure also provides closure and healing. In addition, disclosure may mitigate against medical malpractice action. It should be emphasized that many injured patients may pursue malpractice action simply as a means of discovering the cause of the adverse event.[28]

Patients and families deserve an apology, if the adverse event was the result of a human error or the system's error. In some cases, patients and their families feel the need for someone to recognize that they may have been harmed and that the involved health care providers are sorry for the unfortunate adverse outcome. They also need to hear that the events leading up to the event will be investigated and that changes will be made to prevent this from happening again to another patient.[29]

Patient support

If a patient has been hurt by a medical error and additional follow-up or care is required after discharge, such health care services need to be provided without submitting the patient to any additional financial burden. In addition, the hospital and physician need to ensure that the transition as an outpatient is made as smoothly as possible.

Peer support

This is the most important resource for a physician after an adverse event. The ability to discuss the medical aspects of the case is very important. According to Dr. Leonard, the medical profession has a moral obligation to take care of caregivers who are involved in an adverse outcome.[30] These health care professionals may become very vulnerable and require and deserve compassion, caring, and respect.[31]

REPORTING AND MEASURING SAFETY

Incident reporting system

Monitoring and measuring adverse events, as well as near misses, are fundamental to patient safety. However, there are great challenges in data collection for producing accurate metrics. The most commonly employed tool is the incident reporting system, which relies on self-reports of errors by health care providers. However, the reporting is usually voluntary and since many other factors influence reporting, including the culture of safety and transparency of the organization, the existing incident reporting systems may not be very reliable.[32]

Patient safety indicators (PSI)

The Agency for HealthCare Research and Quality (AHRQ) has recommended measurement of several important PSI.[32] These PSIs consist of outcomes or process measures that designed to measure or assess patient safety. The 2010 National Healthcare Quality Report (NHQR) from AHRQ includes the following patient safety indicators specific to maternal–child health care service[32]: (a) birth trauma injury to neonate per 1000 selected live births; (b) obstetric trauma per 1000 vaginal deliveries without instrument assistance; (c) obstetric trauma per 1000 instrument-assisted deliveries; and (d) obstetric trauma per 1000 cesarean deliveries.

However, it should be noted that PSI measures are frequently extracted from administrative datasets which may present various limitations. These limitations include undercoding, inconsistencies in the use of diagnostic coding and lack of comprehensive clinical details. Retrospective chart review, although more exhaustive and labor intensive, has been traditionally considered the gold standard for identification of errors and adverse events.[11]

Global trigger tools

The use of trigger tools can improve the sensitivity and specificity of detecting adverse events. Trigger tools can be tracked and in some cases they can uncover adverse events. The Institute for Healthcare Improvement (IHI) has developed a list of global trigger tools that are widely accepted.[33] Examples of IHI global trigger tools include readmissions within 30 days, return to surgery, and the use of naloxone. Obstetrical trigger tools include use of terbutaline, third or fourth degree perineal lacerations, platelet count less than 50,000, estimated blood loss greater than 500 cc for vaginal delivery or 1000 cc for cesarean, specialty consults, administration of oxytocin, instrumental delivery, and administration of general anesthesia

Obstetric core measures

It has always been challenging and controversial to develop the appropriate quality metrics relevant to the practice of obstetrics. However, the Joint Commission has recently recommended two Obstetric Core measures such as number of elective deliveries prior to 39 completed weeks of gestation, cesarean delivery rate in the low-risk nulliparous at term with a singleton vertex, and rate of antenatal corticosteroid administration in infants born between 24 and 34 weeks gestation.[34]

Howell et al. reviewed New York City birth certificate data from 2010 and found that elective delivery rates before 39 completed weeks of gestation and cesarean delivery rates in low-risk nulliparous vary widely and that there was no correlation between these quality indicators and maternal or neonatal morbidity; the authors questioned whether or not these quality indicators are sufficiently valid to guide quality improvement management in obstetrics.[35]

MISCELLANEOUS

Hospitalists

Since first defined in 1996, hospitalist and laborist models continue to evolve. The need for high-value inpatient care combining safety with reduced costs has led to the development of the subspecialty of OB/Gyn hospitalists. OB/Gyn hospitalists provide continuous coverage of labor and delivery and initial promising results have shown a safe reduction in the primary cesarean delivery rate, an increase in the vaginal birth after cesarean (VBAC) rate and a lower rate of adverse neonatal outcomes.[36]

In addition, there is some suggestion that malpractice claims, adverse events, and sentinel evens are decreased.[36] Hospitalist fellowship programs are now beginning to emerge in the United States as an option for OB/Gyn physicians, especially targeting recent residency graduates, who want to obtain training as hospital safety officers and at the same time strengthen their clinical skills.[37]

Simulation

The 1999 IOM report advised health care organizations to look toward the aviation industry and their simulation techniques as a means of providing team training in medicine.[2] The Institute of Medicine, Joint Commission on Accreditation of Health Care Organizations, and numerous professional societies and authoritative bodies have advised simulation training. In 2004, the Joint Commission on Accreditation of Healthcare Organizations released a sentinel alert:

> Since the majority of perinatal death and injury cases reported root causes related to problems with organization culture and with communication among caregivers, it is recommended that organizations, 1) conduct team training in perinatal areas to teach staff to work together and communicate more effectively, and 2) for high-risk events, such as shoulder dystocia, emergency cesarean delivery, maternal hemorrhage, maternal cardiac arrest and neonatal resuscitation, conduct clinical drills to help staff prepare for when such events actually occur, and conduct debriefings to evaluate team performance and identify areas for improvement.[5]

While medicine is a far more complex discipline than any of the others managed by High Reliability Organizations, simulations do offer the opportunity for staff to perform in a predictable manner when faced with an infrequent or emergent situation.

Currently the American College of Obstetricians and Gynecologists support simulation-based training in obstetric emergency drills in order to reduce communicating errors and improve interdisciplinary teamwork.[15] Over the past 5 years, there have been an increasing number of studies which have demonstrated decreased rates of brachial plexus injury damage[38,39] and decreased rates in Apgar scores less than 7 in the setting of prolapsed cord.[40] A combined team training of multiple disciplines simultaneously was shown to be superior.[23] Simulations quickly identify process failures or deficiencies such as delays in accessing medications or need for additional staff. In summary, simulations teach obstetrical skills and maneuvers, foster teamwork and communication, and identify flaws in existing processes.[41] According to Ziv,[42] there is a moral imperative to utilize simulation training because it teaches and rehearses the medical staff without compromising the patient.

Patient safety in postgraduate education

The Council for Resident Education (CREOG) has established guidelines for graduate medical education as it applies to OB/Gyn residents. Programs must be committed to for promoting patient safety. Program directors must ensure that residents are integrated and actively participate in interdisciplinary clinical quality improvement and patient safety programs. The program director must ensure that a culture of professionalism exists and an environment that supports patient safety and personal accountability. The CREOG specifically addresses transitions of care charging programs to ensure that there is a structured hand over processes to facilitate both continuity of care and patient safety. Residency programs are responsible for monitoring all transitions of care.

Patient safety in clinical research articles

Peer-reviewed journals are a rich source of new information. This new information may be used as hypothesis generating for future research or can be used to improve clinical practice. Since only few of the published articles are "practice changers", it is imperative that physicians do not misunderstand the conclusion or conclusions of the article. In order to avoid misunderstandings between authors and practitioners, Vintzileos et al.[4] have suggested that the practice implications and patient safety issues for each published article should be addressed by the authors and placed prominently in a text box so that communication among authors and health care providers is clear regarding the implications for practice changes and safety.[4] It is our belief that if, in the future, all medical journals follow this suggestion this can only lead to better patient care.

REFERENCES

1. Emanuel L, Berwick D, Conway J, et al. What exactly is patient safety? In Henriksen K, Battles JB, Keyes, MA et al. (eds), *Advances in Patient Safety: New Directions and Alternative Approaches.* Rockville, MD: AHRQ, 2008.
2. Kohn L, Corigan JM, Donaldson, MS, Institute of Medicine. *To Err Is Human: Building a Safer Health System.* Washington, DC: National Academy Press, 2000.
3. Institute of Medicine (IOM). *Crossing the Quality Chasm: A New Health System For The Century* (21st edition). Washington, DC: National Academy Press, 2001.
4. Vintzileos A, Finamore P, Sicuranza G, Cande A. Patient safety in clinical research articles. *Int J Gynecol Obstet* 2013; 123: 93–95.
5. American College of Obstetricians and Gynecologist. ACOG committee opinion number 286, October 2003: Patient safety in obstetrics and gynecology. *Obstet Gynecol* 2009; 114: 424–427.
6. Geller S, Rosenberg D, Cox S, et al. The continuum of maternal morbidity and mortality: Factors associated with severity. *Obstet Gynecol* 2004; 191: 939–944.
7. Grober E, Bohnen J. Defining medical error. *Can J Surg* 2005; 48: 339–344.
8. Leape L. Preventing medical injury. *Qual Rev Bull* 1993; 19: 144–149.
9. Reason J. Human error: Models and management. *BMJ* 2000; 320.
10. Meltzoff J. *Research Questions and Hypotheses. Critical Thinking about Research: Psychology and Related Fields.* Washington, DC: American Psychological Association 1998; 13–30.
11. Lyndon A, Johnson M, Bingham D, et al. Transforming communication and safety culture in intapartum care. A multi-organization blueprint. *Obstet Gyn* 2015; 125: 5.
12. Myers S, Patient Safety and Hospital Accreditation. *A Model for Ensuring Success.* New York, NY: Springer Publishing Company, 2012.
13. Agency for Healthcare Research and Quality. *TeamSTEPPS: Strategies and Tools to Enhance Performance and Patient Safety.* Available at http://teamstepps.ahrq.gov/abouttoolsmaterials.html. Accessed October 1, 2015.
14. Dadiz R, Weinschreider J, Schriefer J, et al. Interdisciplinary simulation-based training in improved delivery room communication. *Simul Healthc* 2013; 8: 279–91.
15. American College of Obstetricians and Gynecologists Committee on Patient Safety and Quality Improvement. ACOG Committee Opinion No. 447: Patient safety in obstetrics and gynecology. *Obstet Gynecol* 2009; 114: 1424–1427.
16. Spath P. *Error Reduction in Health Care* (2nd edition). San Francisco, CA: Jossey-Bass, 2011.
17. Wachter R. *Understanding Patient Safety* (2nd edition). New York, NY: McGraw Hill Medical, 2012.
18. Clay-William R, Colligan L, Back to basics: Checklist in aviation and healthcare. *BMJ Qual Saf* 2015; 1–4.
19. Shields L, Wiesner S, Fulton J, Pelletreau B. Patient Safety Series. Comprehensive maternal hemorrhage protocols reduce the use of blood products and improve patient safety. *Am J Obstet Gynecol* 2015; 212: 272–280.
20. Frequently Asked Questions about the Universal Protocol for Preventing Wrong Site, Wrong Procedure, Wrong Patient Surgery. 2004. Available from www.JCAHO.org. Accessed on October 1, 2015
21. National Patient Safety Foundation. Partnership for Clear Health Communication Ask Me 3. Available from http://www.NPSF.org/askme3. Accessed on October 1, 2015
22. Main E, Goffman D, Scavone B, et al. National partnership for maternal safety consensus bundle on obstetric hemorrhage. *Ob Gyn* 2015; 126: 155–162.
23. Gosman G, Baldisseri M, Stern K, et al. Introduction of an obstetric-specific medical emergency team for obstetric crisis team; implementation and experience. *Am J Obstet Gynecol* 2008; 198: 367.
24. Leape L, Brennan TA, Laird N, et al. The nature of adverse events in hospitalized patients: Results of the Harvard Medical Practice Study II. *N Engl J Med* 1991; 324: 377–384.
25. Marx D. *Whack-a-Mole: The Price we Pay for Expecting Perfection.* Plano TX: By Your Studios, 2009.
26. Marx D. *Patient Safety and the "Just Culture:" A Primer for Healthcare Executives.* New York, NY: Columbia University, 2001.
27. Rosenthal A, O'Daniel M. A survey of the impact of disruptive behavior and communication defects on patient safety. *Jt Com J Qual Patient Saf* 2008; 34: 464–471.
28. Hogbood C, Weiner B, Tamyao-Sarver J. Medical error identification disclosure, and reporting: Do emergency medicine provider groups differ? *Acad Emer Med* 2006; 13: 443–451.
29. Gibson R, Singh J. *Wall of Silence.* Washington, DC: Lifeline Press, 2003; 58.
30. Leonard M, Graham S, Bonacum D. The human factor: The critical importance of effective teamwork and communication in providing safe care. *Quality Safe Health Care* 2004; 13: 85–90.
31. Denham C. Trust: The 5 rights of the second victim. *J Patient Safety* 2002; 2: 107–119.
32. Agency for Healthcare Research and Quality. Improving patient safety in hospitals. Available at http://www.ahrq.gov/professionals. Accessed October 1, 2015.
33. Institute for Healthcare Improvement. *Innovation Series: IHI Global trigger Tool for Measuring Adverse Events* (2nd edition). Cambridge, MA: Institute for Healthcare Improvement, 2009.

34. ACOG committee opinion: Antenatal corticosteroid therapy for fetal maturation. *Obstet Gynecol* 2002; 99: 871–873.
35. Howell E, Zeitlin J, Paul H, Balbierz A, Egorova N. Association between hospital-level obstetric indicators and maternal and neonatal morbidity. *JAMA* 2014; 152: 1531–1541.
36. Tessmer-Tuck J, McCue B. Ob/Gyn hospitalists and patient safety. *Contemporary Ob/Gyn* 2015; 05: 25–32.
37. Vintzileos AM. Obstetrics and Gynecology hospitalist fellowships. *Obstet Gynecol Clin N Am* 2015; 42: 541–548.
38. Ingles S Feier, N, Chetiyaar J, et al. Effects of shoulder dystocia training on the incidence of brachial plexus injury. *Am J Obstet Gynecol* 2011; 204: 322.e1–6.
39. Draycott T, Crofts J, Ash J, et al. Improving neonatal outcome through practical shoulder dystocia training. *Obstet Gynecol* 2008; 112: 14–20.
40. Siassakos D, Hasafa Z, Sibanda T, et al. Retrospective cohort study of diagnosis-delivery interval with umbilical cord prolapse: The effect of team training. *BJOG* 2009; 116: 1089–1096.
41. Howell E, Zeitlin J, Paul H, Balbierz A, Egorova N. Association between hospital-level obstetric indicators and maternal and neonatal morbidity. *JAMA* 2014; 312: 1531–1541.
42. Ziv A, Small S, Wolpe P. Patient safety and simulation-based medical education. *Med Teacher* 2000; 22: 489–495.

Index